Annual Update
in Intensive Care
and Emergency Medic

C000092916

Edited by J.-L. Vincent

Annual Update in Intensive Care and Emergency Medicine 2012

Edited by J.-L. Vincent

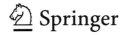 Springer

**The series *Annual Update in Intensive Care and Emergency Medicine*
is the continuation of the series entitled *Yearbook of Intensive Care
Medicine* in Europe and *Intensive Care Medicine: Annual Update* in the
United States.**

Editor:
Prof. Jean-Louis Vincent
Head, Department of Intensive Care
Erasme Hospital, Université libre de Bruxelles
Route de Lennik 808, B-1070 Brussels, Belgium

ISBN 978-3-642-25715-5   eISBN 978-3-642-25716-2

DOI 10.1007/978-3-642-25716-2

ISSN 2191-5709

Springer Heidelberg Dordrecht London New York

© Springer-Verlag Berlin Heidelberg 2012

Cover Design: WMXDesign GmbH, Heidelberg

Printed on acid-free paper

Springer is part of Springer Science+Business Media (www.springer.com)

Table of Contents

IV Endocrine Support

V Acute Respiratory Distress Syndrome

VI Respiratory Support

VII Pneumonia

VIII Fungal Infections

IX Hemodynamic Optimization

X Fluids and Blood Transfusion

XI Pulmonary Edema

XII Emergencies

List of Contributors

AGBEDJRO A
Department of Anesthesia and
Intensive Care
Cattinara Hospital
Strada di Fiume 447
34149 Trieste
Italy

AIRADO C
Department of Neurotraumatology and
Neurosurgery Research Unit
Vall d'Hebron University Hospital
Paseo Vall d'Hebron 119–129
08035 Barcelona
Spain

ALBAICETA GM
Department of Functional Biology,
Physiology Area
University of Oviedo, Faculty of Medicine
Julian Claveria s/n
33006 Oviedo
Spain

ALLAOUCHICHE B
Department of Anesthesia and
Intensive Care
Hospices Civils
CHU Edouard Herriot
Place d'Arsonval
69437 Lyon
France

AMARAL KAJDACSY-BALLA AC
Department of Critical Care Medicine
Sunnybrook Health Sciences Center
2075 Bayview Ave
Office D1 34
Toronto, ON M4N 3M5
Canada

ANDREWS P
Center for Clinical Brain Sciences
University Hospital
Edinburgh, EH4 2XU
United Kingdom

ANTONELLI M
Department of Anesthesiology and
Intensive Care
Catholic University School of Medicine
Largo Gemelli 8
00168 Rome
Italy

ARTIGAS A
Department of Intensive Care
Sabadell Hospital
Parc Tauli
08208 Sabadell
Spain

AYA HD
General Intensive Care Department
St George's Hospital
London, SW17 0QT
United Kingdom

AZUELOS I
Meakins Christie Laboratory and
Respiratory Division
McGill University Health Care Center
Montreal, QC H2X 2P2
Canada

BAGSHAW SM
Division of Critical Care Medicine
University of Alberta Hospital
3C1.16 Walter C. Mackenzie Center
8440–112 Street
Edmonton, AB T6G 2B7
Canada

BAKKER J
Department of Adult Intensive Care
Erasmus MC University Medical
Center
PO Box 2040, Room H-625
3000 CA Rotterdam
Netherlands

BASSETTI M
Infectious Diseases Division
Santa Maria della Misericordia
University Hospital
Piazzale Santa Maria della
Misericordia 15
33100 Udine
Italy

BASSFORD CR
Division of Health Sciences
Clinical Trials Unit
University of Warwick
Coventry, CV4 7AL
United Kingdom

BEIN B
Department of Anesthesiology and
Intensive Care Medicine
Schleswig-Holstein University
Hospital
Schwanenweg 21
24105 Kiel
Germany

BELLANI G
Department of Perioperative Medicine
and Intensive Care
San Gerardo Hospital
Via Pergolesi 33
20900 Monza
Italy

BELLOMO R
Department of Intensive Care
Austin Hospital
Studley Road
Heidelberg, VIC 3084
Australia

BENDJELID K
Intensive Care Unit
Geneva University Hospital
Rue Gabrielle Perret-Gentil 4
1211 Geneva 14
Switzerland

BENES J
Department of Anesthesiology and
Intensive Care
Charles University Hospital
Alej Svobody 80
304 60 Plzen
Czech Republic

BERGER MM
Adult ICU and Burns Center
CHUV
Rue du Bugnon 46
1011 Lausanne
Switzerland

BERLOT G
Department of Anesthesia and
Intensive Care
Cattinara Hospital
Strada di Fiume 447
34149 Trieste
Italy

BERNARDI M
Department of Clinical Medicine
S. Orsola-Malpighi Polyclinic
Via Albertoni 15
40138 Bologna
Italy

BERRA L
Department of Anesthesia, Critical
Care and Pain Medicine
Massachusetts General Hospital
55 Fruit St
Boston, MA 02114
USA

BEZEMER R
Department of Translational
Physiology
Academic Medical Center
Meibergdreef 9
1105 AZ Amsterdam
Netherlands

BISSCHOPS LLA
Department of Intensive Care
Medicine
Radboud University Medical Center
PO Box 9101
6500 HB Nijmegen
Netherlands

BITTNER EA
Department of Anesthesia, Critical
Care and Pain Medicine
Massachusetts General Hospital
55 Fruit St
Boston, MA 02114
USA

BOS LDJ
Department of Intensive Care
Medicine
Academic Medical Center
G3–228
Meibergdreef 9
1105 AZ Amsterdam
Netherlands

BRANDENBURG K
Department of Biophysics
Forschungszentrum
Parkallee 10
23845 Borstel
Germany

BRINDLEY PG
Division of Critical Care Medicine
3c1.04 University of Alberta Hospital
8440–112 Street
Edmonton, AB T6G 2B7
Canada

BRUNO M-A
Coma Science Group
Cyclotron Research Centre and
Neurology Department
University of Liège-Sart Tilman (B30)
4000 Liège
Belgium

BRUSASCO C
Department of Surgical Sciences and
Integrated Diagnostics
University Hospital
Largo Rosanna Benzi 8
16132 Genoa
Italy

BRUYERE R
Department of Medical Intensive Care
Bocage Central Hospital, C.H.U.
14 rue Gaffarel
B.P. 77908
21079 Dijon
France

BURNOD A
Department of Anesthesia, Intensive
Care and Prehospital Emergency
Medicine
Beaujon University Hospital
100 Boulevard du Général Leclerc
92110 Clichy
France

BUSANI S
Department of Anesthesiology and
Intensive Care
University Hospital
Via del Pozzo 71
41100 Modena
Italy

CABRINI L
Department of Cardiothoracic
Anesthesia and Intensive Care
San Raffaele Scientific Institute
Via Olgettina 60
20132 Milan
Italy

CARSON IV WF
Department of Pathology
University of Michigan Medical
School
109 Zina Pitcher Place, 4710 BSRB
Ann Arbor, MI 48109
USA

CAVALLARO F
Department of Anesthesiology and
Intensive Care
Catholic University School of
Medicine
Largo Gemelli 8
00168 Rome
Italy

CECCONI M
General Intensive Care Department
St George's Hospital
London, SW17 0QT
United Kingdom

CHARLES P-E
Department of Medical Intensive Care
Bocage Central Hospital, C.H.U.
14 rue Gaffarel
B.P. 77908
21079 Dijon
France

CHAWLA LS
Department of Critical Care Medicine
and Anesthesiology
George Washington University
Medical Center
900 23rd Street, NW
Room G-105
Washington, DC 20037
United States

CHYTRA I
Department of Anesthesiology and
Intensive Care
Charles University Hospital
Alej Svobody 80
304 60 Plzen
Czech Republic

CLAASSEN J
Division of Neurocritical Care
Neurological Institute
Columbia University Medical Center
710 W. 168th St
New York, NY 10032
USA

CLIFFORD L
Multidisciplinary Epidemiology
Translational Research in Intensive
Care (METRIC)
Division of Critical Care Medicine
Mayo Clinic
200 First St S.W.
Rochester, MN 55905
USA

COHEN J
Department of Intensive Care
Princess Alexandra and Wesley
Hospitals
University of Queensland
Ipswich Road
QLD 4102, Woolloongabba
Australia

COPPADORO A
Department of Anesthesiology and
Intensive Care
San Gerardo Hospital
Via Pergolesi 33
20052 Monza
Italy

CORRADI F
Department of Surgical Sciences and
Integrated Diagnostics
University Hospital
Largo Rosanna Benzi 8
16132 Genoa
Italy

CORREDOR C
General Intensive Care Department
St George's Hospital
London, SW17 0QT
United Kingdom

CORTES GA
Department of Pulmonary and
Critical Care Medicine
Regions Hospital, Office E3844
640 Jackson Street
St. Paul, MN 55101
USA

DALLE F
Laboratory of Parasitology-Mycology,
Bocage Central Hospital, C.H.U.
14 rue Gaffarel
B.P. 77908
21079 Dijon
France

DAVISON DL
Department of Critical Care Medicine
and Anesthesiology
George Washington University
Medical Center
900 23rd Street, NW
Room G-105
Washington, DC 20037
United States

DE LANGE DW
Department of Intensive Care
Medicine, F06.135
University Medical Center
3584 CX Utrecht
Netherlands

DEMOULE A
Medical Intensive Care Unit and
Respiratory Division
Groupe Hospitalier Pitie-Salpetrière
47–83 Boulevard de l'Hôpital
75013 Paris
France

DÍAZ-MARTÍN A
Intensive Care Unit
Virgen del Rocio University Hospital
Avd Manual Siuort s/n
41013 Seville
Spain

DIETZ S
Department of Medicine III
Martin-Luther University
Ernst-Grube-Str. 40
06096 Halle (Saale)
Germany

DRIES DJ
Department of Pulmonary and
Critical Care Medicine
Regions Hospital, Office E3844
640 Jackson Street
St. Paul, MN 55101
USA

DUCHATEAU F-X
Department of Anesthesia, Intensive
Care and Prehospital Emergency
Medicine
Beaujon University Hospital
100 Boulevard du Général Leclerc
92110 Clichy
France

DURANTEAU J
Department of Anesthesiology and
Intensive Care
AP-HP Hôpitaux Universitaires Paris-
Sud
78 avenue du Général Leclerc
94275 Le Kremlin-Bicêtre
France

ERTMER C
Department of Anesthesiology and
Intensive Care
University Hospital
Albert-Schweitzer-Campus 1, Bld. A1
48149 Muenster
Germany

ESPERATTI M
Department of Pneumology
Hospital Clinic
Villaroel 170
08036 Barcelona
Spain

ESTEBAN A
Department of Intensive Care
University Hospital
Carretera de Toledo km 12.500
28905 Madrid
Spain

FARNAN PA
Department of Family Practice
University of British Columbia
Suite 303–4180 Lougheed Hwy
Burnaby, BC V5C 6A7
Canada

FERRI M
Department of Critical Care Medicine
University of Calgary
3134 Hospital Drive NW
McCaig Tower
Calgary, AB T2N 4Z6
Canada

FLOCCARD B
Department of Anesthesia and
Intensive Care
Hospices Civils
CHU Edouard Herriot
Place d'Arsonval
69437 Lyon
France

FOGAS J
Department of Anesthesia and
Intensive Therapy
University of Szeged
6 Semmelweis St
6725 Szeged
Hungary

FOREMAN B
Comprehensive Epilepsy Center
Neurological Institute
Columbia University Medical Center
710 W. 168th St
New York, NY 10032
USA

FORNI LG
Department of Critical Care
Western Sussex Hospitals Trust
Worthing, BN11 2DH
United Kingdom

GARNACHO-MONTERO J
Intensive Care Unit
University Hospital Virgen del Rocio
Avd Manual Siuort s/n
41013 Seville
Spain

GEUKENS P
Department of Intensive Care
Medicine
University Hospital and Faculty of
Biology and Medicine
CHUV-BH 08.623
1011 Lausanne
Switzerland

GILMORE A
Department of Musculoskeletal
Biology, Institute of Ageing & Chronic
Disease
Faculty of Health & Life Sciences
University of Liverpool
Duncan Building, UCD
Daulby Street
Liverpool L69 3GA
United Kingdom

GIRARDIS M
Department of Anesthesiology and
Intensive Care
University Hospital
Via del Pozzo 71
41100 Modena
Italy

GIRAUD R
Intensive Care Unit
University Hospital
Rue Gabrielle Perret-Gentil 4
1211 Geneva 14
Switzerland

GOLDBERG AD
Department of Internal Medicine
Division of Critical Care
Mayo Clinic
200 First Street S.W.
Rochester, MN 55905
USA

GONZÁLEZ-LÓPEZ A
Department of Functional Biology,
Physiology Area
Faculty of Medicine, University of
Oviedo
Julian Claveria s/n
33006 Oviedo
Spain

GOODWIN HE
Department of Neurocritical Care
Johns Hopkins Hospital
600 North Wolfe Street
Carnegie 180
Baltimore, MD 21287
USA

GOUEL A
Department of Anesthesia and
Intensive Care
Hospices Civils
CHU Edouard Herriot
Place d'Arsonval
69437 Lyon
France

GRAESNER J-T
Department of Anesthesiology and
Intensive Care Medicine
Schleswig-Holstein University
Hospital
Schwanenweg 21
24105 Kiel
Germany

GRASSI A
Department of Perioperative Medicine
and Intensive Care
San Gerardo Hospital
Via Pergolesi 33
20900 Monza
Italy

GRIFFITHS RD
Department of Musculoskeletal
Biology, Institute of Ageing & Chronic
Disease
Faculty of Health & Life Sciences,
University of Liverpool
Duncan Building, UCD
Daulby Street
Liverpool, L69 3GA
United Kingdom

HAASE M
Department of Nephrology and
Hypertension, Diabetology and
Endocrinology
Otto-von-Guericke University
Leipziger Strasse 44
39120 Magdeburg
Germany

HARDY G
Faculty of Medical and Health
Sciences
University Hospital
Private Bag 92019
Auckland
New Zealand

HARDY I
5 Grahame Street
Auckland
New Zealand

HARROIS A
Department of Anesthesiology and
Intensive Care
AP-HP Hôpitaux Universitaires Paris-
Sud
78 avenue du Général Leclerc
94275 Le Kremlin-Bicêtre
France

HAUTIN E
Department of Anesthesia and
Intensive Care
Hospices Civils
CHU Edouard Herriot
Place d'Arsonval
69437 Lyon
France

HERRERO R
Department of Intensive Care
Sabadell Hospital
Parc Tauli
08208 Sabadell
Spain

HOEDEMAEKERS CWE
Department of Intensive Care
Medicine
Radboud University Medical Center
PO Box 9101
6500 HB Nijmegen
Netherlands

HOFER S
Anesthesiology Department
University Hospital
Im Neuenheimer Feld 110
69120 Heidelberg
Germany

HOLLEY AD
Department of Intensive Care
Medicine
Royal Brisbane & Women's Hospital
Herston, QLD 4029
Australia

HOMMERS CE
Department of Anesthesia and
Intensive Care
University Hospital
Upper Maudlin Street
Bristol, BS2 8HW
United Kingdom

HONORÉ PM
Department of Intensive Care
University Hospital
Laarbeeklaan 101
1090 Brussels
Belgium

HRAVNAK M
Department of Critical Care Medicine
606 Scaife Hall
3550 Terrace Street
Pittsburgh, PA 15261
USA

INCE C
Department of Translational
Physiology
Academic Medical Center
Meibergdreef 9
1105 AZ Amsterdam
Netherlands

IZQUIERDO-GARCÍA JL
Department of Chemistry-Physics II
Faculty of Pharmacy
Complutense University
Plaza de Ramón y Cajal
28040 Madrid
Spain

JABER S
Department of Intensive Care,
Anesthesiology and Critical Care
Saint Eloi Teaching Hospital
80 Avenue Augustin Fliche
34295 Montpellier
France

JACOBS R
Department of Intensive Care
Medicine
University Hospital
Laarbeeklaan 101
1090 Brussels
Belgium

JANSEN TC
Department of Adult Intensive Care
Medicine
Erasmus MC University Medical
Center
PO Box 2040, Room H-625
3000 CA Rotterdam
Netherlands

JONES C
Intensive Care Unit
Whiston Hospital
Warrington Road
Prescot, L35 5DR
United Kingdom

JUNG B
Department of Intensive Care,
Anesthesiology and Critical Care
Saint Eloi Teaching Hospital
80 Avenue Augustin Fliche
34295 Montpellier
France

KAPLAN LJ
Department of Surgery
Section of Trauma, Surgical Critical
Care and Surgical Emergencies
Yale University School of Medicine
330 Cedar Street, BB-310
New Haven, CT 06520
USA

KESECIOGLU J
Department of Intensive Care
Medicine, F06.135
University Medical Center
3584 CX Utrecht
Netherlands

KINSEY GR
Division of Nephrology and Center
for Immunity, Inflammation and
Regenerative Medicine
University of Virginia
PO Box 800133
Charlottesville, VA 22908
USA

KOKKORIS S
Center for Clinical Brain Sciences
University Hospital
Edinburgh, EH4 2XU
United Kingdom

KOR DJ
Department of Anesthesiology
Mayo Clinic
200 First St S.W.
Rochester, MN 55905
USA

KRUGER PS
Department of Intensive Care
Princess Alexandra Hospital
Ipswich Road, Woolloongabba
Brisbane 4102
Australia

KUNKEL SL
Department of Pathology
University of Michigan Medical
School
109 Zina Pitcher Place, 4710 BSRB
Ann Arbor, MI 48109
USA

LANDONI G
Department of Cardiothoracic
Anesthesia and Intensive Care
San Raffaele Scientific Institute
Via Olgettina 60
20132 Milan
Italy

LAUREYS S
Coma Science Group, Cyclotron
Research Center and Neurology
Department
University of Liège-Sart Tilman (B30)
4000 Liège
Belgium

LEDOUX D
Coma Science Group, Cyclotron
Research Center and Neurology
Department
University of Liège-Sart Tilman (B30)
4000 Liège
Belgium

LEPAPE A
Department of Intensive Care
Pierre Bénite Hospital
165 Chemin du Grand Revoyet
69310 Pierre-Bénite
France

LEWIN III JJ
Department of Critical Care and
Surgery Pharmacy Services
Johns Hopkins Hospital
600 North Wolfe Street
Carnegie 180
Baltimore, MD 21287
USA

LIPPMANN MJ
Department of Surgery and
Emergency Medicine
University of Texas Southwestern
Medical Center
5323 Harry Hines Boulevard
Mail Code 8579
Dallas, TX 75390
USA

López-Giraldo A
Department of Pneumology
Hospital Clinic
Villaroel 170
08036 Barcelona
Spain

Lorente JA
Department of Intensive Care
University Hospital
Carretera de Toledo km 12,500
28905 Madrid
Spain

Luckianow G
Department of Surgery
Section of Trauma, Surgical Critical
Care and Surgical Emergencies
Yale University School of Medicine
330 Cedar Street, BB-310
New Haven, CT 06520
USA

Lui FY
Department of Surgery
Section of Trauma, Surgical Critical
Care and Surgical Emergencies
Yale University School of Medicine
330 Cedar Street, BB-310
New Haven, CT 06520
USA

Maggioli C
Department of Clinical Medicine
S. Orsola-Malpighi Polyclinic
Via albertoni 15
40138 Bologna
Italy

Malbrain M
Intensive Care and High Care Burn
Unit
Antwerp Hospital Network, ZNA
Stuivenberg
Lange Beeldekensstraat 267
2060 Antwerp 6
Belgium

Mantz J
Department of Anesthesia, Intensive
Care and Prehospital Emergency
Medicine
Beaujon University Hospital
100 Boulevard du Général Leclerc
92110 Clichy
France

Manzanares W
Department of Critical Care Medicine
University Hospital
Avenida Italia, 14th Floor
Montevideo
Uruguay

Marini JJ
Department of Pulmonary and
Critical Care Medicine
Regions Hospital MS11203B
640 Jackson Street
St. Paul, MN 55101
USA

Marment SKM
Department of Intensive Care
Princess Alexandra Hospital
Ipswich Road, Woolloongabba
Brisbane 4102
Australia

Márquez-Vácaro JA
Intensive Care Unit
Virgen del Rocio University Hospital
Avd Manual Siuort s/n
41013 Seville
Spain

Martin-Loeches I
Department of Intensive Care
Joan XXIII University Hospital
Dr. Mallafré i Guasch, 4
43007 Tarragona
Spain

Marx G
Department of Intensive Care
University Hospital
Pauwelsstr. 30
52074 Aachen
Germany

MERINO M-A
Department of Neurotraumatology
and Neurosurgery Research Unit
Vall d'Hebron University Hospital
Paseo Vall d'Hebron 119–129
08035 Barcelona
Spain

MEYBOHM P
Department of Anesthesiology and
Intensive Care Medicine
Schleswig-Holstein University
Hospital
Schwanenweg 21
24105 Kiel
Germany

MIRSKI MA
Department of Anesthesiology and
Critical Care Medicine
Johns Hopkins Hospital
600 North Wolfe Street
Carnegie 180
Baltimore, MD 21287
USA

MOLNÁR Z
Department of Anesthesia and
Intensive Therapy
University of Szeged
6 Semmelweis St
6725 Szeged
Hungary

MONNET X
Department of Intensive Care
Medicine
AP-HP Hôpitaux Universitaires Paris-
Sud
94270 Le Kremlin-Bicêtre
France

MOORE J
Department of Critical Care Medicine
606 Scaife Hall
3550 Terrace Street
Pittsburgh, PA 15261
USA

MULLENS W
Department of Cardiovascular
Medicine
Oost-Limburg Hospital
3600 Genk
Belgium

NANAS S
Department of Critical Care Medicine
Evangelismos General Hospital
Ipsilantou 45–47
10675 Athens
Greece

NIN N
Department of Intensive Care
Medicine
University Hospital
Carretera de Toledo km 12.500
28905 Madrid
Spain

NOLAN JP
Department of Anesthesia and
Intensive Care Medicine
Royal United Hospital
Combe Park
Bath, BA1 3NG
United Kingdom

NOLAND B
Alere
9975 Summers Ridge Road
San Diego, CA 92121
USA

ODDO M
Department of Intensive Care
Medicine
CHUV-BH 08.623
1011 Lausanne
Switzerland

OKUSA MD
Division of Nephrology and Center
for Immunity, Inflammation and
Regenerative Medicine
University of Virginia
PO Box 800133
Charlottesville, VA 22908
USA

Ostermann M
Department of Critical Care and
Nephrology
Guy's and St Thomas' Hospital
Westminster Bridge Road
London, SE1 7EH
United Kingdom

Pan A
Infectious Risk Area
Regional Health and Social Agency of
Emilia-Romagna
Viale aldo Moro 21
40127 Bologna
Italy

Päsler M
Department of Medicine III
Martin-Luther University
Ernst-Grube-Str. 40
06096 Halle (Saale)
Germany

Patel B
Department of Critical Care
Mayo Hospital
5777 East Mayo Boulevard
Phoenix, AZ 85054
USA

Peacock WF
Department of Emergency Medicine,
Desk E19
Cleveland Clinic
9500 Euclid Ave
Cleveland, OH 44195–0001
USA

Pelosi P
Department of Surgical Sciences and
Integrated Diagnostics
University Hospital
Largo Rosanna Benzi 8
16132 Genoa
Italy

Pepe PE
Department of Surgery and
Emergency Medicine
University of Texas Southwestern
Medical Center
5323 Harry Hines Boulevard
Mail Code 8579
Dallas, TX 75390
USA

Perkins GD
Lung Injury and Fibrosis Treatment
Program
School of Clinical and Experimental
Medicine
University of Birmingham
Birmingham, B15 2TH
United Kingdom

Philips BJ
Department of Critical Care
St George's Hospital
Blackshaw Road
London, SW17 0QT
United Kingdom

Pichard C
Nutrition Unit
University Hospital
Rue Gabrielle-Perrret-Gentil 4
1211 Geneva 14
Switzerland

Pinsky MR
Department of Critical Care Medicine
606 Scaife Hall
3550 Terrace Street
Pittsburgh, PA 15261
USA

Pradl R
Department of Anesthesiology and
Intensive Care
Charles University Hospital
Alej Svobody 80
304 60 Plzen
Czech Republic

PROWLE JR
Intensive Care Unit
Royal London Hospital
Whitechapel Road
London, E1 1BB
United Kingdom

RACT C
Department of Anesthesia and
Intensive Care
CHU de Bicêtre, APHP
78 rue du Général Leclerc
94275 Le Kremlin Bicêtre
France

RAPHAEL J
Department of Anesthesiology
University of Virginia Health Sciences
Center
PO Box 800710
Charlottesville, VA 22908–0710
USA

READE MC
Department of Intensive Care
Medicine
Royal Brisbane & Women's Hospital
Herston, QLD 4029
Australia

REHBERG S
Department of Anesthesiology and
Intensive Care
University Hospital
Albert-Schweitzer-Campus 1, Bld. A1
48149 Muenster
Germany

RHODES A
General Intensive Care Department
St George's Hospital
London, SW17 0QT
United Kingdom

ROBERTS DJ
Departments of Surgery and
Community Health Sciences
University of Calgary and the
Foothills Medical Center
Intensive Care Unit
3134 Hospital Drive Northwest
Calgary, AB T2N 5A1
Canada

RONCO C
Department of Nephrology Dialysis
and Transplantation
International Renal Research Institute
IRRIV
St. Bortolo Hospital
Viale Rodolfi 37
36100 Vicenza
Italy

RUBENFELD GD
Department of Critical Care Medicine
Sunnybrook Helath Sciences Centre
2075 Bayview Ave
Office D1 34
Toronto, ON M4N 3M5
Canada

SAHUQUILLO J
Department of Neurosurgery,
Neurotraumatology and Neurosurgery
Research Unit
Vall d'Hebron University Hospital
Paseo Vall d'Hebron 119–129
08035 Barcelona
Spain

SALAZAR GA
Department of Surgery and
Emergency Medicine
University of Texas Southwestern
Medical Center
5323 Harry Hines Boulevard
Mail Code 8579
Dallas, TX 75390
USA

SANDRONI C
Department of Anesthesiology and
Intensive Care
Catholic University School of
Medicine
Largo Gemelli 8
00168 Rome
Italy

SCHMIDT M
Medical Intensive Care Unit and
Respiratory Division
Groupe Hospitalier Pitie-Salpetrière
47–83 Boulevard de l'Hôpital
75013 Paris
France

SCHUERHOLZ T
Department of Intensive Care
University Hospital
Pauwelsstr. 30
52074 Aachen
Germany

SCHUIJT TJ
Center for Experimental and
Molecular Medicine
Room G2–130
University Hospital
Meibergdreef 9
1105 AZ Amsterdam
Netherlands

SCHULTZ MJ
Laboratory of Experimental Intensive
Care and Anesthesiology
Academic Medical Center
Meibergdreef 9
1105 AZ Amsterdam
Netherlands

SEMARK AJ
Department of Intensive Care
Princess Alexandra Hospital
Ipswich Road, Woolloongabba
Brisbane 4102
Australia

SHAW AD
Department of Anesthesiology and
Critical Care Medicine
Duke University Health Center
DUMC Box 3094
Durham, NC 27710
USA

SIEGENTHALER N
Intensive Care Unit
University Hospital
Rue Gabrielle Perret-Gentil 4
1211 Geneva 14
Switzerland

SIMILOWSKI T
Medical Intensive Care Unit and
Respiratory Division
Groupe Hospitalier Pitie-Salpetrière
47–83 Boulevard de l'Hôpital
75013 Paris
France

SPAPEN HD
Department of Intensive Care
Medicine
University Hospital
Laarbeeklaan 101
1090 Brussels
Belgium

STELFOX HT
Department of Critical Care Medicine
University of Calgary
3134 Hospital Drive NW
McCaig tower
Calgary, AB T2N 4Z6
Canada

STERK PJ
Department of Respiratory Care
Academic Medical Center
Meibergdreef 9
1105 AZ Amsterdam
Netherlands

TANAKA S
Department of Anesthesiology and
Intensive Care Medicine
AP-HP Hôpitaux Universitaires Paris-
Sud
78 avenue du Général Leclerc
94275 Le Kremlin-Bicêtre
France

TAZAROURTE K
Service d'Aide Médicale Urgente
(SAMU) 77
Pôle urgences
Hôpital Marc Jacquet
Rue Fréteau-de-Peny
77000 Melun
France

TEBOUL J-L
Department of Intensive Care
Medicine
AP-HP Hôpitaux Universitaires Paris-
Sud
94270 Le Kremlin-Bicêtre
France

TEREK M
Department of Critical Care Medicine
and Anesthesiology
George Washington University
Medical Center
900 23rd Street, NW
Room G-105
Washington, DC 20037
United States

THICKETT DR
Critical Care Unit
Heart of England NHS Foundation
Trust
Bordesley Green East
Birmingham, B9 5SS
United Kingdom

THIELE RH
Department of Anesthesiology and
Critical Care Medicine
Duke University Health Center
DUMC Box 3094
Durham, NC 27710
USA

TOMASINI A
Department of Anesthesia and
Intensive Care Medicine
Cattinara Hospital
Strada di Fiume 447
34149 Trieste
Italy

TORRES A
Department of Pneumology
Hospital Clinic
Villaroel 170
08036 Barcelona
Spain

VAN DER HOEVEN JG
Department of Intensive Care
Medicine
Radboud University Medical Center
PO Box 9101
6500 HB Nijmegen
Netherlands

VAN DER POLL T
Center for Experimental and
Molecular Medicine
Room G2–130
University Hospital
Meibergdreef 9
1105 AZ Amsterdam
Netherlands

VENKATESH B
Department of Intensive Care
Princess Alexandra and Wesley
Hospitals
University of Queensland
Ipswich Road
QLD 4102, Woolloongabba
Australia

VERBRUGGE FH
Department of Cardiovascular
Medicine
Oost-Limburg Hospital
3600 Genk
Belgium

VERGRAGT J
Department of Intensive Care
Medicine, F06.135
University Medical Center
3584 CX Utrecht
Netherlands

VIGUÉ B
Department of Anesthesia and
Intensive Care
CHU de Bicêtre, APHP
78 rue du Général Leclerc
94275 Le Kremlin-Bicêtre
France

VILLA G
Infectious Diseases Division
Santa Maria della Misericordia
University Hospital
Piazzale Santa Maria della
Misericordia 15
33100 Udine
Italy

WEIGAND MA
Department of Anesthesiology,
Surgical Intensive Care and Pain
Therapy
Giessen and Marburg University
Hospital
Rudolf-Buchheim-Str. 7
35392 Giessen
Germany

WEISMÜLLER K
Department of Anesthesiology,
Surgical Intensive Care and Pain
Therapy
Giessen and Marburg University
Hospital
Rudolf-Buchheim-Str. 7
35392 Giessen
Germany

WERDAN K
Department of Medicine III
Martin-Luther University
Ernst-Grube-Str. 40
06096 Halle (Saale)
Germany

WESTPHAL M
Department of Anesthesiology and
Intensive Care
University Hospital
Albert-Schweitzer-Campus 1, Bld. A1
48149 Muenster
Germany

WIERSINGA WJ
Center for Experimental and
Molecular Medicine
Room G2–130
University Hospital
Meibergdreef 9
1105 AZ Amsterdam
Netherlands

WILLIAMS DW
School of Dentistry
Cardiff University
Cardiff, CF14 4XY
United Kingdom

WISE MP
Adult Critical Care
University Hospital of Wales
Cardiff, CF14 4XW
United Kingdom

YURUK K
Department of Translational
Physiology
Academic Medical Center
Meibergdreef 9
1105 AZ Amsterdam
Netherlands

ZACCHERINI G
Department of Clinical Medicine
S. Orsola-Malpighi Polyclinic
Via Albertoni 15
40138 Bologna
Italy

ZAMBELLI V
Department of Experimental Medicine
University of Milan-Bicocca
Via Cadore 48
20900 Monza
Italy

ZANGRILLO A
Department of Cardiothoracic
Anesthesia and Intensive Care
San Raffaele Scientific Institute
Via Olgettina 60
20132 Milan
Italy

ZYGUN DA
Departments of Surgery and
Community Health Sciences
University of Calgary and the
Foothills Medical Center
Intensive Care Unit
3134 Hospital Drive Northwest
Calgary, AB T2N 5A1
Canada

Common Abbreviations

AKI	Acute kidney injury
ALI	Acute lung injury
APACHE	Acute Physiology and Chronic Health Evaluation
ARDS	Acute respiratory distress syndrome
AUROC	Area under the receiver operating characteristic curve
BAL	Bronchoalveolar lavage
COPD	Chronic obstructive pulmonary disease
CPB	Cardiopulmonary bypass
CPP	Cerebral perfusion pressure
CPR	Cardiopulmonary resuscitation
CRP	C-reactive protein
CRRT	Continuous renal replacement therapy
CT	Computed tomography
CVP	Central venous pressure
DO_2	Oxygen delivery
EKG	Electrocardiogram
GFR	Glomerular filtration rate
ICP	Intracranial pressure
ICU	Intensive care unit
IFN	Interferon
IL	Interleukin
LPS	Lipopolysaccharide
MAP	Mean arterial pressure
MRI	Magnetic resonance imaging
NF-κB	Nuclear factor-kappa B
NGAL	Neutrophil gelatinase-associated lipocalin
NO	Nitric oxide
NOS	Nitric oxide synthase
PAOP	Pulmonary artery occlusion pressure
PCT	Procalcitonin
PEEP	Positive end-expiratory pressure
PPV	Pulse pressure variation
RBC	Red blood cell
RCT	Randomized controlled trial
ROS	Reactive oxygen species
$ScvO_2$	Central venous oxygen saturation
SIRS	Systemic inflammatory response syndrome
SOFA	Sequential organ failure assessment
SvO_2	Mixed venous oxygen saturation
TBI	Traumatic brain injury
TLR	Toll-like receptor
TNF	Tumor necrosis factor
VAP	Ventilator-associated pneumonia

I Mechanisms of Sepsis and Critical Illness

Molecular Mechanisms Underlying Severe Sepsis: Insights from Epigenetics

W.F. CARSON IV and S.L. KUNKEL

Introduction

Recent investigations into the pathogenesis of severe sepsis, septic shock, burn, stroke and ischemia/reperfusion injury have identified common patterns of disease. Despite their disparate etiologies, these syndromes share many similar immunological outcomes. In particular, survivors of life-threatening shock syndromes often exhibit decreased long-term survival rates as compared to the healthy age-matched population [1]. This decrease in survival often correlates with an increased susceptibility to secondary, nosocomial and opportunistic infections [2, 3]. In addition, survivors of severe shock and trauma often exhibit immunosuppressive phenotypes, particularly in regards to cellular immune activation and effector function. These phenotypes can be observed both in human patients and in animal models of severe inflammation and injury, specifically in animal models of severe sepsis [4]. Severe injury and inflammation are often associated with widespread apoptosis; the immunosuppression observed following these events is often ascribed to this loss of immune cells [5]. However, these deficiencies often persist despite the eventual return of immune cells to pre-injury levels in peripheral blood and immune organs [6]. The focus of current research into sepsis and shock-induced immunosuppression has been to elucidate the molecular mechanisms underlying the persistent immunosuppressive state in cells that have survived both the acute phase of the disease, and have recovered after the widespread apoptotic event.

The challenges from a patient care perspective stem from the proper diagnosis and treatment of immunosuppression both during the acute phase of inflammation and long-term following recovery. Despite advances in the understanding of severe inflammatory responses and subsequent immunosuppression, there remains a paucity of viable biomarkers for the diagnosis of immunosuppression, except for functional analysis of leukocyte function. Additionally, the link between severe inflammation and immunosuppression remains a 'black box', whereby the specific molecular pathways connecting the two remain to be elucidated. Therefore, it becomes challenging to develop treatments to block the development of immunosuppression in these diseases. Additionally, treatments aimed at the immune system in an attempt to improve long-term outcomes (i.e., immunosuppression) may have a deleterious effect on the short-term survival of the patient through deleterious modulation of the immune response. Ultimately, the goal of present research in severe inflammatory diseases is to identify the links between the physiological stresses of the acute phase response and the long-term immunological outcomes of patients that survive the life-threatening inflammatory episode.

J.-L. Vincent (ed.), *Annual Update in Intensive Care and Emergency Medicine 2012*
DOI 10.1007/978-3-642-25716-2 © Springer-Verlag Berlin Heidelberg 2012

Recent advances in the field of epigenetics have provided some insight into the link between severe inflammation, gene regulation and immune cell function. Epigenetics is a relatively broad field of study encompassing any and all molecular mechanisms that can regulate gene expression without changing the underlying genomic content of an organism [7]. Examples of epigenetic mechanisms include the silencing of gene expression via DNA methylation, the modulation of gene expression via histone modifications, and the post-transcriptional regulation of mRNA translation via micro-RNA (miRNA) expression. Epigenetics plays a central role in developmental biology, especially in governing the development of differentiated cells from multipotent progenitor cells – therefore, epigenetic mechanisms also govern hematopoiesis [8], as well as the activation and lineage commitment of mature leukocytes [9]. Productive immune responses require the concerted function of all three epigenetic mechanisms to direct gene expression for functional immunity; as a corollary, improper epigenetic regulation of gene expression can have a deleterious effect on immune function. Modulation in epigenetic regulation of gene expression in immune cells has been linked to numerous disease states, including autoimmune diseases [10] and immunosuppression [6]. Epigenetics is also playing an increasingly important role in our understanding of the pathogenesis of severe sepsis, shock and trauma, and recent studies have identified many epigenetic mechanisms underlying both disease pathogenesis and post-septic immunosuppression [11].

The following sections will summarize the current understanding of the role of epigenetics in the context of life-threatening inflammatory events, specifically in severe sepsis and septic shock. Particular focus will be on the role of histone modifications in governing immune responses post-sepsis. In addition, recent investigations of the role of histone modifications and histone modifying enzymes in the pathogenesis of severe sepsis will be discussed. Ultimately, the goal of this review is to highlight the important role of epigenetic mechanisms in governing the severity of sepsis responses and the immunosuppression that follows, in the hopes of promoting further research into epigenetic regulation of life-threatening inflammation and cellular immunosuppression.

Epigenetic Mechanisms Govern the Function of Leukocytes Post-sepsis

Mortality rates remain high in patients diagnosed with severe sepsis and septic shock, despite advances in the diagnosis and treatment of the disease. This is due in part to the nature of the sepsis response, as the 'cytokine storm' driving multiorgan dysfunction and tissue damage is by nature a multifactorial response encompassing numerous pro-inflammatory chemokines and cytokines [12]. In addition, cells of both the innate and adaptive immune systems play critical roles in the initiation of the inflammatory event, with multiple stimuli driving the activation and effector function of each immune cell subset [13]. Therefore, treatments and therapies aimed at specific pro-inflammatory mediators often fail to adequately control the inflammatory response in sepsis. One particularly striking example of this phenomenon is the usage of anti-tumor necrosis factor alpha (TNF-α) antibodies to blunt the hyperinflammatory response during sepsis. Despite TNF's central role in the 'cytokine storm' of sepsis, blockade of this cytokine in patients does not result in improved clinical outcomes, unless provided in an extremely short (and therefore relatively impractical) time window during the onset of disease [14]. These results highlight the multifactorial nature of the septic response, and underscore the need to address multiple pro-inflammatory mediators at concurrent timepoints to effectively regulate life-threatening inflammation.

In a similar fashion, the immune system of a patient suffering from severe sepsis must control the expression of numerous pro-inflammatory mediators, expressed by numerous cell types, if the physiological stresses of the systemic inflammatory response syndrome (SIRS) are to be overcome. Many of the molecular mechanisms governing the shift from SIRS to the immunosuppressive "compensatory anti-inflammatory response syndrome (CARS)" are, therefore, broad-spectrum in nature, such as the global increase in anti-inflammatory cytokines, like interleukin (IL)-10 and transforming growth factor (TGF)-β, and the increase in T-helper type 2 (Th2) cytokines, like IL-13, which counter the predominantly T-helper type 1 (Th1) response of sepsis [15]. However, these mechanisms do not actively address the continuing overexpression of pro-inflammatory chemokines and cytokines during sepsis; rather, they seek to actively suppress their pro-inflammatory functions. Recent studies have identified epigenetic modifications that occur following the onset of severe sepsis; these modifications can have a direct effect on the ability of both innate and adaptive immune cells to produce pro-inflammatory cytokines [11]. Whereas these epigenetic modifications may have a beneficial role in the short-term through their ability to suppress inflammation-induced pathology, their persistence can lead to the development of immunosuppression, both in the short-term and in the long-term following recovery. Therefore, current research aimed at identifying epigenetic modifications following sepsis has two important outcomes for patient care. First, by identifying endogenous epigenetic mechanisms involved with gene silencing, it may be possible to identify new molecular targets (such as histone-modifying enzymes) that may be promising candidates for pharmacological intervention. Second, identification of the epigenetic 'marks' associated with the development of CARS and post-septic immunosuppression may provide clinicians with new diagnostic tools for the correct diagnosis of patients at high risk of developing immunosuppression following recovery from severe sepsis.

One of the hallmarks of CARS and post-septic immunosuppression is the reduced activation potential of myeloid and lymphoid cells in response to secondary stimuli (e.g., Toll-like receptor [TLR] ligands, antigens in the context of MHC complexes, etc) [16]. This decreased activation is evidenced by the reduced production of pro-inflammatory cytokines following secondary stimuli, and is postulated to play a central role in the susceptibility of septic patients to secondary, nosocomial and opportunistic infections. For example, dendritic cells produce significantly less IL-12 following sepsis, resulting in impaired immune responses to opportunistic pathogens such as the fungus *Aspergillus fumigatus* [17]. Macrophages also exhibit a reduction in pro-inflammatory cytokine production following sepsis, in particular IL-12 and TNF-α [18]. For CD4+ T cells, the cytokine phenotype is more complicated, and manifests as a dysregulation of T-helper cytokine production both *in vitro* and *in vivo* [19]. Additionally, the lineage commitment of CD4+ T cells following sepsis is altered, with observable deficiencies in Th1 and Th2 cytokine phenotypes, as well as an increased propensity for naïve effector CD4+ T cells to become regulatory T cells [20]. In each case, specific epigenetic modifications have been shown to correlate with these changes in activation and effector function, and these epigenetic modifications provide a molecular mechanism whereby cell-intrinsic immunosuppression and immunomodulation can be maintained at timepoints distal from the onset of severe sepsis.

Much of what is understood regarding epigenetic modification of macrophage function comes from studies of lipopolysaccharide (LPS) tolerance, whereby cells exhibit refractory responses to secondary LPS challenge following an initial high dose exposure either *in vivo* or *in vitro* [21]. These refractory responses are characterized by a decrease in pro-inflammatory cytokine production following secondary challenge with LPS. Interestingly, increases in repressive H3K9 methylation levels in the promoter regions of *Il1b* and *Tnfa* correlate with decreased production of both the inflammatory cytokines (IL-1β and TNF-α, respectively) [22, 23]. Additional studies have observed the coordinated function of the histone methyltransferase G9a and the DNA methyltransferase Dnmt3a/b at the promoter region of *Tnfa* during the induction of LPS tolerance, an important observation as DNA methylation is a potent epigenetic mechanism of mediating gene suppression [23]. Increases in repressive histone modifications can also be observed in macrophages following sepsis directly *ex vivo*. In animal models of severe sepsis, pulmonary macrophages exhibit decreases in activating histone acetylation (specifically H4) and methylation (H3K4) in the promoter region of *TNFα*, *Il12p35* and *Nos2*, correlating with decreased production of the respective proteins [18]. These modulations in histone modifications at genes important for the antimicrobial function of macrophages are hypothesized to play an important role in mediating post-septic immunosuppression.

Dendritic cells, another immune cell of the myeloid lineage, share similar cytokine phenotypes to macrophages, in particular a reduction in IL-12 production in response to TLR stimulation [17]. This reduction in IL-12 production has a significant effect on the ability of the post-septic immune system to mount Th1-type immune responses, as IL-12 is critical for the Th1 lineage commitment of CD4+ T cells [24]. This suppression of IL-12 production is observable in animal models of sepsis long after recovery from severe sepsis, and is partly responsible for the susceptibility of post-septic animals to opportunistic infections of the lung [6, 17]. This reduction in IL-12 production also correlates with changes in the histone methylation patterns observed in the promoter regions of *Il12p35* and *Il12p40*. Specifically, dendritic cells from post-septic animals exhibit decreased activating histone methylation (H3K4me) and increased repressive histone methylation (H3K27me) in the promoter regions of *Il12a* and *Il12b* [6]. These epigenetic modifications are thought to play an important role in the decreased IL-12 production observed in post-septic dendritic cells.

Histone modifications also play an important role in governing CD4+ T cell responses following recovery from sepsis. Whereas severe sepsis is often considered an immune syndrome primarily encompassing the innate immune system, through activation of TLR signaling pathways via exposure to microbes, microbial products and/or dead and dying cells and tissues, the adaptive immune system plays an important role in the development of both SIRS and CARS. For example, T cell-derived cytokines such as IL-2, interferon (IFN)-γ and IL-17A play an important role in the cytokine storm of sepsis through promoting lymphocyte proliferation, Th1 activation, and the generation/accumulation of neutrophils, respectively [25]. Also, the switch from SIRS to CARS correlates with the increase in T-cell derived immunomodulatory cytokines, such as IL-10 and IL-4, both of which can suppress and/or deviate the Th1 responses central to sepsis

[26]. Additionally, the switch from SIRS to CARS is correlated with an increase in peripheral regulatory T cells [27], which can serve as a double-edged sword; regulatory T cells can suppress the unchecked inflammation of SIRS, but can also leave the host vulnerable to secondary infections. Importantly, the adaptive immune system is critical for host defense against a wide variety of pathogens, and modulations in adaptive immunity can result in immunosuppression. Previous studies have identified numerous deficiencies in CD4+ T cell function following sepsis, from decreased proliferative responses [28], to modulated cytokine production [19], to increased apoptosis within lymphoid tissues [29]. Recent studies have begun to associate modulations in histone modifications with these activation defects, and have also provided a molecular mechanism for the changes in T helper lineage commitment observed in human patients and in animal models post-sepsis [19].

Following the onset of sepsis, and during the switch from SIRS to CARS, CD4+ T cells exhibit a general shift away from Th1-type cytokine responses, instead exhibiting Th2-type responses [30]. Part of this phenomenon can be ascribed to the decrease in IL-12 production by post-septic dendritic cells; however, these deficiencies persist even when the cells are restimulated *in vitro* in the absence of accessory cells. These studies point to a cell-intrinsic mechanism inhibiting the generation of Th1 responses. Interestingly, CD4+ T cells from post-septic animals exhibit increase H3K27 (repressive) methylation at the promoter region of *Ifng*, a gene critical for Th1 cell function. This increase in repressive histone methylation correlates with decreased production of IFN-γ by post-septic CD4+ T cells that have been skewed to the Th1 lineage *in vitro*. In addition, modulations in histone modifications in the promoter regions of lineage-specific transcription factors can have a dramatic effect on the function of post-septic CD4+ T cells. For example, increases in H3K27 methylation in the promoter region of *Gata3* (an important Th2-specific transcription factor) correlate with incomplete Th2 lineage commitment, as measured by *in vitro* cytokine production following skewing. In addition, increases in H3K9 acetylation (an activating epigenetic mark) in the promoter region of *Foxp3* (an important regulatory T cell transcription factor) correlate with increased regulatory T cells and regulatory T cell function in post-septic CD4+ T cells. In both cases, modulations in transcription factor expression mediated by epigenetic mechanisms can have a dramatic effect on the function of post-septic CD4+ T cells [19, 20].

Clearly, severe life-threatening inflammatory responses can have a significant effect on the long-term function of the immune system. Modulations in the epigenetic signature of myeloid and lymphoid cells play a central role in this long-term immune dysfunction, through the suppression of cytokine production and the modulation of lineage commitment decisions. Of particular interest is the role of histone-modifying enzymes in governing the modulation of histone modifications following sepsis. For example, increases in the H3K9 acetyltransferase, Kat2a, are observed in post-septic CD4+ T cells, correlating with the increase in H3K9 acetylation in the *Foxp3* promoter seen in these cells [20]. However, little is understood about the mechanisms governing the up- or down-regulation of histone modifying enzymes in response to severe sepsis and severe inflammatory processes. Additionally, little is understood about the role of epigenetic mechanisms, and histone-modifying enzymes in particular, in governing the septic response.

Histone Modifying Enzymes and Sepsis: Regulation of Leukocyte Function and Disease Severity

The observation of modulations in histone modifications following severe sepsis suggests that the expression and/or activity of histone modifying enzymes can be affected by widespread inflammation. Additionally, as histone modification is a critical step in transcriptional accessibility, it is interesting to hypothesize that histone-modifying enzymes play a critical role in the initiation of the cytokine storm through activation of pro-inflammatory gene loci. Unfortunately, the techniques available to directly study histone-modifying enzymes in disease models such as severe sepsis remain limited. As histone modifications (and epigenetic mechanisms in general) are critical for developmental biology, genetic models of histone-modifying enzyme function (i.e., gene knockouts) are often impractical, as deletion of these genes can result in embryonic lethality. Additionally, small molecule inhibitors and other pharmacological tools often have broad-spectrum activity, making it difficult to discern the role of specific enzymes in diseases and disease models.

Despite these difficulties, recent experimental studies have indicated that sepsis and sepsis-associated immune cell functions can be modulated via modulation of histone-modifying enzymes. Among the many different types of observed histone modifications (e.g., methylation, phosphorylation, acetylation, etc.), there has been measurable success in developing inhibitors of histone deacetylase enzymes (HDACs). Histone deacetylase inhibitors (HDACIs) that have both wide spectrum activity (i.e., inhibition of numerous HDACs) and specific inhibitory properties (i.e., directed inhibition of specific HDACs) are available for experimental studies. Studies using human peripheral blood cells indicate that certain HDACIs can inhibit the production of pro-inflammatory cytokines in response to LPS [31]. Similar results can be observed in animal models of sepsis, where in vivo administration of HDACIs can increase survival rates and decrease many biomarkers of disease severity, including cellular infiltration and serum cytokine levels [32]. Inhibition of HDAC function can, therefore, have a dramatic effect on the severity of the septic response, and these studies highlight an important role for histone deacetylation in mediating the intensity of the cytokine storm of sepsis.

As mentioned previously, the knowledge base concerning epigenetics and sepsis is largely focused on instances of histone acetylation and methylation. The abundance of pharmacological inhibitors of histone deacetylation allow for the design of experiments aimed at elucidating the role of acetylation in mediating sepsis and sepsis-induced immunosuppression. However, the paucity of reagents available to inhibit histone methylation (and histone methyltransferases/demethylases) makes the study of methylation more challenging. Nevertheless, the recent development of conditional knockouts of histone methyltransferase enzymes has provided insight into the role of these enzymes in mediating the severity of polymicrobial sepsis.

The histone methyltransferase enzyme, mixed-lineage leukemia (MLL), is responsible for the addition of the H3K4me mark, a critical activating epigenetic modification that can be modulated in leukocytes following sepsis [18]. In addition, genetic deficiencies of MLL (i.e., haploinsufficiency, or the loss of a single copy of the gene) can have dramatic effects on the activation of immune cells, and CD4+ T cells in particular [33]. Interestingly, MLL appears to have an impor-

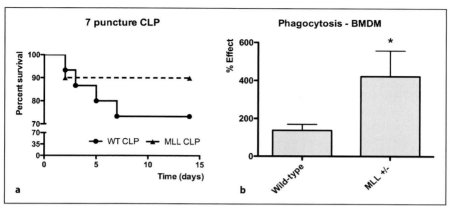

Fig. 1. Mixed-lineage leukemia (MLL)[+/-] mice are protected from sepsis-induced mortality. **a** MLL[+/-] mice exhibit decreased mortality following experimental sepsis (cecal ligation and puncture [CLP]) compared to littermate control animals (MLL[+/+]). **b** MLL[+/-] bone-marrow derived macrophages (BMDM) exhibit increased phagocytosis compared to littermate controls in response to *in vitro* challenge with fluorescently labeled *E. coli.*

tant role in mediating the severity of the septic response as well, as mice haploinsufficient for MLL (MLL[+/-]) appear to be resistant to sepsis-induced mortality (**Fig. 1a**). MLL[+/-] mice also exhibit decreased levels of pro-inflammatory cytokines and chemokines *in vivo*, suggesting that the cytokine storm is suppressed when MLL activity is reduced. Of particular interest is the effect of MLL haploinsufficiency on the function of bone marrow-derived macrophages (BMDM), as MLL[+/-] BMDM exhibit increased phagocytosis *in vitro* as compared to BMDM from littermate control animals (MLL[+/-]) (**Fig. 1b**). The specific role of MLL in governing phagocytosis remains to be elucidated; however, these preliminary results suggest that inhibition of MLL function may be a promising therapeutic target for sepsis.

Much work remains to be done concerning the role of histone modifying enzymes in mediating sepsis and sepsis-induced immunosuppression. However, the identification of specific histone modifications following sepsis – H3K9ac, H3K4me, H3K27me, etc. – provides a framework for the design of future experiments. For example, the identification of H3K9ac in post-septic CD4+ T cells correlated with the upregulation of the H3K9ac-specific acetyltransferase, Kat2a. Studies correlating the up- or down-regulation of histone modifying enzymes with their associated histone modifications can provide a mechanism for the epigenetic regulation of genes following sepsis, and provide useful biomarkers of disease severity and for diagnosis of post-septic immunosuppression in patients.

Conclusion

Severe sepsis and septic shock are characterized by the unchecked production of pro-inflammatory chemokines and cytokines that result in widespread inflammation, leading to tissue damage and significant mortality in affected patients. Epigenetic mechanisms of gene regulation play a central role in the septic response,

I

through their ability to license gene expression during the acute phase of the disease and their association with post-septic immunosuppression. Studies identifying the modulation of specific epigenetic marks, and the enzymes responsible for these marks, can provide valuable insight into the molecular mechanisms governing SIRS and CARS. In addition, identification of epigenetic marks associated with disease severity may serve as useful biomarkers for the diagnosis of patients at high risk of succumbing to sepsis-induced mortality, or for developing long-term immunosuppression following recovery. Further research into the role of epigenetics in sepsis will hopefully provide new clues into the molecular mechanisms governing the disease, as well as providing novel targets for the development of pharmacological treatments.

Acknowledgement: This work was supported in part by NIH grant HL31237

References

1. Winters BD, Eberlein M, Leung J, et al (2010) Long-term mortality and quality of life in sepsis: a systematic review. Crit Care Med 38: 1276–1283
2. Landelle C, Lepape A, Francais A, et al (2008) Nosocomial infection after septic shock among intensive care unit patients. Infect Control Hosp Epidemiol 29: 1054–1065
3. Landelle C, Lepape A, Voirin N, et al (2010) Low monocyte human leukocyte antigen-DR is independently associated with nosocomial infections after septic shock. Intensive Care Med 36: 1859–1866
4. Benjamim CF, Hogaboam CM, Kunkel SL (2004) The chronic consequences of severe sepsis. J Leukoc Biol 75: 408–412
5. Tinsley KW, Grayson MH, Swanson PE, et al (2003) Sepsis induces apoptosis and profound depletion of splenic interdigitating and follicular dendritic cells. J Immunol 171: 909–914
6. Wen H, Dou Y, Hogaboam CM, Kunkel SL (2008) Epigenetic regulation of dendritic cell-derived interleukin-12 facilitates immunosuppression after a severe innate immune response. Blood 111: 1797–1804
7. Delcuve GP, Rastegar M, Davie JR (2009) Epigenetic control. J Cell Physiol 219: 243–250
8. Fisher AG (2002) Cellular identity and lineage choice. Nat Rev Immunol 2: 977–982
9. Smale ST, Fisher AG (2002) Chromatin structure and gene regulation in the immune system. Annu Rev Immunol 20: 427–462
10. Patel DR, Richardson BC (2010) Epigenetic mechanisms in lupus. Curr Opin Rheumatol 22: 478–482
11. Carson WF, Cavassani KA, Dou Y, Kunkel SL (2011) Epigenetic regulation of immune cell functions during post-septic immunosuppression. Epigenetics 6: 273–283
12. Wang H, Ma S (2008) The cytokine storm and factors determining the sequence and severity of organ dysfunction in multiple organ dysfunction syndrome. Am J Emerg Med 26: 711–715
13. Oberholzer A, Oberholzer C, Moldawer LL (2001) Sepsis syndromes: understanding the role of innate and acquired immunity. Shock 16: 83–96
14. Kox WJ, Volk T, Kox SN, Volk HD (2000) Immunomodulatory therapies in sepsis. Intensive Care Med 26 (Suppl 1):S124–128
15. Ward NS, Casserly B, Ayala A (2008) The compensatory anti-inflammatory response syndrome (CARS) in critically ill patients. Clin Chest Med 29: 617–625
16. Kimura F, Shimizu H, Yoshidome H, Ohtsuka M, Miyazaki M (2010) Immunosuppression following surgical and traumatic injury. Surg Today 40: 793–808
17. Wen H, Hogaboam CM, Gauldie J, Kunkel SL (2006) Severe sepsis exacerbates cell-mediated immunity in the lung due to an altered dendritic cell cytokine profile. Am J Pathol 168: 1940–1950
18. Lyn-Kew K, Rich E, Zeng X, et al (2010) IRAK-M regulates chromatin remodeling in lung macrophages during experimental sepsis. PLoS One 5:e11145

19. Carson WF, Cavassani KA, Ito T, et al (2010) Impaired CD4+ T-cell proliferation and effector function correlates with repressive histone methylation events in a mouse model of severe sepsis. Eur J Immunol 40: 998–1010
20. Cavassani KA, Carson WF 4th, Moreira AP, et al (2010) The post sepsis-induced expansion and enhanced function of regulatory T cells create an environment to potentiate tumor growth. Blood 115: 4403–4411
21. Fujihara M, Muroi M, Tanamoto K, et al (2003) Molecular mechanisms of macrophage activation and deactivation by lipopolysaccharide: roles of the receptor complex. Pharmacol Ther 100: 171–194
22. Chan C, Li L, McCall CE, Yoza BK (2005) Endotoxin tolerance disrupts chromatin remodeling and NF-kappaB transactivation at the IL-1beta promoter. J Immunol 175: 461–468
23. El Gazzar M, Yoza BK, Chen X, et al (2008) G9a and HP1 couple histone and DNA methylation to TNFalpha transcription silencing during endotoxin tolerance. J Biol Chem 283: 32198–32208
24. Trinchieri G (2003) Interleukin-12 and the regulation of innate resistance and adaptive immunity. Nat Rev Immunol 3: 133–146
25. Kasten KR, Tschop J, Adediran SG, Hildeman DA, Caldwell CC (2010) T cells are potent early mediators of the host response to sepsis. Shock 34: 327–336
26. Miller AC, Rashid RM, Elamin EM (2007) The "T" in trauma: the helper T-cell response and the role of immunomodulation in trauma and burn patients. J Trauma 63: 1407–1417
27. Venet F, Chung CS, Kherouf H, et al (2009) Increased circulating regulatory T cells (CD4(+)CD25 (+)CD127 (-)) contribute to lymphocyte anergy in septic shock patients. Intensive Care Med 35: 678–686
28. Heidecke CD, Hensler T, Weighardt H, et al (1999) Selective defects of T lymphocyte function in patients with lethal intraabdominal infection. Am J Surg 178: 288–292
29. Oberholzer C, Oberholzer A, Clare-Salzler M, Moldawer LL (2001) Apoptosis in sepsis: a new target for therapeutic exploration. FASEB J 15: 879–892
30. Mack VE, McCarter MD, Naama HA, Calvano SE, Daly JM (1996) Dominance of T-helper 2-type cytokines after severe injury. Arch Surg 131: 1303–1308
31. Brogdon JL, Xu Y, Szabo SJ, et al (2007) Histone deacetylase activities are required for innate immune cell control of Th1 but not Th2 effector cell function. Blood 109: 1123–1130
32. Zhang L, Jin S, Wang C, Jiang R, Wan J (2010) Histone deacetylase inhibitors attenuate acute lung injury during cecal ligation and puncture-induced polymicrobial sepsis. World J Surg 34: 1676–1683
33. Yamashita M, Hirahara K, Shinnakasu R, et al (2006) Crucial role of MLL for the maintenance of memory T helper type 2 cell responses. Immunity 24: 611–622

The Neuroendocrine Axis: The Nervous System and Inflammation

K. Weismüller, M.A. Weigand, and S. Hofer

Introduction

Inflammation is the physiological answer of the organism to damage affecting its integrity, such as infection or trauma. In inflammation, cells of the immune system release cytokines and other mediators, which contribute to the destruction of bacteria and tissue repair. We distinguish here between pro-inflammatory cytokines, e.g., interleukin-1 (IL-1), IL-6 and tumor necrosis factor (TNF)-α, and anti-inflammatory cytokines, e.g., IL-10 and IL-4. Local mechanisms regulate the extent of the inflammatory answer needed to remove the source of the damage and to maintain homeostasis. Humoral as well as neuronal mediators contribute to the regulation of inflammation. Humoral anti-inflammatory mediators, e.g., IL-10 and glucocorticoids, inhibit the release or effect of pro-inflammatory cytokines whereas lipoxins and resolvins contribute to tissue repair. Humoral mediators reach their target cells in distant organs by diffusion or transport by blood flow. Substances which are released by nerves, e.g., norepinephrine and acetylcholine, reach specific cell groups of distant organs rapidly [1].

Sepsis is the complex and systemic inflammatory answer to a mainly bacterial infection. In the early stage, dysregulation and imbalance in favor of pro-inflammatory cytokines provoke tissue damage, organ damage and death. The excessive release of pro-inflammatory cytokines leads to the activation of vasoactive amines and chemokines as well as to the activation of the complement system, coagulation and release of reactive oxygen species (ROS). These mediators are responsible for increased vascular permeability, hypotension and septic shock. Late onset mediators, e.g., high mobility group box 1 protein (HMGB1), allow the inflammatory reaction to continue [1].

It is generally acknowledged that the immune system can be influenced by neurological status and the neurological status of the organism can be influenced by the immune system [2]. Accordingly, pro-inflammatory cytokines (e.g., TNF-α, IL-1 and IL-6) released peripherally in sepsis can increase the permeability of the blood brain barrier and provoke an inflammatory reaction in the brain itself as well as sepsis related behavior [3, 4]. Pro-inflammatory molecules from the peripheral circulation and the autonomic nervous system play an important role in the neuroimmune pathogenesis of sepsis [5].

Bidirectional communication between the central nervous system (CNS) and the immune system increases the effectiveness of both systems in the context of diverse inflammatory diseases, including sepsis. Two pathways connecting the immune system with the CNS are the autonomic nervous system (ANS) and the

J.-L. Vincent (ed.), *Annual Update in Intensive Care and Emergency Medicine 2012*
DOI 10.1007/978-3-642-25716-2 © Springer-Verlag Berlin Heidelberg 2012

hypothalamo-pituitary-adrenal (HPA) system. The activation of these two pathways plays an important role in the pathogenesis of sepsis [6].

The Sympathetic Nervous System (SNS)

Preganglionic efferent fibers leaving the CNS in thoracic and lumbar spinal nerves belong to the SNS or thoracolumbar system. The preganglionic fibers synapse with postganglionic fibers either in the sympathetic chain or in prevertebral ganglia. The postganglionic fibers innervate the organs from these ganglia. The SNS innervates all lymphoid organs and its transmitters, epinephrine and norepinephrine, modulate the immune system [7, 8]. Pro-inflammatory cytokines are able to activate the HPA axis as well as the SNS [4, 9, 10]. The resulting increase in norepinephrine in the CNS [11, 12] and in the peripheral circulation [13] can cause a lasting activation of the SNS including the N. splenicus and provoke increased norepinephrine turnover in the spleen [14].

Various cells of the innate immune system express α- or β-adrenergic receptors. Usually, α-receptors cannot be found on the surface of leukocytes in the peripheral blood but in pathological condition their expression is inducible in certain compartments [15, 16]. Norepinephrine interacting with α-receptors can stimulate macrophages to release TNF-α [17] and thus contribute to the maintenance of sepsis. In contrast, interaction with β-receptors decreases the release of IL-1 and TNF-α and increases the secretion of IL-10 from macrophages [18, 19] and thus mediates anti-inflammatory effects.

The Hypothalamo-pituitary-adrenal Axis

The release of cytokines as a result of infection or injury precipitates vagal afferents. Synaptic connections to the rostroventral medulla and to the locus coeruleus as well as to the hypothalamic nuclei activate the SNS and the HPA axis. Pro-inflammatory cytokines activate also the perivascular cells of the blood brain barrier. Those cells then release inflammatory molecules, e.g., eicosanoids, which affect the hypothalamus. Circulating cytokines are also able to affect circumventricular organs, e.g., the area postrema, which do not have a direct blood brain barrier. The pro-inflammatory cytokines induce the expression of corticotropin releasing hormone (CRH) or arginine vasopressin (AVP) in the hypothalamus and of adrenocorticotropic hormone (ACTH) in the pituitary gland [9]. ACTH causes an increase in cortisol release in the adrenal cortex. Cortisol displays its anti-inflammatory effects in suppression of nuclear factor-kappa B (NF-κB) activation and in activation of IL-4 and IL-10 synthesis. Pro-opiomelanocortin (POMC) is a precursory peptide not only of ACTH but also of α-melanocyte stimulating hormone (α-MSH). α-MSH suppresses NF-κB and increases release of IL-10 and thus inhibits pro-inflammatory activity [20]. In septic shock, α-MSH is relevant as the release of α-MSH after CRH stimulation is impaired in patients who do not survive. In these patients, dexamethasone is also not able to suppress α-MSH release. Accordingly, this phenomenon indicates a dysfunction of the anti-inflammatory system [21]. The systemic anti-inflammatory reaction is essential for an effective immunologic response in sepsis [22]. Various clinical studies have shown that pro-inflammatory cytokines can directly activate the HPA axis and thus induce the release of cortisol [23].

I

Cholinergic Control of Inflammation

Some years ago, the so-called cholinergic anti-inflammatory pathway was described as a mechanism of neuronal inflammation control via the efferent nervus (N.) vagus [1, 24]. Acetylcholine decreases the release of pro-inflammatory cytokines in activated macrophages *in vitro* [25]. *In vivo*, electrical stimulation of the vagal nerve decreases the release of HMGB1 and increases survival [26]. Furthermore, acetylcholine also inhibits the release of TNF-α by binding to the α7-subunit of the acetylcholine receptor [27]. In addition, splenectomy in polymicrobial, experimental sepsis decreases the release of HMGB1 and increases survival in animals [28]. It was also shown that pharmaceutically preventive sympathicolysis by means of clonidine and dexmedetomidine protects from experimental, lethal polymicrobial sepsis [29]. The inhibition of the adrenergic pro-inflammatory pathway which induces the release of pro-inflammatory cytokines by activating α-adrenergic receptors may be the cause of this observation [30].

The immune system gains information from the peripheral organs and acts as a sensory organ which provides information of inflammatory processes for the brain [31, 32]. IL-1 receptors of the afferent neurons of the vagal nerve are involved in this process [33–35]. The afferent fibers of the N. vagus reach the medulla oblongata and end in the nucleus (Ncl.) solitarius. The information is conducted to the Ncl. dorsalis n. vagi, which is the origin of the preganglionic neurons. The axons of those preganglionic neurons constitute the efferent part of the N. vagus. The cholinergic anti-inflammatory pathway, the efferent arm of the inflammatory reflex, consists of the efferent N. vagus, the neurotransmitter acetylcholine and the α7-subunit of the nicotinergic acetylcholine receptor [1]. It has been shown that the spleen is essential for inflammation control by the vagal nerve [36]. Furthermore, there is evidence that the N. splenicus is essential for decreasing serum TNF levels by the N. vagus [37]. The fibers involved in this process presumably originate from the plexus celiacus [38–40]. The route of neuronal impulse conduction is composed of two synapsing neurons. One of these originates from the Ncl. dorsalis n. vagi and the second, postganglionic neuron, originates from the plexus celiacus and reaches the spleen in the N. splenicus. The N. splenicus mainly consists of catecholaminergic, postganglionic sympathetic fibers [41], which terminate in direct proximity of the immune cells from the white pulpa, marginal zone and red pulpa [42]. Reserpine empties the stored catecholamines and thus inhibits the TNF-suppressive effect of stimulation of the N. vagus [37]. This leads to the conclusion that this effect is norepinephrine-mediated because norepinephrine is set free from the terminating fibers of the N. splenicus. Catecholamines can increase or decrease the production of pro-inflammatory cytokines, depending on whether they act on α- or β-adrenergic receptors [17, 43]. There is recent evidence that β2-adrenergic receptors of regulatory T-cells are critical for the anti-inflammatory potential of the vagus nerve [44, 45]. But this phenomenon does not explain the role of the α7-subunit in the context of stimulation of the N. vagus. It is possible that acetylcholine released from the N. vagus affects neurons in the plexus celiacus expressing the α-7-subunit and thus enables the release of norepinephrine from fibers terminating in the spleen [46, 47] (**Fig. 1**).

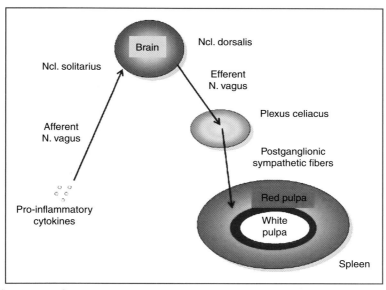

Fig. 1. The inflammatory reflex

Pharmacological Relevance and Perspective

Cholinergic activation by inhibition of cholinesterase with peripherally and centrally acting cholinesterase inhibitors has been used clinically for years in various indications. The interesting question here is whether these substances are also able to influence the cholinergic anti-inflammatory pathway and thus the progress of sepsis in an advantageous way [29].

It was shown that cholinesterase inhibition by physostigmine increased survival in murine experimental sepsis [29] and was as effective as the established model of direct stimulation of acetylcholine receptors by nicotine [48]. Physostigmine weakens the activation of NF-κB, the production of pro-inflammatory mediators and the activation of macrophages. The observed decreased transactivation of NF-κB is possibly the relevant mechanism for increased survival in murine experimental sepsis by controlling excessive inflammation. However, although the levels of TNF-α, IL-1β and IL-6 in plasma were significantly decreased, they were still considerable. However, these cytokine concentrations possibly reflect a sufficient and adequate reaction to infection without an excessive immunological response and all its consequences and thus a functionally directed inflammatory reaction.

If the animals' treatment started six hours after the induction of experimental sepsis and not directly after induction there was a trend for increased survival in the treated animals but this was not significant [29]. If the treatment started later than six hours after the induction of sepsis it had no impact on survival. Hence, there may be a positive effect in clinically manifest sepsis but the use of physostigmine can only lead to positive results when administered as early as possible. This result emphasizes once more the importance of early diagnosis of sepsis and the resulting efficient and consequent therapy [29]. In another trial with rats suf-

I

fering from experimental endotoxemia induced by lipopolysaccharide (LPS), physostigmine was able to reduce capillary leakage and the interaction between leukocytes and endothelium [49].

As inflammation is a basically uniform process that displays immensely differing responses of the organism to various types of damage in terms of quantity and quality and as inflammation is important in the pathophysiology of many diseases, inhibition of cholinesterase could be a useful therapeutic concept not only in sepsis but also in other inflammatory diseases, e.g., pancreatitis or chronic inflammatory bowel disease [50, 51].

The assessment of potential adverse effects is very relevant in this context. Gastrointestinal spasms, bradycardia, hypotension, hypersalivation, hyperthermia and sweating are the main adverse effects of therapy with cholinesterase inhibitors. These effects are even more important because cholinesterase inhibitors would be used in patients with the most serious disease. An experimental study on mice showed that low dose neostigmine could not inhibit the histopathologic damage after endotoxemia but, at a higher dose, neostigmine led to the animals' death, presumably by cardiovascular reactions [50]. Here, further investigation about the adverse effects of cholinesterase inhibitors in septic disease is required. This will include investigation of the various substances, their dosage and their timely administration.

Conclusion

The neuroendocrine axis with the HPA system and the cholinergic anti-inflammatory reflex plays an important role in restriction of the pro-inflammatory reaction in sepsis. Cholinesterase inhibitors make these effects pharmacologically usable. The animal model of murine experimental sepsis suggests that the early use of theses substances may decrease mortality in sepsis. Importantly, early administration of cholinesterase inhibitors seems to be required. As central and peripheral cholinesterase inhibitors have been in clinical use for various indications for many years, it is possible that these substances may have a place in the multimodal concept of sepsis therapy in a few years.

References

1. Rosas-Ballina M, Tracey KJ (2009) Cholinergic control of inflammation. J Intern Med 265: 663–679
2. Sternberg E (2006) Neural regulator of innate immunity: A coordinated nonspecific host response to pathogens. Nat Rev Immunol 6: 318–328
3. Dantzer R, O'Connor JC, Freund GC, Johnson RW, Kelley KW (2008) From inflammation to sickness and depression: When the immune subjugates the brain. Nat Rev Neurosci 9: 46–56
4. Woiciechowsky C, Schoning B, Lanksch WR, Volk H-D, Docke WD (1999). Mechanisms of brain-mediated systemic anti-inflammatory syndrome causing immunodepression. J Mol Med 77: 769–780
5. Ebersoldt M, Sharshar T, Annane D (2007) Sepsis associated delirium. Intensive Care Med 33: 941–950
6. Kumar V, Sharma A (2010) Is neuroimmunomodulation a future therapeutic approach for sepsis? Int Immunopharmacol 10: 9–17
7. Madden K, Sanders V, Felten D (1995) Catecholamine influences and sympathetic neural modulation of immune responsiveness. Annu Rev Pharmacol Toxicol 35: 417–448

8. Weihe E, Nohr D, Michel S, et al (1991) Molecular anatomy of the neuro-immune connection. Int J Neurosci 59: 1–23
9. John C, Buckingham J (2003) Cytokines: Regulation of hypothalamo-pituitary-adrenocortical axis. Curr Opin Pharmacol 3: 378–384
10. Woiciechowsky C, Ruprecht S, Docke WD, Volk HD (2000) Role of the sympathetic nervous system and hypothalamic-pituitary-adrenal axis in brain-mediated compensatory anti-inflammatory response. Biomed Rev 11: 29–38
11. Dunn A, Wang J, Ando T (1999) Effects of cytokines on cerebral neurotransmission. Comparison with the effects of stress. Adv Exp Med Biol 461: 117–127
12. Zhang J, Swiergiel AH, Palamarchouk VS, Dunn A (1998) Intracerebroventricular infusion of CRF increases extracellular concentrations of norepinephrine in the hippocampus and cortex as determined by in vivo voltammetry. Brain Res Bull 47: 277–284
13. Berkenbosch F, de Goeij D, del Rey AE, Besedovsky HO (1989) Neuroendocrine sympathetic and metabolic responses induced by interleukin-1. Neuroendocrinology 50: 570–576
14. Shimizu N, Hori T, Nakane H (1994) An interleukin-1beta-induced noradrenaline release in the spleen is mediated by brain corticotropin-releasing factor. Brain Behav Immun 8: 14–23
15. Elenkov I, Wilder RL, Chrousos GP, Vizi ES (2000) The sympathetic nerve – an integrative interface between to super systems: The brain and the immune system. Pharmacol Rev 52: 595–638
16. Miksa M, Das P, Zhou M, et al (2009) Pivotal role of the a2A-adrenoceptor in producing inflammation and organ injury in a rat model of sepsis. PLoS ONE 4:e5504
17. Spengler R, Allen RM, Demick DG, Strieter RM, Kunkel SL (1990) Stimulation of alpha-adrenergic receptor augments the production of macrophage-derived tumor necrosis factor. J Immunol 145: 1430–1434
18. Hasko G, Nemeth ZH, Szabo C, Zsilia G, Salzman AL, Vizi ES (1998) Isoproterenol inhibits IL-10, TNF-alpha, and nitric oxide production in RAW 264.7 macrophages. Brain Res Bull 45: 183–187
19. Siegmund B, Eigler A, Hartmann G, Hacker U, Endres S (1998) Adrenaline enhances LPS-induced IL-10 synthesis: Evidence for protein kinase A-mediated pathway. Int J Immunopharmacol 20: 57–69
20. Bornstein S, Chrousos G (1998) Adrenocorticotrophin (ACTH)- and non-ACTH-mediated regulation of adrenal cortex: neural and immune inputs. J Clin Endocrinol Metab 84: 1729–1736
21. Matejec R, Löcke G, Mühling J, et al (2008) Release of melanotroph- and corticotroph-type proopiomelanocortin derivates in blood after administration of corticotropin-releasing hormone in patients with septic shock without adrenocortical insufficiency. Shock 31: 553–560
22. Munford R, Levine J (2001) The crucial role of the systemic response in the innate (non-adaptive) host defense. J Endotoxin Res 7: 327–332
23. Besedovsky H, Del RE, Sorkin E, Dinarello C (1986) Immunoregulatory feedback between interleukin-1 and glucocorticoid hormones. Science 233: 652–654
24. Tracey KJ (2002) The inflammatory reflex. Nature 420: 853–859
25. Borovikova L, Ivanova S, Zhang M, et al (2000) Vagus nerve stimulation attenuates the systemic inflammatory response to endotoxin. Nature 405: 458–462
26. Huston J, Gallowitsch-Puerta M, Ochani M, et al (2007) Transcutaneous vagus nerve stimulation reduces serum high mobility group box 1 levels and improves survival in murine sepsis. Crit Care Med 35: 2762–2768
27. Wang H, Yu M, Ochani M, et al (2003) Nicotinic actylcholine receptor α7 subunit is an essential regulator of inflammation. Nature 421: 384–388
28. Huston J, Ochani M, Rosas-Ballina M, et al (2008) Splenectomy protects against sepsis lethality and reduces serum HMGB1 levels. J Immunol 181: 3535–3539
29. Hofer S, Eisenbach C, Lukic IK, et al (2008) Pharmacologic cholinesterase inhibition improves survival in experimental sepsis. Crit Care Med 36: 404–408
30. Rittirsch D, Flierl M, Ward P (2008) Harmful molecular mechanisms in sepsis. Nature 8: 776–787

31. Blalock J (1984) The immune system as a sensory organ. J Immunol 132: 1067–1070
32. Blalock J (2005) The immune system as the sixth sense. J Intern Med 257: 126–138
33. Goehler L, Gaykema RP, Hammack SE, Maier SF, Watkins LR (1998) Interleukin-1 induces c-Fos immunoreactivity in primary afferent neurons of the vagus nerve. Brain Res 804: 306–310
34. Goehler L, Relton JK, Dripps D, et al (1997) Vagal paraganglia bind biotinylated interleukin-1 receptor antagonist: A possible mechanism for immune-to-brain communication. Brain Res Bull 43: 357–364
35. Maier SF, Goehler LE, Fleshner M. Watkins LR (1998) The role of the vagus nerve in cytokine-to-brain communication. Ann NY Acad Sci 840: 289–300
36. Huston J, Ochani M, Rosas-Ballina M, et al (2006) Splenectomy inactivates the cholinergic antiinflammatory pathway during lethal endotoxemia and polymicrobial sepsis. J Exp Med 203: 1623–1628
37. Rosas-Ballina M, Ochani M, et al (2008) Splenic nerve is required for cholinergic antiinflammatory pathway control of TNF in endotoxemia. Proc Natl Acad Sci USA 105: 11008–11013
38. Bellinger D, Felten SY, Lorton D, Felten DL (1989) Origin of noradrenergic innervation of the spleen in rats. Brain Behav Immun 3: 291–311
39. Cano G, Sved AF, Rinaman L, Rabin BS, Card JP (2001) Characterization of the central nervous system innervation of the rat spleen using viral transneuronal tracing. J Comp Neurol 439: 1–18
40. Nance D, Burns J (1989) Innervation of the spleen in the rat: Evidence for absence of afferent innervation. Brain Behav Immun 3: 281–290
41. Klein R, Wilson SP, Dzielak DJ, Yang WH, Viveros OH (1982) Opioid peptides and noradrenaline co-exist in large dense-cored vesicles from sympathetic nerve. Neuroscience 7: 2255–2261
42. Felten D, Ackermann KD, Wiegand SJ, Felten SY (1987) Noradrenergic sympathetic innervation of the spleen: I. Nerve fibres associate with lymphocytes and macrophages in specific compartments of the splenic white pulp. J Neurosci Res 18: 28–36
43. Deng J, Muthu K, Gamelli R, Shankar R, Jones SB (2004) Adrenergic modulation of splenic macrophage cytokine release in polymicrobial sepsis. Am J Physiol Cell Physiol 287:C730–736
44. Pena G, Cai B, Ramos L, Vida G, Deitch EA, Ulloa L (2011) Cholinergic regulatory lymphocytes re-establish neuromodulation of innate immune responses in sepsis. J Immunol 187: 718–725
45. Vida G, Pena G, Kanashiro A, et al (2011) β2-Adrenoreceptors of regulatory lymphocytes are essential for vagal neuromodulation of the innate immune system. FASEB J 25: 4476–4485
46. Bulloch K, Damavandy T, Badamchian M (1994) Characterization of choline O-actyltransferase (ChAT) in the BALB/C mouse spleen. Int J Neurosci 76: 141–149
47. Lips K, König P, Schatzle K, et al (2006) Coexpression and spatial association of nicotinic acytlcholine receptor subunit alpha7 and alpha 10 in rat sympathetic neurons. J Mol Neurosci 30: 15–16
48. Wang H, Liao H, Ochani M, et al (2004) Cholinergic agonists inhibit HMGB1 release and improve survival in experimental sepsis. Nat Med 10: 1216–1221
49. Peter C, Schmidt K, Hofer S, et al (2010) Effects of physostigmine on microcirculatory alterations during experimental endotoxemia. Shock 33: 405–411
50. Ghia J, Blennerhassett P, Kumar-Ondiveeran H, Verdu EF, Collins SM (2006) The vagus nerve: A tonic inhibitory influence associated with inflammatory bowel disease in a murine model. Gastroenterology 131: 1122–1130
51. van Westerloo DJ, Giebelen IA, Florquin S, et al (2006) The vagus nerve and nicotinic receptors modulate experimental pancreatitis severity in mice. Gastroenterology 130: 1822–1830

The mHLA-DR System in the Critically Ill

A. Gouel, A. Lepape, and B. Allaouchiche

I

Introduction

Nosocomial infections represent a major public health problem, with an incidence of about 12 % in the intensive care unit (ICU) in 2005 [1]. Such infections are responsible for a substantial level of morbidity and mortality, and increased length of stay in the ICU and healthcare-associated costs. A new risk factor for nosocomial infection, immunosuppression, has recently been identified in critically ill patients. It is well accepted that every severe inflammatory stress state is accompanied by a hyper-inflammation state, followed by secondary immunosuppression induced by anti-inflammatory mechanisms dedicated to control the initial inflammatory response. This immunosuppressive mechanism has been found in numerous circumstances, such as sepsis, severe trauma, or invasive surgery. In the absence of clinical signs of immune status, various biological parameters have been evaluated. Among the biomarkers studied, monocyte expression of human leukocyte antigen (HLA-DR), or mHLA-DR, has provided the most satisfactory results in representing immune function. The goal of this review is to present an overview of mHLA-DR in the ICU, in terms of its prognostic value for mortality and secondary infections and its potential in the monitoring of new immune treatments in septic shock.

Presentation of the HLA system

Mapping and Nomenclature

The HLA system is located on the centromeric region of the short arm of chromosome 6 (band 6p21.3) [2]. HLA-DR belongs to the class II HLA system which is constitutively expressed on the surface of antigen-presenting cells (monocytes, macrophages, dendritic cells, B lymphocytes). HLA-DR expression depends on a unique transcription factor, CIITA (class II transactivator). HLA-DR is a glycoprotein consisting of a non-covalently associated dimer that presents an extracellular binding site for the antigen peptide.

Functions and Polymorphism of the HLA-DR System

The classical molecules of the class II HLA system are involved in the presentation of antigens to CD4+ T lymphocytes. Antigen-presenting cells internalize circulating antigens. After various steps, the endosomes containing antigens fuse with vesicles containing the class II HLA, permitting their binding. The peptides

J.-L. Vincent (ed.), *Annual Update in Intensive Care and Emergency Medicine 2012*
DOI 10.1007/978-3-642-25716-2 © Springer-Verlag Berlin Heidelberg 2012

I

are then delivered to the surface of the cell, leading to the interaction of the class II HLA-peptide with the T lymphocyte-associated T cell receptor permitting the activation of T lymphocytes and the initiation of the adaptive immune response. The HLA system is characterized by its considerable polymorphism, which is expressed at the level of the peptide niche. For a given individual, a larger diversity in the HLA system corresponds to a greater ability for class II HLA to present different antigens and trigger an effective defense against a new pathogen.

Measurement Techniques for mHLA-DR

The measurement of mHLA-DR is performed using a standardized flow cytometry technique, which was validated in a multicenter European study in 2005 [3]. The collection of the sample is the determining factor for the reliability of the results. Blood samples are collected in EDTA-anticoagulated tubes (ethylenediaminetetraacetic acid). They must be kept at 4 °C and stained within 2 hours after collection, as mHLA-DR is a very sensitive marker and its expression is rapidly regulated *in vitro*. Flow cytometric analysis can be performed using various techniques during the subsequent 24 hours – if the tubes are kept at 4 °C – without causing variation in the results.

The procedure consists of an initial double labeling of the cells with two antibodies: Anti-CD14 – a specific marker for monocytes – and anti-HLA-DR, usually coupled with phycoerythrin. Analysis by flow cytometry allows for identification of monocytes based on CD14 expression. mHLA-DR expression is then evaluated in these cells using the fluorescence of phycoerythrin (**Fig. 1**).

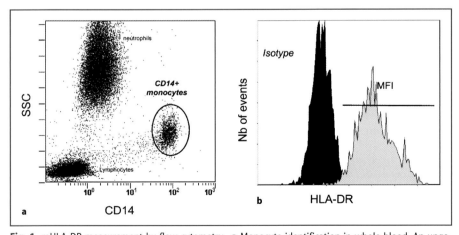

Fig. 1. mHLA-DR measurement by flow cytometry . **a** Monocyte identification in whole blood. An ungated leukocyte biparametric representation on the basis of side scatter characteristics (SSC, y-axis) and CD14 expression (FITC-CD14, x-axis) is shown. The CD14-expressing population is easily distinguishable as gating region 'CD14+ monocytes'. **b** Gated cells from 'CD14+ monocytes' in **a** are expressed on the basis of HLA-DR expression (monoparametric histogram, PE-HLA-DR). The black histogram depicts isotype control, whereas the blue one represents patient expression (illustrative example). FITC, fluorescein isothiocyanate; MFI: mean fluorescence intensity; PE, phycoerythrin. From [28] with permission.

The results can be expressed in three ways:

- As a percentage of HLA-DR-positive monocytes within the total monocyte population (threshold defined by an isotype control antibody);
- Using the Mean of Fluorescence Intensity, or MFI, with respect to the total monocyte population, which reflects the cell density of HLA-DR;
- Using the number of HLA-DR antibodies (also called sites) bound to the monocytes, which also reflects the cell density of HLA-DR. In this case, calibration beads are used: Quantibrite (BD Biosciences, Mississauga, Canada). The use of calibration beads allows for the conversion of MFI into the number of antibodies fixed per cell and approximately indicates the number of HLA-DR molecules per monocyte.

mHLA-DR as a Marker of Immune Function

mHLA-DR: A Reflection of Monocyte Deactivation

The first hours after an acute stress event are characterized by a storm of pro-inflammatory molecules, corresponding to the initiation of a systemic inflammatory response syndrome (SIRS). A strong compensatory anti-inflammatory response syndrome (CARS) inducing a state of immunosuppression follows very rapidly in order to limit inflammation and to prevent the detrimental effects of inflammation at the systemic level (**Fig. 2**). This state translates into the inability of the organism to fight off the initial infection but also an increased sensitivity to nosocomial infections. The compensatory mechanisms are induced in the 10 hours following the onset of stress. Among them, monocyte deactivation is characterized by an alteration of antigen presentation by the monocytes because of the reduction or disappearance of HLA-DR, reduction of the induction of specific antigen responses by T cells following a reduction in antigen presentation, and change in the secretion of pro-inflammatory cytokines in response to various pathogens.

Functional studies have shown an association between weak levels of mHLA-DR expression and alteration in monocyte function. mHLA-DR characterized the inflammatory phenotype of circulating monocytes and is the link between innate and adaptative immunity. In addition, the major advantage of measuring a cell-surface marker like mHLA-DR is that its level of expression is the sum of the effects of multiple mediators involved in the response of the organism to different stress situations, particularly different cytokines. Therefore, the expression level

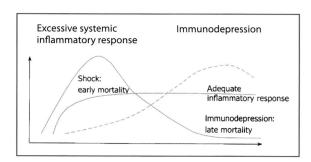

Fig. 2. Presumed immunological phases of sepsis. From [40] with permission.

of mHLA-DR is considered to be a global reflection of the functionality of the immune system.

Factors Influencing the Expression of mHLA-DR

In a study conducted on 77 healthy volunteers [4], monocytes expressed HLA-DR with minimal variability in respect to age, sex, ethnicity, time of day or year, or serum alcohol level. The various therapies used in intensive care do not seem to have an effect on the expression of mHLA-DR, including corticotherapy, exogenous catecholamines, immunosuppressive treatments used after transplantation, transfusions of blood components and antibiotics.

Expression of mHLA-DR is finely regulated by the various cytokines produced during immune responses. mHLA-DR is stimulated by various mediators, such as granulocyte macrophage colony stimulating factor (GM-CSF) [5], interferon (IFN)-γ, and G-CSF, and is negatively regulated by interleukin (IL)-10 [6], transforming growth factor (TGF)-β, prostaglandins, and lipopolysaccharide (LPS, desensitization).

Expression of mHLA-DR in Sepsis

Prediction of the Development of Secondary Infections

Monocyte expression of HLA-DR is altered during the course of sepsis [7]. The reference value for the decrease in mHLA-DR expression during sepsis was defined by Volk et al. as 39.5 % [8], with a nadir corresponding to the onset of sepsis. The loss of mHLA-DR expression is related to the severity of sepsis (septic shock versus severe sepsis or sepsis) [6, 9]. mHLA-DR expression seems to be negatively correlated with the sequential organ failure assessment (SOFA) score [10, 11] and simplified acute physiology score (SAPS) II, and with biological variables such as procalcitonin (PCT) [10]. Observational studies of mHLA-DR expression during sepsis showed that after an initial decrease, mHLA-DR expression changed in two distinct ways: Patients who presented a spontaneous increase in mHLA-DR expression, reaching levels comparable to control groups, had favorable outcomes; patients who maintained low mHLA-DR expression or in whom levels decreased even further developed secondary infections. We can assume that persisting low mHLA-DR expression, i.e., a low efficiency of innate immunity, may expose patients to an increased risk of secondary infections [12, 13]. Researchers are, therefore, interested in using mHLA-DR as a predictor of outcome in two ways: By measuring mHLA-DR expression on a particular day or by comparing mHLA-DR expression over several days.

Prediction of Mortality

The predictive value of a low level of mHLA-DR expression remains controversial. Monneret et al. studied 86 patients with septic shock (global mortality rate of 29 % at day 28) [11]. There was a significant difference in mHLA-DR expression between survivors and non-survivors (43 % versus 18 %, p<.001) on days 3–4 with a threshold value of 30 % (**Fig. 3**). The predictive role of mHLA-DR expression regarding mortality was confirmed in septic ICU patients (whatever severity) at different time points [10, 14–16].

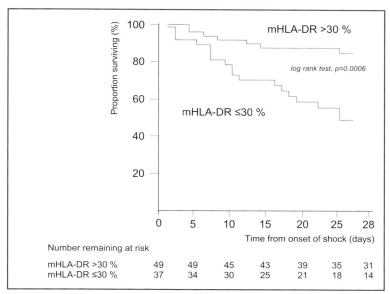

Fig. 3. Survival of patients following septic shock according to mHLA-DR at days 3–4. From [11] with permission.

However, other studies in a large ICU population [13] or in septic patients [17] have reported that mHLA-DR at a given time point was not a predictive marker of outcome. Others found that other biomarkers or scores were better predictors of mortality than mHLA-DR expression, e.g., LPS-induced tumor necrosis factor (TNF)-α production [18] or APACHE II and SOFA scores [19].

These studies have limitations that make comparisons difficult, including the populations studied (severity, number of patients included), the length of monitoring and most importantly the mHLA-DR measurement techniques, which were not all comparable. In conclusion, it seems that the predictive role of mHLA-DR expression for nosocomial infection after sepsis development is well accepted, although the time point needs to be better defined (ranging from day 0 to day 4). A threshold value of 30 % for mHLA-DR expression is presently agreed on in most studies [7, 11, 17]. With respect to mortality, there seems to be a tendency towards a role of mHLA-DR as a predictive marker, but additional studies need to be performed to confirm these results.

Tracking the Effectiveness of Immune-stimulating Treatments

The justification for immune-stimulating treatments stands in the loss of innate and adaptative immunity functions in septic patients [20]. Various studies have focused chiefly on the administration of IFN-γ [21] and CSF growth factors (particularly GM-CSF in comparison with G-CSF, which has been seldom studied). The beneficial effects of IFN-γ treatment were originally proposed in ICU patients at the end of the 1980s [22]; the patients exhibited significant increases in mHLA-DR expression *in vitro* after treatment. Later studies did not demonstrate a clini-

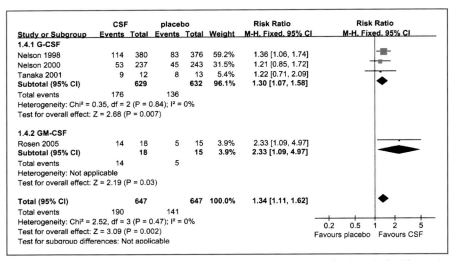

Fig. 4. Reversal rate from infection of G-CSF or GM-CSF therapy *versus* placebo. From [26] with permission.

cal effect after *in vivo* administration of IFN-γ versus placebo [7], despite a trend toward a decrease in the number of infectious episodes among the treated groups. Some studies were conducted without immune monitoring, with no clinical effectiveness [23, 24]. In two recent case reports, a beneficial effect of altered mHLA-DR expression was observed in patients suffering from refractory septic shock with severe immunosuppression [13].

Administration of *in vitro* GM-CSF to monocytes from healthy patients promoted an increase in the expression of mHLA-DR and in the production of proinflammatory cytokines [5]. In septic patients, the *in vitro* stimulation of monocytes by GM-CSF permitted restoration of their function, as for *in vivo* studies [25]. A recent meta-analysis demonstrated a significantly increased reversal rate from infection, with no significant reduction in all cause mortality [26] (**Fig. 4**).

No major adverse effects linked to IFN-γ, except for fever, or to GM-CSF administration have been reported. Considering these results, it seems essential that alterations of the immune status in patients should be followed in order to evaluate the effectiveness of treatments. Despite the encouraging *in vitro* results, *in vivo* studies have not demonstrated clinical effectiveness. It seems likely that patients should be stratified based on mHLA-DR expression, allowing for the selection of patients who could benefit from IFN-γ or GM-CSF treatment. Patients without a sufficient change in mHLA-DR expression would be unlikely to benefit from such therapy. Conversely, immunostimulation would be beneficial for patients exhibiting a significant loss in mHLA-DR expression.

Evaluation of mHLA-DR in Other ICU Patients

Following Severe Trauma

Severe injury is characterized by a sepsis-like immune response. The magnitude of immunosuppression generated by trauma varies in studies, with an early aver-

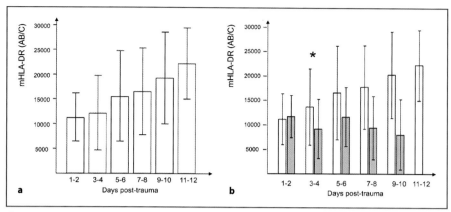

Fig. 5. mHLA-DR expression in trauma patients (*p<.01). **a** In the whole trauma population. **b** Patients with (blue bars) or without (white bars) sepsis. From [28] with permission.

age mHLA-DR expression of between 32 % [22] and 70 % [27]. The amplitude of the decrease in mHLA-DR expression seems to be linked to the severity of the trauma [27]. As with septic patients, mHLA-DR expression can be used to predict infection in trauma patients. In injured patients with an uneventful outcome, mHLA-DR expression returned to normal within a week. In contrast, in patients who developed infection, mHLA-DR levels remained low or decreased even further. In 105 severely injured patients (injury severity score [ISS] $\geq$ 25), a slope of mHLA-DR expression below 1.2 between days 1–2 and days 3–4 was associated with the development of sepsis after adjustment for usual clinical confounders (adjusted OR 5.41, 95 %CI 1.42; 20.52, p = .013) (**Fig. 5**) [28]. This link between the reduction in mHLA-DR expression and the occurrence of post-traumatic nosocomial infections has been confirmed in numerous studies [29, 30].

After Invasive Surgery

Stress induced by a major surgical intervention is also responsible for a transitory suppression of the immune response [13]. Resultant variations in mHLA-DR expression have been found after different surgical procedures, including cardiac, thoracic, abdominal, neurologic, and kidney or liver transplants [10, 31]. The magnitude of the immunosuppression differs between studies, ranging from 40 % [10] to 80 % [31]. Return to normal mHLA-DR levels in patients with favorable outcomes occurred most often in the five to seven days after surgery. In a study by Allen et al., the initial reduction in mHLA-DR expression was more marked for infants who developed secondary sepsis, with a significant difference compared to the non-infected group [31]. The relationship between loss of mHLA-DR expression and postoperative nosocomial infections has been confirmed in various surgical circumstances [10, 17], but no threshold value for mHLA-DR can yet be established. As with sepsis, it seems that variations in mHLA-DR expression over the course of hospitalization are more informative than numerical values [13].

I

During Acute Pancreatitis

The initial phase of medium or severe acute pancreatitis is marked by a negative effect on immune function. Four studies have reported a link between a reduction in mHLA-DR expression, the severity of pancreatitis (severe *versus* moderate), and clinical scores [32–35]. One of these studies established a threshold value of 60 % for the predictiveness of mHLA-DR for sepsis, with a sensitivity of 100 % and a specificity ranging from 91.3 % at day 1 to 98.2 % at day 14 [33]. In contrast to patients with multiple trauma and surgery, infections occur late in these patients, most often in the third to fifth week of disease development, which explains the prolonged reductions in mHLA-DR expression.

In Severe Burns

As in trauma, severe burns induce a major inflammatory response, followed by an anti-inflammatory state. The nadir for mHLA-DR expression occurs later in burn patients compared with trauma patients, between day 7 and day 10. This nadir was later and more marked in patients whose outcome was complicated by sepsis development [36, 37].

In Stroke

A reduction in mHLA-DR expression in the initial phase of a stroke has been shown by two teams, with a nadir at day 3 and values of approximately 55 % [38] or 20,000 antibodies per monocyte [39]. During the first week following the stroke, the reduction in mHLA-DR expression was more marked in patients who later developed a secondary infection, with the establishment of a threshold value for mHLA-DR of 57.8 % at day 2 as a predictive marker for sepsis development, with a sensitivity of 96 % and a specificity of 80 %.

Conclusion

The expression of mHLA-DR is a useful marker of immunosuppression in ICU patients. mHLA-DR expression appears to be an independent predictive factor for infections in all the groups of patients discussed in this review, although its role with respect to the prediction of mortality in septic patients remains to be confirmed. Forthcoming studies should be conducted in order to determine a mHLA-DR threshold value for the prediction of the risk of nosocomial infections. This threshold would allow identification of at-risk patients who could benefit from preventive strategies, such as the immune-stimulating treatments that are presently being evaluated in septic shock.

References

1. REA-RAISIN (2006) Surveillance des infections nosocomiales en réanimation adulte en France – Résultats 2005. Available at: http://www.ladocumentationfrancaise.fr/var/storage/rapports-publics//064000852/0000.pdf Accessed Jan 2012
2. Moalic V, Ferec C (2005) HLA typing, analysis methods, and clinical applications. Presse Med 34: 1101–1108

I

3. Döcke WD, Hoflich C, Davis KA, et al (2005) Monitoring temporary immunodepression by flow cytometric measurement of monocytic HLA-DR expression: a multicenter standardized study. Clin Chem 51: 2341–2347

4. Cheadle WG, Hershman MJ, Wellhausen SR , Polk HC Jr (1991) HLA-DR antigen expression on peripheral blood monocytes correlates with surgical infection. Am J Surg 161: 639–645

5. Nierhaus A, Montag B, Timmler N, et al (2003) Reversal of immunoparalysis by recombinant human granulocyte-macrophage colony-stimulating factor in patients with severe sepsis. Intensive Care Med 29: 646–651

6. Fumeaux T, Pugin J (2002) Role of interleukin-10 in the intracellular sequestration of human leukocyte antigen-DR in monocytes during septic shock. Am J Respir Crit Care Med 166: 1475–1482

7. Döcke WD, Randow F, Syrbe U, et al (1997) Monocyte deactivation in septic patients: restoration by IFN-gamma treatment. Nat Med 3: 678–681

8. Volk HD, Reinke P, Krausch D, et al (1996) Monocyte deactivation--rationale for a new therapeutic strategy in sepsis. Intensive Care Med 22 (Suppl 4): 474–481

9. Schinkel C, Sendtner R, Zimmer S, Faist E (1998) Functional analysis of monocyte subsets in surgical sepsis. J Trauma 44: 743–748

10. Tschaikowsky K, Hedwig-Geissing M, Schiele A, Bremer F, Schywalsky M, Schuttler J (2002) Coincidence of pro- and anti-inflammatory responses in the early phase of severe sepsis: Longitudinal study of mononuclear histocompatibility leukocyte antigen-DR expression, procalcitonin, C-reactive protein, and changes in T-cell subsets in septic and postoperative patients. Crit Care Med 30: 1015–1023

11. Monneret G, Lepape A, Voirin N, et al (2006) Persisting low monocyte human leukocyte antigen-DR expression predicts mortality in septic shock. Intensive Care Med 32: 1175–1183

12. Landelle C, Lepape A, Voirin N, et al (2010) Low monocyte human leukocyte antigen-DR is independently associated with nosocomial infections after septic shock. Intensive Care Med 36: 1859–1866

13. Lukaszewicz AC, Grienay M, Resche-Rigon M, et al (2009) Monocytic HLA-DR expression in intensive care patients: interest for prognosis and secondary infection prediction. Crit Care Med 37: 2746–2752

14. Caille V, Chiche JD, Nciri N, et al (2004) Histocompatibility leukocyte antigen-D related expression is specifically altered and predicts mortality in septic shock but not in other causes of shock. Shock 22: 521–526

15. Monneret G, Debard AL, Venet F, et al (2003) Marked elevation of human circulating CD4+CD25+ regulatory T cells in sepsis-induced immunoparalysis. Crit Care Med 31: 2068–2071

16. Saenz JJ, Izura JJ, Manrique A, Sala F, Gaminde I (2001) Early prognosis in severe sepsis via analyzing the monocyte immunophenotype. Intensive Care Med 27: 970–977

17. Perry SE, Mostafa SM, Wenstone R, Shenkin A, McLaughlin PJ (2003) Is low monocyte HLA-DR expression helpful to predict outcome in severe sepsis? Intensive Care Med 29: 1245–1252

18. Ploder M, Pelinka L, Schmuckenschlager C, et al (2006) Lipopolysaccharide-induced tumor necrosis factor alpha production and not monocyte human leukocyte antigen-DR expression is correlated with survival in septic trauma patients. Shock 25: 129–134

19. Hynninen M, Pettila V, Takkunen O, et al (2003) Predictive value of monocyte histocompatibility leukocyte antigen-DR expression and plasma interleukin-4 and -10 levels in critically ill patients with sepsis. Shock 20: 1–4

20. Hotchkiss RS, Opal S (2010) Immunotherapy for sepsis--a new approach against an ancient foe. N Engl J Med 363: 87–89

21. Turina M, Dickinson A, Gardner S, Polk HC Jr (2006) Monocyte HLA-DR and interferon-gamma treatment in severely injured patients--a critical reappraisal more than a decade later. J Am Coll Surg 203: 73–81

22. Hershman MJ, Appel SH, Wellhausen SR, Sonnenfeld G, Polk HC Jr (1989) Interferon-gamma treatment increases HLA-DR expression on monocytes in severely injured patients. Clin Exp Immunol 77: 67–70

23. Wasserman D, Ioannovich JD, Hinzmann RD, Deichsel G, Steinmann GG (1998) Interferon-gamma in the prevention of severe burn-related infections: a European phase III multicenter trial. The Severe Burns Study Group. Crit Care Med 26: 434–439
24. Dries DJ, Perry JF Jr (2002) Interferon-gamma: titration of inflammation. Crit Care Med 30: 1663–1664
25. Meisel C, Schefold JC, Pschowski R, et al (2009) Granulocyte-macrophage colony-stimulating factor to reverse sepsis-associated immunosuppression: a double-blind, randomized, placebo-controlled multicenter trial. Am J Respir Crit Care Med 180: 640–648
26. Bo L, Wang F, Zhu J, Li J, Deng X (2011) Granulocyte-colony stimulating factor (G-CSF) and granulocyte-macrophage colony stimulating factor (GM-CSF) for sepsis: a meta-analysis. Crit Care 15: R58
27. Giannoudis PV, Smith RM, Windsor AC, Bellamy MC, Guillou PJ (1999) Monocyte human leukocyte antigen-DR expression correlates with intrapulmonary shunting after major trauma. Am J Surg 177: 454–459
28. Cheron A, Floccard B, Allaouchiche B, et al (2010) Lack of recovery in monocyte human leukocyte antigen-DR expression is independently associated with the development of sepsis after major trauma. Crit Care 14: R208
29. Giannoudis PV, Smith RM, Perry SL, Windsor AJ, Dickson RA, Bellamy MC (2000) Immediate IL-10 expression following major orthopaedic trauma: relationship to anti-inflammatory response and subsequent development of sepsis. Intensive Care Med 26: 1076–1081
30. Walsh DS, Thavichaigarn P, Pattanapanyasat K, et al (2005) Characterization of circulating monocytes expressing HLA-DR or CD71 and related soluble factors for 2 weeks after severe, non-thermal injury. J Surg Res 129: 221–230
31. Allen ML, Peters MJ, Goldman A, et al (2002) Early postoperative monocyte deactivation predicts systemic inflammation and prolonged stay in pediatric cardiac intensive care. Crit Care Med 30: 1140–1145
32. Gotzinger P, Sautner T, Spittler A, et al (2000) Severe acute pancreatitis causes alterations in HLA-DR and CD14 expression on peripheral blood monocytes independently of surgical treatment. Eur J Surg 166: 628–632
33. Satoh A, Miura T, Satoh K, et al (2002) Human leukocyte antigen-DR expression on peripheral monocytes as a predictive marker of sepsis during acute pancreatitis. Pancreas 25: 245–250
34. Yu WK, Li WQ, Li N, Li JS (2004) Mononuclear histocompatibility leukocyte antigen-DR expression in the early phase of acute pancreatitis. Pancreatology 4: 233–243
35. Richter A, Nebe T, Wendl K, et al (1999) HLA-DR expression in acute pancreatitis. Eur J Surg 165: 947–951
36. Sachse C, Prigge M, Cramer G, Pallua N, Henkel E (1999) Association between reduced human leukocyte antigen (HLA)-DR expression on blood monocytes and increased plasma level of interleukin-10 in patients with severe burns. Clin Chem Lab Med 37: 193–198
37. Venet F, Tissot S, Debard AL, et al (2007) Decreased monocyte human leukocyte antigen-DR expression after severe burn injury: Correlation with severity and secondary septic shock. Crit Care Med 35: 1910–1917
38. Zhang DP, Yan FL, Xu HQ, Zhu YX, Yin Y, Lu HQ (2009) A decrease of human leucocyte antigen-DR expression on monocytes in peripheral blood predicts stroke-associated infection in critically-ill patients with acute stroke. Eur J Neurol 16: 498–505
39. Harms H, Prass K, Meisel C, et al (2008) Preventive antibacterial therapy in acute ischemic stroke: a randomized controlled trial. PLoS ONE 3: e2158
40. Kox WJ, Volk T, Kox SN, Volk HD (2000) Immunomodulatory therapies in sepsis. Intensive Care Med 26 (Suppl 1): 124–128

Gut Microbiome and Host Defense Interactions during Critical Illness

I

T.J. Schuijt, T. van der Poll, and W.J. Wiersinga

Introduction

For many years it has been hypothesized that the gut has an important detrimental role in promoting systemic inflammation and infection in the critically ill. During stress and mucosal hypoxia, the mucosa is damaged and host defenses break down causing translocation of bacteria and bacterial toxins which are thought to contribute to the overwhelming inflammation associated with sepsis and multiorgan failure [1, 2]. New emerging data on the role of the microbiome have forced us to reassess the old 'gut as motor of sepsis' hypothesis. The gut microbiome consists of a diverse and vast population of microbes that has an

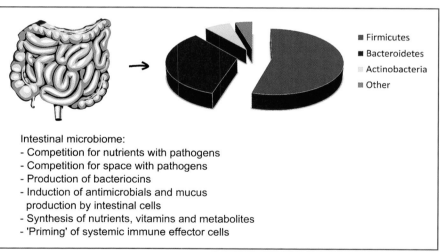

- Firmicutes
- Bacteroidetes
- Actinobacteria
- Other

Intestinal microbiome:
- Competition for nutrients with pathogens
- Competition for space with pathogens
- Production of bacteriocins
- Induction of antimicrobials and mucus production by intestinal cells
- Synthesis of nutrients, vitamins and metabolites
- 'Priming' of systemic immune effector cells

Fig. 1. The intestinal microbiome. The intestinal microbiome is dominated by three phyla: the *Firmicutes* (Gram-positive), *Bacteroides* (Gram-negative) and *Actinobacteria* (Gram-positive). It should be mentioned that significant inter-individual differences in microbiome composition exist. A healthy balanced microbiome is important for the host defense against invading pathogens by preventing pathogenic microorganisms from colonization of the intestine through competition for essential nutrients, space and attachment sites on the epithelium. In addition, members of the intestinal microbiome secrete bacteriocins, defined as toxins produced by bacteria to inhibit the growth of other bacteria, and toxins in order to compete with intestinal pathogens. Other roles of the intestinal microbiome include stimulation of the intestinal immune system, digestion of food, synthesis of essential nutrients for the host and constitutive priming of systemic immune cells.

J.-L. Vincent (ed.), *Annual Update in Intensive Care and Emergency Medicine 2012*
DOI 10.1007/978-3-642-25716-2 © Springer-Verlag Berlin Heidelberg 2012

important protective impact on immune effector functions during both health and disease (**Fig. 1**). It has become clear that the intestinal microbiome, consisting of more bacteria than the total number of cells in the human body, can be seen as an exteriorized organ that exerts numerous functions in the host response against infections [3, 4]. In addition to the more localized influence of the microbiome on the intestinal immune system, recent data show that the microbiome also plays a key role in systemic activation of the immune system contributing to the effective killing of invading pathogens [5]. The clinical relevance of these new insights is underscored by the notion that antibiotic treatment – which on any given day is received by almost three quarters of all patients on the intensive care unit (ICU) [6] – can largely deplete the microbiome. This review focuses on key aspects of the role of the intestinal microbiome in the immune response against pathogens and the importance of intestinal homeostasis for critically ill patients.

The Intestinal Microbiome during Health

The total bowel surface is ~400 m^2 and provides an important habitat for intestinal microorganisms. In addition to the intestinal microbiome, the intestinal epithelium and the mucosal barrier are regarded as the other major entities of the gut [7].

The Intestinal Epithelium and the Mucosal Barrier

The intestinal epithelium is a major hurdle for invading pathogens and is composed of several cell types; key intestinal epithelial cells (IEC) include the enterocytes, Paneth cells, enterochromaffin cells (ECCs), microfold cells and goblet cells which are tightly bound together by tight junctions (**Fig. 2**). Epithelial tight junctions regulate the permeability of the intestinal barrier and control the passage of large molecules. Paneth cells are found throughout the small intestine primarily in the crypts of Lieberkühn [8]. When exposed to bacteria or bacterial antigens, Paneth cells, characterized by large cytoplasmatic granules, secrete innate immune effector molecules such as defensins, but also lysozyme, phospholipase A2 and tumor necrosis factor (TNF)-α, all of which have antimicrobial activity [8]. ECCs are enteroendocrine cells that secrete hormones,

$\triangleright$

Fig. 2. a The intestinal epithelium is composed of enterocytes (pink), goblet cells (green), Paneth cells (red), microfold (M) cells (orange) and enterochromaffin (ECC) cells (blue). Goblet cells continuously produce and secrete mucins which form a thick mucus layer (green layer). The mucus layer consists of two layers; only the upper layer is inhabited by members of the intestinal microbiome. Paneth cells contain granules with antimicrobials such as defensins and lectins which are released into the mucus layer. M cells facilitate the transport of microbes to the underlying Peyer's patches which are aggregated lymphoid nodules. To facilitate ingestion of bacteria by M cells these cells are not covered by the thick mucus layer. The intestinal epithelial cells (IECs) are packed tightly together by tight junctions. Strict regulation of the tight junctions makes the epithelial tissue a selectively permeable barrier. ECCs are enteroendocrine cells that secrete various hormones, like serotonin, in response to several stimuli including toxins produced by bacteria. **b** Several bidirectional relationships between the host and the intestinal microbiome and between bacteria within the microbiome take place in the intestine. Intestinal bacteria provide the human body with metabolites such as short-chain fatty acids, but also with vitamins and other nutrients. Strong mutualism exists between bacteria within the microbiome as well.

Major entities of the gut

Mutualism

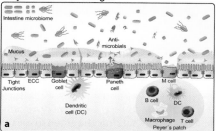

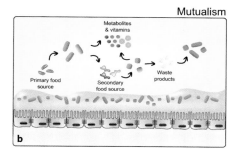

Crosstalk with immune system

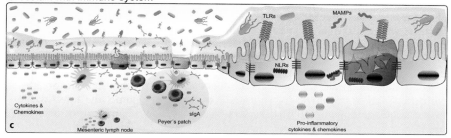

Systemic effects of the gut flora on the host's defense system

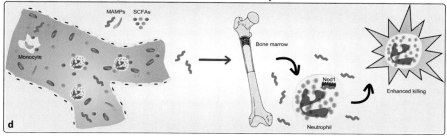

While some intestinal bacteria can process a primary food source, other bacteria are dependent on metabolic products (secondary food source) produced by these bacteria. Other members of the microbiome play a role in the removal of waste products. **c** Components of the microbiome express conserved molecular structures termed microorganism-associated molecular patterns (MAMPs) which are sensed are sensed by pattern recognition receptors (PRRs) – such as Toll-like receptors (TLR) – expressed on IECs, which continuously respond to these compounds in order to orchestrate the immune response. MAMP and metabolite release are a signal for intestinal cells to continuously produce and secrete mucus, antimicrobials and cytokines. Nutrients are also able to activate the immune system directly. M cells are the most important cells in sampling antigens and bacteria from the gut lumen by transferring the material to the underlying Peyer's patches. Dendritic cells (DCs) process and present antigens of T-cells and B-cells in the Peyer's patch or migrate to mesenteric lymph nodes to do this. B-cells that mature become IgA-secreting plasma cells. This dimeric soluble IgA (sIgA) is transported through epithelial cells into the mucosal surface. sIgA is not only important in eradication of pathogens but also in transporting antigens back into the gut lumen in order to maintain hemostasis. Besides M cells, intraepithelial DCs are also involved in direct uptake of antigens and bacteria from the mucosal surface. **d** The impact of the intestinal microbiome does not stop at the gut. Metabolites, such as short-chain fatty acids (SCFA), are partly taken up by IECs while another portion enters the systemic circulation. SCFAs and butyrate have an anti-inflammatory effect on leukocytes. Additionally, components of the intestinal microbiome are translocated into the systemic circulation and continuously prime neutrophils leading to enhanced capability of these cells to kill pathogens.

I

such as serotonin in response to various stimuli including bacterial toxins. Microfold cells can transport bacteria and secreted parts of bacteria across the intestinal barrier to immune cells located in Peyer's patches. Peyer's patches, which are lymphoid follicles, contain antigen presenting cells such as dendritic cells and macrophages. Peyer's patches are part of the gut-associated lymphoid tissue (GALT) of which the other components are the mesenteric lymph nodes and lamina propria lymphocytes.

Before potential intruders meet the intestinal epithelium, they are first awaited by the mucosal barrier. Epithelial and, in particular, goblet cells produce and secrete mucins, which are major components of a thick mucus layer. This layer coats the epithelial surface to protect against pathogens and other irritants such as enzymes, chemicals and mechanical damage. The mucosal barrier itself consists of an inner and outer mucus layer. The outer mucus layer is inhabited by commensal bacteria whereas the inner layer is sterile under normal conditions [9].

Composition of the Intestinal Microbiome

The human intestinal microbiota is composed of 10^{13} to 10^{14} microorganisms whose collective genome ('microbiome') contains at least 100 times as many genes as our own genome [10]. The gut hosts ~1 x 10^{14} bacteria from 500–1,000 different species of which three bacterial divisions – the *Firmicutes* (Gram-positive), *Bacteroides* (Gram-negative) and *Actinobacteria* (Gram-positive) – dominate (**Fig. 1**) [11]. Although the majority of the intestinal microbiome is composed of bacteria, other members have also been identified, including viruses (5.8 %), archaea (0.8 %) and eukaryotes (0.5 %) [12]. Significant differences in the composition of the intestinal microbiome exist between individuals, which can be explained by host genetic and environmental factors [13]. Recent metagenomic studies, that combined 22 sequenced fecal metagenomes of individuals from four countries, have stratified the differences in gut microbiome composition into three robust clusters, termed enterotypes, which are not nation or continent specific [12]. This remarkable finding demonstrates the existence of only a very limited number of well-balanced host-microbial symbiotic states [12]. Differences in gut flora composition may not only contribute to variations in normal physiology as seen among individuals but most probably also affect susceptibility to infection and variations seen in the subsequent immune response [10, 11]. It is anticipated that the identification of enterotypes in patients might allow classification of human groups that respond differently to diet or drug intake [12].

Bidirectional Relationship Between the Immune System and the Intestinal Microbiome

Insight into the close and intense relationship between the intestinal microbiome and the cells of the intestinal epithelium is just beginning to emerge. A role of the microbiome in protection against epithelial cell injury, optimization of host immune systems and resistance against colonization by pathogens have all been described [14, 15]. Furthermore, intestinal bacteria are of importance in the development of mucosal immunity. Germ-free mice, which lack the intestinal microbiome, have underdeveloped Peyer's patches, immature germinal centers, reduced epithelial antimicrobial production and diminished antibody responses [16].

Secretion of Antimicrobials and Competition for Nutrition

Members of the intestinal microbiome secrete antimicrobials and compete for nutrients and space with pathogens. In health, secretion of toxins and antimicrobials such as bacteriocins by bacteria will outcompete pathogens in the intestinal microbiome [17]. For instance, bacteriocins, defined as toxins produced by bacteria to inhibit the growth of similar or closely related bacterial strains, that are produced and secreted by Gram-negative bacteria in the intestine, can inhibit enteropathogenic bacteria such as *Salmonella, Shigella, Klebsiella, Enterobacter,* and *Escherichia* [17]. Competing nutrition is an alternative strategy used by both the 'good' bacteria and the host in order to prevent pathogen invasion [18]. Not surprisingly, diet and nutrition contribute to microbiome composition and immune function [8]. This is the rationale used by those who propagate a prebiotic diet consisting of non-digestible ingredients that can stimulate the health and survival of these 'good' bacteria in order to keep or restore a healthy microbial balance and immune homeostasis. Humans also need certain enzymes from intestinal bacteria that humans themselves do not have; e.g., to digest polysaccharides derived from plant cell walls, enzymes derived from intestinal microbes are essential (**Fig. 2**). Other much needed metabolites such as the short-chain fatty acids (SCFAs), acetate, propionate and butyrate, are main end-products of bacterial metabolism in the intestine as well. Butyrate is an important energy source for enterocytes [19] and plays an important role in the regulation of enterocyte immune effector functions as discussed below.

Interactions between MAMPs and PRRs

Bacteroides, Firmicutes, and *Actinobacteria* and all other components of the microbiome express conserved molecular structures termed microorganism-associated molecular patterns (MAMPs) [20]. Examples of MAMPs include lipopolysaccharide (LPS), peptidoglycan, lipoteichoic acid (LTA) and flagellin. MAMPs are recognized by pattern recognition receptors (PRRs), such as Toll-like receptors (TLRs) and nucleotide oligomerization domain-like receptors (NLRs) [21, 22]. Thirteen TLRs have been identified in mammals. TLR4 is regarded as the LPS receptor, whereas TLR2 is seen as the most important receptor for Gram-positive bacteria (e.g., LTA is recognized by TLR2). TLR5 recognizes flagellin. The recognition of MAMPs by PRRs results in the activation of signaling cascades that in turn lead to activation of the nuclear factor-kappa B (NF-κB) pathway and initiation of the antibacterial immune response [21, 22] (**Fig. 2**). The intracellular NLRs, Nod1 and Nod2, respond to the peptidoglycan components, meso-diaminopimelic acid (DAP) and muramyl dipeptide (MDP), respectively [20]. Nod1 is expressed in many cell lines, including IECs. Nod2, however, is not expressed in enterocytes, but is expressed by Paneth cells in the small intestine [20, 23]. TLRs are expressed on, among other cells, neutrophils, macrophages and enterocytes [21, 22]. Of note, not only the composition of the microbiome but also the expression of PRRs varies considerably in different parts of the lower gastrointestinal tract [20, 24]. As a consequence, cross-talk between the intestinal microbiome and the immune system will be different in the colon compared to the small intestine [20]. IECs of the human small intestine express TLR1, TLR2, TLR3, TLR4, TLR5 and TLR9 at low levels, which will in general increase during inflammation [24]. In addition, the polarity of enterocytes also implies different TLR expression at the apical and basolateral surface of these cells. TLR9 activation through apical and basolateral surface domains of IECs has distinct transcriptional responses: Basolateral TLR9 signals IκBα degradation and activation of the NF-κB pathway, while apical TLR9 stimulation invokes a unique response in which ubiquitinated IκBα accumulates in the cytoplasm preventing NF-κB activation [25]. Furthermore, apical TLR9 stimulation confers intracellular tolerance to subsequent TLR challenges, which implies that polarized IECs are in the unique position to maintain colonic homeostasis and regulate tolerance and inflammation [25]. The differentiated expression of TLR5 on IECs is another example of the polarized function of IECs. TLR5 is expressed only on the basolateral surface of enterocytes, where it can trigger the production of cytokines and chemokines, such as interleukin (IL)-8 and CC-chemokine ligand (CCL)-20 in response to flagellin [24, 25]. Of note, TLR5-deficient mice develop spontaneous colitis and show a large increase in intestinal bacteria density [26]. Just recently it was found that TLR5 deficiency induced changes in gut microbiome composition in mice leading to a full blown metabolic syndrome, including hyperlipidemia, hypertension, insulin resistance, and increased adiposity [27]. Excitingly, transfer of the gut microbiota from TLR5-deficient mice to wild-type germ-free mice conferred many features of metabolic syndrome to the recipients [27]. Lastly, MAMPs also trigger mucin release in order to increase the thickness of the mucosal barrier [9]. In line, PRR mediated responses towards MAMPs will lead to the release of antimicrobials, such as defensins, lectins and lysozymes, into the mucus layer [9].

Microbiome-derived Antigen-induced Production of Antibodies

In humans, the majority of activated B cells reside in the gastrointestinal tract making the gut the largest antibody-producing organ in the human body (reviewed in [20]). Bacteria and their antigenic wall fragments can cross the intestinal barrier primarily through microfold cells that transfer these antigens to immune cells located in Peyer's patches. Dendritic cells in the Peyer's patches present antigens to T cells and B cells either directly in the Peyer's patch or they migrate to the mesenteric lymph nodes to do so. B cells that are located in the lamina propria constantly produce and secrete IgA and IgG after which enterocytes transport and secrete the antibodies into and through the mucus layer [28]. sIgA recognize and bind several pathogens and are, therefore, often named 'natural IgA', whereas infection with a particular pathogen results in production and secretion of specific high-affinity sIgA antibodies [28].

Distant Effects of the Gut Flora on the Host Defense

Perhaps not surprisingly, the impact of the intestinal microflora on the innate immune system does not stop at the gut. Recently it was very elegantly shown that peptidoglycan from the intestinal microbiota constitutively translocates to the circulation and remotely primes bone marrow neutrophils via the NLR, Nod1 [5] (**Fig. 2**). These constitutively primed neutrophils then show an increased capacity to kill microorganisms [5]. In other words, MAMPs – such as peptidoglycan – are released into the circulation from gut bacteria, are sensed by PRRs and subsequently help host defense mechanisms by positively priming distant immune effector cells in order to be prepared in the case of an invasion by pathogens. In addition to MAMPs, metabolites produced by intestinal bacteria, such as

SCFAs, vitamins and ATP, are absorbed from the gut and released systemically (**Fig. 2**). These compounds are known to directly affect several parts of both the innate and adaptive immune system. As an example, butyrate has a broad influence on various immune cells and pathways both in the intestine and systemically [19, 29]. Depending on the cell type and concentration of butyrate, SCFA exert anti-inflammatory activities by inhibiting histone deacetylase (HDAC) and thus NF-κB signaling [29].

The Intestinal Microbiome during Critical Illness

The importance of the gut microbiome in maintaining homeostasis during health has led to a reappraisal of the function – and potential dysfunction – of the gut microbiome during severe illness and infection.

Disturbed Intestinal Homeostasis in the Critically Ill

Both the composition and performance of the gut microbiome, the intestinal epithelium, and the mucosal barrier are all severely affected during critical illness. Studies performed by Shimuzu et al. have shown that the composition of the intestinal microbiome is significantly changed in patients with severe systemic inflammatory response syndrome (SIRS) and that these changes are associated with septic complications and mortality [30, 31]. Using simple Gram-stains to classify the fecal flora into three patterns (diverse, single, depleted), it was shown that mortality due to multiple organ dysfunction syndrome (MODS) for the single pattern (52 %) and the depleted pattern (64 %) was significantly higher than that for the diverse pattern (6 %) [32]. Depletion of the normal gut flora can give

Disturbed intestinal homeostasis   Antibiotics

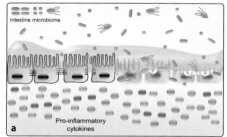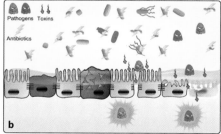

Fig. 3. Altered intestinal homeostasis and the effect of antibiotics on the gut microbiome during critical illness. **a** Pro-inflammatory mediators increase the mucosal permeability by altering the integrity of tight-junctions between enterocytes. Increased apoptosis of intestinal epithelial cells is correlated with sepsis-induced mortality. Loss of the intestinal epithelial barrier function potentially results in translocation of the intestinal microbiome into the circulation. **b** Use of antibiotics can kill members of the intestinal microbiome either directly or indirectly. Indirectly, if these bacteria are dependent on a food source derived from bacteria that are directly affected by antibiotics. Antibiotic treatment decreases the number of intestinal bacteria resulting in diminished release of MAMPs and other metabolites. As a result, fewer antimicrobial molecules, such as defensins and lectins, are produced by Paneth cells, less mucus is produced by goblet cells etc., which makes the host more susceptible to invasion by intestinal pathogens.

rise to pathogenic bacteria. Pro-inflammatory mediators released during critical illness are able to increase epithelial permeability by influencing the regulation of tight junctions between enterocytes [7] (**Fig. 3**). Disruption of tight junction barriers results in increased intestinal permeability, infiltration of luminal antigens and the induction of intestinal inflammation [7]. Of note, pathogenic bacteria, such as enteropathogenic *Escherichia coli*, are also known to be capable of increasing tight junction permeability [7]. Increased apoptosis of gut epithelial cells is another characteristic element observed during critical illness. Autopsy studies among patients who died from sepsis have shown a marked increased in intestinal epithelial apoptosis [33]. Inhibition of intestinal epithelial apoptosis in mice showed a survival advantage, although the mechanism underlying this survival advantage is still poorly understood [7, 34]. Finally, it should be emphasized that many treatment modalities that are standard of care for the treatment of critically ill patients on the ICU are also known to affect the composition of the intestinal microflora: Vasopressors can cause splanchnic ischemia and thus local hypoxia and a lower pH; acid suppressive therapies also alter intraluminal pH; highly processed enteral nutrition or parental nutrition can cause a nutrient deficient milieu in the bowel; long term opiate use is associated with bacterial overgrowth and, lastly, antibiotic use causes depletion of the gut flora and potential selection of resistant organisms [2, 35].

The Effect of Antibiotics on the Gut Flora

Several studies have shown that antibiotic therapy has long lasting alterations and implications for the microbial community structure of the intestine [36, 37]. A study among 14,414 patients in 1,265 ICUs in 75 countries, estimated that on any given day 71 % of patients on the ICU receive antibiotic treatment mostly to cover infections considered to originate in the respiratory tract [6]. Antibiotic treatment – which is standard of care for all patients with sepsis – depletes the gut microbiome and is associated with diminished cytokine production in the gut [37, 38] (**Fig. 3**). Eradication of a specific group of bacteria by antibiotics can indirectly kill other members of the intestinal microbiome that are dependent on food sources provided by these bacteria [39] (**Fig. 3**). Other members of the intestinal microbiome remove toxic waste products of bacterial fermentation [39]. Of clinical importance, alterations of the intestinal microbiome are associated with nosocomial infections, such as vancomycin-resistant *Enterococcus* and *Clostridum difficile* [15, 40]. Targeted depletion of the gut flora can also be used to preemptively eradicate potential pathogens such as *Enterobacteriaceae, Pseudomonas aeruginosa* and *Staphylococcus aureus* in patients on the ICU. Indeed, several studies have shown that selective decontamination of the digestive tract (SDD), in which broad spectrum non-absorbable antibiotics that target yeasts, Gram-positive and Gram-negative pathogens are used to decontaminate the gastrointestinal tract and/or the oropharynx, can decrease ICU and hospital mortality in critically ill patients [41,42]. Worldwide implementation of SDD, however, is hampered by fears of an increase in drug-resistant bacterial strains [43].

Beyond Antibiotics: Therapeutic Modulation of the Gut Microbiome during Critical Illness

During health, the gut microbiome is important in the host defense against invading pathogens. Therefore, manipulation of the gut flora during critical illness in order to restore immune functions is considered an attractive adjunctive therapy for patients on the ICU. One option is to completely renew the gut microbiome. Indeed, recent findings have demonstrated that it is possible to engraft new microbiota from a donor source, resulting in restoration of gut functionality and improvement in health [44, 45]. As an example, fecal transfers have become a serious treatment option for patients with recurrent severe *C. difficile* infections, with a reported cure rate of around 90 % [44, 45]. Another treatment strategy could be to selectively restore gut flora composition by selective administration of MAMPs or whole non-pathogenic bacteria. Traditionally, sepsis is seen as the overwhelming pro-inflammatory host response to invading pathogens; as a consequence, treatment strategies have always aimed to block pro-inflammatory mediators. However, it is now well recognized that most non-survivors from sepsis die in a state of hyporesponsiveness and severe immunosuppression resulting from triggered counter-regulatory anti-inflammatory loops [46]. One could hypothesize that during sepsis depletion of the microbiome – and thus diminished release of adequate amounts of MAMPs into the circulation – attributes to the detrimental state of immunosuppression seen in septic patients. On the flip side, this observation also illustrates that rational targeting of the gut microbiome could hold great therapeutic potential [47]. As an example, a recent study showed that targeting the gut microbiome with *Lactobacillus rhamnosus* administration is safe in critically ill patients and efficacious for the prevention of ventilator-associated pneumonia on the ICU [48]. In line with this, several studies demonstrated that the use of probiotics can result in a better outcome for critically ill patients, including patients with sepsis [49]. However, the findings of the Dutch Acute Pancreatitis Study Group, in which an increase in mortality was observed among patients with severe pancreatitis who received probiotic prophylaxis, have raised important questions as to whether probiotics can be used safely in critically ill patients [35, 50].

Conclusion

Recent breakthroughs in our understanding of the role of the gut microbiome in both health and diseases are of considerable importance for the fields of immunology, infectious diseases and intensive care medicine. In addition to its local contribution in the host defense against infections, it has become clear that the intestine also plays a role in systemic immune responses. Release of gut nutrients and microbial components termed MAMPs continuously primes and supports distant systemic immune cells. The exact role of the intestine in the pathogenesis of SIRS and multiple organ dysfunction syndrome has been further dissected. Breakdown of the intestinal epithelium and mucosal barriers will cause leakage of bacteria and bacterial toxins into the systemic compartment, while depletion of the gut microbiome probably leads towards a more vulnerable mucosal defense system, selection of more virulent microorganisms and reduced positive priming of the systemic immune system. Nonetheless, the notion that the gut microbiome exerts numerous beneficial effects in the host defense against severe infections has forced us to re-evaluate the old 'gut as motor of sepsis' hypothesis. The balance between continuous leakage of bacterial toxins through the gut barriers and the beneficial effects of the intestinal microbiome on our host defense system probably determines the net effect of the gut flora on systemic inflammation in the critically ill. Manipulating the intestinal microbiome by gut flora replacement or the use of specific bacterial components and/or metabolites is an interesting new treatment modality in order to restore gut homeostasis and possibly prevent septic complications and multiple organ dysfunction syndrome in critically ill patients.

Acknowledgement: We would like to thank Dr. M. Nieuwdorp, Department of Endocrinology at our institution and Prof. Dr. Willem de Vos, Laboratory of Microbiology, Wageningen University, the Netherlands, for fruitful discussions leading to this article. W. J. Wiersinga is supported by a VENI grant from the Netherlands Organization for Scientific Research.

References

1. Taylor DE (1998) Revving the motor of multiple organ dysfunction syndrome. Gut dysfunction in ARDS and multiorgan failure. Respir Care Clin N Am 4: 611–631
2. Alverdy JC, Chang EB (2008) The re-emerging role of the intestinal microflora in critical illness and inflammation: why the gut hypothesis of sepsis syndrome will not go away. J Leukoc Biol 83: 461–466
3. Turnbaugh PJ, Hamady M, Yatsunenko T, et al (2009) A core gut microbiome in obese and lean twins. Nature 457: 480–484
4. Qin J, Li R, Raes J, et al (2010) A human gut microbial gene catalogue established by metagenomic sequencing. Nature 464: 59–65
5. Clarke TB, Davis KM, Lysenko ES, et al (2010) Recognition of peptidoglycan from the microbiota by Nod1 enhances systemic innate immunity. Nat Med 16: 228–231
6. Vincent JL, Rello J, Marshall J, et al (2009) International study of the prevalence and outcomes of infection in intensive care units. JAMA 302: 2323–2329
7. Clark JA, Coopersmith CM (2007) Intestinal crosstalk: a new paradigm for understanding the gut as the "motor" of critical illness. Shock 28: 384–393
8. Kau AL, Ahern PP, Griffin NW, Goodman AL, Gordon JI (2011) Human nutrition, the gut microbiome and the immune system. Nature 474: 327–336
9. McGuckin MA, Linden SK, Sutton P, Florin TH (2011) Mucin dynamics and enteric pathogens. Nat Rev Microbiol 9: 265–278
10. Gill SR, Pop M, Deboy RT, et al (2006) Metagenomic analysis of the human distal gut microbiome. Science 312: 1355–1359
11. Eckburg PB, Bik EM, Bernstein CN, et al (2005) Diversity of the human intestinal microbial flora. Science 308: 1635–1638
12. Arumugam M, Raes J, Pelletier E, et al (2011) Enterotypes of the human gut microbiome. Nature 473: 174–180
13. Zoetendal EG, Rajilic-Stojanovic M, de Vos WM (2008) High-throughput diversity and functionality analysis of the gastrointestinal tract microbiota. Gut 57: 1605–1615
14. Rakoff-Nahoum S, Paglino J, Eslami-Varzaneh F, Edberg S, Medzhitov R (2004) Recognition of commensal microflora by toll-like receptors is required for intestinal homeostasis. Cell 118: 229–241
15. Manges AR, Labbe A, Loo VG, et al (2010) Comparative metagenomic study of alterations to the intestinal microbiota and risk of nosocomial Clostridum difficile-associated disease. J Infect Dis 202: 1877–1884
16. Tlaskalova-Hogenova H, Stepankova R, Kozakova H, et al (2011) The role of gut microbiota (commensal bacteria) and the mucosal barrier in the pathogenesis of inflammanory

and autoimmune diseases and cancer: contribution of germ-free and gnotobiotic animal models of human diseases. Cell Mol Immunol 8: 110–120

17. Gillor O, Etzion A, Riley MA (2008) The dual role of bacteriocins as anti- and probiotics. Appl Microbiol Biotechnol 81: 591–606

18. Schaible UE, Kaufmann SH (2005) A nutritive view on the host-pathogen interplay. Trends Microbiol 13: 373–380

19. Hamer HM, Jonkers D, Venema K, et al (2008) Review article: the role of butyrate on colonic function. Aliment Pharmacol Ther 27: 104–119

20. Wells JM, Rossi O, Meijerink M, van Baarlen P (2011) Epithelial crosstalk at the microbiota-mucosal interface. Proc Natl Acad Sci USA 108 (Suppl 1): 4607–4614

21. Abreu MT, Thomas LS, Arnold ET, et al (2003) TLR signaling at the intestinal epithelial interface. J Endotoxin Res 9: 322–330

22. Akira S, Uematsu S, Takeuchi O (2006) Pathogen recognition and innate immunity. Cell 124: 783–801

23. Lala S, Ogura Y, Osborne C, et al (2003) Crohn's disease and the NOD2 gene: a role for paneth cells. Gastroenterology 125: 47–57

24. Abreu MT (2010) Toll-like receptor signalling in the intestinal epithelium: how bacterial recognition shapes intestinal function. Nat Rev Immunol 10: 131–144

25. Lee J, Mo JH, Katakura K, et al (2006) Maintenance of colonic homeostasis by distinctive apical TLR9 signalling in intestinal epithelial cells. Nat Cell Biol 8: 1327–1336

26. Vijay-Kumar M, Sanders CJ, et al (2007) Deletion of TLR5 results in spontaneous colitis in mice. J Clin Invest 117: 3909–3921

27. Vijay-Kumar M, Aitken JD, Carvalho FA, et al (2010) Metabolic syndrome and altered gut microbiota in mice lacking Toll-like receptor 5. Science 328: 228–231

28. Strugnell RA, Wijburg OL (2010) The role of secretory antibodies in infection immunity. Nat Rev Microbiol 8: 656–667

29. Meijer K, de Vos P, Priebe MG (2010) Butyrate and other short-chain fatty acids as modulators of immunity: what relevance for health? Curr Opin Clin Nutr Metab Care 13: 715–721

30. Shimizu K, Ogura H, Hamasaki T, et al (2011) Altered gut flora are associated with septic complications and death in critically ill patients with systemic inflammatory response syndrome. Dig Dis Sci 56: 1171–1177

31. Shimizu K, Ogura H, Goto M, et al (2006) Altered gut flora and environment in patients with severe SIRS. J Trauma 60: 126–133

32. Shimizu K, Ogura H, Tomono K, et al (2011) Patterns of Gram-stained fecal flora as a quick diagnostic marker in patients with severe SIRS. Dig Dis Sci 56: 1782–1788

33. Hotchkiss RS, Swanson PE, Freeman BD, et al (1999) Apoptotic cell death in patients with sepsis, shock, and multiple organ dysfunction. Crit Care Med 27: 1230–1251

34. Coopersmith CM, Stromberg PE, Dunne WM, et al (2002) Inhibition of intestinal epithelial apoptosis and survival in a murine model of pneumonia-induced sepsis. JAMA 287: 1716–1721

35. Morowitz MJ, Carlisle EM, Alverdy JC (2011) Contributions of intestinal bacteria to nutrition and metabolism in the critically ill. Surg Clin North Am 91: 771–785

36. Sommer MO, Dantas G (2011) Antibiotics and the resistant microbiome. Curr Opin Microbiol 14: 556–563

37. Hill DA, Hoffmann C, Abt MC, et al (2010) Metagenomic analyses reveal antibiotic-induced temporal and spatial changes in intestinal microbiota with associated alterations in immune cell homeostasis. Mucosal Immunol 3: 148–158

38. Brandl K, Plitas G, Mihu CN, et al (2008) Vancomycin-resistant enterococci exploit antibiotic-induced innate immune deficits. Nature 455: 804–807

39. Willing BP, Russell SL, Finlay BB (2011) Shifting the balance: antibiotic effects on host-microbiota mutualism. Nat Rev Microbiol 9: 233–243

40. Ubeda C, Taur Y, Jenq RR, et al (2010) Vancomycin-resistant Enterococcus domination of intestinal microbiota is enabled by antibiotic treatment in mice and precedes bloodstream invasion in humans. J Clin Invest 120: 4332–4341

41. de Jonge E, Schultz MJ, Spanjaard L, et al (2003) Effects of selective decontamination of digestive tract on mortality and acquisition of resistant bacteria in intensive care: a randomised controlled trial. Lancet 362: 1011–1016

42. de Smet AM, Bonten MJ (2008) Selective decontamination of the digestive tract. Curr Opin Infect Dis 21: 179–183
43. Vincent JL, Jacobs F (2011) Effect of selective decontamination on antibiotic resistance. Lancet Infect Dis 11: 337–338
44. Palmer R (2011) Fecal matters. Nat Med 17: 150–152
45. Khoruts A, Sadowsky MJ (2011) Therapeutic transplantation of the distal gut microbiota. Mucosal Immunol 4: 4–7
46. de Jong HK, van der Poll T, Wiersinga WJ (2010) The systemic pro-inflammatory response in sepsis. J Innate Immun 2: 422–430
47. Philpott DJ, Girardin SE (2010) Gut microbes extend reach to systemic innate immunity. Nat Med 16: 160–161
48. Morrow LE, Kollef MH, Casale TB (2010) Probiotic prophylaxis of ventilator-associated pneumonia: a blinded, randomized, controlled trial. Am J Respir Crit Care Med 182: 1058–1064
49. Morrow LE (2009) Probiotics in the intensive care unit. Curr Opin Crit Care 15: 144–148
50. Besselink MG, van Santvoort HC, Buskens E, et al (2008) Probiotic prophylaxis in predicted severe acute pancreatitis: a randomised, double-blind, placebo-controlled trial. Lancet 371: 651–659

II Metabolomics

The Metabolomic Approach to the Diagnosis of Critical Illness

N. Nin, J.L. Izquierdo-García, and J.A. Lorente

II

Introduction

Advances in molecular and cell biology over the last two decades, including most notably the sequencing of the human genome, have undoubtedly determined a better understanding of disease pathophysiology, and a more precise identification of populations at risk for certain conditions. However, many questions remain unanswered using the genomic approach alone, including what the gene products and the cell responses to certain insults are, given a certain genetic abnormality. The study of the metabolome offers a unique opportunity to answer some of these questions. The metabolome represents a combination of all the metabolites and intermediate products of metabolism in a biological organism. The study of the metabolome, further down the line from gene structure and function, more closely reflects the activities of the cell at the functional level and magnifies events that occur at the level of the genome, transcriptome and proteome (**Fig. 1**).

The development of chromatographic separation techniques in the early 1970s marked the origin of the metabolite identification field [1]. The ^{1}H-nuclear magnetic resonance (NMR) technique was first used for metabolic studies in 1977, when a range of compounds, such as lactate, creatine and alanine, was detected in a red blood cell suspension [2]. During the 1980s, analysis of the plethora of metabolites detected in ^{1}H-NMR spectra boosted the development of new techniques to classify samples according to their biological status [3, 4]. Thus, the

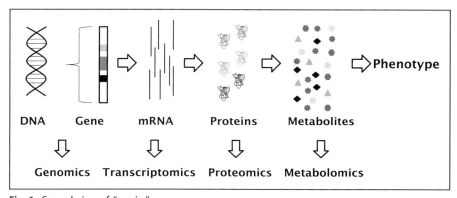

Fig. 1. General view of "-omics".

J.-L. Vincent (ed.), *Annual Update in Intensive Care and Emergency Medicine 2012*
DOI 10.1007/978-3-642-25716-2 © Springer-Verlag Berlin Heidelberg 2012

concept of metabolomics was born, when complex data from biological samples were interpreted using multivariate statistics. Metabolomics is the scientific study of the metabolic response of living systems to pathophysiological stimuli or genetic modification. Transcriptomics, proteomics, and metabolomics comprise what is referred to as systems biology.

The potential for metabolomic analysis in critical illness is based on its ability to detect changes in phenotypes that may be helpful for early diagnosis, prognosis or prediction of response to therapy. In the present chapter, we first describe the principles of metabolomic analysis, including different analytical platforms and data interpretation tools, and then focus on the application of metabolomic sciences in critical care medicine.

Analytical Techniques

Metabolomic data sets are currently generated mainly through NMR spectroscopy (MRS), mostly ^{1}H-MRS, and mass spectrometry (MS). Other structural or analytical methods, such as Fourier transform infra-red (FTIR) spectroscopy or high performance liquid chromatography (HPLC), have the disadvantage of yielding a low level of detailed molecular identification.

NMR Spectroscopy

MRS is a non-destructive technique that provides detailed information on molecular structure as well as information on absolute or relative concentrations. NMR is a phenomenon in which magnetic nuclei in a magnetic field absorb and re-emit electromagnetic radiation. MRS is based on the fact that similar isotopes do not resonate at the same frequency because nuclei are surrounded by a cloud of diamagnetic electrons which generate a local magnetic field. Depending on the local chemical environment, different protons in a molecule resonate at slightly different frequencies. The resultant molecular detection and quantification are acquired as a spectral data set (**Fig. 2**). The horizontal axis is NMR frequency (or chemical shift in parts per million (ppm), relative to a reference chemical at 0 ppm (rather than in the absolute Hertz units), and the vertical axis is signal strength (in arbitrary units). Based on their unique chemical structure, biochemical groups (CH_3, CH_2, OH, etc.) of each molecule originate different peaks in the spectrum which appear at a known frequency. MRS using high-resolution magic angle spinning (HR-MAS) [5, 6] allows the acquisition of high resolution NMR spectra on intact tissue samples with minimal sample preparation. The main limitation of MRS is that this technique is much less sensitive than MS. Recent development of cryogenic probes has provided an improvement in resolution by reducing the thermal noise in the electronics of the spectrometer. MRS, by means of HR-MAS, is the only technique available for studying intact tissues.

Two-dimensional MRS can be very useful for elucidating the connectivity between signals, resulting in unbiased metabolite identification. Experiments using correlation spectroscopy (COSY) [7] and total correlation spectroscopy (TOCSY) [8] provide ^{1}H-^{1}H spin-spin coupling connectivity, informing about which proton signals are close in chemical bond terms. Other heteronuclear correlation NMR experiments can be important to help assign NMR peaks. The interaction between ^{13}C and ^{1}H nuclei [9] is very useful for identification purposes.

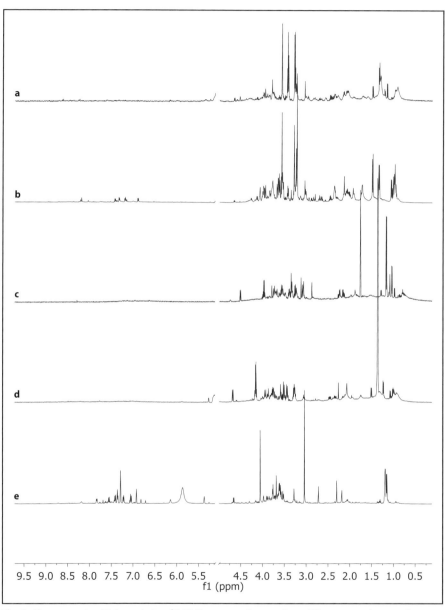

Fig. 2. Representative high-resolution ¹H-NMR spectra. Spectra from different samples are shown: **a** intact lung tissue; **b** intact renal cortex; **c** bronchoalveolar lavage fluid; **d** serum; **e** urine. Spectra **a** and **b** were obtained by high-resolution magic-angle-spinning ¹H-MRS. Spectra **c**, **d** and **e** were obtained by high-resolution liquid ¹H-MRS. All spectra were acquired using a Bruker 500 MHz spectrometer.

Mass Spectroscopy

MS is a destructive analytical technique that measures the mass-to-charge ratio of charged particles. Although the sample preparation requirements of this technique are usually more intensive, MS is considerably more sensitive than MRS, thus allowing the metabolomic analysis of low concentration samples, such as exhaled breath condensate fluid [10]. In general, this technique has been coupled to other pre-separation methods such as gas chromatography (GC) [11], capillary electrophoresis (CE) [12], ion mobility or FTIR spectroscopy [13]. The most common tandem in MS-based metabolomics is liquid chromatography (LC)-MS, which includes HPLC [14] and ultra-high-pressure LC (UHPLC) [15]. LC-MS provides three-dimensional metabolic data (**Fig. 3**), where at each sampling point in the chromatogram (retention time) there is a full mass spectrum (mass vs. intensity).

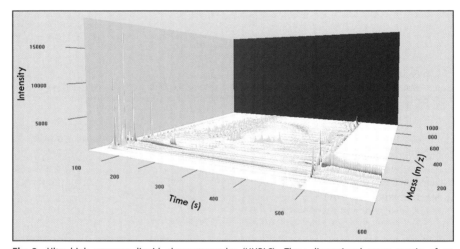

Fig. 3. Ultra-high pressure liquid chromatography (UHPLC). Three-dimensional mass matrix of an exhaled breath condensate from a healthy subject. UHPLC is coupled to a time-off light mass spectrometer. m/z: mass to charge ratio.

Spectral Data Analysis

Regardless of the analytical platform used, the spectral data can be thought of as a complex multi-dimensional set of metabolic coordinates. Interpretation of metabolic data is complicated and requires the application of unsupervised and supervised chemometric tools (**Fig. 4**). Prior to statistical analysis, spectral data have to be preprocessed. Data preprocessing is a necessary step between the acquisition of raw spectra and multivariate analysis of a metabolomic data set. For metabolomic studies, the preprocessing methods are designed to reduce variances and possible influences that might interfere with data analysis (such as possible variations in sample concentrations or variable sample dilutions), phase distortions and rolling baselines in the NMR spectrum and retention time misalignment in LC-MS data.

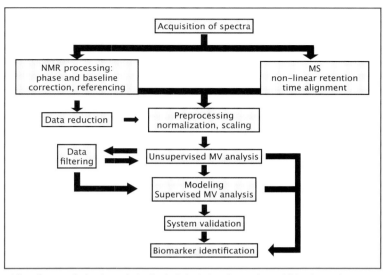

Fig. 4. Basic workflow for metabolomic analysis. Analysis includes: Spectral acquisition by nuclear magnetic resonance spectroscopy (MRS) or mass spectrometry (MS), raw spectra pre-processing, spectral data post-processing, unsupervised multivariate (MV) statistical analysis and modeling.

The multivariate statistical or pattern recognition methods provide a means of collecting relevant information on differences or similarities between the metabolic pathways [16, 17]. These methods include multivariate projection methods, in which principal component analysis (PCA) and partial least square discriminant analysis (PLS-DA) are the most widely used techniques.

PCA is one of the most common exploratory techniques in multivariate analysis [18]. Its most important use is to represent multivariate data in a low-dimensional space (**Fig. 5a**). The first principal component is defined by the spectral profile (loading) in the data which describes most of the variation. The second principal component, orthogonal to the first one, is the second best profile describing the variation, and so on. The principal components are composed of so-called scores and loadings. Loadings contain information about the variables (chemical shifts) in the data set and the scores hold information about sample classes. Score plots (**Fig. 5b**) are used to distinguish the metabolite profile of control from diseased subjects, or to evaluate the progression rate of the disease. Loading plots (**Fig. 5c**) highlight the most significant variables. In other words, the chemical shifts (metabolic signals) with the highest loading values in the right direction would be selected as potential biomarkers (**Fig. 5d**).

PLS-DA is a supervised linear regression method whereby the latent variables constructed with the multivariate variables corresponding to the observations (spectral descriptors) are associated with the class membership for each sample [19]. The aim of PLS-DA is to find in the spectral regions those components that significantly describe relevant variations in the spectra and have maximum covariance with the class information vector. PLS-DA can also be expressed by scores and loadings matrices, and results interpretation is similar as for PCA.

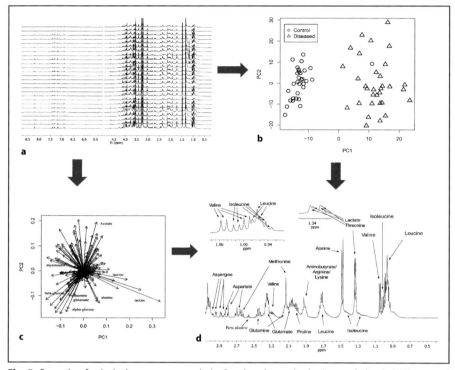

Fig. 5. Example of principal component analysis. Panel **a** shows the basic metabolomic NMR spectral data that can be expressed by a linear combination of a scores matrix **b** and a loadings matrix **c**. The scores matrix summarizes the sample variation (sample classification) and the loadings matrix summarizes the spectral variable variation (biomarker detection). The analysis of both plots will help identify the potential biomarker of the condition under study in the original NMR spectrum.

Metabolomic Analysis and Critical Illness

^{1}H-MRS analysis of biofluids provides a tool for the understanding of biochemical processes associated with critical care illness [20]. ^{1}H-MRS, by means of HR-MAS, is an excellent option to study unprocessed fluids [15–17]. A number of ^{1}H-MRS metabolomic studies of different tissues can be cited as examples for diagnosis in acute animal models and in human illness [21–23].

Critical illness is characterized by a severe disruption of metabolic homeostasis and signal transduction pathways. Metabolomics can define specific phenotypes of acute syndromes that potentially may help understand pathophysiology, perform early diagnosis, identify patients at risk, determine disease severity and prognosis, and predict response to therapy. In this way, metabolomics in critical illness can change the concept of biomarkers. For instance, metabolomics can define a specific metabolomic biomarker associated with progression to acute respiratory distress syndrome (ARDS) in patients at risk, or with infections in patients with severe burns [20, 24].

Sepsis

Xu et al. [25] constructed a prognostic model based on serum analysis by HPLC-MS-based metabolomics in rats undergoing cecal ligation and puncture (CLP). HPLC-MS analysis discriminated between rats that survived and those that did not after CLP and sham-procedure with an accuracy of 94 %. Six metabolites were related to outcome, including linoleic acid, linolenic acid, oleic acid, stearic acid, docosahexaenoic acid and docosapentaenoic acid. In a subsequent study performed by the same group with a different technique, serum samples from septic rats were analyzed using ^{1}H-MRS [26]. Six characteristic metabolites involved in energy metabolism (lactate, alanine, acetate, acetoacetate, hydroxybutyrate and formate) changed in septic rats, more markedly in non-survivors. A prognostic predictive model constructed with these metabolites showed an accuracy of 87 %. In another study [27], LC-MS analysis of plasma samples from thermally injured and septic rats revealed nine characteristic metabolites (hypoxanthine, indoxyl sulfate, glucuronic acid, gluconic acid, proline, uracil, nitrotyrosine, uric acid, and trihydroxy cholanoic acid) discriminating septic from non-septic animals. These biomarkers are mainly related to oxidative stress and tissue damage.

We have recently reported that ^{1}H-MRS of lung tissue, bronchoalveolar lavage (BAL) fluid and serum samples showed different concentrations of characteristic metabolites in rats undergoing CLP as compared to control rats: Alanine, creatine, phosphoethanolamine and myoinositol concentrations increased in lung tissue; creatine increased and myoinositol decreased in BAL fluid; and alanine, creatine, phosphoethanolamine, acetoacetate and two unidentified fatty acids increased whereas formate decreased in serum [23]. We constructed a model that was 100 % predictive of the diagnosis of sepsis, using all the samples combined or the serum samples only (**Fig. 6**). One of the novel findings of our study was the different metabolite behavior in the various samples analyzed.

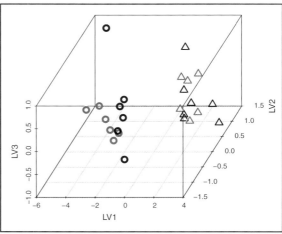

Fig. 6. Partial least square (PLS) discriminant analysis score plot performed on ^{1}H-NMR spectra. Analysis was performed on serum samples (black) from sham operated (Δ) and CLP (O) rats. The model was validated by a new set of samples (blue), showing 100 % sensitivity and specificity.

II

Acute Lung Injury (ALI) and ARDS

Currently the diagnosis of ALI and ARDS is based on the presence of non-specific criteria, such as physiologic and radiologic parameters [28, 29]. Thus there is a need for biomarkers of these conditions. Although several serum proteins and genomic profiles have been proposed as diagnostic biomarkers [30-32] they lack sufficient sensitivity and specificity.

Serkova et al. [22] used ^{1}H-MRS analysis of lung tissue samples from rats receiving an intra-tracheal administration of interleukin (IL)-1β and tumor necrosis factor (TNF)-α. In this model of inflammation-induced ALI, the high energy phosphates (ATP, ADP, energy balance and energy change) and the lactate-to-glucose ratio were biomarkers of the condition. In addition, there was a strong temporal association between MRS-based metabolomics and histological indexes of lung injury.

More recently, Stringer et al. [33] studied serum samples from patients with sepsis-induced ALI using ^{1}H-MRS. They found significant differences in the concentration of total glutathione, myoinositol, adenosine, phosphatidylserine and sphingomyelin between patients with sepsis-induced ALI and healthy subjects. In addition, myoinositol and total glutathione levels were associated with changes in physiologic parameters, such as acute physiologic scores and ventilator-free days.

We have recently used an ^{1}H-MRS-based metabolomic approach for the diagnosis of ventilator-induced lung injury (VILI) in rats. Six metabolites (lactate, glucose, acetate, creatine, glycine and hydroxybutyrate) changed significantly in lung tissue and BAL fluid from rats with VILI [34]. Based on these results, it can be hypothesized that MRS could be useful for the diagnosis of biotrauma in patients receiving mechanical ventilation.

Acute Kidney Injury (AKI)

Traditional biomarkers of AKI include blood urea nitrogen (BUN) concentration and creatinine serum concentration, which are known to lack sensitivity for early decline in kidney function. New biomarkers such as neutrophil gelatinase-associated lipocalin (NGAL) and IL-18 are being studied with encouraging results [35].

There are so far no studies on the role of metabolomics for the diagnosis or prognosis of critically ill patients with AKI. In a murine model of cisplatin-induced acute renal failure, ^{1}H-MRS [36] showed significant changes in the urine concentration of glucose, alanine, lactate, leucine, methionine, 2-oxoglutarate, pyruvate and valine. Moreover cisplatin-treated mice exhibited a time-dependent increase in non-esterified fatty acids and triglyceride levels in serum, urine and kidney tissue. The authors proposed that this metabolomic profile related to AKI could be used as a novel biomarker of kidney injury. Future studies should elucidate the role of metabolomics for the early detection and prognosis of AKI.

Trauma

A metabolomic approach has been used in two studies in trauma patients. A higher lactate plasma concentration assessed by ^{1}H-MRS discriminated trauma patients who developed multiple organ dysfunction syndrome from those who did not [37]. In another study, a decreased plasma concentration of three lipids was a major predictor of outcome in patients with trauma, whereas glucose and glutamate plasma concentrations were intermediate predictors [38].

Conclusion

Sensitive and specific biomarkers for early diagnosis and prognostication are needed for critical illnesses, such as sepsis, ALI/ARDS, AKI and trauma. A metabolomic approach using ^{1}H-MRS can identify metabolic phenotypes specific to certain conditions or outcomes, which can be useful as disease biomarkers. In addition, the analysis of the specific metabolic and signal transduction pathways involved may shed light on the pathophysiology of these conditions.

References

1. Pauling L, Robinson AB, Teranishi R, Cary P (1971) Quantitative analysis of urine vapor and breath by gas-liquid partition chromatography. Proc Natl Acad Sci USA 68: 2374–2376
2. Brown FF, Campbell ID, Kuchel PW, Rabenstein DC (1977) Human erythrocyte metabolism studies by 1H spin echo NMR. FEBS Lett 82: 12–16
3. Bales JR, Higham DP, Howe I, Nicholson JK, Sadler PJ (1984) Use of high-resolution proton nuclear magnetic resonance spectroscopy for rapid multi-component analysis of urine. Clin Chem 30: 426–432
4. Nicholson JK, Wilson ID (1989) High-resolution proton magnetic-resonance spectroscopy of biological-fluids. Prog Nucl Magn Reson Spectrosc 21: 449–501
5. Bollard ME, Garrod S, Holmes E, et al (2000) High-resolution H-1 and H-1-C-13 magic angle spinning NMR spectroscopy of rat liver. Magn Reson Med 44: 201–207
6. Cheng LL, Chang IW, Smith BL, Gonzalez RG (1998) Evaluating human breast ductal carcinomas with high-resolution magic-angle spinning proton magnetic resonance spectroscopy. J Magn Reson 135: 194–202
7. Marion D, Wuthrich K (1983) Application of phase sensitive two-dimensional correlated spectroscopy (COSY) for measurements of 1H-1H spin-spin coupling constants in proteins. Biochem Biophys Res Commun 113: 967–974
8. Spraul M, Nicholson JK, Lynch MJ, Lindon JC (1994) Application of the one-dimensional TOCSY pulse sequence in 750 MHz 1H-NMR spectroscopy for assignment of endogenous metabolite resonances in biofluids. J Pharm Biom Anal 12: 613–618
9. Xi Y, de Ropp JS, Viant MR, Woodruff DL, Yu P (2008) Improved identification of metabolites in complex mixtures using HSQC NMR spectroscopy. Anal Chim Acta 614: 127–133
10. Izquierdo-Garcia JL, Peces-Barba G, Heili S, Diaz R, Want E, Ruiz-Cabello J (2011) Is NMR-based metabolomic analysis of exhaled breath condensate accurate? Eur Respir J 37: 468–470
11. Yang J, Xu GW, Zheng YF, Kong HW, Pang T, Lv S, Yang Q (2004) Diagnosis of liver cancer using HPLC-based metabonomics avoiding false-positive result from hepatitis and hepatocirrhosis diseases. J Chromatogr B 813: 59–65
12. Soga T, Ohashi Y, Ueno Y, Naraoka H, Tomita M, Nishioka T (2003) Quantitative metabolome analysis using capillary electrophoresis mass spectrometry. J Proteome Res 2: 488–494
13. Kaderbhai NN, Broadhurst DI, Ellis DI, Goodacre R, Kell DB (2003) Functional genomics via metabolic footprinting: monitoring metabolite secretion by Escherichia coli tryptophan metabolism mutants using FT-IR and direct injection electrospray mass spectrometry. Comp Funct Genomics 4: 376–391
14. Wilson ID, Plumb R, Granger J, Major H, Williams R, Lenz EM (2005) HPLC-MS-based methods for the study of metabonomics. J Chromatogr B 817: 67–76
15. Wilson ID, Nicholson JK, Castro-Perez J, et al (2005) High resolution "Ultra performance" liquid chromatography coupled to oa-TOF mass spectrometry as a tool for differential metabolic pathway profiling in functional genomic studies. J Proteome Res 4: 591–598
16. Winning H, Larsen FH, Bro R, Engelsen SB (2008) Quantitative analysis of NMR spectra with chemometrics. J Magn Reson 190: 26–32
17. Trygg J, Holmes E, Lundstedt T (2007) Chemometrics in metabonomics. J Proteome Res 6: 469–479

II

18. Lindon JC, Holmes E, Nicholson JK (2001) Pattern recognition methods and applications in biomedical magnetic resonance. Prog Nucl Magn Reson Spectrosc 39: 1–40
19. Brereton RG (2007) Applied Chemometrics for Scientists. John Wiley & Sons, Hoboken
20. Serkova NJ, Standiford TJ, Stringer KA (2011) The emerging field of quantitative blood metabolomics for biomarker discovery in critical illnesses. Am J Respir Crit Care Med 184: 647–655
21. Lin ZY, Xu PB, Yan SK, et al (2009) A metabonomic approach to early prognostic evaluation of experimental sepsis by HNMR and pattern recognition. NMR Biomed 22: 601–608
22. Serkova NJ, Van Rheen Z, Tobias M, Pitzer JE, Wilkinson JE, Stringer KA (2008) Utility of magnetic resonance imaging and nuclear magnetic resonance-based metabolomics for quantification of inflammatory lung injury. Am J Physiol Lung Cell Mol Physiol 295: 152–161
23. Izquierdo-García JL, Nin N, Jesús Ruíz-Cabello J (2011) A metabolomic approach for the diagnosis of experimental sepsis. Intensive Care Med (in press)
24. Lacy P (2011) Metabolomics of sepsis-induced acute lung injury: A new approach for biomarkers. Am J Physiol Lung Cell Mol Physiol 300: 1–3
25. Xu PB, Lin ZY, Meng HB, et al (2008) A metabonomic approach to early prognostic evaluation of experimental sepsis. J Infect 56: 474–481
26. Lin ZY, Xu PB, Yan SK, et al (2009) A metabonomic approach to early prognostic evaluation of experimental sepsis by (1)H NMR and pattern recognition.NMR Biomed 22: 601–608
27. Liu XR, Zheng XF, Ji SZ, et al (2010) Metabolomic analysis of thermally injured and/or septic rats. Burns 36: 992–998
28. Ferguson ND, Frutos-Vivar F, Esteban A, et al (2005) Acute respiratory distress syndrome: underrecognition by clinicians and diagnostic accuracy of three clinical definitions.Crit Care Med 33: 2228–2234
29. Esteban A, Fernández-Segoviano P, Frutos-Vivar F, et al (2004) Comparison of clinical criteria for the acute respiratory distress syndrome with autopsy findings. Ann Intern Med 141: 440–445
30. Chang DW, Hayashi S, Gharib SA, et al (2008) Proteomic and computational analysis of bronchoalveolar proteins during the course of the acute respiratory distress syndrome. Am J Respir Crit Care Med 178: 701–709
31. Bowler RP, Duda B, Chan ED, et al (2004) Proteomic analysis of pulmonary edema fluid and plasma in patients with acute lung injury. Am J Physiol Lung Cell Mol Physiol 286: L1095–1104
32. Howrylak JA, Dolinay T, Lucht L (2009) Discovery of the gene signature for acute lung injury in patients with sepsis. Physiol Genomics 37: 133–139
33. Stringer KA, Serkova NJ, Karnovsky A, Guire K, Paine R 3rd, Standiford TJ (2011) Metabolic consequences of sepsis-induced acute lung injury revealed by plasma "H-nuclear magnetic resonance quantitative metabolomics and computational analysis. Am J Physiol Lung Cell Mol Physiol 300: L4-L11
34. Nin N, Izquierdo JL, Lorente JA, et al (2011) Metabolomic analysis of pulmonary tissue in an experimental model of ventilator induced lung injury. Am J Respir Crit Care Med 183: A1153 (abst)
35. Siew ED, Ware LB, Ikizler TA (2011) Biological markers of acute kidney injury. J Am Soc Nephrol 22: 810–820
36. Portilla D, Schnackenberg L, Beger RD (2007) Metabolomics as an extension of proteomic analysis: study of acute kidney injury. Semin Nephrol 27: 609–620
37. Mao H, Wang H, Wang B et al (2009) Systemic metabolic changes of traumatic critically ill patients revealed by an NMR-based metabonomic approach. J Proteome Res 8: 5423–5430
38. Cohen MJ, Serkova NJ, Wiener-Kronish J, Pittet JF, Niemann CU (2010) 1h-NMR-based metabolic signatures of clinical outcomes in trauma patients--beyond lactate and base deficit. J Trauma 69: 31–40

Metabolomics in Critically ill Patients: Focus on Exhaled Air

L.D.J. Bos, P.J. Sterk, and M.J. Schultz

Introduction

The lungs of critically ill patients are under constant threat. Critically ill patients may develop acute lung injury (ALI) or its more severe form, acute respiratory distress syndrome (ARDS). Development of ALI/ARDS frequently mandates tracheal intubation for mechanical ventilation [1]. Tracheal intubation, however, carries the risk of ventilator–associated pneumonia (VAP) [2], whereas mechanical ventilation has the potential to cause so–called ventilator–associated lung injury (VALI) [3]. ALI/ARDS and VALI are diagnosed according to the American–European consensus criteria, which include bilateral pulmonary infiltrates on chest radiography and hypoxia [4]. VAP is suspected when sputum production increases or changes, in combination with new or changed pulmonary infiltrates on chest radiography and hypoxia [2]. Unfortunately, these signs and symptoms are all far from specific and occur at a relatively late stage of disease, hampering accurate and early diagnosis.

It is likely that the above–mentioned diagnostic signs and symptoms of ALI/ ARDS, VALI and VAP are preceded by local (i.e., pulmonary) production of specific molecules [5–9]. Monitoring of these so–called biological markers may improve the diagnostic process in many ways. Ideally a biological marker is sensitive to early pathophysiologic changes and specific for disease. Assessment of biological markers should preferably be rapid as well as non–invasive and cheap, to allow for frequent monitoring. Several biological markers have been suggested to have potential to assist in diagnosing ALI/ARDS, VALI and VAP [10–12]. Most of these biological markers, unfortunately, have been shown to have an unacceptably low diagnostic accuracy [10–12].

In the Middle Ages, physicians depended heavily on their senses: Color, taste, and smell were their biological markers [13]. Although outdated, this approach provided a quick, non–invasive and integrative view on biochemical processes without additional costs, processing or analysis. Facing the seemingly huge challenges with the use of hundreds to thousands of biological markers, in particular when measured in blood, we warmly welcome the emerging possibilities of 'smelling' exhaled air to diagnose pulmonary diseases in intubated and mechanically ventilated critically ill patients.

Systemic Biological Markers

Numerous studies have tested the diagnostic accuracy of systemic biological markers for pulmonary diseases in critically ill patients. Only rarely have combi-

J.-L. Vincent (ed.), *Annual Update in Intensive Care and Emergency Medicine 2012*
DOI 10.1007/978-3-642-25716-2 © Springer-Verlag Berlin Heidelberg 2012

nations of biological markers been tested. In addition, most studies were restricted to single measurements or at best, repeated measurements on consecutive days. Except for procalcitonin, which was found to have some diagnostic value for VAP [14], other candidate biological markers in blood were found to have an unacceptably low diagnostic accuracy [10–12]. This finding may not come as a surprise because blood levels of biological markers may only partly, if at all, reflect pulmonary changes for several reasons.

First, pulmonary inflammatory responses with ALI/ARDS, VALI and VAP are highly compartmentalized. Whereasd strong and early pro–inflammatory reactions are seen in bronchoalveolar lavage (BAL) fluid in ALI/ARDS [5], VALI [6, 7] and VAP [8, 9], systemic levels of inflammatory mediators change hardly, if at all, before clinical manifestation of ALI/ARDS, VALI or VAP [5–9].

Second, one or two systemic biological markers may not sufficiently capture the complexity of ALI/ARDS, VALI or VAP. The pathophysiology of ALI/ARDS, VALI and VAP comprises numerous biological processes, including but not restricted to inflammation, coagulation and apoptosis [3, 15]. Traditional studies on single proteins or pathways may, therefore, have very limited potential because the complexity of pulmonary disease cannot be captured.

Third, a single measurement of a systemic biological marker heavily disregards the rapid dynamics of (development of) pulmonary diseases [16]. Whereas use of multiple biological markers may improve diagnostics, the rapid dynamics of critical illness remain ignored. Although blood is relatively easily available, frequent blood sampling and analysis in all patients at risk for ALI/ARDS, VALI and VAP are too expensive and too time-consuming.

Pulmonary Biological Markers

The lungs, rather than the blood, should be assessed when aiming for early and accurate diagnosis of ALI/ARDS, VALI or VAP. BAL fluid can be obtained in intubated and mechanically ventilated patients using directed or non-directed techniques [17]. Directed BAL fluid provides detailed information on biological processes in specific compartments of the lung but requires specialized personnel, investment of time and is not without risk for the critically ill patient. Non-directed lung lavage is relatively fast and easy to perform but may still be too invasive for frequent assessment.

As in blood, a single biological marker in BAL fluid may not capture the complexity of ALI/ARDS, VALI or VAP. Different biological pathways should be investigated simultaneously to acquire a balanced view [18]. Recently, proteins in BAL fluid have been profiled collectively using new analytical techniques (proteomics), allowing for biological marker discovery and better understanding of the host response [19].

'-Omics' and Systems Biology

'-Omics' studies represent the integrated view of the biochemistry within a domain of complex organisms (genomics, transcriptomics, proteomics, metabolomics). These techniques are not hypothesis driven (i.e., unbiased) and can be used to discover biological markers of pathophysiological pathways [20]. Systems biology focuses on combinations of different '-omics' domains seeking a deeper understanding in complex biological systems by providing a top-down view of biochemical processes combined with mathematical and computational methods for modeling of structures and processes. The importance of hypothesis-free biological marker discovery is well illustrated by glycosylated hemoglobin (HbA1c) in diabetic glucose control. Discovered by chromatography and serendipitously connected to diabetes mellitus, it was shown to be a major biological marker [21]. Because of low *a priori* biological plausibility, HbA1c would not have been discovered without global assessment by chromatography.

Serkova et al. recently described metabolomics as "the global assessment of endogenous metabolites within a biologic system" representing "a 'snapshot' reading of gene function, enzyme activity and physiological landscape" [22]. The metabolome is very sensitive to physiological and pathophysiological changes because it is an end-product of the genome, transcriptome and proteome combined. Nuclear magnetic resonance (NMR) spectroscopy and liquid-chromatography/mass-spectrometry (LC-MS) can be used to identify hundreds of metabolites in any biological material. As with any '-omics' technique, it remains a challenge to avoid false discoveries when applying metabolomics. Therefore, recommendations concerning bias, sample size, multiple testing and model fitting should be followed strictly [23]. Since metabolism is an ancient and highly conserved biological mechanism, results can easily be translated between mammalian species [24].

So far, little research has focused on metabolomics in critically ill patients. Mao et al. described an NMR-based metabolomic method to aid detection of the systemic inflammatory response syndrome (SIRS) versus multiorgan failure (MOF) based on abnormal metabolic signatures [25]. These authors were able to clearly discriminate patients with SIRS and MOF, suggesting that an NMR-based metabolomic approach can be developed to diagnose the progress of disease in critically ill patients. More recently, Stringer et al. expanded on earlier work on metabolites in the lungs of mice with pulmonary injury [26], by showing that NMR could generate quantitative data sets that revealed differences in the level of several metabolites between patients with ALI/ARDS and healthy subjects [27]. Importantly, some metabolites were associated with acute physiology scores and ventilator-free days. This study clearly demonstrates the feasibility of quantitative plasma NMR metabolomics since it yields a physiologically relevant metabolite data set that distinguished disease from health. Of note, several metabolites are volatile and, therefore, eliminated via the lung.

Breathomics

Breath contains thousands of volatile organic compounds (VOCs), metabolites in gas-phase produced by both physiological and pathophysiological processes [28, 29]. VOC patterns identified by smell have been used to diagnose disease and intoxication for a long time (e.g., scent of acetone in diabetes mellitus) [30]. Alteration of exhaled VOCs can be the consequence of changed systemic metabolism (e.g., diabetes mellitus) or due to pulmonary metabolomic shift. Microorganisms (e.g., bacteria) present in the airways also produce volatile molecules, which may be species specific [31, 32]. A variety of techniques has been used to link disease to changed VOC composition of the exhaled air, including gas-chromatography mass-spectrometry (GC–MS), ion-mobility spectrometry (I-MS), and electronic nose techniques [33].

II Gas-chromatography Mass-spectrometry

GC-MS is considered the gold standard for the detection, separation and identification of large volatile organic compounds. With gas-chromatography volatile molecules are carried with an inert gas (e.g., helium) through a column and separated by volatility. Mass-spectrometry then further separates the molecules based on mass-to-charge ratio: Components are ionized into charged particles, carried though an electromagnetic field and quantitatively detected.

Pre-concentration, storage and transport of air samples is required for GC-MS analysis. The lower limit of detection can be improved using pre-concentration, however storage bears the risk of decomposition and/or loss of compounds. Considering the rapid dynamics of critically ill patients, test results should be available within minutes after measurement. This is still not feasible, limiting the clinical applicability of GC-MS in monitoring critically ill patients. Nevertheless, GC-MS remains essential for VOC identification and, therefore, for the understanding of pathophysiological pathways.

Schubert et al. investigated several volatile metabolites detected by GC–MS in intubated and mechanically ventilated patients (**Table 1**). These authors found a decrease in isoprene production in ALI patients and an increased n-pentane/isoprene ratio during the development of VAP [34]. Increased isoprene concentration is considered a marker of activation of neutrophils [35]. The authors suggest that impaired cholesterol synthesis late in the course of ALI could explain the surprisingly low levels of isoprene. N-pentane is an end product of lipid peroxidation and could reflect an increase in oxidative stress. Although isoprene, pentane and acetone are about the most abundant VOCs in exhaled breath, focusing on just these compounds disregards the '-omics' strategy. All detected molecules should be presented to data reduction and classification algorithms in order to perceive the complexity of the biological material and to obtain maximal diagnostic accuracy while limiting bias [23].

Table 1: Volatile organic compounds detected in exhaled air of mechanically ventilated patients, as described in literature. Adapted from [34] with permission

Compound	Suspected origin
Acetone	Enhanced metabolism
2,3-Dimethylbutane	Unknown
2,4-Dimethylpentane	Unknown
N-hexane	Respiratory delivery system
Isoflurane	Anesthesia
Isoprene	Cholesterol metabolism
Methanol	Unknown
2-Methylbutane	Respiratory delivery system
N-Pentane	Lipid peroxidation

Ion-mobility Spectrometry

I-MS has been proposed as a fast and sensitive alternative analytical method for the detection of molecules in gas-phase [33]. With I-MS, volatile molecules are ionized and moved towards a detector by means of an external electrical field. At specific intervals, the ionized gas is let into a tube in which the ions collide with drift gas molecules travelling in the opposite direction. Based on size and shape, ions are decelerated resulting in different ion drift times [36].

The fast reaction time, on-site application and continuous registration bring I-MS closer to clinical applicability. However, I-MS should not yet be considered an alternative for GC-MS analyses because identification of novel volatile organic compounds based on ion mobility remains very challenging. An extended library on ion mobility could assist in rapid identification of new volatile biomarkers [36].

The potential of I-MS for breath analysis in mechanically ventilated patients was illustrated recently. Dolch et al. reported on continuous analyses of air from the ventilatory circuit, identifying and quantifying several VOCs for up to 120 minutes [37]. Unfortunately, the authors did not perform comparative analyses between relevant patient groups.

Another method to analyze I-MS chromatograms is to use pattern-recognition software. This is based on the concept that diagnostic assessment does not require identification of individual molecular components, rather being dependent on accurate pattern recognition. By using I-MS, all peaks and intensities are combined into one algorithm, which is subsequently used for diagnostic purposes. Recently, Westhoff et al. reported 100 % correct classification of lung cancer patients compared to healthy controls using this approach [38]. No comparative study on I-MS in mechanically ventilated patients has been published yet.

Electronic Nose

Electronic noses (eNose), named after their similarities with the mammalian olfactory system [33], integratively capture complex VOC mixtures using an array of different sensors [33]. Sensors have individual sensitivity and specificity for VOCs. The composite signal of all sensors can be analyzed using pattern-recognition algorithms. eNose analysis of breath results in a unique fingerprint of exhaled metabolites, called a breath-print. Subsequently, these breath-prints can be used for diagnostic and monitoring purposes.

Metal oxides, conducting polymers, optical and infra-red spectroscopy have been used as sensors. As mentioned above, peaks and intensities obtained by I-MS can also be presented to pattern-recognition algorithms, hereby virtually converting every detected mass into a 'sensor'. Pattern-recognition can also be applied to concentrations of masses acquired with GC-MS.

eNoses can be miniaturized and might allow for continuous analyses. Data are available in real-time and eNoses are relatively easy to use. Indeed, eNoses are very attractive from a clinician's point of view [39]. Identification and quantification of specific compounds is not necessary for diagnosis and monitoring as long as patterns are specific for particular conditions. Although promising, several technical issues need to be considered regarding eNoses, including the fact that sensors in use at present have limited sensitivity and specificity for specific VOCs and could 'drift' over time. Sampling techniques should be adapted to the clinical setting and the disease of interest.

II

Several volatile organic compounds have been linked to the metabolic activity of bacterial species: For example 1-undecane to *Pseudomonas aeruginosa* and acetoin to *Staphylococcus aureus* [31]. Assessment of a large quantity of VOCs combined with pattern recognition software leads to good discrimination between bacterial species [32]. Different species of bacteria can be discriminated *in vitro* based on integrative analysis of volatile metabolites using an eNose [40–42]. More recently, Carey et al. reported on distinct metabolic alterations in methicillin-resistant *S. aureus* (MRSA) and vancomycin-resistant *Enterococcus faecalis* as compared to antibiotic susceptible bacteria of the same species [43].

Patterns of VOCs in exhaled breath of intubated and mechanically ventilated patients undergoing surgery are associated with the clinical pneumonia infection score, a sensitive marker for VAP [44]. Shih et al. described real-time pathogen detection in mechanically ventilated critically ill patients with pneumonia, showing good *in vivo* discrimination between *Klebsiella pneumoniae*, *P. aeruginosa*, *S. aureus*, *Acinetobacter baumanii* and *Acinetobacter lwoffi* [45] (**Fig. 1**). Air was

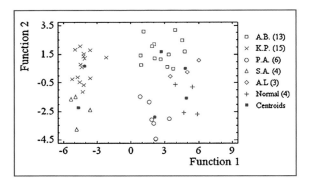

Fig. 1. Discrimination between pathogens in intubated and mechanically ventilated pneumonia patients by electronic nose analysis. The x- and y-axes represent vectors obtained by data reduction. Each point represents an infected patient, infected with: □, *Acinetobacter baumanii*; x, *Klebsiella pneumoniae*; ○, *Pseudomonas aeruginosa*; △, *Staphylococcus aureus*; ◇, *Acinetobacter lwoffi*; +, normal pharyngeal fauna; ■, centroids. Reprinted from [45] with permission.

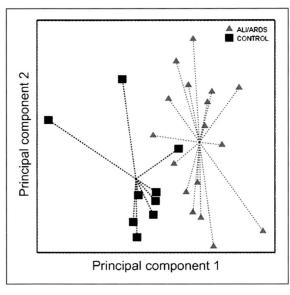

Fig. 2. Discrimination between acute lung injury patients and controls by electronic nose analysis. The x- and y-axes represent principal components obtained by data reduction. Each point represents a critically ill patient: ■, controls; ▲, acute lung injury patients. Each group is connected to a centroid.

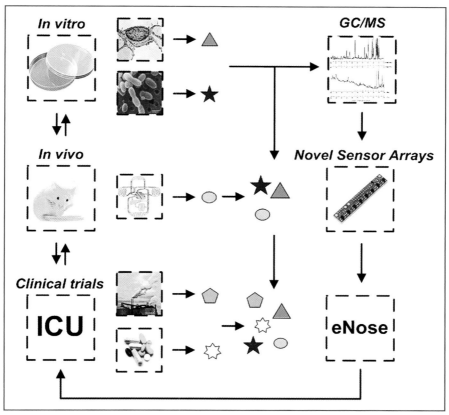

Fig. 3. Translational biology and technology. Translational biology (left panels): Volatile biological markers are discovered *in vitro* (bacteria and alveolar cells). These findings should be reproduced in an *in vivo* model. Animals have a circulation that contributes volatile molecules to the breath. Validation in large clinical trials is essential for future clinical application. The origin of volatile organic compounds (VOCs) found in patients can be investigated in *in vivo* or *in vitro* models. Samples obtained from patients are contaminated by exogenous metabolites and comorbidities. Symbols represent specific but unknown VOCs. Translational technology (right panels): Once volatile biological markers associated with pathophysiological processes are identified with gas-chromatography (GC) and mass-spectrometry (MS), tailor made sensor arrays and customized settings for ion-mobility can be developed. Electronic noses containing these sensor arrays and ion-mobility spectrometry can immediately be applied in clinical trials.

acquired through a suction catheter for the purpose of this study, thus including the non-invasiveness of breath sampling and the possibility of continuous analysis. Although GC-MS analysis of exhaled breath was not performed (i.e., the specific compounds remained unknown), these studies illustrate the diagnostic potential of volatile metabolites generated by airway pathogens and/or host response.

We recently presented an abstract on the potential to discriminate ALI/ARDS patients from critically ill patients without lung injury using eNose analysis (**Fig. 2**) [46]. This was confirmed when comparing ALI/ARDS patients with patients at high-risk for the development of ALI/ARDS [47]. With ROC-analysis, the area under the curve (AUC) was 0.75 for exhaled breath analysis, equal to the AUC of the PaO2/FiO$_2$ (P/F) ratio (0.75). Combination of exhaled breath analysis and P/F ratio resulted in an AUC of 0.84, which is very promising since the patient groups were small and highly heterogeneous. In this study, air was collected for one minute via a disposable T-piece connector placed between the endotracheal tube and the heat-moist exchanger. This methodology allowed for fully non-invasive and continuous sampling, suggesting eNose technology may already be very close to clinical applicability.

Road Map for Future Research

Future research on exhaled breath analysis in intubated and mechanically ventilated patients should approach volatile biomarker discovery using translational biology and translational technology (from bench to bedside and *vice versa*) (**Fig. 3**). VOCs can be discovered *in vitro*, as demonstrated by head-space analysis of bacteria [31]. These findings can be confirmed using 'clean' *in vivo* animal models (e.g., models of pneumonia or lung injury). Clinical trials are than necessary to validate the diagnostic accuracy of breathomics in patients with comorbidities and exposure to exogenous VOCs following STARD (STAndards for the Reporting of Diagnostic accuracy studies) guidelines [48]. Tailor-made eNoses and/or diagnostic algorithms need to be produced when VOCs associated with disease have been identified and validated [49].

Conclusion

Exhaled breath analysis has potential as a diagnostic and monitoring tool in intubated and mechanically ventilated critically ill patients. Breath analysis can be fully non-invasive and as such has the advantage that it can be performed continuously, especially when using eNoses or I-MS. If it is confirmed that breath contains specific composite information about complex metabolic pulmonary processes, breathomics has the potential to become an important diagnostic tool for those who care for the critically ill. After all, adequate and early phenotyping may be the first step to more effective interventions.

References

1. Hudson LD, Steinberg KP (1999) Epidemiology of acute lung injury and ARDS. Chest 116 (Suppl 1): 74S-82S
2. Chastre J, Fagon JY (2002) Ventilator-associated pneumonia. Am J Respir Crit Care Med 165: 867–903
3. Slutsky AS (1999) Lung injury caused by mechanical ventilation. Chest 116 (Suppl 1): 9S-15S
4. Bernard GR, Artigas A, Brigham KL, et al (1994) The American-European Consensus Conference on ARDS. Definitions, mechanisms, relevant outcomes, and clinical trial coordination. Am J Respir Crit Care Med 149: 818–824
5. Pugin J, Verghese G, Widmer MC, Matthay MA (1999) The alveolar space is the site of intense inflammatory and profibrotic reactions in the early phase of acute respiratory distress syndrome. Crit Care Med 27: 304–312
6. Choi G, Wolthuis EK, Bresser P, et al (2006) Mechanical ventilation with lower tidal volumes and positive end-expiratory pressure prevents alveolar coagulation in patients without lung injury. Anesthesiology 105: 689–695

7. Wolthuis EK, Choi G, Dessing MC, et al (2008) Mechanical ventilation with lower tidal volumes and positive end-expiratory pressure prevents pulmonary inflammation in patients without preexisting lung injury. Anesthesiology 108: 46–54

8. Millo JL, Schultz MJ, Williams C, et al (2004) Compartmentalisation of cytokines and cytokine inhibitors in ventilator-associated pneumonia. Intensive Care Med 30: 68–74

9. Schultz MJ, Millo J, Levi M, et al (2004) Local activation of coagulation and inhibition of fibrinolysis in the lung during ventilator associated pneumonia. Thorax 59: 130–135

10. Palazzo SJ, Simpson T, Schnapp L (2011) Biomarkers for ventilator-associated pneumonia: Review of the literature. Heart Lung 40: 293–298

11. Tzouvelekis A, Pneumatikos I, Bouros D (2005) Serum biomarkers in acute respiratory distress syndrome an ailing prognosticator. Respir Res 6: 78

12. Frank JA, Parsons PE, Matthay MA (2006) Pathogenetic significance of biological markers of ventilator-associated lung injury in experimental and clinical studies. Chest 130: 1906–1914

13. Nicholson JK, Lindon JC (2008) Systems biology: Metabonomics. Nature 455: 1054–1056

14. Duflo Fdr, Debon R, Monneret G, Bienvenu J, Chassard D, Allaouchiche B (2002) Alveolar and serum procalcitonin: diagnostic and prognostic value in ventilator-associated pneumonia. Anesthesiology 96: 74–79

15. Ware LB, Matthay MA (2000) The acute respiratory distress syndrome. N Engl J Med 342: 1334–1349

16. Frey U, Maksym G, Suki B (2011) Temporal complexity in clinical manifestations of lung disease. J Appl Physiol 110: 1723–1731

17. Pugin J, Auckenthaler R, Mili N, Janssens JP, Lew PD, Suter PM (1991) Diagnosis of ventilator-associated pneumonia by bacteriologic analysis of bronchoscopic and nonbronchoscopic "blind" bronchoalveolar lavage fluid. Am Rev Respir Dis 143: 1121–1129

18. Martin TR (1997) Cytokines and the acute respiratory distress syndrome (ARDS): a question of balance. Nat Med 3: 272–273

19. Chang DW, Hayashi S, Gharib SA, et al (2008) Proteomic and computational analysis of bronchoalveolar proteins during the course of the acute respiratory distress syndrome. Am J Respir Crit Care Med 178: 701–709

20. Auffray C, Adcock IM, Chung KF, Djukanovic R, Pison C, Sterk PJ (2010) An integrative systems biology approach to understanding pulmonary diseases. Chest 137: 1410–1416

21. Deigner HP, Baranova AV (2010) Current methods and perspectives in biomarker discovery. Curr Mol Med 10: 113–114

22. Serkova NJ, Standiford TJ, Stringer KA (2011) The emerging field of quantitative blood metabolomics for biomarker discovery in critical illnesses. Am J Respir Crit Care Med 184: 647–655

23. Broadhurst D, Kell DB (2006) Statistical strategies for avoiding false discoveries in metabolomics and related experiments. Metabolomics 2: 171–196

24. Salek RM, Maguire ML, Bentley E, et al (2007) A metabolomic comparison of urinary changes in type 2 diabetes in mouse, rat, and human. Physiol Genomics 29: 99–108

25. Mao H, Wang H, Wang B, et al (2009) Systemic metabolic changes of traumatic critically ill patients revealed by an nmr-based metabonomic approach. J Proteome Res 8: 5423–5430

26. Serkova NJ, Van Rheen Z, Tobias M, Pitzer JE, Wilkinson JE, Stringer KA (2008) Utility of magnetic resonance imaging and nuclear magnetic resonance-based metabolomics for quantification of inflammatory lung injury. Am J Physiol Lung Cell Mol Physiol 295: L152–161

27. Stringer KA, Serkova NJ, Karnovsky A, Guire K, Paine R 3rd, Standiford TJ (2011) Metabolic consequences of sepsis-induced acute lung injury revealed by plasma (1)H-nuclear magnetic resonance quantitative metabolomics and computational analysis. Am J Physiol Lung Cell Mol Physiol 300: L4-L11

28. Pauling L, Robinson AB, Teranishi R, Cary P (1971) Quantitative analysis of urine vapor and breath by gas-liquid partition chromatography. Proc Natl Acad Sci USA 68: 2374–2376

29. Moser B, Bodrogi F, Eibl G, Lechner M, Rieder J, Lirk P (2005) Mass spectrometric profile of exhaled breath--field study by PTR-MS. Respir Physiol Neurobiol 145: 295–300

30. Manolis A (1983) The diagnostic potential of breath analysis. Clin Chem 29: 5–15

II

31. Zechman JM, Aldinger S, Labows JN Jr (1986) Characterization of pathogenic bacteria by automated headspace concentration-gas chromatography. J Chromatogr 377: 49–57

32. Shnayderman M, Mansfield B, Yip P, et al (2005) Species-specific bacteria identification using differential mobility spectrometry and bioinformatics pattern recognition. Anal Chem 77: 5930–5937

33. Röck F, Barsan N, Weimar U (2008) Electronic nose: current status and future trends. Chem Rev 108: 705–725

34. Schubert JK, Muller WP, Benzing A, Geiger K (1998) Application of a new method for analysis of exhaled gas in critically ill patients. Intensive Care Med 24: 415–421

35. Mendis S, Sobotka PA, Euler DE (1995) Expired hydrocarbons in patients with acute myocardial infarction. Free Radic Res 23: 117–122

36. Vautz W, Nolte J, Fobbe R, Baumbach JI (2009) Breath analysis-performance and potential of ion mobility spectrometry. J Breath Res 3: 036004

37. Dolch ME, Frey L, Hornuss C, et al (2008) Molecular breath-gas analysis by online mass spectrometry in mechanically ventilated patients: a new software-based method of CO2-controlled alveolar gas monitoring. J Breath Res 2: 037010

38. Westhoff M, Litterst P, Freitag L, Urfer W, Bader S, Baumbach JI (2009) Ion mobility spectrometry for the detection of volatile organic compounds in exhaled breath of patients with lung cancer: results of a pilot study. Thorax 64: 744–748

39. Friedrich MJ (2009) Scientists seek to sniff out diseases: electronic "noses" may someday be diagnostic tools. JAMA 301: 585–586

40. Dutta R, Hines EL, Gardner JW, Boilot P (2002) Bacteria classification using Cyranose 320 electronic nose. Biomed Eng Online 1: 4

41. Fend R, Kolk AH, Bessant C, Buijtels P, Klatser PR, Woodman AC (2006) Prospects for clinical application of electronic-nose technology to early detection of Mycobacterium tuberculosis in culture and sputum. J Clin Microbiol 44: 2039–2045

42. Humphreys L, Orme RM, Moore P, et al (2011) Electronic nose analysis of bronchoalveolar lavage fluid. Eur J Clin Invest 41: 52–58

43. Carey JR, Suslick KS, Hulkower KI, et al (2011) Rapid identification of bacteria with a disposable colorimetric sensing array. J Am Chem Soc 133: 7571–7576

44. Hanson CW, III, Thaler ER (2005) Electronic nose prediction of a clinical pneumonia score: biosensors and microbes. Anesthesiology 102: 63–68

45. Shih C-H, Lin Y-J, Lee K-F, Chien P-Y, Drake P (2009) Real-time electronic nose based pathogen detection for respiratory intensive care patients. Sens Actuators B Chem 148: 153–157

46. Bos LDJ, Fens N, van der Schee MP, Sterk PJ, Schultz MJ (2010) Fast assessment of ALI/ARDS in the ICU using exhaled breath analysis. Am J Respir Crit Care Med 181: A2583 (abst)

47. Bos LDJ, Sterk PJ, Schultz MJ (2011) Exhaled breath analysis in the diagnosis of acute lung injury. Am J Respir Crit Care Med 183: A1163 (abst)

48. Bossuyt PM, Reitsma JB, Bruns DE, et al (2003) Towards complete and accurate reporting of studies of diagnostic accuracy: the STARD initiative. BMJ 326: 41–44

49. Peng G, Tisch U, Adams O, et al (2009) Diagnosing lung cancer in exhaled breath using gold nanoparticles. Nat Nanotechnol 4: 669–673

III Sepsis Management

Cardiovascular Effects of Norepinephrine in Septic Shock

X. Monnet and J.-L. Teboul

III

Introduction

Septic shock is characterized by numerous cardiovascular abnormalities including absolute and relative hypovolemia, vascular tone depression, myocardial dysfunction, derangements in regional blood flow distribution and microcirculation disorders. The degree of severity of each of these abnormalities is variable from patient to patient. Although volume resuscitation is the most urgent therapy, current international guidelines recommend administering a vasopressor early to sustain life and maintain perfusion in the face of life-threatening hypotension, even when hypovolemia has not yet been resolved [1]. Indeed, if the mean arterial pressure (MAP) is markedly reduced, the perfusion pressure of critical organs (e.g., kidney, brain, myocardium, liver) may be lower than the lower threshold of autoregulation so that the ability of autoregulation to maintain vital organ blood flow may be lost. This can result in organ ischemia and eventually in organ failure, even if the systemic blood flow is high. The decrease in organ blood flow may be particularly marked in those patients with pre-existing renal, carotid, coronary or mesenteric atherosclerotic lesions as well as in those with pre-existing hypertension. In these conditions, increasing MAP above a certain critical level can restore organ perfusion even in the absence of an increase in cardiac output. Clinical evidence of such a pressure effect has been provided in the context of septic shock in studies where correction of severe hypotension with a vasoconstrictor was associated with improved renal function in the absence of any change in cardiac output [2–4]. It is currently recommended to achieve at least an MAP value of 65 mmHg [1]. However, in patients with pre-existing long-standing hypertension or other vascular comorbidities, the optimal MAP level may be higher. In septic patients with acute kidney failure, it has been suggested that the optimal MAP could be higher than in septic patients presenting without acute kidney insufficiency [5]. Therefore, an individual evaluation of the value of MAP to target with vasopressors is necessary.

Norepinephrine is now considered as the first-line vasopressor in septic shock [1, 6]. For a long time, it was only used as second choice (after dopamine) because of its potential vasoconstrictive effects on regional circulations. However, harmful regional effects have not been found in clinical studies [2, 3, 7–9]. Importantly, norepinephrine seems to be a more powerful α-agonist agent than dopamine. In a randomized study, Martin et al. showed that the goal of maintaining an MAP of 80 mmHg over six hours was achieved in only five out of 16 patients receiving dopamine compared to 15 out of 16 patients receiving norepinephrine [10]. Moreover, 10 of the 11 patients who did not respond to dopamine

J.-L. Vincent (ed.), *Annual Update in Intensive Care and Emergency Medicine 2012*
DOI 10.1007/978-3-642-25716-2 © Springer-Verlag Berlin Heidelberg 2012

were treated successfully when norepinephrine was added [10]. It is noteworthy that in this study, achievement of the MAP goal with norepinephrine was associated with improved urine output and decreased lactate level.

Results of recent randomized clinical trials (RCTs) suggest the superiority of norepinephrine over dopamine as the first-line vasopressive agent in septic shock patients. In a multicenter RCT, De Backer et al. compared norepinephrine and dopamine in the treatment of shock [11]. Although, there was no significant difference in the mortality rate, use of dopamine was associated with a greater number of adverse events, in particular of arrhythmias [11], compared to use of norepinephrine. Similar results were found in a single-center RCT in which administration of norepinephrine and dopamine were compared in septic shock patients [12].

Norepinephrine exerts its main beneficial effects in septic shock through its effect on arterial tone, but also has other cardiovascular effects, which deserve to be reviewed.

Effects of Norepinephrine on Arterial Tone

Norepinephrine is the predominant endogenous sympathetic amine. It is the physiologic mediator released by the postganglionic adrenergic nerves. It is also a hormone released by the adrenal medulla. Exogenous norepinephrine is a pharmacologic agent commonly used intravenously to reverse severe hypotension in shock states. Norepinephrine increases arterial pressure mainly through an increase in arterial tone after binding to α-receptors on the endothelial surface of peripheral arterioles. Binding to the α-receptor activates phospholipase C. This results in splitting of phosphatidyl inositol into inositol triphosphate-3 and 1,2-diacylglycerol. Inositol triphosphate-3 stimulates the release of calcium ions from the sarcoplasmic reticulum into the cytosol. An additional effect of activation of the α-receptor is the opening of receptor-operated non-selective cation channels that allows influx of extracellular calcium ions into the vascular smooth muscle cell. Calmodulin, which is a cytoplasmic regulatory protein related to troponin C, can then bind four calcium ions to activate the myosin light chain kinase. This results in phosphorylation of myosin heads that cause crossbridge formation with actin and then contraction of the vascular smooth muscle. Relaxation of the vascular smooth muscle cell results from the decrease in the concentration of cytosolic calcium ion, either by expulsion of calcium ion to the extracellular space or by its reuptake into the sarcoplasmic reticulum.

Sepsis is characterized by vascular hyporesponsiveness to vasoconstrictor agents [13]. Overproduction of nitric oxide (NO) induced by activation of inducible NO synthase (NOS), is assumed to play an important role [14]. The molecular target of NO in the vascular smooth muscle cell is soluble guanylate cyclase. This enzyme activates the transformation of GTP into cyclic GMP, which is responsible for vasorelaxation. Inhibitors of NOS have been demonstrated to reverse hyporesponsiveness to norepinephrine induced by endotoxin [15]. Abnormal vasorelaxation and hyporesponsiveness to vasoconstrictors could also involve increased production of prostacyclin [16], of peroxynitrite [17], of superoxide anion [18] or excessive activation of ATP-sensitive potassium channels [19].

Hyporesponsiveness to vasoconstrictors has been evidenced in septic shock patients by Annane et al. who reported a leftward shift of the dose-response curves to norepinephrine in septic patients compared to controls [20]. Clearly, this implies the use of high doses of norepinephrine to achieve a sufficient level of MAP in septic shock. Consequently, clinicians should not be reluctant to use high doses of norepinephrine to achieve an adequate MAP level, if necessary. In this regard, a retrospective study reported a survival rate of 35 % in a series of very severe septic shock patients receiving norepinephrine doses higher than 4 µg/kg/min [21].

III

Effects of Norepinephrine on Venous Return, Cardiac Preload and Preload Responsiveness

The effects of norepinephrine on the venous compartment of the cardiovascular circuit have been explored to a much lesser extent than have its effects on the arterial and microcirculatory compartments. Peripheral veins are thin-walled compliant vessels containing roughly two-thirds of the circulating blood in normal humans. This blood reservoir can be physiologically recruited to increase venous return and cardiac output. Venous return has two determinants: The pressure gradient between the mean systemic pressure and the right atrial pressure on the one hand and the resistance to venous return on the other hand. The backward pressure of the venous return itself depends upon the venous capacitance and compliance. The net effect of any vasoactive drug on the venous return thus depends on the balance between its action on the pressure gradient and the resistance to the venous return. Evidence is growing that the venous effects of norepinephrine may have some important clinical consequences.

Experimental Studies

An increase in venous return induced by norepinephrine has been reported in a few animal studies [22–26]. This effect is mainly related to α-adrenergic stimulation. Indeed, the sympathetic stimulation of the α-adrenergic receptors of the venous wall induces potent constriction [27], as on the arterial side of the circulation. As an α-adrenergic stimulator, norepinephrine may act on both determinants of the venous return, i.e., the pressure gradient and the resistance to the venous return. On the one hand, norepinephrine-induced venoconstriction increases the stress exerted by the venous wall on the vessel contents and thus transforms some part of the unstressed volume into stressed volume. This decrease in venous capacitance has been demonstrated in animals [28]. In a porcine model of endotoxic shock and using the physiological concept developed by Guyton et al. [29], Datta and Magder elegantly demonstrated that administering norepinephrine increased the mean systemic pressure [22], which promotes venous return. On the other hand, norepinephrine-induced venoconstriction could increase the resistance to venous return, which would impede venous return. However, Datta and Magder did not show such an increase in the resistance to the venous return with norepinephrine so that the net effect of norepinephrine was an increase in venous return and cardiac output [22]. An older study in dogs, yielded some contradictory results by showing that norepinephrine decreased the resistance to venous return [24]. The authors hypothesized that this effect was due to some vasodilating β-adrenergic stimulation by norepinephrine. The discrepant results between these two studies could be explained by different methodology and by species differences.

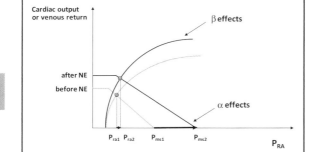

Fig. 1. Schematic effects of norepinephrine (NE) on cardiac output and venous return. Norepinephrine (NE) exerts its effects through α- and β-adrenergic stimulation. The α-stimulation of the venous compartment induces an increase in mean systemic pressure (from Pms1 to Pms2). Provided that it does not increase the resistance to venous return to too large an extent, norepinephrine increases the venous return. The β-stimulation increases cardiac contractility (the slope of the cardiac function curve becomes steeper). As a result of both effects, cardiac output increases while right atrial pressure increases only a little from Pra1 to Pra2

It is important to consider that the effect of norepinephrine on venous return and cardiac preload could be highly dependent on the prior level of venous capacitance. For example, if venous capacitance is already low because of endogenous sympathetic stimulation, as in cardiogenic shock, the effect of norepinephrine on venous capacitance may be less marked than in septic shock. **Figure 1** illustrates the effects of norepinephrine on the venous return curve during sepsis via its α-adrenergic stimulation action: Norepinephrine increases the mean systemic pressure while increasing the resistance to venous return (decrease in the slope of the curve). The resulting effect is a beneficial effect on venous return.

Clinical Evidence

In a clinical cohort study, our group examined the hemodynamic effects of an increase in the dose of norepinephrine in 105 septic shock patients monitored with a transpulmonary thermodilution device [30]. Increasing the dose of norepinephrine induced a significant increase in the global end-diastolic volume (i.e., the volume of blood contained in the four cardiac chambers at end-diastole) [30]; it also significantly increased cardiac output [30]. In another recent study [31], we included 25 septic shock patients in whom the dose of norepinephrine was increased because of profound hypotension. Importantly, all these patients were in a preload-dependent state, as evidenced by a positive passive leg raising test at baseline. We observed that norepinephrine increased the cardiac preload, as assessed by the global end-diastolic volume (GEDV) and the central venous pressure (CVP) [31]. Cardiac output increased in all patients, likely as a consequence of the preload increase in these preload-dependent patients and perhaps also because of an increase in cardiac inotropism. Importantly, when the dose of norepinephrine was increased, the degree of preload-dependence decreased, as assessed by the response of cardiac output to a fluid challenge [31]. In other words, some patients in whom cardiac output would have increased with fluid administration at the lowest dose of norepinephrine no longer responded to volume expansion once the dose of norepinephrine had been increased. This result is in accordance with previous studies showing that another indicator of preload-dependence, namely the respiratory variation of arterial pulse pressure, decreased with norepinephrine administration [30, 32, 33].

These effects of norepinephrine on preload and preload responsiveness may have some important clinical implications. Increasing the dose of norepinephrine in a patient with acute circulatory failure may be physiologically equivalent to infusing fluids; this could lead to a reduction in the total volume of fluid administered. Using a model of endotoxinic shock in rats, Sennoun et al. provided a clear confirmation of this hypothesis [33]. Indeed, compared to fluid administration alone, early use of norepinephrine was associated with less delivered fluid without any adverse effects on either systemic or regional hemodynamics or tissue perfusion [33].

Reducing the total volume of fluid administered may have beneficial prognostic effects. Indeed, the degree of positive fluid balance has been demonstrated to be of poor prognosis in septic patients [34, 35] as well as in critically ill patients with acute renal failure [36] and conservative fluid management has been demonstrated to be beneficial during acute respiratory distress syndrome (ARDS) [37]. In addition, compared to fluid, norepinephrine does not increase the intravascular pressure of the capillaries, which may reduce capillary leak in septic shock patients [22]. Thus, limiting fluid administration by increasing norepinephrine could have some potential benefits that need to be demonstrated in future clinical studies.

Effects of Norepinephrine on Cardiac Contractility

Norepinephrine may improve cardiac contractility through two different effects. First, it should improve myocardial perfusion by increasing not only the MAP but also the diastolic arterial pressure. MAP is the driving pressure for the right coronary circulation, whereas diastolic arterial pressure is the driving pressure for the left coronary circulation. Diastolic pressure is particularly low in septic shock because of the depressed arterial tone [38]. Thus increases in both mean and diastolic arterial pressure may result in an improved contractility in the case of myocardial ischemia. This effect may be even more important in the case of pre-existing coronary stenosis. Second, norepinephrine could theoretically increase cardiac contractility because of its β-adrenergic activity. Evidencing the effects of norepinephrine on cardiac contractility is challenging since the left ventricular ejection fraction (LVEF), i.e., the indicator of left ventricular systolic function that is used in clinical practice, is highly dependent on cardiac preload and afterload conditions [39]. However, the few clinical studies that have investigated this effect of norepinephrine suggest a significant inotropic effect of the drug. For instance, we observed that the LVEF did not change when the dose of norepinephrine was increased whereas the systolic arterial pressure increased [31]. Given the physiological relationship between LVEF and left ventricular systolic pressure [39], this suggests that contractility actually increased with norepinephrine augmentation.

Resultant Effect of Norepinephrine On Cardiac Output

Clinical studies have reported various effects of norepinephrine on cardiac index, some studies showing no change [2-4, 10, 40-43] and others significant increases [9, 30, 31, 44-49] in cardiac index. In fact, these conflicting results may be explained by the diversity of the patients included in these studies in terms of preload-dependence. In the case of preload-dependence, norepinephrine is more likely to increase cardiac output as a result of its effect on cardiac preload and also, to a lesser extent, to increased cardiac contractility (**Fig. 1**). In the case of preload-independence, for example because of massive prior fluid administration, no beneficial effect is expected from any preload effect. It has to be noted that no study reported a decreased cardiac output suggesting that the MAP targets used in clinical practice – usually between 65 and 85 mmHg – are not high enough to reduce cardiac output in relation to an increased left ventricular afterload.

Effects of Norepinephrine on Regional Blood Flow and Microcirculation

Because norepinephrine is a vasoconstrictive agent, its use theoretically carries a risk of inducing peripheral organ/tissue hypoperfusion, especially when high doses are used. However, the literature does not provide much evidence of such a deleterious effect when norepinephrine is titrated to achieve subnormal MAP values, as currently recommended during septic shock. In reality, two different clinical situations should be distinguished in septic shock: (1) Administration of norepinephrine in patients with life-threatening hypotension in order to restore a sufficient organ perfusion pressure; and (2) administration of norepinephrine in moderately hypotensive patients.

In Patients with Life-threatening Hypotension

Improved regional and/or microcirculatory blood flow is expected to occur after reaching an MAP value above the putative lower threshold of organ blood flow autoregulation. In line with this hypothesis, several studies in septic patients with high cardiac output and very low baseline MAP (between 45 and 55 mmHg) demonstrated that restoring MAP with norepinephrine could improve urine output and renal function, in spite of unchanged cardiac output [2–4, 7]. Albanese et al. provided a nice illustration of such a mechanism by using norepinephrine to elevate MAP in two different groups of patients [2]. In a group of septic shock patients, norepinephrine increased MAP from 51 ± 3 mmHg to 79 ± 7 mmHg; renal blood flow and renal function indices improved and cardiac output was unchanged [2]. In a group of head trauma patients, norepinephrine, administered in order to maintain a cerebral perfusion pressure > 70 mmHg, increased MAP from 81 ± 7 mmHg to 98 ± 3 mmHg, but did not change renal function indices or cardiac output [2]. This suggests that the initial value of MAP was below the lower autoregulation threshold of renal blood flow in septic patients but above this threshold in head trauma patients. In addition to the effects on perfusion pressure, it has also been suggested that norepinephrine can exert beneficial effects on intra-renal vasculature in septic conditions. Bellomo et al. showed in animals that norepinephrine infusion at clinically relevant dosages increased renal blood flow by decreasing the vascular closing pressure in endotoxic conditions, whereas it increased the vascular closing pressure in control conditions [50].

The beneficial effect on the microcirculation of restoring MAP with norepinephrine in septic patients with life-threatening hypotension has been illustrated in a study in which the subcutaneous microcirculation was assessed using near-infrared spectroscopy (NIRS) at the thenar eminence [49]. NIRS technology allows measurement of muscle tissue oxygen saturation (StO_2) and its change during a vascular occlusion test, which assesses the recruitment of subcutaneous microvessels in response to the hypoxic stimulus induced by upstream arterial occlusion. Administration of norepinephrine in septic shock patients resulted in increases in MAP from 54 ± 8 to 77 ± 9 mmHg, in cardiac index from 3.1 ± 1.0 to 3.6 ± 1.3 l/min/m^2 and in StO_2 from 75 ± 9 to 78 ± 9 % [49]. Importantly, administration of norepinephrine also resulted in an increased StO_2 recovery slope measured during a vascular occlusion test, suggesting a better recruitment of microvessels in response to local hypoxia. This finding was in agreement with the hypothesis that restoration of MAP allowed recruitment of previously closed microvessels in areas where perfusion depends on pressure.

In Moderately Hypotensive Patients

The regional and/or local vascular effects of norepinephrine are more variable. Recent studies evaluated the effects on cardiac output and organ perfusion indices of using norepinephrine to increase MAP from 60 (or 65) mmHg to 85 (or 90) mmHg in septic shock patients [9, 47, 48, 51]. In 11 septic shock patients, Deruddre et al. showed that increasing MAP from 65 to 75 mmHg with norepinephrine was associated with significant increases in cardiac output and urinary output and a significant decrease in the renal vascular resistance assessed with Doppler ultrasonography [9]. The combined effect of increasing cardiac output and MAP above the autoregulation threshold could be responsible for the putative increase in renal blood flow. It has to be noted that in this study, in which only one patient was being treated for chronic hypertension, no change in renal indices was observed when MAP was further increased from 75 to 85 mmHg [9]. Other clinical studies have shown that increasing MAP above 60 (or 65) mmHg overall was not associated with improved organ perfusion, in spite of the increased cardiac output. In 10 patients with septic shock, who had been previously stabilized after fluid loading and norepinephrine administration, LeDoux et al. reported no change in regional perfusion parameters (gastric mucosal carbon dioxide pressure, skin capillary blood flow and red blood cell velocity, urine output) when MAP was gradually increased from 65 to 85 mmHg [51]. In 16 septic shock patients with an MAP stabilized at 60 mmHg, Jhanji et al. gradually increased the dose of norepinephrine to achieve MAP values of 70, 80 and 90 mmHg [48]. Increase in norepinephrine dose was associated with increases in cutaneous tissue oxygen tension measured using a Clark electrode and in cutaneous red blood cell flux measured using laser Doppler flowmetry but with no change in sublingual microvascular flow using sidestream darkfield (SDF) imaging [48]. These findings emphasize the fact that in sepsis, which is characterized by disparities in microcirculation disturbances within and among organs [52], the microcirculatory response to norepinephrine may differ between organs. Dubin et al. also measured sublingual microcirculatory indices using SDF imaging in septic shock patients already resuscitated with fluid and norepinephrine [47]. Overall, no significant changes in microcirculatory indices were found when the dose of norepinephrine was gradually increased to achieve MAP values of 75 and 85 mmHg. Nevertheless, the most striking result was the correlation between the degree of severity of the microcirculatory disorders at baseline and the positive microcirculatory response to the norepinephrine-induced increase in MAP from 65 to 85 mmHg [47]. Thus, septic patients with normalized microcirculation (after initial hemodynamic resuscitation) may not benefit from any additional increase in MAP above 65 mmHg. In contrast, septic patients with persistently altered microcirculation in spite of achievement of the recommended endpoints, may benefit from a further increase in MAP beyond the value of 65 mmHg.

This hypothesis may explain the results recently reported by Thooft et al. in 13 patients with septic shock [53]. The gradual increase in MAP from 65 to 85 mmHg with norepinephrine was associated with increased cardiac output and mixed venous blood oxygen saturation (SvO_2) and decreased blood lactate [53]; importantly, this was also associated with an overall improvement of the microcirculation. Indeed, the increase in MAP from 65 to 85 mmHg was associated with an increased StO_2 recovery slope assessed by NIRS at the thenar eminence. Unlike Dubin et al. [47], Thooft and colleagues showed an increase in the perfused vessel density and the microvascular flow, which are both relevant sublingual microcirculation indices [54], in the subgroup of 6 patients in whom SDF imaging was also performed [53]. This suggests that microvessel recruitment and microcirculatory blood flow both increased at the MAP of 85 mmHg. These findings could be the result either of a proper perfusion pressure effect in some pressure-dependent areas or of the increase in systemic blood flow observed at the highest level of MAP.

Overall, results of these clinical studies suggest that: (1) regional and/or local vascular effects of norepinephrine aimed at increasing MAP beyond 65 mmHg are variable and not easy to predict in a given patient; (2) titration of norepinephrine to target an 'optimal' MAP needs to be carefully evaluated in each individual patient; and (3) norepinephrine does not have deleterious effects on tissue perfusion provided that 'reasonable' MAP values ($\leq$ 85 – 90 mmHg) are targeted.

Conclusion

Norepinephrine should be used as the first choice vasopressor in hypotensive septic patients. Its first beneficial hemodynamic effect is to restore MAP by constricting the arterial compartment. Norepinephrine could also restore the hemodynamic status by recruiting the venous blood reservoir and increasing cardiac preload, which may increase cardiac output in the case of preload-dependence. Provided that MAP is not increased above normal values, norepinephrine is not harmful to the microcirculation or to tissue perfusion. It is essential to carefully adjust the norepinephrine dose to achieve the optimal MAP level in each individual patient.

References

1. Dellinger RP, Levy MM, Carlet JM, et al (2008) Surviving Sepsis Campaign: international guidelines for management of severe sepsis and septic shock: 2008. Crit Care Med 36: 296 – 327
2. Albanese J, Leone M, Garnier F, et al (2004) Renal effects of norepinephrine in septic and nonseptic patients. Chest 126: 534 – 539
3. Desjars P, Pinaud M, Bugnon D, Tassaud F (1989) Norepinephrine therapy has no deleterious renal effects in human septic shock. Crit Care Med 17: 426 – 429
4. Redl-Wenzl EM, Armbruster C, Edelmann G, et al (1993) The effects of norepinephrine on

hemodynamics and renal function in severe septic shock states. Intensive Care Med 19: 151–154

5. Badin J, Boulain T, Ehrmann S, et al (2011) Relation between mean arterial pressure and renal function in the early phase of shock: a prospective, explorative cohort study. Crit Care 15: R135

6. Pottecher T, Calvat S, Dupont H, et al (2006) Haemodynamic management of severe sepsis: recommendations of the French Intensive Care Societies (SFAR/SRLF) Consensus Conference, 13 October 2005, Paris, France. Crit Care 10:311

7. Albanese J, Leone M, Delmas A, et al (2005) Terlipressin or norepinephrine in hyperdynamic septic shock: a prospective, randomized study. Crit Care Med 33: 1897–1902

8. Marik PE, Mohedin M (1994) The contrasting effects of dopamine and norepinephrine on systemic and splanchnic oxygen utilization in hyperdynamic sepsis (1994) JAMA 272: 1354–1357

9. Deruddre S, Cheisson G, Mazoit JX, Vicaut E, Benhamou D, Duranteau J (2007) Renal arterial resistance in septic shock: effects of increasing mean arterial pressure with norepinephrine on the renal resistive index assessed with Doppler ultrasonography. Intensive Care Med 33: 1557–1562

10. Martin C, Papazian L, Perrin G, et al (1993)Norepinephrine or dopamine for the treatment of hyperdynamic septic shock? Chest 103: 1826–1831

11. De Backer D, Biston P, Devriendt J, et al (2010) Comparison of dopamine and norepinephrine in the treatment of shock. N Engl J Med 362: 779–789

12. Patel GP, Grahe JS, Sperry M, et al (2010) Efficacy and safety of dopamine versus norepinephrine in the management of septic shock. Shock 33: 375–380

13. Levy B, Collin S, Sennoun N, et al (2010) Vascular hyporesponsiveness to vasopressors in septic shock: from bench to bedside. Intensive Care Med 36: 2019–2029

14. Julou-Schaeffer G, Gray GA, Fleming I, et al (1990) Loss of vascular responsiveness induced by endotoxin involves L-arginine pathway. Am J Physiol 259: H1038–1043

15. Gray GA, Schott C, Julou-Schaeffer G, et al (1991) The effect of inhibitors of the L-arginine/nitric oxide pathway on endotoxin-induced loss of vascular responsiveness in anaesthetized rats. Br J Pharmacol 103: 1218–1224

16. Hocherl K, Schmidt C, Kurt B, et al (2008) Activation of the PGI(2)/IP system contributes to the development of circulatory failure in a rat model of endotoxic shock. Hypertension 52: 330–335

17. Szabo C, Zingarelli B, Salzman AL (1996) Role of poly-ADP ribosyltransferase activation in the vascular contractile and energetic failure elicited by exogenous and endogenous nitric oxide and peroxynitrite. Circ Res 78: 1051–1063

18. Macarthur H, Westfall TC, Riley DP, et al (2000) Inactivation of catecholamines by superoxide gives new insights on the pathogenesis of septic shock. Proc Natl Acad Sci USA 97: 9753–9758

19. Landry DW, Oliver JA (1992) The ATP-sensitive K+ channel mediates hypotension in endotoxemia and hypoxic lactic acidosis in dog. J Clin Invest 89: 2071–2074

20. Annane D, Bellissant E, Sebille V, et al (1998) Impaired pressor sensitivity to noradrenaline in septic shock patients with and without impaired adrenal function reserve. Br J Clin Pharmacol 46: 589–597

21. Katsaragakis S, Kapralou A, Theodorou D, et al (2006) Refractory septic shock: efficacy and safety of very high doses of norepinephrine. Methods Find Exp Clin Pharmacol 28: 307–313

22. Datta P, Magder S (1999) Hemodynamic response to norepinephrine with and without inhibition of nitric oxide synthase in porcine endotoxemia. Am J Respir Crit Care Med 160: 1987–9193

23. Emerson TE Jr (1966) Effects of angiotensin, epinephrine, norepinephrine, and vasopressin on venous return. Am J Physiol 210: 933–942

24. Imai Y, Satoh K, Taira N (1978) Role of the peripheral vasculature in changes in venous return caused by isoproterenol, norepinephrine, and methoxamine in anesthetized dogs. Circ Res 43: 553–561

25. Rose JC, Freis ED, Hufnagel CA, et al (1955) Effects of epinephrine and nor-epinephrine in dogs studied with a mechanical left ventricle; demonstration of active vasoconstriction in the lesser circulation. Am J Physiol 182: 197–202

26. Rose JC, Kot PA, Cohn JN, et al (1962) Comparison of effects of angiotensin and norepinephrine on pulmonary circulation, systemic arteries and veins, and systemic vascular capacity in the dog. Circulation 25: 247–252
27. De Mey J, Vanhoutte PM (1981) Uneven distribution of postjunctional alpha 1-and alpha 2-like adrenoceptors in canine arterial and venous smooth muscle. Circ Res 48: 875–884
28. Greenway CV, Seaman KL, Innes IR (1985) Norepinephrine on venous compliance and unstressed volume in cat liver. Am J Physiol 248: H468–476
29. Guyton AC, Lindsey AW, Abernathy B, et al (1957) Venous return at various right atrial pressures and the normal venous return curve. Am J Physiol 189: 609–615
30. Hamzaoui O, Georger JF, Monnet X, et al (2010) Early administration of norepinephrine increases cardiac preload and cardiac output in septic patients with life-threatening hypotension. Crit Care 14: R142
31. Monnet X, Jabot J, Maizel J, et al (2011) Norepinephrine increases cardiac preload and reduces preload dependency assessed by passive leg raising in septic shock patients Crit Care Med 39: 689–694
32. Nouira S, Elatrous S, Dimassi S, et al (2005) Effects of norepinephrine on static and dynamic preload indicators in experimental hemorrhagic shock. Crit Care Med 33: 2339–2343
33. Sennoun N, Montemont C, Gibot S, et al (2007) Comparative effects of early versus delayed use of norepinephrine in resuscitated endotoxic shock. Crit Care Med 35: 1736–1740
34. Boyd JH, Forbes J, Nakada TA, et al (2011) Fluid resuscitation in septic shock: a positive fluid balance and elevated central venous pressure are associated with increased mortality. Crit Care Med 39: 259–265
35. Vincent JL, Sakr Y, Sprung CL, et al (2006) Sepsis in European intensive care units: results of the SOAP study. Crit Care Med 34: 344–353
36. Payen D, de Pont AC, Sakr Y, et al (2008) A positive fluid balance is associated with a worse outcome in patients with acute renal failure. Crit Care 12: R74
37. Wiedemann HP, Wheeler AP, Bernard GR, et al (2006) Comparison of two fluid-management strategies in acute lung injury. N Engl J Med 354: 2564–2575
38. Lamia B, Chemla D, Richard C, Tebould JL (2005) Clinical review: Interpretation of arterial pressure wave in shock states. Crit Care 9: 601–606
39. Robotham JL, Takata M, Berman M, Harasawa Y (1991) Ejection fraction revisited Anesthesiology 74: 172–183
40. De Backer D, Creteur J, Silva E, Vincent JL (2003) Effects of dopamine, norepinephrine, and epinephrine on the splanchnic circulation in septic shock: which is best? Crit Care Med 31: 1659–1667
41. Edwards JD, Brown GC, Nightingale P, et al (1989) Use of survivors' cardiorespiratory values as therapeutic goals in septic shock. Crit Care Med 17: 1098–1103
42. Martin C, Viviand X, Arnaud S, et al (1999) Effects of norepinephrine plus dobutamine or norepinephrine alone on left ventricular performance of septic shock patients. Crit Care Med 27: 1708–1713
43. Meadows D, Edwards JD, Wilkins RG, et al (1988) Reversal of intractable septic shock with norepinephrine therapy. Crit Care Med 16: 663–666
44. Hesselvik JF, Brodin B (1989) Low dose norepinephrine in patients with septic shock and oliguria: effects on afterload, urine flow, and oxygen transport. Crit Care Med 17: 179–180
45. Martin C, Saux P, Eon B, et al (1990) Septic shock: a goal-directed therapy using volume loading, dobutamine and/or norepinephrine. Acta Anaesthesiol Scand 34: 413–417
46. Winslow EJ, Loeb HS, Rahimtoola SH, et al (1973) Hemodynamic studies and results of therapy in 50 patients with bacteremic shock. Am J Med 54: 421–432
47. Dubin A, Pozo MO, Casabella CA, et al (2009) Increasing arterial blood pressure with norepinephrine does not improve microcirculatory blood flow: a prospective study. Crit Care 13: R92
48. Jhanji S, Stirling S, Patel N, et al (2009) The effect of increasing doses of norepinephrine on tissue oxygenation and microvascular flow in patients with septic shock. Crit Care Med 37: 1961–1966

49. Georger JF, Hamzaoui O, Chaari A, et al (2010) Restoring arterial pressure with norepinephrine improves muscle tissue oxygenation assessed by near-infrared spectroscopy in severely hypotensive septic patients. Intensive Care Med 36: 1882–1889
50. Bellomo R, Kellum JA, Wisniewski SR, et al (1999) Effects of norepinephrine on the renal vasculature in normal and endotoxemic dogs. Am J Respir Crit Care Med 159: 1186–1192
51. LeDoux D, Astiz ME, Carpati CM, et al (2000) Effects of perfusion pressure on tissue perfusion in septic shock. Crit Care Med 28: 2729–2732
52. Boerma EC, Kuiper MA, Kingma WP, et al (2008) Disparity between skin perfusion and sublingual microcirculatory alterations in severe sepsis and septic shock: a prospective observational study. Intensive Care Med 34: 1294–1298
53. Thooft A, Favory R, D Ribeiro Salgado, et al (2011) Effects of changes in arterial pressure on organ perfusion during septic shock. Crit Care 15: R222
54. De Backer D, Hollenberg S, Boerma C, et al (2007) How to evaluate the microcirculation: report of a round table conference. Crit Care 11: R101

Vasopressin Therapy in Septic Shock

S. Rehberg, M. Westphal, and C. Ertmer

Introduction

Catecholamine-resistant arterial hypotension associated with severe impairment of tissue oxygenation plays a pivotal role in the development of multiple organ failure (MOF) and is associated with increased mortality in septic shock [1]. Therefore, alternative, non-adrenergic treatment strategies are urgently warranted. During recent years, research has increasingly focused on the use of vasopressinergic agents, such as arginine vasopressin (AVP) and terlipressin. Contrary to adrenergic receptors, the sensitivity of vasopressin receptors increases in septic shock [2]. This phenomenon may be explained by autonomic insufficiency, baroreceptor dysfunction [3] and the relative deficiency of endogenous vasopressin that is linked to increased receptor expression and sensitivity [4]. Mechanisms of action further include stimulation of vasopressin 1a receptors (V1aR), inhibition of nitric oxide (NO) synthesis [5], inhibition of ATP-dependent potassium channels [6] and restoration of adrenergic receptor sensitivity [7]. As a consequence, low doses of vasopressin analogs have been shown to increase mean arterial pressure (MAP) in catecholamine-resistant septic shock in numerous experimental [8, 9] and clinical studies [10–13]. In addition, these studies demonstrated a significant reduction in catecholamine requirements and attenuated renal dysfunction in septic shock patients.

However, the Vasopressin in Septic Shock Trial (VASST), a multicenter randomized controlled trial (RCT), failed to demonstrate a reduction in overall mortality in patients treated just with norepinephrine compared to a combination of norepinephrine and AVP [14]. In addition to the currently discussed value of large RCTs in proving the effectiveness of therapeutic interventions in septic shock [15], these results suggest that we do not take full advantage of the therapeutic potential of vasopressin analogs at the present time.

This review article, therefore, critically discusses potential modifications in the currently recommended therapeutic approach to vasopressin analogs in septic shock.

'State of the Art' Hemodynamic Support

The current guidelines of the Surviving Sepsis Campaign recommend a continuous infusion of low-dose AVP (up to 0.03 U/min), in addition to norepinephrine, as a rescue therapy, i.e., when norepinephrine alone is not effective [16]. This dose is based on the rationale that it is necessary to compensate for a relative

J.-L. Vincent (ed.), *Annual Update in Intensive Care and Emergency Medicine 2012*
DOI 10.1007/978-3-642-25716-2 © Springer-Verlag Berlin Heidelberg 2012

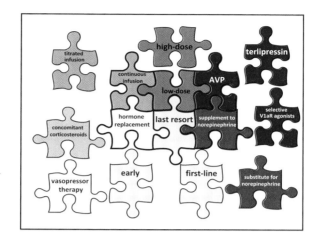

Fig. 1. Jigsaw of the recommended treatment approach for arginine-vasopressin (AVP) in septic shock with alternative pieces for every position. V1aR, vasopressin 1a-receptor

vasopressin deficiency in septic shock as compared to other shock states and, therefore, reflects a type of hormone replacement therapy [17]. The safety of this approach was demonstrated in the VASST trial [14]. **Figure 1** illustrates the recommended therapy as a jigsaw consisting of multiple 'pieces' that are all exchangeable with potential alternatives. The challenge is to find the perfect combination for the individual patient in the intensive care unit (ICU).

One problem with the current recommendation is that AVP is not available in some countries. Therefore, the synthetic, long-acting vasopressin analog, terlipressin, is increasingly used instead of AVP. Despite important pharmacological differences between the two drugs (e.g., receptor selectivity, effective half-life) the use of either substance was (and still is) determined mainly by local availability and institutional inventory. Hence, Leone asked in an editorial, whether it is "terlipressin or europressin" [18]. However, there are no official recommendations for the use of terlipressin in septic shock, mainly because of the lack of large, randomized multicenter studies. Based on its longer elimination half-life of approximately 50 min (vs. 6 min for AVP), terlipressin was first administered as a bolus of 1(-2) mg, resulting in severe adverse effects, such as reduction in cardiac output and global oxygen transport, as well as mesenteric ischemia [13, 19, 20]. In this context, Lange et al. reported that a continuous, low-dose infusion of 2 mg/24h terlipressin was more effective in stabilizing hemodynamics than repeated bolus administration (1 mg every 6 h) and was associated with a significant reduction in unwanted adverse effects [21]. Continuous, low-dose infusion of 1.3 µg/kg/h terlipressin in addition to norepinephrine has been shown to be feasible, safe and effective in stabilizing hemodynamics in patients with septic shock [12].

Furthermore, when using vasopressin agonists, it is critical to treat hypovolemia with adequate fluid resuscitation to minimize the risk of ischemic complications. In this regard, Asfar and colleagues even reported improved splanchnic blood flow in response to terlipressin infusion and effective volume therapy, whereas terlipressin infusion without appropriate fluid substitution was harmful [22, 23].

Time Point of Treatment Initiation

In a retrospective analysis of 316 patients in advanced vasodilatory shock, Luckner et al. noticed that norepinephrine requirements > 0.5 µg/kg/min before initiation of treatment with AVP represented an independent risk factor for mortality [11]. This finding suggested that early use of AVP in the course of septic shock may be more beneficial than the currently recommended last resort strategy. This hypothesis was supported by a predefined subgroup analysis of the VASST study. The combination of AVP and norepinephrine was more effective in stabilizing hemodynamics than norepinephrine alone in patients with a lower dose of norepinephrine (< 15 µg/min vs > 15 µg/min) at the time of treatment initiation of AVP [14]. However, the time from the onset of shock to AVP initiation was not significantly different between the two sub-cohorts. Based on these findings and in line with several therapeutic approaches for the treatment of septic shock (e.g., antibiotic therapy, volume resuscitation), use of AVP early in the course of the disease rather than as a rescue therapy appears reasonable. In addition, from a pathophysiological point of view, a therapy is more likely to be successful when the patient does not already suffer from MOF. The most beneficial time for treatment initiation of vasopressin analogs, however, remains to be determined.

Of note, some studies have even investigated the effects of AVP as well as terlipressin as first-line therapies. In an established ovine model of fecal peritonitis-induced septic shock, our group demonstrated efficacy in maintaining MAP and safety of a continuous, low-dose infusion of AVP (0.5 mU/kg/min) or terlipressin (1 µg/kg/h) supplemented with titrated norepinephrine [8]. Our findings were confirmed by an experimental study in a pig model of septic shock two years later [9]. First-line therapy with AVP up to 5 ng/kg/min (equivalent to ~0.18 U/min) supplemented with norepinephrine was not only safe in respect to myocardial function and global oxygen transport, but also attenuated renal dysfunction and reduced catecholamine requirements as compared to first-line norepinephrine [9]. These experimental results were supported by an open-label RCT in patients with early (12 h) hyperdynamic septic shock. First-line AVP up to 0.2 U/min increased and maintained MAP ≥ 70 mmHg without negatively affecting mesenteric oxygenation. Notably, renal function and sequential organ failure assessment (SOFA) scores were improved compared to patients who received first-line norepinephrine [24]. Despite these promising data, the use of vasopressin analogs as a first-line infusion should be restricted to controlled studies at the present time.

Dose and Treatment Endpoints

The currently recommended low dose of 0.03 U/min AVP for use in septic shock has been questioned in recent studies [25, 26]. This dose recommendation is based mainly on the safety issue. Extremely high doses of up to 0.47 U/min have been shown to be associated with a reduction in global oxygen transport, and with peripheral and myocardial ischemia [20, 27]. Since these doses are more than 15-fold higher than the recommended one, these results are not really surprising. However, there is a wide range between 0.03 and 0.47 U/min. Several studies have provided evidence that with doses of 0.06 U/min the risk of complications is not higher than with norepinephrine, if bolus infusions are omitted and sufficient fluid resuscitation is guaranteed. Dunser et al. already reported in 2003 that a combined infusion of norepinephrine and AVP (4 U/h ~ 0.067 U/min) was more effective and associated with a lower incidence of new-onset tachyarrhythmias than was norepinephrine alone [10]. The same group directly compared the effects of the established dose of 0.03 U/min with a dose of 0.06 U/min AVP in a retrospective analysis of 78 patients as well as in an RCT in 50 patients with vasodilatory shock [25, 26]. In both trials, there was no increased incidence of unwanted adverse effects, such as mesenteric ischemia, with the higher dose compared to norepinephrine and 0.03 U/min of AVP. Restoration of cardiovascular function, however, was more effective with 0.06 U/min AVP. According to these results, AVP in the VASST study may have been not only started too late, but also at too low a dose.

Because of the presumed risk of myocardial ischemia, patients with coronary artery disease were excluded from the VASST trial. However, AVP is also used to treat post-cardiopulmonary bypass vasodilatory shock [28]. Interestingly, the doses of AVP (usually 0.1 U/min) in these high risk cardiovascular patients are three times higher than those recommended in patients with septic shock. Against this background, it does not appear justified to generally withhold therapy with vasopressin analogs from patients with coronary artery disease.

The second argument for the recommendation of 0.03 U/min is the restoration of plasma levels of AVP to the levels seen in other shock states (usually around 100 pg/ml). This so-called hormone replacement therapy is based on the fact that AVP levels in septic shock have been reported to be inappropriately low as compared to other shock states, such as cardiogenic shock [29]. Using higher doses of AVP would represent a vasopressor dose rather than hormone replacement therapy [30]. This therapeutic strategy was tested in two experimental studies of ovine septic shock that are currently under review and, therefore, only published as abstracts [31, 32]. In both studies, titrated, first-line AVP without concomitant norepinephrine was able to keep MAP within the therapeutic range for 24 h. AVP doses were increased up to 0.06 U/min.

In this context, Lauzier et al. performed a very interesting open-label RCT study in 23 patients with early (12 h) septic shock [24]. The administration of titrated AVP (up to 0.2 U/min) failed to increase MAP in the first hour but maintained it above 70 mmHg in two-thirds of patients at 48 h. In addition, norepinephrine requirements, renal dysfunction and SOFA scores were reduced compared to treatment with norepinephrine alone.

Selective vs. Non-selective V1aR Agonists

AVP is a mixed vasopressin 1a/2 receptor (V1aR/V2R) agonist with a selectivity of 1:1 for each of these receptors. Whereas particular attention has been paid to vasoconstriction mediated by vascular V1aRs [4], the effects of AVP stimulation of V2R have been neglected, probably because the most familiar anti-diuretic effect mediated by renal V2Rs is compensated for by an V1aR-mediated increase in glomerular filtration pressure [33]. There is increasing evidence that stimulation of extrarenal (endothelial) V2Rs may aggravate sepsis-induced vasodilation [34], fluid accumulation [31], leukocyte rolling [35] and pro-coagulant effects [36]. In this context, our research group demonstrated, in an established ovine model of septic shock, that a V2R antagonist supplemented with norepinephrine improved cardiovascular, metabolic, liver and renal functions and prolonged survival as compared to AVP or placebo [37].

The use of more selective V1aR agonists may, therefore, be superior to AVP for two reasons: More pronounced vasoconstriction and a reduction in V2R-mediated unwanted effects. In line with this theory, our research group was able to provide experimental [8] and clinical evidence [12] that a continuous, low-dose infusion of terlipressin (1 or 1.3 μg/kg/h, respectively), with a selectivity of 2.2:1 for the V1aR versus the V2R, was more effective than AVP (0.03 U/min) and norepinephrine alone in stabilizing cardiopulmonary hemodynamics in septic shock. Following these promising results, the use of two highly selective V1aR agonists with only negligible intrinsic activity at the V2R was tested in experimental studies. Phe2-Orn8-Vasotocin (POV) has a more than 220 times higher selectivity for the V1aR than AVP [38]. Because of its similar potency compared to AVP [39], POV was administered in an equivalent dose as a first-line continuous infusion in ovine septic shock. POV improved vascular, pulmonary, and renal functions, increased oxygen delivery and slightly prolonged survival as compared to first-line AVP and standard treatment with norepinephrine [40]. Traber titrated the highly selective V1aR agonist, FE 202158, with a selectivity of 1107:1 for the V1aR vs. the V2R, to target an MAP above baseline-10 mmHg. FE 202158 kept MAP within the target range at lower doses and for a longer time period compared to AVP [31].

A very interesting finding of these studies was the fact that net fluid balance was significantly lower in animals treated with highly selective V1aR agonists compared to those treated with AVP, suggesting that V1aR stimulation might attenuate capillary leakage. This hypothesis was tested in an established ovine model of septic shock using a POV infusion titrated to maintain MAP [32]. This study demonstrated an immediate reduction in net fluid balance after the start of the compound. Vascular endothelial growth factor (VEGF) and angiopoietin-2, two established markers of capillary leakage, were significantly reduced in pulmonary tissue samples of animals treated with the highly selective V1aR agonist as compared to those treated with AVP. At the same time, the fluid volume in the thoracic cavity measured during necropsy at the end of the 24 h study period was significantly lower in the POV group than in the control and AVP groups. In addition, urine output increased after the start of POV infusion and cumulative net fluid balance was almost balanced at 24 h. In contrast, cumulative net fluid balance was more than 5000 ml in control animals and almost 3000 ml in AVP-treated animals. Since positive fluid balance represents an independent risk factor for mortality in septic shock [41], this effect of highly selective V1aR agonists may be of critical importance. Interestingly, the beneficial effects of FE 202158 on fluid balance were abolished if it was combined with the selective V2R agonist, desmopressin [31]. This finding further supports the hypothesis that V1aR stimulation attenuates, and V2R activation aggravates, vascular leakage, providing another argument for the use of highly selective V1aR agonists instead of AVP. However, clinical studies are needed to verify these promising results in patients with septic shock. In this regard, it is noteworthy that FE 202158 is currently undergoing a phase II trial.

Combination of AVP with Corticosteroids

From a physiological point of view, combining AVP with corticosteroids for the treatment of septic shock is likely to be beneficial, because these endogenous hormones promote synergistic effects. Whereas AVP increases the secretion of adrenocorticotropin releasing hormone [42], corticosteroids increase the sensitivity of V1aRs [43]. In addition, endogenous plasma levels of AVP and corticosteroids have been reported to be reduced or inappropriately low in septic shock. These physiological rationales may have been one reason why Dr. Annane called the combination of AVP and corticosteroids in his editorial for a post-hoc analysis of the VASST study, "The shock duo" [44]. Russell et al. reported that in septic shock patients who received corticosteroid treatment, AVP was associated with a significantly lower mortality compared to sole norepinephrine (35.9 % vs. 44.7 %) [45]. In addition, the authors pointed out that corticosteroids increased plasma vasopressin levels compared to AVP infusion without corticosteroids by 67 % at 24 h. In contrast, AVP infusion was associated with a higher mortality than sole norepinephrine in the subcohort of patients who did not receive corticosteroids. This positive interaction between AVP and corticosteroids in the treatment of septic shock had already been suggested by a retrospective, case control study by Bauer et al. in 2008 [46]. The addition of corticosteroids to supplementary AVP increased the proportion of patients alive without vasopressor therapy at day 7 of their ICU stay. These results were confirmed by another, recent retrospective study of Torgersen and colleagues, who investigated 159 patients with supplementary AVP infusion [47]. They concluded that "concomitant AVP and hydrocortisone may be associated with a survival benefit in septic shock".

Based on the retrospective and post-hoc character of these studies, these positive findings are only hypothesis generating and sufficiently powered RCTs are warranted. The comment of Dr. Lauzier, in an editorial related to the most recent study [47], that AVP and corticosteroids are "engaged but not yet married" [48] hit the nail on the head. Whether the beneficial effect of combining AVP with corticosteroids also applies to vasopressin analogs, like terlipressin or selective V1aR agonists, remains to be determined.

Patient Selection

The best therapeutic approach is worthless if it is applied to the wrong patient population. In this context, it is well-known that vasopressin deficiency only occurs in one third of septic shock patients [49]. The absence of 'relative vasopressin deficiency' may be one reason for the failure of AVP to decrease mortality in the overall population of the VASST trial. This phenomenon only represents one example of the need to better identify patients who will potentially benefit from a therapeutic approach. The goal should be to have several pharmacogenomic biomarkers that provide information about the probability of success for the individual compound, similar to the treatment of cancer. Regarding the use of AVP, Dr. Nakada and colleagues reported that a specific genetic variation in leucyl/cystinyl aminopeptidase (= vasopressinase, the enzyme that metabolizes AVP) is associated with 28-day mortality in septic shock and with biologic effects on AVP clearance [50]. By determining this genetic variation, the probability of success of AVP therapy could be specified. In addition, dose selection of AVP might be guided by this knowledge. For example, if a patient has an increased AVP clearance, higher doses might be chosen than for a patient with a low AVP clearance.

Conclusion

Based on the current guidelines, vasopressin analogs are recommended for treatment as continuous and low-dose AVP supplementation of first-line norepinephrine infusion in combination with sufficient fluid resuscitation. Recent experimental studies, however, suggest parting with the concepts of hormone replacement and rescue strategy. Instead, the use of vasopressin analogs early in the course of sepsis and a titration of vasopressinergic agents to keep MAP within the therapeutic range may represent potential alternatives. However, the former approach inevitably results in higher doses than currently recommended. In this context it should be considered that such 'high' doses are used anyway in cardiac surgery patients to treat postoperative vasoplegic shock.

Of note, highly selective V1aR agonists may represent a promising alternative to AVP. These compounds are not only characterized by a more pronounced vasoconstriction but also reduce the potential adverse effects of V2R. In addition, a reduction in capillary leakage and subsequent positive fluid balance has been repeatedly reported with the use of highly selective V1aR agonists. Furthermore, recent clinical studies suggest the combination of AVP with corticosteroids and use of genetic analysis to identify patient cohorts that will be most likely to respond to this therapy. However, these very interesting hypotheses and new pieces in the jigsaw of vasopressin therapy in septic shock still need to be evaluated in large clinical, randomized trials before the puzzle can be completed.

References

1. Engel C, Brunkhorst FM, Bone HG, et al (2007) Epidemiology of sepsis in Germany: results from a national prospective multicenter study. Intensive Care Med 33: 606–618
2. Landry DW, Levin HR, Gallant EM, et al (1997) Vasopressin pressor hypersensitivity in vasodilatory septic shock. Crit Care Med 25: 1279–1282
3. Williams TD, Da Costa D, Mathias CJ, Bannister R, Lightman SL (1986) Pressor effect of arginine vasopressin in progressive autonomic failure. Clin Sci (Lond) 71: 173–178
4. Barrett LK, Singer M, Clapp LH (2007) Vasopressin: mechanisms of action on the vasculature in health and in septic shock. Crit Care Med 35: 33–40
5. Yamamoto K, Ikeda U, Okada K, Saito T, Shimada K (1997) Arginine vasopressin inhibits nitric oxide synthesis in cytokine-stimulated vascular smooth muscle cells. Hypertens Res 20: 209–216
6. Vincent JL, Su F (2008) Physiology and pathophysiology of the vasopressinergic system. Best Pract Res Clin Anaesthesiol 22: 243–252
7. Holmes CL, Landry DW, Granton JT (2004) Science Review: Vasopressin and the cardiovascular system part 2 – clinical physiology. Crit Care 8: 15–23
8. Rehberg S, Ertmer C, Kohler G, et al (2009) Role of arginine vasopressin and terlipressin as first-line vasopressor agents in fulminant ovine septic shock. Intensive Care Med 35: 1286–1296
9. Simon F, Giudici R, Scheuerle A, et al (2009) Comparison of cardiac, hepatic, and renal effects of arginine vasopressin and noradrenaline during porcine fecal peritonitis: a randomized controlled trial. Crit Care 13: R113
10. Dunser MW, Mayr AJ, Ulmer H, et al (2003) Arginine vasopressin in advanced vasodnla tory shock: a prospective, randomized, controlled study. Circulation 107: 2313–2319

11. Luckner G, Dunser MW, Jochberger S, et al (2005) Arginine vasopressin in 316 patients with advanced vasodilatory shock. Crit Care Med 33: 2659–2666
12. Morelli A, Ertmer C, Rehberg S, et al (2009) Continuous terlipressin versus vasopressin infusion in septic shock (TERLIVAP): a randomized, controlled pilot study. Crit Care 13: R130
13. Albanese J, Leone M, Delmas A, Martin C (2005) Terlipressin or norepinephrine in hyperdynamic septic shock: a prospective, randomized study. Crit Care Med 33: 1897–1902
14. Russell J, Walley K, Singer J, et al (2008) Vasopressin versus Norepinephrine Infusion in Patients with Septic Shock. N Engl J Med 358: 877–887
15. Vincent JL (2011) We should abandon randomized controlled trials in the intensive care unit. Crit Care Med 38: S534–538
16. Dellinger RP, Levy MM, Carlet JM, et al (2008) Surviving Sepsis Campaign: international guidelines for management of severe sepsis and septic shock: 2008. Crit Care Med 36: 296–327
17. Vincent JL (2002) Endocrine support in the critically ill. Crit Care Med 30: 702–703
18. Leone M (2009) Terlipressin or europressin? Crit Care 13: 192
19. O'Brien A, Clapp L, Singer M (2002) Terlipressin for norepinephrine-resistant septic shock. Lancet 359: 1209–1210
20. Ertmer C, Rehberg S, Westphal M (2008) Vasopressin analogues in the treatment of shock states: potential pitfalls. Best Pract Res Clin Anaesthesiol 22: 393–406
21. Lange M, Morelli A, Ertmer C, et al (2007) Continuous versus bolus infusion of terlipressin in ovine endotoxemia. Shock 28: 623–629
22. Asfar P, Hauser B, Ivanyi Z, et al (2005) Low-dose terlipressin during long-term hyperdynamic porcine endotoxemia: effects on hepatosplanchnic perfusion, oxygen exchange, and metabolism. Crit Care Med 33: 373–380
23. Asfar P, Pierrot M, Veal N, et al (2003) Low-dose terlipressin improves systemic and splanchnic hemodynamics in fluid-challenged endotoxic rats. Crit Care Med 31: 215–220
24. Lauzier F, Levy B, Lamarre P, Lesur O (2006) Vasopressin or norepinephrine in early hyperdynamic septic shock: a randomized clinical trial. Intensive Care Med 32: 1782–1789
25. Luckner G, Mayr VD, Jochberger S, et al (2007) Comparison of two dose regimens of arginine vasopressin in advanced vasodilatory shock. Crit Care Med 35: 2280–2285
26. Torgersen C, Dunser MW, Wenzel V, et al (2010) Comparing two different arginine vasopressin doses in advanced vasodilatory shock: a randomized, controlled, open-label trial. Intensive Care Med 36: 57–65
27. Klinzing S, Simon M, Reinhart K, Bredle DL, Meier-Hellmann A (2003) High-dose vasopressin is not superior to norepinephrine in septic shock. Crit Care Med 31: 2646–50
28. Lavigne D (2010) Vasopressin and methylene blue: alternate therapies in vasodilatory shock. Semin Cardiothorac Vasc Anesth 14: 186–189
29. Landry DW, Levin HR, Gallant EM, et al (1997) Vasopressin deficiency contributes to the vasodilation of septic shock. Circulation 95: 1122–1125
30. Rehberg S, Enkhbaatar P, Traber DL (2009) Arginine vasopressin in septic shock: supplement or substitute for norepinephrine? Crit Care 13: 178
31. Traber DL (2007) Selective V1a receptor agonists in experimental septic shock. Crit Care 11: P51 (abst)
32. Rehberg S, Enkhbaatar P, Yamamoto Y, Hasselbach AK, Traber LD, Traber DL (2010) Selective V_{1a} agonism reduces vascular leakage and cardiopulmonary dysfunction in MRSA sepsis. Crit Care 14: P397 (abst)
33. Edwards RM, Trizna W, Kinter LB (1989) Renal microvascular effects of vasopressin and vasopressin antagonists. Am J Physiol 256: F274–278
34. Kaufmann JE, Lezzi M, Vischer UM (2003) Desmopressin (DDAVP) induces NO production in human endothelial cells via V2 receptor- and cAMP-mediated signaling. J Thromb Haemost 1: 821–828
35. Kanwar S, Woodman RC, Poon MC, et al (1995) Desmopressin induces endothelial P-selectin expression and leukocyte rolling in postcapillary venules. Blood 86: 2760–2766
36. Rehberg S, Laporte R, Enkhbaatar P, et al (2009) Arginine vasopressin increases plasma levels of von Willebrand factor in sheep. Crit Care 13: A182

III

37. Rehberg S, Ertmer C, Lange M, et al (2010) Role of selective V2-receptor antagonism in septic shock: a randomized, controlled, experimental study. Crit Care 14: R200
38. Berde B, Boissonnas RA, Huguenin RL, Sturmer E (1964) Vasopressin analogues with selective pressor activity. Experientia 20: 42–43
39. Mihara T, Tarumi T, Sugimoto Y, Chen Z, Kamei C (1999) [Arg8]-vasopressin-induced increase in intracellular Ca2+ concentration in cultured rat hippocampal neurons. Brain Res Bull 49: 343–347
40. Rehberg S, Ertmer C, Vincent JL, et al (2011) Role of selective V1a receptor agonism in ovine septic shock. Crit Care Med 39: 119–125
41. Boyd JH, Forbes J, Nakada TA, Walley KR, Russell JA (2010) Fluid resuscitation in septic shock: a positive fluid balance and elevated central venous pressure are associated with increased mortality. Crit Care Med 39: 259–265
42. Weidenfeld J, Yirmiya R (1996) Effects of bacterial endotoxin on the glucocorticoid feedback regulation of adrenocortical response to stress. Neuroimmunomodulation 3: 352–357
43. Murasawa S, Matsubara H, Kizima K, Maruyama K, Mori Y, Inada M (1995) Glucocorticoids regulate V1a vasopressin receptor expression by increasing mRNA stability in vascular smooth muscle cells. Hypertension 26: 665–669
44. Annane D (2009) Vasopressin plus corticosteroids: the shock duo! Crit Care Med 37: 1126–1127
45. Russell JA, Walley KR, Gordon AC, et al (2009) Interaction of vasopressin infusion, corticosteroid treatment, and mortality of septic shock. Crit Care Med 37: 811–818
46. Bauer SR, Lam SW, Cha SS, Oyen LJ (2008) Effect of corticosteroids on arginine vasopressin-containing vasopressor therapy for septic shock: a case control study. J Crit Care 23: 500–506
47. Torgersen C, Luckner G, Schroder DC, et al (2011) Concomitant arginine-vasopressin and hydrocortisone therapy in severe septic shock: association with mortality. Intensive Care Med 37: 1432–1437
48. Lauzier FLesur O (2011) Arginine-vasopressin and corticosteroids in septic shock: engaged but not yet married! Intensive Care Med 37: 1406–1408
49. Sharshar T, Blanchard A, Paillard M, Raphael JC, Gajdos P, Annane D (2003) Circulating vasopressin levels in septic shock. Crit Care Med 31: 1752–1758
50. Nakada TA, Russell JA, Wellman H, et al (2011) Leucyl/cystinyl aminopeptidase gene variants in septic shock. Chest 139: 1042–1049

Antimicrobial Peptides and their Potential Application in Inflammation and Sepsis

T. Schuerholz, K. Brandenburg, and G. Marx

Introduction

Starting treatment early is key to increasing survival in patients with severe sepsis and septic shock. The crucial significance of timing has been demonstrated for the treatment of circulatory failure [1], use of antibiotics [2] and use of activated protein C as adjunctive therapy [3]. Whereas it is of vital importance not only to begin anti-infective therapy as soon as possible but to also choose the adequate anti-infective drug [4], the impending problem is the growing number of multi-resistant bacteria [5]. Therefore, there is an increasing interest in the identification and development of new anti-infective agents.

Antimicrobial peptides (AMPs) are found in species ranging from bacteria and insects to mammals. They were identified over 100 years ago as an important part of innate immunity and can be isolated in body fluids and on body surfaces either constitutively or after inflammatory stimulation [6]. Compared to conventional anti-infective agents, some AMP may kill bacteria but also simultaneously neutralize released pathogenic factors, like lipopolysaccharide (LPS) or lipoprotein (LP), thus preventing the devastating consequences of the pro-inflammatory cascades in severe sepsis and septic shock. The obstacle in the application of naturally occurring AMPs is their high toxicity, promoting hemolysis, nephrotoxicity and neurotoxicity [7]. The challenge is, therefore, to develop synthetic peptide-based drugs on the basis of naturally occurring AMPs in order to effectively treat septic patients without causing harm.

Naturally Occurring Antimicrobial Peptides in Inflammation

It has been realized for decades that AMPs have anti-Gram-positive and -negative effects [8] as well as anti-viral and anti-yeast effects. These effects are limited by several mechanisms including modulation of the surface charge and the use of active extrusion [9–11]. Compared to resistance against AMPs, the bacterial mechanisms to defeat conventional anti-infective agents are more evident [12].

The majority of studies have addressed the so-called 'defensins', consisting of an alpha and beta subgroup. There are six different human alpha-defensins [6]. Three, highly homologous human defensins are most important: The human neutrophil peptides (HNP)1-3. HNP1-3 are stored in the azurophilic granules of polymorphonuclear leukocytes (PMN). HNP1-3 deliver approximately 5 % of total PMN protein and comprise about 99 % of the total defensin content of the neutrophils. Their antimicrobial activity is directed against bacteria (Gram-positive

J.-L. Vincent (ed.), *Annual Update in Intensive Care and Emergency Medicine 2012*
DOI 10.1007/978-3-642-25716-2 © Springer-Verlag Berlin Heidelberg 2012

and Gram-negative) and viruses (herpes simplex virus [HSV], cytomegalovirus [CMV], human immunodeficiency virus [HIV]-1). HNP1-3 are chemotactic and regulate the release of cytokines and complement [6].

A comparable range of efficacy with potent antimicrobial activity against bacteria and fungi is described for LL-37. LL-37 is generated by the cleavage of hCAP18, the human cationic antimicrobial peptide of 18 kDa and is isolated by neutrophils and epithelial tissues in respiratory, gastrointestinal and urogenital tracts [6].

The human beta-defensins (HBD)1-3 come from a variety of epithelial cells in different organs. HBD1-3 have broad antimicrobial activity. They are directed against bacteria, viruses and fungi, inducing chemokines and cytokines and thus recruiting cells of the adaptive immune system [6]. HBD3 downregulates pro-inflammatory cytokines, like tumor necrosis factor (TNF)-α or interleukin (IL)-6, in human and mouse macrophages after exposure to LPS *in vitro* and *in vivo*, suggesting a role for this defensin in the resolution of inflammatory processes. In contrast to other naturally occurring or synthetic peptides, this effect is not mediated through direct LPS-peptide LPS binding [13]. Deficits in the production of AMP usually expressed by human epithelial cells may lead to increased susceptibility to bacterial or viral infections [14]. These deficits may be caused by immunosuppressive drugs preventing the induction of AMP, such as HBD2, thus promoting infections [15]. The importance of HBD2 for protection against infections was demonstrated by Milner and Ortega who detected normal levels of HBD1 in burn patients, but the burn-associated loss of epithelium led to a decrease in HBD2 [16]. Since HBD2 effectively kills *Escherichia coli*, *Staphylococcus aureus* and other bacteria, reduced levels of this AMP may result in local bacterial proliferation [17].

Recently, these findings were confirmed in patients with multiple trauma [18]. The authors noted that despite open bone fractures and severe soft tissue trauma in multiple trauma, the rate of bacterial infection is surprisingly low and hypothesized that this may be related to serum concentrations of AMPs. Concentrations of HBD2, HBD3 and LL-37 were elevated after trauma suggesting a higher antibacterial effect compared to healthy donors thus explaining the relatively low infection rates [18].

Moreover, an increase or decrease in susceptibility to inflammation may be related to the highly variable inter-individual composition of AMPs in body fluids [19]. Surprisingly, the capsular polysaccharide production in multiple Group A streptococci strains is upregulated by LL-37, thus increasing virulence [20]. LL-37 itself has functions other than chemotaxis, as shown by investigations of the effects of LL-37 on human omental arteries and veins [21]. In these studies, LL-37 induced endothelium-dependent relaxation by involvement of nitric oxide (NO) of endothelial origin. A localized increase in LL-37 can be mediated by degranulation of granulocytes following the process of granulocyte 'rolling' and 'sticking' on the endothelium [22]. Despite this possible negative consequence, therapeutic application of AMPs may have positive effects in a variety of inflammatory diseases. In experimental sepsis, the administration of AMP in certain doses was associated with increased survival [23]; the effective application of AMPs in animals was not confirmed in human trials. Iseganan, an analog of protegrin-1, a naturally occurring peptide with broad-spectrum microbicidal activity, was not shown to be beneficial in reducing stomatitis in patients receiving chemotherapy [24].

In recent years, an increasing number of synthetic (cationic) peptides have been developed, but none has been approved for human use. Omiganan pentahydrochloride (synthetic cationic peptide; MBI 226), administered at insertion sites, was superior to povidone iodine in preventing central venous catheter-related bloodstream infections in a phase III trial; however, although the study was completed many years ago, the results have not been published in a peer-reviewed journal.

Local treatment of diabetic ulcer with AMPs had at least an equipotent anti-inflammatory effect compared to antibiotics [12]. In recent years, there have been at least 20 different peptides in several steps of development scheduled for anti-infective trials [23]. Two studies on human lactoferrin 1-11 peptide (hLF1-11) were aborted at Phase I and II stages. The purpose of these studies was to establish tolerance to treatment with hLF1-11 administered intravenously as a single daily dose for 10 consecutive days. The target population was patients with bacteremia due to *Staphylococcus epidermidis* (clinicaltrials.gov-identifier NCT00509847) or patients with proven candidemia (clinicaltrials.gov-identifier NCT00509834). The reasons given for withdrawal were that recruitment was not feasible within the timeframe (bacteremia) or the patient population was not available (candidemia).

Development and Anti-LPS Effects of Synthetic Antimicrobial Peptides

Compounds to neutralize bacterial endotoxins were originally synthesized based on the binding region of the Limulus anti-LPS factor (LALF) [25]. Ried et al. were the first authors to report synthesis of peptides based on this domain. These authors found that the complete binding sequence, a cyclic peptide called cLALF22, had the greatest ability to bind to the lipid A part of LPS, its "endotoxic principle" [26]. Analogs shortened down to cLALF10 were much less active. In biophysical studies by Andrä et al., interaction of the complete LALF (called ENP = endotoxin-neutralizing protein in its recombinant form) and of part structures with endotoxins was studied, and considerable inhibition of the biological activity of LPS was found at protein [ENP]:[LPS] ratios greater than 20 to 200:1 molar [27–29].

Data on the supramolecular structure of LPS were indicative of a change of the lipid A cubic aggregate structure into a multilamellar one. This is of considerable interest, since it has been shown that the cubic aggregate structure of lipid A is its bioactive form, whereas some non-enterobacterial biologically inactive LPS/lipid A structures with a different acylation pattern adopt multilamellar aggregates [30]. In subsequent studies, LALF-derived cyclic peptides were analyzed, starting with cLALF22 and various shortened analogs [27, 29]. Consistently in all these investigations, a change in the endotoxin aggregate structure from a preferentially cubic into a multilamellar one was described, as well as a change in the morphologies of the LPS Re aggregates, as evidenced by freeze-fracture electron microscopy, from 'open egg-shells' (i.e., spherical particles in the range 100 to 200 nm), into large stacks of some 1000 nm. The binding of the peptides to LPS was characterized in all cases as an exothermic process by isothermal titration calorimetry (ITC), driven by the Coulomb interaction of the positive charges of peptides with the negative charges of the endotoxins [27, 29].

Pan et al. synthesized the terminal part of the shrimp anti-LPS-factor, a peptide with 24 amino acids, in a cyclic and linear form. Pre-treatment of mice with

III

the cyclic compound led to considerably enhanced survival of mice infected with approximately 10^6 colony-forming units (cfu) of *Pseudomonas aeruginosa*. Parallel to this, the peptides were able to reduce the bacteria-induced production of TNF-α in the animals. However, already at a concentration of 2 μg/ml the peptides exhibited significant cytotoxicity in HeLa, MCF-7, and HT1080 cell lines, impeding their use as an anti-infective drug [31].

Because of the insufficient specificity of the above described peptides, we used a new approach, constructing a new series of peptides of amino acid lengths in the range 17 to 23. The systematic study of various peptides differing in their amino acid chain lengths from 9 to 12 and 17 to 19 showed that the basic sequence, as given by Pep9 (FRRLKWKFW), was already able to confer significant inhibition of LPS-induced cytokine production. Relatively high concentrations of the peptides, however, were still necessary to inhibit cytokine production. Therefore, longer peptides were constructed to adapt to the physico-chemistry of the lipid A part of endotoxins. For this process, the composition of the N-terminal side of the peptide was preferentially provided by polar and basic amino acids, and the C-terminal by more hydrophobic ones. Furthermore, the exact number and type and sequence of amino acids was shown to be important, as deduced from the comparison of the peptides with different chain lengths [32–35].

Additional improvements were obtained by constructing the amino acid sequences on the basis of optimal binding to the lipid A moiety of bacterial LPS. Modifications of the sequences (for amino acid sequences see **Table 1**) led to a nearly complete inhibition of LPS-induced cytokine secretion at a [Pep]:[LPS] 3:1 molar ratio [33, 34]. This was particularly evident in the case of the lead structure, Pep19-2.5, which protected mice in a model of sepsis already at a [Pep]:[LPS] ratio of 50:1 weight % (1250 ng peptide and 25 ng LPS).

More experiments were performed in an *in vitro* assay of human mononuclear cells, studying the peptide-induced inhibition of TNF-α induction by LPS, alone and in the presence of common antibiotics as a model for combination therapy in septic patients. The data for the peptide alone (**Fig. 1**) were indicative of the strong inhibition capacity of Pep19–2.5, whereas the antibiotic alone (streptomycin, see **Fig. 2**) showed nearly no action. The combination of streptomycin with Pep19–2.5 at a 1:1 weight ratio, however, was associated with strong inhibition of cytokine production, exceeding that of the peptide alone indicative of a synergistic action (**Fig. 2**, right hand side). Therefore, from these data, use of a combination of antibiotic and peptide in septic patients seems promising.

Furthermore, for therapeutic use, it is important that inhibition of LPS-induced cytokine release also takes place in the presence of proteases that are known to decompose peptides. Therefore, the peptides were incubated in 20 % AB serum for different time periods. As illustrated in **Fig. 3**, the inhibition of TNF-α production decreased with increasing time of serum incubation; however, even after 2 hours incubation there was still considerable inhibition of cytokine release.

Table 1. Synthetic antimicrobial peptide sequences and molecular weights

Pep19-2.5	GCKKYRRFRWKFKGKFWFWG	2711
Pep19-2.5Dup	GWFWFKGKFKWRFRRYKKCG-GCKKYRRFRWKFKGKFWFWG	5405
Pep19-2.5short	GCKKYRRFRWKFKGK	1988

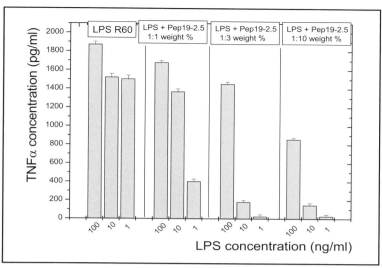

Fig. 1. Inhibition in human mononuclear cells of tumor-necrosis-factor (TNF)-α, induced by lipopoly-saccharide (LPS) from *Salmonella minnesota* Ra (strain R60), by the lead peptide Pep19-2.5 at three different [LPS]:[Pep] weight ratios. Stimulation was performed as described before [34]. Briefly, mononuclear cells (MNC) were isolated from heparinized blood of healthy donors. For stimulation, 200 µl MNC (1x10⁶cells) were transferred into each well of a 96-well culture plate. LPS R60 and the LPS:peptide mixtures were preincubated for 30 min at 37 °C, and added to the cultures at 20 µl per well and incubated for 4 h at 37 °C under 5 % CO_2. Supernatants were collected after centrifugation of the culture plates for 10 min at 400xg and stored at −20 °C until immunological determination of TNF-α, carried out in a Sandwich ELISA using a monoclonal antibody against TNF. The [LPS]:[Pep19-2.5] 1:1 weight% corresponds to 1.5:1 M/M, the 1:3 weight% to 1:2 M/M, and the 1:10 weight% to 1:6.7 M/M.

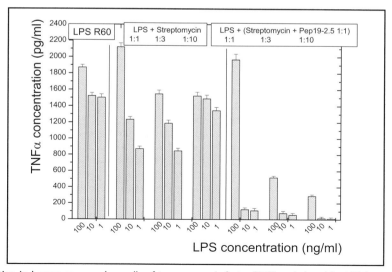

Fig. 2. Inhibition in human mononuclear cells of tumor-necrosis-factor (TNF)-α, induced by LPS from *Salmonella minnesota* Ra (strain R60), by streptomycin alone and in combination with the lead peptide Pep19-2.5 (streptomycin:Pep19-2.5 1:1 weight%) at three different [LPS]:[Streptomycon:Pep] weight ratios. The stimulation was performed as described in the legend of **Fig. 1**.

III

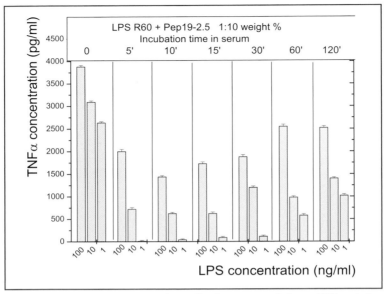

Fig. 3. Inhibition in human mononuclear cells of tumor-necrosis-factor (TNF)-α, induced by LPS from *Salmonella minnesota* Ra (strain R60), by the lead peptide Pep19-2.5 at three different [LPS]:[Pep] weight ratios. Before addition of the peptide, it was incubated for the given times in 20 % AB serum. The stimulation was performed as described in the legend of **Fig. 1.**

Additional experiments were performed with sequence variants of Pep19–2.5, i.e., the duplicated form, Pep19-2.5Dup, the variant with all amino acids in a D-configuration (Pep19-2.5D-AA), and a variant in which the final sequence at the C-terminus is lacking (for sequences see **Table 1**). As demonstrated in **Fig. 4**, duplication of the amino acid sequence did not lead to improvement in the inhibition activity of the peptide, and the peptide with D-configured amino acids still had good inhibitory activity. This latter information is important with respect to the activity of proteases in blood serum, which rapidly decompose L-configuration peptides. A further sequence variation, the peptide Pep19-2.5short, lacking the C-terminal hydrophobic sequence FWFWG, led to a near complete abrogation of any inhibitory activity (**Fig. 5**). This finding is of importance since the driving force between the peptides and LPS was shown to be the Coulomb interaction between the basic residues of the peptides (R and K), and the negative charges of LPS [33]. In a second step of the interaction, however, intercalation of the C-terminal proximal hydrophobic peptide part into the lipid A hydrophobic moiety was described [34]. As can be deduced from the lack of inhibition of the shortened variant, the latter process has considerable impact on understanding the high binding constant of the Pep19-2.5-LPS interaction [34].

Therefore, from these and earlier data, the change of lipid A/LPS cubic aggregate into a multilamellar structure is an important step in the ability of the peptides to neutralize endotoxins, associated with an extremely low saturation value of binding at [peptide]:[LPS] = 0.3 M/M, corresponding to the binding saturation of 3 peptides with 10 LPS molecules [33, 34]. Thus, human binding proteins, such as LPS binding protein (LBP) and CD14, are impeded from binding to LPS epi-

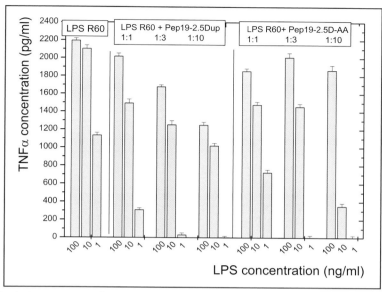

Fig. 4. Inhibition in human mononuclear cells of tumor-necrosis-factor (TNF)-α, induced by LPS from *Salmonella minnesota* Ra (strain R60), by Pep19-2.5Dup and Pep19-2.5D-AA at three different [LPS]:[Pep] weight ratios. The stimulation was performed as described in the legend of **Fig. 1**.

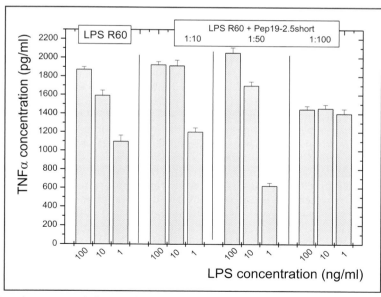

Fig. 5. Inhibition of tumor-necrosis-factor-α (TNF) in human mononuclear cells, induced by LPS from *Salmonella minnesota* Ra (strain R60), by a shortened variant of Pep19-2.5, Pep19-2.5short (sequence see **Table 1**), at three different [LPS]:[Pep] weight ratios. The stimulation was performed as described in the legend of **Fig. 1**.

topes, the charged head groups, and thus cannot initiate the inflammatory reaction. It has been found, furthermore, that the peptides still exert their effect when they are added in a time-delayed mode, i.e., when they are administered up to 3 hours after LPS addition [36]. This observation is indicative of a membrane process of the interaction, in accordance with recent findings that the peptides readily intercalate into membranes made from phosphatidylcholine and phosphatidylserine as characteristic of eukaryotic cells [34]. After membrane incorporation, the peptides apparently act at the site of membrane receptors such as CD14 and the TLR4/MD2-system, thus competitively inhibiting the interaction with LPS. The details of these processes are currently under investigation. Detailed descriptions of the newest aspects of the use of AMPs compared to other therapeutic approaches are summarized in a recent review [35].

Naturally Occurring and Synthetic Antimicrobial Peptides in Human and Experimental Sepsis

Certain anti-microbial peptides kill bacteria without causing cell disruption. Patients with septic shock, in particular, would benefit because antibiotics are known to promote the liberation of pro-inflammatory cell components and thus augment the severity of septic shock [37, 38]. A promising therapeutic approach would involve either the combination of AMP analogs with antibiotic therapy or the combination of AMPs with antibiotic drugs. The resultant synergism between the two antimicrobial components may be especially important for the treatment of critically ill patient with severe infections.

Studies on AMPs in patients with severe sepsis or septic shock are limited. LBP and bactericidal/permeability increasing (BPI) protein are comparable with respect to a high-affinity binding domain for the lipid A component of LPS. The difference is that signal transduction is not hampered by LBP, because it binds to CD14 after CD14 has itself formed complexes with endotoxin. In contrast, BPI prevents endotoxin binding to CD14, hence inhibiting cytokine liberation.

In 49 patients with abscesses, peritonitis or uninfected body fluids, LBP and neutrophil granular BPI protein were investigated. In abscesses, compared to peritoneal fluids and non-infected fluids, the BPI/LBP ratio was significantly elevated. Moreover, BPI concentration was increased more in abscesses with Gram-positive compared to those with Gram-negative organisms. BPI may weaken local and systemic effects in response to an inflammatory stimulus induced by endotoxin release [37]. A comparison of BPI bound to the leukocyte surface and BPI and LBP in plasma in healthy volunteers after endotoxin challenge and in patients with Gram-negative sepsis was performed several years ago [39]. In both groups, there was an increase in leukocyte-bound BPI and plasma LBP. Plasma BPI was significantly elevated as a sign of inadequate competition compared to the more frequently detected LBP [39].

A further study investigated BPI levels and BPI/neutrophil ratios in 42 healthy controls and 34 patients with severe sepsis defined according to the ACCP/SCCM consensus conference [40]. BPI was elevated in sepsis compared to controls (median 15.3, range $< 1.6-205$ µg/l vs 5.2; $< 1.6-24$ µg/l; $p < 0.001$). Moreover, sepsis due to Gram-negative compared to Gram-positive pathogens was associated with higher levels of BPI (16.8, range $< 1.6-205$ µg/l vs. 16.0, $< 1.6-60$ µg/l; $p = 0.05$). Because of a possible association with decreased mean arterial pressure, the authors concluded that BPI may reflect the severity of organ dysfunction in sepsis [40].

The development of a recombinant fragment of human BPI (rBPI21) triggered a large study on the therapeutic use of AMPs in pediatric meningococcal infection. Three hundred and ninety-five children with suspected meningococcal sepsis were randomly assigned to receive rBPI21 within 8 hours of diagnosis [41]. Overall, the study failed to demonstrate a significantly reduced mortality after rBPI21 compared to placebo (7.4 % vs. 9.9 %; $p = 0.48$). Adjusted for patients with incomplete infusion of study drug, the mortality was non-significantly lower in the intervention group (rBPI21 2.2 % vs. placebo 6.2 %; $p = 0.07$). Furthermore, the rate of amputations decreased non-significantly (rBPI21 3.2 % vs. placebo 7.4 %; $p = 0.067$) and significantly more children regained pre-illness performance when treated with rBPI21 (77.3 % vs. 66.3 %, odds ratio 1.75 [95 % CI 1.08 – 2.83]; $p = 0.019$). The study may have failed to reach its target to reduce mortality because of lower than expected placebo group mortality (9.9 % vs. 25 % expected), but the authors hypothesized that an increased benefit may be possible by using parallel and immediate treatment of rBPI21 and anti-infective agents [41].

A prospective case-control study investigated plasma HBD2 in 16 patients with severe sepsis compared to 18 controls [42]. HBD2 was significantly higher in severe sepsis compared to non-septic critically ill patients and to healthy controls. Additionally, HBD2 gene expression in non-septic patients and healthy controls was significantly higher after induction with LPS compared with sepsis patients. Survival status was independent of the inducibility of HBD2 gene expression. This may be understood as a sign of exhaustion after severe infections and may be related to the complex dysfunction of the innate and adaptive immune system in patients suffering from severe sepsis [43]. Administration of intravenous hydrocortisone as adjunctive therapy in septic shock reduced HBD3 expression in contrast to undisturbed HBD2-inducibility [43].

An additional study in children with sepsis and critically ill control patients revealed that levels of HNP1-3 (α-defensins) were increased with onset of sepsis in plasma of non-neutropenic septic patients (median 450 [range 194 – 1031] ng/ml) compared to neutropenic septic patients and controls (50 [0 – 238] ng/ml and 150 [0 – 275] ng/ml; $p < 0.05$). However, HNP1-3 levels were not related to organ failure or outcome of sepsis [44]. Lactoferrin, derived from neutrophils, was elevated in non-neutropenic sepsis (332 [137 – 938] ng/ml) whereas lactoferrin in neutropenic sepsis was decreased compared to control patients (20 [0 – 117] ng/ml vs 176 [39 – 312] ng/ml; $p < 0.05$). Furthermore, lactoferrin was associated with renal and hematologic organ failure. The levels of lactoferrin and HNP1-3 were significantly correlated in this study [44].

Recently, Berkestedt et al. demonstrated that levels of HNP1-3, lactoferrin, BPI and heparin-binding protein (HBP) were higher in 31 patients with sepsis compared to 25 non-septic controls [45]. Out of these AMP, only BPI was associated with outcome, revealing significantly higher levels in non-survivors compared to survivors. The neutrophil granula-derived HBP, BPI and HNP1-3 and lactoferrin were increased in sepsis, thus reflecting the ongoing battle of the innate immunity against invading organisms [45].

The use of polymyxin B and polymyxin E (colistin), cationic polypeptides that neutralize the lethal effects of endotoxin, was abandoned, because nephrotoxicity and neurotoxicity were reported. However, these adverse effects observed in early

III

clinical studies were most likely due to a limited understanding of the pharmacokinetics, pharmacodynamics, and toxicodynamics of these agents, and the use of incorrect quantities [46]. Use was reinstated in a recent study of hemoperfusion with polymyxin-B loaded cartridges in patients with abdominal septic shock (EUPHAS) [47]. In this Italian multicenter trial, 64 patients were assigned to receive standard of care or standard of care plus 2 sessions of polymyxin-B hemoperfusion within 72 hours after the surgical procedure. In addition to improvements in mean arterial pressure and organ dysfunction, 28-day mortality was lower in the polymyxin B group compared to conventional therapy alone (32 % vs. 53 %, unadjusted hazard ratio [HR] 0.43; 95 % CI 0.20 – 0.94; adjusted HR, 0.36; 95 % CI 0.16 – 0.80). In view of the mortality reduction the study was stopped by the ethics committee. To confirm the findings in other patients and to address concerns raised after publication of the EUPHAS study, two further studies are underway (EUPHRATES: clinicaltrials.gov-identifier NCT01046669 and EUPHAS 2 [48]).

Recently, it was demonstrated that a single 25 mg/kg dose of a synthetic peptide protected mice from infection with *P. aeruginosa* and *E. coli* [49]. The application of the AMP led to elimination of bacteria in the blood 18 hours after infection, and the bacterial count was significantly lower in other specimens (peritoneal fluid, spleen and liver) compared to control animals. After an additional 22 hours all tested samples were free of bacteria [49]. A further synthetic AMP, named s-thanatin, showed activity against Gram-positive and -negative bacteria [50]. After combination with the antimicrobial peptide it was demonstrated that the minimum inhibitory concentration (MIC) of various antibiotics was decreased by a factor of 2 to 8 (1 – 3 dilution steps). Moreover, survival after intraperitoneal bacterial challenge was increased after treatment with s-thanatin, in a dose-dependent manner [50]. The most recent study is investigating talactoferrin alfa in a phase III study in patients with severe sepsis (OASIS; clinicaltrials.gov identifier NCT01273779).

Conclusion

Investigations of the past decade show increasing interest in antimicrobial peptides as a tool for sepsis diagnosis and furthermore as a possible therapeutic intervention. Newly designed peptides with decreased toxicity and a broader range of efficacy may have the potential to provide significant improvements in the treatment of infections.

Acknowledgements: The authors are indebted to the German ministry (Ministerium für Bildung und Forschung, BMBF) for financial help in the frame of a preclinical study 'Therapy of infectious diseases with special regards to bacterial sepsis' (project: 01GU0824 and 01GU0826).

References

1. Rivers E, Nguyen B, Havstad S, et al (2001) Early goal-directed therapy in the treatment of severe sepsis and septic shock. N Engl J Med 345: 1368 – 1377
2. Kumar A, Roberts D, Wood KE, et al (2006) Duration of hypotension before initiation of effective antimicrobial therapy is the critical determinant of survival in human septic shock. Crit Care Med 34: 1589 – 1596
3. Vincent JL, Bernard GR, Beale R, et al (2005) Drotrecogin alfa (activated) treatment in

severe sepsis from the global open-label trial ENHANCE: further evidence for survival and safety and implications for early treatment. Crit Care Med 33: 2266–2277

4. Valles J, Rello J, Ochagavia A, Garnacho J, Alcala MA (2003) Community-acquired bloodstream infection in critically ill adult patients: impact of shock and inappropriate antibiotic therapy on survival. Chest 123: 1615–1624

5. Kresken M, Hafner D, Schmitz F-J, Wichelhaus TA, Studiengruppe FD (2009) Resistenzsituation bei klinisch wichtigen Infektionserregern gegenüber Antibiotika in Deutschland und im mitteleuropäischen Raum. Antiinfectives Intelligence, Rheinbach

6. Steinstraesser L, Kraneburg UM, Hirsch T, et al (2009) Host defense peptides as effector molecules of the innate immune response: a sledgehammer for drug resistance? Int J Mol Sci 10: 3951–3970

7. Gordon YJ, Romanowski EG, McDermott AM (2005) A review of antimicrobial peptides and their therapeutic potential as anti-infective drugs. Curr Eye Res 30: 505–515

8. Skarnes RC, Watson DW (1957) Antimicrobial factors of normal tissues and fluids. Bacteriol Rev 21: 273–294

9. Shafer WM, Qu X, Waring AJ, Lehrer RI (1998) Modulation of Neisseria gonorrhoeae susceptibility to vertebrate antibacterial peptides due to a member of the resistance/nodulation/division efflux pump family. Proc Natl Acad Sci USA 95: 1829–1833

10. Yount NY, Bayer AS, Xiong YQ, Yeaman MR (2006) Advances in antimicrobial peptide immunobiology. Biopolymers 84: 435–458

11. Peschel A (2002) How do bacteria resist human antimicrobial peptides? Trends Microbiol 10: 179–186

12. Hancock RE, Sahl HG (2006) Antimicrobial and host-defense peptides as new anti-infective therapeutic strategies. Nat Biotechnol 24: 1551–1557

13. Semple F, Webb S, Li HN, et al (2010) Human beta-defensin 3 has immunosuppressive activity in vitro and in vivo. Eur J Immunol 40: 1073–1078

14. Rieg S, Steffen H, Seeber S, et al (2005) Deficiency of dermcidin-derived antimicrobial peptides in sweat of patients with atopic dermatitis correlates with an impaired innate defense of human skin in vivo. J Immunol 174: 8003–8010

15. Meyer JE, Harder J, Gorogh T, et al (2004) Human beta-defensin-2 in oral cancer with opportunistic Candida infection. Anticancer Res 24: 1025–1030

16. Milner SM, Ortega MR (1999) Reduced antimicrobial peptide expression in human burn wounds. Burns 25: 411–413

17. Tao R, Jurevic RJ, Coulton KK, et al (2005) Salivary antimicrobial peptide expression and dental caries experience in children. Antimicrob Agents Chemother 49: 3883–3888

18. Lippross S, Klueter T, Steubesand N, et al (2012) Multiple trauma induces serum production of host defence peptides. Injury (in press)

19. Gryllos I, Tran-Winkler HJ, Cheng MF, et al (2008) Induction of group A Streptococcus virulence by a human antimicrobial peptide. Proc Natl Acad Sci USA 105: 16755–16760

20. Berkestedt I, Nelson A, Bodelsson M (2008) Endogenous antimicrobial peptide LL-37 induces human vasodilatation. Br J Anaesth 100: 803–809

21. Fukumoto K, Nagaoka I, Yamataka A, et al (2005) Effect of antibacterial cathelicidin peptide CAP18/LL-37 on sepsis in neonatal rats. Pediatr Surg Int 21: 20–24

22. Torossian A, Gurschi E, Bals R, Vassiliou T, Wulf HF, Bauhofer A (2007) Effects of the antimicrobial peptide LL-37 and hyperthermic preconditioning in septic rats. Anesthesiology 107: 437–441

23. Zhang L, Falla TJ (2006) Antimicrobial peptides: therapeutic potential. Expert Opin Pharmacother 7: 653–663

24. Giles FJ, Rodriguez R, Weisdorf D, et al (2004) A phase III, randomized, double-blind, placebo-controlled, study of iseganan for the reduction of stomatitis in patients receiving stomatotoxic chemotherapy. Leuk Res 28: 559–565

25. Vallespi MG, Glaria LA, Reyes O, Garay HE, Ferrero J, Arana MJ (2000) A Limulus antilipopolysaccharide factor-derived peptide exhibits a new immunological activity with potential applicability in infectious diseases. Clin Diagn Lab Immunol 7: 669–675

26. Ried C, Wahl C, Miethke T, et al (1996) High affinity endotoxin-binding and neutralizing peptides based on the crystal structure of recombinant Limulus anti-lipopolysaccharide factor. J Biol Chem 271: 28120–28127

III

27. Andrä J, Lamata M, Martinez de Tejada G, Bartels R, Koch MH, Brandenburg K (2004) Cyclic antimicrobial peptides based on Limulus anti-lipopolysaccharide factor for neutralization of lipopolysaccharide. Biochem Pharmacol 68: 1297–1307

28. Andrä J, Garidel P, Majerle A, et al (2004) Biophysical characterization of the interaction of Limulus polyphemus endotoxin neutralizing protein with lipopolysaccharide. Eur J Biochem 271: 2037–2046

29. Andrä J, Howe J, Garidel P, et al (2007) Mechanism of interaction of optimized Limulus-derived cyclic peptides with endotoxins: thermodynamic, biophysical and microbiological analysis. Biochem J 406: 297–307

30. Brandenburg K, Schromm AB, Gutsmann T (2010) Endotoxins: Structure, function, and recognition: Relationship between structure, function, and activity. Subcell Biochem 53: 53–67

31. Pan CY, Chao TT, Chen JC, et al (2007) Shrimp (Penaeus monodon) anti-lipopolysaccharide factor reduces the lethality of Pseudomonas aeruginosa sepsis in mice. Int Immunopharmacol 7: 687–700

32. Kowalski I, Kaconis Y, Andrä J, et al (2010) Physicochemical and biological characterization of anti-endotoxin peptides and their influence on lipid properties. Protein Pept Lett 17: 1328–1333

33. Gutsmann T, Razquin-Olazaran I, Kowalski I, et al (2010) New antiseptic peptides to protect against endotoxin-mediated shock. Antimicrob Agents Chemother 54: 3817–3824

34. Kaconis Y, Kowalski I, Howe J, et al (2011) Biophysical mechanisms of endotoxin neutralization by cationic amphiphilic peptides. Biophys J 100: 2652–2661

35. Brandenburg K, Andrä J, Garidel P, Gutsmann T (2011) Peptide-based treatment of sepsis. Appl Microbiol Biotechnol 90: 799–808

36. Martinez de Tejada G, Sánchez-Gómez S, Razquin-Olazaran I, et al (2011) Bacterial cell wall compounds as promising targets of antimicrobial agents I. Antimicrobial peptides and lipopolyamines. Curr Drug Targets (in press)

37. Opal SM, Palardy JE, Marra MN, Fisher CJ Jr, McKelligon BM, Scott RW (1994) Relative concentrations of endotoxin-binding proteins in body fluids during infection. Lancet 344: 429–431

38. Marra MN, Wilde CG, Griffith JE, Snable JL, Scott RW (1990) Bactericidal/permeability-increasing protein has endotoxin-neutralizing activity. J Immunol 144: 662–666

39. Calvano SE, Thompson WA, Marra MN, et al (1994) Changes in polymorphonuclear leukocyte surface and plasma bactericidal/permeability-increasing protein and plasma lipopolysaccharide binding protein during endotoxemia or sepsis. Arch Surg 129: 220–226

40. Rintala E, Peuravuori H, Pulkki K, Voipio-Pulkki LM, Nevalainen T (2000) Bactericidal/permeability-increasing protein (BPI) in sepsis correlates with the severity of sepsis and the outcome. Intensive Care Med 26: 1248–1251

41. Levin M, Quint PA, Goldstein B, et al (2000) Recombinant bactericidal/permeability-increasing protein (rBPI21) as adjunctive treatment for children with severe meningococcal sepsis: a randomised trial. rBPI21 Meningococcal Sepsis Study Group. Lancet 356: 961–967

42. Duits LA, Rademaker M, Ravensbergen B, et al (2001) Inhibition of hBD-3, but not hBD-1 and hBD-2, mRNA expression by corticosteroids. Biochem Biophys Res Commun 280: 522–525

43. Book M, Chen Q, Lehmann LE, et al (2007) Inducibility of the endogenous antibiotic peptide beta-defensin 2 is impaired in patients with severe sepsis. Crit Care 11: R19

44. Thomas NJ, Carcillo JA, Doughty LA, Sasser H, Heine RP (2002) Plasma concentrations of defensins and lactoferrin in children with severe sepsis. Pediatr Infect Dis J 21: 34–38

45. Berkestedt I, Herwald H, Ljunggren L, Nelson A, Bodelsson M (2010) Elevated plasma levels of antimicrobial polypeptides in patients with severe sepsis. J Innate Immun 2: 478–482

46. Li J, Nation RL, Turnidge JD, et al (2006) Colistin: the re-emerging antibiotic for multidrug-resistant Gram-negative bacterial infections. Lancet Infect Dis 6: 589–601

47. Cruz DN, Antonelli M, Fumagalli R, et al (2009) Early use of polymyxin B hemoperfusion in abdominal septic shock: the EUPHAS randomized controlled trial. JAMA 301: 2445–2452

48. Martin EL, Cruz DN, Monti G, et al (2010) Endotoxin removal: how far from the evidence? The EUPHAS 2 Project. Contrib Nephrol 167: 119–125

49. Pini A, Falciani C, Mantengoli E, et al (2010) A novel tetrabranched antimicrobial peptide that neutralizes bacterial lipopolysaccharide and prevents septic shock in vivo. FASEB J 24: 1015–1022

50. Wu G, Fan X, Li L, et al (2010) Interaction of antimicrobial peptide s-thanatin with lipopolysaccharide in vitro and in an experimental mouse model of septic shock caused by a multidrug-resistant clinical isolate of Escherichia coli. Int J Antimicrob Agents 35: 250–254

Hypogammaglobulinemia in Sepsis

M. Päsler, S. Dietz, and K. Werdan

Introduction

Immunoglobulin (Ig) preparations are widely used as adjunctive sepsis therapies. The rationale for this treatment concept is the hypothesis that low endogenous serum levels of IgG, IgM or IgA may dispose to severe infection and sepsis, and that substitution with the respective immunoglobulins – either one of the many intravenous IgG preparations or the intravenous IgGMA preparation, Pentaglobin®, might improve prognosis. The following article offers an overview on adjunctive immunoglobulin therapy in adult patients with severe sepsis. For prophylaxis of sepsis in adults see [1], for prophylaxis and therapy of sepsis in neonates and infants see [1, 2].

Treatment of Critically Ill Patients with Immunoglobulin Preparations

In addition to adjunctive therapy in severe sepsis, there are several other evidence based indications for immunoglobulin therapy in critical care medicine. The guidelines of the German Federal Physicians' Chamber for therapy with blood components and plasma derivatives [3] give the following recommendations:

- Recommendation 1A "shall" (strong recommendation, valid for most patients)
  - Autoimmune thrombocytopenic purpura
  - Guillain-Barré-Syndrome
- Recommendation 1C+ "shall" (strong recommendation)
  - Post-transfusion purpura
- Recommendation 2A "should" (medium – strong recommendation)
  - Seronegative and antibody-positive myasthenia gravis, Lambert-Eaton myasthenic syndrome
- Recommendation 2B "can" (weak recommendation)
  - Sepsis and septic shock
- Recommendation 2C+ "can" (weak recommendation)
  - Toxic epidermal necrolysis (Lyell-Syndrome)
- Recommendation 2C "could" (very weak recommendation)
  - Prophylaxis and therapy of cytomegalovirus (CMV) infection (with the current state of knowledge IVIG or CMV-Ig cannot be recommended for therapy of CMV-infection without simultaneous administration of virosta-

J.-L. Vincent (ed.), *Annual Update in Intensive Care and Emergency Medicine 2012*
DOI 10.1007/978-3-642-25716-2 © Springer-Verlag Berlin Heidelberg 2012

tics and has no advantage over exclusive antiviral therapy. There is no approval for this indication).

Is Hypogammaglobulinemia a Negative Prognostic Factor in Severe Sepsis and Septic Shock?

Earlier data pointed towards a higher incidence of infections as well as an impaired prognosis in patients with low immunoglobulin serum levels [1]. Data for patients with severe sepsis and septic shock are shown in **Table 1**.

A considerable proportion of patients have hypogammaglobulinemia G and/or M in the initial state of severe sepsis with rates of 30–50 % and 20 %, respectively, whereas the fraction of patients with decreased IgA levels seems negligible, with a rate of only 2 %. With respect to IgG, the largest of the studies presented in **Table 1** – the Score-based immunoglobulin G therapy of patients with sepsis

Table 1. Frequency of hypogammaglobulinemia G and M in sepsis and septic shock and correlation with prognosis.

Trial Population	Number of patients	Total mortality	Class of Ig	Percentage of hypogamma-globulinemic patients	28-day mortality	Comment
Community-acquired septic shock [7]	N = 21	28.5 %	IgG	48 %	IgG ↓: 6/12 IgG ↔: 0/9 (p = 0.01)	16/21 (76 %) with reduced Ig (IgG ↓ = 7; IgM ↓ = 4; IgG+IgM ↓ = 3; No IgG-therapy
			IgM	33 %	IgM ↓: 3/9 IgM ↔: 3/12: (p = 0.65)	
Severe sepsis and septic shock (APACHE II 20–35) (SBITS-Study) [4, 5]	N = 270 (SBITS-Study, placebo-group)	37.3 %	IgG	27 %	IgG ↓: 39 % IgG ↔: 41 % (p = not significant)	No IgG –therapy
Severe sepsis and septic shock (APACHE II ≥ 20). Resuscitated as well as neutrope-nic patients were excluded [6]	N = 84	50 %	IgG	33 %	IgG ↓: 50 % IgG ↔: 48 % (p= not significant)	All patients treated with 0.25 g/kg bw/day IgGMA from day 1 to 3 (Penta-globin®) (Σ 0.75 g/kg bw)
			IgM	19 %	IgM ↓: 68 % IgM ↔: 45 % (p = not significant)	
			IgA	2 %	IgA ↓: 50 % IgA ↔: 50 % (p = not significant)	

Hypogammaglobulinemia: IgA < 70 mg/dl, IgG < 650 mg/dl, IgM < 40 mg/dl; Ig: Immunoglobulin; IgA: immunoglobulin A; IgG: immunoglobulin G; IgM: immunoglobulin M.

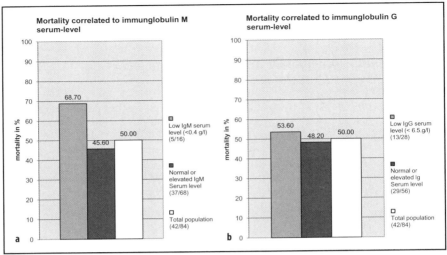

Fig. 1. Correlation of hypogammaglobulinemia M and G with mortality in a cohort of 84 patients with severe sepsis and septic shock. **a** Mortality rates (%) correlated with immunoglobulin M serum levels; **b** Mortality rates (%) correlated with immunoglobulin G serum levels. From [6]

(SBITS) study [4] – did not show any negative influence of a low IgG-level on the 28-day mortality for the 270 patients of the placebo group [5]. The same results were noted in our retrospective analysis of a cohort of 84 patients [6] (**Fig. 1**). In contrast, Taccone et al. [7] demonstrated a significantly higher mortality for patients with hypogammaglobulinemia G in a smaller study (21 patients) with community-acquired septic shock.

For low serum IgM levels, our retrospective analysis [6] demonstrated a considerable but not significant increase in 28-day mortality (**Table 1** and **Fig. 1**), with no effects on mortality at day 4 or 7. In the study by Taccone et al. [7], hypogammaglobulinemia M was of no predictive value with respect to mortality (**Table 1**).

In summary, the rather frequent hypogammaglobulinemia G seems not be correlated with a higher mortality in patients with severe sepsis and septic shock. On the other hand, hypogammaglobulinemia M may be correlated with higher mortality; however, at present, statistically documented proof of this effect is still lacking.

Immunoglobulin Pharmacotherapy in Sepsis: It Works!

The question whether administration of immunoglobulins leads to a sustainable rise in serum levels can be answered with a clear 'yes'. Administration of an intravenous IgG preparation in septic patients at a dose of 0.6 g/kg body weight (bw) on day 1 and 0.3 g/kg bw on day 2 led to a significant increase in the serum IgG level from 10 g/l to 20 g/l in about 24–48 hours, with only a slight later decrease of about 3 g/l till day 4 [4]. Accordingly, an even higher dosage of 2 g/kg, also in use, should cause even higher increases in IgG levels.

With the only available intravenous IgGMA preparation, Pentaglobin®, at the recommended dose of 0.75 g/kg bw (0.25 g/kg bw on three consecutive days), similar increases in IgG levels, from 8 g/l to a maximum of 17 g/l on day two, were achieved [8], with a subsequent decline of about 3 g/l, to 14 g/l, on day four being comparable to the decline seen with the application of intravenous IgG preparations (see above). The IgM level increased from 1.0 g/l to 2.2 g/l on day 3, with only a slight subsequent decline to 1.8 g/l on the fourth day after treatment initiation [8].

Hence, both IgG and IgM serum levels can be kept in, or even above, the upper normal range for several days by intravenous administration of immunoglobulin preparations. However, it has to be mentioned that the total IgG-dosage for adjunctive sepsis therapy at about 1 g/kg bw is only half the dosage given for other indications, like hematological or inflammatory disorders, at about 2 g/kg bw. The rationale for this is hard to see, although one may argue that the 1 g/kg bw dosage seems to trigger a substantial and sufficient (?) rise in IgG serum levels.

Adjunctive Sepsis Therapy: 'Pros and Cons' are the Rule, Not the Exception!

Study approaches to adjunctive sepsis therapy with intravenous immunoglobulins go back to the 1980s [1, 9]; small controlled studies with polyvalent immunoglobulins competed with much larger sepsis studies that tested the effects of monoclonal antibodies against endotoxins and cytokines. The latter all failed, whereas at least some of the smaller immunoglobulin studies showed a reduction in mortality [1, 2, 9]. The situation became more complicated by the fact that in addition to several 5 % intravenous IgG preparations, some trials used an intravenous IgGMA preparation (5 % solution with 3.8g IgG, 0.6g IgA and 0.6g IgM per 100ml; Pentaglobin®). This preparation and its effects may differ substantially from the intravenous IgG preparations [1, 2, 9], supposedly because of the 12.5 % IgM component in this preparation.

Which Meta-analyses can we 'Trust'?

With the exception of the large, multi-centered SBITS study ([4]; see below) only relatively small randomized studies of intravenous immunoglobulin (IVIG) have been performed. Accordingly, numerous meta-analyses [10] have tried to evaluate the effects of intravenous Ig administration in severe sepsis and septic shock. All these analyses found reduced mortality rates in the treated compared to the placebo groups. However, apart from the Cochrane meta-analysis (see [10]), only one other analysis [2] differentiated between the use of intravenous IgG and intravenous IgGMA. This analysis [2] concluded, on the basis of 1500 analyzed patients, that intravenous IgG preparations reduced mortality by 15 % (relative risk 0.85) whereas the intravenous IgGMA preparation reduced mortality by 34 % (relative risk 0.66) (**Table 2**). A similar result was obtained even after including only the high-quality randomized controlled trials (RCTs) in the analysis (IgG: relative risk 0.86; IgGMA: relative risk 0.40 [2]).

Table 2. Meta-analysis for immunoglobulin G and GMA in sepsis: Overview of studies (for detail see [2])

	Number of Studies	Patients included (Treatment/Control)	Relative Risk of Mortality for Treatment-Group
IgGMA	8	279/281	0.66 (0.51 – 0.84)
IgG	7	477/455	0.85 (0.73 – 0.99)

III

Adjunctive Sepsis Therapy: Can we Expect More from Intravenous IgGMA than from Intravenous IgG?

According to the meta-analyses, the intravenous IgGMA preparation seems to be more effective in severe sepsis and septic shock compared with the intravenous IgG preparations. The effect of IgG is, at the most, small. Furthermore, from the two largest intravenous IgG-trials – the SBITS study that included 653 patients with severe sepsis [4] and the Early Supplemental Severe SIRS Treatment With IVIG in Score-Identified High-Risk Patients After Cardiac Surgery (ESSICS) Study that included from 6,984 cardiac surgery patients 244 patients with severe postoperative systemic inflammatory response syndrome (SIRS) [11] – one has to assume that treatment with intravenous IgG at a total dose of 0.9 g/kg bw (0.6 g/kg bw on the first day and 0.3 g/kg bw on the second day) fails to reduce mortality (**Fig. 2**; SBITS Study), and also fails to reduce morbidity to a considerable degree, if at all: The APACHE II score, as a measure of severity of disease, improved from day one to day five by just 0.1 points in the ESSICS study [11] and 1.2 points in the SBITS study [4] (**Table 3**).

This lack of success is not surprising, as administration of intravenous IgG has no anti-inflammatory effect on serum levels of pro-inflammatory cytokines, like interleukin (IL)-6, tumor necrosis factor (TNF)-α and soluble TNF receptors [4, 11], even though, *in vitro*, the production of these cytokines by endotoxin-stimulated cells of the immune system can be inhibited by IgG (literature in [1]).

But why should an intravenous IgGMA preparation be more effective in severe sepsis than the intravenous IgG preparations [12, 13]? To reply, we must consider the quantitative and qualitative differences in characteristics and functions (**Table 3**):

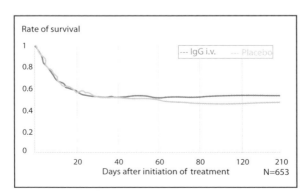

Fig. 2. Kaplan-Meier survival curves from the SBITS study [4] for the intravenous immunoglobulin G group (IgG i.v.) and the placebo group (placebo).

Table 3. Different effects of immunoglobulin G and GMA preparations, particularly with regard to adjunctive sepsis therapy.

	i.v. IgG	i.v. IgGMA
Reduction of mortality in clinical trials		
– meta-analyses [2, 10]	+	++
– SBITS study [4]; ESSICS study [11]	∅	
Prevention of critical illness polyneuropathy [17]	?	+
Inhibition of complement activation [15]	+	++
(Endo) toxin-neutralization [14]	+	++
Anti-inflammatory effects [4, 11]	∅	?
Improvement of impaired microcirculation [16]	+	++
Improvement of disease severity	∅/+	++
Decline in APACHE II score day 1 → day 5		
SBITS study [4]	−1.2	
ESSICS study [11]	−0.1	
septic shock with endotoxemia [18]		−5.0

i.v.: intravenous

- Higher antibody content for (endo-) toxins [14] and more intense complement inhibition [15] of the intravenous IgGMA preparation may be responsible for the better effect, especially in early sepsis.
- Breakdown of microcirculatory perfusion in a sepsis model was attenuated by intravenous IgGMA more than by intravenous IgG [16].
- Neither the SBITS study [4] nor the ESSICS study [11] showed an intravenous IgG-mediated suppression of pro-inflammatory cytokines, like IL-6, TNF-α or the soluble TNF-receptors, sTNFRP55/75 [4, 11] (**Table 3**); for intravenous IgGMA these data are not yet available.
- Critical illness polyneuropathy occurred less frequently in patients with Gram-negative septic shock when treated with intravenous IgGMA [17]
- The meta-analyses showed a stronger reduction in mortality rates for intravenous IgGMA compared to intravenous IgG. Also, the reduction in morbidity seems to be more pronounced with intravenous IgGMA as demonstrated by the decline in APACHE II score within 4 days of therapy (**Table 3**). For intravenous IgGMA, a reduction of 5.0 points was shown [18], whereas intravenous IgG reduced the APACHE II score only slightly (1.2 points in the SBITS study [4]) or not at all (0.1 points in the ESSICS study [11]).

Proof of Concept: The CIGMA Trial

The above mentioned findings suggest that intravenous IgGMA may indeed have a more favorable effect in sepsis than intravenous IgG. The use of an immunoglobulin preparation with a higher concentration of IgM than the currently available preparation with 12 % IgM (Pentaglobin®) may provide more conclusive and less speculative proof. This proof of concept is under way: The purpose of the CIGMA trial (Safety and Efficacy Study of BT086 to Evaluate Adjunctive Therapy in sCAP; ClinicalTrials.gov Identifier: NCT01420744) is to determine whether use of BT086 – a newly developed intravenous IgGMA preparation (Biotest) with a mean IgM content of 23 % – as adjunctive therapy to standard antibiotic treatment is safe and effective in decreasing the number of days patients require endotracheal ventilation due to severe community-acquired pneumonia. The CIGMA trial is a randomized, double-blind, pacebo-controlled, multicenter, parallel-group, adaptive group-sequential phase II study. The estimated enrollment is 82 patients. The trial started in August 2011 and the estimated primary completion date is September 2012.

The intravenous IgGMA preparation, BT086, contains a sufficient number of antibodies against the most frequent pathogens as well as antibodies against lipopolysaccharides and lipid A. Therefore, it can be assumed that administration of BT086 early in the clinical course of a severe infection such as severe community-acquired pneumonia may provide an effective adjunctive treatment to standard antibiotic therapy. BT086, with a mean IgM content of 23 %, is given as an intravenous infusion of 3.65 ml/kg bw/day over a 5-day period. The placebo medication is 1 % albumin given in the same way. The primary outcome measure is ventilator free days in the time frame of 28 days. Secondary outcome measures are, among others, 28-day all-cause mortality and 28-day pneumonia-cause mortality.

Pure Evidence-based Medicine!

What consequences can we draw from the meta-analyses for adjunctive sepsis treatment with IVIG in our daily practice? Even though the majority of analyses found a reduction in mortality in adult patients with severe sepsis or septic shock treated with intravenous IgG (**Table 2**) [2, 10], most stated that larger studies are needed to verify these results. This is of little help for critical care physicians who have to treat their patients now, and need to know what level of evidence the statements from the meta-analyses have. In this context, the meta-analysis of Kreymann et al. [2] is a helpful analysis, as it tells us that the intravenous IgGMA-trials are level II studies. These level II studies are relatively small RCTs with poor statistical quality, and they only justify a level C recommendation – a weak recommendation – for the use of intravenous IgGMA as adjunctive therapy in severe sepsis and septic shock. Nevertheless, this is a higher level of recommendation than pure expert opinion without explicit critical appraisal (Level E = weakest level of recommendation). Consequently, Kreymann et al. [2] state: "Our data showed that the IgGMA preparation can reduce mortality in adults by 34 % ... as long as there is no better evidence, the results demonstrated should be sufficient reason to use such a preparation for adjunctive therapy of sepsis or septic shock."

What conclusions do official guidelines draw from the available literature data and meta-analyses (**Table 4**)? The German Federal Physicians' Chamber guidelines [3] give a weak recommendation for the use of immunoglobulins, the third out of four levels of recommendation (**Table 4**, see also above). The guidelines mention that the evidence for intravenous IgGMA is more convincing than for intravenous IgG, but the recommendation is nevertheless given for both preparations together [3].

The Guideline of the German Sepsis Society [19] distinguishes between intravenous IgG and intravenous IgGMA (**Table 4**): The use of intravenous IgG preparations is rejected with a level B recommendation (A-E) and a level of evidence Ia

Table 4. Recommendation and levels of evidence for adjunctive therapy with immunoglobulin preparations in adult sepsis patients.

	Meta-analyses [2, 10]	SBITS study [4]	Guidelines of the German Sepsis Society [19]	Guidelines of the German Federal Physician Chamber [3]	Guidelines of the Surviving Sepsis Campaign [20]
	Yes/No; LoE	Yes/No; LoE	Yes/No; LoE	Yes/No; LoE	
i.v. IgG	Yes (+); C	No; B	No; B	"can"	No statement
i.v. IgGMA	Yes (++); C		"can"; C	"can"	No statement

Yes/No: Results of the analyses and guideline assessments for the adjunctive use of immunoglobulins in severe sepsis and septic shock; LoE: level of evidence; i.v.: intravenous

("systematic overview of RCTs"; highest of five levels of evidence). The use of the intravenous IgGMA preparation for adjunctive sepsis therapy on the other hand is suggested with a weak level C recommendation (only studies with an evidence level II = RCTs of minor quality) and a level of evidence Ia ("The application of intravenous IgGMA in the treatment of adult patients with severe sepsis and septic shock can be taken into consideration"). However, only 7 of 14 experts voted for this statement, 7 experts were opposed [19].

The guidelines of the international Surviving Sepsis Campaign [20] mention only adjunctive sepsis therapy with immunoglobulins in children (weak recommendation). The Committee does not offer an opinion on the significance of this therapy in adults. It has to be added that the Committee is headed by an American colleague (RP Dellinger) and that intravenous IgGMA preparations are not in use in the USA. Therefore, our American colleagues have no experience with the use of intravenous IgGMA in the treatment of sepsis.

Hard-to-reach for evidence based medicine are rare septic diseases, like meningococcal sepsis and streptococcal toxic shock syndrome. These conditions are characterized by a fulminant toxin burden and a foudroyant clinical course. High levels of toxin neutralizing antibodies should have a favorable effect on the course of the disease. Because of the rare occurrence of these diseases, it is hard to obtain proof of effectiveness in randomized trials (**Table 5**): two of the listed trials are based on comparison with a historical control group [21, 22], the third, a European randomized trial [23], was stopped prematurely due to slow recruitment. It is worth mentioning that the two streptococcal toxic shock syndrome trials treated their patients with total intravenous IgG dosages $\geq$ 2 g/kg – more than twice as high as usually given in sepsis therapy; e.g., in the trial by Darenberg et al. [23] the dosage was 1 g/kg bw on day 1 and 0.5 g/kg bw on days 2 and 3.

At present, the use of immunoglobulins for these two disease entities is not standard therapy. Whether results will ever be available from satisfactory large RCTs seems doubtful. The members of the StreptIg Study Group [23] recommend the use of immunoglobulins in streptococcal toxic shock syndrome until further notice.

Our Practical Approach

So far, sepsis research has not spoiled us with effective adjunctive therapeutics for sepsis [19]! This explains why it is not possible to treat sepsis using just therapeutics of the highest level of evidence! The question is whether we should fill these gaps with expert opinion alone or also use therapeutics with a lower evidence level? We vote for the latter approach [24]:

III

- We treat patients in early stages of severe sepsis and septic shock (our threshold for organ failure: APACHE II score ≥ 20) with 0.25 g/kg bw of the immunoglobulin GMA preparation, Pentaglobin®, for three consecutive days, resulting in a total dose of 0.75 g/kg bw. We can assume that this approach leads to a lasting increase in IgG and IgM serum levels (see above, [8]). If a decreased IgM serum level is indeed linked to a higher mortality (**Table 1**), IgM supplementation may improve prognosis. We exclude septic patients after cardiac arrest and also neutropenic cancer patients; the former have *per se* a very poor prognosis independent of sepsis, and for the latter the use of intravenous IgGMA has shown no positive effects on prognosis [25]. We are aware of the fact that our approach has no high level of evidence but we feel that practical medicine cannot stop at this border, when considering the high mortality rates of patients with severe sepsis.
- In patients with severe sepsis and septic shock we no longer use any intravenous IgG preparations. The main reason for this is the negative result of the placebo controlled SBITS study [4] with 653 patients, the only immunoglobulin RCT with a narrow confidence interval.
- For two rare septic entities – meningococcal sepsis and streptococcal toxic shock syndrome (see above and **Table 5**) – we use intravenous IgGMA in the mentioned dosage in any case, even though convincing RCTs are not yet available and will be – due to the rare occurrence of these diseases – rather hard to accomplish.

Table 5. Use of immunoglobulin preparations in rare sepsis subgroups: Meningococcal sepsis and streptococcal toxic shock syndrome.

Sepsis subgroup	n	IVIG	Mortality Placebo		Risk reduction by IVIG	p	Study design (placebo group)
Meningococcal sepsis							
[21]	32	IgGMA	15/21	3/11	–62 %	0.019	Historical
Streptococcal toxic shock syndrome							
[22]	53	IgG	14/21	11/32	–49 %	0.009	Historical
[23]	21	IgG	4/11	1/11	–72 %	0.3	Prospective

Historical: historical control group; Prospective: prospective study design; IVIG: intravenous immunoglobulin

Conclusion

Hypogammaglobulinemia G in severe sepsis is unlikely to be coupled to an even more unfavorable prognosis (**Table 1**). In contrast, 28-day-mortality of patients with severe sepsis and hypogammaglobulinemia M has been found in one case series to be higher than in patients with normogammaglobulinemia M (**Table 1,**

Fig. 1). This finding coincides with some experimental and clinical evidence of superiority of intravenous IgGMA compared to intravenous IgG in animal sepsis models as well as in patients with severe sepsis. The German sepsis guidelines [19] give a weak recommendation for the treatment of patients with severe sepsis and septic shock with intravenous IgGMA. A newly developed intravenous IgGMA preparation with a larger IgM content (23 %) is under clinical investigation (ClinicalTrials.gov Identifier: NCT01420744).

III

Acknowledgements: The authors thank N. Köhler for her help in processing the data.

References

1. Werdan K (2001) Intravenous immunoglobulin therapy for prophylaxis and therapy of sepsis. Curr Opin Crit Care 7: 354–361
2. Kreymann KG, de Heer G, Nierhaus A, Kluge S (2007) Use of polyclonal immunoglobulins as adjunctive therapy for sepsis or septic shock. Crit Care Med 35: 2677–2685
3. German Federal Physicians' Chamber based on recommendations of its scientific council: [Guidelines on therapy with blood components and plasma derivatives: Chapter 9: Human Immunoglobulins.] Deutscher Ärzteverlag, Köln, 2009: 195–220
4. Werdan K, Pilz G, Bujdoso O, et al, for the Score-Based Immunoglobulin Therapy of Sepsis (SBITS) Study Group (2007) Score-based immunoglobulin G therapy of patients with sepsis: The SBITS study. Crit Care Med 35: 2693–2701
5. Dietz S, Lautenschläger C, Mueller-Werdan U, Werdan K (2010) Low levels of immunoglobulin G in patients with sepsis or septic shock: a signum mali ominis? Crit Care 14 (Suppl1): P26
6. Dietz S, Päsler M, Köhler N, et al (2011) [Is a low serum level of immunoglobulin a preditor of increased mortality in sepsis and septic shock?] Intensivmed 48: 351 (P12)
7. Taccone FS, Stordeur P, de Backer D, Creteur J, Vincent JL (2009) γ-Globulin levels in patients with community-acquired septic shock. Shock 32: 379–385
8. Pilz G, Appel R, Kreuzer E, Werdan K (1997) Comparison of early IgM enriched immunoglobulin vs polyvalent IgG administration in score-identified post-cardiac surgical patients at high risk for sepsis. Chest 111: 419–426
9. Esen F & Tugrul S (2009) IgM-enriched immunoglobulins in sepsis. In: Vincent J-L (ed) 2009 Yearbook of Intensive Care and Emergency Medicine. Springer, Heidelberg, pp 102–110
10. Werdan K (2007) Mirror, mirror on the wall, which is the fairest meta-analysis of all? Crit Care Med 35: 2852–2854
11. Werdan K, Pilz G, Mueller-Werdan U, et al, for the Early Supplemental Severe SIRS Treatment With IVIG In Score-identified High-risk Patients After Cardiac Surgery (ESSICS) Study Group (2008) Immunoglobulin G treatment of postcardiac surgery patients with score-identified severe systemic inflammatory response syndrome – the ESSICS Study. Crit Care Med 36: 716–723
12. Kazatchkine MD, Kaveri SV (2001) Immunomodulation of autoimmune and inflammatory diseases with intravenous immune globulin. N Engl J Med 345: 747–755
13. Vassilev T, Mihaylova N, Voynova E, Nikolova M, Kazatchkine M, Kaveri S (2006) IgM-enriched human intravenous immunoglobulin suppresses T lymphocyte function in vitro and delays the activation of T lymphocytes in hu-SCID mice. Clin Exp Immunol 145: 108–115
14. Trautmann M, Held TK, Susa M, et al (1998) Bacterial lipopolysaccharide (LPS) specific antibodies in commercial human immunoglobulin preparations: superior antibody content of an IgM-enriched product. Clin Exp Immunol 111: 81–90
15. Rieben R, Muizert Y, Gerritsen AF, Daha MR (1999) Immunoglobulin M enriched human intravenous immunoglobulin prevents complement activation in vitro and in vivo in a rat model of acute inflammation. Blood 93: 942–951

16. Hoffmann JN, Fertmann JM, Vollmar B, Laschke MW, Jauch KW, Menger MD (2008) Immunoglobulin M-enriched human immunoglobulins reduce leucocyte-endothelial interactions and attenuate microvascular perfusion failure in normotensive endotoxemia. Shock 29: 133–139

17. Mohr M, Englisch L, Roth A, Burchardi H, Zielmann S (1997) Effects of early treatment with immunoglobulin on critical illness polyneuropathy following multiple organ failure and gram-negative sepsis. Intensive Care Med 23: 1144–1149

18. Schedel I, Dreikhausen U, Nentwig B, et al (1991) Treatment of Gram-negative septic shock with an immunoglobulin preparation: A prospective, randomized clinical trial. Crit Care Med 19: 1104–1113

19. Reinhart K, Brunkhorst FM, Bone H-G, et al (2010) Prävention, Diagnose, Therapie und Nachsorge der Sepsis. 1. Revision der S-2k Leitlinien der Deutschen Sepsis-Gesellschaft e.V. (DSG) und der Deutschen Interdisziplinären Vereinigung für Intensiv- und Notfall-medizin (DIVI) Intensiv- und Notfallbehandlung 35: 56–104

20. Dellinger PR, Carlet JM, Masur H, et al, for the International Surviving Sepsis Campaign Guideline Committee (2008) Surviving Sepsis Campaign: International guidelines for management of severe sepsis and septic shock: 2008. Crit Care Med 36: 296–327

21. Thomson A, Sills J, Hart CA, Harris F (1989) Anti-endotoxin therapy for fulminant meningococcal septicaemia: pilot study. Arch Dis Child 64: 1217–1218

22. Kaul et McGeer A, Norrby-Teglund A, et al, and the Canadian Streptococcal Study Group (1999) Intravenous immunoglobulin therapy for streptococcal toxic shock syndrome – a comparative observational study. Clin Infect Dis 28: 800–807

23. Darenberg J, Ihendyane N, Sjölin J, et al, and the StreptIg Study Group (2003) Intravenous immunoglobulin G therapy in streptococcal toxic shock syndrome: a european random-ized, double-blind, placebo-controlled trial. Clin Infect Dis 37: 333–340

24. Werdan K (2006) Immunoglobulin treatment in sepsis – is the answer "no"? Crit Care Med 34: 1542–1544

25. Hentrich M, Fehnle K, Ostermann H, et al (2006) IgMA-enriched immunoglobulin in neu-tropenic patients with sepsis syndrome and septic shock: a randomized, controlled multi-center trial. Crit Care Med 34: 1319–1325

Timing IgM Treatment in Sepsis: Is Procalcitonin the Answer?

Z. Molnár and J. Fogas

III

Introduction

Modern intensive care therapy could, with a small stretch of the imagination, be argued to equal severe sepsis and septic shock therapy. This does not mean that every patient on the intensive care unit (ICU) is septic, but every critically ill patient certainly has the potential risk of acquiring sepsis. Furthermore, almost everything that we know today about critical illness is somehow linked to what we have learned from experimental and clinical sepsis studies. However, after decades of intense research we are still struggling to improve mortality on our ICUs, although there is a tendency towards some improvement (from 37 to 30.7 %) [1, 2]. So, is it 'much ado about nothing'? Absolutely not! The devil, as always, lies in the details. We keep forgetting that what we call 'sepsis' is not a definitive disease, or diagnosis, but a syndrome, for which the criteria were defined by consensus by a group of scientists led by the late Roger Bone in a Las Vegas hotel room back in the 1980s, and a few years later on at a consensus conference [3–5]. In the case of definitive conditions such as, for example, fractured neck of femur or myocardial infarction, we have specific tools for diagnosis, and treatment. Unfortunately, this is not the case for sepsis. There is no exact diagnostic measure to capture the moment when systemic inflammatory response syndrome (SIRS), infection, sepsis, severe sepsis or septic shock occurs, nor to precisely differentiate between them. This uncertainty will inevitably lead to inhomogeneous groups of patients with selection bias, sampling error in our studies, and eventually failure to produce significant results [6–8].

Out of the more than 70 prospective randomized trials designed to investigate the treatment effect on mortality in sepsis over the last 20 years, most have ended in great disappointment. The results were either negative or have not been implemented into clinical practice as they failed to reach the highest evidence based standard of two controlled trials with high statistical power [8, 9]. The best examples are the results of adjunctive therapies in sepsis including activated protein C, intravenous immunoglobulins (IVIG), selenium, steroids, etc [9]. Lack of proven benefit, and the fact that some of these therapies are expensive has meant that these treatment modalities are either challenged or seldom used in many ICUs and their routine use remains controversial.

The role of IVIG in sepsis treatment has been studied for more than 25 years in adults and pediatric patients. Several reviews and meta-analyses have been published recently, and agree that there is a tendency towards better survival rates when IgM and IgA enriched preparations (IgGMA) were used [10, 11]. The aim of this current review is to give a short overview of the most important

J.-L. Vincent (ed.), *Annual Update in Intensive Care and Emergency Medicine 2012*
DOI 10.1007/978-3-642-25716-2 © Springer-Verlag Berlin Heidelberg 2012

research milestones with polyclonal immune globulins, and then to provoke thoughts on how to proceed in clinical research, and clinical practice with IgM-preparations so that we may eventually be able to answer the questions we have been left with: "To use or not to use?", "For which patients?", "At what time?" [12].

III   Milestones of Research with IgM-preparations

After more than two decades of clinical research, IVIG is still looking for its place in the treatment of severe sepsis and septic shock as an adjunctive therapy. However, several recent reviews and meta-analyses [10, 11] suggest a clearly demonstrable benefit, including greater mortality reduction with the use of IgM-enriched immunoglobulin preparations compared with the standard IVIG treatment. Clinical studies have been conducted since the early 1990s with IgM-preparations, especially in mixed populations of septic patients, and more homogeneous groups for prophylactic use (primarily after cardiac surgery). Most of these studies demonstrated a trend toward reduced morbidity and mortality. The results were promising but not entirely convincing, which was attributed in part to the small number of patients included in the studies.

Intravenous IgM-enriched immunoglobulin was first investigated in 1991, in a homogeneous (medical) septic patient population [13]. Sixty-nine patients in septic shock with high endotoxin levels were randomized and the treatment group received IgM-preparation within 24 hours of the onset of septic shock. The study was discontinued after interim analysis of data because the difference between the mortality rates (4 % vs. 32 %) was statistically significant in favor of the therapy. Another group conducted a prospective, randomized controlled study in a mixed medical and surgical ICU with the aim of evaluating the effect of treatment with an IgM-preparation on progression of organ failure and septic shock in patients with severe sepsis [14]. Progress was followed by serial measures of procalcitonin (PCT) levels, APACHE II and sequential organ failure assessment (SOFA) scores over 8 days. Because of the limited number of patients included in this study, mortality was not an endpoint. PCT levels decreased significantly in the treatment group ($p < 0.001$); however, an improvement in SOFA scores could not be demonstrated. PCT levels and SOFA scores did not change significantly in the control group. Differences in the incidence of septic shock (38 % versus 57 %) or in 28-day mortality rates (23.8 % versus 33.3 %) were not significant between the treated and the control groups. There were no differences in serial APACHE II scores either. The authors concluded that they were not able to demonstrate any beneficial effects of polyclonal immunoglobulin treatment on organ dysfunction, septic shock incidence or mortality rate in patients with severe sepsis. In a similar study including 68 patients with septic shock, a significant mortality reduction (22.4 % vs. 40 %) in the IgM-preparation treated arm was reported [15]. Patients in the treatment group had higher APACHE II scores as compared to controls (21.3 ± 7.2 vs. 10.5 ± 4.6), which may explain the difference in mortality between these two studies [14, 15]. Rodríguez et al. [16] assessed the impact on outcome of adjuvant therapy with a high-dose IgM-preparation in critically ill patients who underwent surgery because of abdominal sepsis. In this multicenter, prospective trial, 56 patients with severe sepsis and septic shock of intra-abdominal origin were randomized within 24 h after the onset of symptoms. The administration of IgM-preparation in addition to antibiotic therapy produced a 20 % mortality reduction in the intent-to-treat analysis. The lack of significant difference in the mortality rate between groups may be attributable to the small sample size. However, in the subgroup of patients with appropriate antibiotic therapy, a significant reduction in the mortality rate was seen in association with the administration of the IgM-preparation. More recently, Hentrich et al. [17] investigated the role of intravenous IgGMA in neutropenic patients with severe sepsis and septic shock. In the largest trial on the use of polyclonal immunoglobulin (n = 211), they failed to document any benefit of IgGMA therapy based on 28-day mortality rate. However, in all patients who survived, there was a trend favoring intravenous IgGMA treatment. The main criticism of this clinical investigation is that most of the patients involved were low grade septic patients with none or one organ failure and a relatively low mortality suggesting that these patients are not a target population for IVIG treatment.

Timing of Treatment

Inclusion criteria and the indication for treatment with IgM-preparations in the above mentioned trials were without exception as per the definition of severe sepsis from the American College of Chest Physicians/Society of Critical Care Medicine (ACCP/SCCM) consensus conference [5]. Although most sepsis trials recruit patients based simply on these consensus definitions, these inclusion criteria may be too general, so it is inevitable that these studies end up with heterogeneous groups of patients. Furthermore, due to the many confounding factors introduced because of the different etiologies of sepsis, the results are likely to be non-conclusive. For example, the PROWESS study, a prospective randomized clinical trial on the effect of activated protein C on mortality from severe sepsis, showed significant improvement in survival in the treatment group [18]. However, after several subgroup analyses, the indications and recommendations for use have been altered [19, 20]. The current Surviving Sepsis Campaign guidelines suggest using activated protein C in adult patients with sepsis-induced organ dysfunction associated with a high risk of death, such as those with an APACHE II ≥ 25 or multiple organ failure, and do not recommend its use in septic patients with a low risk of death [20]. In other words, from the heterogeneous patient cohort defined as 'severe sepsis', a more homogeneous subgroup was defined on the basis of organ dysfunction, which benefit most from the treatment.

When considering trials that have investigated the effects of IVIG in severe sepsis, only one has applied this concept to any degree – the 'Score-based Immunoglobulin Treatment in Sepsis' (SBITS) study [21]. Unfortunately, although this is the largest prospective randomized immunoglobulin study to date (n = 653), the drug investigated was IgG and not IgM. Another limitation of the results is that the study was performed in the early 1990s (published years later in 2007), during which time many therapeutic and diagnostic concepts had changed fundamentally; therefore, the results are difficult to apply to our current practice.

A recent retrospective study found that patients who survived received treatment with IgM-preparation significantly earlier than those who died (23 vs. 62 h) [22]. We all agree that timing is crucial in critical care, but how can we define the term 'early' in this context? Furthermore, is there a way to identify more homogeneous groups of patients, within this large cohort of severe sepsis, who will bene-

III

fit most from adjunctive therapies? The answer has to be at this moment in time: not yet. However, there is a promising marker that is able to diagnose and differentiate between SIRS, infection, sepsis, severe sepsis and septic shock with good sensitivity and specificity, and which also has good prognostic value: PCT [21, 23, 24]. This fast-reacting marker of bacterial infection, especially when measured regularly with evaluation of dynamic changes in concentrations, has been proposed as a tool to warn clinicians, and thereby help them to deliver interventions with proven efficacy to septic patients [25, 26]. Most studies in this context have investigated the effect of PCT-guided antibiotic therapy [27–30]. These studies did not show any effect on outcome, but patients in the PCT-group received significantly less antibiotic and for a shorter duration.

There is only one outcome trial that has investigated the effect of PCT-guided antibiotic treatment on survival, the Procalcitonin and Survival Study (PASS) [31]. Although the main results showed significantly longer times on mechanical ventilation and prolonged use of antibiotics in the PCT-group, the study design had several limitations, detailed discussion of which is far beyond the scope of this review. However, there is one important point to comment on. The percentage of surgical patients was around 40 % in both groups, and the PCT value indicating the need for an intervention, the so called 'alert-PCT', was ≥ 1 ng/ml. This level of PCT is far too low for intervention in surgical patients. It has been shown in several studies that PCT levels 'normally' increase after surgery, and require no intervention at all [32–34]. Furthermore, it has also been shown that there is a significant difference in PCT values accompanying the same severity of sepsis between medical and surgical patients [34]. Clec'h et al. found that the median PCT value in medical versus surgical patients with noninfectious SIRS was 0.35 (0.13–1) vs. 5.70 (2.65–8.35), and in septic shock medical patients 8.4 (3.63–76) versus 34 (7.1–76) ng/ml in surgical septic shock patients [34]. These authors also found that the best cutoff values to differentiate between survivors and nonsurvivors in medical and surgical patients were: 1 ng/ml (80 % sensitivity, 94 % specificity) and 6 ng/ml (76 % sensitivity, 72.7 % specificity) respectively. Therefore, in the PASS study, unnecessary antibiotic use and antibiotic escalation were inevitable in the PCT-group because of the generally low alert-PCT levels in the study protocol [31]. However, the concept of identifying high risk patients by their PCT values, and targeting adjunctive treatment to these patients is just a hypothesis at the moment and should be investigated further in the future.

This concept could also be applied to use of IgM-preparations as treatment in sepsis. There is some evidence that in septic patients treated with IgM-preparations, PCT levels decrease significantly when compared to controls (**Fig. 1**) [14, 35]. In two recent studies, admission PCT levels were high (4.0–5.5 [33] and 7–10 ng/ml [35]), and decreased significantly with time in the IgM-group. In a recent pilot study, we could not find any change in PCT levels over the first 8 days of treatment, or any difference between IgM- and placebo- treated patients [36]. However, PCT levels on recruitment were substantially lower (1.0–1.6 ng/ml) than in the two studies mentioned earlier, indicating that we treated a different patient population compared to the previous trials. This observation suggests that IgM-preparations should be given to patients with higher PCT values in order to observe any treatment effect.

There is no recommendation for the use of IgM-preparations in adults in the Surviving Sepsis Campaign Guidelines, but it received a grade C recommendation in the German Sepsis Society's guidelines, suggesting that it may be considered

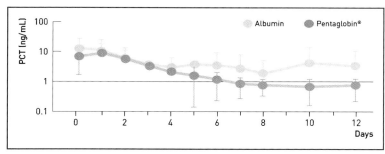

Fig. 1. Procalcitonin levels in the IgM-preparation and placebo treated patients over the first 8 days of treatment. Data from [35].

for treatment of adult patients with severe sepsis or septic shock [37]. However, clinicians are still left with the uncertainty of what to do in everyday practice. Identifying patients who will benefit most from IgM-treatment is the task that we have to accomplish in the future. According to the Surviving Sepsis Guidelines, the treatment algorithm for the septic patient should start with the 'Resuscitation Bundle', followed by the 'Management Bundle' [20]. Because of the concept of early goal-directed resuscitation, more and more patients stabilize after resuscitation, and never receive the low dose steroids or activated protein C included in the 'Management Bundle'. In theory, IgM may have a role in this early phase: After resuscitation and before the 'Management Bundle' is indicated. Targeting IgM-treatment to those who do not fulfill the indication for activated protein C after resuscitation, but are at higher risk as indicated by high PCT levels, may be of benefit.

Conclusion

Sepsis is not a definitive disease, therefore more specific and detailed inclusion criteria should be applied in sepsis research in which etiology, medical or surgical origin, organ dysfunction scores and biomarker levels are all taken into account. Procalcitonin levels with certain cut-off values may be helpful for identifying patients who are not sick enough to receive the full 'Management Bundle' but who are still at a high enough risk to benefit from treatment with IgM-preparations.

Naturally, this hypothesis has to be tested in randomized trials – the stereotype sentence that most papers finish with, but in this case it may be justified as a trial has never been done using this concept. The positive results of the small clinical trials published so far suggest that IgM-preparations have a role in sepsis treatment, but we have not quite found their place yet. There is a long and exciting road ahead of us but we must persevere if we want to give the final answer with a clear conscience.

References

1. Alberti C, Brun-Buisson C, Burchardi H, et al (2002) Epidemiology of sepsis and infection in ICU patients from an international multicentre cohort study. Intensive Care Med 28: 108–121
2. Levy MM, Dellinger RP, Townsend SR (2010) The Surviving Sepsis Campaign: results of an international guideline-based performance improvement program targeting severe sepsis. Intensive Care Med 36: 222–231
3. Bone RC, Fisher CJ, Clemmer TP, et al (1987) A controlled clinical trial of high dose methylprednisolone in the treatment of severe sepsis and septic shock. N Engl J Med 317: 654–658
4. Marshall JC, Aarts MA (2001) From Celsus to Galen to Bone: The illnesses, syndromes, and diseases of acute inflammation. In: Vincent JL (ed), Yearbook of intensive care and emergency medicine, Springer-Verlag, Berlin, pp: 3–12
5. American College of Chest Physicians – Society of Critical Care Medicine (1992) Consensus Conference: Definitions for sepsis and organ failure and guidelines for the use of innovative therapies in sepsis. Crit Care Med 20: 864–875
6. Natanson C, Esposito CJ, Banks St (1998) The sirens' songs of confirmatory sepsis trials: Selection bias and sampling error. Crit Care Med 26: 1927–1931
7. Cohen J (1999) The "failure" of clinical trials in sepsis. Curr Opinion Crit Care 330: 339–340
8. Vincent JL (2010) We should abandon randomized controlled trials in the intensive care unit. Crit Care Med 38 (Suppl): S534–S538
9. Werdan K (2007) Mirror, mirror on the wall, which is the fairest meta-analysis of all? Crit Care Med 35: 2852–2854
10. Kreymann KG, Geraldine H, Nierhaus A, Kluge S (2007) Use of polyclonal immunoglobulins as adjunctive therapy for sepsis or septic shock. Crit Care Med 35: 2677–2685
11. Alejandria MM, Lansang MAD, Dans LF, Mantaring III JB (2001) Intravenous immunoglobulin for treating sepsis, severe sepsis and septic shock. Cochrane Database Syst Rev CD001090
12. Neugebauer EAM (2007) To use or not to use? Polyclonal intravenous immunoglobulins for the treatment of sepsis and septic shock. Crit Care Med 35:2855
13. Schedel I, Dreikhausen U, Nentwig B, et al (1991) Treatment of gram-negative septic shock with an immunoglobulin preparation: A prospective, randomised clinical tial. Crit Care Med 19: 1104–1113
14. Tugrul S, Ozcan P E, Akinci O, et al (2002) The effects of IgM-enriched immunoglobulin preparations in patients with severe sepsis. Crit Care 6: 357–362
15. Karatzas S, Boutzouka E, Venetsanou K, et al (2002) The effect of IgM-enriches immunoglobilin preparations in patients with severe sepsis: another pont of view. Crit Care 6: 543–544
16. Rodríguez A, Rello J, Neira J, et al (2005) Effects of high dose of intravenous immunoglobulin and antibiotics on survival for severe sepsis undergoing surgery. Shock 23: 298–304
17. Hentrich M, Fehnle K, Ostermann H, et al (2006) IgMA-enriched immunoglobulin in neutropenic patients with sepsis syndrome and septic shock: A randomized, controlled, multiple-center trial. Crit Care Med 34: 1319–1325
18. Bernard GR, Vincent JL, Laterre PF, et al (2001) Efficacy and safety of recombinant human activated protein c for severe sepsis. N Engl J Med 344: 699–709
19. Ely EW, Laterre PF, Angus DC, et al (2003) Drotrecogin alfa (activated) administration across clinically important subgroups of patients with severe sepsis. Crit Care Med 31: 12–19
20. Dellinger RP, Levy MM, Carlet JM, et al (2008) Surviving Sepsis Campaign: International guidelines for management of severe sepsis and septic shock: 2008. Intensive Care Med 34: 17–60
21. Simon L, Gauvin F, Amre DK, et al (2004) Serum procalcitonin and C-reactive protein levels as markers of bacterial infection: a systematic review and meta-analysis. Clin Infect Dis 39: 206–217

22. Berlot G, Vassallo MC, Busetto N, et al (2012) Relationship between the timing of administration of IgM and IgA enriched immunoglobulins in patients with severe sepsis and septic shock and the outcome: A retrospective analysis. J Crit Care (in press)
23. Castelli GP, Pognani C, Meisner M, et al (2004) Procalcitonin and C-reactive protein during systemic inflammatory response syndrome, sepsis and organ dysfunction. Crit Care 8: R234-R240
24. Jensen JU, Heslet L, Jensen TH, et al (2006) Procalcitonin increase in early identification of critically ill patients at high risk of mortality. Crit Care Med 34: 2596–2602
25. Ventetuolo CE, Levy MM (2008) Biomarkers: Diagnosis and risk assessment in sepsis. Clin Chet Med 29: 591–603
26. Molnar Z, Bogar L (2006) Let's go dynamic with procalcitonin! Crit Care Med 34: 2687–2688
27. Christ-Crain M, Jaccard-Stolz D, Bingisser R, et al. Effect of procalcitonin-guided treatment on antibiotic use and outcome in lower respiratory tract infections: cluster randomised, single blinded intervention trial. Lancet 363: 600–607
28. Müller F, Christ-Crain M, Bregenzer T, et al. Procalcitonin levels predict bacteremia in patients with community-acquired pneumonia: a prospective cohort trial. Chest 138: 121–129
29. Nobre V, Harbarth S, Graf JD, Rohner P, Pugin J (2008) Use of procalcitonin to shorten antibiotic treatment duration in septic patients. Am J Respir Crit Care Med 177: 498–505
30. Bouadma L, Luyt CE, Tubach F, et al (2010) Use of procalcitonin to reduce patients' exposure to antibiotics in intensive care units (PRORATA trial): a multicentre randomised controlled trial. Lancet 375: 463–474
31. Jensen JU, Hein L, Lundgren B, et al (2011) Procalcitonin-guided interventions against infections to increase early appropriate antibiotics and improve survival in the intensive care unit: A randomized trial. Crit Care Med 39: 2048–2058
32. Szakmany T, Molnar Z (2003) Procalcitonin levels do not predict mortality following major abdominal surgery. Can J Anaesth 50: 1082–1083
33. Lindberg M, Hole A, Johnsen H, et al (2002) Reference intervals for procalcitonin and C-reactive protein after major abdominal surgery. Scand J Clin Lab Invest 62: 189–194
34. Clec'h C, Fosse JP, Karoubi P, et al (2006) Differential diagnostic value of procalcitonin in surgical and medical patients with septic shock. Crit Care Med 34: 102–107
35. Reith HB, Rauchschwalbe SK, Mittelkötter U, et al (2004) IgM-enriched immunoglobulin (Pentaglobin) positively influences the course of post-surgical intra-abdominal infections. Eur J Med Res 9: 479–484
36. Szakmany T, Toth I, Molnar Z, Leiner T, Mikor A, Bogar L (2006). Effects of polyclonal IGM in septic shock accompanied by severe respiratory failure: a randomized trial. Intensive Care Med 32 (Suppl 1): S226 (abst)
37. Reinhart K, Brunkhorst FM, Bone Hg, et al (2010) Prevention, diagnosis, therapy and follow-up care of sepsis: 1st revision of S-2k guidelines of the German Sepsis Society (Deutsche Sepsis-Gesellschaft e.V. (DSG)) and the German Interdisciplinary Association of Intensive Care and Emergency Medicine. Ger Med Sci 8: Doc 14

Sepsis Stewardship Programs: Methods and Results

M. Girardis, S. Busani, and A. Pan

III

Introduction

Hospital mortality in patients with severe sepsis and septic shock is still unacceptably high despite advances in understanding of the physiopathology and the numerous clinical trials on potential therapies. Even with optimal treatment, the mortality rate of patients with septic shock exceeds 40 % and has not varied significantly in the last 5 years [1, 2]. Early identification and proper management of patients with sepsis are key factors for reducing the observed mortality and have been the main goal of the Surviving Sepsis Campaign (SSC) by the development of evidence-based guidelines and the recommendation of specific bundles of care [3, 4]. Some studies have reported a potential benefit on patient outcome by implementing guidelines and bundle care strategies in clinical practice but wide adoption of these approaches is rare. Moreover, it is still unclear whether the observed benefit is more due to the effect of the recommended treatments or to a general increase in the awareness of the sepsis problem as a result of specific educational and stewardship programs.

Sepsis Stewardship Programs: Education and Process-Changes Analysis

Numerous multifaceted programs (sepsis stewardship programs, SSP) aimed to improve the management of septic patients in emergency departments (EDs) and in intensive care units (ICUs) have been instituted around the world in the last few years. Most published papers on SSP relate to prospective observational pre-post single center/unit studies and report the effects of educational programs on compliance to sepsis bundles and on patient outcome (**Table 1**). The strategy used for the implementation of a stewardship program is an important element for achieving positive results [5] but, unfortunately, the methods used for education and process-care improvement are described in detail in only a few of the papers dealing with SSP. As is well known, numerous barriers need to be overcome to implement new methods and evidence-based guidelines in clinical practice. Lack of knowledge and acceptance among staff members, shortage of resources and structural obstacles are frequent problems that impede quality improvement programs [6]. Therefore, the description of the techniques used for developing, spreading and maintaining a SSP may provide useful information for other institutions in planning and realizing similar initiatives.

United States Experience: One of the first reported experiences was the Multiple Urgent Sepsis Therapies (MUST) protocol from the Beth Israel Deaconess

J.-L. Vincent (ed.), *Annual Update in Intensive Care and Emergency Medicine 2012*
DOI 10.1007/978-3-642-25716-2 © Springer-Verlag Berlin Heidelberg 2012

Table 1. Setting, type of education and population and key messages of six sepsis stewardship programs

	Setting	Education	Population	Key Messages
Shapiro et al. [7]	Local, single center, USA	Nurse and physician education: grand rounds, teaching sessions and conferences	ED patients with severe sepsis or septic shock	Improvement in time to antibiotic administration, intravenous fluid delivery and vasopressor use in the first 6 hrs
Nguyen et al. [8]	Local, single center, USA	Conference lectures, bedside teaching, and in-services to physicians and nurses	ED patients with severe sepsis or septic shock	EGDT associated with decreased mortality. In-hospital mortality lower in patients with bundle completed.
Ferrer et al. [9]	National, 59 ICUs, Spain	Oral and slide presentations; translation of the guidelines and posters	ICU patients with severe sepsis or septic shock	Improvement in staff knowledge and hospital processes of care. Lower risk of death in post-intervention cohort.
Castellanos-Ortega et al. [10]	Local, 3 ICUs, Spain	Conference lectures, teaching sessions, posters and pocket cards. 'Sepsis profile' to facilitate an early diagnosis. Feedback during the first study year. Educational refresher program	ICU patients with septic shock	Compliance with six or more interventions of the 6-hr bundle as predictor of survival.
Cardoso et al. [11]	National, 17 ICUs, Portugal	Three regional teaching sessions	ICU patients with community acquired sepsis	Full completion of the core bundle associated with a decrease in 28-day mortality
Moro et al [12]	Regional, 30 hospitals, Italy	Regional educational package, hospital sepsis multidisciplinary team formation, local education	Hospital patients	Wide regional education over a 3 year period. Improvement in processes for patient identification and microbiological diagnosis

EGDT: early goal-directed therapy; ED: emergency department

Medical Center in Boston [7]. Education in correct application of the protocol involved physicians and nurses from the ED and the medical/surgical ICUs. Nursing education consisted of four 3-hour classes whereas physician education was carried out by grand rounds, resident teaching sessions and departmental conferences. In the protocol, nurses were responsible for identification of patients and once an ED patient was defined as eligible, a "code sepsis" was sent to the members of the hospital sepsis team, which included ICU and ED physicians with a nurse bed facilitator. The protocol was initiated by the triage nurse, the ED nurse, or the ED physician caring for the patient. A bedside protocol packet, including a nursing sepsis flow-sheet, a standardized order set for the protocol therapies and a short protocol guide was placed in a strategic place in the ED and became

III

part of the patient's medical record. Hospital implementation of the MUST protocol was associated with more fluids and vasopressor being given to the 79 protocol patients with septic shock, and earlier and more adequate antibiotic therapy compared with 51 historical controls. In addition, protocol patients had tighter glucose control and a more frequent assessment of adrenal function. The absolute mortality risk reduction (RR) of MUST patients was 9.1 % (- 6.2 % to 24.5 %) compared to historical controls, but the small number of patients included in the study did not allow the authors to demonstrate that this protocol resulted in significant benefit for the patients.

In Loma Linda Medical Center, Nguyen et al. [8] implemented a 2-year program for ED doctors and nurses, subdivided into 3-month quartiles that included baseline, education and operational, followed by five quality improvement (QI) phases. The baseline phase served to evaluate the initial level of care by applying a standardized checklist. In the education phase, a physician champion and nurse educator provided conference lectures, bedside teaching, and in-services to physicians and nurses. The operational phase consisted of a 5 intervention bundle delivered in the ED setting including initiation of central venous pressure (CVP)/ venous oxygen saturation measurement within 2 hours, broad-spectrum antibiotic therapy within 2 hours, early goal-directed therapy (EGDT) in 6 hours, steroids in shocked patients and monitoring of lactate clearance. Physicians and nurses used a sepsis toolkit and pocket cards as reminders of the processes involved in the bundle delivery. During the QI phase (5 quartiles), the healthcare staff were provided with an interval summary that included the number of septic patients, percentage compliance with the bundle and patient outcome. In addition, individual cases were discussed and a formal reminder was given to physicians with low bundle adherence. This strategy allowed a progressive improvement in bundle compliance from the baseline phase (0 %) to the end of the 5th QI phase (51 %). In-hospital mortality was lower (absolute RR 18.7 %) in patients in whom the bundle was completed compared to patients without bundle compliance. A multivariate regression analysis including the five bundle elements indicated that only completion of EGDT was independently related to a decrease in hospital mortality. The quality improvement effort required 2 years to achieve ≥ 50 % rate of successful completion of the bundle. The authors indicated EGDT completion within 6 hours as the main limiting factor in the ED and proposed a 'shock team' approach to overcoming this barrier.

Spanish Experience: In 2008, Ferrer et al. [9] reported the experience of a multifaceted educational program in 59 spanish hospitals (Edusepsis Study). In each hospital, a local multidisciplinary team, involving physicians and nurses from ICU, infectious diseases, emergency and internal medicine departments, shared and implemented a homogeneous educational program based on the SSC guidelines. Training and educational material consisted of: i) Oral and slide presentations; ii) a translation of the SSC guidelines; iii) posters focused on the early recognition of sepsis with the definitions of sepsis and its grade; and iv) audit and feedback from the general coordinating center with local and general data. The average time spent at each hospital for lectures was around 10 hours and a multidisciplinary team was active only in half of the centers. The local coordinator estimated that this approach increased staff knowledge and improved the care process in 96 % and 87 % of the hospitals, respectively. Compliance for the sepsis resuscitation bundle (from 5.3 % to 10.0 %) and all its elements improved significantly after the educational program, except for the early administration of broad spectrum antibiotics, which remained stable (from 66.5 % to 68.9 %). Similarly, adherence to the sepsis management bundle improved (from 10.9 % to 15.7 %), except for control of plateau pressure, which did not vary after program implementation. The hospital mortality rate in the 1465 post-intervention patients was lower (absolute RR 4.3 %) than in the 854 pre-intervention patients and the multivariate logistic regression adjusted for possible confounders confirmed that the post-intervention cohort was independently associated witho lower hospital mortality (OR 0.81, 95 % CI 0.67 – 0.98). The long term effects of the program were evaluated in 23 centers one year after the educational program was started. At the follow up, adherence to resuscitation bundles had returned to pre-intervention values, whereas compliance with management measures and hospital mortality remained similar to those observed immediately after education. These findings were in some way expected as a stewardship program has to be continuously supported, particularly in very busy areas like the ED or in hospitals with a high-turnover of healthcare personnel like university hospitals.

Castellanos-Ortega et al. [10] recently reported the results of the SSP established at the Marques de Valdecilla university hospital in Spain, which was based on 4 main elements. First, an educational program based on the SSC guidelines was implemented over a 3-month period by conference lectures and teaching sessions. Posters and pocket cards with the sepsis definitions and the SSC bundles were provided in the emergency, surgery, internal medicine, gynecology and obstetrics, anesthesia, and intensive care departments. All the teaching material was also available on the intranet. Second, a "sepsis profile" including two blood cultures, lactate, procalcitonin, arterial/venous blood gas analysis, hemogram and basic biochemistry was established as an optional tool to facilitate early sepsis diagnosis and grading. Third, repeated audit and feedback activities were carried out during the first SSP year. Last, an educational refresher program was established in the last year of the SSP that included a daily visit from an intensive care specialist to the ED for educational purposes, audit and bedside feedback. After institution of the SSP, adherence to the 6-hour resuscitation and 24-hour management bundles increased from 1 % to 11.3 %. Patients in the historical group (n = 94 over a 1-year period) had a significantly higher hospital mortality rate compared with patients in the intervention group (n = 384 over a 3-year period) (from 57.3 % to 37.5 %, absolute RR = 19.8 %) and the improvement in survival rates was related to the number of bundle interventions completed.

Portuguese Experience: A national multicenter study on community-acquired sepsis was performed in Portuguese ICUs (SACiUCI study) from 2004 to 2005 [11]. Web-based prospective data collection started in 17 Portuguese ICUs using a slightly modified version of the 6-hour SSC bundle (no indications for CVP and central venous oxygen saturation ($SvcO_2$) thresholds and dobutamine use). Training on data collection, SSC recommendations and bundles was organized in three regional sessions (in the north, south and center of Portugal) and was attended by a responsible investigator from each center. No feedback data on adherence to bundles was provided during the study period. In the 778 patients investigated, full completion of the 6 elements of the bundle occurred only in 94 patients (12 %) and was associated with a decrease in 28-day mortality (from 34 % to 25 %, absolute RR 9 %) that remained significant after adjustment for type of sepsis, SAPS II score, type of hospital and ICU.

Italian Experience: In 2006, the Emilia-Romagna Regional Health Agency (ARS-ER) launched a multifaceted regional program (LaSER project) with the

III

aim of improving the early recognition of the septic patient, correct microbiological diagnosis, early and appropriate antibiotic treatment, and initial resuscitation. A multidisciplinary group of experts on behalf of the ARS-RE prepared an educational package consisting of scientific literature, electronic presentations for lectures, clinical cases for practice training, posters and booklets [12]. In the second semester of 2006, 18 multidisciplinary teams, including microbiologists, pharmacists, doctors and nurses from infectious disease wards, intensive care and emergency departments from different regional hospitals shared the educational package. The objective was to promote, in their own hospital, a sepsis program devoted to education of healthcare personnel and specific changes in care processes. At the end of 2008, a SSP had been instituted in around 80 % of the Emilia-Romagna hospitals and more than 4000 nurses and 1800 physicians have been trained according to the regional educational package. In addition, specific protocols for patient identification and management, changes in processes for early microbiological diagnosis, and audit activity for evaluating clinical performance have been implemented in the majority of the regional hospitals. The effects of the LaSER project on patients' outcomes have been evaluated by analyzing the trend in hospital mortality of adult patients admitted for at least one night in six hospitals between October 2003 and October 2009. In comparison with the pre-LaSER period, the relative risk of death was around 0.90 (p < 0.05) for patients admitted after implementation of the hospital sepsis programs [13].

The experiences described above consistently indicate that a national, regional or local SSP, combining education with process changes in sepsis care levels, significantly increased clinical performance of the healthcare staff and this was associated with a significant reduction in mortality of patients with severe sepsis and septic shock. However, which strategies are most effective in overcoming implementation barriers and what implementation model (e.g., ED, ICU centralized model or multidisciplinary team) provides the better outcome benefit remain to be clarified.

Antibiotic and Sepsis Stewardship Programs: A Synergistic Cooperation

Along with aggressive fluid resuscitation and microbiological diagnosis, antimicrobial therapy is one mainstay of the sepsis resuscitation bundle [14]. Two aspects of antibiotic therapy are of paramount importance: Timing and correct antibiotic(s) choice. In fact, delayed therapy and the use of antibiotics that are not effective against the causal microorganism(s) have been associated with an increased risk of mortality [15]. One of the aims of the antimicrobial stewardship program (ASP) is to improve the knowledge of the healthcare staff to ensure prescriptions of the right antibiotic, at the right moment, at the optimum dose, via the right route and for the optimum time period [3, 16]. ASPs also target minimizing antibiotic toxicity and controlling against the selection of pathogenic organisms and the emergence of resistance [16]. Hospital sepsis programs usually include educational material and indications for antibiotic therapy and, thus, they can be considered a sort of ASP. Different from standard ASP, control of antimicrobial resistance and cost containment are not common targets of sepsis programs because of the high risk of death of patients with severe sepsis and septic shock. The guidelines for hospital implementation of ASPs [16] share 4 major strategies with the SSC guidelines: 1) Prospective audit with interventions and feed-back (strength of recommendation A-I); 2) education within an active intervention program (A-III); 3) guidelines and clinical pathways (A-I); and 4) antibiotic dose optimization (A-II).

The results of the SSC international improvement program based on the guidelines [17] showed that the compliance with the recommendation for early antibiotic administration (i.e., starting antimicrobials within 3 hours from admission to the emergency department or 1 hour for the in-hospital patient) increased from 60 % to 68 % over the study period. A sub-analysis performed in the Netherlands, a country well known for its long tradition in antimicrobial use, observed adherence to antimicrobial prescribing of around 50 %, with no significant improvement over the 2-year study period [18]. In the Edusepsis study, compliance with the recommendation for early antibiotic therapy did not vary after the educational program (66 % vs 69 %), although an improvement in both resuscitation and management sepsis bundles, with a reduction in overall mortality, was observed [9]. The reported data indicate that there is still room for a 30 – 50 % improvement in this theoretically simple task. Moreover, few data are available on the quality of antibiotic prescription in patients with severe sepsis. The current rate of appropriate antibiotic use in terms of activity against the causative pathogen and dose, is unknown and remains an important area to study [19]. Data regarding junior doctors show that there has been a significant improvement over the last years regarding understanding of sepsis and choice of antibiotic [20] and that antimicrobial resistance is perceived as a national problem by the majority of them [21]: The next generation will probably manage sepsis and antibiotic therapy better than we are currently able to.

In addition to education, organizational aspects are central elements of any ASP and may allow a significant improvement in antibiotic use. For instance, a computer-based protocol has been shown to increase overall adherence to SSC bundles and to timely antibiotic administration, with a reduction in the mortality rate [22]. Storing broad-spectrum antibiotics in a special dedicated cabinet has also been shown to improve door-to-antibiotic time in an emergency department [23].

A multidisciplinary team should be in charge of both stewardship programs (i.e., antibiotic and sepsis), as knowledge about patients' risk factors, microbiological resistance, antibiotic pharmacokinetics and pharmacodynamics is required to choose the correct antimicrobial agent, particularly in the empiric therapy of a critically ill patient.

Sepsis Bundles and Beyond

The application of a sepsis bundle strategy is consistently associated with an improvement in patient outcome, but whether this is due to some elements of the bundles rather than to others or to all bundle(s) application is still a matter of debate. A recent meta-analysis [24] including eight clinical trials published from 2001 to 2008 highlighted that sepsis bundle application was associated with a consistent and significant increase in survival compared with no bundle care (OR 1.91, 95 % CI 1.49 – 2.45). The analysis also observed marked heterogeneity among the different trials in the implementation of bundle components. Shorter time from diagnosis to antibiotic administration and more appropriate antibiotics administered were homogenously correlated with bundled care whereas all the other treatments (i.e., use of crystalloids, vasopressors, inotropes, red blood cells, corticosteroids and activated protein C) were not consistently increased across the studies. The authors concluded that such heterogeneity makes the impact of these treatments on patient survival uncertain; therefore, as recommended by the Joint Commission and Institute for Healthcare Improvement, they could not yet be considered components of a bundle of care.

Two large trials not included in the above meta-analysis analyzed the effectiveness of the sepsis treatments and bundles. Using a propensity score method, a sub-analysis of the Edusepsis study (2796 patients) [25] showed that very early administration (within 1 h) of antibiotic therapy (OR 0.67, 95 % CI 0.50–0.90) and activated protein C in patients with multiple organ failure (OR 0.59, 95 % CI 0.41–0.84) were the only interventions responsible for reduction in mortality of patients with severe sepsis and septic shock. The relationship between bundle treatments and hospital mortality was also analyzed in the 15022 patients of the SSC database [17]. A risk-adjustment logistic regression model including baseline characteristics of the patients indicated that: i) In all the patients, administration of broad spectrum antibiotics (OR 0.86, 95 % CI 0.79–0.93), blood culture before antibiotics (OR 0.76, 95 % CI 0.70–0.84) and blood glucose control (OR 0.67, 95 % CI 0.62–0.71) were associated with decreased hospital mortality; ii) in shocked patients (n = 7854), the use of activated protein C in the first 24 hours improved survival (OR 0.81, 95 % CI 0.68–0.96); and iii) in patients receiving mechanical ventilation (n = 7860), control of plateau pressure was associated with a better outcome (OR 0.59, 95 % CI 0.41–0.84).

In addition to the interventions suggested by the guidelines of the SSC and included in the sepsis bundles, other therapeutic options have been proposed and tested for patients with severe sepsis and septic shock. The recent guidelines of the German Sepsis Society [26] include as possible effective therapies in patients with severe sepsis: i) The use of albumin for volume therapy (recommendation level E, evidence level V); ii) therapy with epinephrine, phosphodiesterase inhibitors or levosimendan in patients with ventricular function impairment despite the administration of dobutamine (E, V); iii) The use of selenium (C, Ia); and iv) the use IgM-enriched immunoglobulins (C, Ia). Among these options, polyclonal IgM-enriched immunoglobulin seems to be an interesting and useful option because of its activity in neutralizing endotoxin and in modulating the host-immune response. A Cochrane systematic review and other meta-analyses [27–29] demonstrated a reduction in all-cause mortality for patients treated with IgM, although the type of infection, patients most likely to benefit, dose and duration of therapy have not yet been well defined by appropriate trials.

In 2004, we started an in-hospital SSP including the institution of a specific rapid response team (i.e., sepsis team) that collaborates to provide early and adequate treatment of septic patients in the ED and in non-ICU wards. The impact of this SSP on clinical practice and outcome has been remarkable: Adherence to evidence-based guidelines increased from 8 % to 35 % of patients and mortality of ICU patients with severe sepsis and septic shock decreased by about 40 % compared to the pre-SSP period [30]. Nevertheless, the hospital mortality of our patients was still unacceptably high (45 %) and we, therefore, introduced in our care protocol other therapeutic options such as the early use (within 24 hours) of IgM-enriched immunoglobulins in adult patients with septic shock. Because of an initial low adherence to protocol application, IgM-enriched immunoglobulins have been correctly used in only around 50 % of patients with septic shock.

Despite similar sequential organ failure assessment (SOFA) and SAPS II scores and sepsis bundle compliance, the hospital mortality was significantly lower (absolute RR 19 %) in patients treated with IgM than in those who were not treated [31]. Another similar positive experience on early use of IgM has been recently published [32] and, therefore, this therapeutic option can be considered as a useful adjunctive therapy in severe sepsis and septic shock. However, the exact time of administration, dosage and duration of therapy should be better clarified by appropriate high-level studies.

III

Conclusion

The hospital implementation of sepsis and antibiotic stewardship programs seems to be an effective strategy for reducing the mortality associated with severe sepsis by improving early patient identification, correct antibiotic therapy and adequate fluid resuscitation. These stewardship programs should involve nurses, physicians, pharmacists, microbiologists and health administrators and need to provide appropriate education and training to all the healthcare personnel. In addition, creation of specific processes of care (e.g., rapid response teams) and the evaluation of quality and effectiveness of clinical practice should be included in SSPs/ASPs. In the near future, simpler methods for earlier patient and microorganism identification and more effective therapies for patients with severe sepsis and septic shock will probably be available. In the meantime a structured multidisciplinary in-hospital approach to managing problems related to infections and sepsis seems to be a winning and mandatory strategy.

References

1. Esteban A, Frutos-Vivar F, Ferguson ND, et al (2007) Sepsis incidence and outcome: contrasting the intensive care unit with the hospital ward. Crit Care Med 35: 1284–1289
2. GiViTI (2010) Margherita Project. Available at http://www.giviti.marionegri.it/ Accessed Oct 2011
3. Dellinger RP, Levy MM, Carlet JM, et al (2008) Surviving Sepsis Campaign: international guidelines for management of severe sepsis and septic shock: 2008. Intensive Care Med 34: 17–60
4. Dellinger RP, Carlet JM, Masur H, et al (2004) Surviving Sepsis Campaign guidelines for management of severe sepsis and septic shock. Intensive Care Med 30: 536–555
5. Kahn JM,Bates DW (2008) Improving sepsis care: the road ahead. JAMA 299: 2322–2323
6. Funk D, Sebat F, Kumar A (2009) A systems approach to the early recognition and rapid administration of best practice therapy in sepsis and septic shock. Curr Opin Crit Care 15: 301–307
7. Shapiro NI, Howell MD, Talmor D, et al (2006) Implementation and outcomes of the Multiple Urgent Sepsis Therapies (MUST) protocol. Crit Care Med 34: 1025–1032
8. Nguyen HB, Corbett SW, Steele R, et al (2007) Implementation of a bundle of quality indicators for the early management of severe sepsis and septic shock is associated with decreased mortality. Crit Care Med 35: 1105–1112
9. Ferrer R, Artigas A, Levy MM, et al (2008) Improvement in process of care and outcome after a multicenter severe sepsis educational program in Spain. JAMA 299: 2294–2303
10. Castellanos-Ortega A, Suberviola B, Garcia-Astudillo LA, et al (2010) Impact of the Surviving Sepsis Campaign protocols on hospital length of stay and mortality in septic shock patients: results of a three-year follow-up quasi-experimental study. Crit Care Med 38: 1036–1043
11. Cardoso T, Carneiro AH, Ribeiro O, Teixeira-Pinto A, Costa-Pereira A (2010) Reducing

mortality in severe sepsis with the implementation of a core 6-hour bundle: results from the Portuguese community-acquired sepsis study (SACiUCI study). Crit Care 14:R83

12. Moro ML RD, Peghetti A, Melotti R (2007) Progetto LaSER Lotta alla sepsi in Emilia-Romagna Razionale, obiettivi, metodi e strumenti. Dossier 143. Available at http://asr.regi one.emilia-romagna.it/wcm/asr/collana_dossier/doss143/link/doss143.pdf Accessed Oct 2011

13. Girardis M, Baricchi R, Caramelli F, et al. (2011) Progetto lotta alla sepsi in Emilia Romagna. Minerva Anestesiol (in press)

14. Levy MM, Pronovost PJ, Dellinger RP, et al (2004) Sepsis change bundles: converting guidelines into meaningful change in behavior and clinical outcome. Crit Care Med 32:S595–7.

15. Kumar A, Roberts D, Wood KE, et al (2006) Duration of hypotension before initiation of effective antimicrobial therapy is the critical determinant of survival in human septic shock. Crit Care Med 34: 1589–1596

16. Dellit TH, Owens RC, McGowan JE, et al (2007) Infectious Diseases Society of America and the Society for Healthcare Epidemiology of America guidelines for developing an institutional program to enhance antimicrobial stewardship. Clin Infect Dis 44: 159–177

17. Levy MM, Dellinger RP, Townsend SR, et al (2010) The Surviving Sepsis Campaign: results of an international guideline-based performance improvement program targeting severe sepsis. Intensive Care Med 36: 222–231

18. Paul M, Shani V, Muchtar E, Kariv G, Robenshtok E, Leibovici L (2010) Systematic review and meta-analysis of the efficacy of appropriate empiric antibiotic therapy for sepsis. Antimicrob Agents Chemother 54: 4851–4863

19. Pea F,Viale P (2009) Bench-to-bedside review: Appropriate antibiotic therapy in severe sepsis and septic shock--does the dose matter? Crit Care 13: 214

20. Ziglam HM, Morales D, Webb K, Nathwani D (2006) Knowledge about sepsis among train-ing-grade doctors. J Antimicrob Chemother 57: 963–965

21. Pulcini C, Williams F, Molinari N, Davey P, Nathwani D (2011) Junior doctors' knowledge and perceptions of antibiotic resistance and prescribing: a survey in France and Scotland. Clin Microbiol Infect 17: 80–87

22. McKinley BA, Moore LJ, Sucher JF, et al (2011) Computer protocol facilitates evidence-based care of sepsis in the surgical intensive care unit. J Trauma 70: 1153–1166

23. Hitti EA, Lewin JJ, 3rd, Lopez J, et al (2011) Improving door-to-antibiotic time in severely septic emergency department patients. J Emerg Med 2011 Jul 5. [Epub ahead of print]

24. Barochia AV, Cui X, Vitberg D, et al. (2010) Bundled care for septic shock: an analysis of clinical trials. Crit Care Med 38: 668–78.

25. Ferrer R, Artigas A, Suarez D, et al (2009) Effectiveness of treatments for severe sepsis: a prospective, multicenter, observational study. Am J Respir Crit Care Med 180: 861–866

26. Reinhart K, Brunkhorst FM, Bone HG, et al (2010) Prevention, diagnosis, therapy and fol-low-up care of sepsis: 1st revision of S-2k guidelines of the German Sepsis Society (Deut-sche Sepsis-Gesellschaft e.V. (DSG)) and the German Interdisciplinary Association of Intensive Care and Emergency Medicine (Deutsche Interdisziplinare Vereinigung fur Intensiv- und Notfallmedizin (DIVI)). Ger Med Sci 8: Doc14

27. Alejandria MM, Lansang MA, Dans LF, Mantaring JB (2002) Intravenous immunoglobulin for treating sepsis and septic shock. Cochrane Database Syst Rev CD001090

28. Laupland KB, Kirkpatrick AW, Delaney A (2007) Polyclonal intravenous immunoglobulin for the treatment of severe sepsis and septic shock in critically ill adults: a systematic review and meta-analysis. Crit Care Med 35: 2686–2692

29. Kreymann KG, de Heer G, Nierhaus A, Kluge S (2007) Use of polyclonal immunoglobulins as adjunctive therapy for sepsis or septic shock. Crit Care Med 35: 2677–2685

30. Girardis M, Rinaldi L, Donno L, et al (2009) Effects on management and outcome of severe sepsis and septic shock patients admitted to the intensive care unit after imple-mentation of a sepsis program: a pilot study. Crit Care 13: R143

31. Cavazzuti I RL, Donno L, Braccini S, Busani S, Girardis M (2010) Early use of immuno-globulin in septic shock. Crit Care 14: P25

32. Berlot G, Vassallo MC, Busetto N, et al (2012) Relationship between the timing of admin-istration of IgM and IgA enriched immunoglobulins in patients with severe sepsis and septic shock and the outcome: A retrospective analysis. J Crit Care (in press)

IV Endocrine Support

The Corticotrophin Test in Critical Illness: Traps and Tricks

B. Venkatesh and J. Cohen

Introduction

The contribution of adrenal insufficiency to the morbidity of critically ill patients is currently under renewed scrutiny. Absolute adrenocortical insufficiency (diagnosed by very low plasma cortisol concentrations) is uncommon in the intensive care population. The diagnosis of relative adrenocortical insufficiency (RAI, elevated basal plasma cortisol with a subnormal increase in plasma concentrations following an adrenocorticotropic hormone [ACTH] stimulus) continues to generate much debate [1–3]. One of the most common dynamic testing procedures for assessment of adrenocortical function is the standard cosyntropin test (also known as the corticotrophin test, synacthen test, and ACTH stimulation test). The test comprises the measurement of plasma cortisol concentrations immediately prior, and at 30 and 60 minute intervals after, the intravenous administration of 250 μg of 1-24 ACTH. The normal response in unstressed volunteers is a rise in serum levels to above 500–550 nmol/l. In the setting of critical illness, the corticotrophin test has become the mainstay of diagnosis for suspected 'relative' adrenal insufficiency [4]. Although many diagnostic thresholds have been advocated, the most recent consensus guidelines suggest that an increase in measured cortisol of less than 250 nmol/l in response to the test is diagnostic of RAI. Early studies using these criteria suggested a strong association between the presence of RAI and poor outcome in patients with septic shock [5]. This observation, in conjunction with the findings of the first randomized controlled trial (RCT) on low dose corticosteroids in septic shock that demonstrated an improved outcome in patients with RAI given steroids [6], formed the basis for the Surviving Sepsis Campaign guidelines endorsing the performance of the corticotrophin test prior to steroid therapy [7]. These findings have not been consistently reproducible. However, the corticotrophin test was originally described in non-stressed subjects, and its applicability and interpretation in the setting of critical illness is controversial. In this chapter, we review the history and the evolution of corticotrophin testing methodology and discuss some of the controversies which continue to plague the test.

Physiological Basis of the Corticotrophin Test

Cortisol secretion is under the control of the hypothalamic-pituitary axis. There are a variety of stimuli to secretion, including stress, tissue damage, cytokine release, hypoxia, hypotension and hypoglycemia. These factors act upon the

J.-L. Vincent (ed.), *Annual Update in Intensive Care and Emergency Medicine 2012*
DOI 10.1007/978-3-642-25716-2 © Springer-Verlag Berlin Heidelberg 2012

hypothalamus to favor the release of corticotrophin releasing hormone (CRH) and vasopressin. These peptide hormones stimulate release of ACTH from the pituitary gland. ACTH in turn stimulates release of cortisol, mineralocorticoids (principally aldosterone) and androgens from the adrenal cortex. Cortisol levels feedback upon both CRH and ACTH to decrease further secretion. During periods of stress, trauma or infection, there is an increase in CRH and ACTH secretion and a reduction in the negative feedback effect, resulting in increased cortisol levels, in amounts roughly proportional to the severity of the illness. This complexity of the cortisol secretory and feedback loops can be taken advantage of in the evaluation of a patient for adrenal insufficiency. The principle behind the corticotrophin test is the demonstration of an *inappropriately* low cortisol production in response to exogenous ACTH, a situation analogous to physiological stress.

History

The corticotrophin test was first described in 1948 using hog pituitary extract as the source of ACTH and assessing changes in plasma cell count and urinary uric acid creatinine ratios as endpoints [8]. The development of purified corticotrophin and ability to measure plasma 17-hydroxycorticosteroids led to the establishment of 25 IU as the dose of corticotrophin which tested the maximal secretory capacity of the adrenal cortex [9]. Recombinant technology allowed the development of synthetic corticotrophin to minimize anaphylactic reactions. Schuler et al., using bioequivalence studies, established that 1 IU of purified corticotrophin = 10 μg of synthetic polypeptide [10]. This formed the basis for the use of 250 μg of synthetic polypeptide (as 25 IU tested the maximal secretory capacity) as the dose used in the dynamic assessment of adrenal function [11].

Interpretation of the Test

In the investigation of adrenal function in the stable outpatient population, it is the peak cortisol value post-stimulation that is used as the threshold value for normality [12, 13]. This is in marked contrast to the use of the test in the critically ill population in which the cortisol increment (the baseline cortisol subtracted from the peak) is used in the majority of studies. This is problematic, as there is evidence to suggest that the cortisol increment is not a valid indicator of adrenal function. May and Carey [14], in a study of 399 patients, demonstrated the dependence of the increment on the basal cortisol level. Speckart et al. observed an increment of less than 200 nmol/l in two out of nine healthy controls, although all the peak values were above 500 nmol/l [15]. A similar observation from Widmer et al. noted that a third of healthy controls did not achieve an increment of over 250 nmol/l, despite the peak cortisol values reaching 500 nmol/l in all cases [16]. Debono et al. investigated the corticotrophin test in patients undergoing cardiac surgery. These authors observed a 57 % incidence of an increment less than 250 nmol/l postoperatively despite the demonstration of a normal increment in all the patients one week beforehand [17]. Reliance on the cortisol increment in this setting raises the confusing scenario of a patient with a high peak cortisol but reduced increment being diagnosed with adrenal insufficiency

Table 1. Corticotropin test endpoint criteria: Use of peak and delta total cortisol and plasma free cortisol

	Total Cortisol Criteria	Free Cortisol Criteria
Peak post-synacthen [nmol/l]	700 [52]	85 [32]
	600 [53]	55 [48]
	550 [54]	33 [56]
	500 [55]	
Increment post-synacthen [nmol/l]	250 [57]	110 [61]
	200 [55]	76 [33]
	100 [58]	55 [48]
Basal [nmol/l]	690 [59]	55 [32]
	280 [57]	22 [48]

IV

whereas a counterpart with a lower peak cortisol but adequate increment is not. Comparison of peak total values versus the increment post-corticotropin is provided in **Table 1**.

Controversies

With widespread use of the test and publication of several studies relating to its use, controversies have emerged in both its conduct and interpretation. These are summarized below:

Methodological Factors

Dose of corticotrophin

As noted, the dose of corticotrophin traditionally used is an intravenous injection of 250 µg. Critics have pointed out that the 250 µg dose of corticotrophin results in supraphysiological plasma concentrations as high as 60000 pmol/l and may override adrenal resistance to ACTH, thus producing a false negative test with mild secondary adrenal insufficiency [18, 19]. Work by Landon et al. has shown that doses of corticotrophin as low as 250 ng are sufficient to test the sensitivity of the adrenal cortex. In contrast the 250 µg dose tests the maximal secretory capacity of the adrenal [20]. Consequently, a 'low-dose' corticotrophin test (1 µg) has been suggested which would result in more physiological concentrations (90 pmol/l) similar to those seen in the insulin hypoglycemia (70–100 pmol/l) and metyrapone tests [21, 22]. Data on what constitutes an appropriate response to 1 µg of corticotrophin in critically ill patients are minimal. Some authors have suggested that many patients in whom adrenal insufficiency is diagnosed on the basis of an abnormal response to a low-dose corticotrophin test (< 20 µg/dl) will have a normal response to the high-dose test, and that 40 % of patients with hypotension and sepsis have adrenal insufficiency diagnosed by the low-dose method. Widmer et al. suggested that there is a dissociation between the response to the high- and low-dose test in situations of high stress [16]. Furthermore, the cortisol response is also similar between the low-dose corticotrophin test and the insulin hypoglycemia test [21]. Data from several authors clearly suggest that the low-dose test is superior for identification of secondary adrenal insufficiency in the non-critically ill patient [23–25]. The low-dose test has also been shown to be more sensitive in the human immunodeficiency virus (HIV) infected critically ill patient population [26], and there are minimal published data in the septic critically ill population [27, 28]. Similar conclusions have been arrived at by Siraux et al. in the critically ill population [29].

Endpoints

The recommended endpoint is plasma total cortisol at 60 min after corticotrophin injection and the cut-off values are a delta cortisol of 250 nmol/l or a peak value > 550 nmol/l. Plasma free cortisol is the biologically active fraction and little heed was paid to changes in its concentrations following corticotrophin. There is a sound pathophysiological basis to consider plasma free cortisol rather than plasma total cortisol. In healthy volunteers, following corticotrophin stimulation, plasma total cortisol changed by 106 %, whereas plasma free cortisol changed by 263 % [30]. Moreover, cortisol binding globulin (CBG) and albumin concentrations decline in acute illness resulting in higher plasma free cortisol levels for the same amount of plasma total cortisol [31]. This finding was confirmed in an elegant study published by Hamrahian et al., in which they demonstrated that, in critically ill patients, despite evidence of RAI based on plasma total cortisol, there were no differences between the groups (RAI vs non-RAI) with respect to plasma free cortisol [32]. The role of free cortisol in interpreting the corticotrophin test remains controversial. Whereas one recent study of 49 patients with sepsis indicated a good correlation between total and free cortisol increments following a high dose corticotrophin test [33], another of 29 patients with septic shock reported no correlation between total and free increments after a low-dose test [28]. A comparison of the endpoints and the differences in the incidence of RAI obtained using total and free as well as the peak and the delta values is illustrated in **Table 1**.

Role of the cortisol assay

Total cortisol is commonly measured using immunoassays. Immunoassays are subject to significant inter-assay variability and endogenous interference by other steroid compounds. This was convincingly demonstrated in a trial by Cohen et al. in which four different assays were compared [34]. The coefficient of variation of cortisol estimations is usually 10–12 %, and the same specimen submitted to different assays can yield significantly different results. Variable plasma cortisol results due to different assays and/or laboratories will greatly influence the interpretation of plasma cortisol and the corticotrophin test [34]. This was subsequently confirmed in the Corticus sub-study [35].

Physiological and Pathophysiological Factors

Effect of protein concentrations

Cortisol is bound to CBG and albumin in the serum. In critical illness, concentrations of these proteins are frequently reduced [31, 32], resulting in altered bound-unbound ratios. This effect has been shown to have a significant impact on the interpretation of the corticotrophin test. For example, a serum albumin < 25 g/l results in significant differences in the threshold response compared to values > 25 g/l (peak cortisol 550 nmol/l vs 410 nmol/l, respectively). Similarly, variations in CBG have also been shown to influence the peak cortisol at 30 min [36].

Is the corticotrophin test a reliable reflector of the stress response?

The rationale behind the corticotrophin test is that if the adrenal gland responds well to an exogenous stimulus, it would be expected to respond in a similar fashion to an endogenous stress factor. Christ-Crain et al. examined changes in plasma total cortisol and plasma free cortisol following a standard corticotrophin test and during an endotracheal extubation process [37]. The increase in plasma free cortisol seen during physiological stress was much higher than that noted with the ACTH test. On the other hand, plasma total cortisol levels were not different between the two tests. The authors concluded that the ACTH test does not reliably identify the plasma free cortisol levels required during severe stress.

IV

Effect of plasma cortisol variability

Venkatesh et al. demonstrated significant fluctuations in plasma total cortisol over a 24 hour period [27]. This finding has significant implications for the interpretation of a random plasma cortisol. By measuring hourly cortisols in individual patients, these authors were able to assess maximal hourly fluctuations in plasma total cortisol. They were able to demonstrate that maximal spontaneous hourly rises in plasma cortisol exceeded those induced by corticotrophin thus raising questions about the validity of the corticotrophin test.

Effect of adrenal blood flow

An important determinant of the cortisol output by the adrenal cortex is the ACTH presentation rate to the zona glomerulosa, which in turn is influenced by adrenal blood flow. For the same plasma concentration of ACTH with differing blood flows to the adrenal gland, the one with the higher blood flow will result in higher cortisol output [38–40]. During shock states, there are reductions in blood flow to the adrenal cortex. This may be a transient phenomenon. The implication of this is that the final measurement of plasma cortisol following corticotrophin is not merely dependent upon the plasma ACTH concentration and the responsiveness of the glomerulosa cells, but is significantly influenced by other factors, such as cardiac output and adrenal blood flow. Consequently the timing of the test becomes critical.

Effect of body composition and endogenous and exogenous sex hormones

Klose et al. investigated the effect of body composition and sex hormones on the results of the corticotrophin test [41]. Central adiposity in men was an independent predictor of the ACTH response. Whereas endogenous sex hormone levels did not influence the test, total and calculated free cortisol responses were significantly influenced by the presence of the oral contraceptive pill.

Reproducibility of the Test

Given the alterations in cortisol production rates and metabolism in critical illness [42] and the dynamic nature of the inflammatory response, the optimal timing of the test has come under scrutiny. Further questions on the reliability of the short corticotrophin test in critically ill patients have been raised by investigations into its reproducibility over the time course of illness. Bouachour et al. performed consecutive short corticotrophin tests on 22 patients with septic shock over two days and found no correlation between the observed cortisol increments [43]. Comparable results were obtained by Loisa et al., who noted that 60 % of patients with septic shock who had an abnormal corticotrophin test result on the first day of testing had a normal result on the second day, whereas 30 % of patients with a normal result on the first day developed an abnormal result on the second [44].

The response of the test to treatment with hydrocortisone is also of interest. Given that the investigation is asserted to indicate a state of adrenal insufficiency, it would be reasonable to hypothesize that treatment with corticosteroids would revert an abnormal test result. Roquilly et al. performed a randomized trial of hydrocortisone in trauma patients with an abnormal corticotrophin test, and repeated the test at day 8 after treatment [45]. Patients who received hydrocortisone were observed to have a lower rate of development of ventilator-associated pneumonia (VAP), but had no reduction in the incidence of abnormal tests, which was significantly higher than in those who received placebo [45].

In summary, repetitive ACTH testing in critically ill patients with septic shock 24 h apart has shown poor reproducibility of the test and raises further questions about the validity of a single measurement of the ACTH response.

Other Dynamic Tests

The insulin tolerance test (ITT) and the metyrapone tests are two other dynamic endocrine investigations used in the non-critically ill patient (**Fig. 1**). These tests are associated with significant adverse effects and thus have no place in *routine* adrenal assessment in the intensive care unit (ICU) patient; their role in the critically ill patient remains to be determined.

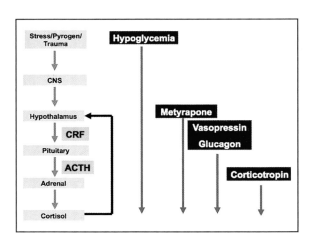

Fig. 1. Postulated sites of assessment of the HPA axis of the various tests during dynamic adrenal testing. From [60] with permission

Insulin Tolerance Test [24, 46]

Induction of hypoglycemic stress through the use of exogenous insulin is a potent stimulus for cortisol secretion through hypothalamic and pituitary activation. The ITT has long been considered the standard for the diagnosis of adrenal insufficiency because it assesses the integrity of the entire hypothalamic-pituitary-adrenal (HPA) axis. The major drawbacks of the ITT are that it is contraindicated in the elderly and in those with cardiovascular disease or seizure history. Short-acting regular insulin is injected intravenously at doses ranging between 0.1 U/kg and 0.15 U/kg. Adequate adrenal function is demonstrated by a peak cortisol level over 18 pg/dl at any time during the test, a cut-off that reliably separates normal controls from patients with adrenal insufficiency. Hypoadrenalism is demonstrated by a peak cortisol level of less than 18 pg/dl with symptomatic hypoglycemia [7]. As noted, there is concordance in the peak cortisol response between the insulin hypoglycemia test and the corticotropin stimulation test [21]. A rare patient will pass the ITT while exhibiting clinical adrenal insufficiency.

Metyrapone Test [47]

The metyrapone test was developed specifically as a test of pituitary reserve. Metyrapone inhibits the adrenal enzyme 11 beta-hydroxylase, which converts 11-desoxycortisol (compound S, 11-S) to cortisol in the final step of adrenal steroidogenesis. 11-S does not have glucocorticoid activity and, therefore, does not inhibit ACTH production. When metyrapone is given to a normal subject, the decline in serum cortisol stimulates ACTH production, driving adrenal steroidogenesis proximal to the enzyme blockade and causing 11-S to accumulate. When metyrapone is given to a patient with adrenal insufficiency of any type, 11-S fails to increase.

The potential limitations of the test include:

a) adverse reactions to metyrapone – mainly gastrointestinal
b) inability to guarantee enteral absorption of metyrapone in critically ill patients (an intravenous formulation is available)
c) interference of the test by concomitant administration of phenobarbitone or phenytoin

There are few published data on the metyrapone test in critical illness. Annane et al. examined the agreement between the corticotropin stimulation test and the metyrapone test in two septic cohorts and a group of non-septic critically ill patients [48]. There was little correlation between the two tests in identifying RAI in either group.

Glucagon Stimulation Test (GST) [49]

Although the GST is thought to be a test of HPA axis integrity and has been shown to be equivalent to the ITT and the corticotropin stimulation test, few data exist on its usefulness in critical illness.

Other Possible Tests

Plasma ACTH and CRH stimulation tests investigate the integrity of the HPA axis. However, few data are available on the usefulness of these tests in critically ill patients. Data from Venkatesh et al. suggest that plasma ACTH has no relationship with sickness severity, total plasma cortisol and urinary free cortisol and thus may not be a useful index of adrenal assessment [27]. Data on radiological investigations such as computed tomography (CT) and magnetic resonance imaging (MRI) of the adrenal cortex are limited at the present time.

Areas Requiring Further Investigation

1. Lack of a longitudinal assessment: Most studies have examined adrenal function at a single time point during a patient's hospitalization. Sepsis and critical illness are dynamic processes with both upregulation and downregulation of inflammation over the course of hospitalization. A longitudinal profile of adrenal function should be obtained to judge the extent of alterations.
2. Tissue cortisol activity: Recent research has identified an enzyme of steroid metabolism, 11β-hydroxysteroid dehydrogenase (HSD), which regulates intracellular concentrations of cortisone (inactive) and active cortisol. Disturbances of this enzyme system have been implicated in the pathogenesis of hypertension, obesity and vascular disease thus highlighting the pivotal role of elevated tissue cortisol concentrations in the genesis of these diseases. Preliminary data in inflammatory and septic states suggest that alterations of this enzyme system may lead to potentially elevated tissue cortisol concentrations, an argument against the adrenal insufficiency hypothesis [28, 42].

IV

Conclusion

The corticotrophin test was developed on sound physiological principles and has found widespread application in the evaluation of adrenocortical function in endocrine clinics. Its role in the critically ill patient to assess adrenocortical status is less well established. Several confounding variables exist, which have been outlined above. To have a 'one size fits all' approach with a single endpoint in the face of several methodological and pathophysiological confounders may be flawed and may result in inappropriate therapy. The results of the most recent RCT of steroids in septic shock by Sprung et al. [50] add further weight to the campaign against the corticotrophin test in its current form, and the revised Surviving Sepsis Campaign guidelines [51] find no benefit in testing for relative adrenal insufficiency and recommendations are that corticotrophin testing not be performed. We urge caution and more research before defining and developing guidelines for adrenal assessment.

References

1. Loriaux DL, Fleseriu M (2009) Relative adrenal insufficiency. Curr Opin Endocrinol Diabetes Obes 16: 392–400
2. Cohen J, Venkatesh B (2010) Relative adrenal insufficiency in the intensive care population; background and critical appraisal of the evidence. Anaesth Intensive Care 38: 425–436
3. Venkatesh B, Prins J, Torpy D, et al (2006) Relative adrenal insufficiency in sepsis: match point or deuce? Crit Care Resusc 8: 376–80
4. Ligtenberg J, Zijlstra J (2002) Relative adrenal insufficiency syndrome. In: Vincent JL (ed) 2002 Yearbook of Intensive Care and Emergency Medicine. Springer, Heidelberg, pp 492–498
5. Annane D, Sebille V, Troche G, Raphael JC, Gajdos P, Bellissant E (2000) A 3-level prognostic classification in septic shock based on cortisol levels and cortisol response to corticotropin. JAMA 283: 1038–1045
6. Annane D, Sebille V, Charpentier C, et al (2002) Effect of treatment with low doses of hydrocortisone and fludrocortisone on mortality in patients with septic shock. JAMA 288: 862–871

7. Dellinger RP, Carlet JM, Masur H, et al (2004) Surviving Sepsis Campaign guidelines for management of severe sepsis and septic shock. Crit Care Med 32: 858–873

8. Thorn GW, Forsham PH, et al (1948) A test for adrenal cortical insufficiency; the response to pituitary andrenocorticotropic hormone. JAMA 137: 1005–1009

9. Eik-Nes K, Sandberg AA, Nelson DH, Tyler FH, Samuels LT (1954) Changes in plasma levels of 17-hydroxycorticosteroids during the intravenous administration of ACTH. I. A test of adrenocortical capacity in the human. J Clin Invest 33: 1502–1508

10. Schuler W, Schar B, Desaulles P (1963) [On the pharmacology of an ACTH-active, fully synthetic polypeptide, beta1–24 corticotropin, Ciba 30920-Ba, Synacthen]. Schweiz Med Wochenschr 93: 1027–1030

11. Wood JB, Frankland AW, James VH, Landon J (1965) A rapid test of adrenocortical function. Lancet 1: 243–245

12. Oelkers W (1996) Adrenal insufficiency. N Engl J Med 335: 1206–1212

13. Arlt W, Allolio B (2003) Adrenal insufficiency. Lancet 361: 1881–1893

14. May ME, Carey RM (1985) Rapid adrenocorticotropic hormone test in practice. Retrospective review. Am J Med 79: 679–684

15. Speckart PF, Nicoloff JT, Bethune JE (1971) Screening for adrenocortical insufficiency with cosyntropin [synthetic ACTH]. Arch Intern Med 128: 761–763

16. Widmer IE, Puder JJ, Konig C, et al (2005) Cortisol response in relation to the severity of stress and illness. J Clin Endocrinol Metab 90: 4579–4586

17. Debono M, Sheppard L, Irving S, et al (2011) Assessing adrenal status in patients before and immediately after coronary artery bypass graft surgery. Eur J Endocrinol 164: 413–419

18. Cunningham SK, Moore A, McKenna TJ (1983) Normal cortisol response to corticotropin in patients with secondary adrenal failure. Arch Intern Med 143: 2276–2279

19. Dickstein G, Shechner C, Nicholson WE, et al (1991) Adrenocorticotropin stimulation test: effects of basal cortisol level, time of day, and suggested new sensitive low dose test. J Clin Endocrinol Metab 72: 773–778

20. Landon J, James VH, Wharton MJ, Friedman M (1967) Threshold adrenocortical sensitivity in man and its possible application to corticotrophin bioassay. Lancet 2: 697–700

21. Nye EJ, Grice JE, Hockings GI, et al (1999) Comparison of adrenocorticotropin [ACTH] stimulation tests and insulin hypoglycemia in normal humans: low dose, standard high dose, and 8-hour ACTH-[1–24] infusion tests. J Clin Endocrinol Metab 84: 3648–3655

22. Nye EJ, Grice JE, Hockings GI, et al (2001) Adrenocorticotropin stimulation tests in patients with hypothalamic-pituitary disease: low dose, standard high dose and 8-h infusion tests. Clin Endocrinol (Oxf) 55: 625–633

23. Dickstein G, Arad, Shechner C (1991) Low dose ACTH stimulation test. Endocrinologist 7: 285–293

24. Abdu TA, Elhadd TA, Neary R, Clayton RN (1999) Comparison of the low dose short synacthen test [1 microg], the conventional dose short synacthen test (250 microg), and the insulin tolerance test for assessment of the hypothalamo-pituitary-adrenal axis in patients with pituitary disease [see comments]. J Clin Endocrinol Metab 84: 838–843

25. Broide J, Soferman R, Kivity S, et al (1995) Low-dose adrenocorticotropin test reveals impaired adrenal function in patients taking inhaled corticosteroids. J Clin Endocrinol Metab 80: 1243–1246

26. Marik PE, Kiminyo K, Zaloga GP (2002) Adrenal insufficiency in critically ill patients with human immunodeficiency virus. Crit Care Med 30: 1267–1273

27. Venkatesh B, Mortimer RH, Couchman B, Hall J (2005) Evaluation of random plasma cortisol and the low dose corticotropin test as indicators of adrenal secretory capacity in critically ill patients: a prospective study. Anaesth Intensive Care 33: 201–209

28. Cohen J, Lassig-Smith M, Deans R, et al (2012) Serial changes in plasma total cortisol, plasma free cortisol and tissue cortisol activity in patients with septic shock. An observational study. Shock 37: 28–33

29. Siraux V, De Backer D, Yalavatti G, et al (2005) Relative adrenal insufficiency in patients with septic shock: comparison of low-dose and conventional corticotropin tests. Crit Care Med 33: 2479–2486

30. Vogeser M, Briegel J, Zachoval R (2002) Dialyzable free cortisol after stimulation with Synacthen. Clin Biochem 35: 539–543

IV

IV

31. Beishuizen A, Thijs L, Vermes I (2001) Patterns of corticosteroid-binding globulin and the free cortisol index during septic shock and multitrauma. Intensive Care Med 27: 1584–1591
32. Hamrahian AH, Oseni TS, Arafah BM (2004) Measurements of serum free cortisol in critically ill patients. N Engl J Med 350: 1629–1638
33. Molenaar N, Groeneveld J, Dijstelbloem H, et al (2011) Assessing adrenal insufficiency of corticosteroid secretion using free versus total cortisol levels in critical illness. Intensive Care Med 37: 1986–1993
34. Cohen J, Ward G, Prins J, Jones M, Venkatesh B (2006) Variability of cortisol assays can confound the diagnosis of adrenal insufficiency in the critically ill population. Intensive Care Med 32: 1901–1905
35. Briegel J, Sprung CL, Annane D, et al (2009) Multicenter comparison of cortisol as measured by different methods in samples of patients with septic shock. Intensive Care Med 35: 2151–2156
36. Dhillo WS, Kong WM, Le Roux CW, et al (2002) Cortisol-binding globulin is important in the interpretation of dynamic tests of the hypothalamic--pituitary--adrenal axis. Eur J Endocrinol 146: 231–235
37. Christ-Crain M, Jutla S, Widmer I, et al (2007) Measurement of serum free cortisol shows discordant responsivity to stress and dynamic evaluation. J Clin Endocrinol Metab 92: 1729–1735
38. Urquhart J (1965) Adrenal blood flow and the adrenocortical response to corticotropin. Am J Physiol 209: 1162–1168
39. Urquhart J, Li CC (1968) The dynamics of adrenocortical secretion. Am J Physiol 214: 73–85
40. Jones CT, Edwards AV, Bloom SR (1990) The effect of changes in adrenal blood flow on adrenal cortical responses to adrenocorticotrophin in conscious calves. J Physiol 429: 377–386
41. Klose M, Lange M, Rasmussen AK, et al (2007) Factors influencing the adrenocorticotropin test: role of contemporary cortisol assays, body composition, and oral contraceptive agents. J Clin Endocrinol Metab 92: 1326–1333
42. Venkatesh B, Cohen J, Hickman I, et al (2007) Evidence of altered cortisol metabolism in critically ill patients: a prospective study. Intensive Care Med 33: 1746–1753
43. Bouachour G, Roy PM, Guiraud MP (1995) The repetitive short corticotropin stimulation test in patients with septic shock. Ann Intern Med 123: 962–963
44. Loisa P, Uusaro A, Ruokonen E (2005) A single adrenocorticotropic hormone stimulation test does not reveal adrenal insufficiency in septic shock. Anesth Analg 101: 1792–1798
45. Roquilly A, Mahe PJ, Seguin P, et al (2011) Hydrocortisone therapy for patients with multiple trauma: the randomized controlled HYPOLYTE study. JAMA 305: 1201–1209
46. Greenwood FC, Landon J, Stamp TC (1966) The plasma sugar, free fatty acid, cortisol, and growth hormone response to insulin. I. In control subjects. J Clin Invest 45: 429–436
47. Liddle GW, Estep HL, Kendall JW Jr, Williams WC Jr, Townes AW (1959) Clinical application of a new test of pituitary reserve. J Clin Endocrinol Metab 19: 875–894
48. Annane D, Maxime V, Ibrahim F, Alvarez JC, Abe E, Boudou P (2006) Diagnosis of adrenal insufficiency in severe sepsis and septic shock. Am J Respir Crit Care Med 174: 1319–1326
49. Rao RH, Spathis GS (1987) Intramuscular glucagon as a provocative stimulus for the assessment of pituitary function: growth hormone and cortisol responses. Metabolism 36: 658–663
50. Sprung CL, Annane D, Keh D, et al (2008) Hydrocortisone therapy for patients with septic shock. N Engl J Med 358: 111–124
51. Dellinger RP, Levy MM, Carlet JM, et al (2008) Surviving Sepsis Campaign: International guidelines for management of severe sepsis and septic shock: 2008. Intensive Care Med 34: 17–60
52. Bourne RS, Webber SJ, Hutchinson SP (2003) Adrenal axis testing and corticosteroid replacement therapy in septic shock patients--local and national perspectives. Anaesthesia 58: 591–596
53. Faber M, Flachs H, Frimodt-Moller N, Lindholm J (1993) Hyponatremia and adrenocortical function in patients with severe bacterial infections. Scand J Infect Dis 25: 101–105

54. Manglik S, Flores E, Lubarsky L, Fernandez F, Chhibber VL, Tayek JA (2003) Glucocorticoid insufficiency in patients who present to the hospital with severe sepsis: a prospective clinical trial. Crit Care Med 31: 1668–1675
55. Bouachour G, Tirot P, Gouello JP, Mathieu E, Vincent JF, Alquier P (1995) Adrenocortical function during septic shock. Intensive Care Med 21: 57–62
56. Lewis JG, Bagley CJ, Elder PA, Bachmann AW, Torpy DJ (2005) Plasma free cortisol fraction reflects levels of functioning corticosteroid-binding globulin. Clin Chim Acta 359: 189–194
57. Marik PE, Pastores SM, Annane D, et al (2008) Recommendations for the diagnosis and management of corticosteroid insufficiency in critically ill adult patients: consensus statements from an international task force by the American College of Critical Care Medicine. Crit Care Med 36: 1937–1949
58. de Jong MF, Beishuizen A, Spijkstra JJ, Groeneveld AB (2007) Relative adrenal insufficiency as a predictor of disease severity, mortality, and beneficial effects of corticosteroid treatment in septic shock. Crit Care Med 35: 1896–1903
59. Marik PE, Zaloga GP (2003) Adrenal insufficiency during septic shock. Crit Care Med 31: 141–145
60. Landon J, James VH, Stoker DJ (1965) Plasma-cortisol response to lysine-vasopressin. Comparison with other tests of human pituitary-adrenocortical function. Lancet 2: 1156–119
61. Ho JT, Al-Musalhi H, Chapman MJ, et al (2006) Septic shock and sepsis: a comparison of total and free plasma cortisol levels. J Clin Endocrinol Metab 91: 105–114

Glitazones: Could They Have a Rosy Future in Critical Care?

S.K.M. Marment, A.J. Semark, and P.S. Kruger

IV

Introduction

The thiazolidinediones (glitazones) are drugs used in the management of diabetes. They are classified as synthetic selective peroxisome proliferator-activated receptor (PPAR) agonists and examples include rosiglitazone, pioglitazone, troglitazone and ciglitazone. The issues that have emerged around rosiglitazone and its cardiovascular side effects have dominated much of the discussion of these agents in the literature.

As the use of these agents increases in patients with type II diabetes, practicing critical care clinicians will require greater familiarity with them. The unintentional discontinuation of medications for chronic illnesses after acute hospital admission and in particular after intensive care unit (ICU) admission has recently been highlighted [1]. Although increased familiarity with the rationale for long-term prescribing may help reduce this problem, it is also realized that some chronic medications may have benefits to patients beyond those of their usual indication. In some cases, this may have particular relevance to the critically ill [2, 3].

In this chapter, we review the role of glitazones in the management of diabetes but also potential roles in neurological injury and inflammatory states such as sepsis.

Glitazones in the Treatment of Type II Diabetes Mellitus

Type II diabetes is a complex disorder characterized by hyperglycemia secondary to peripheral insulin resistance and pancreatic beta cell dysfunction. Activation of PPARγ by glitazones enhances the action of insulin by increasing glucose uptake in skeletal muscle and adipose tissue and inhibiting hepatic gluconeogenesis and glycolysis. In addition to their role as PPAR agonists, glitazones also increase pancreatic beta cell function.

Glitazones were approved in 1999 for the treatment of type II diabetes after large scale clinical trials demonstrated improvements in glucose control as manifested by lower glycosylate hemoglobin (HbA1c) values [4]. Their approval and subsequent large scale use based solely on trials showing improvement in a surrogate endpoint has generated considerable controversy. Current consensus guidelines from the American Diabetes Association and the European Association for the Study of Diabetes recommend pioglitazone as a second line option if HbA1c targets are not met despite lifestyle modification and metformin, and the risk of hypoglycemia with insulin or sulphonylureas is undesirable [5].

J.-L. Vincent (ed.), *Annual Update in Intensive Care and Emergency Medicine 2012*
DOI 10.1007/978-3-642-25716-2 © Springer-Verlag Berlin Heidelberg 2012

In patients with impaired glucose tolerance, glitazones have recently been shown to reduce the development of diabetes [6] and may be superior to metformin in this regard [7]. The two currently available glitazones are pioglitazone and rosiglitazone.

The Peroxisome Proliferator-Activated Receptors

The PPARs are a super family of nuclear receptors for steroid, thyroid and retinoid hormones. They are dependent on ligand binding for activation and three isoforms have been indentified: Alpha (α), beta/delta (β/δ) and gamma (γ). The alpha receptor is largely expressed in the liver and is involved in the regulation of fatty acid oxidation. Beta/delta receptors are ubiquitously expressed in the gut, epidermis, placenta, skeletal muscle, and adipose tissues; they function as a key regulator of energy homeostasis. PPARγ receptors are essential for glucose metabolism. Initially the synthetic PPARγ agonists were introduced as insulin sensitizers in the management of type II diabetes.

The γ receptor in fact has numerous isoforms and is expressed on vascular endothelial cells, smooth muscle cells, B and T lymphocytes, monocytes, macrophages and cardiac myocytes. Recent literature suggests that through PPARγ stimulation, glitazones affect the transcription of pro-inflammatory cytokines as well as factors affecting angiogenesis, vascular tone and cell growth and differentiation [8]. These so called pleiotropic effects of glitazones may provide the basis for novel therapeutic indications including a role in attenuating the inflammatory response associated with sepsis.

The PPARγ receptor functions through transrepression. Transrepression is a protein-protein interaction which results in the inhibition of gene expression. Usually a transcription factor for genetic upregulation is inhibited. Ligand binding and stimulation of the PPARγ receptor results in inhibition of genetic transcription.

Pharmacology and Safety

Glitazones have been studied in several large scale clinical trials and over a decade of post-marketing experience. Each particular glitazone agent has very different receptor interactions and pharmacodynamic effects. This likely affects both their therapeutic and their toxic effects. Rosiglitazone is 10 times more potent than pioglitazone at activating PPARγ. Pioglitazone is also a partial agonist of PPARα.

At present, only oral formulations are available. Both drugs are well absorbed with good bioavailability. Both glitazones are metabolized by cytochrome P450 enzymes, mainly 2C8 with lesser contributions from 3A4 in the case of pioglitazone and 2C9 for rosiglitazone. Neither has been shown to cause clinically significant enzyme induction or inhibition. There are few active metabolites and dose adjustment is not necessary in renal impairment.

Adverse Effects

Many side effects of glitazones seem to be drug specific, which may relate to their different patterns of gene modulation [9]. A recognized complication of the use of glitazones is the finding of fluid retention and associated heart failure in some patients prescribed glitazones [10]. Glitazones are associated with reduced sodium excretion and increased sodium and water retention as well as increased endothelial permeability. Studies utilizing echocardiography have shown no change in left ventricular mass or function with glitazone use and thus a direct toxic effect on cardiac myocytes is thought to be unlikely [10]. A meta-analysis published in 2007 cast doubt over the safety of rosiglitazone showing a 43 % increase in myocardial infarction and 64 % increase in cardiovascular related death [12]. This meta-analysis included previously unpublished trials and led to rosiglitazone being withdrawn across the European Union and its use restricted in the United States and Australia. Pioglitazone has a dramatically different cardiovascular profile, associated with a significant reduction in death, myocardial infarction and stroke in the recent PROactive trial [11]. The reason for the different cardiovascular effects between rosiglitazone and pioglitazone is unclear but could be related to their differing effects on lipid profiles. Rosiglitazone use is associated with increased low density lipoproteins and triglycerides while pioglitazone causes a reduction in both triglycerides and high density lipoproteins and a lesser increase in low density lipoproteins [13]. In addition, rosiglitazone has also been shown to activate matrix metalloprotease 3, an enzyme linked to plaque rupture [14].

The first glitazone approved for clinical use, troglitazone, was withdrawn due to cases of severe hepatotoxicity. The incidence of hepatic dysfunction in clinical trials of pioglitazone and rosiglitazone has not been different to those in the placebo groups [10]. It is still recommended that glitazones are not initiated in patients with an elevated alanine aminotransferase (ALT, greater than 2.5 times normal) and should be stopped if the ALT rises to greater than three times normal [15]. Rosiglitazone is not recommended in Child's B or C cirrhosis due to evidence of decreased clearance. Other reported side effects include macular edema and osteoporosis [13]. Recent commentaries suggest that given similar efficacy in diabetes and the differing side effect profile, no role currently exists for prescribing rosiglitazone [10].

Role in inflammation

Glitazones appear to influence the inflammatory pathway at several levels (**Fig. 1**). PPARγ activation in immune cells results in the inhibition of pro-inflammatory gene expression. Glitazones reduce synthesis of pro-inflammatory cytokines in macrophages, T cells and endothelial cells. *In vitro* studies demonstrate that PPARγ agonists reduce the secretion of cytokines including tumor necrosis factor (TNF)-α, interleukin (IL)-1β, and IL-6 [16]. Elevated IL-6 and TNF-α levels predict mortality in sepsis [17]. Further anti-inflammatory actions of glitazones are mediated through the suppression of nuclear factor-kappa B (NF-κB) [18] and transrepression of genes encoding inducible nitric oxide synthase (iNOS). Activated NF-κB activates an array of genes encoding acute phase proteins, cytokines and iNOS. The inhibition of NF-κB is achieved by reducing the quantity of cofactors that function to activate NF-κB.

IV

Fig. 1. Glitazone interaction with the peroxisome proliferator-activated receptor (PPAR) and the biological consequences. ⊕ denotes stimulation, ⊘ denotes inhibition, ↑ denotes an increase, and ↓ a decrease. RxR: Retinoid X receptor; HSP: heat shock protein; ROS: reactive oxygen species; MMP: matrix metalloproteinases: TNF-α tumor necrosis factor alpha; NF-κB: nuclear factor-kappa B; iNOS: inducible nitric oxide synthase; HDL: high density lipoproteins; LDL: low density lipoproteins

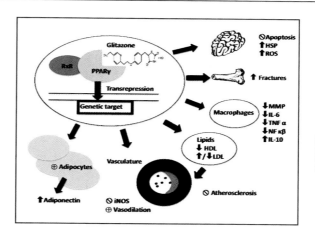

Atherosclerosis is well established as an inflammatory disease and experimental evidence from animal models shows that glitazones reduce inflammation, foam cell formation, smooth muscle proliferation and increased plaque stability [19]. In early clinical studies, pioglitazone was shown to reduce atheroma progression in both coronary and carotid vessels whereas mixed results were seen with rosiglitazone. The recently published PROactive study demonstrated a significant improvement in a composite secondary endpoint of death, myocardial infarction and stroke, in diabetic patients treated with pioglitazone [11]. This contrasts with rosiglitazone, which has been linked to increased rates of myocardial infarction and cardiovascular related mortality [12]. Recent studies suggest the reduced atheroma progression could be related to changes in lipid profile associated with pioglitazone use [21].

How Adiponectin Might Fit Into The Picture?

Adiponectin is a protein secreted by adipocytes, which increases insulin sensitization and has potent anti-inflammatory properties. Diabetes and obesity are known to be associated with lower levels of adiponectin and the experimental models suggest a possible protective effect of adiponectin. Adiponectin synthesis is increased by both rosiglitazone and pioglitazone and is reduced by glucocorticoids and catecholamines [22–25]. It has a central role in the pathophysiology of the metabolic syndrome and is of increasing interest in critical illness [26]. Studies demonstrate that high circulating levels of TNF-α and IL-6 inhibit the secretion of adiponectin. Adiponectin has a direct inhibitory affect on the secretion of these pro-inflammatory cytokines and increases levels of the anti-inflammatory cytokine, IL-10. The anti-inflammatory effects of adiponectin are, at least in part, due to the direct suppression of mature macrophage TNF-α secretion and the inhibition of the maturation of macrophage precursors [27]. Low levels of adiponectin are associated with vasodilatation and may contribute to the vasoplegic shock of sepsis [28].

Studies of adiponectin levels in sepsis yield conflicting results. Adiponectin levels in ICU patients have been reported to be lower [29, 30] or no different [31] than levels in healthy controls. In a study of 170 critically patients, those with diabetes or obesity had reduced adiponectin levels although, interestingly, low adiponectin levels at ICU admission were also independent positive predictors of short-term and overall survival [31].

Use in Other Diseases

IV

Recognition of the potential anti-inflammatory effects of glitazones has led to interest in a number of other diseases. Many experimental studies and early clinical trials have recently been published on the effects of glitazones in a diverse range of conditions including multiple sclerosis, Alzheimer's disease, Parkinson's disease, non-alcoholic steatohepatitis and inflammatory bowel disease. Potential roles in the treatment of several cancers have also been suggested based on experimental evidence showing that glitazones cause cell cycle arrest, induce apoptosis and inhibit tumor angiogenesis [32]. Several trials have also suggested a role in treating lipoatrophy associated with highly active antiretroviral therapy for human immunodeficiency virus (HIV) infection [33]. A role in modulating allergy has been postulated in animal studies [34] and a small randomized trial has shown improved lung function in smoking asthmatics taking rosiglitazone compared to inhaled betamethasone [35]

Studies in Sepsis

Sepsis and the systemic inflammatory response syndrome are associated with leukocyte activation and the release of several pro-inflammatory cytokines and oxygen free radicals. These substances are involved in the pathogenesis and manifestations of sepsis as they interact with various biological substrates inducing membrane dysfunction, tissue damage and organ injury.

Animal Studies in Sepsis

Glitazones have been studied in a number of different animal models of sepsis and inflammation. In rodent cecal ligation and puncture models of polymicrobial sepsis, glitazones have been shown to reduce mortality, ameliorate hypotension, reduce expression of inflammatory markers, such as TNF-α and IL-6 [36, 37], and reduce neutrophil infiltration of major organs [38]. Uji et al. were able to demonstrate that these beneficial effects were absent in adiponectin knock-out rodents providing further support for the close association between PPARγ, adiponectin and TNF-α [39]. Wu and colleagues exposed rodents to bacterial endotoxin and demonstrated a significant reduction in TNF-α and IL-6 and interestingly an amelioration of renal dysfunction, with lower urea and creatinine and improved hemodynamics in rodents exposed to glitazones [40]. Beneficial effects of glitazones have also been found in rodent models of pancreatitis and burns with attenuated organ dysfunction and reduced inflammatory markers [20, 41].

Human Studies in Sepsis

There is a paucity of research into the effects of glitazones in human sepsis. In a small study of children with septic shock, both PPARγ activity in peripheral blood monocytes and high molecular weight adiponectin levels were higher in comparison with matched controls [42]. In a small placebo controlled study of healthy humans injected with endotoxin, pioglitazone mitigated the hypotension but had no effect on IL-6 or TNF-α levels [43].

Studies are not all positive, with a recent meta-analysis of data from randomized controlled trials suggesting that long term use of glitazones is associated with a modestly increased risk of pneumonia (number needed to harm 239 patients) [44]. This data provides an interesting paradox, particularly in regard to the data surrounding long term statin use. A recent study has suggested that much of the long term benefit associated with statin use is due to a reduction in infections and pneumonia more than to a reduction in cardiovascular morbidity [3]. This is an evolving field in which further studies are required to clarify the biological impact of glitazone therapy beyond glucose control.

Perhaps the most interesting study of glitazones in infection relates to their potential use in malaria. In a small pilot study by Boggild and colleagues [45], patients with uncomplicated *Plasmodium falciparum* malaria who received rosiglitazone had higher rates of parasite clearance and lower levels of IL-6. At least part of this beneficial effect can be explained by the fact that PPARγ agonists have been shown to increase levels of CD36, a molecule that mediates macrophage clearance of malarial parasites [45].

Role in Traumatic Brain Injury, Spinal Cord Injury and Stroke

Recent experimental work has also suggested a role for glitazones in improving outcome from focal and global cerebral ischemia, spinal cord injury and traumatic brain injury (TBI). Propagation of secondary injury in TBI and ischemic insults is related to multiple processes including glutamate excitotoxicity, apoptosis, inflammation, edema, ionic imbalance and oxidative stress [46]. PPARγ expression in the brain is localized to microglia and astrocytes, cells that play a crucial role in inflammation. In animal models, glitazones reduce the expression of pro-inflammatory cytokines and macrophage infiltration of injured central nervous system (CNS) tissue [47, 48].

Glitazones have several other potentially beneficial actions in addition to their anti-inflammatory effects. They reduce apoptosis in injured CNS tissue, increase the expression of heat shock proteins, which are known to reduce glutamate release and oxidative stress, and increase anti-oxidant proteins [47]. Their ability to affect multiple processes may give glitazones an advantage over other agents that target only single pathways.

Despite its lower potency with regards to PPARγ agonism, pioglitazone has a theoretical advantage given its better CNS penetration compared to rosiglitazone. Not all the beneficial effects of glitazones may be mediated through the PPARγ receptor, with some investigators postulating that partial agonism of the PPARα receptor by pioglitazone may be important [48]. The clinical relevance of these differences is currently unclear.

A meta-analysis of animal studies of glitazones in ischemic stroke found that they reduced infarct volume and improved neurological outcome [49]. Both pioglitazone and rosiglitazone were effective. The beneficial effects were seen even when treatment was delayed up to 24 hours following the injury. Beneficial effects on motor function have also been found for both glitazones in rodent models of

IV

spinal cord injury when given at the time of injury [50]. In rodent models of TBI, pioglitazone and rosiglitazone have been found to reduce contusion size and improve neurological outcomes [47, 48].

Conclusion

IV

The thiazolidinediones have undergone extensive laboratory and clinical study as an adjunct to the management of type II diabetes. Some of the more notable adverse effects are most likely specific to individual drugs rather than the class of agents in general. At present, pioglitazone appears to have an increasing role in preventing vascular complications and improving outcomes for patients with diabetes or impaired glucose tolerance. Preliminary studies have suggested a more general modulation of inflammation that may have future clinical relevance. Promising animal and laboratory data now warrant additional clinical studies, particularly in patients with infection and neurological injury. Potential concerns regarding adverse effects, such as fluid retention, heart failure and liver dysfunction, require clarification in critically ill patients. This is an evolving field and further studies are required to clarify the biological impact of glitazone therapy beyond glucose control.

References

1. Bell CM, Brener SS, Gunraj N, et al (2011) Association of ICU or hospital admission with unintentional discontinuation of medications for chronic diseases. JAMA 306: 840–847
2. Kruger PS (2006) Statins: the next anti-endotoxin. Crit Care Resusc 8: 223–226
3. Sever PS, Chang CL, Gupta AK, Whitehouse A, Poulter NR (2011) The Anglo-Scandinavian Cardiac Outcomes Trial: 11-year mortality follow-up of the lipid-lowering arm in the UK. Eur Heart J 32: 2525–2532
4. Sherifali D, Nerenberg K, Pullenayegum E, Cheng JE, Gerstein HC (2010) The effect of oral antidiabetic agents on A1C levels: a systematic review and meta-analysis. Diabetes Care 33: 1859–1864
5. Nathan DM, Buse JB, Davidson MB, et al (2009) Medical management of hyperglycemia in type 2 diabetes: A consensus algorithm for the initiation and adjustment of therapy. Diabetes Care 32: 193–203
6. DeFronzo RA, Tripathy D, Schwenke DC, et al (2011) Pioglitazone for diabetes prevention in impaired glucose tolerance. N Engl J Med 364: 1104–1115
7. DeFronzo RA, Abdul-Ghani M (2011) Type 2 diabetes can be prevented with early pharmacological intervention. Diabetes Care 34 (Suppl 2): S202-S209
8. Kalaitzidis RG, Sarafidis PA, Bakris GL (2009) Effects of thiazolidinediones beyond glycaemic control. Curr Pharm Des 15: 529–536
9. Hsiao A, Worrall DS, Olefsky JM, Subramaniam S (2004) Variance-modeled posterior inference of microarray data: detecting gene-expression changes in 3T3-L1 adipocytes. Bioinformatics 20: 3108–3127
10. Tolman KG (2011) The safety of thiazolidinediones. Expert Opin Drug Saf 10: 419–428
11. Dormandy JA, Charbonnel B, Eckland DJ, et al (2005) Secondary prevention of macrovascular events in patients with type 2 diabetes in the PROactive Study (PROspective pioglitAzone Clinical Trial In macroVascular Events): a randomised controlled trial. Lancet 366: 1279–1289
12. Nissen SE, Wolski K (2007) Effect of rosiglitazone on the risk of myocardial infarction and death from cardiovascular causes. N Engl J Med 356: 2457–2471
13. Shah P, Mudaliar S (2010) Pioglitazone: side effect and safety profile. Expert Opin Drug Saf 9: 347–354

14. Wilson KD, Li Z, Wagner R, et al (2008) Transcriptome alteration in the diabetic heart by rosiglitazone: implications for cardiovascular mortality. PLoS One 3: e2609
15. MacIsaac R, Jerums G (2004) Clinical Indications for thiazolidinediones. Australian Prescriber 27: 70–74
16. Jiang C, Ting AT, Seed B (1998) PPAR-gamma agonists inhibit production of monocyte inflammatory cytokines. Nature 391: 82–86
17. Pierrakos C, Vincent JL (2010) Sepsis biomarkers: a review. Crit Care 14: R15
18. Ghanim H, Garg R, Aljada A, et al (2001) Suppression of nuclear factor-kappaB and stimulation of inhibitor kappaB by troglitazone: evidence for an anti-inflammatory effect and a potential antiatherosclerotic effect in the obese. J Clin Endocrinol Metab 86: 1306–1312
19. Wang N, Yin R, Liu Y, Mao G, Xi F (2011) Role of peroxisome proliferator-activated receptor-γ in atherosclerosis. Circ J 75: 528–535
20. Sener G, Sehirli AO, Gedik N, Dulger GA (2007) Rosiglitazone, a PPAR-gamma ligand, protects against burn-induced oxidative injury of remote organs. Burns 33: 587–593
21. Nicholls SJ, Tuzcu, EM, Wolski, K, et al (2011) Lowering the triglyceride/high-density lipoprotein cholesterol ratio is associated with the beneficial impact of pioglitazone on progression of coronary atherosclerosis in diabetic patients: insights from the PERISCOPE (Pioglitazone Effect on Regression of Intravascular Sonographic Coronary Obstruction Prospective Evaluation) study. J Am Coll Cardiol 57: 153–159
22. Fasshauer M, Klein J, Neumann S, Eszlinger M, Paschke R (2001) Adiponectin gene expression is inhibited by beta-adrenergic stimulation via protein kinase A in 3T3-L1 adipocytes. FEBS Lett 507: 142–146
23. Fasshauer M, Klein J, Neumann S, Eszlinger M, Paschke R (2002) Hormonal regulation of adiponectin gene expression in 3T3-L1 adipocytes. Biochem Biophys Res Commun 290: 1084–1089
24. Lihn AS, Richelsen B, Pedersen SB, et al (2003) Increased expression of TNF-alpha, IL-6, and IL-8 in HALS: implications for reduced adiponectin expression and plasma levels. Am J Physiol Endocrinol Metab 285: E1072–1080
25. Coletta DK, Sriwijitkamol A, Wajcberg E, et al (2009) Pioglitazone stimulates AMP-activated protein kinase signalling and increases the expression of genes involved in adiponectin signalling, mitochondrial function and fat oxidation in human skeletal muscle in vivo: a randomised trial. Diabetologia 52: 723–732
26. Robinson K, Kruger PS, Prins J, Venkatesh B (2011) The metabolic syndrome in critically ill patients. Best Pract Res Clin Endocrinol Metab 25: 835–845
27. Yokota T, Oritani K, Takahashi I, et al (2000) Adiponectin, a new member of the family of soluble defense collagens, negatively regulates the growth of myelomonocytic progenitors and the functions of macrophages. Blood 96: 1723–1732
28. Ouchi N, Ohishi M, Kihara S, et al (2003) Association of hypoadiponectinemia with impaired vasoreactivity. Hypertension 42: 231–234
29. Hillenbrand A, Knippschild U, Weiss M, et al (2010) Sepsis induced changes of adipokines and cytokines – septic patients compared to morbidly obese patients. BMC Surg 10: 26
30. Venkatesh B, Hickman I, Nisbet J, Cohen J, Prins J (2009) Changes in serum adiponectin concentrations in critical illness: a preliminary investigation. Crit Care 13: R105
31. Koch A, Sanson E, Voigt S, et al (2011) Serum adiponectin upon admission to the intensive care unit may predict mortality in critically ill patients. J Crit Care 26: 166–174
32. Galli A, Mello T, Ceni E, Surrenti E, Surrenti C (2006) The potential of antidiabetic thiazolidinediones for anticancer therapy. Expert Opin Investig Drugs 15: 1039–1049
33. Raboud J, Diong C, Carr A, et al (2010) A meta-analysis of six placebo-controlled trials of thiazolidinedione therapy for HIV lipoatrophy. HIV Clin Trials 11: 39–50
34. Wang W, Zhu Z, Zhu B, Ma Z (2010) Pioglitazone attenuates allergic inflammation and induces production of regulatory T lymphocytes. Am J Rhinol Allergy 24: 454–458
35. Spears M, Donnelly I, Jolly L, et al (2009) Bronchodilatory effect of the PPAR-gamma agonist rosiglitazone in smokers with asthma. Clin Pharmacol Ther 86: 49–53
36. Uji Y, Yamamoto H, Maeda K, et al (2010) Adiponectin deficiency promotes the production of inflammatory mediators while severely exacerbating hepatic injury in mice with polymicrobial sepsis. J Surg Res 161: 301–311
37. Zingarelli B, Sheehan M, Hake PW, et al (2003) Peroxisome proliferator activator receptor-

gamma ligands, 15-deoxy-Delta(12,14)-prostaglandin J2 and ciglitazone, reduce systemic inflammation in polymicrobial sepsis by modulation of signal transduction pathways. J Immunol 171: 6827–6837

38. Haraguchi G, Kosuge H, Maejima Y, et al (2008) Pioglitazone reduces systematic inflammation and improves mortality in apolipoprotein E knockout mice with sepsis. Intensive Care Med 34: 1304–1312

39. Uji Y, Yamamoto H, Tsuchihashi H, et al (2009) Adiponectin deficiency is associated with severe polymicrobial sepsis, high inflammatory cytokine levels, and high mortality. Surgery 145: 550–557

40. Wu WT, Lee CC, Lee CJ, et al (2011) Rosiglitazone ameliorates endotoxin-induced organ damage in conscious rats. Biol Res Nurs 13: 38–43

41. Cuzzocrea S, Pisano B, Dugo L, et al (2004) Rosiglitazone, a ligand of the peroxisome proliferator-activated receptor-γ, reduces the development of nonseptic shock induced by zymosan in mice. Crit Care Med 32: 457–466

42. Kaplan JM, Denenberg A, Monaco M, et al (2010) Changes in peroxisome proliferator-activated receptor-gamma activity in children with septic shock. Intensive Care Med 36: 123–130

43. Schaller G, Kolodjaschna J, Pleiner J, et al (2008) Pioglitazone does not affect vascular or inflammatory responses after endotoxemia in humans. Horm Metab Res 40: 549–555

44. Singh S, Loke YK, Furberg CD (2011) Long-term use of thiazolidinediones and the associated risk of pneumonia or lower respiratory tract infection: systematic review and meta-analysis. Thorax 66: 383–388

45. Boggild AK, Krudsood S, Patel SN, et al (2009) Use of peroxisome proliferator-activated receptor γ agonists as adjunctive treatment for Plasmodium falciparum malaria: A randomized, double-blind, placebo-controlled trial. Clin Infect Dis 49: 841–849

46. Kunz A, Dirnagl U, Mergenthaler P (2011) Acute pathophysiological processes after ischaemic and traumatic brain injury. Best Pract Res Clin Anaesthesiol 24: 495–509

47. Yi JH, Park SW, Brooks N, Lang BT, Vemuganti R (2008) PPAR agonist rosiglitazone is neuroprotective after traumatic brain injury via anti-inflammatory and anti-oxidative mechanisms. Brain Res 1244: 164–172

48. Sauerbeck A, Gao J, Readnower R, et al (2011) Pioglitazone attenuates mitochondrial dysfunction, cognitive impairment, cortical tissue loss, and inflammation following traumatic brain injury. Exp Neurol 227: 128–135

49. White AT, Murphy AN (2010) Administration of thiazolidinediones for neuroprotection in ischemic stroke: a pre-clinical systematic review. J Neurochem 115: 845–853

50. Park SW, Yi JH, Miranpuri G, et al (2007) Thiazolidinedione class of peroxisome proliferator-activated receptor agonists prevents neuronal damage, motor dysfunction, myelin loss, neuropathic pain, and inflammation after spinal cord injury in adult rats. J Pharmacol Exp Ther 320: 1002–1012

IV

V Acute Respiratory Distress Syndrome

V

The Complex Interaction between Sepsis and Lung Injury

R. Herrero, I. Martin-Loeches, and A. Artigas

Introduction

V

Sepsis is a major cause of acute lung injury (ALI) and its more severe form, the acute respiratory distress syndrome (ARDS) [1, 2]. In addition, sepsis frequently complicates the clinical course of patients with ALI of other etiologies. The most common cause of ALI/ARDS is pneumonia (bacterial, viral or fungal), followed by severe sepsis from pulmonary or non-pulmonary infections [2, 3]. Sepsis accounts for approximately 25 to 40 % of cases of ALI/ARDS, the risk of ALI being especially high in the presence of intense systemic inflammatory response, shock and multiorgan dysfunction. The association of sepsis with disseminated intravascular coagulation (DIC) also increases the risk of progression to ALI/ARDS [3, 4].

Sepsis is a clinical condition characterized by systemic inflammation in the setting of severe infection. In the intensive care unit (ICU), the incidence and mortality of sepsis are 12 % and 40 %, respectively [5]. ALI/ARDS is one of the most frequent organ dysfunctions to develop in patients with severe sepsis [2]. The Surviving Sepsis Campaign (SSC) provided guidelines for the care of patients with severe sepsis and septic shock, and compliance with these recommendations has been associated with reduced mortality. Lung protective strategies in patients who required mechanical ventilation, in particular the use of low tidal volumes and pressure limitation, have been clearly associated with a better outcome in patients with ALI/ARDS [5–8].

Patients with sepsis-related ALI have been reported to have higher mortality and more severe multiorgan dysfunction than patients with ALI from other causes. However, sepsis is not an independent predictor of mortality. Instead, the development of multiorgan dysfunction is considered the main factor explaining the higher mortality of patients with ALI associated with sepsis [9].

Pathogenesis of Sepsis-Induced Acute Lung Injury

ALI/ARDS is characterized by widespread neutrophilic alveolitis with important disruption of the alveolar endothelial and epithelial barriers, which leads to protein-rich edema formation in the interstitium and alveolar spaces [10]. The mechanisms by which sepsis causes ALI are not completely understood. Endotoxin has been detected in plasma samples and in bronchoalveolar (BAL) fluid of patients with established ARDS, who also show an upregulation of endotoxin recognition pathways in the lungs [11, 12]. These observations suggest that endotoxin is

J.-L. Vincent (ed.), *Annual Update in Intensive Care and Emergency Medicine 2012*
DOI 10.1007/978-3-642-25716-2 © Springer-Verlag Berlin Heidelberg 2012

involved in the development of ARDS. Intra-tracheal instillation of bacterial lipopolysaccharide (LPS) in healthy subjects causes an acute inflammatory response in the lungs with neutrophil migration. In experimental animals, the intravenous or intratracheal administration of LPS causes lung injury with increased pulmonary protein permeability and edema formation associated with alveolar inflammation and damage of cells in the alveolar wall [13, 14]. Exoproducts of bacteria, such as elastase and *Pseudomonas* exoenzyme U, also cause injury to the lung [15]. Similar results have been found in experimental sepsis induced by intravenous administration of live *Pseudomonas aeruginosa* and acute peritonitis secondary to cecal ligation and puncture [16].

Mechanical ventilation has been shown to interact with infectious agents to increase lung injury and inflammation in laboratory animals [17]. A synergistic effect on the development of lung injury with the combination of endotoxin and mechanical ventilation was observed in adult mice but not in juvenile mice, suggesting that such synergism develops with age [18]. Mechanical ventilation also reduces bacterial clearance and contributes to the translocation of bacteria and their products from the alveoli to the bloodstream, which may contribute to the development of systemic infection and multiorgan dysfunction [19].

Fever associated with sepsis may be an additional factor that increases the degree of lung damage. In animal models of ALI induced by live bacteria or exogenous bacterial products, hyperthermia increased mortality and augmented lung damage by enhancing apoptotic and inflammatory signaling through the tumor necrosis factor (TNF)-receptor superfamily [20].

Mechanisms of Sepsis-induced Acute Lung Injury

The mechanisms by which infection and sepsis injure the lungs are not totally understood. The direct cytotoxic effect of bacteria and other microorganisms does not seem to be sufficient to cause lung injury, indicating that other factors are probably involved. Infection- and sepsis-induced alterations of the inflammatory response, coagulation and cell death pathways are likely to contribute to the development of ALI (**Fig. 1**).

Pathogen Recognition

The rapid response of the innate immune system to infection occurs through the recognition of pathogen-associated molecular patterns (PAMPs), which are molecules associated to groups of pathogens. Examples of PAMPs include LPS, a component of the outer membrane of Gram-negative bacteria, and lipoteichoic acid (LTA), a major constituent of Gram-positive bacteria. Phagocytic cells involved in host defense express receptors in the cell surface that recognize these PAMPs. Activation of these pattern recognition receptors (PRRs) results in endocytosis of the offending pathogen and/or activation of intracellular signaling cascades with release of inflammatory mediators, leading to the activation and recruitment of inflammatory cells to the site of infection. Two of these PRRs are the Toll-like receptors (TLRs) and CD14. Endotoxin induces lung inflammation via TLR4, whereas LTA activates inflammatory responses via TLR2 [21]. CD14 is a receptor on the surface of monocytes and macrophages and, in association with TLRs, mediates responses to LPS and to other cell-wall products from Gram-negative

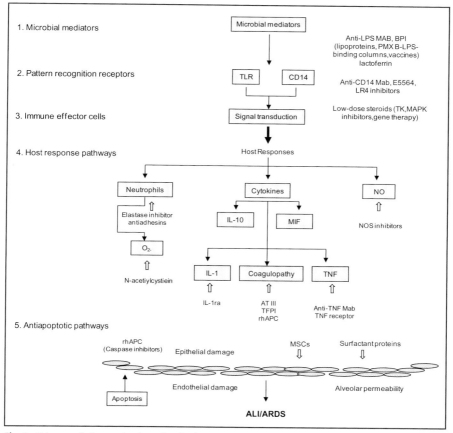

Fig. 1. Scheme of the mechanisms involved in sepsis-induced acute lung injury (ALI), and proposed therapeutic strategies. TLR: Toll-like receptor; IL: interleukin; NO: nitric oxide; LPS: lipopolysaccharide; TNF: tumor necrosis factor; BPI: bactericidal/permeability-increasing protein; MIF: macrophage migration inhibitory factor. Adapted from [50]

and -positive bacteria [12]. Inhibition of these receptors blocks systemic cytokine responses, reduces lung protein leak, and improves survival in experimental models [22]. Genetic factors also influence the susceptibility and severity of sepsis and ALI. Some single nucleotide polymorphisms (SNPs) in genes related to pathogen receptors (CD14 and TLRs) have been associated with increased incidence and higher mortality rates in sepsis and sepsis-induced ALI [23].

Inflammation

Cellular and humoral inflammatory responses are activated in sepsis. These inflammatory responses are essential in early host defense, but also contribute to later organ injury, including ALI. The degree of activation of this protective host inflammatory response, rather than the precipitating insult, seems to be the major factor influencing patient outcome in ALI/ARDS [24].

Neutrophils

Migration of polymorphonuclear neutrophils (PMNs) into the lung occurs within hours after a septic insult. In animal models of sepsis-induced ALI, endotoxin stimulates innate immunity cells and causes an overexpression of cytokines and chemokines, which mediate migration of neutrophils into the lung. Activated PMNs release toxic mediators including proteases (e.g., elastase, collagenase, metalloproteinases), cationic peptides (defensins), reactive oxygen (O_2^-, H_2O_2, OH^-, HOCl) and nitrogen (NO and $ONOO^-$) species, pro-inflammatory cytokines and procoagulant molecules. These toxic mediators may damage both the alveolar-epithelial and -endothelial barriers. Patients with neutropenia, however, also develop ARDS, indicating that a neutrophil-independent mechanism also occurs [25, 26].

Pulmonary migration of PMNs toward alveolar spaces requires first the adhesion of PMNs to the lung endothelial and epithelial cells. This intercellular communication between infiltrating neutrophils, endothelium and epithelium is mediated by cell-surface adhesion molecules. The most important of these adhesion molecules expressed in PMNs and endothelial cells are selectins (L-selectin in PMN and E-selectin in endothelial cells) and B_2-integrins (CD11/CD18, in the surface of PMNs). The intercellular adhesion molecule-1 (ICAM-1), expressed on the surface of endothelial cells, binds to the integrin receptors CD11/CD18 of the activated neutrophils to maintain tight adherence between neutrophils and endothelial cells [26]. Sepsis has been shown to increase the expression of CD11b and CD11b/c on leukocytes from blood, lung tissue and BAL fluid [26]. New evidence indicates that the way that endothelial cells interact with PMNs might be different in patients with sepsis and patients with other risk factors (no sepsis) for ARDS. In this context, Moss et al observed that the serum concentrations of ICAM-1 and E-selectin were higher in patients with sepsis compared to trauma patients at risk of ARDS [27].

At sites of vascular damage, adherent platelets interact with circulating neutrophils and release factors into the circulation, including cytokines, which may have deleterious local and systemic effects on blood and endothelial cells [28]. Other lines of evidence based on experimental endotoxin-induced lung injury show that lymphocytes, in contrast, may contribute to the resolution of lung injury [29].

Cytokines

Following an endotoxin challenge, the biological activity of BAL fluid is known to increase, due in part to the release of cytokines (TNF-α, TNF receptors, interleukin [IL]-1, IL-1 receptor antagonist [IL-1ra], IL-6, and granulocyte-colony stimulating factor [G-CSF]) and chemokines (IL-8, endothelial nitric oxide synthase-associated protein [ENAP]-78, monocyte chemotactic protein [MCP]-1, macrophage inflammatory protein [MIP]-1) to the alveolar space. These cytokines and chemokines are produced locally in the lung by endothelial cells, epithelial cells, alveolar macrophages and neutrophils. TNF-α and IL-1β are major cytokines released into the alveolar spaces of patients with ARDS, which propagate the inflammatory response initiated by endotoxin. The cytokine levels in patients with sepsis-induced ALI differ from those in patients with non-sepsis-induced ALI. Comparing sepsis-induced ALI with trauma-induced ALI, patients with sepsis had higher increases in TNF-α and IL-6 in blood. Large amounts of TNF-α and IL-6 in patients with septic shock correlate with fatal outcome [9, 30]. The combination of ARDS and pneumonia was also associated with higher levels of

IL-8 compared with ARDS or pneumonia alone. Excessive or unregulated release of cytokines results in disruption of the alveolar-capillary membrane and can also lead to adverse systemic effects. Although measurement of cytokine levels in plasma or BAL fluid does not clearly predict the development of ARDS, persistently elevated cytokine concentrations (TNF-α, IL-1β, IL-6, IL-8) in BAL fluid or plasma in patients with ARDS are associated with poor prognosis [31]. In patients with sepsis and ALI/ARDS, several SNPs in genes related to inflammatory markers (TNF-α, IL-6, IL-1ra, pre-B-cell colony-enhancing factor) also correlate with more severe illness and mortality [23].

Coagulation

Alterations of the coagulation system have long been recognized to be an integral part of inflammation, sepsis and ALI. Coagulation is activated as a result of systemic and local injury, and participates in the innate response to bacterial infection. An intense activation of coagulation plays a critical role in the pathogenesis of severe sepsis and ALI, diseases in which it is a strong independent predictor of mortality [3].

BAL fluid from patients with ALI reflects an increase in procoagulant activity with elevated levels of soluble tissue factor (TF), activated factor VII (FVIIa), TF-dependent factor X, thrombin, fibrinopeptide A and D-dimer. Concomitantly, there is a decrease in fibrinolytic activity, as shown by decreased BAL levels of urokinase and increased levels of the fibrinolysis inhibitors, plasminogen activator inhibitor (PAI) and α2-antiplasmin. In addition, the BAL fluid from patients with ARDS shows impaired natural anticoagulant mechanisms, manifested by a reduction in activated protein C levels. This reduction in activated protein C levels is one of the strongest predictors of an adverse outcome and mortality in patients with sepsis or ALI. In patients with ALI, elevated levels of PAI-1 in the plasma and pulmonary edema fluid are also predictive of mortality [32].

In patients with sepsis-induced ALI, plasma protein C levels are lower and Von Willebrand factor (vWF) antigen levels are higher compared to those with ALI not related to sepsis [27]. This pro-coagulant environment contributes to the pathophysiology of ALI by causing intra-alveolar, interstitial and endovascular fibrin deposition. This intravascular fibrin deposition contributes to organ failure as a direct result of obstructive thrombus in small vessels and via enhancement of endothelial-PMN interactions. Alveolar interstitial accumulation of fibrin promotes pulmonary neutrophil migration, surfactant dysfunction, and pro-fibrotic processes, all of which contribute to lung injury [33]. The intrapulmonary fibrin deposition in patients with ARDS is thought to be mediated by the interaction of TF and FVIIa. In sepsis, a similar procoagulant environment develops rapidly in the vascular space when bacteria enter the circulation. In animal models of sepsis induced by *Escherichia coli*, the TF-FVIIa complex contributes to lung injury in part through selective stimulation of pro-inflammatory cytokine release and fibrin deposition [34]. Specific SNPs of coagulation factor genes (α-thrombin, fibrinogen, factor V, protein C, endothelial protein C receptor, and PAI-1) appear to increase the risk of coagulation in the vascular spaces and airspaces of the lung, thus influencing the risk of ALI in patients with sepsis [23].

Cell Death

Necrosis of alveolar epithelial cells in the lungs of patients who die with ALI/ARDS is thought to be caused by mechanical factors, local ischemia, bacterial products (toxins released by *Pseudomonas* sp., *E. coli* or *Staphylococcus aureus*) and/or lytic viruses in the airspaces. Apoptotic cells have also been found in the alveolar wall of these patients, especially in patients who died from ARDS [10]. One of the consequences of necrosis and apoptosis is loss of cellular attachment, resulting in exposure of the underlying alveolar epithelial basement membrane to inflammatory products, such as oxidants, proteinases, and inflammatory factors. Exposure to these factors increases the alveolar damage and contributes to fibroblast activation and collagen deposition, which can lead to lung fibrosis [10]. Evidence of extensive alveolar epithelial cell apoptosis has been described in murine models of LPS-induced lung injury [35]. In the acute phase of lung injury in septic ARDS patients, there is upregulation of the Fas ligand/Fas system, one of the major apoptotic pathways (**Fig. 2**) [36, 37].

Fas is a death receptor on the cell surface that is activated by its natural ligand, Fas ligand (FasL). Activation of Fas induces apoptosis and modulates the inflammatory response in experimental models of sepsis-induced ALI [13, 35]. Fas is

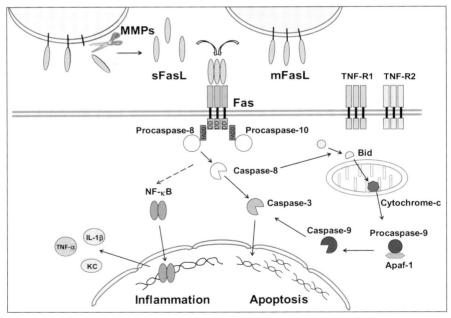

Fig. 2. Cellular pathways of apoptosis and inflammation in sepsis and ALI. A family of death receptors including the Fas/FasL system and the tumor necrosis factor (TNF)-receptors (TNFR1 and TNFR2) can initiate apoptosis and inflammation. Membrane FasL can be cleaved by the proteolytic action of metalloproteinases 7 and 3 (MMP-7, MMP-3) into a soluble form. Both membrane FasL (mFasL) and the soluble FasL (sFasL) can aggregate and activate Fas receptor on the cell surface of target cells. Aggregation of Fas is followed by a series of intracellular molecular interactions that coordinate the activation of caspases and cell death, as well as nuclear factor-kappa B (NF-κB) and inflammation. IL: interleukin; Apaf: apoptotic protease activating factor

detectable in airway epithelial cells (Clara cells) and alveolar type II cells, and the expression of Fas in epithelial cells increases in response to LPS. Soluble FasL is released into the alveolar spaces of patients with ARDS at concentrations that induce apoptosis in human lung distal epithelial cells cultured *in vitro* [36]. Cells recovered from the airspaces of patients with ARDS release soluble FasL, which further increases after stimulation with LPS. This is particularly relevant, since LPS is also present in the BAL fluid of patients with ARDS [12]. Moreover, FasL mRNA is increased in the cellular component of BAL fluid retrieved from patients with early septic ARDS [38]. This suggests that FasL is produced or released locally in the airspace compartment in sepsis-induced ALI. In murine models of sepsis-induced ALI, a functional Fas/FasL system was required for the development of alveolar wall permeability changes, apoptosis and inflammation (neutrophil migration and cytokine production) in the lung, as lung injury was significantly attenuated in Fas-deficient mice [14]. In other studies, Fas-deficient mice had significantly reduced mortality from hypoxia-induced lung injury during *Legionella* pneumonia [39]. Apoptosis in the alveolar epithelial cells and activation of inflammatory responses in the lung can also be induced through activation of TNF and angiotensin II receptors on the cell surface [40, 41]. Following exposure to LPS, live bacteria, and sepsis, therefore, apoptotic pathways appear to play an important role for the development of ALI by inducing apoptosis and inflammation in the lungs. In addition, factors such as hypoxia, hyperoxia (high FiO_2) and mechanical ventilation, may also contribute to apoptosis of pulmonary epithelial cells in patients with sepsis and ALI.

Alveolar Endothelial and Epithelial Permeability

As a result of widespread endothelial damage, increased vascular permeability typically develops in patients with sepsis and leads to microvascular leak and tissue edema, which may impair the function of the lungs and other organs. After the recognition of bacteria or bacterial products, released cytokines activate endothelial cells by upregulating their adhesion receptors, inducing the binding of neutrophils, monocytes, macrophages and platelets to endothelial cells. These effector cells release further inflammatory mediators, proteases, oxidants, prostaglandins and leukotrienes that can damage the structure and function of the vascular endothelium. Indeed, they can induce gaps between endothelial cells by disassembly of intercellular adherence junctions, by altering the cellular cytoskeletal structure, or by directly inducing endothelial cell death [42]. In the development of ALI/ARDS, endothelial cell damage is one of the initial events and is usually accompanied by alveolar epithelial cell damage. The alteration of both the endothelial and epithelial barrier will lead to alveolar flooding and formation of protein-rich edema inside the alveoli, resulting in acute respiratory failure [10]. In sepsis, there is also an increase in the activity of inducible nitric oxide synthase (iNOS) leading to the synthesis of nitric oxide (NO) [43]. Increased NO promotes further vasodilation that may also contribute to more edema formation. Therefore, early restoration of the vascular integrity in sepsis and ALI might be critical for the prevention or improvement of sepsis and ALI.

Treatment of Sepsis-Induced Acute Lung Injury

Lung-protective ventilation techniques have reduced the mortality of ALI from 40 % to 25 % in the last decade. In addition, the use of a fluid-conservative strategy in patients with ARDS has reduced the duration of mechanical ventilation. New pharmacological therapies have been evaluated in patients with sepsis and ALI/ARDS [33]. Some of these therapies are exogenous surfactants, glucocorticoids, inhaled NO, intravenous prostaglandin E1, antioxidants (N-acetylcysteine), inflammatory inhibitors, protease inhibitors, some anticoagulants (antithrombin III or tissue factor pathway inhibitor) or TLR-4 inhibitors. However, none of these therapies has been shown to be fully effective [44, 45].

Given that sepsis is a major cause of lung injury, studies of new therapies for sepsis could be directly relevant for the treatment of lung injury. Based on their beneficial effects in sepsis, clinical trials testing the therapeutic value of statins in patients with ALI are currently in progress. Activated protein C, a molecule with anticoagulant, anti-inflammatory, fibrinolytic and antiapoptotic effects, is a novel therapy approved for the treatment of patients with severe sepsis, based on the results of the Recombinant Human Activated Protein C Worldwide Evaluation in Severe Sepsis (PROWESS) clinical trial [46]. Activated protein C lowered mortality rates and reduced circulatory dysfunction and respirator-dependent days in patients with severe sepsis, but its therapeutic value on the progression of ARDS remains to be determined [33, 44, 46]. The complex mechanisms involved in the development of ALI/ARDS make it difficult to find a successful pharmaceutical therapy. Future studies may require a greater focus on the early identification of patients at risk for ALI/ARDS, as well as those patients who are at the earliest phase of the disease by using more sensitive and specific biomarkers. New therapies targeting specific populations of patients with ALI according to their mechanisms of injury (sepsis vs non-sepsis ALI) and degree of severity are also important. Finally, optimizing therapy may also require a combination of different therapeutic agents as well as evaluation of their local administration directly into the lung.

One promising new treatment for ALI is transplantation of bone-marrow derived mesenchymal stem cells (MSCs). Recent studies in mice indicate that MSCs may be of value in treating ALI as well as sepsis. MSCs possess the ability to differentiate into many types of cells, including vascular endothelium and alveolar epithelium. MSCs also secrete paracrine factors, including keratin growth factors, which can be protective for the lung. In experimental models of sepsis-induced ALI, the direct intrapulmonary administration of MSCs decreased lung injury and mortality. It has been suggested that these beneficial effects are independent of the MSCs and derive instead from their paracrine actions. It is thought that paracrine factors from MSCs can regulate barrier permeability and modulate inflammation in injured lungs by decreasing pro-inflammatory response and increasing anti-inflammatory cytokines, particularly IL-10 levels [47]. Several investigators are working on translating these experimental studies into phase I and II clinical trials in patients with severe ALI.

Utilization of new therapies for sepsis could contribute directly and indirectly to limit the progression of ALI/ARDS. In this line, lactoferrin, phospholipid LPS binders, methods of filtration/absorption of LPS or other microbial components (polymyxin B column), and other new therapeutic strategies with different anti-infective activities are currently being tested [48, 49].

Conclusion

Sepsis remains the leading cause of ALI/ARDS. Although numerous studies have provided valuable information on the pathogenesis of sepsis and ALI/ARDS, the mechanisms that directly link these two clinical conditions have not been fully defined. A better understanding of the initial mechanisms by which sepsis induces ALI and of how they might differ from those involved in ALI not related to sepsis could be essential for finding effective therapeutic targets for each condition. In this line, the development of new specific pharmacologic or cell-based therapies is currently a major focus of research in sepsis and ALI/ARDS.

Acknowledgement: This work was funded by the CIBER Network of Pulmonary Diseases and the Instituto de Salud Carlos III (Fondo de Investigación Sanitaria, FISPI080646).

V

References

1. Gajic O, Dabbagh O, Park PK, et al (2011) Early identification of patients at risk of acute lung injury: evaluation of lung injury prediction score in a multicenter cohort study. Am J Respir Crit Care Med 183: 462–470
2. Hudson LD, Steinberg KP (1999) Epidemiology of acute lung injury and ARDS. Chest 116: 74S-82S
3. Iscimen R, Cartin-Ceba R, Yilmaz M, et al (2008) Risk factors for the development of acute lung injury in patients with septic shock: an observational cohort study. Crit Care Med 36: 1518–1522
4. Fein AM, Calalang-Colucci MG (2000) Acute lung injury and acute respiratory distress syndrome in sepsis and septic shock. Crit Care Clin 16: 289–317
5. Dellinger RP, Levy MM, Carlet JM, et al (2008) Surviving Sepsis Campaign: international guidelines for management of severe sepsis and septic shock: 2008. Intensive Care Med 34: 17–60
6. Suarez D, Ferrer R, Artigas A, Azkarate I, et al (2011) Cost-effectiveness of the Surviving Sepsis Campaign protocol for severe sepsis: a prospective nation-wide study in Spain. Intensive Care Med 37: 444–452
7. Ferrer R, Artigas A, Suarez D, et al (2009) Effectiveness of treatments for severe sepsis: a prospective, multicenter, observational study. Am J Respir Crit Care Med 180: 861–866
8. Ferrer R, Artigas A, Levy MM, et al (2008) Improvement in process of care and outcome after a multicenter severe sepsis educational program in Spain. JAMA 299: 2294–2303
9. Sheu CC, Gong MN, Zhai R, et al (2010) Clinical characteristics and outcomes of sepsis-related vs non-sepsis-related ARDS. Chest 138: 559–567
10. Ware LB, Matthay MA (2000) The acute respiratory distress syndrome. N Engl J Med 342: 1334–1349
11. Martin TR, Rubenfeld GD, Ruzinski JT, et al (1997) Relationship between soluble CD14, lipopolysaccharide binding protein, and the alveolar inflammatory response in patients with acute respiratory distress syndrome. Am J Respir Crit Care Med 155: 937–944
12. Martin TR (2000) Recognition of bacterial endotoxin in the lungs. Am J Respir Cell Mol Biol 23: 128–132
13. Matute-Bello G, Winn RK, Martin TR, Liles WC (2004) Sustained lipopolysaccharide-induced lung inflammation in mice is attenuated by functional deficiency of the Fas/Fas ligand system. Clin Diagn Lab Immunol 11: 358–361
14. Perl M, Chung CS, Lomas-Neira J, et al (2005) Silencing of Fas, but not caspase-8, in lung epithelial cells ameliorates pulmonary apoptosis, inflammation, and neutrophil influx after hemorrhagic shock and sepsis. Am J Pathol 167: 1545–1559
15. Kudoh I, Wiener-Kronish JP, Hashimoto S, Pittet JF, Frank D (1994) Exoproduct secretions of Pseudomonas aeruginosa strains influence severity of alveolar epithelial injury. Am J Physiol 267: L551–556

16. Brigham KL, Woolverton WC, Blake LH, Staub NC (1974) Increased sheep lung vascular permeability caused by pseudomonas bacteremia. J Clin Invest 54: 792–804
17. Altemeier WA, Matute-Bello G, Frevert CW, et al (2004) Mechanical ventilation with moderate tidal volumes synergistically increases lung cytokine response to systemic endotoxin. Am J Physiol Lung Cell Mol Physiol 287: L533–542
18. Smith LS, Gharib SA, Frevert CW, Martin TR (2010) Effects of age on the synergistic interactions between lipopolysaccharide and mechanical ventilation in mice. Am J Respir Cell Mol Biol 43: 475–486
19. Kurahashi K, Ota S, Nakamura K, et al (2004) Effect of lung-protective ventilation on severe Pseudomonas aeruginosa pneumonia and sepsis in rats. Am J Physiol Lung Cell Mol Physiol 287: L402–410
20. Lipke AB, Matute-Bello G, Herrero R, et al (2010) Febrile-range hyperthermia augments lipopolysaccharide-induced lung injury by a mechanism of enhanced alveolar epithelial apoptosis. J Immunol 184: 3801–3813
21. Faure E, Equils O, Sieling PA, et al (2000) Bacterial lipopolysaccharide activates NF-kappaB through toll-like receptor 4 (TLR-4) in cultured human dermal endothelial cells. Differential expression of TLR-4 and TLR-2 in endothelial cells. J Biol Chem 275: 11058–11063
22. Seki H, Tasaka S, Fukunaga K, et al (2010) Effect of Toll-like receptor 4 inhibitor on LPS-induced lung injury. Inflamm Res 59: 837–845
23. Reddy AJ, Kleeberger SR (2009) Genetic polymorphisms associated with acute lung injury. Pharmacogenomics 10: 1527–1539
24. Monchi M, Bellenfant F, Cariou A, et al (1998) Early predictive factors of survival in the acute respiratory distress syndrome. A multivariate analysis. Am J Respir Crit Care Med 158: 1076–1081
25. Martin TR (2002) Neutrophils and lung injury: getting it right. J Clin Invest 110: 1603–1605
26. Pittet JF, Mackersie RC, Martin TR, Matthay MA (1997) Biological markers of acute lung injury: prognostic and pathogenetic significance. Am J Respir Crit Care Med 155: 1187–1205
27. Moss M, Gillespie MK, Ackerson L, Moore FA, Moore EE, Parsons PE (1996) Endothelial cell activity varies in patients at risk for the adult respiratory distress syndrome. Crit Care Med 24: 1782–1786
28. Li Z, Yang F, Dunn S, Gross AK, Smyth SS (2011) Platelets as immune mediators: their role in host defense responses and sepsis. Thromb Res 127: 184–188
29. Venet F, Chung CS, Huang X, Lomas-Neira J, Chen Y, Ayala A (2009) Lymphocytes in the development of lung inflammation: a role for regulatory CD4+ T cells in indirect pulmonary lung injury. J Immunol 183: 3472–3480
30. Martin C, Boisson C, Haccoun M, Thomachot L, Mege JL (1997) Patterns of cytokine evolution (tumor necrosis factor-alpha and interleukin-6) after septic shock, hemorrhagic shock, and severe trauma. Crit Care Med 25: 1813–1819
31. Meduri GU, Kohler G, Headley S, Tolley E, Stentz F, Postlethwaite A (1995) Inflammatory cytokines in the BAL of patients with ARDS. Persistent elevation over time predicts poor outcome. Chest 108: 1303–1314
32. Welty-Wolf KE, Carraway MS, Ortel TL, Piantadosi CA (2002) Coagulation and inflammation in acute lung injury. Thromb Haemost 88: 17–25
33. Matthay MA, Zemans RL (2011) The acute respiratory distress syndrome: pathogenesis and treatment. Annu Rev Pathol 6: 147–163
34. Miller DL, Welty-Wolf K, Carraway MS, et al (2002) Extrinsic coagulation blockade attenuates lung injury and proinflammatory cytokine release after intratracheal lipopolysaccharide. Am J Respir Cell Mol Biol 26: 650–658
35. Kitamura Y, Hashimoto S, Mizuta N, et al (2001) Fas/FasL-dependent apoptosis of alveolar cells after lipopolysaccharide-induced lung injury in mice. Am J Respir Crit Care Med 163: 762–769
36. Matute-Bello G, Liles WC, Steinberg KP, et al (1999) Soluble Fas ligand induces epithelial cell apoptosis in humans with acute lung injury (ARDS). J Immunol 163: 2217–2225
37. Albertine KH, Soulier MF, Wang Z, et al (2002) Fas and fas ligand are up-regulated in pul-

monary edema fluid and lung tissue of patients with acute lung injury and the acute respiratory distress syndrome. Am J Pathol 161: 1783–1796

38. Hashimoto S, Kobayashi A, Kooguchi K, Kitamura Y, Onodera H, Nakajima H (2000) Upregulation of two death pathways of perforin/granzyme and FasL/Fas in septic acute respiratory distress syndrome. Am J Respir Crit Care Med 161: 237–243

39. Tateda K, Deng JC, Moore TA, et al (2003) Hyperoxia mediates acute lung injury and increased lethality in murine Legionella pneumonia: the role of apoptosis. J Immunol 170: 4209–4216

40. Liu L, Qiu HB, Yang Y, Wang L, Ding HM, Li HP (2009) Losartan, an antagonist of AT1 receptor for angiotensin II, attenuates lipopolysaccharide-induced acute lung injury in rat. Arch Biochem Biophys 481: 131–136

41. Lipke AB, Matute-Bello G, Herrero R, Wong VA, Mongovin SM, Martin TR (2011) Death receptors mediate the adverse effects of febrile-range hyperthermia on the outcome of lipopolysaccharide-induced lung injury. Am J Physiol Lung Cell Mol Physiol 301: L60–70

42. Lee WL, Slutsky AS (2010) Sepsis and endothelial permeability. N Engl J Med 363: 689–691

43. Russell JA (2006) Management of sepsis. N Engl J Med 355: 1699–1713

44. Raghavendran K, Pryhuber GS, Chess PR, Davidson BA, Knight PR, Notter RH (2008) Pharmacotherapy of acute lung injury and acute respiratory distress syndrome. Curr Med Chem 15: 1911–1924

45. Rice TW, Wheeler AP, Bernard GR, et al (2010) A randomized, double-blind, placebo-controlled trial of TAK-242 for the treatment of severe sepsis. Crit Care Med 38: 1685–1694

46. Vincent JL, Angus DC, Artigas A, et al (2003) Effects of drotrecogin alfa (activated) on organ dysfunction in the PROWESS trial. Crit Care Med 31: 834–840

47. Matthay MA, Goolaerts A, Howard JP, Lee JW (2010) Mesenchymal stem cells for acute lung injury: preclinical evidence. Crit Care Med 38: S569–573

48. Manzoni P, Rinaldi M, Cattani S, et al (2009) Bovine lactoferrin supplementation for prevention of late-onset sepsis in very low-birth-weight neonates: a randomized trial. JAMA 302: 1421–1428

49. Cruz DN, Antonelli M, Fumagalli R, et al (2009) Early use of polymyxin B hemoperfusion in abdominal septic shock: the EUPHAS randomized controlled trial. JAMA 301: 2445–2452

50. Cross AS, Opal SM (2003) A new paradigm for the treatment of sepsis: is it time to consider combination therapy? Ann Intern Med 138: 502–505

Biomarkers of Acute Lung Injury

J.A. Lorente, N. Nin, and A. Esteban

V Introduction

A biomarker is "any substance, structure or process that can be measured in the body or its products and influence or predict the incidence or outcome of disease" [1]. A biomarker can be useful for several purposes, including diagnosis, prognostication, identification of patients at risk, or prediction of response to therapy. In the case of acute lung injury (ALI) and acute respiratory distress syndrome (ARDS), a biomarker may help answer one or several of the following questions: How likely is this at risk patient to develop ALI/ARDS? Does this patient have hyperpermeability or cardiogenic pulmonary edema? What is the mortality of this patient with ALI/ARDS? How is this patient responding to therapy?

In addition, biomarkers may reflect the pathophysiology of the disease, and thus be useful to determine the degree of the pathophysiological derangement and its time course. For instance, the determination of a marker of alveolar type I cell injury will help define the degree of epithelial injury, a hallmark of ALI. In addition, it can help track patients' responses to therapy. Ideally, changes in this biomarker should precede obvious changes in other commonly measured variables (e.g., oxygenation, x-ray changes), so that physiological improvement or deterioration, or the development of complications (e.g., ventilator-induced lung injury [VILI], infection) can be detected in a timely fashion.

The availability of biomarkers that characterize different populations within a diagnostic category may help the enrollment of more homogeneous patient populations in clinical trials. Likewise, biomarkers sensitive to changes in disease activity or severity over time may serve as surrogate markers for other outcomes such as mortality, making more feasible the demonstration of efficacy of certain therapeutic interventions [2].

In the case of ALI, the control group to test the characteristics of the biomarkers under study is usually a group of normal subjects or a group of patients with cardiogenic pulmonary edema. However, sepsis is the context in which ALI most commonly develops, and sepsis by itself changes the concentration of most of the biomarkers analyzed. Thus, it would probably be appropriate to use patients with sepsis but without ALI as a control group. On the other hand, the issue is not whether a biomarker identifies a group of patients with a given diagnosis, or predicts the disease, but rather whether the use of the biomarker adds anything to what is already known just using tools already commonly available. For instance, if we are testing a marker of alveolar type I cell injury, the relevant question is not whether the concentration of that protein increases in patients with ALI and not in patients with cardiogenic pulmonary edema? The question should be whether

J.-L. Vincent (ed.), *Annual Update in Intensive Care and Emergency Medicine 2012*
DOI 10.1007/978-3-642-25716-2 © Springer-Verlag Berlin Heidelberg 2012

the determination of that protein helps make the diagnosis earlier than applying commonly used criteria, or whether it helps differentiate ALI from cardiogenic pulmonary edema more accurately than applying currently used criteria.

ALI and ARDS: Operational and Pathophysiological Definitions

In humans, the definition of ALI is based on clinical criteria developed by the American European Consensus Conference: Acute onset, radiological evidence of diffuse bilateral pulmonary infiltrates, a ratio of the partial pressure of arterial oxygen to the fraction of inspired oxygen (PaO_2/FiO_2) of less than 300, and no clinical evidence of elevated pulmonary arterial pressure [3]. The more severe form, ARDS, is characterized by a PaO_2/FiO_2 of less than 200. The pathological correlate of ALI is 'diffuse alveolar damage' (DAD), characterized by inflammatory infiltrates, thickened alveolar septae and deposition of hyaline membranes [4].

The main features of experimental ALI, according to a panel of experts [5], include rapid onset (within 24 hours) and three of the four following features: Histological evidence of tissue injury, alteration of the alveolar capillary barrier, an inflammatory response, and evidence of physiological dysfunction. Of these, the most relevant features were considered to be evidence of tissue injury, and evidence of alteration of the alveolar capillary barrier.

The presence of the main features of experimental lung injury can be established with the following measurements, which were categorized by the experts either as "very relevant" or as "somewhat relevant":

1. Measurements of histological evidence of tissue injury. *Very relevant*: Accumulation of neutrophils in the alveolar or the interstitial space, formation of hyaline membranes, presence of proteinaceous debris in the alveolar space (such as fibrin strands), thickening of the alveolar wall, enhanced injury as measured by a standardized histology score. *Somewhat relevant*: Evidence of hemorrhage, areas of atelectasis, gross macroscopic changes such as discoloration of the lungs.

2. Measurements of alteration of the alveolar capillary barrier. *Very relevant*: An increase in extravascular lung water (EVLW) content, accumulation of an exogenous protein or tracer in the airspaces or the extravascular compartment, increase in total bronchoalveolar (BAL) protein concentration, increase in BAL fluid concentration of high molecular weight proteins, increase in the microvascular filtration coefficient. *Somewhat relevant*: Increase in lung weight, translocation of a protein from the airspaces into plasma, increased lung lymph flow, high lymph protein concentration.

3. Measurements of the inflammatory response. *Very relevant*: Increase in the absolute number of neutrophils in BAL fluid, increase in lung myeloperoxidase (MPO) activity, increase in the concentrations of pro-inflammatory cytokines. *Somewhat relevant*: Increase in pro-coagulatory activity, increased expression of adhesion molecules, conversion of the neutrophilic alveolitis into a mononuclear alveolitis with time, increased levels of complement factors and matrix metalloproteinase.

4. Measurements of physiological dysfunction. *Very relevant*: Hypoxemia, increased alveolar-arterial oxygen difference. *Somewhat relevant*: PaO_2/FiO_2 < 200, increase in minute ventilation, increase in respiratory frequency.

Therefore, the criteria for diagnosis in humans reflect the concept of ALI and ARDS as a non-cardiogenic (hyperpermeability) pulmonary edema. The criteria for animal models of ALI emphasize the inflammatory nature of the underlying pathophysiological process, and pinpoint specific measurements that investigators believe are appropriate to assess the pulmonary inflammatory response.

Biomarkers of Acute Lung Injury

Biomarkers for ALI have been tested to predict the diagnosis in at risk patient populations, diagnose the condition or predict certain outcomes, most notably mortality (**Table 1**).

Table 1. Biomarkers of acute lung injury

Inflammation and Cytokines
IL-2, IL-6, IL-8, IL-10, IL-1beta, IL-1ra, TNF-alpha; sTNFR-1, sTNFR-2
Decoy receptor 3
Lipopolysaccharide (LPS)-binding protein (LBP)
High-mobility group box 1 protein (HMGB1)
Markers of Coagulation and Fibrinolysis
PAI-1
Protein C
Markers of Epithelial Injury
Receptor for advanced glycation products (RAGE)
Surfactant proteins A, B, D
Clara cell protein
Laminin-5
Rat type I cell 40-kDa protein/type I cell alpha protein
Human hTIa-2 and gp36
Human type I cell 56-kDa protein
Caveolin-1 and -2
Alpha 2-Isoform of sodium/potassium-exchanging ATPase
Aquaporin 5
Cytochrome P450 2B1
Carboxypeptidase M
Markers of Endothelial Injury
Angiopoietin-2
Vascular endothelial growth factor
von Willebrand factor antigen
Selectins
Intercellular Adhesion Molecule (ICAM)-1
Extracellular Matrix
Procollagen peptide type III

Inflammation and Cytokines

ALI is characterized by intra-alveolar inflammation, and many cytokines and cytokine receptors (interleukins [IL]-2, IL-6, IL-8, IL-10, and IL-1beta, IL-1 receptor antagonist [IL-1ra], tumor necrosis factor [TNF]-α and its soluble receptors [sTNFR-1 and sTNFR-2]) have been implicated in its pathogenesis. Thus it can be anticipated that the local (as determined in the BAL fluid) and systemic determination of cytokines may precede the development of ALI, potentially making these proteins useful biomarkers as predictors of ALI. However, most studies have failed to show a relationship between the concentration of these cytokines and the development of ALI in at risk patients. For instance, plasma levels of IL-10 and IL-1ra did not predict the development of ALI [6]. IL-6 or IL-8 concentrations in plasma or BAL fluid did not predict the development of ARDS in patients at risk [7], nor did TNF-α levels in BAL fluid [8].

Although their predictive ability for ALI is poor, cytokines seem to be good prognostic markers. In one study in 593 patients with ALI [9], an independent association with mortality, ventilator dependence and organ failure was shown for IL-6, IL-8, and sTNF-R1 serum concentrations.

Decoy receptor 3 (DcR 3) is a member of the TNF superfamily that binds Fas ligand and LIGHT (a lymphotoxin receptor). In a study measuring a large number of potential biomarkers in 88 patients with ARDS (including TNF-α, IL-6, and soluble triggering receptor expressed on myeloid cells 1 [sTREM]) [10], DcR 3 was the biomarker that best discriminated non-survivors from survivors.

Lipopolysaccharide (LPS)-binding protein (LBP) mediates the transduction of the biological response to LPS, and is produced as an acute-phase reactant by alveolar type II cells. In a recent study, sustained elevations of plasma LBP at 48 hours post-admission to an intensive care unit (ICU) were associated with ARDS [11].

High-mobility group box 1 protein (HMGB1) is an inflammatory cytokine that binds the receptor for advanced glycation end products (RAGE). In one study in trauma patients in the emergency department, HMBG1 was released early (within 30 minutes) into the circulation and correlated with the development of acute organ dysfunction, including ALI [12].

Markers of Coagulation and Fibrinolysis

ALI and ARDS are characterized by intraalveolar fibrin deposition and inhibition of fibrinolysis. Plasminogen activator inhibitor-1 (PAI-1) is an antiprotease inhibitor of fibrinolysis that promotes fibrin deposition. Plasma and pulmonary edema fluid levels of PAI-1 are increased in patients with early ALI compared with patients with severe hydrostatic pulmonary edema [13].

PAI-1 levels are also good prognostic markers of mortality and organ failure-free days [35]. Low protein C plasma levels, indicating activation of the coagulation system, are also prognostic markers in patients with ALI [14].

Markers of Epithelial Injury

Epithelial injury in ALI interferes with edema fluid clearance, surfactant synthesis, normal host defense mechanisms and alveolar repair processes, and facilitates bacterial translocation. As damage to alveolar type I and II cells is central to the pathophysiology of ALI, markers of alveolar epithelial injury could be predictive or diagnostic of ALI.

The RAGE is a transmembrane protein of the immunoglobulin superfamily and multiligand receptor that binds modified glycoproteins, including HMGB-1, involved in intracellular pro-inflammatory signaling via nuclear factor-kappa B

(NF-κB). It is ubiquitously expressed, but expression levels are highest in the lung. The protein is anchored on the basolateral membrane of alveolar type I cells. RAGE levels are increased in the plasma and pulmonary edema fluid of patients with ALI compared to patients with hydrostatic pulmonary edema [15]. RAGE was the best performing biomarker out of a panel of 21 biomarkers for distinguishing patients with ALI from those without ALI in patients with severe trauma [16], and was associated with outcome in patients from the ARDSNet trial in the higher tidal volume arm of the study [17].

Surfactant protein (SP)-A and SP-D are hydrophilic proteins involved in the innate immune response, whereas SP-B and SP-C are hydrophobic proteins with biophysical properties. In one study in patients at risk for ALI, BAL fluid levels of SP-A were low, and high levels were negatively predictive for ALI [18]. In a subsequent study, high plasma SP-A levels were found in an at-risk cohort who developed ARDS secondary to sepsis and aspiration but not trauma [19]. Thus leaking of SP-A into the circulation may be a marker of ALI. However, in a large series of 54 cases at risk for ALI, it was found that elevated plasma levels of SP-B, but not SP-A, predicted ALI [20]. In another study, it was shown that SP-D is a prognostic marker, as higher plasma SP-D levels were independently associated with 180-day mortality and reduced ventilator-free and organ-failure free days in 565 patients [21].

Clara cell protein (CC-16) is a small 16-kDa anti-inflammatory protein secreted almost exclusively by Clara cells of the terminal bronchial epithelium. It inhibits the phospholipase A2 second messenger pathway. In a study on 22 at-risk patients with ventilator-associated pneumonia (VAP), an acute elevation in plasma CC-16 anticipated the development of ALI [22]. On the other hand, in a subsequent study [23], it was found that plasma and pulmonary edema fluid CC-16 levels were lower in patients with ALI/ARDS than in control patients with cardiogenic pulmonary edema. Thus more studies are needed to solve these discrepancies and determine the role of CC-16 in the diagnosis of ALI.

Laminin-5 is a polymorphic, polyfunctional epithelial cell adhesion molecule. Laminins play an important role in cell adhesion, growth, and differentiation. The degradation product of laminin-5, G2F, the terminal active portion of its g2-chain, was significantly increased in the plasma of ALI patients compared to the plasma of patients with cardiogenic pulmonary edema [24]. High levels were maintained in non-surviving patients. Thus it seems that laminin-5 could be a diagnostic and prognostic marker of ALI.

Markers of Endothelial Injury

Lung endothelial injury is central to the pathophysiology of ALI and ARDS. The expression of adhesion molecules for neutrophils favors the migration of circulating inflammatory cells to the interstitium, causing parenchymal cell damage, vascular hyperpermeability, and coagulation activation. Thus markers of endothelial activation or injury could be potential biomarkers to predict or diagnose ALI.

The angiopoietins regulate vascular permeability. Ang-1 is constitutively expressed and binds Tie 2, a tyrosine kinase receptor present on the endothelial cell surface. Ang-2, up regulated after vessel injury, inhibits Tie-2, and activates Rho kinase. This in turn activates NF-κB and inhibits the cell protective pathway phosphoinositide-3 kinase/Akt signaling. Intercellular junctions are lost, and capillary leak and inflammatory cell migration ensue. Ang-2 serum concentrations in

63 at risk surgical ICU patients were higher in those who developed ARDS than in those who did not [25], and levels were also predictive of survival.

Vascular endothelial growth factor (VEGF) has a role in vascular permeability, angiogenesis and tissue repair. Studies have not found different serum or BAL fluid VEGF concentrations in patients who developed ALI or ARDS [26].

von Willebrand factor antigen (vWF) is involved in hemostasis by binding platelets to the endothelium and as a transport protein for factor VIII. It is synthesized in endothelial cells (where it is present in the Weibel-Palade bodies) and to a lesser extent in platelets. One study found a relationship between serum vWF levels above 450 % of control and the development of ALI in a group of 45 patients with non-pulmonary sepsis [27]. However, these findings were not reproduced in later studies. vWF has been proven, however, to be a good prognostic marker. Elevations in plasma levels of vWF were independently associated with hospital mortality in 559 patients with ALI, even after controlling for illness severity, sepsis, and ventilator strategy [28].

Selectins are cell-surface adhesion molecules involved in the early phase of neutrophil rolling and homing to a site of inflammation. In 50 unselected patients with systemic inflammatory response syndrome (SIRS) admitted to an emergency department, higher levels of E-selectin had a positive predictive value of 68 % and negative predictive value of 86 % for the development of ALI [29]. The assay was also predictive for other organ failures. In another study in 82 at risk patients with trauma, pancreatitis, or perforated bowel, soluble L-selectin (sL-selectin) was significantly lower in those patients who progressed to ARDS than in those who did not [30].

Intercellular adhesion molecule (ICAM)-1 mediates intercellular adhesion of leukocytes to the endothelium and epithelium, and is upregulated in inflammatory conditions. In one study, ICAM-1 levels were high in pulmonary edema fluid from patients with ALI [31]. A more recent study found that plasma and BAL fluid ICAM-1 concentrations were elevated in patients with ALI as compared to patients with cardiogenic pulmonary edema [32]. ICAM-1 is also a potential prognostic marker, as it was independently associated with mortality in a group of 778 patients [38].

The measurement of the protein concentration in the lung edema fluid, in relation to the plasma protein concentration, is a measure of the permeability of the alveolar-capillary membrane and therefore of the epithelial-endothelial integrity. Pulmonary hyperpermeability is a pathophysiological hallmark of ALI and ARDS. Measurements have to be performed early after intubation, as fluid resorption mechanisms will alter protein concentration in the alveolar space, giving rise to false positive results for the diagnosis of hyperpermeability.

In a large group of 390 patients, measurement of the edema fluid to plasma ratio [33], taking expert clinical diagnosis as the gold standard, had an area under the curve (AUC) in receiver operating characteristic curve (ROC) analysis for discriminating ALI from cardiogenic edema of 0.81, increasing to 0.85 for measurements taken within 3 hours of endotracheal intubation.

Extracellular Matrix

Procollagen peptide type III (PCP III) is a marker of collagen synthesis. Two small studies [34, 35] have suggested an association of higher edema fluid levels of PCP III with ALI. In a study on trauma patients testing a large panel of biomarkers [16], PCP III was the second-best performing biomarker for distinguishing patients with ALI from severely injured controls without ALI.

Multiple Biomarkers in Combination

In a panel of 21 biomarkers tested for diagnosis of ALI in trauma patients [16], the top 7 were: RAGE, PCP III, brain natriuretic peptide (BNP), angiopoietin-2 (Ang-2), TNF-α, IL-10, and IL-8, with an AUC in ROC analysis for the model including these 7 biomarkers of 0.86 for differentiating ALI/ARDS from a group of critically ill trauma patients without ALI who had normal chest radiographs or hydrostatic pulmonary edema.

A panel of biomarkers has also been used for mortality prediction. In one study, the use of a panel of 8 biomarkers previously associated with mortality (vWF, SP-D, TNF-R1, IL-6, IL-8, ICAM-1, protein C, and PAI-1) improved the mortality predictive ability of the model only slightly compared to a model using only clinical variables (AUC increased from 0.815 to 0.834 in the ROC analysis) [36]. The best performing biomarkers were markers of alveolar epithelial injury (SP-D) and inflammation/neutrophil chemotaxis (IL-8). Finally, using the method of risk reclassification, a panel of 5 biomarkers (ICAM, vWF, IL-8, SP-D, and sTNF-R1) significantly improved risk prediction for mortality when compared with a clinical prediction model using APACHE III scores only [37].

Genetic Polymorphisms and Gene Expression Studies

Two approaches are used in genetic studies of ALI: The candidate gene approach and the genome-wide approach. Only 31 genetic associations with ALI [38] have been reported, including *TNFA*, *IL6*, and *IL8*, *IL10*, *SP-B*, mannose-binding lectin (*MBL*), and *NF-κB1*. The most widely replicated polymorphisms are in the genes for IL-6, SP-B, and angiotensin 1 converting enzyme [39]. Genome-wide association studies require a larger sample size and cost is higher. Genome-wide association studies identify genes that are in turn candidates that can be supported by other genome-wide approaches, such as expression array and proteomic profiling.

Polymorphisms in the Ang-2 gene (*ANGPT2*) are associated with susceptibility to trauma-induced ALI [40, 41]. Using a large-scale candidate gene platform, the two single nucleotide polymorphisms most strongly associated with ALI were present in the Ang-2 gene. These findings were validated in two separate populations. One of the *ANGPT2* polymorphisms was associated with higher levels of a variant Ang-2 isoform in plasma [42].

A set of 8 genes uniquely activated in ALI (the gene signature of ALI) [43] has been reported in patients with ALI due to sepsis, with a high within-study (100 %) and external (89 %) accuracy.

Proteomics

Proteomics is the large-scale study of proteins, particularly their structures and functions. The proteome is the entire complement of proteins, including the modifications made to a particular set of proteins, produced by an organism or system. A variety of approaches has been used, including 2-D electrophoresis methods as well as liquid chromatography-tandem mass spectrometry. Using this methodology, the relationship between insulin-like growth factor–binding protein 3, a marker of apoptosis, and S100 proteins A8 and A9 (markers of inflammation) with ALI was found [44, 45].

Metabolomics

The metabolome represents a combination of all the metabolites and intermediate products of metabolism in a biological organism. Metabolomics allows real-time integration of upstream genomic and proteomic data. Metabolomic data sets are currently generated mainly through nuclear magnetic resonance (NMR) spectroscopy (MRS), mostly ^{1}H-MRS, and mass spectrometry (MS). The role of metabolomics as diagnostic or prognostic biomarkers in ALI is still in its infancy. Serkova et al. [46] found decreased high-energy phosphates and increased lactate-to-glucose ratio in a model of inflammation-induced ALI in mice. In patients with sepsis-induced ALI, total glutathione, adenosine, phosphatidylserine and sphingomyelin in plasma discriminated samples from patients from samples from healthy subjects [47]. We have recently used ^{1}H-MRS in different biological samples (lung tissue, BAL fluid and serum) from rats with VILI, and have found a metabolomic pattern that discriminates rats with VILI from controls with a 100 % accuracy (unpublished data).

Conclusion

In summary, although ALI is an inflammatory condition, measurement of proinflammatory cytokines has a weak correlation with the development of ALI in at risk patients, although those measurements correlate with mortality. Markers of endothelial and epithelial injury, alveolar-epithelial integrity or collagen synthesis can be diagnostic or prognostic markers. However, some of these proteins (IL-8, IL-6, vWF, protein C, PAI-1, and SP-D) need large scale validation studies, whereas others (Ang-2, CC-16, DcR 3) need further confirmation. Finally, new methodologies such as genomics, proteomics and metabolomics, in combination with bioinformatics, will help integrate vast arrays of information in a systems biology approach.

References

1. WHO Task Group on Environmental Health Criteria for Biomarkers in Risk Assessment: Validity and Validation (2001) International Programme on Chemical Safety. Biomarkers in risk assessment: validity and validation (EHC 222). Available at: http://www.inchem.org/documents/ehc/ehc/ehc222.htm. Accessed October, 2011
2. Barnett N, Ware LB (2011) Biomarkers in acute lung injury – Marking forward progress. Crit Care Clin 27: 661–683
3. Bernard GR, Artigas A, Brigham KL, et al (1994) Report of the American-European consensus conference on ARDS: definitions, mechanisms, relevant outcomes and clinical trial coordination. The Consensus Committee. Intensive Care Med 20: 225–232
4. Katzenstein AL, Bloor CM, Leibow AA (1976) Diffuse alveolar damage--the role of oxygen, shock, and related factors. Am J Pathol 85: 209–228

5. Matute-Bello G, Downey G, Moore BB (2011) Acute Lung Injury in Animals Study Group. An official American Thoracic Society workshop report: features and measurements of experimental acute lung injury in animals. Am J Respir Cell Mol Biol 44: 725–738

6. Parsons PE, Moss M, Vannice JL, et al (1997) Circulating IL-1ra and IL-10 levels are increased but do not predict the development of acute respiratory distress syndrome in at-risk patients. Am J Respir Crit Care Med 155: 1469–1473

7. Bouros D, Alexandrakis MG, Antoniou KM, et al (2004) The clinical significance of serum and bronchoalveolar lavage inflammatory cytokines in patients at risk for Acute Respiratory Distress Syndrome. BMC Pulm Med 17: 4–6

8. Suter PM, Suter S, Girardin E, et al (1992) High bronchoalveolar levels of tumor necrosis factor and its inhibitors, interleukin-1, interferon, and elastase, in patients with adult respiratory distress syndrome after trauma, shock, or sepsis. Am Rev Respir Dis 145: 1016–1022

9. Parsons PE, Eisner MD, Thompson BT, et al (2005) Lower tidal volume ventilation and plasma cytokine markers of inflammation in patients with acute lung injury. Crit Care Med 33: 1–6

10. Chen CY, Yang KY, Chen MY, et al (2009) Decoy receptor 3 levels in peripheral blood predict outcomes of acute respiratory distress syndrome. Am J Respir Crit Care Med 180: 751–760

11. Villar J, Perez-Mendez L, Espinosa E, et al (2009) Serum lipopolysaccharide binding protein levels predict severity of lung injury and mortality in patients with severe sepsis. PLoS One 4: e6818

12. Cohen MJ, Brohi K, Calfee CS, et al (2009) Early release of high mobility group box nuclear protein 1 after severe trauma in humans: role of injury severity and tissue hypoperfusion. Crit Care 13: R174

13. Prabhakaran P, Ware LB, White KE, et al (2003) Elevated levels of plasminogen acti- vator inhibitor-1 in pulmonary edema fluid are associated with mortality in acute lung injury. Am J Physiol Lung Cell Mol Physiol 285: L20–28

14. Ware LB, Matthay MA, Parsons PE, et al (2007) Pathogenetic and prognostic signifi- cance of altered coagulation and fibrinolysis in acute lung injury/acute respiratory distress syndrome. Crit Care Med 35: 1821–1828

15. Uchida T, Shirasawa M, Ware LB, et al (2006) Receptor for advanced glycation end- products is a marker of type I cell injury in acute lung injury. Am J Respir Crit Care Med 173: 1008–1015

16. Fremont RD, Koyama T, Calfee CS, et al (2010) Acute lung injury in patients with traumatic injuries: utility of a panel of biomarkers for diagnosis and pathogenesis. J Trauma 68: 1121–1127

17. Calfee CS, Ware LB, Eisner MD, et al (2008) Plasma receptor for advanced glycation end products and clinical outcomes in acute lung injury. Thorax 63: 1083–1089

18. Greene KE, Wright JR, Steinberg KP, et al (1999) Serial changes in surfactant- associated proteins in lung and serum before and after onset of ARDS. Am J Respir Crit Care Med 160: 1843–1850

19. Greene KE, Ye S, Mason RJ, et al (1999) Serum surfactant protein-A levels predict development of ARDS in at-risk patients. Chest 116: 90S–91S

20. Bersten AD, Hunt T, Nicholas TE, et al (2001) Elevated plasma surfactant protein-B predicts development of acute respiratory distress syndrome in patients with acute respiratory failure. Am J Respir Crit Care Med 164: 648–652

21. Eisner MD, Parsons P, Matthay MA, et al (2003) Plasma surfactant protein levels and clinical outcomes in patients with acute lung injury. Thorax 58: 983–988

22. Determann RM, Millo JL, Waddy S, et al (2009) Plasma CC16 levels are associated with development of ALI/ARDS in patients with ventilator-associated pneumonia: a retrospective observational study. BMC Pulm Med 9: 49

23. Kropski JA, Fremont RD, Calfee CS, et al (2009) Clara cell protein (CC16), a marker of lung epithelial injury, is decreased in plasma and pulmonary edema fluid from patients with acute lung injury. Chest 135: 1440–1447

24. Katayama M, Ishizaka A, Sakamoto M, et al (2010) Laminin gamma2 fragments are increased in the circulation of patients with early phase acute lung injury. Intensive Care Med 36: 479–486

V

25. Gallagher DC, Parikh SM, Balonov K, et al (2008) Circulating angiopoietin 2 correlates with mortality in a surgical population with acute lung injury/adult respiratory distress syndrome. Shock 29: 656–661
26. van der Heijden M, van Nieuw Amerongen GP, Koolwijk P, et al (2008) Angiopoietin-2, permeability oedema, occurrence and severity of ALI/ARDS in septic and non- septic critically ill patients. Thorax 63: 903–909
27. Rubin DB, Wiener-Kronish JP, Murray JF, et al (1990) Elevated von Willebrand factor antigen is an early plasma predictor of acute lung injury in nonpulmonary sepsis syndrome. J Clin Invest 86: 474–480
28. Ware LB, Eisner MD, Thompson BT, et al (2004) Significance of von Willebrand factor in septic and nonseptic patients with acute lung injury. Am J Respir Crit Care Med 170: 766–772
29. Donnelly SC, Haslett C, Dransfield I, et al (1994) Role of selectins in development of adult respiratory distress syndrome. Lancet 344: 215–219
30. OkajimaK, HaradaN, SakuraiG, et al (2006) Rapid assay for plasma soluble E-selectin predicts the development of acute respiratory distress syndrome in patients with systemic inflammatory response syndrome. Transl Res 148: 295–300
31. Conner ER, Ware LB, Modin G, et al (1999) Elevated pulmonary edema fluid concentrations of soluble intercellular adhesion molecule-1 in patients with acute lung injury: biological and clinical significance. Chest 116: 83S–84S
32. Calfee CS, Eisner MD, Parsons PE, et al (2009) Soluble intercellular adhesion molecule-1 and clinical outcomes in patients with acute lung injury. Intensive Care Med 35: 248–257
33. Ware LB, Fremont RD, Bastarache JA, et al (2010) Determining the aetiology of pulmonary oedema by the oedema fluid-to-plasma protein ratio. Eur Respir J 35: 331–337
34. Pugin J, Verghese G, Widmer MC, et al (1999) The alveolar space is the site of intense inflammatory and profibrotic reactions in the early phase of acute respiratory distress syndrome. Crit Care Med 27: 304–312
35. Chesnutt AN, Matthay MA, Tibayan FA, et al (1997) Early detection of type III procollagen peptide in acute lung injury. Pathogenetic and prognostic significance. Am J Respir Crit Care Med 156: 840–845
36. Ware LB, Koyama T, Billheimer DD, et al (2010) Prognostic and pathogenetic value of combining clinical and biochemical indices in patients with acute lung injury. Chest 137: 288–296
37. Calfee CS, Ware L, Glidden DV, et al. (2011) Use of risk reclassification with multiple biomarkers improves mortality prediction in acute lung injury. Crit Care Med 39: 711–717
38. Gao L, Barnes KC (2009) Recent advances in genetic predisposition to clinical acute lung injury. Am J Physiol Lung Cell Mol Physiol 296: L713–725
39. Lam E, dos Santos CC (2008) Advances in molecular acute lung injury/acute respiratory distress syndrome and ventilator-induced lung injury: the role of genomics, proteomics, bioinformatics and translational biology. Curr Opin Crit Care 14: 3–10
40. Christie JD, Wurfel MM, Keefe GE, et al (2010) Genome wide association (gwa) iden- tifies functional susceptibility loci for trauma-induced acute lung injury. Am J Respir Crit Care Med 181: A1205 (abst)
41. Meyer NJ, Li M, Shah CV, et al (2010) Large scale genotyping in an African American trauma population identifies angiopoeitin-2 variants associated with ALI. Am J Respir Crit Care Med 179: A3879 (abst)
42. Meyer NJ, Li M, Feng R, et al (2011) ANGPT2 genetic variant is associated with trauma-associated acute lung injury and altered plasma angiopoietin-2 isoform ratio. Am J Respir Crit Care Med 183: 1344–1353
43. Howrylak JA, Dolinay T, Lucht L, et al (2009) Discovery of the gene signature for acute lung injury in patients with sepsis. Physiol Genomics 37: 133–139
44. Schnapp LM, Donohoe S, Chen J, et al (2006) Mining the acute respiratory distress syndrome proteome: identification of the insulin-like growth factor (IGF)/IGF- binding protein-3 pathway in acute lung injury. Am J Pathol 169: 86–95
45. de Torre C, Ying SX, Munson PJ, et al (2006) Proteomic analysis of inflammatory biomarkers in bronchoalveolar lavage. Proteomics 6: 3949–3957
46. Serkova NJ, Van Rheen Z, Tobias M, Pitzer JE, Wilkinson JE, Stringer KA (2008) Utility of

V

magnetic resonance imaging and nuclear magnetic resonance-based metabolomics for quantification of inflammatory lung injury. Am J Physiol Lung Cell Mol Physiol 295: 152–161

47. Stringer KA, Serkova NJ, Karnovsky A, Guire K, Paine R 3rd, Standiford TJ (2011) Metabolic consequences of sepsis-induced acute lung injury revealed by plasma "H-nuclear magnetic resonance quantitative metabolomics and computational analysis. Am J Physiol Lung Cell Mol Physiol 300: L4-L11

V

Role of the Renin-Angiotensin System in ARDS

V. Zambelli, A. Grassi, and G. Bellani

Introduction

V

The renin-angiotensin system (RAS) is a powerful biological system that plays an important role in regulation of systemic blood pressure through the maintenance of fluid and salt homeostasis. It is a multifactorial system since it includes different components (**Fig. 1**): The first, renin, was discovered in 1898 [1], whereas the discovery of the last component, angiotensin-converting enzyme 2 (ACE 2), is relatively recent, from 2000 [2, 3]. Three kinds of RAS are known: A) circulating, B) local, and C) intracellular.

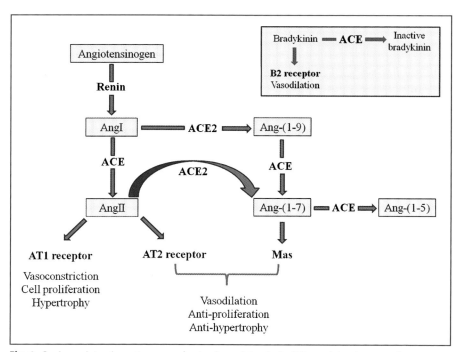

Fig. 1. Renin-angiotensin system cascade. AngI: angiotensin I; ACE: angiotensin-converting enzyme; AT1 receptor: AngII type 1 receptor; AT2 receptor: AngII type 2 receptor; Mas: Ang-(1-7) receptor; B2 receptor: bradykinin receptor.

J.-L. Vincent (ed.), *Annual Update in Intensive Care and Emergency Medicine 2012*
DOI 10.1007/978-3-642-25716-2 © Springer-Verlag Berlin Heidelberg 2012

a) The circulating RAS acts at a systemic level: Its substrate is angiotensinogen, which is released from the liver and cleaved, to form angiotensin I (AngI), by renin, an enzyme secreted from the juxtaglomerular cells of the kidney. The main effector peptide of the system is angiotensin II (AngII), generated from AngI by ACE and acting as a powerful vasoconstrictor.

b) Local tissue RASs, described in several organs and tissues, can synthesize AngII locally, since they possess the whole RAS enzymatic machinery.

c) More recent studies have revealed an intracellular complete RAS, which can produce AngII.

The RAS can, therefore, be considered an endocrine, paracrine and intracrine system [4].

V

RAS and Inflammation

The endothelium is a continuous layer of simple squamous epithelial cells (endo-thelial cells), which contributes to systemic homeostasis through different func-tions: Barrier, maintenance of coagulation and thrombolytic processes, participa-tion in immune reactions, and synthesis of different vasoactive compounds [5]. Direct injury (mechanical, chemical or infective) of the endothelium exposes the basement membrane components to the blood, leading to a series of events (the so called inflammatory cascade), including alteration of vascular integrity and production and release of cytokines, adhesion molecules, procoagulant agents and reactive oxygen species (ROS). In addition to its well-known regulatory role in hemodynamic homeostasis, RAS, and in particular AngII (**Fig. 2**), is also involved in the modulation of the inflammatory process [6]. Indeed AngII can regulate vascular permeability, the first step of the inflammatory response, by inducing the synthesis of prostaglandins and vascular endothelial cell growth fac-tor (VEGF) [7, 8]. Moreover, RAS participates in leukocyte extravasation, a criti-cal step in the inflammatory response, at different levels. AngII activates leuko-cytes and increases their adhesion to endothelial cells [9] via the induction of pro-inflammatory mediators like selectins, adhesion molecules, chemokines, cytokines and other factors (e.g., transforming growth factor [TGF]-β). AngII effects are mediated by its receptor angiotensin receptor 1 (AT1R), which leads to the activation of transcription factors, including activating protein-1 (AP-1) and nuclear factor-κB (NF-κB), and the ensuing expression of genes involved in inflammation and tissue injury [10]. In patients with cardiovascular disease, the increased selectin expression and plasma chemokine levels are attenuated by treatment with losartan (AT1R antagonist) [11]. Experimental studies have dem-onstrated that AngII infusion (at dosages unable to induce vasoconstriction) increases leukocyte transmigration, and that treatment with angiotensin receptor antagonists suppresses this leukocytes response [12]. Finally RAS participates in the last phase of inflammation: Cell growth and tissue repair. Preclinical studies on the kidney [13] have revealed that AngII induces cellular growth and release of several growth factors, resulting in organ hypertrophy, massive matrix synthe-sis and formation of scarring. Further studies demonstrated that AngII also induces fibrosis in other tissues, such as heart [14] and lung [15].

It is now well known that RAS is involved in the pathophysiology of several diseases, occurring in different organs (e.g., heart and kidney). Overactivation of RAS is linked with the development of atherosclerosis, hypertension and cardio-

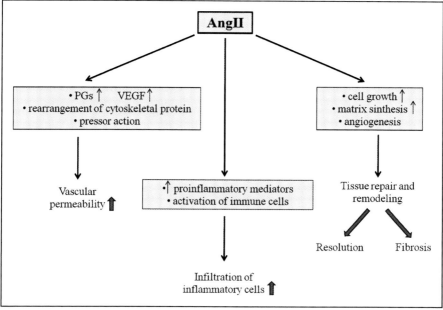

Fig. 2. Pro-inflammatory effects of angiotensin II (AngII). PGs: prostaglandins; VEGF: vascular endothelial cell growth factor.

vascular and renal events, such as myocardial infarction, stroke, congestive heart failure, diabetes, nephrosclerosis [16] and tumorigenesis [17]. Several studies have focused on lung diseases, such as pulmonary hypertension and pulmonary fibrosis, in order to better understand the role of RAS in this field. Capillaries in the lungs are one of the main sites of ACE expression [18], and thereby lungs are considered an important source of AngII. Pulmonary hypertension is characterized by increased vascular resistances and endothelial remodeling, eventually leading to right heart failure and death. In this context, AngII seems to mediate pro-inflammatory signaling (rather than vasoconstriction), resulting in pulmonary vascular remodeling [19]. Indeed AngII can induce smooth muscle cells proliferation [20], with consequent increase in pulmonary artery wall thickness. Evidence has demonstrated the involvement of RAS in the pathophysiology of pulmonary fibrosis. AngII upregulates the expression of TGF-β, thus the differentiation of fibroblasts to myofibroblasts and increase in extracellular matrix deposition [21], as well as alveolar epithelial cells apoptosis [22].

Among the various scenarios in which RAS can have a role, this chapter focuses on current knowledge of the role of RAS in acute lung injury (ALI) and acute respiratory distress syndrome (ARDS).

Angiotensin-converting Enzyme: The 'Dark Side' of RAS

ACE is a dipeptidylcarboxypeptidase, which converts AngI to AngII by cleavage of C-terminal dipeptides (**Fig. 3**). ACE is also responsible for the breakdown of the

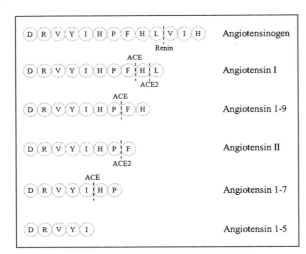

Fig. 3. Amino acid sequences and cleavage sites of components of the renin-angiotensin system (RAS). D: aspartic acid; R: arginine; V: valine; Y: tyrosine; I: isoleucine; H: histidine; P: proline; F: phenylalanine; L: leucine; ACE: angiotensin-converting enzyme

V

nonapeptide of bradykinin (**Fig. 1**). ACE is the key enzyme of the RAS and is highly expressed on lung endothelial cells, where it represents an ectoenzyme uniformly distributed along the luminal surface, with its catalytic site exposed to the blood-borne substrates [5].

Some clinical data seem to indicate that ACE activity is related to ALI pathogenesis and outcome. In 1987, Idell et al. [23] found that ACE levels were augmented in bronchoalveolar lavage (BAL) fluid of ARDS patients, compared to normal subjects and to patients affected by sarcoidosis and fibrosis. In particular ACE levels were highest in BAL fluid from patients with ARDS of infectious origin. The authors speculated that ACE in BAL fluid could be a marker of endothelial damage. Two years earlier, in 1985, Fourrier et al. [24] had performed sequential measurements of ACE levels in the serum of patients with ARDS or with sepsis (without ARDS). They found that, in ARDS survivors, ACE levels had a biphasic evolution, decreasing in the early phases of the illness, and increasing at the time of weaning. Conversely, ACE levels in ARDS non-survivors decreased in the early phases without the later increase. Finally, in patients with sepsis without ARDS the levels of ACE remained elevated. The authors postulated that a low level of circulating ACE was an index of pulmonary endothelial injury correlating with the presence and severity of ARDS.

ARDS appears to have a relatively low incidence compared to the number of subjects who are potentially at risk of developing this syndrome. Thus, some genetic background predisposing to the illness has been postulated. The ACE gene is located on chromosome 17q23 and contains a restriction fragment length polymorphism consisting of the insertion or deletion of an Alu repeated sequence in intron 16. Deletion of the Alu sequence is associated with greater ACE activity in plasma and peripheral blood mononuclear cells [25]. Marshall et al. [26] performed a retrospective study in 2002 comparing patients with ARDS to patients with non-ARDS respiratory failure. They found that the deletion of the Alu sequence in the ACE gene was associated with a higher incidence of ARDS and increased mortality in the ARDS group, suggesting that an increase in ACE activity correlates with the risk and outcome of ARDS.

Different results were obtained by Orfanos et al. in 2000 [27]. In order to assess whether pulmonary capillary endothelium bound (PCEB)-ACE activity could be a marker of endothelial injury, thus predicting the development and severity of ALI, patients were grouped according to lung injury score (LIS) and PCEB-ACE activity was measured. The authors observed that PCEB-ACE activity was decreased in patients with ALI/ARDS compared with non-ARDS patients, with an inverse correlation with LIS and APACHE II score. These data suggest that PCEB-ACE dysfunction is an early marker of the presence and severity of endothelial cell damage.

The fact that deletion of the Alu sequence, which leads to a higher activity of ACE, is related to the pathogenesis of ARDS, appears in contrast with the fact that PCEB-ACE activity is reduced as a consequence of pulmonary endothelial dysfunction. Maniatis et al. [28] interpreted this paradox by inferring that increased ACE and AngII activity could generate superoxide anions. The interactions between ROS and nitric oxide (NO) lead to the synthesis of reactive nitrogen species, that damage the pulmonary endothelium. The consequent reduction in ACE activity counterbalances its pro-inflammatory activity. Another hypothesis is that the crude losses of endothelium result in reduced PCEB-ACE activity, whereas it is normally, or even more than normally, active in healthy zones of the lungs.

Angiotensin II

The main biological activity of ACE is the cleavage of AngI to give AngII, which thus appears the main effector through which ACE is responsible for ARDS pathogenesis. AngII is an octapeptide with several biological activities, many of which have been already described in this review. Its action is mediated by two different receptors, AT1R and AT2R, that show opposite biological effects (**Fig. 2**). The role of AngII in the pathogenesis of ALI/ARDS seems to be strongly linked to its pro-inflammatory properties.

Kuba et al. [29] showed that in a murine model of ALI caused by acid aspiration or by the injection of severe acute respiratory syndrome (SARS) coronavirus spike proteins, the levels of AngII in the lungs were increased, and the degree of increase was proportional to the degree of lung injury assessed by histopathology (AngII levels were significantly higher in the lungs of mice subjected to a double injury, acid aspiration and viral infection). However, pulmonary edema, the hallmark of ALI/ARDS, can be due to increased hydrostatic pressure (the typical effect of AngII is augmentation of systemic pressure, which may promote pulmonary edema) or to enhanced permeability: Some studies [6, 30] demonstrated that local AngII was able to act directly on vascular permeability by stimulating VEGF and prostaglandins, thus exerting a primarily pro-inflammatory effect, not mediated by hemodynamic alterations, yielding important evidence in the assessment of the role of AngII in the pathogenesis of ALI/ARDS. The same group [29] demonstrated that the receptor implicated in AngII action during development of ALI is AT1R: Inhibition of AT1R attenuated ALI, as shown by increased compliance and attenuated pulmonary edema.

Ang II may also play a role in the regulation of apoptosis of type II pneumocytes, an important phenomenon in the late phases of ARDS. In fact, while proliferation of type II pneumocytes is characteristic of the early phases of ALI as a reparative phenomenon, their apoptosis indicates evolution towards a fibrotic phase of the disease [31]. AngII seems to promote apoptosis by modulating the Fas/Fas ligand system [32], which bears major implications in the pathogenesis and evolution of ALI by apoptosis of alveolar epithelial cells. Wang et al. [22] confirmed the role of AngII in modulation of apoptosis: Alveolar epithelial cells were cultured in a medium supplemented with different doses of AngII or angiotensinogen. Both these proteins were able to induce apoptosis in alveolar epithelial cells in a concentration-dependent manner. Moreover, the authors observed that the non-selective angiotensin receptor antagonist, saralasin, could inhibit apoptosis induced by both proteins, while lisinopril, an ACE-inhibitor, blocked apoptosis induced by angiotensinogen but not by AngII. These data showed the relationship between AngII and alveolar epithelial cell apoptosis. Although alveolar epithelial cells express mRNAs for both AngII receptors (AT1R and AT2R), only selective inhibition of AT1 blocked apoptosis caused by AngII [33]. Other findings by Marshall et al. showed that AngII could influence the progression of ALI towards a fibrotic disease: AngII is mitogenic for human adult fibroblasts via the AT1 receptor and stimulates the autocrine release of TGF-β (a pro-fibrotic cytokine) and pro-collagen production from fetal lung fibroblasts [34]. Finally, in a rat model of pulmonary fibrosis, bleomycin augmented lung AngII concentration, whereas treatment with an ACE inhibitor or an AT1 inhibitor was able to attenuate lung collagen accumulation and TGF-β expression [34].

Several animal models [33, 35, 36] helped to disclose the relationship between lipopolysaccharide (LPS)-induced ALI and AngII mainly by using selective inhibitors of AT1 receptors. First, sepsis-induced ALI was characterized by increased levels of AngII in lung tissue. Treatment with an inhibitor of AT1 led to improvements in permeability index *in vivo*, such as wet/dry weight ratio, quantification of Evans blue dye extravasation, histological evidence of edema. *In vitro* studies [35] supported these data, since monolayers of rat pulmonary microvascular endothelial cells had increased permeability following exposure to AngII; this increase in permeability was partially corrected by adding an inhibitor of AT1 to the culture medium. The role of AngII in the inflammatory cascade and endothelial dysfunction was further demonstrated by cytokine levels: Sepsis induced the secretion of several pro-inflammatory cytokines in the lungs and plasma, including tumor necrosis factor (TNF)-α, interleukin (IL)-1β, IL-6; this secretion was partially inhibited by the infusion of an AT1 inhibitor. Two groups [33, 36] performed additional studies to understand the mechanisms underlying AngII's pro-inflammatory actions: Both groups found that inhibition of AT1 led to a lesser activation of the NF-κB pathway, mediated by increased levels of IκB (inhibitor of NF-κB). Signal transduction through the mitogen-activated protein kinase (MAPK) cascade, c-jun N-terminal kinase (JNK) and AP-1 seems also to be involved in the pro-inflammatory effects of AngII.

Angiotensin-converting Enzyme 2: The 'Bright Side' Of RAS

In 2000, ACE2, the first human homolog of ACE, was discovered by two independent groups [2, 3]. Human ACE2 is expressed in the endothelium, but predominantly in the heart, kidney and testis [2], although its expression is also distributed to lung, liver, small intestine and brain [37]. Human ACE2 consists of 805 amino acids and is a type I integral membrane glycoprotein with an extracellular domain, containing a potential metalloprotease zinc binding site, a single transmembrane domain, and a cytoplasmic tail. It has only one catalytic domain, which shows 42 % identity with the amino domain of ACE. ACE2 is a carboxypeptidase, since it cleaves only one C-terminal residue from its substrate, rather than a dipeptide, as ACE does (**Fig. 3**). This particular difference between the two enzymes makes ACE2 resistant to the action of ACE inhibitors, since they mimic the dipeptidyl C-terminal binding sites of ACE substrates. ACE2 converts AngI to Ang 1-9 and AngII to Ang 1-7 [2, 3]. Ang 1-9 can be converted by ACE to Ang 1-7 [2]. Rice and colleagues [38] demonstrated that ACE2 hydrolyzed AngII more efficiently than AngI; therefore, the production of Ang 1-7, a powerful vasodilator, is believed to be the primary goal of ACE2 activity (Ang 1-7 will be discussed in depth later in the chapter). Moreover, other vasoactive peptides are substrates of ACE2 catalytic activity, such as neurotensin, kinetensin, des-Arg bradykinin and apelin-13 [2, 3].

ACE2 is present in the lungs of healthy and diseased humans; it is expressed by type I and type II alveolar epithelial cells and in bronchiolar epithelial cells [30, 39]. ACE2 may play an important role in ALI as shown by experimental studies. Imai et al. [30] examined extensively ACE2-induced protection from severe acute lung failure in two murine models of ALI (acid aspiration and sepsis). Loss of *Ace2* (*Ace2* knockout mice) resulted in decreased compliance, pulmonary edema and leukocyte infiltration in both animal models. The pulmonary edema seemed to be predominantly due to the altered vascular permeability (as demonstrated by Evans blue accumulation), rather than to hemodynamic causes. Indeed no differences in heart contractility or pulmonary vascular tone were found, although the authors did not exclude a potential effect of AngII on blood vessels. To further underline the protective action of ACE2, which counterbalances ACE functions, Imai et al. demonstrated that ACE, AngII and AT1R promoted ALI in different types of knockout mice, whereas ACE2 and AT2R protected against it. ACE2 negatively regulates AngII levels, which, if ACE2 is lacking, increase both in lungs and plasma.

ACE2 appears to play a role also in the pathogenesis of SARS [29]. ACE2 is now considered the SARS virus receptor: The interaction of ACE2 and the virus leads to endocytosis of viral particles and to viral fusion with cells. The absence of ACE2, in *Ace2* knockout mice, results in a dramatic reduction in SARS-coronavirus infection, with subsequent reduced histologic alterations and leukocyte infiltration. Kuba et al. [29] demonstrated *in vivo* the mechanism underlying the elevated severity and mortality of the viral infection: SARS-coronavirus infection downregulated ACE2 expression. During SARS infection, the protective arm of the RAS is impaired by the loss of ACE2 and of its ability to negatively regulate AngII, the levels of which are significantly increased in lung tissue. These authors demonstrated that the inhibition of AT1R, thus inhibition of AngII activity, attenuated the severity of lung injury, in terms of lung mechanical properties and pulmonary edema, in SARS-coronavirus challenged mice.

Angiotensin-(1 – 7) and Mas Receptor

Ang-(1-7) is a biologically active heptapeptide (**Fig. 3**) released from AngI or AngII by different peptidases, of which ACE2 is one of the most important. Ang-(1-7) exerts its action via the receptor, Mas, an 'orphan' G protein-coupled receptor [40] although it can also bind AT2R, but the affinity with AT2R is modest as compared to that of AngII. The ACE2-Ang-(1-7)-Mas arm is now consid-

V

ered the principal counterregulatory mechanism for the other RAS arm, ACE-AngII-AT1R. Indeed the two arms of the system act in opposite ways, the first leading to formation of Ang-(1-7) and simultaneously decreasing AngII, and the second forming the powerful vasoconstrictor AngII and catabolizing Ang-(1-7) and bradykinin [41]. Ang-(1-7) is both substrate and inhibitor of ACE, since it is cleaved by the N-domain of ACE to form Ang-(1-5) but it can also inhibit the function of ACE C-domain [42]. Ang-(1-7) acts as a vasodilator through the inhibition of ACE and, in addition, through the release of NO achieved by the indirect potentiation of bradykinin [43].

In addition to its vasodilatory properties, Ang-(1-7) interaction with the receptor Mas exerts an antiproliferative effect on vascular smooth muscle cells, fibromuscular tissue, and lung cancer cells. Moreover, it can reduce organ remodeling by limiting hypertrophy and collagen deposition, and thus fibrosis, with subsequent improvement in organ functions [41]. A recent study on experimental models of arthritis [44] showed the anti-inflammatory effects of the Ang-(1-7) Mas receptor. The activation of Mas, through the use of a Mas agonist, decreased the release of cytokines (TNF-α and IL-1β), and the rolling and adhesion of leukocytes to the endothelium at the injured site. It also decreased histological abnormalities and classical signs of inflammation, such as pain and edema. The authors suggested that Mas receptor agonists may be a novel therapeutic approach for the treatment of arthritis in humans.

Limited information is available concerning the role of Ang-(1-7) and its receptor in healthy or diseased lungs. Uhal et al. [45] recently demonstrated the protective effects of Ang-(1-7) on alveolar epithelial cell survival via the Mas-mediated inhibition of apoptosis. In fact, Ang-(1-7) inhibits JNK phosphorylation, caspase activation and nuclear fragmentation, acting through Mas receptors, blockade of which, conversely, favors apoptosis.

Therapeutic Strategies

The previously reviewed data show that RAS has a role in ALI/ARDS pathogenesis. For this reason, several experimental studies have been performed to evaluate the therapeutic role of RAS modulation in this setting. For example, Hagiwara et al. [46] developed a model of LPS-induced ALI in rats and showed that therapy with ACE inhibitors could diminish interstitial edema, alveolar cellular infiltration and cytokine release, probably via a reduction of Ang II levels and inhibition of the NF-κB pathway. In a different model of ALI [47], induced by the association of chronic ethanol ingestion and endotoxemia, alveolar epithelial permeability was improved by therapy with lisinopril or losartan. The same drugs were able to reduce TGF-β levels in lung tissue and avoid glutathione depletion, thus limiting epithelial dysfunction and oxidative stress. Finally, an experimental model of oleic acid-induced ALI [48] confirmed that captopril could attenuate pulmonary injury by protecting the vascular endothelium: The number of circulating endothelial cells in the captopril-treated group was reduced as compared to the control group, in addition to a decreased expression of intercellular adhesion molecule (ICAM)-1 and activation of the NF-κB pathway. Captopril treated rats also had a better PaO_2/FiO_2 ratio and less edema.

No clinical trial has been performed to investigate the effects of RAS modulation in ARDS patients. However, a retrospective cohort study [49] has been conducted to assess the effects on survival of prior use of ACE inhibitors in patients hospitalized with community acquired pneumonia. Prior use of ACE inhibitors was associated with a lower 30-day mortality.

As far as the ACE2-Ang(1-7)-Mas arm is concerned, the anti-inflammatory properties of ACE2 have been proposed as therapy for ALI/ARDS. The injection of recombinant human ACE2 (rhACE2) in *Ace2* knockout mice (rescue of phenotype) decreased the severity of ALI, and improved ALI/ARDS symptoms in wild type mice, suggesting that rhACE2 administration may be a novel potential therapeutic strategy for ARDS [30]. A study evaluating the therapeutic potential of rhACE2 in an animal model of LPS-induced lung injury [50] showed that treatment with rhACE2 reduced plasma TNF-α and AngII levels, improving the inflammatory response and pulmonary edema. Control animals receiving LPS infusion developed pulmonary hypertension, whereas in the treatment group, mean pulmonary arterial pressure was reduced (without changes in pulmonary artery occlusion pressure), indicating a pulmonary vasodilatory function of ACE2. In addition, rhACE2 treatment improved LPS-induced arterial hypoxemia, probably because of a more homogeneous perfusion in ACE2 treated animals.

Conclusion

In this chapter, we have reviewed the main evidence concerning the role of RAS components in ALI/ARDS. In addition to its well known cardiovascular and renal regulatory properties, the RAS participates in the different phases of inflammation, from the release of cytokines and the extravasation of leukocytes to matrix deposition and tissue repair. ALI/ARDS is characterized by a powerful inflammatory response that persists over time and, while attempting to repair the injury, results in the formation of scar tissue. Although RAS modulation appears a promising therapeutic strategy, more data need to be collected to elucidate whether it would be a feasible and clinically effective means of attenuating lung injury. Enhancement of the effects of the recently discovered ACE-AngII-AT1R arm may be a potential strategy to decrease the deleterious effects of AngII.

References

1. Tigerstedt R, Bergman P (1898) Niere und Kreislauf. Scand Arch Physiol 8: 223–271
2. Donoghue M, Hsieh F, Baronas E, et al (2000) A novel angiotensin-converting enzyme-related carboxypeptidase (ACE2) converts angiotensin I to angiotensin 1–9. Circ Res 87: E1–9
3. Tipnis SR, Hooper NM, Hyde R, Karran E, Christie G, Turner AJ (2000) A human homolog of angiotensin-converting enzyme. Cloning and functional expression as a captopril-insensitive carboxypeptidase. J Biol Chem 275: 33238–33243
4. Fyhrquist F, Saijonmaa O (2008) Renin-angiotensin system revisited. J Intern Med 264: 224–236
5. Orfanos SE, Mavrommati I, Korovesi I, Roussos C (2004) Pulmonary endothelium in acute lung injury: from basic science to the critically ill. Intensive Care Med 30: 1702–1714
6. Suzuki Y, Ruiz-Ortega M, Lorenzo O, Ruperez M, Esteban V, Egido J (2003) Inflammation and angiotensin II. Int J Biochem Cell Biol 35: 881–900
7. Gimbrone MA, Alexander RW (1975) Angiotensin II stimulation of prostaglandin production in cultured human vascular endothelium. Science 189: 219–220
8. Reddy HK, Sigusch H, Zhou G, Tyagi SC, Janicki JS, Weber KT (1995) Coronary vascular hyperpermeability and angiotensin II. J Lab Clin Med 126: 307–315

9. Krejcy K, Eichler HG, Jilma B, et al (1996) Influence of angiotensin II on circulating adhesion molecules and blood leukocyte count in vivo. Can J Physiol Pharmacol 74: 9–14

10. Barnes PJ, Karin M (1997) Nuclear factor-kappa B: A pivotal transcription factor in chronic inflammatory diseases. N Engl J Med 336: 1066–1071

11. Prasad A, Koh KK, Schenke WH, et al (2001) Role of angiotensin II type 1 receptor in the regulation of cellular adhesion molecules in atherosclerosis. Am Heart J 142: 248–253

12. Piqueras L, Kubes P, Alvarez A, et al (2000) Angiotensin II induces leukocyte-endothelial cell interactions in vivo via AT(1) and AT(2) receptor-mediated P-selectin upregulation. Circulation 102: 2118–2123

13. Wolf G, Neilson EG (1993) Angiotensin II as a renal growth factor. J Am Soc Nephrol 3: 1531–1540

14. Linz W, Schölkens BA, Ganten D (1989) Converting enzyme inhibition specifically prevents the development and induces regression of cardiac hypertrophy in rats. Clin Exp Hypertens A 11: 1325–1350

15. Ward WF, Molteni A, Ts'ao CH (1989) Radiation-induced endothelial dysfunction and fibrosis in rat lung: modification by the angiotensin converting enzyme inhibitor CL242817. Radiat Res 117: 342–350

16. Ferrario CM, Strawn WB (2006) Role of the renin-angiotensin-aldosterone system and proinflammatory mediators in cardiovascular disease. Am J Cardiol 98: 121–128

17. Deshayes F, Nahmias C (2005) Angiotensin receptors: a new role in cancer? Trends Endocrinol Metab 16: 293–299

18. Studdy PR, Lapworth R, Bird R (1983) Angiotensin-converting enzyme and its clinical significance--a review. J Clin Pathol 36: 938–947

19. Kuba K, Imai Y, Penninger JM (2006) Angiotensin-converting enzyme 2 in lung diseases. Curr Opin Pharmacol 6: 271–276

20. Morrell NW, Morris KG, Stenmark KR (1995) Role of angiotensin-converting enzyme and angiotensin II in development of hypoxic pulmonary hypertension. Am J Physiol 269: H1186–1194

21. Guo W, Shan B, Klingsberg RC, Qin X, Lasky JA (2009) Abrogation of TGF-beta1-induced fibroblast-myofibroblast differentiation by histone deacetylase inhibition. Am J Physiol Lung Cell Mol Physiol 297: L864-L870

22. Wang R, Zagariya A, Ibarra-Sunga O et al (1999) Angiotensin II induces apoptosis in human and rat alveolar epithelial cells. Am J Physiol 276: L885–889

23. Idell S, Kueppers F, Lippmann M, Rosen H, Niederman M, Fein A (1987) Angiotensin converting enzyme in bronchoalveolar lavage in ARDS. Chest 91: 52–56

24. Fourrier F, Chopin C, Wallaert B, Mazurier C, Mangalaboyi J, Durocher A (1985) Compared evolution of plasma fibronectin and angiotensin-converting enzyme levels in septic ARDS. Chest 87: 191–195

25. Rigat B, Hubert C, Alhenc-Gelas F, Cambien F, Corvol P, Soubrier F (1990) An insertion/deletion polymorphism in the angiotensin I-converting enzyme gene accounting for half the variance of serum enzyme levels. J Clin Invest 86: 1343–1346

26. Marshall RP, Webb S, Bellingan GJ, et al (2002) Angiotensin converting enzyme insertion/deletion polymorphism is associated with susceptibility and outcome in acute respiratory distress syndrome. Am J Respir Crit Care Med 166: 646–650

27. Orfanos SE, Armaganidis A, Glynos C, et al (2000) Pulmonary capillary endothelium-bound angiotensin-converting enzyme activity in acute lung injury. Circulation 102: 2011–2018

28. Maniatis NA, Kotanidou A, Catravas JD, Orfanos SE (2008) Endothelial pathomechanisms in acute lung injury. Vascul Pharmacol 49: 119–133

29. Kuba K, Imai Y, Rao S, et al (2005) A crucial role of angiotensin converting enzyme 2 (ACE2) in SARS coronavirus-induced lung injury. Nat Med 11: 875–879

30. Imai Y, Kuba K, Rao S, et al (2005) Angiotensin-converting enzyme 2 protects from severe acute lung failure. Nature 436: 112–116

31. Bardales RH, Xie SS, Schaefer RF, Hsu SM (1996) Apoptosis is a major pathway responsible for the resolution of type II pneumocytes in acute lung injury. Am J Pathol 149: 845–852

32. Martin TR, Nakamura M, Matute-Bello G (2003) The role of apoptosis in acute lung injury. Crit Care Med 31: S184–188

33. Wang F, Xia ZF, Chen XL, Jia YT, Wang YJ, Ma B (2009) Angiotensin II type-1 receptor antagonist attenuates LPS-induced acute lung injury. Cytokine 48: 246–253
34. Marshall RP, Gohlke P, Chambers RC, et al (2004) Angiotensin II and the fibroproliferative response to acute lung injury. Am J Physiol Lung Cell Mol Physiol 286: L156–164
35. Zhang H, Sun GY (2005) LPS induces permeability injury in lung microvascular endothelium via AT(1) receptor. Arch Biochem Biophys 441: 75–83
36. Shen L, Mo H, Cai L, et al (2009) Losartan prevents sepsis-induced acute lung injury and decreases activation of nuclear factor kappa B and mitogen-activated protein kinases. Shock 31: 500–506
37. Hamming I, Cooper ME, Haagmans BL, et al (2007) The emerging role of ACE2 in physiology and disease. J Pathol 212: 1–11
38. Rice GI, Thomas DA, Grant PJ, Turner AJ, Hooper NM (2004) Evaluation of angiotensin-converting enzyme (ACE), its homologue ACE2 and neprilysin in angiotensin peptide metabolism. Biochem J 383: 45–51
39. Hamming I, Timens W, Bulthuis ML, Lely AT, Navis GJ, van Goor H (2004) Tissue distribution of ACE2 protein, the functional receptor for SARS coronavirus. A first step in understanding SARS pathogenesis. J Pathol 203: 631–637
40. Santos RA, Simoes e Silva AC, Maric C, et al (2003) Angiotensin-(1–7) is an endogenous ligand for the G protein-coupled receptor Mas. Proc Natl Acad Sci USA 100: 8258–8263
41. Santos RA, Ferreira AJ, Simões E Silva AC (2008) Recent advances in the angiotensin-converting enzyme 2-angiotensin(1–7)-Mas axis. Exp Physiol 93: 519–527
42. Deddish PA, Marcic B, Jackman HL, Wang HZ, Skidgel RA, Erdös EG (1998) N-domain-specific substrate and C-domain inhibitors of angiotensin-converting enzyme: angiotensin-(1–7) and keto-ACE. Hypertension 31: 912–917
43. Li P, Chappell MC, Ferrario CM, Brosnihan KB (1997) Angiotensin-(1–7) augments bradykinin-induced vasodilation by competing with ACE and releasing nitric oxide. Hypertension 29: 394–400
44. da Silveira KD, Coelho FM, Vieira AT, et al (2010) Anti-inflammatory effects of the activation of the angiotensin-(1–7) receptor, MAS, in experimental models of arthritis. J Immunol 185: 5569–5576
45. Uhal BD, Li X, Xue A, Gao X, Abdul-Hafez A (2011) Regulation of alveolar epithelial cell survival by the ACE-2/angiotensin 1–7/Mas axis. Am J Physiol Lung Cell Mol Physiol 301: L269–274
46. Hagiwara S, Iwasaka H, Matumoto S, Hidaka S, Noguchi T (2009) Effects of an angiotensin-converting enzyme inhibitor on the inflammatory response in in vivo and in vitro models. Crit Care Med 37: 626–633
47. Bechara RI, Pelaez A, Palacio A, et al (2005) Angiotensin II mediates glutathione depletion, transforming growth factor-beta1 expression, and epithelial barrier dysfunction in the alcoholic rat lung. Am J Physiol Lung Cell Mol Physiol 289: L363–370
48. He X, Han B, Mura M, et al (2007) Angiotensin-converting enzyme inhibitor captopril prevents oleic acid-induced severe acute lung injury in rats. Shock 28: 106–111
49. Mortensen EM, Restrepo MI, Anzueto A, Pugh J (2005) The impact of prior outpatient ACE inhibitor use on 30-day mortality for patients hospitalized with community-acquired pneumonia. BMC Pulm Med 5: 12
50. Treml B, Neu N, Kleinsasser A, et al (2010) Recombinant angiotensin-converting enzyme 2 improves pulmonary blood flow and oxygenation in lipopolysaccharide-induced lung injury in piglets. Crit Care Med 38: 596–601

The Rise and Fall of β-Agonists in the Treatment of ARDS

C.R. Bassford, D.R. Thickett, and G.D. Perkins

V Introduction

The acute respiratory distress syndrome (ARDS) is a severe inflammatory condition of the lung, which can be triggered by a number of different pulmonary and extra-pulmonary insults [1]. The characteristic pathological changes of ARDS include an exudative phase, with the accumulation of fluid within the lung, the release of pro-inflammatory cytokines and infiltration of inflammatory cells, especially neutrophils, into the lung parenchyma. Damage to the alveolar epithelium and pulmonary capillary endothelium occur and patients develop the characteristic histological appearance of diffuse alveolar damage [1]. This manifests clinically as non-cardiogenic pulmonary edema, which reduces lung compliance and impairs gas exchange.

Pharmacological interventions to date have had limited success in improving outcomes [2]. Improvements to supportive care (protective ventilation [3] and conservative fluid management [4]) are thought to have contributed to the improved outcomes observed in recent years [5]. β-adrenoceptor agonists (β-agonists) are well established in the treatment of airflow obstruction. In addition to actions as bronchodilators, they have anti-inflammatory properties, promote the clearance of alveolar fluid, and promote epithelial and endothelial repair [6]. The scientific rationale for a potential role in the treatment of ARDS is summarized in **Figure 1**. The clinical effectiveness of β-agonists has been the subject of clinical trials spanning the last 25 years. Despite early studies showing promise, two large scale randomized controlled trials have recently been terminated on the basis of

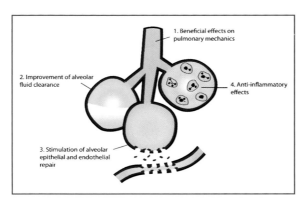

Fig. 1. Schematic diagram showing potential therapeutic effects of β-agonists in acute respiratory distress syndrome (ARDS)

J.-L. Vincent (ed.), *Annual Update in Intensive Care and Emergency Medicine 2012*
DOI 10.1007/978-3-642-25716-2 © Springer-Verlag Berlin Heidelberg 2012

futility and concerns about safety. In this review, we will outline the pre-clinical evidence for β-agonists and discuss the results of recent clinical trials.

The β-Adrenoceptor in the Lung

The β-adrenoceptor is a transmembrane G-protein-coupled receptor linked to adenylate cyclase (AC). Activation of the β-adrenoceptor stimulates an increase in the production of cAMP from adenosine triphosphate by this enzyme [7]. There are three distinct β-adrenoceptor subtypes: β1, β2 and β3, with different distributions, effects and genetics. β1 receptors are primarily present within the heart, and β3 receptors present principally in adipocytes, but also found on lung endothelial cells. β2 receptors are the most important pulmonary adrenoceptor subtype, present in increasing numbers with each generation of airway branching; greatest amounts are, therefore, present in the distal airways and alveoli where they are expressed on the surface of alveolar type I and type II cells [8].

β-Agonists Improve Alveolar Fluid Clearance

The presence of non-cardiogenic pulmonary edema is central to the pathophysiology and outcome of ARDS [9]. The most well studied mechanism for the clearance of alveolar fluid is the active transport of ions across the alveolar epithelium, creating an osmotic gradient for the subsequent movement of fluid. There is good evidence that transported sodium ions are the main driver for this process, entering the alveolar cell through amiloride-sensitive Na^+ channel (ENaC) or other cationic channels on the apical alveolar cell surface, and actively transported out by Na^+-K^+-ATPase on the basal surface [10]. The role of chloride ions is less well characterized; although they must follow sodium ions to maintain electro-neutrality, the pathway through which they move is as yet unidentified. Until recently, alveolar type II cells were thought to be responsible for the majority of ion transport. Sodium and chloride channels have recently been found on the more numerous alveolar type I cells, which may indicate a significant functional role. A contribution to this process may also be made by the distal airway epithelium.

β-agonists up-regulate the transport of both sodium and chloride ions through the increase in intracellular cAMP caused by β-adrenoceptor stimulation. A number of mechanisms have been proposed by which ion transport is increased by raised cAMP levels, including a greater sodium channel open probability, changes in the phosphorylation of the Na^+-K^+-ATPase α-subunit, greater delivery of ENaC and Na^+-K^+-ATPase, and increased chloride transport by the cystic fibrosis transmembrane conductance regulator [6, 10].

A higher rate of alveolar fluid clearance following β-agonist administration has been demonstrated in a number of experimental animal models [6], as well as the *ex vivo* human lung [11]. Additionally, over-expression of the epithelial β-adrenoceptor induced a higher rate of lung edema clearance in a rat lung injury model, increasing sensitivity to endogenous catecholamines [12].

The Anti-Inflammatory Effects of β-Agonists

There is a well recognized interaction between the sympathetic nervous system and the immune response, and β-adrenoceptors are present on many of the cells that have relevance in the development of ARDS, including macrophages, T-lymphocytes and neutrophils. ARDS is usually associated with an intense alveolar neutrophilia. Neutrophils migrate into the lungs, within hours of the causative insult, and their numbers correlate with severity of disease, and with mortality when persistently high numbers are seen [13]. β-agonists decrease neutrophil-related inflammation, and this may therefore confer a therapeutic benefit [6, 14]. β-agonists reduce neutrophil adhesion to bronchial epithelial and endothelial cells [15], which may contribute to the reduced neutrophil accumulation within the alveolar space. β-agonists also decrease neutrophil production of cytotoxic reactive oxygen species (ROS) *in vitro*. In a human model of acute lung injury (ALI), pre-treatment of health volunteers with inhaled salmeterol prior to lipopolysaccharide (LPS) inhalation attenuated neutrophil infiltration into the lung, myeloperoxidase (MPO) release and tumor necrosis factor (TNF)-α production [16].

Pro-inflammatory stimulation in the pathogenesis of ARDS is mediated within individual cells through the transcription factor, nuclear factor-κB (NF-κB). This cytosolic protein relocates to the nucleus under the influence of pro-inflammatory cytokines, where it binds to specific regions of DNA and in so doing increases the transcription of various inflammatory gene products. To allow movement into the nucleus, the endogenous inhibitor of this protein; inhibitor-κB (I-κB), must dissociate from the protein. During tissue inflammation cytosolic levels of I-κB decrease and increased activity of NF-κB is seen. This decrease in I-κB levels is reversed by the action of β-agonists. In the setting of LPS stimulation of human mononuclear cells, β-agonists act in a protein kinase A and cAMP dependent manner to increase cytosolic I-κB and thereby inhibit the pro-inflammatory action of NF-κB [17].

The interaction between β-agonists and the inflammatory response is, however, not straightforward. Although in the presence of inflammation, β-agonists have anti-inflammatory properties, in the absence of pro-inflammatory stimulation they themselves can be pro-inflammatory. *In vitro*, unstimulated macrophages exposed to β-agonists, increase their production of pro-inflammatory cytokines, such as interleukin (IL)-1β and IL-6 [18]. Increases in inflammatory mediator concentrations are also seen in β-agonist stimulation of skeletal muscle, fibroblasts and adipocytes, through β-adrenoceptor and non-β-adrenoceptor pathways.

β-Agonist Effects on Alveolar Epithelial and Endothelial Repair

The alveolar capillary barrier is comprised of the capillary endothelium, the interstitial space including the basement membrane and the extracellular matrix, and the alveolar epithelium. During ALI there is significant damage to all three structures. The clinical importance of this is highlighted by the findings that markers of endothelial damage (von Willebrand factor [vWF]) and epithelial cell damage (KL-6 or receptor for advanced glycation end products [RAGE]) are elevated in those who die from ARDS. Efficient alveolar epithelial repair is therefore important for ARDS patients' recovery.

Several different lines of research suggest that β-agonists may reduce endothelial damage or enhance repair in models of lung injury. Evidence for endothelial protection comes from the findings that in experimental acid-induced lung injury, β-agonists and cAMP donors significantly reduced lung endothelial cell permeability. *In vitro* thrombin-induced pulmonary endothelial permeability is reduced by β-agonists by directly maintaining actin filaments and the shape of endothelial cells [19]. Ischemia-reperfusion injury of the pulmonary endothelium is attenuated by agents that increase intracellular cAMP such as β-agonists, a feature that is of specific interest in the prevention of damage to the lung in non-heart beating organ donation, but is also relevant to all conditions that involve injury to the alveolar-capillary membrane [20].

Evidence for a role of β-agonists in epithelial repair comes from *in vitro* studies showing that β agonists stimulate the closure of mechanically induced wounds of epithelial monolayers by increasing cAMP and activating protein kinase A (PKA). Incubating bronchoalveolar lavage (BAL) fluid from patients with ARDS who had received treatment with intravenous salbutamol enhanced *in vitro* epithelial wound repair [21].

Clinical Studies Of β-Agonists In ARDS

Early Studies

The key elements of each trial are summarized in **Table 1**. The first clinical trial of β-agonists took place over 25 years ago. Basran et al. conducted an open label trial which examined the effect of a 7 μg/kg infusion of terbutaline on lung vascular permeability in 10 ventilated patients with ARDS [22]. Lung vascular permeability was measured by recording the pulmonary accumulation of radio-labelled transferrin. There was no overall change in lung vascular permeability; however, the five patients who demonstrated a reduction in plasma protein accumulation index survived as opposed to the five patients who showed no improvement (or worsening) of plasma protein accumulation index.

Subsequent trials focused on the effects of β-agonist therapy on pulmonary mechanics. The increase in cAMP levels caused by β-adrenoceptor stimulation promotes bronchial smooth muscle relaxation which results in bronchodilation, reducing airways resistance and the pressures required for adequate mechanical ventilation. Pesenti et al. studied the effect of an intravenous infusion of salbutamol in seven mechanically ventilated, paralyzed patients with ARDS [23]. Inspiratory resistance (maximal [total] and minimum [ohmic airway resistance]) and respiratory system compliance were measured at different levels of positive end-expiratory pressure (PEEP) before and 30 minutes after a continuous intravenous infusion of 15 μg/min salbutamol. Treatment with salbutamol reduced maximum and minimum inspiratory resistances (from 6.48 ± 2.56 to 4.67 ± 1.74 and from 4.06 ± 2.12 to 2.07 ± 0.95 $cmH_2O/l/sec$, respectively) but had no effect on effective additional resistance or respiratory system compliance.

Wright et al. conducted the first randomized controlled crossover trial of β-agonists in the treatment of ARDS [24]. In this study, eight patients with ARDS were randomized to receive 1 ml of 0.5 % metaproterenol solution mixed with 3 ml of normal saline solution, or 4 ml solution of normal saline solution (placebo). Six hours later, treatment arms were crossed over and the opposite regime administered to the same patient. Lung mechanics, shunt fraction, dead space

V

Table 1. Summary of clinical trials of β-agonists in patients with acute respiratory distress syndrome (ARDS)

First author	Basran [22]	Pesenti [23]	Wright [24]	Morina [25]	Manocha [26]	Perkins [27]	Licker [28]	Matthay [31]	Smith [33]
Publication year	1986	1993	1994	1997	2006	2006	2008	2011	2012
Patient population	Adult ARDS	Adult ARDS	Adult ARDS	Adult ARDS	Adult ARDS	Adult ARDS	Lung resection patients at risk of ARDS	Adult ARDS	Adult ARDS
Setting	ICU	ICU	ICU	ICU	ICU	ICU	Intermediate care	ICU	ICU
Age, years (mean [SD])	Range 23–79	Range 17–55	51 [7]	49 [6]	Low dose 54.7 [16.6]; high dose 65.7 [15.1], p< 0.05	Salbutamol arm 68.7 [16]; placebo 57 [14.7], p = 0.021	69 [7]		Salbutamol 55.8 [17.2]; placebo 54.2 [17.5]
Total sample size	10	7	8	11	86	40	24	282	326
Trial type	Non randomized interventional study	Non randomized interventional study	Randomized controlled crossover trial	Non randomized interventional study	Retrospective, observational study	Randomized, double blind, placebo controlled trial	Randomized, blinded cross over trial	Randomized, double blind, placebo controlled trial	Randomized, double blind, placebo controlled trial
Randomized?	No	No	Yes	No	No	Yes	Yes	Yes	Yes
Randomization and concealment	N/A	N/A	Computer generated	N/A	N/A	1:1 sealed envelope	Random number tables, sealed envelopes	Web based. Stratified by hospital and shock (1:1)	Telephone. Stratified by hospital, age and P/F ratio
Drug	Terbutaline	Salbutamol	Metaproterenol	Salbutamol	Salbutamol	Salbutamol	Salbutamol	Salbutamol	Salbutamol
Route	i.v.	i.v.	Nebulized	Nebulized	Nebulized	i.v.	Nebulized	Nebulized	i.v.

Table 1. (*cont.*)

Dose	7 µg/kg over 30 min	15 µg/ml	1 ml 0.5% solution	5 mg	High dose > 2.2 mg/day; low dose < 2.2 mg/day	15 µg/kg/h	5 mg salbutamol, 0.5 mg ipratropium bromide	5 mg	15 µg/kg/h
Number of patients	10	7	8	11	22 high dose, 68 low dose	19 salbutamol 21 placebo	24	152 salbutamol, 130 saline	162 salbutamol, 164 saline
Outcome	Reduced lung accumulation of radio-labeled transferrin in responder group (n = 5)	Max and min airway resistance reduced. No effect on compliance or effective additional resistance	Reduced resistance, peak/plateau airway pressures; increased Cdyn. No effect on deadspace, Cstat or oxygenation	Reduced resistance, peak and plateau airway pressures. No effect on compliance or oxygenation	More days alive and free from ALI in high dose arm (12.2 ± 4.4 days versus 7.6 ± 1.9 days, p = 0.02)	Reduced extravascular lung water and plateau airway pressures. No effect on lung injury score	Reduced lung water and permeability index and improved P/F ratio on postoperative day 1 following salbutamol	No difference in VFD, mortality, cytokines or plateau airway pressures	Increased 28-day mortality. Reduced VFD and OFFD.
28-day mortality	50 % survival	Not reported	Not reported	Not reported	46.9 % low dose arm, 50.0 % high dose arm	66 % placebo, 58 % salbutamol	N/A	90-day mortality 24.3 % salbutamol, 18.5 % placebo	Salbutamol 34.2 %, placebo 23.3 % (risk ratio 1.47, 95 % CI, 1.03 to 2.08)
Adverse effects	None reported	None reported	Tachycardia and hypertension	None reported	None reported	Trend to greater tachycardia and arrhythmia in salbutamol arm	Increased heart rate and stroke volume, reduced SVRI and increased CI and Dp/dtmax	Increased heart rate	Termination of infusion due to tachycardia, new arrhythmia, or lactic acidosis greater in salbutamol arm

ALI: acute lung injury; VFD: ventilator-free days; OFFD: organ failure-free days; i.v.: intravenous; CI: confidence interval; P/F: PaO$_2$/FiO$_2$; N/A: not available/applicable; Cstat: static compliance; Cdyn: dynamic compliance and oxygenation were measured at baseline, 30, 60 and 120 minutes. Aerosolized metaproterenol promptly reduced peak and plateau airway pressure and airway resistance whereas dynamic compliance increased. The effects persisted over the 2 hours of the study. Total compliance also increased as did oxygenation but the changes did not reach statistical significance. There was no effect on minute ventilation, pulmonary shunt fraction or deadspace.

In a subsequent cohort study, the effect of 1 mg nebulized salbutamol was examined in 11 patients with ARDS [25]. Compared to baseline, nebulized salbutamol was associated with modest reduction in peak and plateau airway pressures (4.9 ± 0.8 cmH$_2$O and 2.1 ± 0.6 cmH$_2$O, respectively), intrinsic PEEP (1.9 ± 0.5 cmH$_2$O) and minimal respiratory resistance (1.9+/-0.3 cmH$_2$O/l/s). Additional resistance, static compliance, oxygenation, heart rate and blood pressure did not change.

V

Recent Studies

A retrospective chart review of 86 adult patients with ALI found that patients with ALI who also received high dose nebulized salbutamol (2.5–6.4 mg/day) had significantly more days alive and free of ALI (n = 22, 12.2 [4.4] days) compared with the group receiving ≤ 2.4 mg/day (n = 64, 7.6 [1.9] days). There were no differences in non-pulmonary organ failure or hospital mortality rates (48 % vs 50 %) [26]. After adjustment for differences in case mix between the groups, high dose salbutamol remained independently associated with the number of days alive and free of ALI in a multivariate model.

The β-agonist Lung Injury Trial (BALTI-1) [27] was a phase II prospective randomized, double blind, placebo-controlled and the first study in humans to evaluate the effect of β-agonists on lung water. This single center study randomized 40 adult patients with ARDS to an intravenous infusion of salbutamol 15 μg/kg/hr for 7 days and serially recorded the effect on extravascular lung water (EVLW). The study demonstrated that salbutamol significantly reduced lung water at day 7 (mean [SD] 9.2 [6] vs. 13.2 [3] ml/kg, p = 0.038), alveolar capillary permeability [21] and plateau airway pressures compared to placebo and showed a trend towards reduced lung injury score (LIS). There were no differences in alveolar neutrophil sequestration or inflammatory cytokines [14]. The study protocol included a dose titration algorithm in the event of new onset tachycardia or arrhythmia. Nineteen patients received intravenous salbutamol for a total of 2,148 hours. Five patients in the salbutamol arm developed new onset of supraventricular arrhythmia compared to two patients in the placebo group (p = 0.2). No patients sustained serious ventricular arrhythmias. Heart rates were higher in the salbutamol group (average difference at day 1 of 11 beats per min [bpm]) although this was not statistically significant. There were no substantial differences in electrolyte or lactate concentrations between salbutamol and placebo arms.

Licker et al. examined the use of nebulized salbutamol compared to ipratropium bromide in a randomized controlled crossover trial in 21 patients following lung resection who were at risk of, but had not developed ALI [28]. These authors found a significant reduction in EVLW, pulmonary vascular permeability index and an improvement in PaO$_2$/FiO$_2$ ratio and increased cardiac output on the first postoperative day in the salbutamol arm. The authors concluded that aerosolized salbutamol accelerates the resolution of lung edema, improves blood oxygenation, and stimulates cardiovascular function after lung resection in high-risk patients. Although EVLW has been shown to be an independent predictor of outcome in ARDS [29], its use as a trial outcome has been criticized as decreases in lung perfusion because of worsening disease and non-linear thermal wash-out present in heterogeneously diseased lung may be erroneously interpreted as an improvement in lung edema [30].

The AlbuteroL for the Treatment of ALI (ALTA) study was a multicenter, randomized controlled trial of nebulized salbutamol in patients with ALI run by ARDSnet investigators [31]. This double blind, placebo controlled trial allocated patients to receive either salbutamol 5 mg every four hours or saline placebo for up to 10 days. The primary outcome for the trial was ventilator-free days. The trial started in August 2007 and set out to recruit up to 1000 patients with ALI. The trial was terminated by the Data Monitoring and Safety Board on the grounds of futility after 282 patients had been enrolled. There were no significant differences in the number of ventilator-free days between salbutamol and placebo arms (14.4 vs 16.6 days, 95 % confidence interval [CI] difference –4.7 to 0.3 days, p = 0.087). There was no difference in hospital mortality rates (23.0 and 17.7 %; 95 % CI difference – 4.0 to 14.7 %, p = 0.30). There were no differences in plateau airway pressure, minute ventilation or oxygenation index between groups. Although heart rates were significantly higher in the salbutamol arm (average 4 bpm), there was no difference in rates of new atrial fibrillation (10 % in both groups) or other cardiac arrhythmias. There were no differences in IL-6 and IL-8 at baseline or on day 3.

The BALTI-2 trial [32, 33] sought to extend the results of BALTI-1 and determine whether treatment with intravenous salbutamol (15 µg/kg/h) early in the course of ARDS would improve clinical outcomes. The trial commenced in December 2006 with the target of recruiting 1334 patients but was terminated in March 2010 due to safety concerns after the second interim analysis showed a significant (p = 0.02) adverse effect of salbutamol on 28-day mortality and the 99.8 % CI excluded a benefit for salbutamol of the size anticipated in the protocol. The final analysis confirmed that intravenous salbutamol increased 28-day mortality (salbutamol group 34.2 % [55/161], placebo group 23.3 % [38/163]; risk ratio 1·47, 95 % CI 1.03–2.08). The increase in mortality was associated with a reduction in the number of ventilator-free days (mean difference -2.7 days, 95 % CI -4.7 to -0.7 days) and organ failure-free days (mean difference -2.3 days, 95 % CI -4.5 to -0.1 days). The risks of developing a tachycardia, new arrhythmia, or lactic acidosis severe enough to warrant stopping the study drug were substantially higher in the salbutamol group (23 [14.3 %] versus 2 [1.2 %]; risk ratio 11·71, 95 % CI 2.81 to 48.88).

Ongoing Clinical Trials

A search of the International Standard Randomized Controlled Trial Number (ISRCTN) register and Clinicaltrials.gov for trials using β-agonists in ARDS identified two additional trials. The BALTI-prevention study is a double blind placebo controlled trial investigating whether inhalation of the long acting β-agonist salmeterol can prevent the development of ALI in patients undergoing esophagectomy (ISRCTN47481946)[34]. The trial completed recruitment in June 2011 and is due to report in 2012 when follow-up is complete. A second study, the Beta-agonists for Oxygenation in Lung Donors (BOLD) is testing the effect of nebulized salbutamol on oxygenation and lung transplantation rates in brain dead organ donors. This study has completed recruitment and is due to report shortly.

What are the Possible Reasons for Failure of β-Agonists to Improve Outcomes in ARDS?

Adverse Cardiac Effects

Salbutamol is known to have arrhythmia- and tachycardia-inducing properties. Traditional teaching is that β–adrenoceptors in the heart are of the β-1 subtype; however up to one third of the β-adrenoceptors in the atria and ventricles are β-2. The electrophysiological changes seen in patients treated with salbutamol are attributed to stimulation of these β-2 receptors. This myocardial stimulation has the potential to result in increased myocardial oxygen demand, with detrimental effects on myocardial function, especially in hypoxic ARDS patients. In a study of patients with acute severe asthma, of the 129 patients given inhaled salbutamol, there was an increase in the incidence of ventricular and supraventricular ectopic beats, but none of the patients had a clinically significant arrhythmia; this study excluded hypoxic patients, however [35]. In a large case-control study which enrolled elderly patients with chronic obstructive pulmonary disease (COPD), a dose response relationship was identified between prescription of a β-agonist and subsequent development of an acute coronary syndrome [36]. Many patients with critical illness have comorbid cardiovascular disease. It is, therefore, possible that some patients experienced adverse cardiovascular events including occult cardiac ischemia. These adverse effects may, therefore, limit any benefit associated with alveolar fluid balance.

Vasodilatation

Salbutamol is known to induce vasodilatation, an effect which precedes its bronchodilatory properties. This phenomenon and the increase in cardiac output cause an increase in ventilation/perfusion mis-match in patients when salbutamol is administered by the intravenous route. In a canine model of ALI, treatment with intravenous terbutaline increased cardiac index, aggravating capillary-alveolar macromolecular leakage [37]. A third possibility is the downregulation of β-agonist receptors (tachyphylaxis) during sustained treatment with β-agonists. Although most experimental studies suggest this is a minor factor it has been described in some models [38].

Biochemical Effects and Lactic Acidosis

Biochemical effects of salbutamol are known to include the induction of hypokalemia and hypomagnesemia. The BALTI-1 trial showed no significant difference in plasma electrolyte concentrations between placebo treated and salbutamol treated groups. The risks of developing a tachycardia, new arrhythmia, or lactic acidosis, severe enough to warrant stopping the study drug, were substantially higher in the salbutamol group than in the placebo group in the BALTI-2 trial [33].

Lactic acidosis is also a recognized side effect of intravenous and nebulized β_2 agonists [39]. This effect is probably mediated by β_2-adrenoreceptors and is thought to be due to an increase in skeletal muscle glycogenolysis and a subsequent rise in peripheral lactate production. Splanchnic glucose production and lactate extraction are also increased, as a result of increases in hepatic glycogenolysis and gluconeogenesis. Acidosis does not develop until the bicarbonate buffering system is saturated, and this usually does not occur until lactate concentrations exceed 5 mmol/l [40]. In the BALTI-1 study there was no significant difference in the incidence of lactic acidosis between the placebo and treatment arms of the study, and no patients had their infusion discontinued because of lactic acidosis. It should be noted however that this study was not statistically powered to detect such a difference in this adverse event.

Dosage and Route of Administration

The nebulized route for administration of β-agonists is better tolerated with fewer adverse side effects than the intravenous route. However, a limitation of the nebulized route is the lack of certainty that the drug reaches the required site of action, particularly in the setting of ALI which is characterized by injured, fluid filled alveoli. Although the ALTA investigators had preliminary evidence that nebulized salbutamol achieved drug concentrations of 10^{-6} M in undiluted pulmonary edema fluid [41], there remains uncertainty as to whether the drug reached the required site of action.

The dose of salbutamol used in the BALTI-2 trial (15 µg/kg/h) was selected after an early dose ranging study identified it to be the maximum dose that critically ill patients could receive without an increase in ventricular, atrial tachycardia or ectopy. This dose was used in the BALTI-1 study and achieved plasma levels of salbutamol (10^{-6} M) [14] which are associated with a 100 % increase in basal alveolar fluid clearance in animal models of ARDS. This dose is at the higher end of the manufacturer's recommended dosing regimen. It is possible, therefore, that a lower dose of salbutamol might have been better tolerated so the conclusions from the BALTI studies only relate to the dose given.

Conclusion

Over three decades of intense research activity has examined the potential role that β-agonists could play in the treatment of ARDS. Pre-clinical trials suggested that these drugs could accelerate alveolar fluid clearance, may have beneficial immunomodulatory effects and may reduce alveolar-epithelial permeability. A small phase 2 randomized controlled trial demonstrated proof of concept by showing that a sustained infusion of intravenous salbutamol reduced EVLW in patients with ARDS. Despite this preliminary evidence, the early promise has not held up to robust testing in the context of multicenter clinical trials. The ALTA trial was terminated on the grounds of futility after it became clear that salbutamol did not affect ventilator-free days. The BALTI-2 trial was terminated for similar reasons alongside concerns about safety and tolerability. Together these findings suggest that the routine administration of β-agonists as a treatment for ARDS should be avoided.

Acknowledgements: We wish to thank Dr Park and Professor Gao for their helpful comments during the development of this review. CR Bassford is funded by the National Institute for Health Research Clinical Lecturer scheme; DR Thickett is funded by the Wellcome Foundation; GD Perkins is funded by a Clinician Scientist Award from the National Institute for Health Research.

References

1. Ware LB, Matthay MA (2000) The acute respiratory distress syndrome. N Engl J Med 342: 1334–1349
2. Adhikari N, Burns KE, Meade MO (2004) Pharmacologic therapies for adults with acute lung injury and acute respiratory distress syndrome. Cochrane Database Syst Rev CD004477
3. The Acute Respiratory Distress Syndrome Network (2000) Ventilation with lower tidal volumes as compared with traditional tidal volumes for acute lung injury and the acute respiratory distress syndrome. N Engl J Med 342: 1301–1308
4. Wiedemann HP, Wheeler AP, Bernard GR, et al (2006) Comparison of two fluid-management strategies in acute lung injury. N Engl J Med 354: 2564–2575
5. Zambon M, Vincent JL (2008) Mortality rates for patients with acute lung injury/ARDS have decreased over time. Chest 133: 1120–1127
6. Perkins GD, McAuley DF, Richter A, Thickett DR, Gao F (2004) Bench-to-bedside review: beta2-Agonists and the acute respiratory distress syndrome. Crit Care 8: 25–32
7. Johnson M (2006) Molecular mechanisms of beta(2)-adrenergic receptor function, response, and regulation. J Allergy Clin Immunol 117: 18–24
8. Mutlu GM, Factor P (2008) Alveolar epithelial beta2-adrenergic receptors. Am J Respir Cell Mol Biol 38: 127–134
9. Ware LB, Matthay MA (2001) Alveolar fluid clearance is impaired in the majority of patients with acute lung injury and the acute respiratory distress syndrome. Am J Respir Crit Care Med 163: 1376–1383
10. Berthiaume Y, Matthay MA (2007) Alveolar edema fluid clearance and acute lung injury. Respir Physiol Neurobiol 159: 350–359
11. Sakuma T, Folkesson HG, Suzuki S, Okaniwa G, Fujimura S, Matthay MA (1997) Beta-adrenergic agonist stimulated alveolar fluid clearance in ex vivo human and rat lungs. Am J Respir Crit Care Med 155: 506–512
12. Dumasius V, Sznajder JI, Azzam ZS, et al. (2001) β2-Adrenergic receptor overexpression increases alveolar fluid clearance and responsiveness to endogenous catecholamines in rats. Circ Res 89: 907–914
13. Grommes J, Soehnlein O (2011) Contribution of neutrophils to acute lung injury. Mol Med 17: 293–307
14. Perkins GD, Nathani N, McAuley DF, Gao F, Thickett DR (2007) In vitro and in vivo effects of salbutamol on neutrophil function in acute lung injury. Thorax 62: 36–42
15. Bloemen PG, van den Tweel MC, Henricks PA, et al (1997) Increased cAMP levels in stimulated neutrophils inhibit their adhesion to human bronchial epithelial cells. Am J Physiol 272: L580-L587
16. Maris NA, de Vos AF, Dessing MC, et al (2005) Antiinflammatory effects of salmeterol after inhalation of lipopolysaccharide by healthy volunteers. Am J Respir Crit Care Med 172: 878–884
17. Farmer P, Pugin J (2000) beta-adrenergic agonists exert their "anti-inflammatory" effects in monocytic cells through the IkappaB/NF-kappaB pathway. Am J Physiol Lung Cell Mol Physiol 279: L675–682
18. Tan KS, Nackley AG, Satterfield K, Maixner W, Diatchenko L, Flood PM (2007) Beta2 adrenergic receptor activation stimulates pro-inflammatory cytokine production in macrophages via PKA- and NF-kappaB-independent mechanisms. Cell Signal 19: 251–260
19. Minnear FL, DeMichele MA, Moon DG, Rieder CL, Fenton JW (1989) Isoproterenol reduces thrombin-induced pulmonary endothelial permeability in vitro. Am J Physiol 257: H1613-H1623
20. Takashima S, Schlidt SA, Koukoulis G, Sevala M, Egan TM (2005) Isoproterenol reduces ischemia-reperfusion lung injury despite beta-blockade. J Surg Res 126: 114–120

V

21. Perkins GD, Gao F, Thickett DR (2008) In vivo and in vitro effects of salbutamol on alveolar epithelial repair in acute lung injury. Thorax 63: 215–220
22. Basran GS, Hardy JG, Woo SP, Ramasubramanian R, Byrne AJ (1986) Beta-2-adrenoceptor agonists as inhibitors of lung vascular permeability to radiolabelled transferrin in the adult respiratory distress syndrome in man. Eur J Nucl Med 12: 381–384
23. Pesenti A, Pelosi P, Rossi N, Aprigliano M, Brazzi L, Fumagalli R (1993) Respiratory mechanics and bronchodilator responsiveness in patients with the adult respiratory distress syndrome. Crit Care Med 21: 78–83
24. Wright PE, Carmichael LC, Bernard GR (1994) Effect of bronchodilators on lung mechanics in the acute respiratory distress syndrome (ARDS). Chest 106: 1517–1523
25. Morina P, Herrera M, Venegas J, Mora D, Rodriguez M, Pino E (1997) Effects of nebulized salbutamol on respiratory mechanics in adult respiratory distress syndrome. Intensive Care Med 23: 58–64
26. Manocha S, Gordon AC, Salehifar E, Groshaus H, Walley KR, Russell JA (2006) Inhaled beta-2 agonist salbutamol and acute lung injury: an association with improvement in acute lung injury. Crit Care 10: R12
27. Perkins GD, McAuley DF, Thickett DR, Gao F (2006) The beta-agonist lung injury trial (BALTI): a randomized placebo-controlled clinical trial. Am J Respir Crit Care Med 173: 281–287
28. Licker M, Tschopp JM, Robert J, Frey JG, Diaper J, Ellenberger C (2008) Aerosolized salbutamol accelerates the resolution of pulmonary edema after lung resection. Chest 133: 845–852
29. Craig TR, Duffy MJ, Shyamsundar M, et al (2010) Extravascular lung water indexed to predicted body weight is a novel predictor of intensive care unit mortality in patients with acute lung injury. Crit Care Med 38: 114–120
30. Effros RM (2006) The beta-agonist lung injury trial (BALTI). Am J Respir Crit Care Med 173: 1290
31. Matthay MA, Brower RG, Carson S, et al (2011) Randomized, placebo-controlled clinical trial of an aerosolized beta-2 agonist for treatment of acute lung injury. Am J Respir Crit Care Med 184: 561–568
32. Perkins GD, Gates S, Lamb SE, McCabe C, Young D, Gao F (2011) Beta Agonist Lung Injury TrIal-2 (BALTI-2) trial protocol: A randomised, double-blind, placebo-controlled of intravenous infusion of salbutamol in the acute respiratory distress syndrome. Trials 12: 113
33. Smith FG, Perkins GD, Gates S, et al (2012) The effect of Intravenous beta-2 agonist therapy on clinical outcomes in the acute respiratory distress syndrome (BALTI-2): a multicentre, randomised controlled trial. Lancet (in press)
34. Perkins GD, Park D, Alderson D, et al (2011) The Beta Agonist Lung Injury TrIal (BALTI)--prevention trial protocol. Trials 12: 79
35. Newhouse MT, Chapman KR, McCallum AL, et al (1996) Cardiovascular safety of high doses of inhaled fenoterol and albuterol in acute severe asthma. Chest 110: 595–603
36. Au DH, Curtis JR, Every NR, McDonell MB, Fihn SD (2002) Association between inhaled beta-agonists and the risk of unstable angina and myocardial infarction. Chest 121: 846–851
37. Briot R, Bayat S, Anglade D, Martiel JL, Grimbert F (2009) Increased cardiac index due to terbutaline treatment aggravates capillary-alveolar macromolecular leakage in oleic acid lung injury in dogs. Crit Care 13: R166
38. Abel SJ, Finney SJ, Brett SJ, Keogh BF, Morgan CJ, Evans TW (1998) Reduced mortality in association with the acute respiratory distress syndrome (ARDS). Thorax 53: 292–294
39. Stratakos G, Kalomenidis J, Routsi C, Papiris S, Roussos C (2002) Transient lactic acidosis as a side effect of inhaled salbutamol. Chest 122: 385–386
40. Day NP, Phu NH, Bethell DP, et al (1996) The effects of dopamine and adrenaline infusions on acid-base balance and systemic haemodynamics in severe infection. Lancet 348: 219–223
41. Atabai K, Ware LB, Snider ME, et al (2002) Aerosolized beta(2)-adrenergic agonists achieve therapeutic levels in the pulmonary edema fluid of ventilated patients with acute respiratory failure. Intensive Care Med 28: 705–711

Repair after Acute Lung Injury: Molecular Mechanisms and Therapeutic Opportunities

A. González-López and G.M. Albaiceta

V Introduction

Acute lung injury (ALI) is a clinical syndrome characterized by impairment in gas exchange and/or lung mechanics that leads to hypoxemia and increased work of breathing (WOB). When respiratory failure occurs, most patients require mechanical ventilation. This clinical scenario is related to high morbidity and mortality rates.

There have been large amounts of research on the pathogenetic mechanisms of lung injury, which include changes in alveolocapillary permeability, the inflammatory response, extracellular matrix remodeling and abnormal alveolar micromechanics. In spite of this knowledge, no effective therapy, other than treating the initial cause of injury and providing supportive treatment, has been shown to have a significant clinical benefit. Fortunately, the cause of ALI is known in most cases, so specific therapy can be initiated (e.g., antibiotics in sepsis, surgery when appropriate). In other cases, the cause is time-limited, such as in aspiration pneumonitis or polytrauma. However, even in these cases, ALI may persist beyond the initial insult. In this setting, restoration of normal lung structure and function is of paramount importance for survival.

There is increasing evidence of the lung's capacity to repair itself. This process involves an interplay between various cellular and molecular mechanisms, including resolution of edema and inflammation, cell proliferation and tissue remodeling. Moreover, it is possible that some of these mechanisms, activated early in the response to injury, are essential for normal repair later on. With this in mind, timing of a therapeutic intervention becomes a critical issue, as blockade of one mediator may prevent injury when administered early, but also impair the repair phase. Moreover, strategies aimed at promoting repair could represent a new alternative for patients with ALI.

Knowledge of the repair mechanisms could, therefore, be the next step to understanding the lung response to injury. In this review, we will summarize some of these mechanisms and discuss their relevance as potential therapeutic targets in ALI.

An Overview of the Repair Process

The lung response to an injurious stimulus involves transduction of the danger signal into a biochemical response. Depending on the cause, there are many pathways that can be activated. For instance, bacterial antigens may trigger an inflam-

J.-L. Vincent (ed.), *Annual Update in Intensive Care and Emergency Medicine 2012*
DOI 10.1007/978-3-642-25716-2 © Springer-Verlag Berlin Heidelberg 2012

matory response by activating any of the Toll-like receptors (TLR). Chemical agents induce cell membrane damage and, in some cases, oxidative stress, leading to the activation of a number of intracellular kinases. Mechanical stress, such as positive pressure ventilation, can also precipitate a biological response after a mechanotransduction process [1].

In addition to exogenous causes, an endogenous system detects tissue and cell damage and triggers the physiological response. Alarmins, a subgroup of molecules of a larger set called DAMPs (damage-associated molecular patterns), lead to this system. Structurally different, these endogenous molecules are released in response to tissue damage by dead cells and local inflammatory cells (alveolar macrophages in the case of lung), activating and recruiting immune cells through binding to different receptors, such as TLR, interleukin-1 receptor (IL-1R) and RAGE (receptor of advanced glycation end-products)[2], thereby activating the pro-inflammatory pathway. Irrespective of the cause, these signals converge in a group of transcription factors (e.g., nuclear factor-kappa B [NF-κB], activator protein [AP]-1), which induce the synthesis of new molecules that ultimately mediate the inflammatory response to the aggression. Hallmarks of this response are the increased alveolocapillary permeability, which causes a protein-rich edema, the neutrophil infiltrate (recruited from the circulation in response to chemokines), and the release of a wide variety of mediators, such as cyto- and chemokines, proteases, eicosanoids and growth factors, into the extracellular space. **Figure 1** summarizes this process. During this stage, pneumocyte death due to apoptosis (in response to released mediators) and/or necrosis (caused by toxins, proteases...) results in exposure of the basement membrane of the alveolar epithelium.

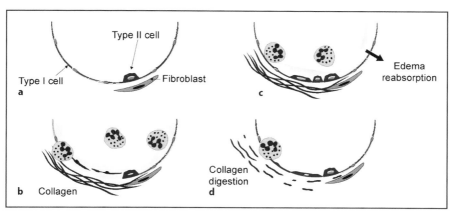

Fig. 1. Overview of the injury and repair mechanisms in an alveolus. **a** The normal alveolus is formed by type I and type II alveolar cells. The former cover the majority of the alveolar area, and the latter are reduced in number. **b** After acute lung injury, the inflammatory response results in the recruitment of neutrophils from the circulation, the development of alveolar edema and the deposition of collagen fibers. The necrotic alveolar cells are detached from the basement membrane. **c** During the repair phase, the alveolar fluid is reabsorbed, the inflammatory response attenuated, and type II alveolar cells (among others) proliferate and differentiate into type I pneumocytes. In this phase, collagen fibers may facilitate cellular migration. **d** Finally, digestion of the collagen scar is needed for complete normalization of lung functions.

One of the key steps in the tissue response is the deposition of collagen fibers at the sites of injury. Similarly to what happens in skin wounds, lung fibroblasts release procollagen peptides into the extracellular space, in order to create a scar. This is probably an attempt to keep the lung structure as intact as possible. So collagen deposition must not be viewed as a late response to abnormal healing, but as an early phenomenon. Some experimental studies corroborate this early onset of collagen deposition [3]. Moreover, patients show an increase in procollagen levels in the first 48 hours after meeting ALI criteria [4].

Tissue repair involves a variety of mechanisms including edema reabsorption, resolution of inflammation and cell proliferation in order to repopulate the alveolar epithelium (**Fig. 1c**). Lung edema clearance is a crucial step. It has been documented that mild alveolar injury results in increased alveolar fluid reabsorption. However, in severe cases, the injured pneumocytes cannot sustain the active transport of ions and water across the epithelium. Therefore, cell integrity is essential for edema clearance. The molecular mechanisms of ion and water transport in lung exceed the scope of this article, and have been reviewed elsewhere [5]. Regulation of the inflammatory response is a complex mechanism that requires interplay between several immune mediators [6]. Some anti-inflammatory cytokines, IL-10 being the most studied, are released even during a pro-inflammatory response as a negative feedback mechanism. When the pro-inflammatory pathways are downregulated (i.e., after cessation of the stimulus), these anti-inflammatory mediators decrease cytokine expression. Apoptosis of inflammatory cells (mainly neutrophils) has also been documented when pro-survival signals, such as granulocyte-colony stimulating factor (G-CSF), disappear. Alveolar macrophages also play a role in this phase engulfing death cells.

Finally, the regeneration of the alveolar structure requires the proliferation and differentiation of some progenitors into type I pneumocytes (**Fig. 2**). Different growth factors (e.g. epidermic [EGF], keratinocyte [KGF] or hepatic growth factor [HGF]), acting through tyrosin-kinase receptors, promote cell proliferation. The cell lines implicated in this step are a matter of research, stimulated by the growing interest in stem cells and regenerative medicine [7]. Endogenous progenitor cells include both resident stem cells and bone marrow-derived cells. Regarding the first, type II pneumocytes proliferate after injury and can originate type I cells. This has been demonstrated after pneumonectomy, hyperoxia or repeated

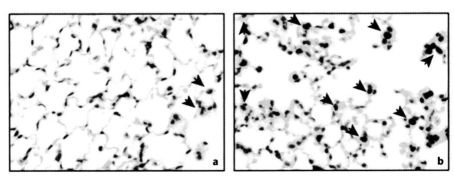

Fig. 2. Cell proliferation in control mice **a** and during the repair phase after ventilator-induced lung injury **b**. Some cells (arrows) show positive staining for Ki-67, a marker of cell proliferation.

bleomycin instillation in mice. Moreover, bone marrow-derived stem cells could also participate in alveolar repair, although data on the engraftment and differentiation of these cells are more focused on their therapeutic use than to clarify their role in the normal repair process. In addition, other cell types may also play a role in alveolar regeneration. Lung mesenchymal cells are activated after ALI and, in addition to collagen synthesis, they may secrete growth factors and even modulate the immune response by secreting anti-inflammatory cytokines [8].

The previously formed collagen scar can facilitate cell attachment to keep the alveolar structure. Again, collagen synthesis should be viewed as part of the normal healing process. However, excessive collagen deposition may impair gas exchange and lung mechanics. So, in order to restore normal respiratory function, the previously formed scar must be processed and removed (**Fig. 1d**). This can be carried out by matrix metalloproteinases (MMPs), a family of enzymes that can digest virtually all types of extracellular fibers [9]. One of the most important sources of MMPs is inflammatory cells (neutrophils and macrophages contain significant amounts of MMP-8 and MMP-9). Therefore, it can be hypothesized that the inflammatory response is important for adequate lung repair, and that MMPs are one of the links between these two phenomena. The underlying mechanisms that regulate this step in ALI are unknown, but knowledge of these mechanisms could help clarify why some patients develop a severe fibrotic response, which can cause long-term disabilities.

The Special Case of Repair after Ventilator-induced Lung Injury

Ventilation with high tidal volumes or transpulmonary pressures may cause severe injury to the lungs. In experimental models, there is a clear causality relationship between ventilatory settings and so-called ventilator-induced lung injury (VILI). Although this relationship is less clear in patients, especially those with previous ALI, the development of ventilatory strategies aimed to avoid further lung injury has been shown to decrease mortality. Therefore, although experimental models of VILI cannot be directly extrapolated to critically ill patients, they highlight the mechanisms of injury and repair involved.

A few studies have focused on repair after VILI, giving some insights into this process. The first was published by Nin et al. in 2008 [10]. These authors submitted Sprague-Dawley rats to injurious ventilation for one hour, reestablishing spontaneous breathing and letting them recover. Histological studies showed a significant reduction in capillary congestion, interstitial edema, type-I pneumocyte necrosis and hyaline membrane formation after 24 hours of recovery, reaching normality after 72 hours. Inflammatory markers showed a similar pattern. Aortic vascular and pulmonary microvessel responses to acetylcholine and norepinephrine were impaired and returned to normal at 168 and 72 hours respectively. This study demonstrated that VILI can revert rapidly after spontaneous breathing is reestablished.

In another study, Gonzalez-Lopez et al. [11] submitted CD1 mice to a combination of two ventilator strategies. One group was ventilated for 90 minutes with high pressures and another group was ventilated with the same strategy followed by up to 4 hours of protective ventilation. Histological score, pulmonary edema, alveolar permeability and tumor necrosis factor (TNF)-α increased during injury and returned to baseline values during repair. Later comparisons of the repair phase showed that survivors had higher pneumocyte proliferation and leukocyte infiltration and lower alveolar permeability and collagen content than non-survivors. MMP-2 levels were also increased in survivors. This MMP improves wound healing in *ex vivo* models using mice and human alveolar epithelial cell lines. Taken together, these studies suggest that an appropriate inflammatory response and tissue remodeling are key events during repair.

The Role of Inflammation In Tissue Damage and Repair

Inflammation is necessary for the development of a proper response to the insult, but it can damage the tissue where it takes place. Inflammation leads initially to an alteration in homeostasis, during which tissue partially sacrifices cellular and extracellular matrix integrity and tissue functionality for the benefit of a quick response. A good example of this compromise is the early recruitment of immune cells to the site of injury. The first cells arriving are neutrophils [12]. Representing 70 % of total circulating leukocytes, these cells are rapid responders to chemokines, appearing in the lungs a few minutes after initial injury. But this recruitment has a price for lung integrity; after migrating through endothelial cells and before arriving in the alveolar space, leukocytes find the basement membrane, a highly organized extracellular matrix mainly composed of four families of glycoproteins (laminin, collagen type IV isoforms, nidogen and heparan sulfate proteoglycans). The basement membrane is actively involved in leukocyte recruitment by its potential to bind and release cytokines and chemotactic factors. The only way neutrophils can cross this barrier is by proteolytic degradation [13], contributing to further damage of lung structure. Once in the lung, the release of a variety of alarmins, free oxygen radicals, leukotrienes, proteases and other pro-inflammatory molecules maintain the inflammatory state, thereby contributing to the ALI phase.

The role of proteases, especially of MMPs, in the pathogenesis of ALI has been controversial. Extracellular matrix processing releases some bioactive molecules. For example, type I collagen degradation generates an acetylated tripeptide with similar chemotactic activity to IL-8 [14]; moreover, MMPs process many immune mediators, like pro- and anti-inflammatory cytokines and chemokines, altering their activity (e.g., IL-1β, transforming growth factor [TGF]β and lipopolysaccharide-induced CXC chemokine [LIX] activation and macrophage inflammatory protein [MIP]-1α inactivation) and bioavailability (TNF-α and TGFβ release from cell surface and extracellular matrix, respectively) [15]. Their ability to regulate the inflammatory mediators and degrade collagen fibers also makes MMPs key elements in the later stages of inflammation, when resolution and repair of the injured tissue are of paramount importance. In a model of liver injury, it has been demonstrated that neutropenic animals develop more severe fibrosis, probably due to the lack of MMPs (released by neutrophils) in the repair phase [16]. A similar dependence between inflammation and collagenolysis in the lung has not been demonstrated, but these findings warrant more research.

Research on models of lung injury using knock-out mice for single MMPs, such as MMP-2, MMP-3, MMP-7, MMP-8 and MMP-9, has shed some light on this issue. MMP-2 [11], MMP-7 [17] and MMP-9 [18] have been shown to be involved in alveolar epithelial repair in experimental models of wound healing. Furthermore, a model of VILI [19] demonstrated that MMP-9 function is worth preserving, given that mice deficient in this protease had increased levels of lung injury. On the other hand, MMP-3 may be detrimental, as mice lacking this MMP were protected against lung injury caused by administration of nonspecific IgG [20] or bleomycin [21]. Regarding MMP-8, this protease has shown different effects depending on the experimental model. It has a detrimental role in models of VILI [22] and lung fibrosis, due to IL-10 cleavage [23]. However, this enzyme may be beneficial after lipopolysaccharide (LPS) or hyperoxia exposition [24]. Moreover, it may have a role in resolution stages of ALI, as it seems to be involved in neutrophil apoptosis through modulation of IL-4 levels [25].

Therefore, this complex family serves not only to regulate the influx and clearance of leukocytes and the inflammatory process itself, but also the removal of excess deposits of collagen fibers released by fibroblasts during ALI. It is becoming clearer that pharmacotherapy should be aimed at blocking specific MMPs during the early stages of ALI, in order to avoid destruction of the basement membrane and extracellular matrix caused by their proteolytic action. Although this could have an initial benefit it may turn detrimental to the repair process if treatment is continued.

Signs of Tissue Repair in Patients

The assessment of lung repair in patients could be of great interest because of its prognostic relevance in ALI patients. However, measurement of any mediator involved in tissue repair has one fundamental limitation: If a patient shows high levels of a given marker, it could be due to ongoing repair and, therefore, associated with a good prognosis. However, the same high levels could also be due to massive injury triggering a full-blown response. In this case, the outcome may not be so good.

Collagen levels illustrate this two-sided interpretation of biomarkers. As mentioned before, collagen deposition is an early event during ALI. Increased levels of procollagen in pulmonary edema fluid may have a prognostic significance in patients with ALI. For instance, Chesnutt et al. [26] reported that a procollagen concentration above 1.75 U/ml had a positive predictive value for death of 0.75. However, a recent article by Quesnel et al. [27] showed that patients with ALI/acute respiratory distress syndrome (ARDS) with fibroblasts in their alveolar fluid had increased levels of type I procollagen, a decreased pro-inflammatory response (lower neutrophil count, decreased IL-8 levels), and improved prognosis, suggesting a switch from inflammation and tissue destruction to alveolar repair.

Research on the prognostic value of MMP-9 has yielded similar conflicting results. Abundance of this protease in bronchoalveolar lavage (BAL) fluid has been related to a worse outcome. However, MMP-9 has shown a protective role in experimental models of lung injury [19, 28], and a clinical study demonstrated that this enzyme could have therapeutic value (see below). Finally, the prognostic value of growth factors in ALI was addressed years ago by Verghese et al. [29]. Lower levels of HGF and KGF were found in survivors. Although these mediators promote cell proliferation, differentiation and, ultimately, alveolar repair, their presence reflects a worse outcome. But, as the authors of the article discussed, the increased levels in non-survivors may be a marker of more severe injury.

Collectively, published results suggest that measurement of a single biomarker in patients can be misleading, as it can reflect both the severity of the injury and the subsequent healing process. An accurate prediction may require complex reasoning that takes into account the initial conditions but also the host's biological response. Therefore, an approach based on multiple markers could offer an alternative to monitor the course of this disease in patients.

Therapeutic Strategies Aimed At Lung Repair

Since identification of the pathways involved in lung injury, most literature has been focused on the use of therapies aimed at reducing ALI by truncating the inflammatory response. Unfortunately, none of these strategies has been successfully applied in the clinical practice. Recently, a significant number of studies have centered their efforts on enhancing the repair process using different approaches, ranging from the use of biocompatible materials or cells to the therapeutic use of mediators aimed at promoting cell proliferation, migration and differentiation. **Figure 3** summarizes the different therapeutic targets aimed at favoring lung repair.

In many cases, these studies are still at the *in vitro* stages, such as the use of vimentin to improve wound repair [30], or just suggest a possible beneficial role (e.g., connexins [31], adrenomedullin [32] or a possible modulation of the transcription factors, FoxM1 and Runx3 [33, 34]) and need further research to prove their viability *in vivo*. Improvement of plasma membrane repair is a possible direct treatment. A recent study in an *ex vivo* model using an amphiphilic macromolecule (Poloxamer 188) with sealing properties showed signs of membrane repair in alveolar resident cells and an improvement in conventional measures of lung injury [35].

Enhancement of the epithelial repopulation is a promising therapeutic target that could be achieved in different ways. In recent years, therapy using stem cells is gaining considerable interest. It has been demonstrated that these cells are active players in lung repair [36]. In spite of doubts about their safety and the

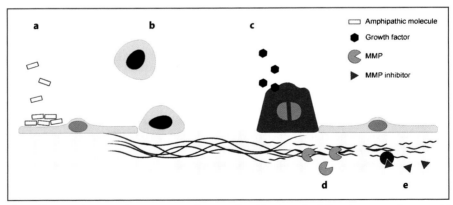

Fig. 3. Therapeutic approaches to promote lung repair. **a** Direct repair of the plasma membrane could be achieved using amphipathic compounds that seal injured membranes. **b** Exogenous stem cells to repair the denuded areas. **c** Administration of growth factors to stimulate the proliferation of endogenous stem cells. **d** and **e** Stimulation (**d**) or selective blockade (**e**) of different matrix metalloproteinases (MMPs) to promote collagen processing or avoid the adverse effects of these enzymes.

best administration route to improve their engraftment, use of stem cells in animal models has been demonstrated to attenuate damage and fibrosis in lungs challenged with endotoxin [37]. In a recent study, Curley et al. [38] submitted a group of rats to VILI followed by an intravenous injection of mesenchymal stem cells; these animals showed less lung injury and increased levels of the anti-inflammatory and anti-fibrotic cytokine, IL-10, than did rats who did not receive the stem cells. The specific mechanisms by which stem cells perform their functions in tissue repair are still under study, but the release of several growth factors and the suppression of pro-inflammatory cytokines seem to be involved.

An alternative approach is the therapeutic use of exogenous growth factors to induce the proliferation of endogenous stem cells. Among these factors, EGF, KGF and HGF have been the most studied. All of them are mitogens in type II pneumocytes, and act synergistically to mediate their maturation and increase surfactant synthesis [8]. EGF had beneficial effects in an animal model of ALI [39], and inhibition of EGF receptor had a detrimental effect during airway epithelium repair [40]. KGF has been linked to upregulation of anti-inflammatory cytokines and modulation of epithelial cell migration [41]. In the same way, HGF attenuates inflammation and showed antifibrotic effects in a murine model of bleomycin-induced fibrosis [42]. Vascular endothelial growth factor (VEGF) could also have a therapeutic effect by its ability to repair damaged endothelium, therefore helping in clearance of lung edema, but animal models have shown disappointing results [43].

Finally, manipulation of tissue remodeling could improve the outcome of ALI patients by favoring re-epithelization or avoiding fibrosis. The use of steroids in ALI has yielded conflicting results, depending on the time of application. These discrepancies can be explained if one takes into account the beneficial effects of inflammation during the repair phase discussed earlier. However, no study has specifically addressed the effects of steroids during lung repair.

MMPs are alternative targets to promote repair. Non-selective MMP inhibitors are available, but the lack of specificity could limit their benefits and none of them has been tested in ALI. Selective blockade or stimulation (depending on the role of the MMP and timing) could be a more promising approach. One of the first examples that has arrived in human trials is the use of beta-2 adrenergic receptor agonists. Intravenous administration of salbutamol decreased the duration and severity of lung injury by reducing lung edema in patients with ARDS [44]. This finding was associated with an upregulation of MMP-9 [18] and, therefore, with better alveolar epithelial repair [45]. Nevertheless, the route of administration could be relevant, as a recent trial has concluded that patients with ALI treated with inhaled salbutamol show no significant improvement in clinical outcomes [46]. On the other hand, blockade of MMP-8 has shown beneficial effects in experimental models of lung injury [22], including decreased lung fibrosis after bleomycin administration [23]. However, no clinical study aimed at modulating this protease has yet been proposed.

Conclusion

The lungs have a substantial potential for recovery after ALI. Of note, the mechanisms that can cause tissue disruption in the early phase also contribute to its repair later on, inflammation and matrix remodeling being paradigmatic examples. Therefore, therapies that disrupt these pathways, such as MMP inhibition, may have a prophylactic value, but their application at a later phase could be detrimental. Knowledge of the mediators involved in tissue repair could lead to new therapeutic strategies being applied after the initial insult has been controlled. Growth factors, exogenous stem cells (including type II pneumocytes) or drugs that promote matrix remodeling could be new alternatives to improve the prognosis of patients with ALI.

Acknowledgement: Supported by Instituto de Salud Carlos III (Fondo de Investigación Sanitaria PI 10/00606) and Universidad de Oviedo (UNOV-09-BECDOC), Spain

References

1. Ventrice EA, Marti-Sistac O, Gonzalvo R, Villagra A, Lopez-Aguilar J, Blanch L (2007) [Molecular and biophysical mechanisms and modulation of ventilator-induced lung injury]. Med Intensiva 31: 73–82
2. Bianchi ME (2007) DAMPs, PAMPs and alarmins: all we need to know about danger. J Leukoc Biol 81: 1–5
3. de Carvalho ME, Dolhnikoff M, Meireles SI, Reis LF, Martins MA, Deheinzelin D (2007) Effects of overinflation on procollagen type III expression in experimental acute lung injury. Crit Care 11: R23
4. Armstrong L, Thickett DR, Mansell JP, et al (1999) Changes in collagen turnover in early acute respiratory distress syndrome. Am J Respir Crit Care Med 160: 1910–1915
5. Berthiaume Y, Matthay MA (2007) Alveolar edema fluid clearance and acute lung injury. Respir Physiol Neurobiol 159: 350–359
6. Bhatia M, Moochhala S (2004) Role of inflammatory mediators in the pathophysiology of acute respiratory distress syndrome. J Pathol 202: 145–156
7. Kubo H (2011) Molecular basis of lung tissue regeneration. Gen Thorac Cardiovasc Surg 59: 231–244
8. Lindsay CD (2011) Novel therapeutic strategies for acute lung injury induced by lung damaging agents: the potential role of growth factors as treatment options. Hum Exp Toxicol 30: 701–724
9. Davey A, McAuley DF, O'Kane CM (2011) Matrix metalloproteinases in acute lung Injury: mediators of injury and drivers of repair. Eur Respir J 38: 959–970
10. Nin N, Lorente JA, de Paula M, et al (2008) Rats surviving injurious mechanical ventilation show reversible pulmonary, vascular and inflammatory changes. Intensive Care Med 34: 948–956
11. Gonzalez-Lopez A, Astudillo A, Garcia-Prieto E, et al (2011) Inflammation and matrix remodeling during repair of ventilator-induced lung injury. Am J Physiol Lung Cell Mol Physiol 301: L500–509
12. Abraham E (2003) Neutrophils and acute lung injury. Crit Care Med 31: S195–199
13. Korpos E, Wu C, Sorokin L (2009) Multiple roles of the extracellular matrix in inflammation. Curr Pharm Des 15: 1349–1357
14. Lin M, Jackson P, Tester AM, et al (2008) Matrix metalloproteinase-8 facilitates neutrophil migration through the corneal stromal matrix by collagen degradation and production of the chemotactic peptide Pro-Gly-Pro. Am J Pathol 173: 144–153
15. Van Lint P, Libert C (2007) Chemokine and cytokine processing by matrix metalloproteinases and its effect on leukocyte migration and inflammation. J Leukoc Biol 82: 1375–1381
16. Harty MW, Muratore CS, Papa EF, et al (2010) Neutrophil depletion blocks early collagen degradation in repairing cholestatic rat livers. Am J Pathol 176: 1271–1281
17. Parks WC (2003) Matrix metalloproteinases in lung repair. Eur Respir J Suppl 44:36s-38s
18. O'Kane CM, McKeown SW, Perkins GD, et al (2009) Salbutamol up-regulates matrix metalloproteinase-9 in the alveolar space in the acute respiratory distress syndrome. Crit Care Med 37: 2242–2249

19. Albaiceta GM, Gutierrez-Fernandez A, Parra D, et al (2008) Lack of matrix metalloproteinase-9 worsens ventilator-induced lung injury. Am J Physiol Lung Cell Mol Physiol 294: L535–543
20. Nerusu KC, Warner RL, Bhagavathula N, McClintock SD, Johnson KJ, Varani J (2007) Matrix metalloproteinase-3 (stromelysin-1) in acute inflammatory tissue injury. Exp Mol Pathol 83: 169–176
21. Yamashita CM, Dolgonos L, Zemans RL, et al (2011) Matrix metalloproteinase 3 is a mediator of pulmonary fibrosis. Am J Pathol 179: 1733–1745
22. Albaiceta GM, Gutierrez-Fernandez A, Garcia-Prieto E, et al (2010) Absence or inhibition of matrix metalloproteinase-8 decreases ventilator-induced lung injury. Am J Respir Cell Mol Biol 43: 555–563
23. Garcia-Prieto E, Gonzalez-Lopez A, Cabrera S, et al (2010) Resistance to bleomycin-induced lung fibrosis in MMP-8 deficient mice is mediated by interleukin-10. PLoS One 5:e13242

24. Quintero PA, Knolle MD, Cala LF, Zhuang Y, Owen CA (2010) Matrix metalloproteinase-8 inactivates macrophage inflammatory protein-1 alpha to reduce acute lung inflammation and injury in mice. J Immunol 184: 1575–1588
25. Gueders MM, Balbin M, Rocks N, et al (2005) Matrix metalloproteinase-8 deficiency promotes granulocytic allergen-induced airway inflammation. J Immunol 175: 2589–2597
26. Chesnutt AN, Matthay MA, Tibayan FA, Clark JG (1997) Early detection of type III procollagen peptide in acute lung injury. Pathogenetic and prognostic significance. Am J Respir Crit Care Med 156: 840–845
27. Quesnel C, Nardelli L, Piednoir P, et al (2010) Alveolar fibroblasts in acute lung injury: biological behaviour and clinical relevance. Eur Respir J 35: 1312–1321
28. Yoon HK, Cho HY, Kleeberger SR (2007) Protective role of matrix metalloproteinase-9 in ozone-induced airway inflammation. Environ Health Perspect 115: 1557–1563
29. Verghese GM, McCormick-Shannon K, Mason RJ, Matthay MA (1998) Hepatocyte growth factor and keratinocyte growth factor in the pulmonary edema fluid of patients with acute lung injury. Biologic and clinical significance. Am J Respir Crit Care Med 158: 386–394
30. Rogel MR, Soni PN, Troken JR, Sitikov A, Trejo HE, Ridge KM (2011) Vimentin is sufficient and required for wound repair and remodeling in alveolar epithelial cells. FASEB J (in press)
31. Losa D, Chanson M, Crespin S (2011) Connexins as therapeutic targets in lung disease. Expert Opin Ther Targets 15: 989–1002
32. Vadivel A, Abozaid S, van Haaften T, et al (2010) Adrenomedullin promotes lung angiogenesis, alveolar development, and repair. Am J Respir Cell Mol Biol 43: 152–160
33. Liu Y, Sadikot RT, Adami GR, et al (2011) FoxM1 mediates the progenitor function of type II epithelial cells in repairing alveolar injury induced by Pseudomonas aeruginosa. J Exp Med 208: 1473–1484
34. Lee JM, Kwon HJ, Bae SC, Jung HS (2010) Lung tissue regeneration after induced injury in Runx3 KO mice. Cell Tissue Res 341: 465–470
35. Plataki M, Lee YD, Rasmussen DL, Hubmayr RD (2011) Poloxamer 188 facilitates the repair of alveolus resident cells in ventilator injured lungs. Am J Respir Crit Care Med 184: 939–947
36. Giangreco A, Arwert EN, Rosewell IR, Snyder J, Watt FM, Stripp BR (2009) Stem cells are dispensable for lung homeostasis but restore airways after injury. Proc Natl Acad Sci USA 106: 9286–9291
37. Yang KY, Shih HC, How CK, et al (2011) IV delivery of induced pluripotent stem cells attenuates endotoxin-induced acute lung injury in mice. Chest 140: 1243–1253
38. Curley GF, Contreras M, Higgins BD, O'Toole DP, Laffey JG (2011) The role of mesenchymal stem cells during repair from ventilator induced lung injury. J Respir Crit Care Med (in press)
39. Plopper CG, St George JA, Read LC, et al (1992) Acceleration of alveolar type II cell differentiation in fetal rhesus monkey lung by administration of EGF. Am J Physiol 262: L313–321
40. Harada C, Kawaguchi T, Ogata-Suetsugu S, et al (2011) EGFR tyrosine kinase inhibition

worsens acute lung injury in mice with repairing airway epithelium. Am J Respir Crit Care Med 183: 743–751

41. Panoskaltsis-Mortari A, Ingbar DH, Jung P, et al (2000) KGF pretreatment decreases B7 and granzyme B expression and hastens repair in lungs of mice after allogeneic BMT. Am J Physiol Lung Cell Mol Physiol 278: L988–999

42. Dohi M, Hasegawa T, Yamamoto K, Marshall BC (2000) Hepatocyte growth factor attenuates collagen accumulation in a murine model of pulmonary fibrosis. Am J Respir Crit Care Med 162: 2302–2307

43. Medford AR, Millar AB (2006) Vascular endothelial growth factor (VEGF) in acute lung injury (ALI) and acute respiratory distress syndrome (ARDS): paradox or paradigm? Thorax 61: 621–626

44. Perkins GD, McAuley DF, Thickett DR, Gao F (2006) The beta-agonist lung injury trial (BALTI): a randomized placebo-controlled clinical trial. Am J Respir Crit Care Med 173: 281–287

45. Perkins GD, Gao F, Thickett DR (2008) In vivo and in vitro effects of salbutamol on alveolar epithelial repair in acute lung injury. Thorax 63: 215–220

46. Matthay MA, Brower RG, Carson S, et al (2011) Randomized, placebo-controlled clinical trial of an aerosolized beta-2 agonist for treatment of acute lung injury. Am J Respir Crit Care Med 184: 561–568

V

VI Respiratory Support

Non-invasive Ventilation Outside the ICU

G. Landoni, A. Zangrillo, and L. Cabrini

Introduction

Non-invasive ventilation (NIV), including both non-invasive positive pressure ventilation (NPPV) and non-invasive continuous positive airway pressure (CPAP), is increasingly applied to prevent or to treat acute respiratory failure [1]. Evidence of benefit has been demonstrated in some common diseases, such as chronic obstructive pulmonary disease (COPD) exacerbations, acute respiratory failure in immunosuppressed patients, and cardiogenic pulmonary edema. There is still no strong scientific evidence on the usefulness of NIV in other settings and more research is required [1, 2]. Nevertheless, NIV is an established, relevant option in the management of acute respiratory failure and the number of publications on this topic is steadily increasing (**Fig. 1**).

Most studies on NIV have been conducted in intensive care units (ICUs), as a logical setting in which expertise on ventilation, staff and equipment are maximal to effectively and safely treat patients with moderate to severe (but potentially fatal) acute respiratory failure. The emergency department (ED) shares many characteristics of the ICU, and NIV has been extensively applied and studied also in the ED. Recently, NIV application outside the ICU and the ED has been reported. NIV use in general wards can be attractive for many reasons, such as cost-effectiveness and the possibility to treat patients at an early stage (**Box 1**,

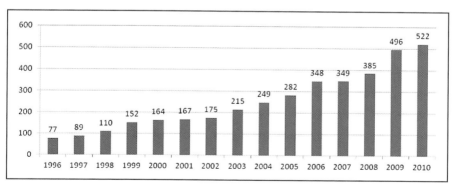

Fig. 1. Number of publications on NIV per year for the last 15 years. Papers were searched for in Scopus from January 1995 to January 2011 according to the following string "non invasive ventilation or non-invasive ventilation or NIV". There has been a steady increase in the number of publications on this topic.

J.-L. Vincent (ed.), *Annual Update in Intensive Care and Emergency Medicine 2012*
DOI 10.1007/978-3-642-25716-2 © Springer-Verlag Berlin Heidelberg 2012

Box 1. Advantages (panel A) and disadvantages (panel B) of performing non-invasive ventilation (NIV) on general wards

Panel A. NIV on general wards: Potential advantages
Patients can be treated at an early, more responsive stage of acute respiratory failure
Reduced costs compared to the intensive care unit
Intensive care unit beds can be used for other critically ill patients
NIV can "buy time" while diagnostic investigations or therapeutic procedures are performed
Patients can avoid the stressful setting of the intensive care unit
Patients for whom intensive care unit admission is considered inappropriate can be treated, and half of them will survive to hospital discharge
NIV can be used to prevent or treat acute respiratory failure in new fields of application

Panel B. NIV on general wards: Potential disadvantages
NIV application can be suboptimal, lowering the efficacy of the treatment compared to on the intensive care unit
NIV failure can be detected with delay
In case of respiratory sudden deterioration, tracheal intubation may be performed less promptly than in an intensive care unit
NIV-related complications may not be immediately detected and treated
Patients with a high risk of failure cannot be treated in inexperienced and under-monitored wards
NIV-related workload can be difficult to manage on under staffed wards; other ward patients can suffer from a reduction in assistance
If NIV is applied without a careful selection of patients, massive overuse is possible and cost-effectiveness can be lost

panel A); however, this setting is very different from an ICU, and might jeopardize patient safety (**Box 1** panel B).

We hereby report published data on NIV use on general wards, describe the pros and cons of this field of use, suggest how to safely introduce NIV in the wards, and anticipate future applications.

Is NIV Already Used on General Wards?

Several papers have reported NIV use on general wards. The first reports were published almost 20 years ago [3]. The pivotal study was performed some years later by Plant et al. [4], who demonstrated the efficacy of NIV in COPD exacerbations; the study took place in a respiratory ward.

A completely different approach was described by Paus-Jenssen et al. a few years later [5]. In response to financial constraints and intensive bed limitations, NIV was introduced in all hospital wards without a formal protocol and without preliminary training. All physicians could order NIV for patients with acute respiratory failure and NIV was initiated and maintained on the original patient ward; 41 % of cases were treated on general wards and the authors concluded that "Patients in whom NIV was initiated outside of a critical care unit did not appear to have worse outcomes" compared to similar patients treated in the ICU.

Two surveys in Canada and the UK showed that NIV was applied in general wards in both countries, although this was not common [6, 7]. Two surveys were conducted in the United States. The first [8] was sent to all the respiratory care directors of the 82 hospitals in Massachusetts and Rhode Island. Responders estimated that 18 % of NIV treatments were started on general wards, and in two thirds of the hospitals, NIV patients were allowed to remain on the general ward. In the second survey [9], sent to physicians and respiratory therapists of 63 Veterans Affairs hospitals, 40 % of respondents reported use of NIV on the wards (42 % of which were with no restriction on location of use).

In a single-center prospective observational study, Schettino et al. [10] reported that among 449 treated patients, NIV was initiated on general units in 33 % of cases, and 35 % (including a few patients in whom NIV was initiated in the ED) of the NIV treatments initiated were then managed on general units: Of these patients, 27.3 % were intubated and 14.9 % died.

A trend toward an increased use of NIV on medical wards to treat mild COPD exacerbations (pH > 7.28) was reported from one experienced center. The percentage of patients managed on the general ward increased from about 15 % to almost 80 % in the eight year study period, with similar outcomes [11]. In a recent national survey performed in Italy and specifically addressing NIV use outside the ICU, 65 % of the respondents reported NIV application on general wards and 28 % allowed NIV use in every ward [12]. Positive effectiveness and feasibility results have also been reported from Spain, China, Turkey and Saudi Arabia [13–16]. A growing number of papers have described the use of NIV in general wards as a resource of a medical emergency team (MET) or a critical care outreach (nurse-managed) team (CCOT) [17]. After an initial experience in a surgical ward in the UK [18], an observational study in a single center on 129 consecutive patients treated by a MET in medical and surgical wards showed a high success rate with few, mild complications; however, the NIV-related workload for the MET was quite intensive and time-consuming [19]. More recently, reports from centers with similar METs or CCOTs have been published from Australia [20] and the UK [21]. An NIV service managed by a MET in a hematologic ward was associated with a reduction in the risk of death in a randomized trial [22].

In conclusion, NIV use in general wards has been widely and increasingly reported and we cannot exclude that in real clinical practice NIV is now mainly applied in this setting. Nevertheless, we must keep in mind that published data on this technique were almost exclusively obtained from studies within the ICU or the ED, with the notable exceptions described above.

Why should NIV be Applied in General Wards?

The ICU is considered the safest setting to deliver NIV. The sophisticated monitoring resources in this environment, the experienced staff and a high nurse:patient ratio allow even critically ill patients to be treated [2]. Nevertheless, ICU beds are expensive and limited; a shortage of available intensive beds is experienced worldwide [23], and triage criteria must frequently be applied to decide which patients should be admitted and which refused. If the use of NIV is only allowed in the ICU, we run the risk of underuse. As stated in the British Thoracic Society Guidelines for Non-invasive Ventilation, "...If an acute NIV service is not provided, the shortage of ICU beds means that some patients will die" [24]. The need to use NIV on general wards to avoid its underuse has been reported from several countries [4, 5, 19].

There is also growing awareness that NIV efficacy is maximal when the treatment is initiated in an early, more responsive stage of acute respiratory failure (a 'window of opportunity') to prevent further deterioration of lung function and

VI

need for tracheal intubation [2, 22, 25]. As a result, if NIV should be applied to patients with mild to moderate acute respiratory failure, we should anticipate a relevant increase in treatments compared to the present situation [26]. There will be insufficient ICU beds to admit all patients requiring NIV. Moreover, new fields of application of NIV have been evaluated with promising results, further increasing the number of potential candidates for NIV. In particular, NIV use to prevent or to treat postoperative acute respiratory failure is very attractive [27–30].

Provided that patient safety and efficacy of the technique are preserved, NIV use in general wards has been demonstrated to be cost-effective. In a prospective randomized study performed in general wards [4], the introduction of an NIV service to treat mild COPD exacerbations saved about 70,000 Euros (118 patients treated with NIV compared to 118 treated with standard therapy); indeed, the mortality rate in the NIV group was halved. The main area of cost saving was in the reduced use of the ICU. Carlucci et al. observed a daily reduction of 90 Euro for each NIV treatment over an eight year period; the saving was due to an increased percentage of patients treated in general wards [11].

NIV application in general wards can be a life-saving option for 'too ill' patients for whom ICU admission is considered inappropriate. NIV can be used as the maximal allowed treatment (patients 'not for intubation'); in this condition, about 50 % of treated patients will survive to hospital discharge [2, 31]. In dying patients, NIV can sometimes be indicated to alleviate respiratory discomfort [31]. Not rarely, NIV application buys time while diagnostic investigations or therapeutic procedures are performed [32]; as an example, during this extra-time, the health care staff can decide whether tracheal intubation is an option or not, and the patient can have the opportunity to express his/her opinion.

Finally, although, to our knowledge, no study has evaluated the patient's perspective when treated with NIV in ICU compared to on the general ward, patients frequently report that their stay in the ICU was very unpleasant [33].

Risks Associated with NIV Misuse and Overuse

Lowered Efficacy

General wards are extremely heterogeneous not only among different hospitals, but also in the same institution. They are also usually dedicated to a specific specialty and health care staff can lack knowledge and experience on other diseases or techniques, like acute respiratory failure and NIV. The reported failure rate (considering the need for tracheal intubation as failure) of NIV in general wards in a mixed population ranges from 19 to 27 % [10, 19, 20]; when applied at an early stage of acute respiratory failure or in highly responsive diseases like COPD, the failure rate seems significantly lower [4, 22, 30]. However, in all the studies, a relevant percentage of patients needed to be transferred to the ICU whereas another subgroup, considered 'not-for-intubation', died on the ward. The perception of physicians and respiratory therapists on NIV success rate (reported as modest by about 50 %) [9, 12] confirms the data. Indeed, these results were always obtained in hospitals with considerable experience of NIV use, and worse outcomes can be expected in other centers. The impact of specific training and experience of the ward staff on NIV efficacy has never been evaluated. Unanimously, training and experience of the staff are considered the most important factors determining NIV efficacy [32]. Training and experience are necessary to correctly select patients in whom NIV is indicated, and to choose the right moment (not too early, not too late) to start and to stop the treatment. Ward personnel must be able to set optimal ventilatory parameters. Even if NIV can be easily applied, its success is strictly dependent on many factors that are not evident, like the ability to motivate the patient and the right tightening of the mask (not too much to avoid discomfort, not too weak to avoid excessive air leaks). Patient intolerance is a common reason for failure, and only trained, expert staff can prevent it by looking for the best patient-ventilator interaction [34]. Above all, ward staff should be able to promptly recognize the failure of the technique without delaying tracheal intubation when this is an option. It is evident that the ward personnel may not reach the required level of knowledge and experience to optimize the efficacy of NIV and consequently a lower efficacy can be expected when compared to the ICU setting (where the personnel is supposed to be more expert).

Patient Safety

Given the limited human and equipment resources, patient monitoring in general wards is less intensive compared to the ICU setting. So far, to the best of our knowledge (and excluding NIV failure – see previous paragraph), only two prospective studies from the same center have reported data on complications during NIV application on general wards [19, 30]. In 214 treated patients, the only major complication was one episode of arterial hypotension that resolved immediately after NIV suspension; nasal skin lesions and patient discomfort were the observed minor complications and occurred in less than 10 % of patients, all without consequences. Technical or organizational problems, such as suboptimal mask positioning with excessive air leaks, ventilator malfunctioning and failure to accomplish the prescribed ventilatory cycles, were more common, but no consequences for the patients were observed. However, two subsequent surveys from the same hospital gave a different picture. Ninety ward nurses reported a high incidence of potentially severe complications such as sudden desaturation and ventilator malfunctioning; more alarming, in the nurses' perception, detection of the problem or the medical intervention had a delay longer than 5 min in one third of the cases [35]. In the same study, nurses reported a very low incidence of staff errors in managing NIV; nevertheless, only 23 % reported that the prescribed NIV cycles were always administered, 18 % said that NIV was often interrupted with some delay, and 6 % reported that NIV was usually interrupted too early. In a twin study performed by interviewing 45 patients after successful NIV treatment, all patients reported at least one complication (with worsening of respiration during NIV in 18 % of the cases); 28 patients reported having suffered a medical emergency, and four noted that they waited for help from staff for more than 3 minutes [36].

Despite the lack of data, there is a general consensus in the literature that wards (with the possible exception of respiratory wards) are commonly inadequate to safely monitor patients on NIV [37, 38]. Nevertheless, it should be noted that there is no consensus on which monitoring is mandatory [39], and so far NIV has commonly been applied to patients with moderate to severe acute respiratory failure. Hypoxemic patients are particularly at risk, as deterioration can be very rapid with fatal consequences [2]. More in general, patients presenting known risk factors for NIV failure such as acute lung injury/acute respiratory distress syndrome (ALI/ARDS), multiple or severe comorbidities, severe acute respiratory failure, low tolerance or no improvement after the first 1–2 hour of treatment, should be considered unfit for a general ward [34]. In addition, general wards are usually inadequate settings for patients unable to maintain spontaneous respiration for at least 15–60 minutes without NIV [2]. In any case, a team able to assist the patient in case of respiratory deterioration and to perform tracheal intubation if required should be immediately available: As a rule, general wards that are unable to guarantee this requirement should be considered inadequate for NIV in patients without a limitation of treatment policy.

Finally, the NIV related workload could negatively affect the safety (and the quality of care) of the other patients present on the wards. Although no study has evaluated this issue, it is likely that in understaffed wards, NIV can 'steal' a significant amount of time from other patients.

Cost-effectiveness

Although two studies reported that NIV in general wards allowed significant savings compared to NIV in the ICU [4, 11], so far several factors related to introduction of NIV in general wards have never been evaluated. It should be noted that training for all ward staff is mandatory, both before introduction of NIV and as periodical education (see dedicated paragraph); indeed, better training seems to be the main request from ward staff [8, 12]. Moreover, there is a risk of over-utilizing NIV. Without strict selection of patients, NIV may be applied too early (when not useful), too late/too long (when tracheal intubation is required), or to patients in whom it is not indicated (for example, unnecessarily prolonging the dying process in terminal patients). The waste of resources of overuse could easily grow out of control. Finally, the workload to the personnel can be considerable.

How To Make NIV a Safe and Effective General Ward Tool

NIV use outside the ICU could be seen as part of the general tendency to treat deteriorating ward patients as early as possible, as a result of the finding that often (if not always) outcomes of critically ill patients depend on a time-sensitive approach; the trend to promptly initiate intensive treatments in ordinary wards has been called "critical care without walls" [17, 40]. Nevertheless, general wards are quite different from the ICU and they cannot be considered an adequate setting for NIV unless some prerequisites are met. The first and most important prerequisite is the presence of a multidisciplinary enthusiastic group (or a minimum of one enthusiastic clinician) that acts as a "clinical champion" [41], working with organizational leaders to introduce the technique in the hospital, promoting training, motivating other clinicians, keeping knowledge on the topic updated, collecting data and publicizing positive outcomes.

Training

Although many centers have applied NIV outside the ICU without any prior educational program [5, 12], to achieve maximal efficacy while preserving patient safety, training about NIV should be considered mandatory before introducing this technique on general wards [41, 42]. Periodical re-training should also be offered, particularly when considering the often elevated staff turn-over, especially among ward nurses [35].

Basic training requirements include understanding the rationale for assisted ventilation, the indications and contraindications of NIV, prevention and treatment of its complications, ventilator functioning and settings, interface choices and fitting, clinical and instrumental monitoring, the importance of patient cooperation and how to increase patient comfort [32, 41, 42]. Patient safety issues should be extensively addressed. While theoretical content can be offered in traditional lessons, workshops may be the best way to train on practical aspects, like mask fitting or ventilator circuit assembly. Finally, troubleshooting and problem solving of serious situations (sudden desaturation, patient intolerance, coma, respiratory deterioration while on NIV...) could be addressed in simulated scenarios. Training should also consider the local organization of the NIV service (that is, if NIV is prescribed by a MET, by a respiratory therapist or by the ward physicians). The decision to initiate treatment is particularly critical, as it must be based on a complex evaluation of patient condition, the ward's human and technical resources and the alternative options, in order to balance risks and benefits. As a consequence, whoever prescribes NIV must be fully trained and experienced on NIV and on local resources/reliability.

After NIV introduction in the wards, periodical surveys should be performed among the ward personnel to determine educational needs and gaps [6, 35]. Finally, whenever possible, if patient status permits, NIV education should be offered to her/him and to her/his family, in order to increase patient compliance and to enable careful monitoring also from the relatives.

VI

Equipment

While treating mild to moderate acute respiratory failure, portable dedicated NIV ventilators are at least as effective as more expensive critical care ventilators [41–44]; a reliable battery power source is mandatory. To deliver CPAP, cheaper 'continuous high flow' devices can be used. A wide range of interfaces must be available, with different sizes and models [2]. Sequential use of interfaces can be very effective in long treatments when skin injuries ensue. If humidification is required, heated humidifiers are preferred [43].

Monitoring should be dictated by the severity of illness of the patient and not by the resources available. In most wards, new monitoring equipment is likely to be needed when NIV is introduced. At a minimum, continuous pulse oximetry and electocardiogram (best if telemetric) should be available for every patient [32], even if, in selected cases, periodical evaluation of vital signs may be sufficient. When more sophisticated monitoring is required, the patient should be transferred to the ICU.

Local Protocols

General wards are extremely heterogeneous. Developing local (valid for all the wards of a hospital or for a limited number, or even specific for a single ward) protocols can help to standardize treatments. Simple, comprehensive practice guidelines should include indications, contraindications, complications, suggested modalities of delivering NIV (how to start, how to continue, when to stop), monitoring, solutions to common problems. An algorithm could help to evaluate whether NIV may be more useful than risky for the specific patient in a specific ward. The main factors to be considered when defining the criteria to initiate NIV in wards include the risks of failure (cause and severity of acute respiratory failure, comorbidities...), the achievable level of patient safety (nurse:patient ratio, monitoring capabilities, staff experience and training, level of consciousness of the patient and his/her autonomy without NIV...) and the concrete alternatives (is the patient considered unfit for the ICU?) [19, 41, 42, 45]. Local protocols can be helpful in educating clinicians and keeping all updated; an accurate description of roles and responsibilities can also avoid unnecessary conflicts among the involved health care workers.

Organization

Two main model of organization have been reported: NIV can be prescribed by ward physicians and fully managed by the ward staff [4, 5]; alternatively, NIV can be prescribed by someone external to the ward and better trained in use of NIV (respiratory therapist, MET, CCOT). Once initiated, treatment is then managed in conjunction with the ward staff [19, 20, 22]. No studies comparing the pros and cons of the two models are available. With the exception of respiratory wards, in our opinion the complexity of NIV and above all the need for an expert evaluation of the risk/benefit balance suggest that the decision to prescribe NIV should be made by a well-trained and experienced group external to the general wards and always present in the hospital. We are not aware of papers describing fully dedicated 'NIV teams', although such highly specialized teams could be justified in large hospitals. Given the recent worldwide trend to introduce rapid response teams in hospitals [17], assigning NIV prescription to them seems a logical solution [19, 20, 22].

In the present review, intermediate care units (also known as step-down units or high dependency units – HDUs) have not been considered. Such units are usually better staffed and equipped than the general ward, offering better monitoring. Although no studies have compared NIV use on HDUs and general wards, an NIV-dedicated HDU could be the optimal setting to treat acute respiratory failure patients who are not so sick as to require ICU admission. In an HDU, the staff could more easily reach a high level of expertise and efficacy and safety could be optimized in a location less expensive than an ICU [2, 45]. However, many hospitals do not have an HDU. Moreover, it would be difficult to transfer all patients potentially benefiting from NIV to an HDU.

Quality Improvement, Cost-Effectiveness and Patient Safety

Data on NIV treatments should be collected and analyzed. So far, we know very little about outcomes of patients treated with NIV in ordinary wards; in a national survey, some form of data collection was performed by only 18 % of hospitals using NIV outside the ICU [12]. As wards and NIV organization are heterogeneous, only analysis of local data can be informative for single centers. A quality improvement program should be implemented to assure that findings from data analysis improve clinical practice and shape the training.

Cost-effectiveness should be continuously evaluated. The determination of costs from supplies and equipment is easy, while estimation of the NIV-related workload is more difficult. Determination of outcomes is quite complex, as it must include an economic evaluation of improvements in mortality rates, lengths of hospital stay, avoidance of transfer to the ICU, avoidance of endotracheal intubation and so on. Delivering NIV in general wards should enable cost savings [4, 11], but it could also have the opposite effect if NIV is misused (lowering its efficacy) or overused (increasing costs without benefit). A careful economic supervision is required [41, 42].

Data on patient safety with NIV use on general wards are almost completely lacking. Local data collection should verify the incidence and consequences of NIV-related adverse events. All commonly applied risk management procedures should form part of NIV management, such as incident reporting, audits, root cause analysis. Questionnaires or interviews should be performed to investigate the point of view of patients and their family [36]. At the same time, preventive tools like checklist, posters, and written protocols should be developed.

Research

Despite hundreds of published studies on NIV, many questions are still without answers. We know very little about NIV efficacy or hazards when applied early in acute respiratory failure other than COPD exacerbations, about optimal NIV protocols (should it be applied continuously or administered in intermittent cycles?), or about patients' perspectives. Above all, we have few data about NIV efficacy and safety when delivered on general wards. Notwithstanding the differences among wards and hospitals, multicenter studies and collaborative networking are urgently needed to explore the limits and the possibilities of NIV outside the ICU.

Next Applications: A Look into the (Possible) Future Of NIV

New Ideas From (and to) Manufacturers

Although in recent years ventilators have been equipped with new diagnostic or therapeutic options, ventilator manufacturers have not yet focused their attention towards NIV application and monitoring on general wards. We anticipate that portable ventilators with new 'ward user-friendly' functions and integrated with telemetric monitoring will make NIV use on the wards safer, easier and more effective. Ventilator displays will guide the user through the correct assembling and application of the interface (and it is likely that dedicated interfaces will be presented); errors will be immediately detected; alarms will alert both ward staff and the MET; patient interactivity will be enhanced ('patient-controlled ventilation') to achieve maximal comfort. Expert NIV clinicians will be, as always, the main source of ideas to the manufacturers.

Novel Applications, Novel Users

NIV use during bronchoscopies has been extensively evaluated. New applications have been recently reported [46, 47] during therapeutic or diagnostic procedures in high-risk patients. As we all become more familiar with NIV, we will test its efficacy in new settings. Likely, in the same way that ultrasonography is now a resource for many specialties and no longer restricted to the hands of radiologists, NIV will become a resource (and a potential risk) for many specialists performing long procedures or administering mild sedatives in patient with labile respiratory function. This could be particularly true if ventilators are more user-friendly and in locations in which NIV 'experts', such as intensivists or pulmonologists, are costly or rare. Finally, NIV could be an emergent lifesaving measure during dangerous respiratory depression; as an example a new interface to be used in such conditions while performing endoscopies has just arrived on the market.

New Organization of NIV Services, New Training Modalities

When a critical mass of data on NIV use on general wards has been gathered, evidence-based guidelines will be developed and organizational aspects optimized. We foresee that multidisciplinary dedicated NIV teams will be considered the standard; they will be available to treat patients in every setting, and will manage an HDU where the small percentage of sicker patients will be admitted. Findings from local data analysis, published studies and collaborative networking will continuously improve clinical practice and will be quickly implemented into local protocols. Training will be improved and will be almost continuous, being based less on traditional lectures and more on interactive workshops, high fidelity simulated scenarios, screen based microsimulation and enhanced virtual reality. A closed loop using data from local quality improvement programs will help focus training on really relevant topics.

Conclusion

NIV is already extensively applied on general wards, and a growing use in this setting is expected with benefits for patients and costs savings for hospitals. To maximize efficacy and patient safety, careful institutional management is required. So far, there is great uncertainty about many fundamental aspects and further research is warranted.

References

1. Keenan SP, Sinuff T, Burns KE, et al (2011) Clinical practice guidelines for the use of noninvasive positive-pressure ventilation and noninvasive continuous positive airway pressure in the acute care setting. CMAJ 183: E195–214
2. Nava S, Hill NH (2009) Non-invasive ventilation in acute respiratory failure. Lancet 374: 250–259
3. Bott J, Carroll MP, Conway JH, et al (1993) Randomised controlled trial of nasal ventilation in acute ventilatory failure due to chronic obstructive airways disease. Lancet 341: 1555–1557
4. Plant PK, Owen JL, Elliott MW (2000) Early use of non-invasive ventilation for acute exacerbations of chronic obstructive pulmonary disease on general respiratory wards: a multicentre randomised controlled trial. Lancet 355: 1931–1935
5. Paus-Jenssen ES, Reid JK, Cockcroft DW, Laframboise K, Ward HA (2004) The use of noninvasive ventilation in acute respiratory failure at a tertiary care center. Chest 126: 165–172
6. Burns KEA, Sinuff T, Adhikari NKJ et al (2005) Bilevel positive pressure ventilation for acute respiratory failure: survey of Ontario practice. Crit Care Med 33: 1477–1483
7. Sulaiman MI, Rodger KA, Hawkins M (2004) A survey of the use of non invasive positive pressure ventilation in critical care units in the United Kingdom. Am J Respir Crit Care Med 169: A522 (abst)
8. Maheshwari V, Paioli D, Rothaar R, Hill NS (2006) Utilization of noninvasive ventilation in acute care hospitals. Chest 129: 1226–1233

VI

9. Bierer GB, Soo Hoo GW (2009) Noninvasive ventilation for acute respiratory failure: a national survey of Veterans Affair Hospitals. Respir Care 54: 1313–1320

10. Schettino G, Altobelli N, Kacmarek RM (2008) Noninvasive positive-pressureventilation in acute respiratory failure outside clinical trials: experience at the Massachusetts General Hospital. Crit Care Med 36: 441–447

11. Carlucci A, Delmastro M, Rubini F, Fracchia C, Nava S (2003) Changes in the practice of non-invasive ventilation in treating COPD patients over 8 years. Intensive Care Med 29: 419–425

12. Cabrini L, Antonelli M, Savoia G, Landriscina M (2011) Non-invasive ventilation outside the intensive care unit: an Italian survey. Minerva Anestesiol 77: 313–322

13. González Barcala FJ, Zamarrón Sanz C, Salgueiro Rodríguez M, Rodríguez Suárez JR (2004) Non-invasive ventilation in chronic obstructive pulmonary disease patients with acute respiratory hypercapnic failure in a conventional hospital ward. An Med Interna 21: 373–377

14. Collaborative Research Group of Noninvasive Mechanical Ventilation for Chronic Obstructive Pulmonary Disease (2005) Early use of non-invasive positive pressure ventilation for acute exacerbations of chronic obstructive pulmonary disease: a multicentre randomized controlled trial. Chin Med J 118: 2034–2040

15. Dikensoy O, Ikidag B, Filiz A, Bayram N (2002) Comparison of non-invasive ventilation and standard medical therapy in acute hypercapnic respiratory failure: a randomised controlled study at a tertiary health centre in SE Turkey. Int J Clin Pract 56: 85–88

16. Al-Mutairi SS, Al-Deen JS (2004) Non-invasive positive pressure ventilation in acute respiratory failure. An alternative modality to invasive ventilation at a general hospital. Saudi Med J 25: 190–194

17. DeVita MA, Bellomo R, Hillman K, et al. (2006) Findings of the first consensus conference on medical emergency teams. Crit Care Med 34: 2463–2478

18. Badiger R, Green M, Hackwood H, Palin C, Shee CD (2004) Non-invasive ventilation in surgical patients in a district general hospital. Anaesthesia 59: 967–970

19. Cabrini L, Idone C, Colombo S, et al (2009) Medical Emergency Team and non-invasive ventilation outside ICU for acute respiratory failure. Intensive Care Med 35: 333–343

20. Schneider AG, Calzavacca P, Mercer I, Hart G, Jones D, Bellomo R (2011) The epidemiology and outcome of medical emergency team call patients treated with non-invasive ventilation. Resuscitation 82: 1218–1223

21. Sumner K, Yadegafar G (2011) The utility and futility of non-invasive ventilation in non-designated areas: can critical care outreach nurses influence practice? Intensive Crit Care Nurs 27: 211–217

22. Squadrone, V, Massaia M, Bruno B, et al (2010) Early CPAP prevents evolution in acute lung injury in patients with hematologic malignancy. Intensive Care Med 36: 1666–1674

23. Edbrooke DL, Minelli C, Mills GH, et al (2011) Implications of ICU triage decisions on patient mortality: a cost-effectiveness analysis. Crit Care 15: R56

24. British Thoracic Society Standards of Care Committee (2002) Non-invasive ventilation in acute respiratory failure. Thorax 57: 192–211

25. Liesching T, Kwok H, Hill NS (2003) Acute applications of noninvasive positive pressure ventilation. Chest 124: 699–713

26. Cabrini L, Monti G, Landoni G, Colombo S, Savia I, Zangrillo A (2011) Non-invasive ventilation, ordinary wards and medical emergency team: maximizing effectiveness while preserving safety. Resuscitation 82: 1464

27. Jaber S, Chanques G, Jung B (2010) Postoperative noninvasive ventilation. Anesthesiology 112: 453–461

28. Chiumello D, Chevallard G, Gregoretti C (2011) Non-invasive ventilation in postoperative patients: a systematic review. Intensive Care Med 37: 918–929

29. Landoni G, Zangrillo A, Cabrini L (2012) Noninvasive ventilation after cardiac and thoracic surgery in adult patients: A review. J Cardiothorac Vasc Anesth (in press)

30. Olper L, Cabrini L, Landoni G, et al (2012) Non-invasive ventilation after cardiac surgery outside the intensive care unit. Minerva Anestesiol 77: 40–45

31. Azoulay E, Demoule A, Jaber S, et al (2011) Palliative noninvasive ventilation in patients with respiratory failure. Intensive care Med 37: 1250–1257

VI

32. Elliott MW, Confalonieri M, Nava S (2002) Where to perform non-invasive ventilation? Eur Respir J 19: 1159–1166
33. Samuelson KA (2011) Unpleasant and pleasant memories of intensive care in adult mechanically ventilated patients--findings from 250 interviews. Intensive Crit Care Nurs 27: 76–84
34. Hess DR (2011) Patient-ventilator interaction during non-invasive ventilation. Respir Care 56: 153–165
35. Cabrini L, Monti G, Villa M, et al (2009) Non-invasive ventilation outside the intensive care unit for acute respiratory failure: the perspective of the general ward nurses. Minerva Anestesiol 75: 427–433
36. Cabrini L, Moizo E, Nicelli E, et al (2012) Non-invasive ventilation outside the intensive care unit from the patient point of view. A pilot study. Respir Care (in press)
37. Chiumello D, Conti G, Foti G, Giacomini M, Braschi A, Iapichino G (2009) Non-invasive ventilation outside the intensive care unit for acute respiratory failure. Minerva Anestesiol 75: 459–466
38. Ambrosino N, Vagheggini G (2008) Noninvasive positive pressure ventilation in the acute care setting: where are we? Eur Respir J 31: 874–886
39. Cabrini L, Silvani P, Landoni G, Monti G, Colombo S, Zangrillo A (2010) Monitoring non-invasive ventilation outside the intensive care unit. Minerva Anestesiol 76: 71
40. Hillman K(2002) Critical care without walls. Curr Opin Crit Care 8: 594–599
41. Hess DR (2009) How to initiate a noninvasive ventilation program: bringing the evidence to the bedside. Respir Care 54: 232–245
42. Davies JD, Gentile MA (2009) What does it take to have a successful noninvasive ventilation program? Respir Care 54: 53–61
43. Schonhofer B, Sortor-Leger S (2002) Equipment needs for noninvasive mechanical ventilation. Eur Respir J 20: 1029–1036
44. Chatburn RL (2009) Which ventilators and modes can be used to deliver noninvasive ventilation? Respir Care 54: 85–101
45. Hill NS (2009) Where should noninvasive ventilation be delivered? Respir Care 54: 62–70
46. Benditt JO (2009) Novel uses of noninvasive ventilation. Respir Care 54: 212–219
47. Guarracino F, Cabrini L, Baldassarri R, et al (2010) Non-invasive ventilation-aided transoesophageal echocardiography in high-risk patients: a pilot study. Eur J Echocardiogr 11: 554–556

VI

Dyspnea in the Mechanically Ventilated Patient

A. Demoule, M. Schmidt, and T. Similowski

Introduction

Over the past decade, growing attention has been given to the detection and treatment of pain in intensive care unit (ICU) patients. Interestingly, during the same period, very little attention has been given to dyspnea. Indeed, data regarding dyspnea in ICU patients are scarce and there are no recommendations regarding the assessment and management of dyspnea in ICU patients. Apart from being a major source of discomfort, dyspnea shares many physiological and clinical features with pain. This factor should make dyspnea a major preoccupation for ICU physicians and nurses whose mission is to relieve symptoms in addition to treating disease processes; this is especially true in conscious mechanically ventilated patients who cannot easily complain of symptoms.

The objective of the present review is to provide information regarding the prevalence and the risk factors of dyspnea in mechanically ventilated ICU patients. We also suggest some approaches to detecting, quantifying and managing dyspnea in these patients.

A Few Words Regarding Physiology

Before exposing the clinical facts, a few physiological points warrant mention. Several mechanisms contribute to the generation of respiratory discomfort. There are two main distinct uncomfortable breathing sensations: Excessive effort and air hunger [1]. These different forms of dyspnea are caused by different afferent mechanisms and are evoked by different physiologic stimuli [2].

Excessive Effort

The sense of breathing effort arises both from muscle receptors and from corollary discharge arising from cerebral motor cortex activation during voluntary respiratory effort [3]. Effort of breathing is perceived when the physical work of breathing (WOB) is increased by an augmentation of respiratory muscle loading (i.e., increased impedance), or when cortical motor drive is increased because of respiratory muscle weakness [2]. Increased impedance can be the result either of deceased compliance or of increased resistance. A respiratory system compliance of less than 40 ml/cmH$_2$O is a common cause of dyspnea. Common causes of low compliance of the respiratory system are disorders involving the parenchyma (fibrosis, pulmonary edema), pleura (large pleural effusions), or chest wall (obe-

J.-L. Vincent (ed.), *Annual Update in Intensive Care and Emergency Medicine 2012*
DOI 10.1007/978-3-642-25716-2 © Springer-Verlag Berlin Heidelberg 2012

VI

sity). Airway obstruction, as reflected by airway resistance values greater than around 10 cmH$_2$O/l/sec, may also generate dyspnea in ventilated patients.

In theory, the ventilated patient should not have to perform excessive respiratory work since the ventilator is supposed to assume a large part of the WOB. However, if the level of assistance provided by the ventilator does not compensate the load excess, there is an imbalance between the patient's demand and the level of assistance, a typical cause of excessive inspiratory effort. Excessive inspiratory effort could also occur if the trigger level is set too high. Finally, dynamic hyperinflation (often called 'intrinsic positive end-expiratory pressure [PEEP]') is a typical cause of excessive work. In this case, the patient must generate inspiratory muscle pressure to overcome the difference between ventilator PEEP and intrinsic PEEP before the ventilator can be triggered. In this way, excessive resistance of the respiratory system may generate excessive effort.

VI

Air Hunger

Air hunger is the conscious perception of the need for more air and is typically described by subjects as "not getting enough air". Air hunger arises from stimulation of arterial chemoreceptors and from other drives to breathe. An increase in PaCO$_2$ or a decrease in PaO$_2$ will evoke air hunger [4, 5]. During volume-control ventilation in healthy subjects and in alert patients ventilated for respiratory muscle paralysis, an acute increase in PaCO$_2$ evokes severely uncomfortable air hunger [6]. It is hypothesized that air hunger is transmitted to the cerebral cortex by a corollary discharge of medullary respiratory center activity (also known as ventilatory drive). Air hunger is not caused by contraction of respiratory muscles. However, mechanoreceptor input arising from the respiratory system can dramatically reduce air hunger; increase in tidal volume is known to decrease dyspnea [7].

Increased resistive or elastic impedance may also contribute to air hunger generation in the ventilated patient by reducing ventilation, thus reducing PaO$_2$ and increasing PaCO$_2$. Excessive resistance may reduce ventilation either by causing patient triggering efforts to fail, or by reducing tidal volumes delivered by pressure-targeted ventilators. Decreased compliance may also reduce ventilation in patients receiving pressure-controlled ventilation.

What Is The Prevalence of Dyspnea in Mechanically Ventilated Patients?

To date, only six studies have been devoted to dyspnea in mechanically ventilated patients [8–13] (**Table 1**). Most of them were small-scale studies. Regarding the incidence of dyspnea, large variations were found between studies. However, the largest and the most recent of these studies found that 47 % of patients reported dyspnea. Three of these six studies quantified dyspnea, either with a visual analog scale (VAS) or using semi-quantitative descriptors [9, 11, 12]. Globally, about 20 % of patients experienced mild to severe dyspnea. In one study patients were asked to characterize the quality of their discomfort and 33 % reported experiencing air hunger, 16 % reported excessive effort, and 13 % experienced both air hunger and excessive effort [12].

One of the major limitations of these studies is the exclusion of patients who cannot answer, generally because of sedation. These patients may indeed

Table 1. Prevalence and severity of dyspnea in six published studies

Author [ref]	Number of patients	Prevalence of dyspnea	Quantification of dyspnea	Severity of dyspnea
Karampela et al. [8]	600	11 %	Qualitative	mild
Knebel et al. [9]	22	NA	VAS	32.2 ± 22.6
Lush et al. [10]	5	NA	No	NA
Powers et al. [11]	26	NA	No	NA
Schmidt et al. [12]	96	47 %	No	NA
Connelly et al. [13]	21	NA	VAS	3.22 ± 2.26

NA: Not available; VAS: Visual analog scale

experience dyspnea, but physicians do not have the appropriate tools to diagnose it.

VI

Consequences of Dyspnea in ICU Patients

There is growing evidence suggesting that dyspnea has a deleterious impact on mechanically ventilated patients. The consequences of dyspnea may occur either immediately during the ICU stay or be delayed.

Immediate Impact of Dyspnea

Dyspnea is a noxious sensation that shares many characteristics with pain. In laboratory experiments, healthy subjects exposed to dyspnea have reported terrifying feelings such as: "it's a feeling... you're going to die because you're not getting enough air"; "if I felt I had to live my life feeling like that I would jump out the window"; "When the shortness of breath was at its extreme I thought I was going to die,"; "... wouldn't want to live if it continued" [14]. Dyspnea seems clearly to be an awful feeling. With VAS ratings of ≥ 4 in most cases, dyspnea appeared to qualify as "moderate to intense" [9, 12]. Similar pain ratings are an indication for analgesia [15].

Patients with dyspnea are also more likely to present with anxiety than non-dyspneic patients (71 % vs. 24 %) and dyspnea is independently associated with anxiety in mechanically ventilated patients (odds ratio [OR] 8.84; 95 % confidence interval [CI], 3.26–24.0; $p < 0.0001$) [12]. This finding is not surprising because the interplay between anxiety and dyspnea is complex and causative relationships can exist in both directions. In healthy subjects, anxiety and fear stimulate ventilation and can thus produce dyspnea [16]. Anxiety-relieving interventions could thus have a positive effect on respiratory rhythm. Reciprocally, dyspnea generates anxiety [17]. Indeed, dyspnea causes anxiety, even in healthy subjects who experience dyspnea in a safe laboratory situation, and relieving dyspnea decreases anxiety [18]. In line with this, in a recent study, anxiety significantly decreased in patients who reported improvements in dyspnea after adjustments of the ventilator settings [12]. Therefore, relieving dyspnea is likely to have positive effects on anxiety.

As with anxiety, pain is more frequently experienced in dyspneic than in non-dyspneic patients [12]. Pain also stimulates ventilation [19] and pain control may have beneficial effects on dyspnea. Because of this interrelationship, we believe that anxiety, dyspnea, and pain should be assessed systematically and together in mechanically ventilated ICU patients.

Delayed Impact of Dyspnea

In addition to the immediate effects of dyspnea that occur during the ICU stay, dyspnea may contribute to the severe neuropsychological sequelae associated with an ICU stay. Indeed, it has been demonstrated over the last decade that survivors of an ICU stay often have extremely negative recollections of the experience. A recent study reported that 15 % of patients recalled feeling at risk of being murdered, 17 % felt betrayed, 39 % felt at risk of imminent death, and 55 % felt they were being suffocated [20]. Regarding dyspnea, a study devoted to patients' recollections of stressful experiences while receiving prolonged mechanical ventilation in an ICU showed that after their stay in the ICU almost 29 % of ventilated patients recalled that they had been moderately to extremely disconcerted by not getting enough air from the endotracheal tube [21]. In addition, it is important to remember that post-traumatic stress disorder (PTSD) is now recognized as a common sequel of the ICU experience [22]. PTSD symptom scores in the post-ICU population are significantly correlated with duration of mechanical ventilation and with recalled memories of respiratory distress [22]. It is therefore likely that dyspnea is one of the traumatizing events leading to PTSD in ICU patients.

Taken together, these arguments suggest that alleviating dyspnea should be a major goal of ICU physicians, as is pain management. A short-term objective might be to relieve patients of this noxious feeling. A longer-term objective might be to prevent recollections of stressful experiences and PTSD. Reaching these goals requires accurate tools to both diagnose and quantify dyspnea.

How to Detect and Measure Dyspnea in a Mechanically Ventilated Patient

There are, unfortunately, no reliable surrogates of dyspnea. A recent study showed that respiratory rate, heart rate and use of accessory muscles were not reliable surrogates of dyspnea [12]. To date, the only reliable tool to detect dyspnea is to ask the patient, but this requires the patient to be alert. Several rating methods have been shown to be feasible in intubated and ventilated patients. By definition, a mechanically ventilated patient cannot speak. However, he/she can provide information through simple number, word, or visual analog scales, similar to those routinely used in clinical pain assessment [8, 10]. In mechanically ventilated patients with dyspnea, the VAS and the Borg scale are highly correlated [10]. Patients can point to the appropriate responses but in some cases the interviewer will need to say or point to responses in succession and stop when the patient indicates with a sign.

Of course, in sedated patients who cannot provide information, there is high risk of underevaluation of dyspnea. Recently, a Respiratory Distress Observation Scale (RDOS) has been developed and validated in spontaneously breathing subjects [23]. This scale comprises measures of heart rate, respiratory rate, accessory muscle use, paradoxical breathing pattern, restlessness, grunting at end-expiration, nasal flaring, and fearful facial display. Adaptation and validation of the scale for ventilated patients is needed. Signs can be very useful when patients are unable to communicate, but they may be misleading [10].

What Causes Dyspnea in ICU Patients?

In the largest study dealing with dyspnea in mechanically ventilated ICU patients, assist control ventilation (ACV) was the principle cause of dyspnea. Indeed, dyspneic patients were more frequently mechanically ventilated with the ACV mode than non-dyspneic patients (69 vs. 45 %), and multivariate analysis showed that the ACV mode was independently associated with dyspnea (OR, 4.77; 95 % CI, 1.60–14.3) [12]. Interestingly, common generators of dyspnea such as hemoglobin, the PaO_2/FiO_2 ratio, or $PaCO_2$ were not significantly associated with dyspnea in this study. The ventilatory mode seems, therefore, to be a major determinant of dyspnea. Five of the seven patients who chose "excessive respiratory effort" as the sole descriptor of their dyspnea received ACV with an inspiratory flow < 60 l/min. In addition, in patients with "air hunger", there was a trend toward more dyspnea in those who received a pressure support ventilatory mode with a pressure support level < 15 cmH_2O [12]. Although these latter differences were not significant, they suggest that in addition to ventilatory mode, ventilatory settings might be involved in the genesis of dyspnea. This is not surprising because ACV leaves almost no room for natural respiratory fluctuations and induces patient-ventilator asynchrony [24]. Conversely, positive pressure assisted ventilation [25], proportional assisted ventilation [25], and negative pressure ventilation [26] induced less dyspnea in healthy subjects.

Although there are few data, the level of assistance also seems to have a major role in the genesis of dyspnea. Indeed, in a study in which ventilatory variables, WOB, and dyspnea were measured at different levels of invasive ventilator support, increasing the percentage of respiratory work done each minute by the ventilator proportionally decreased ratings of "difficulty breathing" [27]. The effect was significant, with breathing difficulty ratings decreasing from 60 % of the scale with no support to 30 % of the scale with 80 % support. Finally, the inspiratory flow delivered by the ventilator is also of importance. Although studies devoted to the impact of inspiratory flow on comfort are sometimes confusing because too many parameters are modified together (e.g., tidal volume and inspiratory flow), it seems that an inspiratory flow below 1 l/sec equates to a risk of generating dyspnea [12, 28–30].

This marked implication of the ventilator in the genesis of dyspnea is reinforced by the fact that, in 35 % of dyspneic patients, at least one intervention on the ventilator significantly reduced the intensity of dyspnea [12]. The intervention that is the most often associated with dyspnea relief is an increase in inspiratory flow. This is in line with data from normal volunteers [28] in which low inspiratory flow is associated with higher inspiratory muscle energy expenditure [31] and high inspiratory flow optimizes respiratory muscle relaxation [29]. Low pressure support levels have also been associated with a sense of excessive inspiratory effort [32], and low tidal volumes are associated with air hunger [33].

VI

Does Dyspnea Have An Impact On Clinical Outcome?

Data regarding the impact of dyspnea on clinical outcome are scarce. Indeed, this issue has been examined in only one study [12]. In this study, the median length of ICU stay was greater in patients reporting dyspnea than in those who did not (8 [4–20] vs. 14 [8–28] days, p < 0.017). The median duration of mechanical ventilation from inclusion to extubation, the rate of successful extubation within the three days after inclusion, and the mortality rate were all comparable between patients with and without dyspnea. The occurrence of successful extubation within three days after dyspnea assessment was significantly less frequent in patients whose dyspnea failed to recede in response to ventilator setting adjustments than in the other patients (non-dyspneic patients and those with a 'responsive' dyspnea). The duration of mechanical ventilation was not statistically different between these two groups, whereas the length of stay in the ICU tended to be longer when dyspnea did not respond to ventilator adjustment [12].

VI   These data, therefore, suggest a clear impact of dyspnea on the outcome of mechanically ventilated patients. However, they do not clearly demonstrate that minimizing dyspnea would improve the prognosis of patients.

What Should We Do In A Mechanically Ventilated Patient Who Complains Of Dyspnea?

Once dyspnea has been diagnosed, it is essential to have a step-by-step procedure to identify the cause of dyspnea and treat it in so far as this is possible (**Fig. 1**).

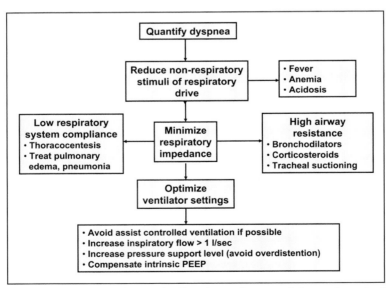

Fig. 1. Step-by-step procedure to identify and treat the cause of dyspnea in mechanically ventilated intensive care unit (ICU) patients. PEEP: positive end-expiratory pressure

Reduce Non-respiratory Stimuli of Respiratory Drive

As previously stated, respiratory drive in excess of achieved ventilation is the cause of air hunger [12]. Although respiratory drive is increased by stimuli arising from various respiratory afferents, many metabolic stimuli, such as fever or hyperthermia, may also stimulate the respiratory drive. We suggest that, when it is either not possible, not advisable or not logical to increase ventilation, factors such as acidosis, hypoxia, hyperthermia, and anemia should be corrected [34].

Minimize Respiratory Impedance

Increased resistance or decreased compliance may promote excessive effort and air hunger. When increased airway resistance is due to chronic obstructive pulmonary disease (COPD) or asthma, bronchodilators and corticosteroids may be used. In the case of reduced compliance because of a large pleural effusion, thoracocentesis might be performed. In other cases, such as reduced pulmonary compliance because of pneumonia or cardiogenic pulmonary edema, there is no other option than to wait for treatment of the causative disease to take effect.

In patients with high intrinsic PEEP (e.g., severe COPD), an important step in achieving relief is to set PEEP to equal the intrinsic PEEP (which reduces the preload the patient must overcome before triggering inspiration) [35].

VI

Dyspnea Associated With Care Activity

Dyspnea is frequently associated with normal care activities, such as planned turns, transfers, bathing, and suctioning [10]. Good oxygenation should be assured before the activity. In some brief procedures generating a high level of dyspnea, such as bronchoscopy, it may be advisable to administer a pre-emptive dose of a very short-acting sedative agent before commencing.

Optimize Ventilator Settings

The present review has stressed the importance of ventilator settings in the pathogenesis of dyspnea. In patients receiving ACV, the first step should be to evaluate the possibility of changing the ventilatory mode. Indeed, because ACV is strongly associated with dyspnea, this mode should be avoided in spontaneously breathing conscious patients and pressure controlled ventilation should be preferred. Other modes such as proportional ventilatory assist or neurally-adjusted ventilatory assist (NAVA) might be beneficial for dyspnea, but this point needs further evaluation.

If the patient needs to stay under ACV, then the inspiratory flow should be optimized and increased to greater than 1 l/sec. If the patient is ventilated in pressure support ventilation, then the pressure support level could be increased, but overdistention should be avoided. Finally, in patients with instrinsic PEEP, the level of external PEEP should be set to compensate intrinsic PEEP, which is not always easy without invasive measurements.

Conclusion

There is growing evidence suggesting that dyspnea is a frequent problem in mechanically ventilated ICU patients. In these patients, dyspnea is highly associated with the presence and degree of anxiety and pain. In addition, the ventilator seems to be a major determinant of dyspnea. Large-scale studies are now needed to further evaluate these issues. These studies should aim to quantify the prevalence of dyspnea in large populations of patients using a multicenter design. They should also study the occurrence and intensity of dyspnea on a longitudinal basis. The results of such studies would help determine whether dyspnea may be a monitoring tool that could predict ongoing complications in an ICU patient (e.g., ventilator-induced pneumonia, pneumothorax). Finally, the long-term impact of dyspnea on ICU patients needs to be evaluated.

VI

References

1. Cherniack NS, Altose MD (1987) Mechanisms of dyspnea. Clin Chest Med 8: 207–214
2. Lansing RW, Im BS, Thwing JI, Legedza AT, Banzett RB (2000) The perception of respiratory work and effort can be independent of the perception of air hunger. Am J Respir Crit Care Med 162: 1690–1696
3. Killian KJ, Gandevia SC (1996) Sense of effort and dyspnea. In: Adams L, Guz A (eds) Respiratory Sensation, 1st edn. Marcel Dekker, New York, pp 181–199
4. Banzett RB, Lansing RW, Reid MB, Adams L, Brown R (1989) 'Air hunger' arising from increased PCO2 in mechanically ventilated quadriplegics. Respir Physiol 76: 53–67
5. Moosavi SH, Golestanian E, Binks AP, Lansing RW, Brown R, Banzett RB (2003) Hypoxic and hypercapnic drives to breathe generate equivalent levels of air hunger in humans. J Appl Physiol 94: 141–154
6. Banzett RB, Lansing RW, Brown R, et al (1990) 'Air hunger' from increased PCO2 persists after complete neuromuscular block in humans. Respir Physiol 81: 1–17
7. Opie LH, Smith AC, Spalding JM (1959) Conscious appreciation of the effects produced by independent changes of ventilation volume and of end-tidal pCO2 in paralysed patients. J Physiol 149: 494–499
8. Karampela I, Hansen-Flachen J, Smith S, Reily D, Fuchs BD (2002) A dyspnea evaluation protocol for respiratory therapists: a feasibility study. Respir Care 47: 1158–1161
9. Knebel AR, Janson-Bjerklie SL, Malley JD, Wilson AG, Marini JJ (1994) Comparison of breathing comfort during weaning with two ventilatory modes. Am J Respir Crit Care Med 149: 14–18
10. Lush MT, Janson-Bjerklie S, Carrieri VK, Lovejoy N (1988) Dyspnea in the ventilator-assisted patient. Heart Lung 17: 528–535
11. Powers J, Bennett SJ (1999) Measurement of dyspnea in patients treated with mechanical ventilation. Am J Crit Care 8: 254–261
12. Schmidt M, Demoule A, Polito A, et al (2011) Dyspnea in mechanically ventilated critically ill patients. Crit Care Med 39: 2059–2065
13. Connelly B, Gunzerath L, Knebel A (2000) A pilot study exploring mood state and dyspnea in mechanically ventilated patients. Heart Lung 29: 173–179
14. O'Driscoll M, Corner J, Bailey C (1999) The experience of breathlessness in lung cancer. Eur J Cancer Care (Engl) 8: 37–43
15. College of Emergency Medicine (2004) Guideline for the Management of Pain in Adults. College of Emergency Medicine, London
16. Smoller JW, Pollack MH, Otto MW, Rosenbaum JF, Kradin RL (1996) Panic anxiety, dyspnea, and respiratory disease. Theoretical and clinical considerations. Am J Respir Crit Care Med 154: 6–17
17. Bergbom-Engberg I, Haljamae H (1989) Assessment of patients' experience of discomforts during respirator therapy. Crit Care Med 17: 1068–1072

18. Twibell R, Siela D, Mahmoodi M (2003) Subjective perceptions and physiological variables during weaning from mechanical ventilation. Am J Crit Care 12: 101–112

19. Borgbjerg FM, Nielsen K, Franks J (1996) Experimental pain stimulates respiration and attenuates morphine-induced respiratory depression: a controlled study in human volunteers. Pain 64: 123–128

20. de Miranda S, Pochard F, Chaize M, et al (2011) Postintensive care unit psychological burden in patients with chronic obstructive pulmonary disease and informal caregivers: A multicenter study. Crit Care Med 39: 112–118

21. Rotondi AJ, Chelluri L, Sirio C, et al (2002) Patients' recollections of stressful experiences while receiving prolonged mechanical ventilation in an intensive care unit. Crit Care Med 30: 746–752

22. Cuthbertson BH, Hull A, Strachan M, Scott J (2004) Post-traumatic stress disorder after critical illness requiring general intensive care. Intensive Care Med 30: 450–455

23. Campbell ML, Templin T, Walch J (2011) A Respiratory Distress Observation Scale for patients unable to self-report dyspnea. J Palliat Med 13: 285–290

24. Russell WC, Greer JR (2000) The comfort of breathing: a study with volunteers assessing the influence of various modes of assisted ventilation. Crit Care Med 28: 3645–3648

25. Gay PC, Hess DR, Hill NS (2001) Noninvasive proportional assist ventilation for acute respiratory insufficiency. Comparison with pressure support ventilation. Am J Respir Crit Care Med 164: 1606–1611

26. Nishino T, Isono S, Ide T (1998) Effects of negative pressure assisted ventilation on dyspnoeic sensation and breathing pattern. Eur Respir J 12: 1278–1283

27. Leung P, Jubran A, Tobin MJ (1997) Comparison of assisted ventilator modes on triggering, patient effort, and dyspnea. Am J Respir Crit Care Med 155: 1940–1948

28. Manning HL, Molinary EJ, Leiter JC (1995) Effect of inspiratory flow rate on respiratory sensation and pattern of breathing. Am J Respir Crit Care Med 151: 751–757

29. Ward ME, Corbeil C, Gibbons W, Newman S, Macklem PT (1988) Optimization of respiratory muscle relaxation during mechanical ventilation. Anesthesiology 69: 29–35

30. Chiumello D, Pelosi P, Croci M, Bigatello LM, Gattinoni L (2001) The effects of pressurization rate on breathing pattern, work of breathing, gas exchange and patient comfort in pressure support ventilation. Eur Respir J 18: 107–114

31. Fernandez R, Mendez M, Younes M (1999) Effect of ventilator flow rate on respiratory timing in normal humans. Am J Respir Crit Care Med 159: 710–719

32. Vitacca M, Bianchi L, Zanotti E et al (2004) Assessment of physiologic variables and subjective comfort under different levels of pressure support ventilation. Chest 126: 851–859

33. Bloch-Salisbury E, Spengler CM, Brown R, Banzett RB (1998) Self-control and external control of mechanical ventilation give equal air hunger relief. Am J Respir Crit Care Med 157: 415–420

34. Schonhofer B, Bohrer H, Kohler D (1998) Blood transfusion facilitating difficult weaning from the ventilator. Anaesthesia 53: 181–184

35. MacIntyre NR, Cheng KC, McConnell R (1997) Applied PEEP during pressure support reduces the inspiratory threshold load of intrinsic PEEP. Chest 111: 188–193

VI

How to Improve Oxygenation before Intubation in Patients at Risk

B. Jung, I. Azuelos, and S. Jaber

Introduction

Airway management is one of the most commonly performed procedures in operating rooms (OR), intensive care units (ICUs), and emergency departments (EDs). Hypoxemia and cardiovascular collapse represent the initial and most serious life-threatening complications associated with difficult airway access, both in planned intubations (e.g., scheduled surgery) and in emergency intubations of critically ill patients [1–3]. To prevent and limit the incidence of hypoxemia following intubation, several pre-oxygenation techniques have been proposed. Nonetheless, these techniques, which usually combine breathing maneuvers and high inspired oxygen fraction (FiO_2), may be associated with adverse effects and may be complicated by post-intubation atelectasis [4]. They may also provoke discomfort for patients and are time consuming in daily practice. The objectives of the present review are to describe the rationale for optimizing pre-oxygenation and associated maneuvers, to discuss the evidence for performing these maneuvers, and finally to propose an algorithm for secure airway management in patients considered 'at risk' of life-threatening complications.

Pre-oxygenation: What is the Rationale?

Cellular Oxygenation

The aim of pre-oxygenation is ultimately to prevent and to limit cellular hypoxia during the intubation process by increasing oxygen stores. Cellular oxygenation depends directly on the arterial delivery of oxygen (DO_2) to the cells and is calculated as follows (Eq1):

$$DO_2 = 10 \times CO \times 1.33 \times [Hb] \times SaO_2 + (0.003 \times PaO_2) \tag{1}$$

where DO_2 is in ml O_2/min, CO is the cardiac output in l/min, [Hb] the plasma hemoglobin concentration in g/l, SaO_2 the arterial oxygen saturation in percentage, and PaO_2 the partial arterial pressure for O_2 in mmHg.

Although blood product transfusions and drugs to increase cardiac output may promote DO_2 to cells, we do not consider these treatments as 'pre-oxygenation maneuvers'. Oxygen stores are limited to what is present in the blood and in the lungs. Since dissolved oxygen (not linked to hemoglobin) represents a minor portion of the arterial oxygen content (Eq 1), the main blood oxygen store will vary based on the hemoglobin concentration and its affinity to oxygen (variables that cannot be simply modified). Even after oxygenation with 100 % oxygen, the

J.-L. Vincent (ed.), *Annual Update in Intensive Care and Emergency Medicine 2012*
DOI 10.1007/978-3-642-25716-2 © Springer-Verlag Berlin Heidelberg 2012

blood stores of oxygen will only increase slightly, from about 850 ml to 950 ml [5]. However, the lungs can store a much larger amount of oxygen. This amount depends on both the patient's functional residual capacity (FRC) and the maximal alveolar pressure of oxygen (PAO_2).

Functional Residual Capacity

The FRC is the volume of air (approximately 3 to 4 l in a healthy adult, less in women) that is present in the lungs after passive expiration, i.e., when the inward elastic recoil of the lungs is counterbalanced by the outward recoil of the chest wall and diaphragm. Indeed, if the lung elastic recoil decreases (age, chronic or acute obstructive lung disease), FRC will increase. If the lung elastic recoil increases (i.e., pulmonary fibrosis), FRC will decrease (**Fig. 1**).

Surgical procedures, anesthesia, intubation and mechanical ventilation are associated with certain factors that may affect FRC, such as the supine position and anesthetic drugs. Supine position decreases FRC (0.8 to 1.0 l on average) through multiple mechanisms, including the lungs' weights on a rigid chest wall, and the heart and chest wall weights decreasing the transverse thoracic diameter [6]. Abdominal contents are also moved upwards, causing a cranial shift of the diaphragm, thereby impairing lung volumes. Obesity is, therefore, also associated with a reduction in FRC [7, 8]. Anesthetic drugs induce a decrease in muscular tone. This will result in a reduction in FRC (0.4 to 0.5 l on average) by shifting the balance between the inward elastic recoil force of the lung (unchanged) and the outward recoil of the chest wall (reduced) [6] towards smaller lung volumes.

VI

Closing Volume

Despite a maximum expiratory effort, the lungs will not empty completely. The remaining lung volume is called the residual volume. There are two main mechanisms explaining why the lungs do not collapse at the end of expiration. First, the chest wall would need to be totally deformed, which is mechanically not possible. Second, in adults, at the end of a forceful expiration, the distal airways close before complete alveolar collapse [9].

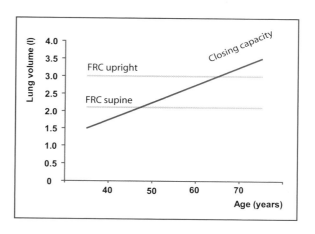

Fig. 1. Figure describing the expected changes in closing capacity and functional residual capacity (FRC) with age. Note how the FRC is lower in the supine position. The FRC approaches the closing capacity around the age of 65 in an upright patient. Adapted from [9]

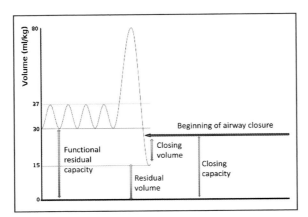

Fig. 2. Figure describing the spirometric nomenclature. Note that the closing capacity is the sum of the residual volume and the closing volume. By definition, at closing capacity, distal airways in the dependent areas start to close which impairs ventilation, possibly resulting in hypoxemia. Adapted from [9]

The volume at which the airways begin to close during expiration is called the closing capacity. The volume of air between the closing capacity and the residual volume is called the closing volume (**Fig. 2**). It is important to note that the distal airways do not close at the same time throughout the lungs during a forceful expiration maneuver. Airways in the dependent areas (located in the lower lobes when upright and in the lower/posterior lobes when supine) close first. This concept can be easily understood when the changes in pleural pressures within the chest are taken into account [9]. In a normal subject at any lung volume, the pleural pressure is slightly more positive in the dependent areas of the thorax due to gravity. For instance, in a healthy standing adult at end-expiration (FRC), the pleural pressure is about -10 cmH$_2$O at the top of the thoracic cavity and about -2 cmH$_2$O at the bottom. During a forceful expiration, the pleural pressure is (voluntarily) increased and becomes positive (more so at the bottom of the chest). This pressure is transmitted to the alveoli and permits exhalation of air via a pressure drop over the course of the larger airways. At low lung volumes, the higher pleural pressure in the lower chest will preferentially compress the lower distal airways, causing some lower airway closure. Airways will be kept patent either due to the cartilage within their walls (larger airways) or due to the traction created by the adjacent parenchyma. Therefore, any process that would decrease lung recoil and parenchymal traction (emphysema, age, edema), weaken the small airways (asthma, bronchitis), or exaggerate the pleural pressure gradient over the chest (obesity, pregnancy in the supine position) will promote earlier closure of the lower airways and thereby increase the closing capacity (**Fig. 1**) [9, 10]. In the above-mentioned cases, the work of breathing (WOB) will necessarily include the work required to open the closed distal airways.

Alveolar Pressure of Oxygen

The PAO$_2$ depends on the inspiratory pressure of oxygen, the alveolar pressure of carbon dioxide (CO$_2$) and the respiratory quotient, which represents the ratio of CO$_2$ production per oxygen consumption (Eq 2):

$$PAO_2 = PiO_2 - PACO_2 / R \tag{2}$$

where PAO$_2$ is in mmHg, PiO$_2$ is the inspiratory pressure of oxygen in mmHg, PACO$_2$ is the alveolar pressure of CO$_2$ in mmHg and R is the respiratory quotient which is 0.8 in most patients.

Equation 2 shows how hypoventilation, which may occur during anesthesia because of difficult airway access and through the effects of anesthetic agents, decreases PAO_2. One effective pre-oxygenation maneuver could be to increase minute ventilation to avoid hypercapnia. Furthermore, pre-oxygenation needs to be performed with an FiO_2 set at 100 % oxygen (maximal PiO_2) to increase PAO_2 as much as possible (usually about 100–150 ml of oxygen). However, if pure oxygen is administered without positive pressure application, the clinician must be aware of the increased risk of atelectasis in the dependent lung areas, a condition labeled denitrogenation-related atelectasis [4]. In fact, the oxygen administered will be rapidly diffused from the alveoli to the blood causing alveolar collapse. In contrast, when positive pressure is applied and/or air is co-administered with oxygen, the nitrogen delivered (which diffuses much more slowly than oxygen) will prevent the alveoli from collapsing.

To summarize, during induction of anesthesia for intubation, several factors contribute to the development of hypoxia: Hypoventilation, decreased lung volumes, and increased airway resistance. Maximizing oxygen stores before induction could delay the onset of hypoxemia, a concept that makes sense.

VI

Who are the Patients 'At Risk'?

The main indication for intubation in the ICU is acute respiratory failure [1–3]. In these cases, the risk of hypoxemia and cardiovascular collapse during the intubation process (often crucial) is particularly elevated. Respiratory muscle weakness ('ventilatory insufficiency') and gas exchange impairment ('respiratory insufficiency') are often present. It is then worth anticipating life-threatening complications that may occur during intubation [4].

Some non-critically ill patients (scheduled for surgery) are also considered 'at risk'. As explained earlier, obesity and pregnancy are the two main situations in which FRC is decreased and the risk of atelectasis is increased [4]. Other 'at risk' patients include those who cannot safely tolerate a mild degree of hypoxemia (epilepsy, cerebrovascular disease, coronary artery disease, sickle cell disease, etc). Finally, patients considered to be 'difficult to intubate' also require adequate pre-oxygenation [11].

Pre-Oxygenation: How to Do It?
Spontaneous Ventilation

Several maneuvers in spontaneous ventilation (e.g., 3–8 vital capacities vs 3 minutes tidal volume breathing) exist and seem to be almost equally effective [5, 12]. Some technical details, however, can make a significant difference. First, the clinician needs to make sure the facemask fits the patient's facial morphology properly. Second, fresh gas flow needs to be set at a high range to homogenize ventilation through the lungs and to decrease the impact of leaks [13, 14]. Third, leaks should be avoided and diagnosed either by flaccid reservoir bag or by the absence of a normal capnograph waveform, since leaks impair the efficacy of pre-oxygenation.

Newer technology may also be useful. In modern anesthesia workstations, end-tidal oxygen concentration is available as a surrogate for PAO_2. The target commonly adopted is 90 % [5]. This target is reached more quickly when pure oxygen is administered. Although the clinician must be aware of the potential complication of denitrogenation-induced atelectasis, the benefit of reaching an end-inspiratory oxygen fraction of 90 % before attempting intubation outweighs the risk of developing atelectatic-related hypoxia in 'at risk patients'.

In critically ill patients, the advantage of a prolonged period of pre-oxygenation has not been clearly demonstrated. Most of these patients present with acute respiratory failure with a certain amount of shunt, a reduced FRC, and do not respond to administration of oxygen as well as patients scheduled for surgery [15]. Mort et al. demonstrated a moderate increase in PaO_2 after a 4 min period of oxygen therapy before intubation (from 62 to 88 mmHg before and after oxygen therapy); despite pre-oxygenation, half of the 34 patients included in the study experienced severe hypoxia during intubation [15].

Position

VI

Patient position is also an important factor and limits the decrease in FRC. Studies have reported that pre-oxygenation in the semi-sitting position or in the 25° head-up position can achieve higher arterial oxygen pressures; it may also prolong the time to hypoxemia in obese patients scheduled for surgery [16, 17]. To our knowledge, only one study performed in non-obese patients scheduled for surgery has reported a beneficial impact of inclined position (20° head up) during pre-oxygenation in terms of time to desaturation [18]. An inclined position seems not to be beneficial in pregnant patients probably because of the gravid uterus constraining the diaphragm in its upper position and because of the detrimental effect of the sitting position on vena caval back flow [19]. There are no pre-oxygenation studies evaluating the inclined versus the supine positions in the critically ill.

Positive Pressure

Positive end-expiratory pressure (PEEP) with high-flow oxygen has been evaluated as a pre-oxygenation method in the morbidly obese. The aim of positive pressure used as a pre-oxygenation method is to increase the proportion of aerated lung, thereby increasing FRC. This increase in FRC will result in an increase in lung oxygen stores, and may also help keep the closing capacity below the FRC.

The first study was performed in the early 2000s and found that applying 7 cmH_2O of continuous positive airways pressure (CPAP) for 3 minutes did not prolong time to desaturation in morbidly obese women. Important limitations of that study were the absence of ventilation between the onset of apnea and the intubation; and the relative brevity of the pre-oxygenation (only 3 minutes) [20]. Later studies, however, showed a benefit of applying CPAP with oxygen during pre-oxygenation in morbidly obese patients [21, 22]. Compared to oxygen alone, CPAP of 10 cmH_2O plus oxygen for 5 min increased the time to desaturate and reduced the amount of atelectasis following intubation [21, 22]. Immediately after intubation, the amount of atelectasis measured by computed tomography (CT) was 10 % in the oxygen group compared to only 2 % in the 10 cmH_2O PEEP group [21].

In a landmark study of morbidly obese patients, Delay et al. showed that pre-oxygenation using non-invasive ventilation (NIV) with pressure support ventilation (PSV, 8 cmH_2O) and PEEP (6 cmH_2O) for 5 minutes was safe, feasible, and effective [23]. They reported that 95 % of patients reached the target of end-expiratory oxygen fraction of 90 % with NIV in comparison with 50 % in patients pre-oxygenated by spontaneously breathing oxygen [23]. Arterial blood gases at both the end of the pre-oxygenation period and at 5 min after intubation were not significantly different between the groups. The impact of the combination of inclined position and NIV in surgical patients needs to be evaluated. Pre-oxygenation with NIV in pregnant patients has never been formally evaluated, as it may be harmful owing to the risk of aspiration in this patient population.

NIV as a pre-oxygenation maneuver has also been evaluated in critically ill patients. Our team reported its superiority compared to administration of oxygen alone [24]. Indeed, in a randomized controlled trial, the incidence of severe hypoxemia (SpO$_2$ below 80 %) within 30 min after intubation was 7 % in the NIV group (PSV 5 – 15 cmH$_2$O, PEEP 5 – 10 cmH$_2$O, FiO$_2$ 100 %), compared to 42 % in the oxygen group. Although NIV seems to be beneficial compared to spontaneous breathing in the critically ill, its impact on outcome has only recently been evaluated in a multiple center randomized controlled trial (RCT) (Preoxygenation Using NIV in Hypoxemic Patients, Clinical Trials.gov identifier NCT00472160) and the results will be presented in the next few months. To perform NIV in critically ill patients, the facial masks available in every ICU room are sufficient. The patient should be in the inclined position, FiO$_2$ set at 100 %, inspiratory pressure set to maintain a tidal volume of 6 to 10 ml/kg and respiratory rate of 10 to 25 cycles/min. The duration of the procedure usually corresponds to the time needed to prepare the drugs and equipment for intubation. Pre-oxygenation with NIV was included in a bundle of interventions, use of which was associated with a decrease in life-threatening hypoxemia following intubation in a multicenter study [1, 2] (**Box 1**).

VI

Box 1. Intubation bundle care management, adapted from [2]

PRE-Intubation
1. Presence of two operators
2. Fluid loading (isotonic saline 500 ml or starch 250 ml) in absence of cardiogenic edema
3. Preparation of long-term sedation
4. Pre-oxygenate for 3 min with NIV in case of acute respiratory failure (FiO$_2$ 100 %, pressure support ventilation level between 5 and 15 cmH$_2$O to obtain an expiratory tidal volume between 6 and 8 ml/kg and PEEP of 5 cmH$_2$O)

PER-Intubation
5. Rapid sequence induction:
   – Etomidate 0.2–0.3 mg/kg or ketamine 1.5–3 mg/kg
   – Succinylcholine 1–1.5 mg/kg (in absence of allergy, hyperkalemia, severe acidosis, acute or chronic neuromuscular disease, burn patient for more than 48h and medullar trauma)
   – Rocuronium: 0.6 mg/kg i.v. in case of contraindication to succinylcholine or prolonged stay in the ICU or risk factor for neuromyopathy
6. Sellick maneuver

POST-Intubation
7. Immediate confirmation of tube placement by capnography
8. Norepinephrine if diastolic blood pressure remains < 35 mmHg
9. Initiate long-term sedation
10. Initial 'protective ventilation': tidal volume 6–8 ml/kg, PEEP < 5 cmH$_2$O and respiratory rate between 10 and 20 cycles/min, FiO$_2$ 100 % for a plateau pressure < 30 cmH$_2$O
11. Recruitment maneuver: CPAP 40 cmH$_2$O during 40s, FiO$_2$ 100 % (if no cardiovascular collapse)
12. Maintain intubation cuff pressure of 25–30 cmH$_2$O

NIV: non-invasive ventilation; PEEP: positive end-expiratory pressure

Recruitment Maneuver

As discussed earlier, the aim of NIV during pre-oxygenation is to recruit lung tissue available for gas exchange ('open the lung'). Conversely, the combination of denitrogenation (with 100 % O_2) and the apneic period associated with the intubation procedure can dramatically decrease the aerated lung volume ratio, thereby causing atelectasis. In obese patients pre-oxygenated without positive pressure, the proportion of atelectasis following intubation can represent 10 % of the total lung volume [21]. One option to limit derecruitment after intubation is to ventilate the patient using a bag-valve balloon. However, it is not possible to measure the pressure delivered when the patients are ventilated with this method.

A recruitment maneuver consists of a transient increase in inspiratory pressure. Several maneuvers exist, but the one best described in this situation consists of applying CPAP of 40 cmH_2O for 30 to 40 s [25–27]. In the ICU, an RCT was conducted in 40 critically ill patients requiring intubation for acute hypoxemic respiratory failure [25]. Compared to no recruitment maneuver, a recruitment maneuver performed immediately after intubation was associated with a higher PaO_2 (under 100 % FiO_2) 5 min after intubation (93 ± 36 vs 236 ± 117 mmHg) and 30 min after intubation (110 ± 39 and 180 ± 79 mmHg).

In the OR, a first study assessed the impact of applying several PEEP (0, 5, 10 cmH_2O) values following intubation in obese and non-obese patients scheduled for surgery [27]. At each step, end-expiratory lung volume, static elastance, gas exchange and dead space were measured. In obese and non-obese patients, PEEP of 10 cmH_2O compared with zero end-expiratory pressure (ZEEP) improved end-expiratory lung volume and elastance without effects on oxygenation. The same team then randomized 66 morbidly obese patients (body mass index 46 +/- 6 kg/m^2) scheduled for surgery into 3 groups: Conventional pre-oxygenation, pre-oxygenation with NIV and pre-oxygenation with NIV + post-intubation recruitment maneuver [26]. These author nicely demonstrated that the combination of preoxygenation with NIV + post-intubation recruitment maneuver helped maintain lung volumes and oxygenation during anesthesia induction more so than pre-oxygenation with either pure oxygen alone or with NIV. One of the main take home messages of that study is that to improve PaO_2 5 min after intubation, a recruitment maneuver added to NIV was needed. Both oxygenation (PaO_2, 234 +/- 73 mmHg vs 128 +/- 54 mmHg) and capnia ($PaCO_2$ 42 +/- 3 vs 40 +/- 3 mmHg) were improved in the recruitment maneuver + NIV group compared to NIV alone.

Bundles

Pre-oxygenation is only one of the procedures that may improve airway safety. Managing the airway of 'at risk' patients poses some unique challenges for the anesthesiologist/intensivist. The combination of a limited physiologic reserve in these patients and the potential for difficult mask ventilation and intubation mandates careful planning with a good working knowledge of alternative tools and strategies, should conventional attempts at securing the airway fail. Pre-oxygenation techniques can be combined to limit the risk of hypoxia during intubation attempts (**Fig. 3**).

To limit the incidence of severe complications occurring after this potentially hazardous procedure, we believe that the whole process (pre-, per- and post-

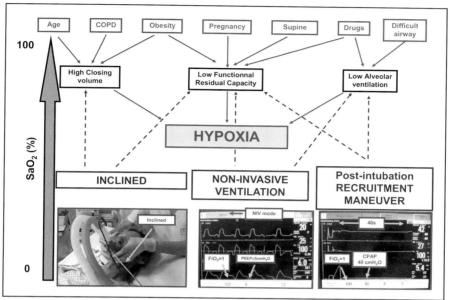

Fig. 3. Patients 'at risk' present several factors, such as obesity, pregnancy, chronic respiratory diseases, which increase closing volume, impair functional residual capacity (FRC) and decrease minute ventilation leading to hypoxia. Pre-oxygenation techniques should be combined in these patients to minimize the risks of life-threatening hypoxia following intubation attempt(s). COPD: chronic obstructive pulmonary disease; NIV: non-invasive ventilation; CPAP: continuous positive airway pressure. Solid arrows: factors which increase the risk of hypoxia; dashed arrows: pre-oxygenation techniques that can improve respiratory parameters and decrease the risk of life-threatening hypoxia following intubation attempt(s).

intubation) should be guided by protocols geared towards patient safety. In the ICU, we designed a multicenter study and described how implementation of such bundle protocols improved the safety of airway management [1, 2]. This bundle is summarized in **Box 1**.

Conclusion

Pre-oxygenation is a standard of care before intubation in ORs and in the ICU, aimed at increasing the lung stores of oxygen. Denitrogenation can be associated with resorption-related atelectasis but the benefit of increasing oxygen stores is higher than the risk of developing atelectasis in patients 'at risk'. These patients include the critically ill but also the obese, the pregnant and those in whom even slight hypoxemia can be life-threatening (mainly those with brain or heart disease). In these patients, the combination of pure oxygen, NIV, denitrogenation and post-intubation recruitment maneuvers outweighs the potential risk of post-intubation atelectasis.

References

1. Jaber S, Amraoui J, Lefrant JY, et al (2006) Clinical practice and risk factors for immediate complications of endotracheal intubation in the intensive care unit: a prospective, multiple-center study. Crit Care Med 34: 2355–2361
2. Jaber S, Jung B, Corne P, et al (2010) An intervention to decrease complications related to endotracheal intubation in the intensive care unit: a prospective, multiple-center study. Intensive Care Med 36: 248–255
3. Martin LD, Mhyre JM, Shanks AM, Tremper KK, Kheterpal S (2011) 3,423 emergency tracheal intubations at a university hospital: airway outcomes and complications. Anesthesiology 114: 42–48
4. Duggan M, Kavanagh BP (2007) Atelectasis in the perioperative patient. Curr Opin Anaesthesiol 20: 37–42
5. Hedenstierna G (2009) Respiratory physiology. In Miller RD (ed) Miller's Anesthesia. Churchill Livingstone, Philadelphia, pp 361–392
6. Hedenstierna G, Edmark L (2005) The effects of anesthesia and muscle paralysis on the respiratory system. Intensive Care Med 31: 1327–1335
7. Reinius H, Jonsson L, Gustafsson S, et al (2009) Prevention of atelectasis in morbidly obese patients during general anesthesia and paralysis: a computerized tomography study. Anesthesiology 111: 979–987
8. Salome CM, King GG, Berend N (2010) Physiology of obesity and effects on lung function. J Appl Physiol 108: 206–211
9. Milic-Emili J, Torchio R, D'Angelo E (2007) Closing volume: a reappraisal (1967–2007). Eur J Appl Physiol 99: 567–583
10. Hedenstierna G (2003) Alveolar collapse and closure of airways: regular effects of anaesthesia. Clin Physiol Funct Imaging 23: 123–129
11. American Society of Anesthesiologists Task Force on Management of the Difficult Airway (2003) Practice guidelines for management of the difficult airway: an updated report. Anesthesiology 98: 1269–1277
12. Tanoubi I, Drolet P, Donati F (2009) Optimizing preoxygenation in adults. Can J Anaesth 56: 449–466
13. Russell EC, Wrench I, Feast M, Mohammed F (2008) Pre-oxygenation in pregnancy: the effect of fresh gas flow rates within a circle breathing system. Anaesthesia 63: 833–836
14. Sum Ping SJ, Makary LF, Van Hal MD (2009) Factors influencing oxygen store during denitrogenation in the healthy patient. J Clin Anesth 21: 183–189
15. Mort TC, Waberski BH, Clive J (2009) Extending the preoxygenation period from 4 to 8 mins in critically ill patients undergoing emergency intubation. Crit Care Med 37: 68–71
16. Altermatt FR, Muñoz HR, Delfino AE, Cortínez LI (2005) Pre-oxygenation in the obese patient: effects of position on tolerance to apnoea. Br J Anaesth 95: 706–709
17. Dixon BJ, Dixon JB, Carden JR, et al (2005) Preoxygenation is more effective in the 25 degrees head-up position than in the supine position in severely obese patients: a randomized controlled study. Anesthesiology 102: 1110–1115
18. Ramkumar V, Umesh G, Philip FA (2011) Preoxygenation with 20° head-up tilt provides longer duration of non-hypoxic apnea than conventional preoxygenation in non-obese healthy adults. J Anesth 25: 189–194
19. Baraka AS, Hanna MT, Jabbour SI, et al (1992) Preoxygenation of pregnant and nonpregnant women in the head-up versus supine position. Anesth Analg 75: 757–759
20. Cressey DM, Berthoud MC, Reilly CS (2001) Effectiveness of continuous positive airway pressure to enhance pre-oxygenation in morbidly obese women. Anaesthesia 56: 680–684
21. Coussa M, Proietti S, Schnyder P, et al (2004) Prevention of atelectasis formation during the induction of general anesthesia in morbidly obese patients. Anesth Analg 98: 1491–1495
22. Gander S, Frascarolo P, Suter M, Spahn DR, Magnusson L (2005) Positive end-expiratory pressure during induction of general anesthesia increases duration of nonhypoxic apnea in morbidly obese patients. Anesth Analg 100: 580–584
23. Delay J, Sebbane M, Jung B, et al (2008) The effectiveness of non invasive positive pressure ventilation to enhance preoxygenation in morbidly obese patients: a randomized controlled study. Anesth Analg 107: 1707–1713

VI

24. Baillard C, Fosse JP, Sebbane M, et al (2006) Noninvasive ventilation improves preoxygenation before intubation of hypoxic patients. Am J Respir Crit Care Med 174: 171–177
25. Constantin JM, Futier E, Cherprenet AL (2010) A recruitment maneuver increases oxygenation after intubation of hypoxemic intensive care unit patients: a randomized controlled study. Crit Care 14: R76
26. Futier E, Constantin JM, Pelosi P, et al (2011) Noninvasive ventilation and alveolar recruitment maneuver improve respiratory function during and after intubation of morbidly obese patients: a randomized controlled study. Anesthesiology 114: 1354–1363
27. Futier E, Constantin JM, Petit A, et al (2010) Positive end-expiratory pressure improves end-expiratory lung volume but not oxygenation after induction of anaesthesia. Eur J Anaesthesiol 27: 508–513

Position and the Compromised Respiratory System

G.A. Cortes, D.J. Dries, and J.J. Marini

Introduction

In the critical care setting, positioning is a fundamental tool for implementing an integrated respiratory care strategy. Conversion from the upright to the near-horizontal position used in intensive care is accompanied by important changes in ventilation, perfusion, oxygenation and secretion clearance. These effects are largely accounted for by the influence of gravity on perfusion distribution and by the shifting of pressure vectors as the tissues surrounding the lungs reconfigure. Re-positioning aids or impairs muscle function, affects secretion drainage, influences gas trapping and alters the development or redistribution of lung collapse. Many of these phenomena hold implications for the expression of disease or its management. Mechanical ventilation, sedation, intra-abdominal and intracranial hypertension – common therapies and problems confronted in the intensive care unit (ICU) – are strongly influenced by body orientation.

Physiology of Recumbent Positioning

Ribcage and Diaphragm

According to results reported by Lumb and Nunn in 1991 [1], repositioning the patient from sitting to supine decreases the average contribution of the ribcage to total ventilation from 69.7 % to 32.3 %. Supine (arms down or up), prone and lateral positions all reduced the relative contribution of the ribcage compared to the sitting position; however, there were no significant differences among them. An explanation might be that recumbent positioning increases the length of the diaphragmatic muscle fibers, which results in stronger contraction that augments the participation of the abdomen-diaphragm component [1].

When interpreting chest radiographs, diaphragm position and shape are commonly interpreted to indicate normal or abnormal lung volume. However, certain non-disease variables are also influential. For example, in the same individual, recumbent postures and increasing body weight clearly predisposes to higher diaphragm position. Across individuals, lower diaphragmatic positions are associated with narrower transverse dimensions and reduced anterior-posterior thoracic diameters [2]. Age (independently associated with lower position) also correlates with diaphragmatic function and anatomy, suggesting that all three variables should be taken into account when deciding optimal patient positions in critical care practice.

J.-L. Vincent (ed.), *Annual Update in Intensive Care and Emergency Medicine 2012*
DOI 10.1007/978-3-642-25716-2 © Springer-Verlag Berlin Heidelberg 2012

Position-associated Lung Volume Changes

In normal subjects, reclining decreases functional residual capacity (FRC), primarily because of the upward pressure of the abdominal contents on the diaphragm and to a lesser extent because of reduced lung compliance [3, 4]. FRC declines in non-obese subjects free of lung disease by approximately 30 % (or 800 ml) in shifting from the sitting to the horizontal supine position. Older subjects experience marginally less positional volume loss than do younger individuals. In normal subjects, the lateral decubitus orientation causes a reduction from sitting FRC of approximately 17 % at 0 degrees, and a decline of 27.4 % at -25 degrees (steep Trendelenburg position) [3]. Because proning simultaneously compresses the ventral while distending the dorsal zones of the lung, conversion from the supine to the prone position is accompanied by a redistribution of lung contents and an overall increase of average resting lung volume $\leq$ 15 % [4]. The effects of proning on lung volume are influenced by body habitus, as well as by the nature of the surface upon which proning occurs. Allowing the abdomen to suspend freely when prone may increase resting FRC [5]. Spontaneously breathing patients with severe airflow obstruction lose less volume when recumbent in either the supine or lateral orientation [3]. Dependent air trapping and the need to maintain hyperinflation to preserve airway caliber and elastic recoil are likely contributors.

VI

Position-associated Lung Hemodynamic Changes

The gravitational model of ventilation-perfusion (V/Q) distribution has motivated therapeutic strategies for many years. However, current research findings defy this schema by highlighting situations that cannot be totally explained by gravity as a determinant of pulmonary blood flow distribution [6]. Heterogeneity of perfusion within isogravitational planes [7] and the inability of the gravitational model to explain V/Q redistribution in distinct positions [8] call the dominant role of gravity on ventilation-perfusion distribution into dispute.

From a purely hydrostatic perspective, higher vascular pressures should exist in both dependent arteries and veins, so that the vascular pressure gradient is theoretically maintained, independent of vertical position within the lung. Whereas higher vascular pressures would tend to distend dependent vascular beds to reduce their resistance to this gradient, such beds may already be fully distended by the pulmonary hypertension of the diseased lungs.

Using a normal canine model, Glenny et al. demonstrated experimentally that under zone 3 conditions, gravity is not the principal determinant of regional perfusion distribution in either the supine or prone position [7]. Perfusion measurements using microspheres indicated that vertical height explained only 20 % of flow variability when supine and 12 % when prone [7]. However, not all work agrees with these microsphere studies. Perfusion measurements performed with a variety of imaging techniques, such as positron emission tomography (PET), single photon emission computed tomography (SPECT) and magnetic resonance imaging (MRI) have demonstrated an important gravitational influence on pulmonary perfusion [9]. Hopkins et al. provided evidence for a "Slinky effect" to explain the vertical perfusion gradient found by imaging but challenged by microsphere experiments. In accordance with this model, a component of the apparent vertical perfusion gradient found by imaging methods is due to compression of dependent lung, which increases local lung density and, therefore, perfusion/volume ratios in the supine position [9]. These authors found apparently significant vertical gradients of perfusion but, when the regional variations in lung density were co-analyzed, these vertical gradients were largely minimized [9], thereby reconciling the findings of microsphere and imaging studies.

Hydrostatic pressures and blood flows distribute preferentially to the dorsal regions in the supine position due in part to the preponderance of lung tissue in those zones [7]. As a partial consequence, there is a linear increase in pulmonary perfusion from anterior to posterior lung fields in the supine position [6–7]. Dependent zones experience less vascular resistance, as their higher hydrostatic pressures recruit capillary beds that may not otherwise open [7,9].

Nyren et al. [8] found that blood distributed more uniformly in the prone posture, whereas a more dependent distribution was detected in the supine posture. Because the distribution of ventilation is also influenced in the same fashion by the shift to the prone orientation, the authors concluded that there is a tendency toward more homogenous V/Q matching along the vertical axis in prone compared with supine posture (**Fig. 1**) [8].

By similar mechanisms, the lateral decubitus position encourages perfusion of the lower lung. This observation has been supported by MRI of lung perfusion using arterial spin tagging (MRI-AST) [10]. Such techniques have shown that in both lateral positions, an increase occurs in the intensity (indicating greater perfusion) of the dependent lung compared with its supine values (229 % for left lateral, 40 % for right lateral) [10]. These perfusion measurements, however, might be influenced to some degree by the aforementioned increase in lung density that occurs in dependent zones, as well [9]. Utilizing similar MRI-AST methods, Prisk et al. [11] conducted a study with the hypothesis that in the supine position greater compression of the most dependent lung could limit regional pulmonary blood flow. Their results showed that conversion from supine to prone position improved density-normalized perfusion distribution (milliliters blood per minute per gram of lung tissue), especially in posterior lung zones within the central part of the lung. Such observations support the idea that conversion to prone position recovers collapsed lung volume [11].

Lung perfusion was assessed for the lateral positions by Lan et al. [12] in pneumonectomized pigs; these authors found that the best position after pneumonectomy was the lateral position with remaining lung uppermost, leading to improved V/Q matching and better gas exchange when compared to the lung dependent position [12]. Rohdin et al. [13] evaluated the effects of gravitational forces on lung diffusing capacity and cardiac output in prone and supine humans. Ten healthy subjects were exposed to centrifuge-generated gravity spins of 1 and

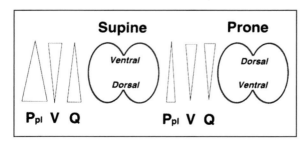

Fig. 1. Components of ventilation/perfusion (V/Q) matching. Transpulmonary pressure (Ppl) gradient differs in the prone and supine positions. A more favorable blood perfusion distribution in the prone position allows efficient irrigation of the zones with better ventilation

5 times normal. Their results indicated a 46 % reduction in diffusing capacity in 5G-hypergravity compared with 1G in the supine position, but a reduction of only 25 % in prone position. The authors considered that reduced pulmonary-capillary blood flow and decreased alveolar volume may explain the impressive reduction of diffusing capacity that occurs when supine. These results support the role of increased lung weight because of tissue edema as a contributor to lung collapse in supine patients with acute lung injury (ALI) and acute respiratory distress syndrome (ARDS) [12]. As a conclusion about the determinants of positional blood flow distribution in the lungs, it may be said that gravity accounts for only 4 – 25 % of observed spatial differences in regional perfusion [9], leaving the remainder to be attributed to specific characteristics of the vascular structure, airway architecture and vasoregulatory factors [14].

Positioning, Pleural Topography, and Ventilation Distribution

During spontaneous breathing, ventilation normally distributes preferentially to the dependent lung zones in the supine, prone, and lateral positions and postural readjustments occur frequently [15]. Approximately 8 to 10 times per hour, the normal subject takes 'sigh' breaths two to four times deeper than the average tidal volume. Microatelectasis and arterial oxygen desaturation tend to develop if breathing remains shallow and uninterrupted by periodic sighs or variations of position [16]. In contrast to spontaneous breathing, the nondependent regions receive relatively more ventilation when the patient is inflated passively by a mechanical ventilator. Dependent regions not only have the least end-expiratory (resting) lung volume but also receive less ventilation than during spontaneous breathing, further promoting atelectasis in those areas [16].

Recumbency redistributes lung volume because it alters the geometry of the thorax. The heart tends to compress the left lower lobe bronchi and is supported partially by the lung tissue beneath. This anatomy helps account for the tendency for atelectasis to develop so commonly in the left lower lobe in postoperative and bedridden patients – especially those with cardiovascular disease [16]. The pleural pressure adjacent to the diaphragm is considerably less negative than at the

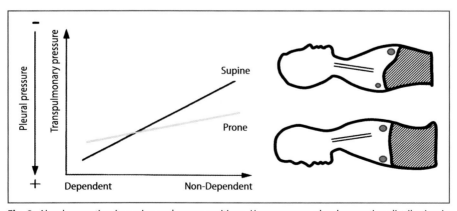

Fig. 2. Alveolar aeration in supine and prone positions. Homogeneous alveolar aeration distribution in the prone position because of a reduction in the pleural pressure gradient.

apex [17]. The vertical gradient of transpulmonary pressure (alveolar minus pleural pressure) is approximately 0.25 cmH$_2$O per cm of vertical height for normal subjects in the erect position and approximately 0.17 cmH$_2$O per cm for normal subjects in supine recumbency [15,18]; therefore, alveolar volumes are greatest in the nondependent regions (**Fig. 2**). For patients with edematous lungs, an intensified gravitational gradient of pleural pressure accentuates dorsal atelectasis and consolidation [19].

Available data indicate that the gradient of pleural pressure is less steep in the prone than in the supine position, perhaps in part because of the shifting weight of the heart and mediastinal contents [15]. The prone position also favors airway drainage [20]. The lateral decubitus position causes the upper lung to assume a resting volume nearly as large as it has in the sitting position and to undergo better drainage, whereas the lower lung tends to pool mucus and is compressed to a size similar to or less than it has in the supine position [20]. As already noted, total FRC is normally greater in the lateral decubitus than in the supine horizontal orientation. Positional losses of lung volume are considerably less in patients with airflow obstruction, in part due to gas trapping in dependent regions [3].

VI

Positioning in Disease Conditions

Ascites

Ascites is a common complicating feature of a variety of pathologic liver, peritoneal and cardiac conditions commonly seen in ICUs. Ascites may increase abdominal elastance and expand the lower rib cage [21]. In a supine canine model, Leduc and De Troyer demonstrated that increments of ascites progressively decreased tidal volume and minute ventilation, causing an elevation of arterial PCO$_2$ and an increase in the parasternal intercostal inspiratory muscle activity [21]. Despite the upward pressure exerted on its dome that should favor diaphragmatic geometry, massive ascites inhibits the diaphragmatic component of lung expansion by dilating the costal ring of its insertion. In so doing, ascites overstretches the diaphragmatic musculature, reducing its contraction capacity and helping to explain the dyspnea associated with this condition. Surprisingly, the expiratory action of the abdominal muscles may also be adversely affected by a very large ascites collection, presumably due to fiber overstretch [22].

Chang et al. [23] evaluated the effects of ascites and body position in 22 men with cirrhosis. The authors reported that single breath-carbon monoxide diffusing capacity (DLco) was greater in the erect (sitting) than in the supine position. However, when DLco was adjusted for alveolar volume (DLco/VA), it was significantly higher in the supine position. When patients in the study underwent large volume paracentesis, the volume-corrected parameter showed an important decrease, indicating that ascites may prevent or attenuate the worsening of gas exchange that otherwise would occur due to postural changes in patients with cirrhosis [23].

Morbid Obesity

Excess adipose tissue reduces both FRC and expiratory reserve volume. These effects augment the risk of expiratory flow limitation and airway closure, producing abnormalities in ventilation distribution, increasing of lung collapse in dependent zones, and altering pulmonary blood flow distribution [24]. In addition, there is an inverse relationship between body mass index (BMI) and PaO_2 values [24, 25]. Pelosi et al. reported that in anesthetized and paralyzed obese patients (BMI > 30 kg/m^2), the prone position improved pulmonary function by increasing FRC, lung compliance and oxygenation [5]. In mechanically ventilated patients, increasing positive end-expiratory pressure (PEEP) to 10 cmH$_2$O significantly reduced the elastance values of the lung, chest wall, and total respiratory system in obese subjects [26]. Valenza et al. evaluated the effect of the beach chair position, PEEP and pneumoperitoneum on respiratory function in morbidly obese patients [27]. The authors concluded that the beach chair position improved the elastance of the respiratory system, almost doubling end-expiratory lung volume (0.83 ± 0.3 and 0.85 ± 0.3 l, beach chair position and PEEP10, respectively) compared with the supine position at zero PEEP (0.46 ± 0.1 l). However, during pneumoperitoneum, only the combination of the two improved oxygenation [27]. Reverse Trendelenburg positioning has been found to be another beneficial posture, especially for morbidly obese patients undergoing bariatric surgery. Perilli et al. found that in this group of patients, the reverse Trendelenburg position narrowed the alveolar-arterial oxygen difference and improved respiratory system compliance [28].

Available data suggest that obesity functionally modifies thoraco-abdominal mechanical interdependence. Obesity augments the tendency of dependent zones to collapse, alters regional perfusion patterns, and adversely affects the roles of the diaphragmatic and abdominal muscles. It follows that the respiratory care strategy in this patient subgroup should be directed toward improving respiratory system and chest wall compliances via prone, reverse Trendelenburg or beach chair positions in conjunction with sufficient PEEP to offset the enhanced tendency for regional lung collapse [24–28].

Pleural Effusion

A variety of diseases that prompt ICU admission are commonly complicated by large pleural effusions, many of which are unilateral. Prominent causes of unilateral pulmonary effusion have been reported to include infection, congestive heart failure and atelectasis [29]. Although not all studies agree [30, 31], convincing data from spontaneously breathing patients (inspired oxygen fraction [FiO$_2$] 0.21) demonstrated better oxygenation when patients with unilateral pulmonary effusion were positioned laterally with the affected lung uppermost [30]. This result is potentially explained by positionally-improved V/Q matching [30]. The absence of significant positional change in PaCO$_2$ has been interpreted to indicate that overall alveolar ventilation was not affected by the positional variations (diseased lung uppermost vs lowermost) [30]. Data from our own experimental study in normal pigs indicated that modest PEEP restored FRC values to their non-pulmonary effusion baseline, predominantly by reversal of lung unit collapse and by preventing intratidal derecruitment with unilateral pulmonary effusion, independent of position [32].

Positional Dyspnea: Heart Failure, Airway Obstruction and Neuromuscular Weakness

Certain positions may relieve or exacerbate dyspnea. Orthopnea, although most emblematic of congestive heart failure, also characterizes severe airflow obstruction, pregnancy, extreme obesity, pericardial tamponade, and diaphragmatic

VI

weakness. Gas trapping and aversion to the work of breathing effectively limit lung volume reduction when patients with severe airflow obstruction assume a supine position [3]. Patients with persistent hypoxemia, hypercapnia and chronic obstructive pulmonary disease (COPD) who required invasive mechanical ventilation were positioned prone and supine for 36 hours, with turns occurring every three hours [33]. PaO_2/FiO_2 remained significantly improved after the first turn back from the prone position, with better values for subsequent supine measurements. $PaCO_2$, however, was not significantly affected by position [33]. Presumed mechanisms by which prone positioning improves PaO_2/FiO_2 values in patients with airflow obstruction include better V/Q matching [8], improved airway drainage [20] and reduction of airway resistance and dynamic hyperinflation [34].

In patients with bilateral diaphragmatic weakness or paralysis, oxygenation and vital capacity usually worsen when moving from upright to supine [35]. In these patients, surgical plication of the diaphragm or avoidance of the supine position are prudent, because ventilation strongly or solely depends on the accessory muscles of respiration, which are better stabilized when upright and should not be loaded by having to displace the abdominal contents cephalad with each inspiration [36]. Conversely, patients with quadriplegia or extreme orthostatic hypotension and those who experience abdominal or back pain accentuated by the upright position may not tolerate sitting without breathlessness. High level spinal cord injuries require the patient to breathe using only the diaphragm. In such patients, the supine position often exerts a positive influence by improving the curvature and performance of the diaphragm [37].

ARDS

For more than 30 years, physiologists, physicians, nurses and respiratory care practitioners have espoused, tested, and at times cautioned against the prone positioning of patients with severe oxygenation problems. There seems to be general agreement that prone positioning is likely to improve the lung's ability to oxygenate more efficiently by inducing a homogeneous V/Q distribution [8], but key nagging questions remain unsettled. For example, does prone positioning reduce the morbidity or mortality of patients with ARDS? Despite a persuasive rationale suggesting that prone ventilation could improve patient outcomes, four large studies from Europe – two Italian [38, 39], one Spanish [40], and one French [41] – each designed to assess proning's effect on survival in patients with ALI/ARDS of varying severity, yielded discouraging results. Although oxygenation markedly improved in most patients when ventilated prone, no change in overall mortality was observed [38, 41]. Yet, a number of weaknesses of study design or execution limit acceptance of the 'no outcome benefit' conclusion; indeed, the question of mortality reduction is still quite active. First, and perhaps most importantly, in two of these studies patients randomized to prone ventilation were not kept that way during most of the period of greatest vulnerability [38, 41]. In one trial, patients were returned to the supine position for more than two thirds of each day [38]. This is of fundamental concern, as numerous animal studies have shown that ventilator-induced lung injury (VILI) can develop within hours, or even minutes, after instituting an adverse ventilatory strategy [42]. Accordingly, any potentially beneficial effect of prone ventilation could have been diluted by the limited period of time the intervention was applied. Second, from a statistical viewpoint, it is probable that these randomized studies, though relatively large, were not sufficiently powered to utilize mortality as an end-point across a patient sample of mixed severity. Interestingly, enrollment was stopped early in two of the three randomized trials, at least in part because many caregivers, influenced by their occasional observation of dramatic response to proning, were eventually unwilling to forgo its use should the patient be allocated to the control group. Third, in all trials, proning was not initiated as soon as possible after the diagnosis of ALI/ARDS was made. Accordingly, VILI could already have developed by the time the patients were enrolled. Good reasons can be enumerated not to prone from the start, but most recruitment from prone positioning is expected to occur early in the process. Finally, the proning intervention was only applied for a restricted number of days. Post-hoc analysis of the first Italian trial results indicated that mortality was strikingly reduced in the subsets of patients with the worst gas exchange, those with severe lung injury, those exposed to very high tidal volumes, and those who improved CO_2 exchange after proning [38]. For such patients at the highest mortality risk from ALI/ARDS or VILI, withholding proning leaves an important therapeutic asset on the table. Such thinking prompted the Italian group to conduct a prospective trial of proning in a targeted high mortality risk subpopulation, with attention to the lessons learned earlier. The results from that trial [39], as well as a recently published pooled meta-analysis of studied ARDS patients from multiple trials [43], reveal that mortality is positively influenced by appropriate prone positioning in the most seriously ill patients.

Several studies have reported conflicting evidence regarding the utility of CT imaging patterns in making the decision to prone [44]. Presently, however, there are no highly reliable predictors of who will or will not respond. If prone ventilation improves mortality among the very critically ill, the question of why benefit accrues remains open. Could it be that improving oxygenation allows us to reduce or withdraw other iatrogenic elements of treatment – the FiO_2 and/or high levels of mean airway pressure, for example? An alternative explanation is that reducing damaging strain mitigates VILI.

The role of periodic partial repositioning (i.e., 15°–°) to the left and right lateral decubitus angles or alternating swimmer's positions when patients are primarily prone rather than supine has not been clarified. Studies conducted in the 1940s established a two-hour turning interval as the standard of everyday practice so as to limit skin breakdown in supine patients. The effect of various frequencies and degrees of periodic partial repositioning has never been studied for the prone posture. Solely from the standpoint of skin ulceration, however, there is no obvious reason to suggest that the positional adjustments should be made less frequently than the 'every two-hour' supine standard. Because some areas exist over anterior body prominences that are predisposed to ulcerate, intermittent partial repositioning might have to be more frequent to limit skin breakdown when prone on a conventional bed surface. Considering only the lungs, however, ventilation is more uniform when oriented prone, so that periodic partial repositioning might be needed a little less often. Among the factors thought to contribute to the development of atelectasis are impaired clearance of secretions from dependent airways and failure to sufficiently expand ventilating regions. Because the forces contributing to dependent atelectasis are reduced and secretion clearance is enhanced when patients are prone, the frequency with which atelectasis develops may be somewhat less (and more ventrally located) in this position. Hemodynamic benefit might also be a characteristic of the prone position. Vieillard-Baron et al. demonstrated that prone positioning effectively countered right ventricular (RV) overload in patients with severe ARDS; in that study, RV function was evaluated by bedside transesophageal echocardiography, before and after 18 h of prone-position ventilation [45].

In summary, most conclusions from experimental, observational, and clinical trial meta-analyses suggest prone positioning is an important therapeutic tool in severe forms of ARDS and in patients with refractory hypoxemic conditions, providing predictively improved oxygenation, 10 % increase in survival in this patient subgroup, and perhaps an appropriate contribution to lung protection [42].

Position as a Therapeutic Tool in Non-ARDS Settings

Other important questions regarding prone positioning are sometimes debated. Does the prone position have a positive role in treating patients with other forms of lung compromise than ARDS? For patients with volume overload secondary to congestive heart failure it definitely does; Nakos and colleagues demonstrated an excellent oxygenation response to prone positioning in left heart failure for multiple reasons, perhaps one of which is augmented lymphatic clearance of edema [46].

With the exception of a single encouraging study in COPD, the effects of prone ventilation have not been systematically studied in patients with severe airflow limitation [33]. Yet, in theory, the prone orientation might help to clear retained secretions from dependent airways. Gas trapping may predominate in the dependent zones in COPD. Although clearly not yet proven, proning has theoretical appeal for improving the clinical course of the ventilated 'blue bloater' subtype of COPD whose progress stalls. Positional reopening of dependent airways might help zonal delivery of bronchodilating aerosols or relieve bronchial compression, and these patients frequently have enlarged hearts from *cor pulmonale* as well as dorsal airway plugging.

Dangers of Repositioning

Well known adverse consequences of prone positioning may include skin ulceration and soft tissue damage, ocular injury, inadvertent catheter and endotracheal tube extraction, and elevation of cerebral pressure secondary to obstructed jugular venous drainage. Repositioning may have other less well documented, but nonetheless potentially hazardous consequences. For example, secretion mobilization through the airway tree has been proposed as one of the mechanisms responsible for injury propagation in patients with ARDS and other regional lung pathologic conditions like pneumonia [47]. The stage of disease is likely to be very important, since once secretions thicken, biofluids are unable to "alveolarize" easily [48].

Secretion mobilization analysis in a swine model, using CT to track contrasted mucus stimulant, concluded that gravity had an important potential to help move moderately viscous fluid either toward or away from the airway opening; ventilation with the rapid inspiratory flows and smaller tidal volumes often used clinically tended to embed the mucus stimulant more peripherally [48]. Despite the current lack of clinical studies to directly support the idea, positioning the diseased region in the dependent orientation seems prudent when confronting the very first phase of ventilating acute non-symmetrical lung disease (even though doing so temporarily impedes secretion clearance). In the earliest stages of inflammation, when biofluids are highly mobile, some attention should be directed toward selecting options for positioning and ventilation that confine noxious fluids to the smallest number of lung segments [47]. Later on, the mandate for such positioning is relaxed or reversed.

Positioning must be carefully regulated in patients with acute brain injury. Good response has been reported in patients with head injury and a Glasgow scale score of 8 or less to 24 hours of enforced, unchanged supine positioning with 30° of head elevation. Ledwith et al. described the effect of body positioning on brain tissue oxygen ($PbtO_2$) and intracranial pressure (ICP) [49]. When supine, ICP decreased with the head of bed elevated to 30 or 45° with the knees bent. In contrast an increase of ICP was detected in both right and left lateral positions with the head of bed at 15°. $PbtO_2$ values showed a downward trend following any change of position compared to the unperturbed baseline in this study [49], emphasizing that the injured brain is very sensitive to hemodynamic changes generated by repetitive repositioning.

VI

Conclusion

Judicious body positioning offers a potent therapeutic tool for use in critical care and emergency medicine. Clinicians must understand the physiologic changes – both helpful and hazardous – that different positions generate when attempting to develop an optimal cardiorespiratory prescription for supporting the ventilated patient.

References

1. Lumb AB, Nunn JF (1991) Respiratory function and ribcage contribution to ventilation in body positions commonly used during anesthesia. Anesth Analg 73: 422–426
2. Suwatanapongched T, Gierada DS, Slone RM, Pilgram TK, Tuteur PG (2003) Variation in diaphragm position and shape in adults with normal pulmonary function. Chest 123: 2019–2027
3. Marini JJ, Tyler ML, Hudson LD, Davis BS, Huseby JS (1984) Influence of head-dependent positions on lung volume and oxygen saturation in chronic air-flow obstruction. Am Rev Respir Dis 129: 101–105
4. Behrakis PK, Baydur A, Jaeger MJ, Milic-Emili J (1983) Lung mechanics in sitting and horizontal body positions. Chest 83: 643–646
5. Pelosi P, Croci M, Calappi E, et al (1996) Prone positioning improves pulmonary function in obese patients during general anesthesia. Anesth Analg 83: 578–583
6. Galvin I, Drummond GB, Nirmalan M (2007) Distribution of blood flow and ventilation in the lung: gravity is not the only factor. Br J Anaesth 98: 420–428
7. Glenny RW, Lamm WJ, Albert RK, Robertson HT (1991) Gravity is a minor determinant of pulmonary blood flow distribution. J Appl Physiol 71: 620–629
8. Nyren S, Radell P, Lindahl S, et al (2010) Lung ventilation and perfusion in prone and supine postures with reference to anesthetized and mechanically ventilated healthy volunteers. Anesthesiology 112: 682–687
9. Hopkins SR, Henderson AC, Levin DL, et al (2007) Vertical gradients in regional lung density and perfusion in the supine human lung: the Slinky effect. J Appl Physiol 103: 240–248
10. Keilholz SD, Knight-Scott J, Christopher JM, Mai VM, Berr SS (2001) Gravity-dependent

VI

perfusion of the lung demonstrated with the FAIRER arterial spin tagging method. Magn Reson Imaging 19: 929–935

11. Prisk G, Yamada K, Cortney A, et al (2007) Pulmonary perfusion in the prone and supine postures in the normal human lung. J Appl Physiol 103: 883–894

12. Lan CH, Hsu H, Wu Ch, et al (2011) Lateral Position with the remaining lung uppermost improves matching of pulmonary ventilation and perfusion in pneumonectomized pigs. J Surg Res 167: e55–e61

13. Rohdin M, Petersson J, Sundblad P, et al (2003) Effects of gravity on lung diffusing capacity and cardiac output in prone and supine humans. J Appl Physiol 95: 3–10

14. Glenny RW (2009) Determinant of regional ventilation and blood flow in the lung. Intensive Care Med 35: 1833–1842

15. Lai-Fook SJ, Rodarte JR (1991) Pleural pressure distribution and its relationship to lung volume and interstitial pressure. J Appl Physiol 70: 967–978

16. Duggan M, Kavanagh BP (2005) Pulmonary atelectasis. Anesthesiology 102: 838–854

17. D'angelo E, Agostoni E (1973) Continuous recording of pleural surface pressure at various sites. Respir Physiol 19: 356–368

18. Hoppin FG, Green ID, Mead J (1969) Distribution of pleural surface pressure in dogs. J Appl Physiol 27: 863–873

19. O'Quin RJ, Marini JJ, Culver BH, Butler J (1985) Transmission of airway pressure to pleural space during lung edema and chest wall restriction. J Appl Physiol 59: 1171–1177

20. Takahashi N, Murakami G, Ishikawa A, Sato TJ, Ito T (2004) Anatomic evaluation of postural bronchial drainage of the lung with special reference to patients with tracheal intubation: which combination of postures provides the best simplification? Chest 125: 935–944

21. Leduc D, De Troyer A (2007) Dysfunction of the canine respiratory muscle pump in ascites. J Appl Physiol 102: 650–657

22. Leduc D, De Troyer A (2008) Impact of acute ascites on the action of the canine abdominal muscles. J Appl Physiol 104: 1568–1573

23. Chang SC, Chang HI, Chen FJ, Shiao GM, Wang SS (1995) Effects of ascites and body position on gas exchange in patients with cirrhosis. Proc Natl Sci Counc Repub China B 19: 143–150

24. Salome CM, King GG, Berend N (2010) Physiology of obesity and effects on lung function. J Appl Physiol 108: 206–211

25. Yamane T, Date T Michifumi T, et al (2008) Hypoxemia in inferior pulmonary veins in supine position is dependent on obesity. Am J Respir Crit Care Med 178: 295–299

26. Pelosi P, Ravagnan I, Giurati G, et al (1999) Positive end-expiratory pressure improves respiratory function in obese but not in normal subjects during anesthesia and paralysis. Anesthesiology 91: 1221–1231

27. Valenza F, Vagginelli F, Tiby A, et al (2007) Effects of the beach chair position, positive end-expiratory pressure, and pneumoperitoneum on respiratory function in morbidly obese patients during anesthesia and paralysis. Anesthesiology 107: 725–732

28. Perilli V, Sollazzi L, Bozza P, et al (2000) The effects of the reverse trendelenburg position on respiratory mechanics and blood gases in morbidly obese patients during bariatric surgery. Anesth Analg 91: 1520–1525

29. Mattison LE, Coppage L, Alderman DF, Herlong JO, Sahn SA (1997) Pleural effusions in the medical ICU: prevalence, causes, and clinical implications. Chest 111: 1018–1023

30. Sonnenblick M, Melzer E, Rosin AJ (1983) Body positional effect on gas exchange in unilateral pleural effusion. Chest 83: 784–786

31. Chang SC, Shiao GM, Perng RP (1989) Postural effect on gas exchange in patients with unilateral pleural effusions. Chest 96: 60–63

32. Graf J, Fomenti P, Santos A, et al (2011) Pleural effusion complicates monitoring of respiratory mechanics Crit Care Med 39: 1–6

33. Reignier J, Lejeune O, Renard B, et al (2005) Short-term effects of prone position in chronic obstructive pulmonary disease patients with severe acute and hypercapnic respiratory failure. Intensive Care Med 31: 1128–1131

34. Mentzelopoulos SD, Roussos C, Zakynthinos SG (2005) Prone position improves expiratory airway mechanics in severe chronic bronchitis. Eur Respir J 25: 259–268

35. Qureshi A (2009) Diaphragm paralysis. Semin Respir Crit Care Med 30: 315–320
36. Celli BR (2002) Respiratory management of diaphragm paralysis. Semin Respir Crit Care Med 23: 275–281
37. Baydur A, Adkins RH, Milic-Emili (2001) Lung mechanics in individuals with spinal cord injury: effects of injury level and posture. J Appl Physiol 90: 405–411
38. Gattinoni L, Tognoni G, Pesenti A, et al (2001) Effect of prone positioning on the survival of patients with acute respiratory failure. N Engl J Med 345: 568–573
39. Taccone P, Pesenti A, Latini R, et al (2009) Prone positioning in patients with moderate and severe acute respiratory distress syndrome. JAMA 302: 1977–1984
40. Mancebo J, Fernandez R, Blanch Ll, et al (2006) A multicenter trial of prolonged prone ventilation in severe acute respiratory distress syndrome. Am J Respir Crit Care Med 173: 1233–1239
41. Guerin C, Gaillard S, Lemasson S, et al (2004) Effects of systematic prone positioning in hypoxemic acute respiratory failure. JAMA 292: 2379–2387
42. Broccard A, Shapiro RS, Schmitz LL, Adams AB, Nahum A, Marini JJ (2000) Prone positioning attenuates and redistributes ventilator-induced lung injury in dogs. Crit Care Med 28: 295–303
43. Gattinoni L, Carlesso E, Taccone P, Polli F, Guérin C, Mancebo J (2010) Prone positioning improves survival in severe ARDS: a pathophysiologic review and individual patient meta-analysis. Minerva Anestesiol 76: 448–454
44. Chung JH, Kradin RL, Greene RE, Shepard JA, Digumarthy SR (2011) CT predictors of mortality in pathology confirmed ARDS. Eur Radiol 21: 730–737
45. Vieillard-Baron A, Charron C, Caille V, Belliard G, Page B, Jardin F (2007) Prone positions unloads the right ventricule in severe ARDS. Chest 132: 1440–1446
46. Nakos G, Batistatou A, Galiatsou E, et al (2006) Lung and 'end organ' injury due to mechanical ventilation in animals: comparison between the prone and supine positions. Crit Care 10: R38
47. Marini JJ, Gattinoni L (2008) Propagation prevention: a complementary mechanism for "lung protective" ventilation in acute respiratory distress syndrome. Crit Care Med 36: 3252–3258
48. Graf J, Mentzelopoulos SD, Adams AB, Zhang J, Tashjian JH, Marini JJ (2009) Semi-quantitative tracking of intra-airway fluids by computed tomography. Clin Physiol Funct Imaging 29: 406–413
49. Ledwith MB, Bloom S, Maloney-Wilensky E, Coyle B, Polomano RC, Le Roux PD (2010) Effect of body position on cerebral oxygenation and physiologic parameters in patients with acute neurological conditions. J Neurosci Nurs 42: 280–287

VI

VII Pneumonia

Severe Community-acquired Pneumonia

J. Vergragt, J. Kesecioglu, and D.W. de Lange

Introduction

Severe community-acquired pneumonia (CAP) is an important disease and on many intensive care units (ICUs) it is one of the most prevalent infectious diseases. Despite advances in antimicrobial therapy, rates of mortality from CAP remain unacceptably high. In fact, mortality rates have not decreased significantly since penicillin became routinely available and CAP remains the seventh leading cause of death in the United States [1, 2]. Estimates of the incidence of CAP range from 4 million to 5 million cases per year in the United States, with about 500,000 patients requiring hospitalization and 45,000 deaths annually [3].

VII

Apart from mortality, the economic burden of CAP is enormous. In Europe the estimated direct costs for CAP are estimated to be 10.1 billion euros annually. Half of the costs are from patients who are admitted to the hospital (5.7 billion euros) [4]. This breaks down to mean direct costs of ~1500 euros per hospitalized patient in Europe [5]. The costs of patients admitted to the ICU are often more than 5-fold higher [6]. In addition, the indirect costs of work days lost amounts to 3.6 billion euros annually.

Furthermore, patients with mild to moderate CAP need 6 to 18 months to fully recover, according to the Medical Outcomes Study 36-item short form (SF-36) questionnaire [7]. However, no such data are available for patients with severe CAP. Patients with severe CAP are very prone to develop complications and have a higher risk of dying. Most of those patients are admitted to the ICU but still have mortality rates of ~25 %. If these patients develop shock, mortality increases to 50 % [8, 9]. Recognition of these severely ill patients is critical and treatment should be prompt and optimal. Here we discuss the difficulties in diagnosis and treatment of patients with severe CAP who are admitted to the ICU.

Predicting Which Patients with Severe Community-acquired Pneumonia need Intensive Care

Although much has been written on the definition of severe CAP, a consensus has yet to be agreed upon. For educational, clinical and scientific purposes, an objective and uniform measure of pneumonia severity is very desirable. Unfortunately, some aspects of pneumonia severity models tend to be self-fulfilling, like the need for intubation, admission to the ICU, being moribund, etc. Basically, two approaches can be used: A sum of clinical findings surmounting a certain threshold that indicates severe pneumonia, or the allocation of certain necessary treat-

J.-L. Vincent (ed.), *Annual Update in Intensive Care and Emergency Medicine 2012*
DOI 10.1007/978-3-642-25716-2 © Springer-Verlag Berlin Heidelberg 2012

ments (like ICU admission or mechanical ventilation) to prove that the pneumonia is severe. It is obvious that most contemporary scoring systems to assess severity of pneumonia are intertwined with the definition of severity.

Most efforts have been directed toward the classification of patients with pneumonia presenting in the emergency department (ED). This has resulted in multiple scoring systems applicable to this heterogeneous population. Most systems incorporate clinical parameters reflecting compromised respiration or circulation, infection, as well as laboratory and radiological criteria. Some also address chronic health items, and all are targeted to predict mortality or the level of care needed. However, since most models use endpoints like 30-day mortality and ICU admission on day three, their clinical use as prediction models for the ED or ICU physician seems modest at best [10].

An ideal scoring system (and accompanying definition) would be easy to learn and apply, would incorporate patient characteristics and progression of disease, and accurately predict the appropriate level of treatment and monitoring, or even palliative care. Commonly used scoring systems have acceptable negative predictive value (91–97 %) (**Table 1**). Although the majority of patients (75–90 %) is initially treated on general wards, an underestimation of the severity in only a small fraction of patients will eventually result in a substantial number of secondary or delayed ICU admissions [11]. The rate of severe CAP patients with such delayed ICU admission varies (12–66 %). This probably reflects differences in local practices [11, 12]. Unfortunately, delayed admission to the ICU results in decreased survival, despite lower 'severity' on initial presentation [11, 12]. These unexpected deteriorations are not measured by existing scoring systems. This could be because of an unknown determinant of disease that is not taken into account, or simply to the fact that to determine the speed of progression one needs at least two assessments on the time axis.

On the other hand, only 17.3–36 % of patients who rank in the highest risk groups according to severity scores are admitted to the ICU [10, 13]. If all of these

Table 1. Characteristics of commonly applied pneumonia severity scores

Name	Validity	PPV (%)	NPV (%)	ICU-Specific	Simplicity	Remarks
mATS/IDSA	++	31–87	88–99	+/–	+/–	Major criteria are self-fulfilling
PSI	++	14–29	87–98	–	–	Includes patients from nursing homes, complex
CURB65	++	10–29	87–96	+/–	+	Has many spin-offs (e.g., CURXO-80, CORB)
SMARTCOP	+/–	20–22	97–98	++	+/–	Superior for younger patients
SEWS	+/–	27	86	+	++	Serial assessments are a fundamental aspect
APACHE	++	22	85–97	+	–	Most useful from ICU perspective

PPV: positive predictive value; NPV: negative predictive value; mATS/IDSA: modified American Thoracic Society/Infectious Diseases Society of America; PSI: Pneumonia Severity Index; CURB65: Confusion, Urea, Respiratory rate, Blood pressure, age> 65yrs; SMARTCOP: Systolic blood pressure, Multilobar infiltrates, Albumin, Respiratory rate, Tachycardia, Confusion, Oxygen low, arterial Ph; SEWS: Standardized Early Warning System; APACHE: Acute Physiology And Chronic Health Evaluation.

'predicted to be very sick patients with pneumonia' were to be admitted to the ICU this would pose a tremendous burden on healthcare resources. This limitation in positive predictive value is a feature of most scoring systems.

Another shortcoming of prognostic models is the advanced age of patients presenting with pneumonia. Such patients often suffer from other important comorbid conditions, resulting in a high mortality that is often unrelated to pneumonia. Furthermore, many such patients with pneumonia are not suitable for or do not want intensified care and are treated with palliative measures only. Mortality is, therefore, a debatable measure of outcome and probably neither reflects quality of care nor severity of the pneumonia.

There are several pneumonia severity scores (see **Table 1**). Most of these models are based upon logistic regression analysis, which has been used to identify (statistically) significant predictors for pneumonia outcome (mostly death). Some models are quite elaborate, incorporating numerous variables, while others are quite simple and can be performed at the bedside. The parameters included in such scores are used to 'earn points' and these points are used for classification of patients into risk groups. Various reviews have been conducted only to come to the same conclusions; performance is reasonable, but improvement is mandatory [11, 14–16]. Another limitation of most of these models is that they do not perform well outside the setting they were developed in. For example, in seasonal influenza, these scoring systems perform suboptimally, as most of these patients were excluded from the initial study populations [17]. The position of viral pneumonia in the spectrum of severe CAP should be re-evaluated and its contribution to the total burden of severe CAP needs further elucidation.

VII

An interesting future development is the application of ubiquitous available biomarkers as predictors of severity of pneumonia, like C-reactive protein (CRP), procalcitonin (PCT), tumor necrosis factor (TNF), interleukin-6 (IL-6), etc. However, the predictive value of most of those markers needs to be elucidated [18]. It is, however, very doubtful whether one biomarker will be able to outperform an entire pneumonia severity model based upon comorbidity and derangements of acute physiology (like the Acute Physiology and Chronic Health Evaluation [APACHE] or Pneumonia Severity Index [PSI]). Most likely, those new biomarkers will be incorporated in updates of already existing pneumonia severity models.

Much is in favor of applying existing pneumonia severity models, such as PSI or the Standardized Early Warning System (SEWS), in the ED in a repetitive fashion. The SEWS was outperformed by CURB65, but only in a single point assessment [19]. The inherent value of these systems is to draw attention to patients who are potentially at risk, and to stick with them until things have become clear. Results of current research on this subject are to be expected in the coming years.

In conclusion, none of the existing scoring systems seems to be universally applicable; not all patients in need of intensive care are correctly and timely detected. Limitations in both negative and especially positive predictive value reflect the dynamic nature of pneumonia, with patients presenting at different stages of development. Furthermore about 50 % of mortality is caused by comorbidities worsening after admission [10]. On the other hand, the dichotomy between ICU and non-ICU no longer seems a sensible approach from the patient's point of view. Treating severe CAP as an emergency, like stroke or myocardial infarction, could and should be accomplished with minimal changes in healthcare infrastructure [10, 11, 14]. Streamlining the process from ED to ICU, while preventing unnecessary admissions to the ICU, will be the challenge of the near future.

Empirical Treatment of Severe Community-acquired Pneumonia

Several national and international guidelines describe which empirical antimicrobial treatment is optimal for patients with severe CAP. Local epidemiology of microorganisms (**Table 2**) and differences in the resistance of pathogens causing severe CAP direct the choice of empirical antimicrobial treatment. It is obvious that local guidelines cannot be extrapolated to all populations or countries without taking these differences into account. Internationally acclaimed guidelines are often unnecessarily broad and aggressive and should be tailored to local epidemiology to prevent occurrence of resistance.

Most guidelines advocate combination antimicrobial therapy for the empirical treatment of severe CAP [20, 21]. Often a beta-lactam is used in combination with either a fluorquinolone or macrolide (mostly azithromycin) to provide coverage for atypical pathogens. The beta-lactam is substituted by an antipseudomonal beta-lactam if *Pseudomonas* infection is suspected. If methicillin resistant *Staphylococcus aureus* (MRSA) is suspected, vancomycin or linezolid are added to the empirical scheme. The addition of aminoglycosides to the abovementioned treatment schemes is associated with increased nephrotoxicity and bothersome pharmacokinetic properties (poor penetration into the lung parenchyma) [21]. However, the increasing rate of extended-spectrum beta-lactamase (ESBL) producing pathogens might resurrect the aminoglycosides in empirical treatment schemes.

However, does adherence to such guidelines result in increased survival? In general, there is low adherence to guidelines (8 – 45.9 %) [22]. Some older, retrospective analyses do show a modest survival benefit when patients are treated according to such guidelines [23, 24]. A prospective randomized trial to evaluate whether adherence to such guidelines influences outcome will for obvious ethical reasons never be performed.

A number of, again, retrospective studies show that combination therapy with a macrolide might improved outcome in comparison to combination therapy with a fluoroquinolone, especially in more severely ill patients [22]. However, a meta-analysis of 23 trials showed the opposite; fluoroquinolones were associated with a greater success of treatment in patients who had to be hospitalized for pneumonia, although a benefit in mortality was not observed [25]. The studies included

VII

Pathogen	ICU	Hospital	Outpatient
Unknown	28 %	41 %	50 %
Streptococcus pneumoniae	2 %	5 %	8 %
Mycoplasma pneumoniae	7 %	6 %	13 %
Chlamydia pneumoniae	4 %	11 %	21 %
Staphylococcus aureus	9 %	3 %	15 %
Enterobacteriaceae	9 %	4 %	0 %
Pseudomonas aeruginosa	4 %	3 %	1 %
Legionella spp.	12 %	5 %	0 %
Coxiella burnetii	7 %	4 %	1 %
Viruses	3 %	12 %	17 %

Table 2. Frequencies of cultured microorganisms in Europe depending on treatment setting

Depicted are the mean percentages. Reproduced from [4] with permission of the BMJ Publishing Group Ltd.

in this meta-analysis included heterogeneous populations and, unfortunately, the minority of studies was double-blinded. Therefore, there is enough equipoise to warrant a prospective trial on the optimal combination therapy in severe CAP.

Most international acclaimed guidelines, like the Surviving Sepsis Campaign, acknowledge the fact that antimicrobial therapy should be given as soon as possible, but preferably within one hour after admission to the ED [26]. This claim appears to be scientifically solid for patients with septic shock [27]. However, whether it holds true for patients with moderate-to-severe CAP without septic shock remains to be proven. The time-to-first-antibiotic-dose (TFAD) has become a core quality measure in several countries. A negative spin-off of this quality parameter is a decrease in the accuracy of the diagnosis of pneumonia without decreasing the mortality [28, 29].

Another important topic in the antimicrobial treatment of severe CAP is the duration of treatment. Most contemporary guidelines advocate a 7–10 day treatment period [20, 21]. However, clinicians often tend to treat patients for 10–11 days and treat patients even longer when they are admitted to the ICU, are hypotensive, have pleural effusions, have multilobar infiltrates, or are given combination therapy (11–15 days) [30]. Recent trials have shown that antibiotic treatment can be safely reduced from an average of 10.7 days to 7.2 days based upon a PCT-guided strategy [31]. In a recent ICU study, the subgroup of patients with CAP was treated for 5.5 days in the PCT-guided group versus 10.4 days in the control group [32]. Because certain subgroups were excluded from these studies, like patients with Legionnaire's disease, the true reduction in antibiotic treatment still needs to be established. The results of the largest PCT-guided ICU study (Safety and Efficacy of Procalcitonin Guided Antibiotic Therapy in Adult Intensive Care Units, ClinicalTrials.gov identifier NCT01139489) are needed to confirm the reduction in antimicrobial therapy duration in patients with severe CAP. Optimal dosing of antimicrobials, based upon pharmacokinetic and pharmacodynamic parameters, may decrease duration of therapy even further. However, this needs to be confirmed by prospective studies [33].

In conclusion, the challenge is to prove which empirical combination therapy leads to improved outcomes in patients with severe CAP. New research may confirm the previous studies that suggested that severe CAP could be treated for 5 days instead of the current 10–14 days.

Adjunctive Therapies

Whereas antibiotics are the cornerstone in the treatment of pneumonia, there is still room for other supportive measures. For example, delayed assessment of oxygenation and subsequent delayed administration of oxygen increases mortality [24, 34]. Although restoration of oxygenation is self evident for the most severely ill patients with pneumonia in the ICU, it should be implemented in the ED as well. Several other adjunctive measures have been proposed and will be discussed below.

'Mechanical Options'

Intubation and mechanical ventilation come at a cost. Patients often have to be sedated and sometimes muscle relaxants are used as well. Therefore, intubation should be avoided whenever possible, leaving upper airway function intact and cough more effective. Non-invasive ventilation (NIV) is a treatment option in selected patients. Interestingly, little research has been published on NIV in pneumonia. Of course, NIV will, at least theoretically, push sputum and debris into the peripheries of the lung without the benefit of endotracheal suction provided by intubation. However, a small Italian study showed that 28 out of 64 patients with severe CAP (43 %) could be successfully treated with NIV. In this study, especially patients with a high severity of illness who failed to improve their oxygenation (PaO_2/FiO_2) while on NIV were likely to end up needing endotracheal intubation and mechanical ventilation. The down-side of this study was that the in-hospital mortality was much higher in patients (35 %) with NIV-failure [35]. Clearly, more research is needed to determine which patients are eligible for a trial of NIV.

Another mechanical measure is postural drainage. Prone positioning has been extensively analyzed and was shown to improve oxygenation and possibly survival in a subgroup of severely hypoxemic patients with acute respiratory distress syndrome (ARDS) [36]. Pneumonia is the commonest cause of ARDS, accounting for 40 % of the ARDS-cases. Because of the need to clear sputum in this condition, one would expect the greatest effect to be found in patients with severe CAP. This observation is, however, not explicitly reported in clinical trials addressing the use of prone positioning [36]. In a very small study (n = 22) in patients with severe CAP and ARDS, prone position improved oxygenation [37]. Of course, this study was not powered to assess differences in mortality. More research is needed to establish whether prone position is beneficial in selected patients with severe CAP. For now, prone positioning can be advised for severely hypoxemic patients without contraindications (e.g., intracranial hypertension) [38].

Postural drainage by rotating the entire bed has been advocated as a preventive tool for ventilator-associated pneumonia (VAP), but the high price of necessary equipment may not be justified. We found no studies that have addressed this technique in severe CAP. Simple lateral positioning is well tolerated by most patients and improves oxygenation especially in unilateral pneumonia, but research on this subject is very limited [39]. Bronchoscopy is used in many ICUs to improve oxygenation by removing debris from the lung, sometimes with spectacular improvements in oxygenation and subsequent avoidance of high peak inspiratory pressures [40]. Whether this approach is superior to postural drainage or prone positioning has never been investigated.

Severe CAP is sometimes accompanied by pleural effusions and this is associated with a worse outcome. Thoracentesis is a logical treatment leading to improved diagnostic yield and results in a change of antimicrobial therapy in 45 % of patients [41, 42]. Whether routine thoracentesis in patients with parapneumonic effusions leads to improved outcome still needs to be established.

In patients with severe CAP or ARDS who cannot be ventilated, extra-corporeal membrane oxygenation (ECMO) might be a measure which could be used as a bridge-to-recovery. In the 2009 H1N1 influenza pandemic, 71 % of the patients with ARDS survived [43]. Whether these numbers and success rates can be extrapolated to patients with severe CAP of bacterial origin is rather speculative.

Pharmacological Options

Several pharmacological options have been explored as adjunctive therapy to antibiotics in the treatment of severe CAP. In septic patients there is a delicate balance between pro-inflammatory mediators and anti-inflammatory mediators; too much inflammation might cause too much collateral damage, while too little inflammation results in decreased clearance of pathogens. Corticosteroids and other immunomodulatory drugs have been considered since 1956 to modulate inflammatory overshoot and thus reduce collateral damage. Although this has been extensively studied in patients with severe sepsis and septic shock only few studies have addressed this question in patients with severe CAP. Two systematic reviews favored the use of corticosteroids in patients with CAP; however, the quality of the included trials was questionable [44]. A recent, nicely performed, randomized trial failed to show a benefit of corticosteroids in patients with CAP [45]. In the corticosteroid-treated patient group, more patients had progression or persistence of disease, a new infiltrate or development of an extra-pulmonary infection. The authors concluded that there was no benefit from corticosteroids and possible harm. Patients with severe CAP were underrepresented in this study. Another recent and well-performed, placebo-controlled, randomized trial showed that dexamethasone was able to reduce the length of stay and improve quality of life at 30-days, but there was no statistically significant effect on in-hospital mortality [46]. Again, less than half of the patients included in this study had severe CAP (PSI class IV and V). At present, it is still undetermined whether corticosteroids are a useful adjunct in patients with severe CAP who are not in septic shock. Differences in corticosteroids (prednisolone versus dexamethasone), in patients (severe CAP on the ICU versus moderate CAP on the ward), and different timing of administration of corticosteroids (immediately in the ED or later in the ICU) may influence effectiveness and these questions still need to be answered.

N-acetylcysteine (NAC) is widely used in respiratory medicine as a mucolytic therapy, especially in patients with chronic obstructive pulmonary disease (COPD). Although it did not prevent exacerbations in COPD patients, it was not associated with many adverse effects [47]. In experimental studies, NAC has immunomodulating properties that, theoretically, would be beneficial in patients with severe CAP. However, this has never been studied in patients with severe CAP.

One cannot be surprised that some attention has been directed at the pleiotropic effects of statins and their possible beneficial effects in CAP patients. This effect was, at least partially, ascribed to the high correlation between myocardial infarction and pneumonia. In 2008, an observational study showed that patients using statins had a 54 % lower 90-day mortality than patients not using statins [48]. A recent observational cohort study in patients with CAP showed that there was no difference in severe sepsis risk between patients with or without prior statins, whether or not those statins were discontinued at admission [49]. However, these were observational studies and 'healthy user bias' seemed to play a role. Nevertheless, in the latter study in patients whose statins were stopped at admission, mortality was doubled compared to those who continued their statins (15.3 versus 7.9 %) [49]. These results still leave room to investigate whether starting a statin in patients who are not using this kind of medication would be beneficial. At present, such trials are underway for a general sepsis population but not specifically in a severe CAP population.

Several observations have revealed an association between CAP and acute myo-cardial infection [50]. Therefore, patients who are using aspirin may have a better outcome. In the previously mentioned observational study, patients using aspirin had an odds ratio for 90-day mortality of 0.63 (confidence interval 0.36 – 1.11, p = 0.11) [48]. Although this difference was not statistically significant it supports the idea that cardioprotection might be beneficial as patients with CAP are often older and have cardiovascular comorbidity [50]. However, in this cohort, co-prescription might have confounded the relationship between aspirin and mortality from CAP; many patients were using statins and aspirin at the same time. So, the relationship between severe CAP and myocardial infarction and the possible beneficial effects of aspirin in these patients is controversial, to say the least.

In a subgroup analysis (n = 850) of the original Recombinant Human Activated Protein C Worldwide Evaluation in Severe Sepsis (PROWESS) trial, investigators looked at whether activated protein C (drotecogin alfa [activated]) reduced mortality in patients with severe CAP [51]. The 90-day mortality was lower (relative risk reduction 14 %) in the patients who had received activated protein C. However, subgroup analyses may lead to wrong conclusions if the study was not intended or powered for it and we should, therefore, consider activated protein C carefully in patients with severe CAP as long as this result has not been confirmed by others.

VII

Outcome

As discussed earlier, ICU mortality or even in-hospital mortality may not be ideal markers of outcome. Approximately 25 – 50 % of patients with severe CAP die [8, 9]. What happens to the survivors after hospital discharge? Most of these patients are elderly, have comorbidities, and already have limited life expectancies. However, do survivors of severe CAP have an increased mortality rate as a result of having been severely ill? This seems very likely, but proper observational studies in patients with severe CAP are lacking. Studies in patients with moderate CAP have shown that it takes 6 – 18 months for these patients to recover in terms of quality of life [7]. However, studies addressing quality of life after severe CAP are lacking. What if certain survivors appear to have a very poor quality of life? Should we withhold intensive treatment in these patients and direct to palliative care at an earlier phase of the treatment? Timely assessment of medical futility and communication with relatives remains a challenging aspect of intensive care medicine.

Conclusion

Severe CAP is a potentially lethal disease and treatment should be immediate and adequate. Unfortunately, current severity models are too focused on a one-point evaluation. Pneumonia is a dynamic disease and patients can deteriorate after scoring has taken place. Therefore, continuous or repeated models are necessary and physicians should be aware that their patients are at risk. Admission to an intermediate or intensive care facility might be a solution [10], treating the patient with severe CAP like treating a patient with a acute coronary syndrome. Although numerous guidelines have provided us with evidence-based treatment options, many questions remain! What is the optimal combination therapy, should we add corticosteroids as an adjunct to antibiotics, does postural drainage help, and which patients benefit from salvation therapies, like ECMO? These and many other questions need to be answered in the near future to optimize the treatment of patients with severe CAP: It is no longer the old man's friend!

References

1. Feikin DR, Schuchat A, Kolczak M, et al (2000) Mortality from invasive pneumococcal pneumonia in the era of antibiotic resistance, 1995–1997. Am J Public Health 90: 223–229
2. Hoyert DL, Heron MP, Murphy SL, et al (2006) Deaths: final data for 2003. Natl Vital Stat Rep 54: 1–120
3. Brown SM, Dean NC (2010) Defining and predicting severe community-acquired pneumonia. Curr Opin Infect Dis 23: 158–164
4. Welte T, Torres A, Nathwani D (2012) Clinical and economic burden of community-acquired pneumonia among adults in Europe. Thorax 67: 71–79
5. Bauer TT, Welte T, Ernen C, et al (2005) Cost analyses of community-acquired pneumonia from the hospital perspective. Chest 128: 2238–2246
6. Angus DC, Marrie TJ, Obrosky DS, et al (2002) Severe community-acquired pneumonia: use of intensive care services and evaluation of American and British Thoracic Society Diagnostic criteria. Am J Respir Crit Care Med 166: 717–723
7. El Moussaoui R, Opmeer BC, de Borgie CA, et al (2006) Long-term symptom recovery and health-related quality of life in patients with mild-to-moderate-severe community-acquired pneumonia. Chest 130: 1165–1172
8. Rodríguez A, Mendia A, Sirvent JM, et al (2007) Combination antibiotic therapy improves survival in patients with community-acquired pneumonia and shock. Crit Care Med 35: 1493–1498
9. Woodhead M, Welch CA, Harrison DA, et al (2006) Community-acquired pneumonia on the intensive care unit: secondary analysis of 17,869 cases in the ICNARC Case Mix Programme Database. Crit Care 10 (Suppl 2): S1
10. Ewig S (2011) Gains and limitations of predictive rules for severe community-acquired pneumonia. Clin Infect Dis 53: 512–514
11. Renaud B, Santin A, Coma E, et al (2009) Association between timing of intensive care unit admission and outcomes for emergency department patients with community-acquired pneumonia. Crit Care Med 37: 2867–2874
12. Restrepo MI, Mortensen EM, Rello J, et al (2010) Late admission to the ICU in patients with community-acquired pneumonia is associated with higher mortality. Chest 137: 552–557.
13. Marrie TJ, Shariatzadeh MR (2007) Community-acquired pneumonia requiring admission to an intensive care unit: a descriptive study. Medicine (Baltimore) 86: 103–111
14. Chalmers JD, Taylor JK, Mandal P, et al (2011) Validation of the Infectious Diseases Society Of America/American Thoracic Society minor criteria for intensive care unit admission in community-acquired pneumonia patients without major criteria or contraindications to intensive care unit care. Clin Infect Dis 53: 503–511
15. Charles PG, Wolfe R, Whitby M, et al (2008) SMART-COP: a tool for predicting the need for intensive respiratory or vasopressor support in community-acquired pneumonia. Clin Infect Dis 47: 375–384
16. Ewig S, Woodhead M, Torres A (2011) Towards a sensible comprehension of severe community-acquired pneumonia. Intensive Care Med 37: 214–223
17. Mulrennan S, Tempone SS, Ling IT, et al (2010) Pandemic influenza (H1N1) 2009 pneumonia: CURB-65 score for predicting severity and nasopharyngeal sampling for diagnosis are unreliable. PLoS One 5: e12849
18. Bloos F, Marshall JC, Dellinger RP, et al (2011) Multinational, observational study of procalcitonin in ICU patients with pneumonia requiring mechanical ventilation: a multicenter observational study. Crit Care 15: R88
19. Barlow G, Nathwani D, Davey P (2007) The CURB65 pneumonia severity score outper-

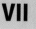

forms generic sepsis and early warning scores in predicting mortality in community-acquired pneumonia. Thorax 62: 253–259

20. Mandell LA, Wunderink RG, Anzueto A, et al (2007) Infectious Diseases Society of America/American Thoracic Society consensus guidelines on the management of community-acquired pneumonia in adults. Clin Infect Dis 44 (Suppl 2): S27–S72

21. Woodhead M, Blasi F, Ewig S, et al (2005) Guidelines for the management of adult lower respiratory tract infections. Eur Respir J 26: 1138–1180

22. Martin-Loeches I, Lisboa T, Rodriguez A, et al (2010) Combination antibiotic therapy with macrolides improves survival in intubated patients with community-acquired pneumonia. Intensive Care Med 36: 612–620

23. Martínez R, Reyes S, Lorenzo MJ, et al (2009) Impact of guidelines on outcome: the evidence. Semin Respir Crit Care Med 30: 172–178

24. Menéndez R, Torres A, Reyes S, et al (2012) Initial management of pneumonia and sepsis. Factors associated with improved outcome. Eur Respir J 39: 156–162

25. Vardakas KZ, Siempos II, Grammatikos A, et al (2008) Respiratory fluoroquinolones for the treatment of community-acquired pneumonia: a meta-analysis of randomized controlled trials. CMAJ 179: 1269–1277

26. Dellinger RP, Levy MM, Carlet JM, et al (2008) Surviving Sepsis Campaign: international guidelines for management of severe sepsis and septic shock: 2008. Crit Care Med 36: 296–327

27. Kumar A, Ellis P, Arabi Y, et al (2009) Initiation of inappropriate antimicrobial therapy results in a fivefold reduction of survival in human septic shock. Chest 136: 1237–1248

28. Bruns AH, Oosterheert JJ, Hustinx WN, et al (2009) Time for first antibiotic dose is not predictive for the early clinical failure of moderate-severe community-acquired pneumonia. Eur J Clin Microbiol Infect Dis 28: 913–919

29. Pines JM, Isserman JA, Hinfey PB (2009) The measurement of time to first antibiotic dose for pneumonia in the emergency department: a white paper and position statement prepared for the American Academy of Emergency Medicine. J Emerg Med 37: 335–340

30. Aliberti S, Blasi F, Zanaboni AM, et al (2010) Duration of antibiotic therapy in hospitalised patients with community-acquired pneumonia. Eur Respir J 36: 128–134

31. Schuetz P, Christ-Crain M, Thomann R, et al (2009) Effect of procalcitonin-based guidelines vs standard guidelines on antibiotic use in lower respiratory tract infections: the ProHOSP randomized controlled trial. JAMA 302: 1059–1066

32. Bouadma L, Luyt CE, Tubach F, et al (2010) Use of procalcitonin to reduce patients' exposure to antibiotics in intensive care units (PRORATA trial): a multicentre randomised controlled trial. Lancet 375: 463–474

33. Ambrose PG (2008) Use of pharmacokinetics and pharmacodynamics in a failure analysis of community-acquired pneumonia: implications for future clinical trial study design. Clin Infect Dis 47 (Suppl 3): S225-S231

34. Blot SI, Rodriguez A, Solé-Violán J, et al (2007) Effects of delayed oxygenation assessment on time to antibiotic delivery and mortality in patients with severe community-acquired pneumonia. Crit Care Med 35: 2509–2514

35. Carron M, Freo U, Zorzi M, et al (2010) Predictors of failure of noninvasive ventilation in patients with severe community-acquired pneumonia. J Crit Care 25: 540.e9–14

36. Gattinoni L, Carlesso E, Taccone P, et al (2010) Prone positioning improves survival in severe ARDS: a pathophysiologic review and individual patient meta-analysis. Minerva Anestesiol 76: 448–454

37. Chan MC, Hsu JY, Liu HH, et al (2007) Effects of prone position on inflammatory markers in patients with ARDS due to community-acquired pneumonia. J Formos Med Assoc 106: 708–716

38. Guerin C, Gaillard S, Lemasson S, et al (2004) Effects of systematic prone positioning in hypoxemic acute respiratory failure: a randomized controlled trial. JAMA 292: 2379–2387

39. Thomas PJ, Paratz JD (2007) Is there evidence to support the use of lateral positioning in intensive care? A systematic review. Anaesth Intensive Care 35: 239–255

40. Marquette CH, Wermert D, Wallet F, et al (1997) [Fibroscopic bronchoscopy in intensive care]. Rev Mal Respir 14: 101–111

41. Fartoukh M, Azoulay E, Galliot R, et al (2002) Clinically documented pleural effusions in medical ICU patients: how useful is routine thoracentesis? Chest 121: 178–184

VII

42. Tu CY, Hsu WH, Hsia TC, et al (2006) The changing pathogens of complicated parapneumonic effusions or empyemas in a medical intensive care unit. Intensive Care Med 32: 570–576
43. The Australia and New Zealand Extracorporeal Membrane Oxygenation (ANZ ECMO) Influenza Investigators (2009) Extracorporeal Membrane Oxygenation for 2009 Influenza A(H1N1) Acute Respiratory Distress Syndrome. JAMA 302: 1888–1895
44. Meduri GU, Rocco PR, Annane D, et al (2010) Prolonged glucocorticoid treatment and secondary prevention in acute respiratory distress syndrome. Expert Rev Respir Med 4: 201–210
45. Snijders D, Daniels JM, de Graaff CS, et al (2010) Efficacy of corticosteroids in community-acquired pneumonia: a randomized double-blinded clinical trial. Am J Respir Crit Care Med 181: 975–982
46. Meijvis SC, Hardeman H, Remmelts HH, et al (2011) Dexamethasone and length of hospital stay in patients with community-acquired pneumonia: a randomised, double-blind, placebo-controlled trial. Lancet 377: 2023–2030
47. Black PN, Morgan-Day A, McMillan TE, et al (2004) Randomised, controlled trial of N-acetylcysteine for treatment of acute exacerbations of chronic obstructive pulmonary disease [ISRCTN21676344]. BMC Pulm Med 4: 13
48. Chalmers JD, Singanayagam A, Murray MP, et al (2008) Prior statin use is associated with improved outcomes in community-acquired pneumonia. Am J Med 121: 1002–1007
49. Yende S, Milbrandt EB, Kellum JA, et al (2011) Understanding the potential role of statins in pneumonia and sepsis. Crit Care Med 39: 1871–1878
50. Pham JC, Kelen GD, Pronovost PJ (2007) National study on the quality of emergency department care in the treatment of acute myocardial infarction and pneumonia. Acad Emerg Med 14: 856–863
51. Laterre PF, Garber G, Levy H, et al (2005) Severe community-acquired pneumonia as a cause of severe sepsis: data from the PROWESS study. Crit Care Med 33: 952–961

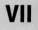

Empiric Therapy of Gram-positive Bloodstream Infections and Pneumonia

M. Bassetti and G. Villa

Introduction

Intensive care units (ICUs) represent high-risk areas for nosocomial infections. One third of hospital-acquired infections are related to the ICU, where a patient has a 5- to 7-fold greater risk of nosocomial infection compared to another hospitalized in a different ward [1]. Gram-positive organisms play an important part in this setting, being a leading cause of morbidity and mortality in ICUs [2]; moreover, several reports have shown an increase in antimicrobial resistance for these isolates in recent years [3].

In this context, methicillin-resistant *Staphylococcus aureus* (MRSA) is a concern [4]; although vancomycin became the drug of choice for its treatment and is still widely used, many studies suggest that when vancomycin minimum inhibitory concentration (MIC) values are at the end of the susceptibility range, it is less effective [5, 6]. Inappropriate antibiotic therapy has been found to be an important determinant of mortality in this setting [7].

The aim of this chapter is to focus attention on Gram-positive infections in ICUs and on new therapeutic approaches for them. Bloodstream infections and pneumonia will be discussed in greater detail, since they represent, in terms of frequency and mortality, high-challenge infectious conditions.

Bloodstream Infections

General Epidemiology

Bloodstream infections (BSIs) represent one of the leading causes of death in the Western World. In hospitalized patients, BSIs are responsible for approximately 150,000 deaths in Europe annually and 210,000 in the United States [8], and typically occur in ICUs. In this setting, crude mortality related to hospital-acquired BSIs ranges from 20 % to 60 %, whereas mortality directly attributable to the BSI ranges from 14 % to 38 % [9]. Furthermore, BSIs are responsible for prolonged hospital stays with greater costs.

The Surveillance and Control of Pathogens of Epidemiologic Importance (SCOPE) study analyzed 24179 nosocomial BSIs in 49 hospitals of various sizes distributed widely across the USA from 1995 through 2002. From this analysis, it emerged that 50.5 % of BSIs occurred in ICUs, and the overall crude mortality rate was 27 %. From a microbiological point of view, of the 20978 monomicrobial BSIs, 65 % were caused by Gram-positive bacteria. Coagulase-negative staphylococci and *S. aureus* were the most commonly isolated organisms both in the ICU

J.-L. Vincent (ed.), *Annual Update in Intensive Care and Emergency Medicine 2012*
DOI 10.1007/978-3-642-25716-2 © Springer-Verlag Berlin Heidelberg 2012

and in non-ICU ward settings, followed by *Enterococcus* spp. [2]. Moreover, this analysis is concordant with other studies that demonstrate how antibiotic resistance has increased over this period of time, with MRSA still playing a major role.

The OASIS multicenter study (In vitrO prospective research on Antimicrobial Susceptibility on Invasive pathogenS) is another, more recent example of a similar analysis. The study was designed to assess the prevalence of bacteria and fungi from blood cultures and the *in vitro* antimicrobial susceptibility; it involved 20 hospital microbiology laboratories located in Northern and Central Italy and investigated blood cultures collected over a 1-year period. This study showed that 67.2 % of the 29481 positive blood cultures represented hospital-acquired BSIs, of which 44 % were due to Gram-positive organisms. Resistance to methicillin was found in 35.8 % of *S. aureus* isolates, whereas vancomycin resistance was found in 4.0 % of *Enterococcus faecalis* and 18.9 % of *Enterococcus faecium* [10].

The results of the OASIS study are concordant with other scientific evidence showing that in recent years Gram-negative organisms have become more common than Gram-positive organisms among blood isolates [11], although more so for community-acquired cases than for hospital-acquired ones. This observation may be due, according to some authors, to the appropriate use of glycopeptides and the recent availability of new drugs for Gram-positive organisms [12], although this is still debated (see below). These two approaches may have had an effective role in controlling infections that are common sources of BSIs, such as low respiratory tract infections, skin and soft tissues infections and infections of intravascular catheters. The high prevalence of elderly individuals in this study population could have also played an important part in determining this epidemiology, since urinary tract infections, frequently caused by enterobacteria, are more common in this subset of patients. Furthermore, greater attention has been given to new guidelines for the correct management of intravascular catheters and their infection, with a focus on the correct use of glycopeptides. From the OASIS study, in terms of species isolated in the ICU setting, *Escherichia coli, S. aureus, Staphylococcus epidermidis* and *Pseudomonas aeruginosa* were the most prevalent [10].

Another study conducted in Canada showed similar results: Of the 8228 positive blood cultures, 51.1 % isolated Gram-positive organisms [13]. *E. coli* and *S. aureus* were the most common pathogens and were responsible for more than 40 % of the bloodstream infections. As far as Gram-positive organisms are concerned, 24.4 % of the *S. aureus* isolated from blood cultures were MRSA, the incidence of which remained constant through the three-year period. Of the 356 MRSA isolates, five had a vancomycin MIC of 2 µg/ml and one had a vancomycin MIC of 4 µg/ml, whereas no resistance was demonstrated for linezolid or for daptomycin. Of the *E. faecalis* and *E. faecium* isolates, 4.6 % were vancomycin resistant, and no resistance to linezolid or daptomycin was observed. During this three-year period, nonetheless, the rate of vancomycin-resistant enterococcus (VRE) increased. In this analysis, patients were stratified according to age group; among the younger ages, there was a predominance of coagulase-negative staphylococci, as previously noted [14], whereas MRSA and *P. aeruginosa* were important causes of bloodstream infections in the adults and the elderly.

VII

Antimicrobial Resistance and the Role of Vancomycin

Recent years have witnessed a rise in the incidence of multi-drug resistance in Gram-positive bacteria causing infections in critically ill patients, and this is particularly evident if one considers the role that MRSA has in this setting [4]. Some evidence indicates that MRSA BSIs are associated with a poorer outcome compared to methicillin-susceptible *S. aureus* BSIs [15]. In Italy, the prevalence of MRSA in ICUs ranges from 50 % to 70 % [16]; this high prevalence of MRSA infection has led to a progressive increase in the use of vancomycin in empirical regimens, a phenomenon that is observed worldwide, and strains with higher MICs have become more common.

The efficacy of vancomycin in the treatment of MRSA infection is directly related to the MIC of the pathogen, even within the range of susceptibility: Therapies with vancomycin for pathogens whose MICs are between 1 and 2 µg/ml have a significantly poorer response compared to those with MICs less than 0.5 µg/ml, and have higher mortality rates [17]. The duration of bacteremia in cases of MRSA BSI with higher MICs is usually longer, and these patients have a higher likelihood of recurrence and a longer hospital stay. A recent analysis of the evolutionary trend among *S. aureus* clinical isolates demonstrated a tendency toward increasing vancomycin MICs in Italy [18] (**Fig. 1**). Because existing findings indicate that the probability of therapy failure is higher for invasive MRSA infections caused by strains with an increased vancomycin MIC [19], and because a 'creep phenomenon' appears to exist in several regions, we suggest that every medical center should examine the local situation of vancomycin MICs in MRSA isolates from blood cultures using Etest. Furthermore, if vancomycin MIC creep is observed in MRSA strains in the patient population of any medical center, the center's decision-makers should include in their discussions the appropriate therapy and the main risk factors associated with patient acquisition of MRSA with elevated vancomycin MICs.

These effects can be explained in terms of the pharmacodynamics of the drug, the efficacy of vancomycin being related to the ratio between the area under the concentration-time curve (AUC) and the MIC; therefore, suboptimal drug concentrations may trigger the development of resistance, such as MIC values as high as 1, by being able to increase this ratio. To improve the AUC/MIC ratio, higher serum trough concentrations of vancomycin should be used, but this is associated

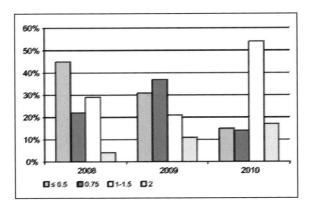

Fig. 1. Minimum inhibitory concentration (MIC) distribution among MRSA bloodstream isolates in the period (2008–2010) in Italy. Data from [18]

with greater renal dysfunction. Regarding this concern, Jeffres at al. studied 94 patients with healthcare-associated pneumonia (HCAP) in order to evaluate the relationship between aggressive vancomycin dosing and nephrotoxicity, demonstrating in this different setting that patients with higher steady-state mean trough serum vancomycin concentrations (20.8 mg/l vs. 14.3 mg/l, $p < 0.001$) had a higher incidence of nephrotoxicity [20]. These authors also demonstrated that longer duration of treatment was associated with a higher risk of renal dysfunction.

On the use of vancomycin in this setting, some authors have postulated that the shift in vancomycin MIC values is associated with a concurrent increase in the MIC values of other anti-MRSA agents. To date, analyses have primarily focused on the correlation between daptomycin and vancomycin. Patel et al. conducted a study in which they examined the correlation between vancomycin MIC values and the MIC values of daptomycin, linezolid, tigecycline and teicoplanin among 120 patients with BSIs in a tertiary care hospital in the USA between January 2005 and May 2007 [21]. Collectively, these authors showed how MIC values increased under the selective pressure of vancomycin in a pool of patients in whom MRSA was isolated from blood cultures on day 1 and subsequently after treatment with vancomycin was initiated. They demonstrated that the MIC values of all the antibiotics under study increased in parallel, in a fashion similar to that demonstrated by Watanabe et al. for linezolid and vancomycin with infections caused by vancomycin-intermediate *S. aureus* (VISA) [22]. Based on all these considerations, alternatives to vancomycin should be considered for critically ill patients in whom an anti-MRSA agent has to be initiated as empirical treatment, or when the MRSA MIC is ≥ 1 µg/ml, in order to avoid an inadequate AUC/MIC ratio and to prevent the phenomenon of MIC 'creep', already described for daptomycin and vancomycin, but possible for other anti-MRSA agents as well.

Another problem that concerns ICUs is the emergence of infections due to *Enterococcus* spp. with limited or full resistance to vancomycin. In the US, the proportion of VRE is high (20 % for *E. faecalis* and 60 % for *E. faecium*) [2], whereas in Italy it is still significantly lower (6 %). As demonstrated for MRSA, it seems that mortality rates in patients with VRE infections is significantly higher than for infections caused by vancomycin-susceptible enterococci (VSE) [23].

The increasing antimicrobial resistance in Gram-positive organisms therefore remains an issue of vital importance, given the decreasing role that vancomycin has in this subset of patients, especially in the ICU setting. New classes of antimicrobial have been developed, and their rational use may help clinicians to make the best empirical choices.

New Approaches to Antimicrobial Therapy: The Role of Daptomycin and Linezolid

When treating a BSI, one should opt for a bactericidal agent with rapid activity, good penetration into the biofilm, an easy mode of administration, a good safety profile and similar microbiological activity against different strains of methicillin-sensitive *S. aureus* (MSSA), MRSA, heteroresistant VISA (hVISA) and VRE [4] (Table 1).

Approved by the FDA for the treatment of MRSA skin and soft tissue infections (SSTIs), bacteremia and right-sided endocarditis, daptomycin, a cyclic lipopeptide antibiotic, is a bactericidal antimicrobial agent that exerts its mechanism of action by creating pores or ion channels into the bacterial cell membrane and

VII

Table 1. Characteristics of new drugs used for empiric therapy in Gram-positive bloodstream infections. Adapted from [4]

Characteristics	Vancomycin	Linezolid	Tigecycline	Daptomycin
Bactericidal activity against MRSA	Yes, but slow	No	No	Yes
Biofilm activity	No	No	No	Yes
Microbiology activity and same eradication rate against MSSA, MRSA, hVISA and VRE	No	Yes	Yes	Yes
Proven efficacy for primary Gram + bacteraemia	Yes	No	No	Yes
Optimal dosage	No	Yes	Yes	Yes
Mode of administration	i.v.	Oral and i.v.	i.v.	i.v.
Good safety profile	No, especially for higher dosage	Yes, rarely causes thrombocytopenia and myelosuppression	Yes, some gastro-intestinal effects	Yes
Resistance described	Yes	Yes, but uncommon	Yes	Yes

MRSA: methicillin-resistant *Staphylococcus aureus*; MSSA: methicillin-sensitive *S. aureus*; VRE: vancomycin-resistant enterococcus; hVISA: heteroresistant vancomycin-intermediate *S. aureus*; i.v.: intravenous

thus causing membrane depolarization and rapid cell death [24]. The antimicrobial spectrum of daptomycin includes the majority of Gram-positive organisms [25]; moreover, this drug possesses great *in vitro* bactericidal activity and synergy with a number of other antibiotics, and is effective also for biofilm producing strains [26]. Daptomycin has a concentration-dependent bactericidal activity, and may sometimes require levels equivalent to eight times the lipopeptide MIC for a given strain [27].

The FDA approved 4 mg/kg of daptomycin for the treatment of complicated SSTIs, and 6 mg/kg for *S. aureus* BSI, including treatment of right-side endocarditis. Although prospective randomized trials claimed that these dosage regimens are safe and effective for their respective indications [28, 29], optimal dose levels still need to be established.

In vitro studies of simulated endocardial vegetations with susceptible and non-susceptible strains of *S. aureus* treated with simulated daptomycin doses of 6 mg/ kg and 10 mg/kg in combination with gentamicin and rifampin have demonstrated rapid bactericidal activity of all doses against susceptible *S. aureus*. Nonetheless, this study demonstrated an increased rate of killing at the higher dose, improved activity with combination therapy against a majority of drug-susceptible strains, and improved activity even against some of the non-susceptible strains [30]. Despite its recent advent in the pharmacological armamentarium, reports on clinical failure and on the emergence of resistance to daptomycin have been raising concerns; these reports have been related to several *S. aureus* and *Enterococcus* spp. strains, and reported either in severely ill patients who had been pre-treated with other antibiotics or during daptomycin treatment at an inappropriate dose [31].

Regimens with higher doses of daptomycin have been proposed to treat difficult infections, such as complicated bacteremia and endocarditis. This approach may be particularly important in the ICU setting, where, aside from the known difficulties with antimicrobial resistance and in-tissue activity of the antimicrobial, clinicians deal with critically ill patients. Pharmacokinetic data from healthy individuals show that daptomycin dosed once daily at 12 mg/kg achieved trough levels of about 20 μg/ml, a level that better guarantees an optimal tissue concentration for organisms with higher MICs [32]. On the basis of the pharmacokinetic profile and concentration-dependent killing, higher doses may be beneficial in treating severe infections as well. Clinical experience with doses greater than 6 mg/kg are limited, but recent studies support the theory that higher doses of daptomycin are more effective and have an adequate safety profile [33, 34].

Linezolid, discussion of which will be developed later, is an alternative, in some circumstances, for the treatment of MRSA infections, since it possesses a good microbiological profile against MSSA, MRSA, hVISA and VRE. Despite its bacteriostatic mechanism of action, there are some reports of clinical and microbiological efficacy for MRSA bacteremia and endocarditis [35, 36]. A recent study showed that linezolid should not be used for the empirical treatment of catheter-related BSIs before isolation and identification of a pathogenic organism, but could be used, depending on the circumstance, once isolates have been identified [35]. A meta-analysis of 144 patients with MRSA bacteremia from five studies that compared vancomycin with linezolid showed no statistical differences in the rate of clinical cure [37]. In this setting, linezolid may play a role in sequential therapy, such as when bacteremia is already resolved and the patient needs to complete a therapeutic cycle at home with oral antibiotics.

VII

Pneumonia

Pneumonia is a common infection in communities and health-care facilities, with mortality rates as high as 76 % reported in some circumstances in ventilated patients [38, 39]. Categories of pneumonia include community-acquired pneumonia (CAP) and nosocomial pneumonia, the latter encompassing HCAP, hospital-acquired pneumonia (HAP), and ventilator-associated pneumonia (VAP) [38].

A distinction can also be made between early-onset and late-onset nosocomial pneumonia, with late-onset infections ($\geq$ 5 days of current hospitalization) more likely to be caused by multi-drug resistant (MDR) pathogens [38]. Additional risk factors for infection with MDR pathogens are antimicrobial therapy in the previous 90 days, current hospitalization of at least 5 days, high frequency of antibiotic resistance in the community or hospital unit, presence of risk factors for HCAP, and immunosuppressive disease and/or therapy [38].

HAP is the second most common nosocomial infection (after urinary tract infection) and the most common nosocomial infection acquired in the ICU [40]. VAP has an estimated incidence of 8 – 28 % [39], and is associated with a prolonged ICU stay, and increased costs and attributable mortality [41]. Etiologic diagnosis of VAP is difficult, and the results of culture and sensitivity testing are often obtained days after the collection of the samples [39]. On the other hand, prompt administration of empirical therapy is essential, since it has been demonstrated that lack of an appropriate antimicrobial therapy from the onset of symptoms is an independent determinant of mortality in patients with VAP [42]. Similar results have been obtained for *S. aureus* respiratory [43] and bloodstream infections [44], as seen above. Kollef et al. [42] demonstrated by multiple logistic regression analysis that inappropriate antimicrobial therapy was independently associated with prior administration of antibiotics (thought to result in subsequent infection with drug-resistant pathogens) in ICU patients. Furthermore, this same study demonstrated that patients infected with MRSA were more likely to receive inappropriate antimicrobial therapy [42].

Initial treatment for VAP should be started right after diagnostic specimens are obtained, even though the optimal antimicrobial agent(s) remains unclear. The timing of the episode, the local ecology of isolates, severity of the illness and previous antibiotic exposure all influence the choice of antibiotic, and recommendations for the treatment of VAP should be flexible enough to allow for all possible different scenarios [38]. The treatment of early VAP is a simpler task, since etiologic agents are usually acquired from the community environment (*Haemophilus influenzae*, *Streptococcus pneumoniae* and MSSA), whereas late VAP or VAP in a patient previously exposed to antibiotic therapy represents a more serious challenge, since these conditions are more likely caused by MDR pathogens, such as MRSA, *P. aeruginosa* or *Acinetobacter* spp. [45].

VII

According to a consensus document written by the GISIG Working Group on Hospital-Associated Pneumonia [46], initial selection of the antimicrobial regimen should be influenced by the local microbial ecology; in populations of patients at low risk of MDR (including MRSA) or difficult-to-treat pathogens, therapy with a single antibiotic may be adequate, whereas patients with HAP at risk of MRSA should receive combination therapy that includes an anti-MRSA agent, such as linezolid or a glycopeptide, which should be adapted later based on culture results. In this setting, the use of pharmacodynamic and pharmacokinetic parameters is recommended, at least for critically ill patients. In this context, the vancomycin target should be a trough serum concentration that allows an AUC/MIC of ≥ 400; since the ratio is unlikely to be reached for MIC > 1 mg/l, for infections caused by isolates of MRSA with this MIC or higher, another agent should be used. Finally, use of a de-escalation strategy in the antimicrobial treatment of HAP based on an institutional protocol that incorporates local resistance patterns is recommended; following initiation of an empirical broad-spectrum antibiotic therapy based on patient risk factors and clinical presentation, therapy is tailored to the specific pathogen once culture results are available, by changing to a narrower spectrum treatment, or antibiotics are stopped if the diagnosis of HAP is not confirmed. Duration of therapy should not be longer than 8 days in patients with a confirmed microbial etiology (≥ 14 days for *P. aeruginosa* and *A. baumannii*) [46].

Antimicrobial Agents and Pneumonia in the ICU: A Focus on MRSA

S. aureus is a major cause of HCAP, HAP and VAP, and increasingly CAP in some countries, especially in the USA [47]. *S. aureus* is uniquely problematic due to its ubiquity, expression of virulence factors and high frequency of resistance to many antimicrobial agents. It was the only pathogen that correlated with mortality in a multiple logistic regression analysis carried out in a large retrospective cohort study of inpatients with culture-positive pneumonia in the USA [48]. MRSA is growing in prevalence and is now endemic in many healthcare facilities and communities.

Among the characteristics that an antimicrobial has to have in order to effectively treat nosocomial pneumonia in the ICU, some are of particular importance: They should be effective against the most common etiologic agents, including MDR pathogens, such as MRSA; bactericidal activity is preferable in order to obtain more rapid resolution of serious infections; they should have good penetration into the site of infection thus reaching microbiologically active concentrations in the lung; and should not be inactivated by pulmonary surfactant, as occurs with daptomycin. Low nephrotoxicity is also important; many patients with MRSA pneumonia are critically ill in the ICU with multiple organ dysfunction [49]. Only vancomycin and linezolid are currently approved in the USA for the treatment of MRSA pneumonia. In some European countries, teicoplanin and quinupristin/dalfopristin (Q/D) are available in addition to vancomycin and linezolid for this indication [43]. In spring 2011, the European Medicines Agency (EMA) approved telavancin for second line treatment of HAP. Telavancin is particularly promising because of its rapid concentration-dependent bactericidal activity against *S. aureus*, its good penetration into human epithelial lining fluid and alveolar macrophages [50], and a low potential for resistance development [51].

Vancomycin, a glycopeptide with a slow bactericidal activity, exerts its killing by disrupting cell wall synthesis in Gram-positive organisms by interfering with peptidoglycan biosynthesis. Vancomycin is less effective than ß-lactams in the treatment of pneumonia caused by MSSA, and penetrates poorly into the lung at therapeutic doses. Theoretically, vancomycin can be combined with rifampin, fusidic acid and fosfomycin for the treatment of MRSA pneumonia, but data from randomized control trials (RCTs) are lacking. A South Korean study showed that when combined with rifampin, vancomycin was more effective in the treatment of MRSA nosocomial pneumonia than when used alone, but more clinical data are required to assess whether such therapy has clinical utility [52].

Although it remains the treatment of choice, the comments already made regarding the efficacy of vancomycin for isolates with a MIC > 1 mg/l can also be applied for nosocomial pneumonia. Moreover, the same considerations can be made concerning its nephrotoxicity, and its frequent combination with other nephrotoxic agents, such as aminoglycosides. In the treatment of pneumonia, vancomycin is frequently combined with ß-lactam antimicrobials. In 2002, a class of MRSA strains that developed vancomycin resistance in the presence of ß-lactam antibiotics (β-lactam-induced vancomycin-resistant methicillin-resistant *S. aureus* [BIVR]) was reported in Japan [53]. Although defined phenotypically, the mechanism of this acquired resistance is not yet understood. Up to 20 % of MRSA strains in a further Japanese study exhibited the BIVR phenotype [54].

Linezolid is a synthetic oxazolidinone that prevents binding of the 30S and 50S ribosomal subunits, thus inhibiting the initiation of protein synthesis. It has a bacteriostatic activity against Gram-positive organisms and limited activity against Gram-negative bacteria. Two retrospective subgroup analyses of ventilated and non-ventilated patients with MRSA [55, 56] from nosocomial pneumonia clinical trials [57, 58] showed that linezolid-treated patients had higher survival rates than vancomycin-treated patients. It has been suggested that this may be due to the favorable intrapulmonary distribution of linezolid [59]. However, the viability and validity of these subset analyses has been questioned [60]. A trial of patients with MRSA VAP failed to show statistical superiority of linezolid over vancomycin, although linezolid-treated patients had numerically better values compared with vancomycin-treated patients with respect to microbiological

VII

eradication (66.7 % vs. 52.9 %, respectively), survival rate (86.7 % and 70.0 %, respectively), length of hospitalization (18.8 days and 20.1 days, respectively), duration of ventilation (10.4 days and 14.3 days, respectively), and length of ICU stay (12.2 and 16.2 days, respectively) [61]. A very recent trial, called Zephyr, of patients with proven MRSA pneumonia (HAP, HCAP and VAP) showed that linezolid achieved a statistically significantly higher clinical success rate compared to vancomycin at the end of the study in the per-protocol population. Similar results were observed for clinical and microbiological response at end of study and end of therapy in both per-protocol and modified intention to treat populations [62]

There are some reports of S. aureus and S. epidermidis strains that are resistant to linezolid. In a recent genetic study, linezolid resistance emerged in multiple clones [63], a similar phenomenon to that observed for E. faecium in patients with prosthetic devices who are receiving extended antibiotic therapy [64]. Among the adverse reactions to linezolid, thrombocytopenia is the most common [65], but others related to the inhibition of mitochondrial protein synthesis have been observed, such as optic and peripheral neuropathy and lactic acidosis. These effects are usually reversible after discontinuation of the drug, but permanent effects have been reported, like blindness [66]. In combination with serotonergic agents, linezolid has been associated with serotonin syndrome, due to its reversible, non-selective monoamine oxidase inhibitory action.

Teicoplanin is another glycopeptide with bactericidal activity against Gram-positive organisms; for the treatment of pneumonia and other Gram-positive infections, linezolid was shown to be superior [67], and equally effective in the critically ill. A retrospective analysis comparing the two drugs also showed clinical superiority of linezolid over teicoplanin, with numerically better response to therapy (although not statistically significant) for S. aureus [68]. Penetration into lung tissue has been demonstrated to be better for teicoplanin than for vancomycin, although still suboptimal, and, therefore, high doses of teicoplanin are required to treat VAP. Resistance patterns follow those of vancomycin, since they share a common target in the bacterial cell wall. Compared with vancomycin, teicoplanin is less nephrotoxic and causes fewer adverse reactions dependent on the release of histamine, such as the red-man syndrome. However, thrombocytopenia is more common, especially when administered at higher doses.

Q/D consists of two streptogramin components that inhibit different stages of protein synthesis. It is active against Gram-negative and Gram-positive organisms, including MRSA, and in some European countries it is licensed for the treatment of MRSA pneumonia. The American Thoracic Society/Infectious Diseases Society Of America (ATS/IDSA) guidelines do not recommend its use because of its inferiority compared to vancomycin for clinical cure of MRSA pneumonia [38].

Tigecycline is a semisynthetic glycylcycline with antimicrobial activity against a broad range of Gram-positive, Gram-negative and anaerobic species, with the exclusion of P. aeruginosa and P. mirabilis. It is a bacteriostatic agent that, like tetracyclines, inhibits protein synthesis. It is approved in the USA and in some European countries for the treatment of complicated SSTIs and complicated intra-abdominal infections, as well as for the treatment of CAP in the USA. Pharmacodynamic and pharmacokinetic studies in humans indicate that it has a good penetration into alveolar cells, but achieves only low levels in epithelial lining fluid [69]. There is some evidence on the use of tigecycline for VAP and/or bacteremia caused by Gram-negative organisms, such as A. baumannii, but development of resistance to tigecycline has been observed in this setting [70].

VII

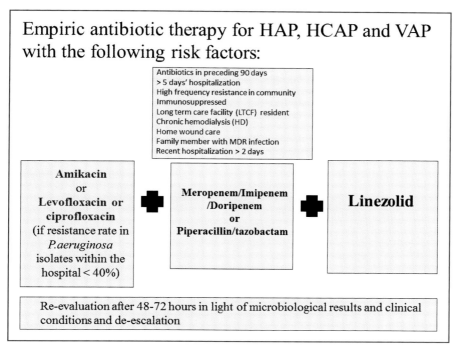

Fig. 2. Empiric antibiotic therapy for nosocomial pneumonia. HAP: hospital-acquired pneumonia; HCAP: healthcare-associated pneumonia; VAP: ventilator-associated pneumonia; MDR: multidrug resistant

At present, it is difficult to establish whether new agents are superior to vancomycin; however, in HAP and VAP linezolid seems better and demonstrated superiority in one RCT study. We believe there are concerns about the future utility of glycopeptides as a first line agent in the empirical treatment of MRSA pneumonia and, therefore, suggest a new antibiotic scheme for nosocomial pneumonia (**Fig. 2**).

Conclusion

Gram-positive infections in the ICU continue to present a challenge for clinicians. In addition to the associated medical conditions in critically ill patients, in recent years the increasing risk of antimicrobial resistance among Gram-positive pathogens has raised additional concerns. New antibiotics have been developed to furnish the pharmaceutical armamentarium, but judicious use is mandatory to avoid the emergence of new resistance. Daptomycin is a highly active agent against bloodstream infections, and should be used in all critical conditions when one suspects a poor response to vancomycin, such as for isolates with MIC > 1 mg/l. For nosocomial pneumonia and VAP, linezolid has exhibited better performance than vancomycin with regard clinical efficacy and pathogen eradication, and is a valid choice for empiric therapy.

References

1. Chen YY, Wang FD, Liu CY, Chou P (2009) Incidence rate and variable cost of nosocomial infections in different types of intensive care units. Infect Control Hosp Epidemiol 30: 39–46
2. Wisplinghoff H, Bischoff T, Tallent SM, Seifert H, Wenzel RP, Edmond MB (2004) Nosocomial bloodstream infections in US hospitals: analysis of 24,179 cases from a prospective nationwide surveillance study. Clin Infect Dis 39: 309–317
3. Wise R (2003) Introduction: treatment of Gram-positive infections. J Antimicrob Chemother 51 (Suppl 2): ii5–ii7
4. Bassetti M, Ginocchio F, Giacobbe DR (2011) New approaches for empiric therapy in Gram-positive sepsis. Minerva Anestesiol 77: 821–827
5. Sakoulas G, Moellering RC, Eliopoulos GM (2006) Adaptation of methicillin-resistant Staphylococcus aureus in the face of vancomycin therapy. Clin Infect Dis 42 (Suppl 1): S40–S50
6. Moise PA, Sakoulas G, Forrest A, Schentag JJ (2007) Vancomycin in vitro bactericidal activity and its relationship to efficacy in clearance of methicillin-resistant Staphylococcus aureus bacteremia. Antimicrob Agents Chemother 51: 2582–2586
7. Rodríguez-Baño J, Millán AB, Domínguez MA, et al (2009) Impact of inappropriate empirical therapy for sepsis due to health care-associated methicillin-resistant Staphylococcus aureus. J Infect 58: 131–137
8. Moreno R, Afonso S, Fevereiro T (2006) Incidence of sepsis in hospitalized patients. Curr Infect Dis Rep 8: 346–350
9. Vallés J, Ferrer R (2009) Bloodstream infection in the ICU. Infect Dis Clin North Am 23: 557–569
10. Luzzaro F, Ortisi G, Larosa M, Drago M, Brigante G, Gesu G (2011) Prevalence and epidemiology of microbial pathogens causing bloodstream infections: results of the OASIS multicenter study. Diagn Microbiol Infect Dis 69: 363–369
11. Albrecht SJ, Fishman NO, Kitchen J, et al (2006) Reemergence of gram-negative health care-associated bloodstream infections. Arch Intern Med 166: 1289–1294
12. Vergidis PI, Falagas ME (2008) New antibiotic agents for bloodstream infections. Int J Antimicrob Agents 32 (Suppl 1): S60-S65
13. Adam HJ, DeCorby M, Rennie R, et al (2011) Prevalence of antimicrobial resistant pathogens from blood cultures from Canadian hospitals: results of the CANWARD 2007–2009 study. Diagn Microbiol Infect Dis 69: 307–313
14. Wilson J, Elgohari S, Livermore DM, et al (2011) Trends among pathogens reported as causing bacteraemia in England, 2004–2008. Clin Microbiol Infect 17: 451–458
15. Cosgrove SE, Sakoulas G, Perencevich EN, Schwaber MJ, Karchmer AW, Carmeli Y (2003) Comparison of mortality associated with methicillin-resistant and methicillin-susceptible Staphylococcus aureus bacteremia: a meta-analysis. Clin Infect Dis 36: 53–59
16. Nicoletti G, Schito G, Fadda G, et al (2006) Bacterial isolates from severe infections and their antibiotic susceptibility patterns in Italy: a nationwide study in the hospital setting. J Chemother 18: 589–602
17. Soriano A, Marco F, Martínez JA, et al (2008) Influence of vancomycin minimum inhibitory concentration on the treatment of methicillin-resistant Staphylococcus aureus bacteremia. Clin Infect Dis 46: 193–200
18. Bassetti M, Mesini, A, Molinari MP, Viscoli C (2011) Vancomycin susceptibility of meticillin-resistant Staphylococcus aureus (MRSA) bacteraemia isolates in an Italian hospital. Int J Antimicrob Agents 38: 453–454
19. Sakoulas G, Moise-Broder PA, Schentag J, Forrest A, Moellering RC, Eliopoulos GM (2004) Relationship of MIC and bactericidal activity to efficacy of vancomycin for treatment of methicillin-resistant Staphylococcus aureus bacteremia. J Clin Microbiol 42: 2398–2402
20. Jeffres MN, Isakow W, Doherty JA, Micek ST, Kollef MH (2007) A retrospective analysis of possible renal toxicity associated with vancomycin in patients with health care-associated methicillin-resistant Staphylococcus aureus pneumonia. Clin Ther 29: 1107–1115
21. Patel N, Lubanski P, Ferro S, et al (2009) Correlation between vancomycin MIC values and those of other agents against gram-positive bacteria among patients with bloodstream

VII

infections caused by methicillin-resistant Staphylococcus aureus. Antimicrob Agents Chemother 53: 5141–5144

22. Watanabe Y, Neoh HM, Cui L, Hiramatsu K (2008) Improved antimicrobial activity of linezolid against vancomycin-intermediate Staphylococcus aureus. Antimicrob Agents Chemother 52: 4207–4208

23. DiazGranados CA, Zimmer SM, Klein M, Jernigan JA (2005) Comparison of mortality associated with vancomycin-resistant and vancomycin-susceptible enterococcal bloodstream infections: a meta-analysis. Clin Infect Dis 41: 327–333

24. Hawkey PM (2008) Pre-clinical experience with daptomycin. J Antimicrob Chemother 62 (Suppl 3): iii7–ii14

25. Streit JM, Jones RN, Sader HS (2004) Daptomycin activity and spectrum: a worldwide sample of 6737 clinical Gram-positive organisms. J Antimicrob Chemother 53: 669–674

26. Smith K, Perez A, Ramage G, Gemmell CG, Lang S (2009) Comparison of biofilm-associated cell survival following in vitro exposure of meticillin-resistant Staphylococcus aureus biofilms to the antibiotics clindamycin, daptomycin, linezolid, tigecycline and vancomycin. Int J Antimicrob Agents 33: 374–378

27. Hanberger H, Nilsson LE, Maller R, Isaksson B (1991) Pharmacodynamics of daptomycin and vancomycin on Enterococcus faecalis and Staphylococcus aureus demonstrated by studies of initial killing and postantibiotic effect and influence of Ca2+ and albumin on these drugs. Antimicrob Agents Chemother 35: 1710–1716

28. Arbeit RD, Maki D, Tally FP, Campanaro E, Eisenstein BI, Daptomycin 98–01 and 99–01 Investigators (2004) The safety and efficacy of daptomycin for the treatment of complicated skin and skin-structure infections. Clin Infect Dis 38: 1673–1681

29. Fowler VG, Boucher HW, Corey GR, et al (2006) Daptomycin versus standard therapy for bacteremia and endocarditis caused by Staphylococcus aureus. N Engl J Med 355: 653–665

30. Rose WE, Leonard SN, Rybak MJ (2008) Evaluation of daptomycin pharmacodynamics and resistance at various dosage regimens against Staphylococcus aureus isolates with reduced susceptibilities to daptomycin in an in vitro pharmacodynamic model with simulated endocardial vegetations. Antimicrob Agents Chemother 52: 3061–3067

31. Boucher HW, Sakoulas G (2007) Perspectives on daptomycin resistance, with emphasis on resistance in Staphylococcus aureus. Clin Infect Dis 45: 601–608

32. Benvenuto M, Benziger DP, Yankelev S, Vigliani G (2006) Pharmacokinetics and tolerability of daptomycin at doses up to 12 milligrams per kilogram of body weight once daily in healthy volunteers. Antimicrob Agents Chemother 50: 3245–3249

33. Figueroa DA, Mangini E, Amodio-Groton M, et al (2009) Safety of high-dose intravenous daptomycin treatment: three-year cumulative experience in a clinical program. Clin Infect Dis 49: 177–180

34. Bassetti M, Nicco E, Elena Nicco, et al (2010) High-dose daptomycin in documented Staphylococcus aureus infections. Int J Antimicrob Agents 36: 459–461

35. Wilcox M, Nathwani D, Dryden M (2004) Linezolid compared with teicoplanin for the treatment of suspected or proven Gram-positive infections. J Antimicrob Chemother 53: 335–344

36. Stevens DL, Herr D, Lampiris H, Hunt JL, Batts DH, Hafkin B (2002) Linezolid versus vancomycin for the treatment of methicillin-resistant Staphylococcus aureus infections. Clin Infect Dis 34: 1481–1490

37. Shorr AF, Kunkel MJ, Kollef M (2005) Linezolid versus vancomycin for Staphylococcus aureus bacteraemia: pooled analysis of randomized studies. J Antimicrob Chemother 56: 923–929

38. American Thoracic Society, Infectious Diseases Society of America (2005) Guidelines for the management of adults with hospital-acquired, ventilator-associated, and healthcare-associated pneumonia. Am J Respir Crit Care Med 171: 388–416

39. Chastre J, Fagon JY (2002) Ventilator-associated pneumonia. Am J Respir Crit Care Med 165: 867–903

40. Richards MJ, Edwards JR, Culver DH, Gaynes RP (1999) Nosocomial infections in medical intensive care units in the United States. National Nosocomial Infections Surveillance System. Crit Care Med 27: 887–892

41. Safdar N, Dezfulian C, Collard HR, Saint S (2005) Clinical and economic consequences of ventilator-associated pneumonia: a systematic review. Crit Care Med 33: 2184–2193
42. Kollef MH, Sherman G, Ward S, Fraser VJ (1999) Inadequate antimicrobial treatment of infections: a risk factor for hospital mortality among critically ill patients. Chest 115: 462–474
43. Zahar JR, Clec'h C, Tafflet M, et al (2005) Is methicillin resistance associated with a worse prognosis in Staphylococcus aureus ventilator-associated pneumonia? Clin Infect Dis 41: 1224–1231
44. Lodise TP, McKinnon PS, Swiderski L, Rybak MJ (2003) Outcomes analysis of delayed antibiotic treatment for hospital-acquired Staphylococcus aureus bacteremia. Clin Infect Dis 36: 1418–1423
45. Rello J, Ausina V, Ricart M, Castella J, Prats G (2009) Impact of previous antimicrobial therapy on the etiology and outcome of ventilator-associated pneumonia. Chest 136: e30
46. Franzetti F, Antonelli M, Bassetti M, et al (2010) Consensus document on controversial issues for the treatment of hospital-associated pneumonia. Int J Infect Dis 14 (Suppl 4): S55–S65
47. Hidron AI, Edwards JR, Patel J, et al (2008) NHSN annual update: antimicrobial-resistant pathogens associated with healthcare-associated infections: annual summary of data reported to the National Healthcare Safety Network at the Centers for Disease Control and Prevention, 2006–2007. Infect Control Hosp Epidemiol 29: 996–1011
48. Kollef MH, Shorr A, Tabak YP, Gupta V, Liu LZ, Johannes RS (2005) Epidemiology and outcomes of health-care-associated pneumonia: results from a large US database of culture-positive pneumonia. Chest 128: 3854–3862
49. Welte T, Pletz MW (2010) Antimicrobial treatment of nosocomial meticillin-resistant Staphylococcus aureus (MRSA) pneumonia: current and future options. Int J Antimicrob Agents 36: 391–400
50. Gotfried MH, Shaw JP, Benton BM, et al (2008) Intrapulmonary distribution of intravenous telavancin in healthy subjects and effect of pulmonary surfactant on in vitro activities of telavancin and other antibiotics. Antimicrob Agents Chemother 52: 92–97
51. Hegde SS, Reyes N, Wiens T, et al (2004) Pharmacodynamics of telavancin (TD-6424), a novel bactericidal agent, against gram-positive bacteria. Antimicrob Agents Chemother 48: 3043–3050
52. Jung YJ, Koh Y, Hong SB, et al (2010) Effect of vancomycin plus rifampicin in the treatment of nosocomial methicillin-resistant Staphylococcus aureus pneumonia. Crit Care Med 38: 175–180
53. Haraga I, Nomura S, Fukamachi S, et al (2002) Emergence of vancomycin resistance during therapy against methicillin-resistant Staphylococcus aureus in a burn patient--importance of low-level resistance to vancomycin. Int J Infect Dis 6: 302–308
54. Hanaki H, Yamaguchi Y, Barata K, Sakai H and Sunakawa K (2004) Improved method of detection of beta-lactam antibiotic-induced VCM-resistant MRSA (BIVR). Int J Antimicrob Agents 23: 311–313
55. Kollef MH, Rello J, Cammarata SK, Croos-Dabrera RV, Wunderink RG (2004) Clinical cure and survival in Gram-positive ventilator-associated pneumonia: retrospective analysis of two double-blind studies comparing linezolid with vancomycin. Intensive Care Med 30: 388–394
56. Wunderink RG, Rello J, Cammarata SK, Croos-Dabrera RV, Kollef MH (2003) Linezolid vs vancomycin: analysis of two double-blind studies of patients with methicillin-resistant Staphylococcus aureus nosocomial pneumonia. Chest 124: 1789–1797
57. Rubinstein E, Cammarata S, Oliphant T, Wunderink R (2001) Linezolid Nosocomial Pneumonia Study Group. Linezolid (PNU-100766) versus vancomycin in the treatment of hospitalized patients with nosocomial pneumonia: a randomized, double-blind, multicenter study. Clin Infect Dis 32: 402–412
58. Wunderink RG, Cammarata SK, Oliphant TH, Kollef MH (2003) Linezolid Nosocomial Pneumonia Study Group. Continuation of a randomized, double-blind, multicenter study of linezolid versus vancomycin in the treatment of patients with nosocomial pneumonia. Clin Ther 25: 980–992
59. Conte JE, Golden JA, Kipps J, Zurlinden E (2002) Intrapulmonary pharmacokinetics of linezolid. Antimicrob Agents Chemother 46: 1475–1480

60. Powers JH, Ross DB, Lin D, Soreth J (2004) Linezolid and vancomycin for methicillin-resistant Staphylococcus aureus nosocomial pneumonia: the subtleties of subgroup analyses. Chest 126: 314–315
61. Wunderink RG, Mendelson MH, Somero MS, et al (2008) Early microbiological response to linezolid vs vancomycin in ventilator-associated pneumonia due to methicillin-resistant Staphylococcus aureus. Chest 134: 1200–1207
62. Kunkel M, Chastre JE, Kollef M, et al (2010) Linezolid vs vancomycin in the treatment of nosocomial pneumonia proven due to methicillin-resistant Staphylococcus aureus. IDSA 48th Annual Meeting, Vancouver Abstract LB49
63. Wong A, Reddy SP, Smyth DS, Aguero-Rosenfeld ME, Sakoulas G, Robinson DA (2010) Polyphyletic emergence of linezolid-resistant staphylococci in the United States. Antimicrob Agents Chemother 54: 742–748
64. Bassetti M, Farrel PA, Callan DA, Topal JE, Dembry LM (2003) Emergence of linezolid-resistant Enterococcus faecium during treatment of enterococcal infections. Int J Antimicrob Agents 2003 6: 593–594
65. Attassi K, Hershberger E, Alam R, Zervos MJ (2002) Thrombocytopenia associated with linezolid therapy. Clin Infect Dis 34: 695–698
66. Azamfirei L, Copotoiu SM, Branzaniuc K, Szederjesi J, Copotoiu R, Berteanu C (2007) Complete blindness after optic neuropathy induced by short-term linezolid treatment in a patient suffering from muscle dystrophy. Pharmacoepidemiol Drug Saf 16: 402–404
67. Wilcox M, Nathwani D, Dryden M (2004) Linezolid compared with teicoplanin for the treatment of suspected or proven Gram-positive infections. J Antimicrob Chemother 53: 335–344
68. Tascini C, Gemignani G, Doria R, et al (2009) Linezolid treatment for gram-positive infections: a retrospective comparison with teicoplanin. J Chemother 21: 311–316
69. Burkhardt O, Rauch K, Kaever V, Hadem J, Kielstein JT, Welte T (2009) Tigecycline possibly underdosed for the treatment of pneumonia: a pharmacokinetic viewpoint. Int J Antimicrob Agents 34: 101–102
70. Anthony KB, Fishman NO, Linkin DR, Gasink LB, Edelstein PH, Lautenbach E (2008) Clinical and microbiological outcomes of serious infections with multidrug-resistant gram-negative organisms treated with tigecycline. Clin Infect Dis 46: 567–570

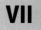

Oral Biofilms, Systemic Disease, and Pneumonia

M.P. Wise and D.W. Williams

Introduction

Physicians are taught at an early stage of training to incorporate inspection of the oral cavity as part of their routine clinical examination. Structures within the mouth may be involved by local disease processes, such as tumor and infection, or demonstrate manifestations of systemic disorders. Medical education usually focuses on the latter, as observation of a pathognomonic sign immediately discloses the diagnosis of an often complex multisystem disorder. Typically this facilitates a focused clinical examination and additional relevant history to be elicited. Unfortunately, patients with the ulceration of Behcet's disease, pigmentation of Addison's disease or the characteristic macules of Peutz-Jeghers syndrome occur infrequently and the oral cavity may receive relatively little further consideration in a patient's well-being. The one notable exception is infective endocarditis, which invariably prompts a close inspection of the teeth for a potential portal of infection entry. Critical care physicians are probably more likely to consider the oral cavity in patient management, but until recently this may have been limited to processes such as a dental abscess as a source of severe sepsis, aspiration pneumonitis, airway foreign body, oropharyngeal candidosis and intubation.

More recently an increasing body of data has emerged demonstrating that poor oral health characterized by excessive dental plaque and periodontitis has an important role in the etiology of systemic diseases such as myocardial ischemia, stroke, diabetes and pneumonia [1–3]. The following review will discuss dental plaque as a biofilm and how this drives disease processes both systemically and locally within the aerodigestive tract.

Dental Plaque: An Archetypal Biofilm

Dental plaque consists of a complex heterogeneous microbial community embedded in an extracellular polymeric matrix derived from bacteria and saliva, and represents the archetypal biofilm [4]. It has been recognized for some time that biofilms are present in device-associated or wound infections but they also occur in less obvious circumstances such as tissue infections caused by pneumococcus. Pneumonia, meningitis or otitis media caused by *Streptococcus pneumoniae* originate from biofilms and switching from planktonic to biofilm phenotype is a key event in the pathogenesis of this microbe [5]. In an animal model of pneumococcal infection, Oggioni and colleagues [5] demonstrated that not only was biofilm formation dependent on competence stimulating peptide (CSP), a quorum sens-

J.-L. Vincent (ed.), *Annual Update in Intensive Care and Emergency Medicine 2012*
DOI 10.1007/978-3-642-25716-2 © Springer-Verlag Berlin Heidelberg 2012

ing peptide, but so too was virulence *in vivo*. Mutants that had defective receptors for CSP were unable to form biofilms and had reduced pathogenicity. The authors concluded that during bacteremic sepsis, pneumococci were more likely to resemble planktonic growth, whilst during tissue infections they existed in a biofilm. Many other pathogens that are common in the critically ill also cause biofilm-mediated diseases; examples include *Pseudomonas aeruginosa, Hemophilus influenzae, Escherichia coli, Staphylococcus aureus* (including methicillin resistant *S. aureus* [MRSA]) and *Acinetobacter baumannii* [6–9]. This fact is especially relevant because one of the diagnostic features of a biofilm infection is often a culture-negative result despite a clinically documented infection [7], a situation fre-

VII

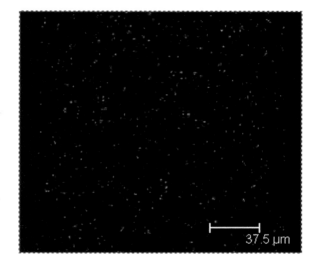

Fig. 1. Live/dead staining of planktonic bacteria treated with a commercially available antimicrobial mouthwash for 3 min. Dead cells (stained with both SYTO® 9 dye and propidium iodide) are shown as red.

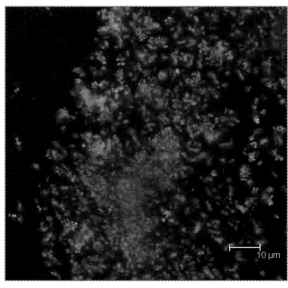

Fig. 2. Live/dead staining of plaque biofilm treated with a commercially available antimicrobial mouthwash for 3 min. A mixture of live cells (stained only with SYTO®-9 dye) depicted green and dead cells (stained SYTO® 9 dye and propidium iodide) shown as red, are present in the preparation.

quently encountered in critical care. Moreover, microbiological culture and sensitivity testing largely depend on planktonic techniques, which may be misleading when treating bacterial infections *in vivo*.

The microbiota of the mouth is the most diverse of any site within the body and contains > 500 cultivable bacterial species and an even greater number of non-cultivable bacteria that can only be detected using molecular techniques. Plaque formation occurs in a stochastic manner [reviewed in 10] and begins within seconds as saliva is exposed to a clean dental surface. Salivary glycoproteins are adsorbed at the tooth surface forming an enamel pellicle, which attracts planktonic pioneer colonizing bacteria, typically mitis-group streptococci that flow over the surface. Initial interactions with the pellicle occur through weak reversible electrochemical interactions and then bacteria bind irreversibly via bacterial adhesins to receptors within the pellicle. Early colonizing bacteria undergo rapid growth and produce metabolites, which alter the microenvironment and favor the growth of facultative anaerobes. Pioneer microbes are soon joined by other bacterial species, with which they have complex interactions, and coaggregate via lectin binding. Eventually the early colonizing bacteria diminish or become replaced in a process called microbial succession. Over time the biofilm matures and division slows, such that bacteria may divide only once or twice a day.

The mature biofilm is an extremely diverse structure in terms of bacterial composition, pH, redox potential and nutritional gradients [4]. Bacteria within the biofilm are sessile and demonstrate resistance to antibiotics and antimicrobials, such as chlorhexidine. This antimicrobial resistance exhibited by the biofilm can be 100–1000 fold greater than the same species in planktonic form [11]. This is shown in **Figures 1** and **2**, which illustrate the effect of a commercially available antiseptic mouthwash containing a variety of essential oils (e.g. eucalyptol and thymol) on putative periodontal pathogens either in planktonic or biofilm culture.

Oral Heath: A Major Health Problem?

Dental plaque is found naturally in the mouth, and in healthy individuals may exclude potentially pathogenic bacteria. However, perturbation of the delicate host-microbial balance results in plaque-mediated disease. Locally this is manifested as diseases such as dental carries, gingivitis and periodontitis. Gingivitis can be reversed by improving oral hygiene, decreasing plaque burden and reducing inflammation. However, unchecked gingivitis can progress to periodontitis, which is characterized by tissue destruction and even tooth loss. Plaque may cause disease beyond the local confines of the oral cavity. Microorganisms are capable of detaching from the biofilm as a result of sheer forces or proteolytic enzymes released in response to environmental stress. Detached bacteria can then colonize other sites including the lower respiratory tract. Periodontitis, driven by excessive plaque, is also involved in the pathogenesis of systemic diseases such as macrovascular disease and diabetes.

Periodontitis, especially when severe, represents an enormous inflammatory burden. If oral hygiene is inadequate and excessive plaque is allowed to accumulate around the gingiva, the host mounts an inflammatory response. This is characterized by an increase in gingival crevicular fluid, which not only recruits host defense molecules into the periodontal space, but also potential nutrients for the causative pathogens. If the inflammatory response fails to adequately control periodontal pathogens and restore homeostasis, a rapid cascade of events occurs. This culminates in a rise in pH and a fall in redox potential of the periodontal pocket, favoring proteolytic Gram-negative anaerobic bacteria. The result is severe inflammation or gingivitis, which may progress further to periodontitis.

Periodontitis is common amongst the adult population, even when effective preventative measures and treatment are available. Severe disease affects 10 – 20 % of adults and the majority of those aged > 65 have at least one tooth involved [12]. The area of inflamed epithelium in periodontitis may be as large as 44 cm^2 [13] and this injured tissue lies in direct contact with the substantial microbial burden present within plaque (> 10^8 bacteria per mm^3). Bacteria within the periodontal pocket, their metabolites and inflammatory mediators are free to access the circulation.

Macrovascular Disease

Many cohort and cross-sectional studies have demonstrated an association between periodontitis and coronary artery disease, peripheral vascular disease and stroke [1]. Clearly there are many confounding factors that are common to both macrovascular disease and periodontitis but a consistent association remains even when these variables are taken into account. Invasive periodontal bacteria such as *Porphyromonas gingivalis* may be directly isolated from diseased vascular specimens [14 – 16]. Although isolation of periodontal bacteria does not prove a causal relationship, this issue has been addressed in a number of animal models. Delbosc et al. demonstrated that repeated injection of *P. gingivalis* in rats promoted abdominal aortic aneurysms with the same pathological characteristics as in humans [17]. In a murine hyperlipidemic apolipoprotein E deficient model, atherosclerosis was accelerated by oral inoculation with *P. gingivalis* and could be prevented by previous immunization [18]. The pro-inflammatory environment within atheromatous vessels appears dependent in part on *P. gingivalis* signaling through Toll-like receptor 2 (TLR2) [19]. Whether treating periodontitis can influence the progression of vascular disease was addressed in a landmark study by Tonetti et al. [20]. One hundred and twenty patients with severe periodontitis were randomized to standard community-periodontal treatment or intensive periodontal treatment, which involved the removal of subgingival plaque. Endothelial function was assessed by measuring brachial artery diameter during flow-mediated dilatation; as well markers of inflammation (C-reactive protein [CRP], interleukin [IL]-6), endothelial activation and coagulation (soluble E-selectin and von Willebrand factor). An early deterioration of endothelial function was observed in the intensive treatment group; however, this function soon recovered and was significantly better than controls even six months after completion of treatment. These results suggest that intensive periodontal treatment may alter the pathogenesis and outcome in patients with macrovascular disease.

Diabetes

Periodontitis has been described as the sixth complication of diabetes, along with nephropathy, retinopathy, neuropathy, vascular disease and impaired wound heal-

VII

ing [21]. There is a complex interaction between the two diseases, such that diabetic patients have around three times the risk of having periodontal disease compared to non-diabetics [22] and there is a dose response relationship between the area of inflamed periodontal epithelium and glycemic control [23]. Several small studies have demonstrated that periodontal treatment can improve glycemic control [24, 25].

Pneumonia

The generally accepted dogma is that the lung is a sterile organ periodically challenged by microbial insults that are resisted by pulmonary defense mechanisms. On occasion, pulmonary infection develops as the balance tips in favor of the pathogen as a consequence of impaired host defense, an overwhelming microbial load or enhanced virulence factors. Recently this dogma has been challenged by Charlson et al. who used quantitative molecular techniques to sample throughout the airway of healthy individuals [26]. Low levels of 16S bacterial DNA were detected in the distal airways and were indistinguishable from community DNA profiles of the upper airway. The authors suggested that when corrections for carriage from the upper airway were taken into account, a continuum of flora from the upper to lower respiratory tract exists. Molecular techniques cannot distinguish whether the low numbers of bacteria detected distally in lung parenchyma are alive or have already been killed by host defense mechanisms. However, these observations suggest that even in normal individuals there is continual aspiration of potential respiratory pathogens into the distal airways and supports previous work showing microaspiration of oropharyngeal secretions in healthy individuals [27].

If one accepts that even in healthy individuals potential respiratory pathogens can transit from the upper to lower aerodigestive tract, it is not too difficult to envisage how an increase in the oral biomass, as a consequence of poor oral hygiene, might increase the incidence of all pulmonary infections. An increasing body of data supports this contention across the spectrum of pneumonia from community-acquired, healthcare-associated, hospital-acquired and ventilator-associated pneumonia.

A population-based cohort study of roughly 860,000 individuals identified 1,336 with community-acquired pneumonia (CAP) who were then matched to control subjects by age, sex and primary center [28]. A number of risk factors were identified for CAP, which may have been anticipated, including overcrowding, contact with children and pets, smoking, frequent alcohol consumption, low body weight, diabetes, renal failure, cardiorespiratory disease, cancer and immunosuppression. Previous immunization with influenza or pneumococcal vaccines decreased the incidence of CAP. Dental dysesthesia and the wearing of a dental prosthesis were also risk factors, whereas visiting a dentist in the previous month was protective.

Several observational studies have examined the role of poor oral hygiene in higher risk populations, such as the elderly, nursing home residents and hospitalized patients, and identified that this predisposes to pneumonia [29, 30]. Individuals in these groups invariably have other comorbidities recognized as risk factors for pulmonary infection, and frequently have difficulty swallowing which increases the risk of aspirating oropharyngeal secretions [29, 30]. In addition to

VII

having poor dentition and higher plaque scores, nursing home residents are more likely to be colonized with potential respiratory pathogens than age-matched controls [31, 32]. Sumi and colleagues examined the dental plaque of 138 dependent elderly individuals and found that 65 % contained bacteria capable of causing pneumonia [32]. Measures aimed at improving oral cleanliness and providing help with feeding could potentially substantially reduce morbidity and mortality in this group of patients. Yoneyama et al. analyzed 366 residents from 11 nursing homes randomized to an oral care package or standard treatment [33]. Those in the treatment group had their teeth and soft tissues, including the tongue, cleaned with a toothbrush after each meal by a caregiver. Plaque and calculus were removed once a week by a dental healthcare professional. In the control group residents administered their own oral care. Follow-up was over a two-year period and events recorded included febrile days and pneumonia. New episodes of pneumonia occurred in 11 % of the intervention group compared to 19 % of those receiving standard care. The effects of the oral intervention were greatest for those who required help with eating. A systematic review of the preventative effects of oral hygiene on pneumonia in elderly nursing home and hospitalized patients concluded there was an absolute risk reduction of 6.6 %–11.7 % and that approximately one in ten deaths from pneumonia were preventable [34].

VII

Ventilator-associated Pneumonia (VAP)

Once a relatively neglected topic in the critically ill intubated patient, oral hygiene now constitutes a part of the care bundle on the prevention of VAP [35]. Critically ill patients have poor oral health and cleanliness compared to healthy individuals [36]. Plaque scores are elevated on admission to critical care and in common with institutionalized individuals are frequently colonized with potentially pathogenic bacteria. In the absence of adequate oral hygiene, colonization rates and plaque scores increase over time [36]. The relationship between host defense and bacteria within plaque is severely disrupted in the critically ill and favors plaque formation. The endotracheal tube facilitating mechanical ventilation has a number of adverse effects on oral health. Normal tongue movements and swallowing are impaired causing pooling of secretions in the oropharynx. Provision of oral care is impeded by both the physical presence of the tube and fear of dislodgement by nursing staff. The endotracheal tube provides an ideal surface on which biofilm formation can occur, further increasing the bacterial biomass in the upper airway. Finally, the endotracheal tube holds the mouth open allowing the mucous membranes to dry out and impairing salivary function. Saliva is extremely important in maintaining oral health and contains more than forty antimicrobial proteins and peptides, which include secretory IgA, lysozyme, histatins, defensins, cathelicidin, lactoperoxidase, secretory leukocyte protease inhibitor and lactoferrin. Salivary volume and flow rate are equally as important as the qualitative properties of saliva as it buffers and washes debris through the oral cavity into the stomach. Salivary volume is greatly impaired in critically ill patients partly as a result of incomplete mouth closure and also because many frequently used drugs reduce production [37].

Prevention of VAP by Improving Oral Hygiene

The role of dental plaque as a reservoir of infection in VAP has been well studied. One of the earliest investigations to reach this conclusion prospectively studied colonization and infection in 86 mechanically ventilated patients. Oropharyngeal or gastric colonization were detected and quantified, as were new episodes of VAP. Using pulsed field electrophoresis, the investigators were able to demonstrate that the bacteria causing VAP originated predominantly from the oral cavity [38]. Given that dental plaque acts as a reservoir for respiratory infection it follows that cleaning the oral cavity is likely to be an important component in reducing the incidence of VAP. This is now recognized in care bundles, developed by consensus, that include measures to improve mouth care [35]. A number of approaches have been adopted in critical care to improve oral hygiene and can be divided into mechanical interventions (tooth brushing) or pharmacological methods (e.g., mouth rinses and antibiotics). A survey of 59 European ICUs found that 88 % of those responding performed oral care with mouthwash (61 % chlorhexidine) and 41 % used a toothbrush, none of which were electric [39]. Interestingly, 23 % felt they had inadequate training, 68 % found it difficult, 32 % difficult and unpleasant and as many as 37 % thought oral hygiene deteriorated over time [39]. An earlier survey of 102 ICUs in the United States found that mouthwashes and foam swabs were used most frequently [40].

The optimal methods for the physical removal of plaque in the critically ill have been poorly studied and this is undoubtedly reflected in the variable use of different methods [39]. Although many studies of mechanically ventilated patients have incorporated tooth brushing as part of a treatment protocol, to date only one study by Needleman and colleagues [41] has adequately addressed the optimal method for mechanically removing plaque in this patient population. Forty-six patients were randomly allocated to having their teeth cleaned with either an electric toothbrush or a sponge toothette four times a day. All patients in the study received 0.2 % chlorhexidine at the time of cleaning. Plaque scores reduced in both groups, but there was a significantly greater reduction in those cleaned with an electric toothbrush. Total viable bacterial count was also measured and was significantly lower in patients whose teeth were cleaned with an electric toothbrush.

Pharmacological methods are not only restricted to antimicrobial mouth rinses but also include the application of non-absorbable antibiotics to the oropharynx. The majority of studies in critically ill patients have focused on pharmacological methods of improving oral hygiene rather than on mechanical methods of removing plaque. Moreover, it is uncommon for studies in intensive care to measure changes in plaque following an oral hygiene intervention, but instead focus on VAP rates. This perhaps reflects the background and focus of the physicians orchestrating the investigations. Logically one would not expect to see a reduction in VAP unless the oral intervention had demonstrated some improvement in oral hygiene. Greater consideration should be given in future studies to documenting the efficacy of oral hygiene protocols.

Most studies of oral cleanliness conducted to date have used antiseptic treatments rather than antibiotics, usually with chlorhexidine. Evidence is accumulating that supports the concept that topically applied oral medication can improve oral cleanliness and reduce VAP, although not all studies demonstrate a benefit. This is probably a reflection of the considerable methodological heterogeneity in these investigations including the use of mechanical techniques of plaque removal. Some studies are in restricted patient groups such as cardiac surgery [42, 43], used variable preparations of chlorhexidine ranging from 0.12 % [42, 43] to 2 % [44, 45], different vehicles (rinse [42, 43, 45], gel [46], petroleum jelly [44]) and frequencies of application. However, the accumulated data have been the subject of a number of systematic reviews and meta-analyses, which also included topical antibiotics [47, 48]. These have concluded that there is a reduction in VAP but no proven mortality benefit.

As a consequence, measures aimed at improving oral hygiene have been recommended to reduce the incidence of VAP, and this often focuses on the use of chlorhexidine mouthwash [39]. Unfortunately, the antimicrobial mechanism of this drug is poorly understood by critical care physicians. Chlorhexidine is an effective antiseptic *in vivo* because of the property of substantivity, which means that it binds to a clean oral surface and is then released over time [49]. Indeed, substantivity makes it a more effective antiseptic *in vivo* than many other agents that show much greater *in vitro* potency [11]. Consequently the main role of chlorhexidine is in preventing the reaccumulation of plaque, rather than eliminating it [49]. This was unambiguously demonstrated by Zannata and colleagues who studied 20 individuals who refrained from all mechanical plaque control for a total of 25 days [49]. In this split-mouth study baseline values were recorded of plaque, gingivitis and gingival fluid volumes, plaque was allowed to accumulate until day 4. Two randomized quadrants were then cleaned to remove all plaque, whilst the remaining two quadrants served as plaque-covered controls. Individuals rinsed twice daily from day 4 with 0.12 % chlorhexidine for the next three weeks. At the conclusion of the study plaque that had accumulated during the 21-day period was measured. Plaque scores were significantly higher in the plaque covered compared to plaque free quadrants. Inflammation, as determined by gingival indices and gingival fluid volumes, were also markedly higher in the plaque-covered quadrants. The inability of chlorhexidine to kill all bacteria within plaque is well known amongst dental practitioners. Biofilms are exceptionally resistant to the actions of antibiotics and antiseptics. Oie et al. tested a variety of antiseptics against MRSA either as bacteria in suspension (planktonic) or as a biofilm [11]. Exposure of planktonic MRSA for as little as 20 seconds resulted in effective eradication, but this could not be achieved for the biofilm even after an hour of continuous exposure.

Adequate mechanical disruption and removal of plaque is, therefore, a prerequisite for chlorhexidine to reduce the risk of VAP. Unfortunately, this is not emphasized by guidelines promoting chlorhexidine use [35].

Conclusion

Previously, oral health was largely overlooked by many physicians but is now recognized as being increasingly important in the management of a number of diverse diseases. Uncontrolled dental plaque is the *sine qua non* of disease mediated by poor oral health and represents the archetypal example of biofilm infection. Biofilms are now regarded as being important components of many infectious diseases in humans and consequently the study of biofilm biology may yield many additional benefits. Dental plaque drives periodontal disease that is implicated in the pathogenesis of both macrovascular disease and diabetes, two major

VII

global diseases. Tackling periodontal disease therefore offers a new potential therapeutic avenue.

Dental plaque appears to be implicated in the etiology of the entire spectrum of pneumonia and consequently represents a major health issue. Strategies to reduce pneumonia in both the community and hospital require effective provision of oral hygiene. Undoubtedly this will require greater collaboration between dental and medical healthcare professionals and new models of service delivery. The optimal methods for delivering oral care, especially in the critically ill, require further refinement and this will be guided by a greater understanding of biofilms. An example of how this is already taking place is the recognition that mechanical disruption and removal of plaque is a prerequisite for chlorhexidine to reduce the risk of VAP.

References

1. Friedewald VE, Kornman KS, Beck JD, et al (2009) (2009) The American Journal of Cardiology and Journal of Periodontology Editors' Consensus: Periodontitis and atherosclerotic cardiovascular disease. Am J Cardiol 104: 59–68
2. Preshaw PM (2009) Periodontal disease and diabetes. J Dent 37: S575–577
3. Raghavendran K, Mylotte JM, Scannapieco FA (2007) Nursing home-associated pneumonia, hospital-acquired pneumonia and ventilator-associated pneumonia: the contribution of dental biofilms and periodontal inflammation. Periodontol 2000 44: 164–177
4. Zijnge V, van Leeuwen MB, Degener JE, et al. (2010) Oral biofilm architecture on natural teeth. PloS One 5:e9321
5. Oggioni MR, Trappetti C, Kadioglu A, et al (2006) Switch from planktonic to sessile life: a major event in pneumococcal pathogenesis. Mol Microbiol 61: 1196–1210
6. Foreman A, Wormald PJ (2010) Different biofilms, different disease? A clinical outcomes study. Laryngoscope 120: 1701–1706
7. Hall-Stoodley L, Stoodley P (2009) Evolving concepts in biofilm infections. Cell Microbiol 1034–1043
8. Telang NV, Satpute MG, Niphadkar KB, Joshi SG (2010) An increased incidence of biofilm-producing multidrug resistant methicillin-resistant Staphylococcus aureus in a tertiary care hospital from India. Am J Infect Control 38: 165–166
9. McQueary CN, Actis LA (2011) Acinetobacter Baumannii biofilms: variations among strains and correlations with other cell properties. J Microbiol 49: 243–250
10. Jakubovics NS, Kolenbrander PE (2010) The road to ruin: the formation of disease associated oral biofilms. Oral Dis 16: 729–739
11. Oie S, Huang Y, Kamiya A, et al (1996) Efficacy of disinfectants against biofilm cells of methicillin-resistant Staphylococcus aureus. Micribios 85: 223–230
12. Pihlstrom BL, Michalowicz BS, Johnson NW (2005) Periodontal diseases. Lancet 366: 1809–1820
13. Hujoel PP, White BA, García RI, Listgarten (MA 2001) The dentogingival epithelial surface area revisited. J Periodontal Res 36: 48–55
14. Nakano K, Wada K, Nomura R, et al (2011) Characterization of aortic aneurysms in cardiovascular disease patients harboring Porphyromonas gingivalis. Oral Dis 17: 370–378
15. Nakano K, Inaba H, Nomura R, et al (2008) Distribution of Porphyromonas gingivalis fimA genotypes in cardiovascular specimens from Japanese patients. Oral Microbiol Immunol 23: 170–172
16. Figuero E, Sanchez-Beltran M, Cuesta-Frechoso S, et al (2011) Detection of periodontal bacteria in atheromatous plaques by nested polymerase chain reaction. J Periodontol 82: 1469–1477
17. Delbosc S, Alsac JM, Journe C, et al (2011) Porphyromonas gingivalis participates in pathogenesis of human abdominal aortic aneurysm by neutrophil activation. Proof of concept in rats. PLoS One 6: e18679
18. Gibson FC 3rd, Hong C, Chou HH, et al (2004) Innate immune recognition of invasive

bacteria accelerates atherosclerosis in apolipoprotein E-deficient mice. Circulation 109: 2801–2806

19. Hayashi C, Madrigal AG, Liu X, et al (2010) Pathogen-mediated inflammatory atherosclerosis is mediated in part via Toll-like receptor 2-induced inflammatory responses. J Innate Immun 2: 334–343

20. Tonetti MS, D'Aiuto F, Nibali L, et al (2007) Treatment of periodontitis and endothelial function. N Engl J Med 356: 911–920

21. Löe H (1993) Periodontal disease. The sixth complication of diabetes mellitus. Diabetes Care 16: 329–334

22. Emrich LJ, Shlossman M, Genco RJ (1991) Periodontal disease in non-insulin-dependent diabetes mellitus. J Periodontol 1991 62: 123–131

23. Nesse W, Linde A, Abbas F, et al (2009) Dose-response relationship between periodontal inflamed surface area and HbA1c in type 2 diabetics. J Clin Periodontol 36: 295–300

24. Koromantzos PA, Makrilakis K, Dereka X, Katsilambros N, Vrotsos IA, Madianos PN (2011) A randomized, controlled trial on the effect of non-surgical periodontal therapy in patients with type 2 diabetes. Part I: effect on periodontal status and glycaemic control. J Clin Periodontol 38: 142–147

25. Navarro-Sanchez AB, Faria-Almeida R, Bascones-Martinez A (2007) Effect of non-surgical periodontal therapy on clinical and immunological response and glycaemic control in type 2 diabetic patients with moderate periodontitis J Clin Periodontol 34: 835–843

26. Charlson ES, Bittinger K, Haas AR, et al (2011) Topographical continuity of bacterial populations in the healthy human respiratory tract. Am J Respir Crit Care Med 184: 957–963

27. Gleeson K, Eggli DF, Maxwell SL (1997) Quantitative aspiration during sleep in normal subjects. Chest 111: 1266–1272

28. Almirall J, Bolíbar I, Serra-Prat M, et al (2008) New evidence of risk factors for community-acquired pneumonia: a population-based study. Eur Respir J 31: 1274–1284

29. Terpenning MS, Taylor GW, Lopatin DE, Kerr CK, Dominguez BL, Loesche WJ (2001) Aspiration pneumonia: dental and oral risk factors in an older veteran population. J Am Geriatr Soc 49: 557–563

30. Quagliarello V, Ginter S, Han L, Van Ness P, Allore H, Tinetti M (2005) Modifiable risk factors for nursing home-acquired pneumonia. Clin Infect Dis 40: 1–6

31. Russell SL, Boylan RJ, Kaslick RS, Scannapieco FA, Katz RV (1999) Respiratory pathogen colonization of the dental plaque of institutionalized elders. Spec Care Dentist 19: 128–134

32. Sumi Y, Miura H, Michiwaki Y, Nagaosa S, Nagaya M (2007) Colonization of dental plaque by respiratory pathogens in dependent elderly. Arch Gerontol Geriatr 44: 119–124

33. Yoneyama T, Yoshida M, Ohrui T, et al (2002) Oral care reduces pneumonia in older patients in nursing homes. J Am Geriatr Soc 50: 430–433

34. Sjögren P, Nilsson E, Forsell M, Johansson O, Hoogstraate J (2008) A systematic review of the preventive effect of oral hygiene on pneumonia and respiratory tract infection in elderly people in hospitals and nursing homes: effect estimates and methodological quality of randomized controlled trials. J Am Geriatr Soc 56: 2124–2130

35. Rello J, Lode H, Cornaglia G, Masterton R (2010) A European care bundle for prevention of ventilator-associated pneumonia. Intensive Care Med 36: 773–780

36. Fourrier F, Duvivier B, Boutigny H, Roussel-Delvallez M, Chopin C (1998) Colonization of dental plaque: a source of nosocomial infections in intensive care unit patients. Crit Care Med 26: 301–308

37. Dennesen P, van der Ven A, Vlasveld M, et al (2003) Inadequate salivary flow and poor oral mucosal status in intubated intensive care unit patients. Crit Care Med 31: 781–786

38. Garrouste-Orgeas M, Chevret S, Arlet G, et al (1997) Oropharyngeal or gastric colonization and nosocomial pneumonia in adult intensive care unit patients. A prospective study based on genomic DNA analysis. Am J Respir Crit Care Med 156: 1647–1655

39. Rello J, Koulenti D, Blot S, et al (2007) Oral care practices in intensive care units: a survey of 59 European ICUs. Intensive Care Med 33: 1066–1070

40. Binkley C, Furr LA, Carrico R, McCurren C (2004) Survey of oral care practices in US intensive care units. Am J Infect Control 32: 161–169

41. Needleman IG, Hirsch NP, Leemans M, et al (2011) Randomized controlled trial of tooth-

VII

brushing to reduce ventilator-associated pneumonia pathogens and dental plaque in a critical care unit. J Clin Periodontol 38: 246–252

42. DeRiso AJ 2nd, Ladowski JS, Dillon TA, Justice JW, Peterson AC (1996) Chlorhexidine gluconate 0.12 % oral rinse reduces the incidence of total nosocomial respiratory infection and nonprophylactic systemic antibiotic use in patients undergoing heart surgery. Chest 109: 1556–1561

43. Segers P, Speekenbrink RG, Ubbink DT, van Ogtrop ML, de Mol BA (2006) Prevention of nosocomial infection in cardiac surgery by decontamination of the nasopharynx and oropharynx with chlorhexidine gluconate: a randomized controlled trial. JAMA 296: 2460–2466

44. Koeman M, van der Ven AJ, Hak E, et al (2006) Oral decontamination with chlorhexidine reduces the incidence of ventilator-associated pneumonia. Am J Respir Crit Care Med 173: 1348–1355

45. Tantipong H, Morkchareonpong C, Jaiyindee S, Thamlikitkul V (2008) Randomized controlled trial and meta-analysis of oral decontamination with 2 % chlorhexidine solution for the prevention of ventilator-associated pneumonia. Infect Control Hosp Epidemiol 29: 131–136

46. Fourrier F, Dubois D, Pronnier P, et al, PIRAD Study Group (2005) Effect of gingival and dental plaque antiseptic decontamination on nosocomial infections acquired in the intensive care unit: a double-blind placebo-controlled multicenter study. Crit Care Med 33: 1728–1735

47. Pileggi C, Bianco A, Flotta D, Nobile CG, Pavia M (2011) Prevention of ventilator-associated pneumonia, mortality and all intensive care unit acquired infections by topically applied antimicrobial or antiseptic agents: a meta-analysis of randomized controlled trials in intensive care units. Crit Care 15: R155

48. Chan EY, Ruest A, Meade MO, Cook DJ (2007) Oral decontamination for prevention of pneumonia in mechanically ventilated adults: systematic review and meta-analysis. BMJ 334: 889

49. Zanatta FB, Antoniazzi RP, Rösing CK (2007) The effect of 0.12 % chlorhexidine gluconate rinsing on previously plaque-free and plaque-covered surfaces: a randomized, controlled clinical trial. J Periodontol 78: 2127–2134

VII

Novel Preventive Strategies for Ventilator-associated Pneumonia

A. COPPADORO, E.A. BITTNER, and L. BERRA

Introduction

Ventilator-associated pneumonia (VAP) is a complication of mechanical ventilation and is defined as the occurrence of pneumonia in patients undergoing mechanical ventilation for at least 48 hours. Clinical suspicion of VAP arises when new infiltrates are present on chest x-ray, and at least one of the following is present: Fever, leukocytosis, or purulent tracheo-bronchial secretions.

VII

The incidence of VAP reported in the literature ranges from 15 to 20 % [1]. However, the real incidence of VAP is difficult to assess, given the extreme variability of the diagnostic criteria for pneumonia, which often rely on bronchoscopic procedures. The specific mortality attributable to VAP is also debated. The reported VAP-associated mortality ranges from 20 to 70 %. Patients with VAP are often critically ill, and survival may be affected both by underlying conditions and the new-onset VAP. A recent study demonstrated a relatively limited attributable intensive care unit (ICU)-mortality of VAP, about 1 – 1.5 %, when adjusting for severity of co-existing diseases [2]. In the last few years, various strategies have been investigated in order to reduce the incidence of VAP. Reducing the duration of intubation, oral and endotracheal tube (ETT) care, positioning, and ETT modifications are aspects that may have a role in the prevention of VAP. Many of these strategies have been incorporated into 'VAP bundles', a set of treatments implemented simultaneously to reduce VAP incidence. Recent studies suggest that the use of bundle treatments can result in substantial reductions in rates of VAP [3].

In this chapter, we will present some novel VAP prevention strategies, explaining the possible mechanisms by which they may be clinically beneficial in reducing the incidence of VAP. A summary of these novel strategies is given in **Table 1**.

Reduce Duration of Intubation

The risk of developing VAP increases with prolonged intubation, and reintubation is a known risk factor [4]. This fact suggests that the presence of the ETT, although necessary for the survival of the patient, interferes with the normal physiological mechanisms that maintain the airways free of bacterial contamination. When the ETT is in place, the cough reflex is impaired and normal mucociliary flow is blocked by the inflated cuff. The ETT itself allows bacteria to drain into the trachea and distal airways leading to pneumonia. Intubated patients may be more prone to develop VAP as compared to tracheostomized patients because the ETT keeps the trachea and the oropharynx in communication, acting as a

J.-L. Vincent (ed.), *Annual Update in Intensive Care and Emergency Medicine 2012*
DOI 10.1007/978-3-642-25716-2 © Springer-Verlag Berlin Heidelberg 2012

Table 1. Most relevant clinical studies supporting the use of novel strategies to prevent ventilator-associated pneumonia (VAP)

First Author [ref]	Journal, Year	Implemented strategy	Summary
Morris [3]	Crit Care Med, 2011	VAP bundle	Before-and-after study, showing that implementation of a 4 item bundle (head elevation, oral chlorhexidine gel, sedation interruptions and a ventilator weaning protocol) reduced VAP rate
Terragni [6]	JAMA, 2010	Tracheostomy	Randomized trial showing that VAP incidence was not significantly different comparing early (7 days after intubation) to late (14 days) tracheostomy
Nseir [20]	Am J Respir Crit Care Med, 2011	Control of ETT cuff pressure	Randomized trial showing VAP rate reduction using a pneumatic device to maintain ETT cuff inflating pressure constant
Lacherade [22]	Am J Respir Crit Care Med, 2010	Intermittent SSD system	Randomized trial; the use of a SSD system resulted in a significant reduction of VAP incidence, including late-onset VAP
Kollef [27]	JAMA, 2008	Silver coated ETT	Randomized trial showing that VAP rates were lower with silver coated ETTs, as compared to standard ETTs
Miller [33]	J Crit Care, 2011	Polyurethane ETT cuff	Retrospective assessment of VAP rate with polyurethane vs. PVC cuffed ETTs, favoring the use of polyurethane ETT cuff
Siempos [44]	Crit Care Med, 2010	Probiotics	Meta-analysis of randomized controlled trials showing an association between the use of probiotics and reduced VAP incidence

ETT: endotracheal tube; SSD: subglottic secretion drainage

VII

bridge for bacteria to move toward the dependent airways. Aspiration of pathogens from the oropharynx in patients with subglottic dysfunction may occur both during extubation and reintubation. The rate of reintubation can be reduced by a variety of measures, including avoiding accidental removal of the ETT, improving planned extubations with weaning protocols designed to improve extubation success, and use of non-invasive ventilation (NIV).

On the basis of the observation that the ETT creates a communication between the oropharynx and airways, early tracheostomy has been advocated as one of the possible preventive measures for VAP. Although tracheostomy reduces duration of ventilation and ICU stay [5], a recent randomized trial failed to demonstrate a reduction in VAP incidence when early tracheostomy (6–8 days after intubation) was performed [6].

Since the ETT is believed to be involved in the pathogenesis of VAP, many clinicians avoid intubation when possible. The early use of NIV with the aim of avoiding intubation may be worth considering, particularly in fragile patients. Although a reduction in VAP incidence has not been demonstrated, the early use of continuous positive airway pressure (CPAP) reduced the need for ICU admission and ventilatory support in a randomized trial in 40 patients with hematological malignancies [7].

Another strategy to indirectly prevent the occurrence of VAP is the reduction of sedative administration. Reduced administration of sedatives is associated with shorter ICU stays and fewer days of intubation. Although no data are currently available to prove that VAP occurrence is decreased by reduced sedative administration, daily suspension of sedative drugs has been suggested as a preventive measure. Similarly, the implementation of a protocol for ventilator weaning may be useful to prevent VAP, as a result of the reduction in unneeded days on the ventilator and need for reintubation [8].

Oral Care

After prolonged intubation, tracheal colonization is frequently demonstrated, and the gastric enzyme, pepsin, may be detected in trachea-bronchial aspirates. In patients affected by VAP, the same bacteria are often present in the distal airways and in the stomach or oropharynx [9]. This suggests that the draining of saliva or gastric contents to below the ETT cuff determines the colonization of the tracheal mucosa, possibly leading to pneumonia.

VII

The use of acid-suppressive medications and the subsequent increase in gastric pH allows bacterial growth in the stomach, increasing the risk of colonization in case of aspiration of gastric contents. A cohort study of more than 60,000 patients showed an increased risk of hospital-acquired pneumonia when acid-suppressive medications were used [10]. However, no definitive recommendation can be provided about the use of acid-suppressive medications in relation to VAP in the ICU setting, and stress-ulcer prophylaxis is still suggested as part of the bundle treatments for VAP prevention published by the Institute for Healthcare Improvement.

To reduce the bacterial load of the fluids that drain into the airways when the ETT is in place, selective digestive tract decontamination (SDD) has been proposed. Decontamination with antibiotics reduces the incidence of VAP [11], but it is not currently recommended because of concern for possible selection of resistant bacteria. Oropharyngeal rinse with chlorhexidine was shown to be effective in reducing tracheal colonization and VAP incidence in a randomized, placebo-controlled study on nearly 400 patients [12], and is now widely used as standard of care for the intubated patient.

Airway Care

Draining of secretions around the ETT cuff is not the only way for bacteria to reach the distal airways and, therefore, lead to pneumonia. Another possible mechanism is the inoculation of bacteria through the inner lumen of the tube. To reduce this occurrence, proper hand hygiene by healthcare workers is a preventive measure that should always be implemented when treating intubated patients [13]. With time and despite routine suctioning, the inner surface of the ETT becomes covered by a layer of mucus and cells soon after intubation, which increases with duration of ETT use. This layer of 'biofilm' is an optimal environment for growth of a wide range of bacterial species [14], through which antibiotics penetrate with difficulty. Biofilm forms on both the internal and the external surface of the ETT. The presence of biofilm is particularly marked in proximity to the cuff, where secretions accumulate. Bacteria in the biofilm may detach to inoculate the lower airways leading to the development of pneumonia [15]. The importance of biofilm in the pathogenesis of VAP is suggested by the finding that about 70 % of patients with VAP show the same pathogens isolated from the biofilm and the tracheal secretions [16].

Tube Care

Care of the inner lumen of the ETT might be a new strategy to prevent VAP. The Mucus Shaver is a device able to keep the ETT free of secretions and biofilm by mechanically removing the deposits. Recently, a randomized clinical study confirmed the efficacy of the device in intubated patients, showing a marked reduction of secretions and contaminants in the treatment group [17]. Although the removal of biofilm with this device may be helpful, no data are yet available showing a reduction in VAP incidence.

Cuff Care

Maintaining adequate cuff pressure is vital to reduce draining of oropharyngeal and gastric secretions around the ETT. An inflating cuff pressure less than 20 cmH$_2$O may favor secretion drainage, while a pressure greater than 30 cmH$_2$O may result in mucosal injury [18]. Despite routine cuff pressure controls, variations in ETT cuff pressure frequently occur, exposing patients to increased risk of VAP [19]. Several devices have been developed to constantly monitor and adjust the ETT cuff inflating pressure. A recent randomized study of 122 patients showed lower levels of pepsin in the tracheal aspirates of the group treated with a device maintaining the cuff pressure constant, confirming the effectiveness of these devices in reducing micro-aspiration. Moreover, the treatment group had lower VAP rate as compared to controls, with no evident adverse effects [20].

Tube Modifications

A number of approaches have been investigated to reduce VAP incidence through modifications of the ETT. These efforts have focused on systems for drainage of subglottic secretions, coating of the ETT with antibacterial materials, and the sealing capacity of the cuff.

Subglottic Secretion Drainage

Despite tracheal suctioning, secretions tend to accumulate around the ETT cuff, where they cannot be removed. Subglottic secretion drainage systems usually consist of an accessory aspiration conduit opening above the ETT cuff and a vacuum source. Secretions may be continuously or intermittently removed from the subglottic space. Continuous aspiration has been shown to cause mucosal injuries in animal models [21], therefore intermittent aspiration systems are generally preferred. Use of an ETT equipped with a subglottic secretion drainage system has been associated with a reduction in VAP incidence. A multicenter study of more than 300 patients showed a decrease in VAP rate in the group treated with intermittent secretion drainage [22]. The beneficial effects of secretion drainage lasted over time, with no significant adverse events. A recent meta-analysis including nearly 2500 patients confirmed the efficacy of ETTs equipped with subglottic secretion drainage systems in preventing VAP, shortening ICU stay and reducing days of ventilation [23].

A different method of secretion drainage is the Mucus Slurper, a modified tube equipped with multiple aspirating holes opening on the tip of the ETT. Secretions are aspirated intermittently in the early expiratory phase, keeping the ETT lumen and the proximal trachea free from secretions [24]. However, no clinical data are available and the effectiveness of this device in VAP prevention remains to be determined.

ETT Coating

The inner surface of coated ETT tubes may be covered by a thin layer of anti-microbial agent(s), to prevent the formation of biofilm and bacterial colonization. Among several coating agents, silver seems to be feasible: It is biologically compatible, easy to employ, and effective in reducing tracheal colonization and bacterial growth in animal models [25]. The silver coating has bacteriostatic properties: Silver ions penetrate into the microbial membrane interfering with DNA synthesis, thereby preventing cell replication. Other agents have shown even greater *in vitro* antibacterial activity as compared to silver, but their clinical use remains to be investigated [26].

Several clinical trials have been conducted evaluating the efficacy of VAP prevention using silver-coated ETTs. In the North American Silver-Coated Endotracheal Tube (NASCENT) study, the use of a silver-coated ETT was associated with lower rates of VAP and of late-onset VAP in more than 2000 patients [27]. Hence, the use of antibacterial coating seems suitable to treat patients expected to be ventilated for more than 48 hours, possibly resulting in VAP prevention and cost-effectiveness [28].

VII

Cuff Seal and Shape

Modified cuffs have been proposed to improve tracheal sealing and reduce secretion drainage. Traditional hi-volume/low-pressure cuffs are made of polyvinyl-chloride (PVC). The surface of a traditional ETT cuff folds when inflated in the trachea, creating potential channels through which secretions can drain and reach the subglottic space. *In vitro* models have shown passage of fluids around a traditional ETT cuff already 1 minute after the beginning of the experiment, whereas modified cuffs provided significantly better sealing [29]. The principal cuff modifications involve changes in cuff shape and materials employed. The tapered shape seems to provide better sealing as compared to the classical cylindrical shape [30], possibly because the tapered cuff maintains better contact with the tracheal wall, resulting in less folding of the cuff surface. The use of materials other than PVC, such as polyurethane, lycra, silicone or latex, also result in better sealing *in vitro* [31]; however, no definitive clinical data are available regarding the material of choice to prevent VAP. ETTs equipped with polyurethane cuffs protected against early postoperative pneumonia in a population of cardiac surgery patients, but the effect on VAP rate was not investigated [32]. A retrospective study on more than 3000 patients showed an association between the use of a polyurethane cuff and a decrease in VAP incidence [33]. A randomized clinical trial showed VAP rate reduction for patients intubated with an ETT equipped with both a subglottic secretion drainage system and a polyurethane cuff, but the contribution of the polyurethane cuff to preventing VAP in this combined system is unclear [34].

Positioning

Positioning of the intubated patient is believed to be a relevant factor for the development of VAP. The 45° semi-recumbent position is widely recommended, but recent data suggest that the lateral position may be superior to prevent VAP.

Semi-recumbent Position

The rationale for keeping patients in the semi-recumbent position is that elevation of the head above the stomach reduces the aspiration of gastric reflux. A clinical cross-over trial demonstrated a greater amount of gastric content in the airways when patients were kept supine compared to a period of head elevation [35]. A later randomized trial showed the effectiveness of the semi-recumbent position in reducing VAP incidence as compared to the supine position [36]. On the basis of these data, many guidelines recommend the semi-recumbent position as a preventive measure for VAP. Recently, however, some investigators have questioned whether this position is optimal for VAP prevention [37, 38]. In the semi-recumbent position, aspiration of subglottic secretions across the tracheal cuff is not prevented and secretions in the lower respiratory tract cannot be cleared. The effects of gravity on aspiration in the semi-recumbent position may be most pronounced in patients intubated for a prolonged period and especially during suctioning because of the pressure drop within the respiratory system with this maneuver. Interestingly, a study using an animal model of long term mechanical ventilation showed that mucus flow was reversed toward the lungs in the semi-recumbent position and that it could be drained out of the lungs in the horizontal position [39]. The animals did not develop VAP if the tracheal tube and trachea were maintained slightly below horizontal. A pilot study of 10 intubated patients placed in the lateral horizontal position compared to 10 patients in the semi-recumbent position showed that the lateral position was feasible and did not cause serious adverse events [40]. Furthermore, the authors found more ventilator free days and a trend toward a lower incidence of VAP in the lateral horizontal position group. A multinational trial is currently ongoing to corroborate these benefits [41].

Kinetic Therapy

Immobility of the intubated critically ill patient may impair mucociliary clearance [42]. Mechanical rotation of patients with 40° turns (kinetic therapy) may improve pulmonary function more than the improvement in function achieved via standard care (i.e., turning patients every 2 hours). Kinetic therapy is believed to improve movement of secretions and to avoid the accumulation of mucus in dependent lung zones. A meta-analysis of 10 studies found that kinetic therapy reduced VAP incidence but did not reduce the duration of mechanical ventilation, ICU stay or mortality [43]. Many of the studies of kinetic therapy are limited by small sample sizes and VAP diagnoses made on a clinical basis without microbiological cultures. In addition, many of the patients in studies of kinetic therapy had complications, which might be associated with the therapy, including intolerance to rotation, unplanned extubation, loss of vascular access and arrhythmias. Based on the limitations of the existing studies and potential complications, a definitive recommendation regarding the use of kinetic therapy cannot be made at this time.

Other Measures

Probiotics

Probiotics are commercially available preparations of live non-pathogenic microorganisms administered to improve microbial balance resulting in health benefits for the host. Administration of probiotics has been advocated as a means of preventing a variety of infections including VAP in the ICU. The potential beneficial effect of probiotics in prevention of VAP may be in their competition with VAP-producing microorganisms in the oropharynx and stomach. In addition, it has been suggested that the benefits of probiotics might be explained by their immunomodulatory properties. A recent meta-analysis of randomized controlled trials comparing probiotics to control in patients undergoing mechanical ventilation found a lower incidence of VAP in the probiotics group compared with control [44]. Administration of probiotics was also found to be beneficial in reducing length of stay in the ICU and colonization of the respiratory tract by *Pseudomonas aeruginosa*.

VII

Early and Enteral Feeding

Enteral feeding may predispose to aspiration of gastric contents and the subsequent development of VAP. It has been suggested that placement of a post-pyloric feeding tube might reduce the risk of aspiration and VAP. A meta-analysis of seven studies found that post-pyloric feeding showed a trend toward lower incidence of VAP and mortality than gastric feeding [45]; however, the differences were not statistically significant. A more recent randomized trial showed a similar non-significant trend [46]. Therefore, a definitive recommendation regarding the routine use of post-pyloric feeding cannot be made. The timing of initiation of enteral feeding has also been reported to be associated with the development of VAP. In a large retrospective multicenter analysis, early feeding (i.e., within 48 hours of onset of mechanical ventilation) was found to be associated with an increased risk of VAP, although ICU and hospital mortality were decreased in the early feeding group [47].

Conclusion

Many factors contribute to the development of VAP. A number of strategies have been proposed for VAP prevention; however, only a few have been demonstrated to be effective, and many others still need evaluation in large randomized clinical trials before definitive recommendations can be made. Among others, modifications to the ETT (e.g., subglottic secretion drainage systems, antimicrobial coating, alternative cuff shapes and materials), continuous maintenance of proper cuff inflating pressures, ETT secretion removal, patient positioning in the lateral horizontal position, kinetic therapy, and administration of probiotics are measures worthy of consideration and further study in the ongoing battle to reduce the rates of VAP.

References

1. American Thoracic Society; Infectious Diseases Society of America (2005) Guidelines for the management of adults with hospital-acquired, ventilator-associated, and healthcare-associated pneumonia. Am J Respir Crit Care Med 171: 388–416
2. Bekaert M, Timsit JF, Vansteelandt S, et al (2011) Attributable mortality of ventilator associated pneumonia: A reappraisal using causal analysis. Am J Respir Crit Care Med 184: 1133–1139
3. Morris AC, Hay AW, Swann DG, et al (2011) Reducing ventilator-associated pneumonia in intensive care: Impact of implementing a care bundle. Crit Care Med 39: 2218–2224
4. Torres A, Gatell JM, Aznar E, et al (1995) Re-intubation increases the risk of nosocomial pneumonia in patients needing mechanical ventilation. Am J Respir Crit Care Med 152: 137–141
5. Griffiths J, Barber VS, Morgan L, Young JD (2005) Systematic review and meta-analysis of studies of the timing of tracheostomy in adult patients undergoing artificial ventilation. BMJ 330: 1243
6. Terragni PP, Antonelli M, Fumagalli R, et al (2010) Early vs late tracheotomy for prevention of pneumonia in mechanically ventilated adult ICU patients: a randomized controlled trial. JAMA 303: 1483–1489
7. Squadrone V, Massaia M, Bruno B (2010) Early CPAP prevents evolution of acute lung injury in patients with hematologic malignancy. Intensive Care Med 36: 1666–1674
8. Blackwood B, Alderdice F, Burns KE, Cardwell CR, Lavery G, O'Halloran P (2010) Proto-colized versus non-protocolized weaning for reducing the duration of mechanical ventilation in critically ill adult patients. Cochrane Database Syst Rev 12: CD006904
9. Torres A, el-Ebiary M, González J, et al (1993) Gastric and pharyngeal flora in nosocomial pneumonia acquired during mechanical ventilation. Am Rev Respir Dis 148: 352–357
10. Herzig SJ, Howell MD, Ngo LH, Marcantonio ER (2009) Acid-suppressive medication use and the risk for hospital-acquired pneumonia. JAMA 301: 2120–2128
11. Bergmans DC, Bonten MJ, Gaillard CA, et al (2001) Prevention of ventilator-associated pneumonia by oral decontamination: a prospective, randomized, double-blind, placebo-controlled study. Am J Respir Crit Care Med 164: 382–388
12. Koeman M, van der Ven AJ, Hak E, et al (2006) Oral decontamination with chlorhexidine reduces the incidence of ventilator-associated pneumonia. Am J Respir Crit Care Med 173: 1348–1355
13. Flanagan ME, Welsh CA, Kiess C, Hoke S, Doebbeling BN (2011) Agency for Healthcare Research and Quality (AHRQ) Hospital-Acquired Infections (HAI) Collaborative. A national collaborative for reducing health care?associated infections: Current initiatives, challenges, and opportunities. Am J Infect Control 39: 685–689
14. Cairns S, Thomas JG, Hooper SJ et al (2011) Molecular analysis of microbial communities in endotracheal tube biofilms. PLoS One 6: e14759
15. Inglis TJ, Millar MR, Jones JG, Robinson DA (1989) Tracheal tube biofilm as a source of bacterial colonization of the lung. J Clin Microbiol 27: 2014–2018
16. Adair CG, Gorman SP, Feron BM, et al (1999) Implications of endotracheal tube biofilm for ventilator-associated pneumonia. Intensive Care Med 25: 1072–1076
17. Berra L, Coppadoro A, Bittner EA, et al (2012) A clinical assessment of the Mucus Shaver: A device to keep the endotracheal tube free from secretions. Crit Care Med 40: 119–124
18. Seegobin RD, van Hasselt GL (1984) Endotracheal cuff pressure and tracheal mucosal blood flow: endoscopic study of effects of four large volume cuffs. Br Med J (Clin Res Ed) 288: 965–968
19. Nseir S, Brisson H, Marquette CH, et al (2009) Variations in endotracheal cuff pressure in

VII

intubated critically ill patients: prevalence and risk factors. Eur J Anaesthesiol 26: 229–234
20. Nseir S, Zerimech F, Fournier C, et al (2011) Continuous control of tracheal cuff pressure and microaspiration of gastric contents in critically ill patients. Am J Respir Crit Care Med 184: 1041–1047
21. Berra L, De Marchi L, Panigada M, Yu ZX, Baccarelli A, Kolobow T (2004) Evaluation of continuous aspiration of subglottic secretion in an in vivo study. Crit Care Med 32: 2071–2078
22. Lacherade JC, De Jonghe B, Guezennec P, et al (2010) Intermittent subglottic secretion drainage and ventilator-associated pneumonia: a multicenter trial. Am J Respir Crit Care Med 182: 910–917
23. Muscedere J, Rewa O, McKechnie K, Jiang X, Laporta D, Heyland DK (2011) Subglottic secretion drainage for the prevention of ventilator-associated pneumonia: A systematic review and meta-analysis. Crit Care Med 39: 1985–1991
24. Li Bassi G, Curto F, Zanella A, Stylianou M, Kolobow T (2007) A 72-hour study to test the efficacy and safety of the "Mucus Slurper" in mechanically ventilated sheep. Crit Care Med 35: 906–911
25. Berra L, Curto F, Li Bassi G, et al (2008) Antimicrobial-coated endotracheal tubes: an experimental study. Intensive Care Med 34: 1020–1029
26. Raad II, Mohamed JA, Reitzel RA, et al (2011) The prevention of biofilm colonization by multidrug-resistant pathogens that cause ventilator-associated pneumonia with antimicrobial-coated endotracheal tubes. Biomaterials 32: 2689–2694
27. Kollef MH, Afessa B, Anzueto A, et al (2008) Silver-coated endotracheal tubes and incidence of ventilator-associated pneumonia: the NASCENT randomized trial. JAMA 300: 805–813
28. Shorr AF, Zilberberg MD, Kollef M (2009) Cost-effectiveness analysis of a silver-coated endotracheal tube to reduce the incidence of ventilator-associated pneumonia. Infect Control Hosp Epidemiol 30: 759–763
29. Zanella A, Scaravilli V, Isgrò S, et al (2011) Fluid leakage across tracheal tube cuff, effect of different cuff material, shape, and positive expiratory pressure: a bench-top study. Intensive Care Med 37: 343–347
30. Dave MH, Frotzler A, Spielmann N, Madjdpour C, Weiss M (2010) Effect of tracheal tube cuff shape on fluid leakage across the cuff: an in vitro study. Br J Anaesth 105: 538–543
31. Kolobow T, Cressoni M, Epp M, Corti I, Cadringher P, Zanella A (2011) Comparison of a novel lycra endotracheal tube cuff to standard polyvinyl chloride cuff and polyurethane cuff for fluid leak prevention. Respir Care 56: 1095–1099
32. Poelaert J, Depuydt P, De Wolf A, Van de Velde S, Herck I, Blot S (2008) Polyurethane cuffed endotracheal tubes to prevent early postoperative pneumonia after cardiac surgery: a pilot study. J Thorac Cardiovasc Surg 135: 771–776
33. Miller MA, Arndt JL, Konkle MA, et al (2011) A polyurethane cuffed endotracheal tube is associated with decreased rates of ventilator-associated pneumonia. J Crit Care 26: 280–286
34. Lorente L, Lecuona M, Jiménez A, Mora ML, Sierra A (2007) Influence of an endotracheal tube with polyurethane cuff and subglottic secretion drainage on pneumonia. Am J Respir Crit Care Med 176: 1079–1083
35. Torres A, Serra-Batlles J, Ros E, et al (1992) Pulmonary aspiration of gastric contents in patients receiving mechanical ventilation: the effect of body position. Ann Intern Med 116: 540–543
36. Drakulovic MB, Torres A, Bauer TT, Nicolas JM, Nogué S, Ferrer M (1999) Supine body position as a risk factor for nosocomial pneumonia in mechanically ventilated patients: a randomised trial. Lancet 354: 1851–1858
37. Panigada M, Berra L (2011) Gravity. It's not just a good idea. It's the law. Minerva Anestesiol 77: 127–128
38. Li Bassi G, Torres A (2011) Ventilator-associated pneumonia: role of positioning. Curr Opin Crit Care 17: 57–63
39. Bassi GL, Zanella A, Cressoni M, Stylianou M, Kolobow T (2008) Following tracheal intubation, mucus flow is reversed in the semirecumbent position: possible role in the pathogenesis of ventilator-associated pneumonia. Crit Care Med 36: 518–525

VII

40. Mauri T, Berra L, Kumwilaisak K, et al (2010) Lateral-horizontal patient position and horizontal orientation of the endotracheal tube to prevent aspiration in adult surgical intensive care unit patients: a feasibility study. Respir Care 55: 294–302
41. Gravity-VAP network (2010) Prospective, randomized, multi-center trial of lateral trendelenburg versus semi-recumbent body position in mechanically ventilated patients for the prevention of ventilator-associated pneumonia. Available at http://www.gravityvaptrial.org/joomla/documents/summaryProtocol.pdf. Accessed November 2011
42. Nakagawa NK, Franchini ML, Driusso P, de Oliveira LR, Saldiva PH, Lorenzi-Filho G (2005) Mucociliary clearance is impaired in acutely ill patients. Chest 128: 2772–2777
43. Delaney A, Gray H, Laupland KB, Zuege DJ (2006) Kinetic bed therapy to prevent nosocomial pneumonia in mechanically ventilated patients: a systematic review and meta-analysis. Crit Care 10: R70
44. Siempos II, Ntaidou TK, Falagas ME (2010) Impact of the administration of probiotics on the incidence of ventilator-associated pneumonia: a meta-analysis of randomized controlled trials. Crit Care Med 38: 954–962
45. Marik PE, Zaloga GP (2003) Gastric versus post-pyloric feeding: a systematic review. Crit Care 7: R46–51
46. White H, Sosnowski K, Tran K, Reeves A, Jones M (2009) A randomised controlled comparison of early post-pyloric versus early gastric feeding to meet nutritional targets in ventilated intensive care patients. Crit Care 13: R187
47. Artinian V, Krayem H, DiGiovine B (2006) Effects of early enteral feeding on the outcome of critically ill mechanically ventilated medical patients. Chest 129: 960–967

VII

Viral-associated Ventilator-associated Pneumonia

M. Esperatti, A. López-Giraldo, and A. Torres

VII

Introduction

Nosocomial pneumonia is the most commonly acquired infection in intensive care units (ICUs). Its frequency is approximately 10 cases/1000 admissions; however, the incidence may increase to 20 times that number in patients undergoing invasive mechanical ventilation [1–3]. The overall incidence of ventilator-associated pneumonia (VAP) may range between 15 % to 20 % [2–6]. This complication prolongs the length of hospital stay, increases healthcare costs and may increase mortality [4, 5, 7, 8].

Classically, the etiology of this entity has been assumed to be bacterial, although in a significant percentage of patients with clinically suspected VAP, no bacteria can be identified. In recent years, introduction of highly sensitive techniques for detecting viruses in the respiratory tract, such as nucleic acid amplification by polymerase chain reaction (PCR), has significantly improved the diagnostic yield of infections such as community-acquired pneumonia (CAP), increasing the isolation rate from less than 10 % (using traditional techniques) to 35 % when using PCR in CAP that requires hospital admission [9].

Recently, new evidence has shown that viral isolation in the respiratory tract of immunocompetent patients undergoing invasive mechanical ventilation is higher than previously thought [10–12]. However, there are several limitations when determining the role of viruses in VAP:

- Difficulty in establishing a causal relationship between the viral isolate in the respiratory tract and pneumonia;
- Lack of an accessible gold standard for establishing the diagnosis;
- Lack of evidence regarding the efficacy of antiviral therapy in the context of suspected viral pneumonia during mechanical ventilation.

Incidence

In critically ill immunocompetent patients undergoing invasive mechanical ventilation, two kinds of virus may cause viral nosocomial pneumonia: Herpesviridae or the 'classic' respiratory viruses (influenza A, parainfluenza, respiratory syncytial virus [RSV], rhinovirus, metapneumovirus, and adenovirus). Although many clinical studies have focused on a particular aspect of the role of viruses in the critically ill patient, few studies have determined the frequency of viral respiratory tract involvement in patients with risk factors or suspected VAP.

J.-L. Vincent (ed.), *Annual Update in Intensive Care and Emergency Medicine 2012*
DOI 10.1007/978-3-642-25716-2 © Springer-Verlag Berlin Heidelberg 2012

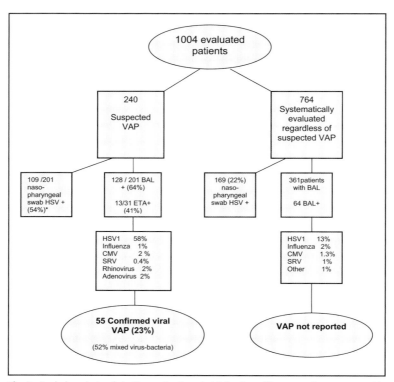

Fig. 1. Pooled analysis of studies evaluating viral infection of lower respiratory tract with more than one diagnostic test, including molecular testing or viral cultures on respiratory samples. BAL: bronchoalveolar lavage; ETA: endotracheal aspirate sample; CMV: cytomegalovirus; HSV1: herpes simplex type 1; SRV: syncytial respiratory virus. * 201 patients were evaluated with naso-pharyngeal swab and BAL [12].

Ideally, a study to address this issue should have an appropriate design (prospective cohort), systematically evaluate samples from the upper and lower respiratory tract, explore a wide range of viruses, and include nucleic acid amplification (PCR) as diagnostic test. After an exhaustive review of the literature, only three studies meet most of these requirements [10, 12, 13]. **Figure 1** shows a pooled analysis of these studies.

Although the presence of viruses in respiratory samples was not always accompanied by a definitive diagnosis of viral VAP and not all these studies reported this final diagnosis, all the studies reported a very low incidence of the 'classic' respiratory viruses. Herpes simplex virus (HSV) and cytomegalovirus (CMV) were the most frequently isolated agents. For this reason, we will focus on the description of the most relevant aspects regarding respiratory tract infections associated with these viruses.

It should be clarified that because viral pneumonia due to HSV and CMV during mechanical ventilation in the majority of cases is assumed to be a reactivation from a previous infection acquired outside the hospital, the term VAP, which implies nosocomial acquisition of the infection, will not be used, instead we will refer to viral reactivated pneumonia.

Herpes Simplex Virus

Initial infection with HSV usually occurs during childhood and is asymptomatic in most cases. A small percentage of patients may present with gingivostomatitis or pharyngitis. HSV type 1 may be isolated in the saliva of between 1 % and 5 % of the healthy population. Several factors such as tissue trauma, radiation therapy, heat exposure and acute bacterial infections may cause reactivation of the infection from a latent state, causing lesions of the skin and mucous membrane [14].

Lower respiratory tract infection with HSV-1 was initially considered as an entity exclusive of immunocompromised patients; however, in the past two decades, different studies have indicated the potential role of HSV-1 in non-immunosuppressed patients who are critically ill.

Incidence and Risk Factors

HSV respiratory infection in non-immunosuppressed critically ill patients was first reported in patients with acute respiratory distress syndrome (ARDS) in 1983 [15]. The presence of HSV in the lower respiratory tract was previously thought to be exceptional. Four studies evaluated a necropsy series of unselected patients between 1966 and 1982 and reported an incidence of 42 cases per 8535 patients (0.5 %) with a very high mortality and mainly affecting patients with underlying malignancies and extensive burns [16]. It was, therefore, assumed that respiratory tract involvement of HSV was very unusual and associated with a poor prognosis. Findings of a high incidence of HSV in patients with ARDS sparked interest in the hypothesis that HSV reactivation may play a role in an unfavorable clinical outcome in non-immunosuppressed critically ill patients. This was reflected in the increased number of publications reporting the frequency of HSV.

The overall incidence reported thereafter ranges between 5 % and 64 % (10, 15, 17–26]. The wide variability of the reported incidence of HSV is due to differences in study designs, study populations and the diagnostic tests used. Despite these differences, particularly susceptible populations, and various risk factors have been identified: Extensive burns, patients with ARDS, intubation and prolonged invasive mechanical ventilation, positive serology for HSV-1 (IgG), appearance of herpetic mucocutaneous lesions, advanced age, high severity scores at admission and use of systemic corticoid therapy during the ICU stay.

It should be noted that, despite the widely varying incidence reported in the literature, the best quality study (in terms of design, adequate number of studied patients, use of highly sensitivity diagnostic tests and consecutive evaluation of non-immunosuppressed critically ill patients) showed high incidences of HSV detection in the lower respiratory tract (64 %) and of HSV bronchopneumonitis (21 %) among patients undergoing mechanical ventilation for more than 5 days [12]. In this study, the presence of herpetic oral-labial lesions, positive pharyngeal swab and macroscopic bronchial lesions were predictors for herpetic bronchopneumonitis.

Table 1 shows a detailed summary of studies evaluating lower respiratory tract infection caused by HSV-1 in critically ill patients since 1982.

VII

Table 1. Summary of studies of lower respiratory tract infections by herpes simplex virus (HSV) 1 in immunocompetent ICU patients.

Year [reference]	Design	Population	HSV 1 + (%)	Risk Factors	Outcomes (HSV+ vs HSV-)	Mortality (%)
1982 [15]	Prospective	ARDS	14/46 (30)	N.A	↑ Days on M.V. ↑ Mortality	57
1982 [16]	Prospective	Suspected VAP	37/308 (12)	Intubation/MV	NA	24
1992 [18]	Retrospective	Mixed	42/42	Intubation/MV	NA	57
1996 (20)	Retrospective	Burned critically ill	27/54 [50]	ARDS	¶	¶
1998 [21]	Retrospective	Sepsis postoperative	8/142 (6)	Thrombocytopenia	↑ Mortality ↑ Bacterial nosocomial infections	63
2000 [22]	Retrospective	Pulmonary infiltrates in trauma patients	4/74 (5)	NA	NA	NA
2003 [23]	Prospective	ICU-LOS > 5 days	11/104 (23)	None	No adverse outcomes	27
2003 [10]	Prospective	ICU-LOS > 3 days	58/361 (16)	HSV+ in pharyngeal swabs SOFA score↑ MV > 7 days	↑ Days on MV ↑ Hospital-LOS	38
2004 [11]	Prospective	Postoperative and trauma patients	106/393 (27)	APACHE II score↑ Elderly	↑ Mortality	41
2007 [12]	Prospective	VAP suspected/ ICU > 5 days	128/201 (64)	HSV + in pharyngeal swab HSV-like skin or mucosa lessions	↑ Days on MV ↑ ICU LOS	48
2008 [24]	Retrospective	Suspected VAP	99/308 (32)	Elderly	↑ Mortality in patients with high HSV load in BAL fluid	26
2009 [25]	Prospective	MV > 48 hour	65/105 (61)	Corticosteroids IgG HSV 1+ at admission	↑ Days on MV ↑ ICU LOS ↑ Hospital-LOS	35
2011 [26]	Prospective	Suspected VAP in mixed population	19/177 (11)	Elderly ↑ Comorbidity and severity index	↑ ICU LOS	76

ARDS: acute respiratory distress syndrome; ICU: intensive care unit; LOS: length of stay; MV: mechanical ventilation; NA: not available; VAP: ventilator-associated pneumonia; SOFA: sequential organ failure assessment; BAL: bronchoalveolar lavage; ¶: retrospective study on lung biopsy samples

VII

Pathogenesis

Reactivation of the latent virus seems to be the initial mechanism of HSV respiratory infection: All patients with herpetic respiratory infection in the ICU have previous HSV-positive serology and, usually, a pharyngeal swab positive for HSV, or oral-labial lesions preceding the lower tract infection [10, 25]. Manipulation and traumatism of the airways predispose patients to viral reactivation in the oropharyngeal mucosa and upper airway, with subsequent micro-aspiration to more distal airways, thereby causing potential lung parenchyma involvement [10, 14]. Therefore, viral reactivation on the tracheobronchial mucosa could explain, in some cases, how respiratory infection presents without any evidence of viruses in the oropharyngeal mucosa [12, 16]. Although hematogenous spread has been described, this mechanism seems to be limited to patients with a major degree of immunosuppression [16].

Typically, viral reactivation begins between day 3 and 5 of mechanical ventilation. This reactivation is followed by an exponential increase in the viral load in the inferior airways, which reaches a peak on day 12. Viral load at this point can reach up to 10^8 copies/ml as measured by PCR performed on tracheobronchial secretions [25]. This viral load corresponds to the viral concentration found in the vesicular lesions of the oral mucosa. This phase is followed by a slow decline of the viral load. This chronology appears relevant when considering the diagnosis of viral VAP on an individual basis.

It should be noted that a high viral load (assessed by viral culture) appears to correlate well with the diagnosis of bronchopneumonitis based on histologic examination (cytology of the bronchoalveolar lavage [BAL] fluid and/or bronchial biopsies are considered as gold standard). A viral load of $8x10^4$ copies/10^6 cells has sensitivity and specificity of 81 % and 83 %, respectively, for the diagnosis of herpetic bronchopneumonitis [12].

In animal models, instillation of HSV into the nostrils causes pneumonia and triggers a strong inflammatory response with extensive tissue damage secondary to induction of inducible nitric oxide synthase (iNOS) on the lung parenchyma. Inhibition of this enzyme improves tissue damage, pulmonary compliance and survival. Interestingly, these effects are independent of the viral load, thus suggesting a mechanism of inflammatory response amplification rather than direct viral pathogenicity [27].

It should be noted that although viral reactivation is the main mechanism of pathogenesis of HSV pneumonia during mechanical ventilation, several cases of HSV clusters due to nosocomial transmission have been reported in the ICU [28].

Clinical Outcomes

The detection of HSV in the lower respiratory tract does not necessarily mean lung infection and, on an individual basis, it is unclear whether it represents viral contamination of the lower respiratory tract from the mouth and/or throat, local tracheobronchial viral excretion or HSV broncho-pneumonitis [14]. For these reasons, the exact role of HSV remains to be clarified: Is it just a marker of disease severity or a real pathogen with its own morbidity and mortality?

The analysis is even more complicated when the association of virus and bacteria in viral VAP (52 % of cases) is taken into consideration [10, 12]. Several studies have reported more days on mechanical ventilation and longer stays in

VII

the ICU and/or hospital in patients infected with HSV [10, 13, 15, 25, 26]. Interestingly, these were prospective studies that evaluated a large number of patients and failed to show an increase in mortality. The only prospective study that is often cited as an example of increased mortality in the group of HSV+ patients did not reach statistical significance when adjusted for severity, assessed by APACHE II [23]. The studies that reported increased mortality in HSV infected patients were retrospective [10, 29] or prospective with a very small sample size and limited to populations with ARDS [15]. As a result, the question of the effects of infection on mortality remains to be clarified.

Treatment

Despite the high incidence and association with adverse clinical outcomes, there are no randomized controlled trials (RCTs) that make it possible to provide definitive recommendations regarding intervention in these patients. In all the studies, treatment was prescribed by clinicians and analysis of clinical outcomes under controlled conditions was not available. The only interventional study was a small randomized trial that evaluated the efficacy and safety of acyclovir for preventing reactivation of HSV in patients with ARDS [29]. Although acyclovir was effective in preventing viral reactivation in the respiratory tract (absolute risk reduction of 65 %), there was no difference in severity of respiratory failure, duration of mechanical ventilation or mortality between the control and intervention arms.

Given the particular characteristics of this phenomenon (high incidence, association with unfavorable clinical outcomes and potential therapeutic interventions), the need for RCTs that could clarify this issue is imperative.

Cytomegalovirus

Most healthy immunocompetent adults have been infected with CMV, a fact that is evidenced by the presence of specific immunoglobulin (Ig) G for this virus [30]. In most cases, the infection remains latent without causing disease. Reactivation and CMV disease has traditionally been described in populations with marked alterations in cellular immunity [31]. However, in the past two decades there has been increasing evidence that reactivation of CMV is a common finding in the immunocompetent critically ill patient [32]. The frequency of CMV varies depending on the diagnostic methods used, from 12 % when cultures are used to 33 % when PCR is used [30].

Viral reactivation begins between days 14 and 21 of the ICU stay. Risk factors for reactivation are prolonged ICU stays, higher severity scores on admission, and severe sepsis. In this group, the incidence may reach up to 36 %. Although a clear cause and effect has not been found, reactivation is associated with increased mortality and longer hospital stay [30, 32]. Viral reactivation in humans can begin in the lung parenchyma [23, 28, 33)]. In animal models with latent CMV, sepsis may produce pulmonary reactivation of the viral infection; this reactivation is associated with a persistent increase in cytokine-mediated inflammatory response in the lung and both findings (reactivation and persistent inflammation) do not occur in the presence of prior ganciclovir treatment [34]. Thus, to the epidemiological evidence of the association of CMV-unfavorable clinical outcomes is added the biological evidence of potential pathogenicity in the lungs.

In 1996, Papazian et al published the first study that showed a high incidence of CMV reactivated pneumonia during mechanical ventilation [33]. The authors studied 85 patients with ARDS, prolonged mechanical ventilation and suspected VAP with negative cultures for bacteria in respiratory specimens (25 open lung biopsies and 60 post mortem biopsies). Conclusive histopathological findings of CMV pneumonia were found in 25 patients (only 3 cases also showed evidence of bacterial pneumonia). The same authors studied the diagnostic value of open lung biopsies on patients with acute lung injury (ALI), suspected VAP and negative cultures of respiratory specimens. Among 100 patients, evidence of CMV infection was found in 30 subjects (3 patients had HSV findings), 4 cases also showed evidence of ARDS in a fibroproliferative phase. With the diagnosis of pulmonary fibrosis, CMV pneumonia was the most frequent finding that conditioned changes in medical treatment [35].

The value of the different diagnostic techniques is not clear; thus, in the first study mentioned, the BAL culture had sensitivity and specificity of 53 % and 92 %, respectively [33]. In another study by the same authors, diagnosis was based on histologic findings after negative cultures and negative pp65 antigenemia [35]. The only study that evaluated PCR assay in BAL in an unselected sample of patients with suspected VAP found 13 % of positive samples without cytoplasmic inclusions and no histological evaluation was performed; it was therefore not possible to reach a definitive diagnosis [12].

VII

The diagnosis of VAP due to CMV may, therefore, be more common than thought, but there are issues that still need to be clarified regarding the appropriate diagnostic tests. Previous studies suggest a low sensitivity of standard diagnostic tests. However, in the populations studied, CMV appears to have a clear pathogenic role, as evidenced by the extensive presence of pneumonitis and of cytoplasmic inclusions in biopsy specimens [33, 35].

Individual management of patients, is further complicated when considering the risk and benefits of treatment with ganciclovir, which has potentially serious adverse effects. For these reasons, RCTs are needed to clarify the role of antiviral treatment in patients with CMV reactivation. Similarly, it is difficult to make a final recommendation regarding the overall approach to individual patients with suspected CMV VAP. It may be suggested that this entity be suspected in patients with risk factors (persistent pulmonary infiltrates with clinical deterioration and no evidence of bacterial infection). If the patient also shows evidence of viral reactivation (preferably assessed by PCR), initiation of antiviral therapy should be considered. Lung biopsy appears to play an important role in this group of patients because it can demonstrate CMV pneumonia even when respiratory specimens are negative.

Mimivirus

Acanthamoeba polyphaga (mimivirus) is a double-stranded DNA virus with the largest viral genome yet described [36]. Although it was thought to be a potential causative agent of pneumonia, the role has not been clearly defined. This microorganism was first described in 1992 as part of a suspected outbreak of *Legionella* pneumonia. Initially categorized as a bacterium, it was finally reclassified as a virus in 2003. Subsequently, serological evidence of mimivirus has been reported in between 7 % and 9 % of patients with community-acquired and nosocomial pneumonia [37, 38].

The potential role of this virus was questioned in a study that evaluated one cohort with pneumonia using different serologies; results were negative in all cases. The nosocomial pneumonia cohort included 71 samples of elderly patients from health care centers; it is not known if any of them received invasive mechanical ventilation [39].

One study systematically evaluated ventilated patients with suspected VAP [40]. Of 300 patients with suspected VAP, 59 had positive serology for mimivirus (19.6 %); 64 % of these had, additionally, positive BAL for bacteria. A comparison of mimivirus-seropositive patients with a seronegative group matched for age, diagnostic category, and severity showed that the positive group experienced increased duration of mechanical ventilation and ICU stay; no differences in mortality were found. It should be noted that the overall effectiveness of matching was 95 % and other relevant variables, such as adequate antibacterial therapy and the bacteremia rate, were similar in the two groups.

Thus, although no definitive recommendations can be made regarding screening for this microbiological agent, there is cumulating evidence of the potential role of this new virus in VAP.

VII

Conclusion

Respiratory viruses are not a common cause of VAP. Herpesviridae (HSV and CMV) are detected frequently in the lower respiratory tract of ventilated patients. HSV is detected between days 7 and 14 of invasive mechanical ventilation; presence of the virus does not necessarily imply pathogenicity, but the association with adverse clinical outcomes supports the hypothesis of a pathogenic role in a variable percentage of patients. Bronchopneumonitis associated with HSV should be considered in patients with prolonged invasive mechanical ventilation, reactivation with herpetic mucocutaneous lesions, and those belonging to a risk population with burn injuries or ALI.

Reactivation of CMV is common in critically ill patients and usually occurs between days 14 and 21 in patients with defined risk factors. The potential pathogenic role of CMV seems clear in patients with ALI and persistent respiratory failure in whom there is no isolation of a bacterial agent as a cause of VAP. The best diagnostic test is not defined although lung biopsies should be considered in addition to the usual methods before starting specific treatment.

Because of the lack of randomized clinical trials, it is not possible to make a definitive recommendation regarding the antiviral treatment for suspected HSV or CMV reactivation pneumonia during mechanical ventilation. The decision to start antiviral treatment should be made on an individual basis, taking into consideration the risk factors mentioned above, a correct interpretation of diagnostic methods and the whole clinical picture of the patient. There is an urgent need for RCTs to address this aspect.

The role of mimivirus is uncertain and yet to be defined, but serologic evidence of this new virus in the context of VAP appears to be associated with adverse clinical outcomes.

References

1. American Thoracic Society and Infectious Diseases Society of America (2005) Guidelines for the Management of Adults with Hospital-acquired, Ventilator-associated, and Health-care-associated Pneumonia. Am J Respir 171: 388–416
2. Celis R, Torres A, Gatell JM, Almela M, Rodriguez-Roisin R, Agustí-Vidal A (1988) Nosocomial pneumonia: A multivariate analysis of risk and prognosis. Chest 93: 318–324
3. Torres A, Aznar R, Gatell JM, et al (1990) Incidence, risk, and prognosis factors of nosocomial pneumonia in mechanically ventilated patients. Am Rev Respir Dis 142: 523–528
4. Koulenti D, Lisboa T, Brun-Buisson C, et al (2009) Spectrum of practice in the diagnosis of nosocomial pneumonia in patients requiring mechanical ventilation in European intensive care units. Crit Care Med 37: 2360–2368
5. Warren DK, Shukla SJ, Olsen MA, et al (2003) Outcome and attributable cost of ventilator-associated pneumonia among intensive care unit patients in a suburban medical center. Crit Care Med 31: 1312–1317
6. Luna CM, Blanzaco D, Niederman MS, et al (2003) Resolution of ventilator-associated pneumonia: prospective evaluation of the clinical pulmonary infection score as an early clinical predictor of outcome. Crit Care Med 31: 676–682
7. Kollef MH (1993) Ventilator-associated pneumonia: A multivariate analysis. JAMA 270: 1965–1970
8. Fagon JY, Chastre J, Hance AJ, Montravers P, Novara A, Gibert C (1993). Nosocomial pneumonia in ventilated patients: A cohort study evaluating attributable mortality and hospital stay. Am J Med 94: 281–288
9. Marcos MA, Esperatti M, Torres A (2009). Viral pneumonia. Curr Opin Infect Dis 22: 143–147
10. Bruynseels P, Jorens PG, Demey HE, et al (2003). Herpes simplex virus in the respiratory tract of critical care patients: a prospective study. Lancet 362: 1536–1541
11. Ong GM, Lowry K, Mahajan S, et al (2004) Herpes simplex type 1 shedding is associated with reduced hospital survival in patients receiving assisted ventilation in a tertiary referral intensive care unit. J Med Virol 72: 121–125
12. Luyt CE, Combes A, Deback C, et al (2007) Herpes simplex virus lung infection in patients undergoing prolonged mechanical ventilation. Am J Respir Crit Care Med 175: 935–942
13. Daubin C, Vincent S, Vabret A, et al (2005) Nosocomial viral ventilator-associated pneumonia in the intensive care unit: a prospective cohort study. Intensive Care Med 31: 1116–1122
14. Simoons-Smit AM, Kraan EM, Beishuizen A, Strack van Schijndel RJ, Vandenbroucke-Grauls CM (2006) Herpes simplex virus type 1 and respiratory disease in critically-ill patients: Real pathogen or innocent bystander? Clin Microbiol Infect 12: 1050–1059
15. Tuxen DV, Cade JF, McDonald MI, Buchanan MR, Clark RJ, Pain MC (1982) Herpes simplex virus from the lower respiratory tract in adult respiratory distress syndrome. Am Rev Respir Dis 126: 416–419
16. Ramsey PG, Fife K, Hackman RC, Meyers JD, Corey L (1982) Herpes simplex virus pneumonia: clinical, virologic, and pathologic features in 20 patients. Ann Intern Med 97: 813–820
17. Tuxen DV, Wilson JW, Cade JF (1987) Prevention of lower respiratory herpes simplex virus infection with acyclovir in patients with the adult respiratory distress syndrome. Am Rev Respir Dis 136: 402–405
18. Prellner T, Flamholc L, Haidl S, Lindholm K, Widell A (1992) Herpes simplex virus--the most frequently isolated pathogen in the lungs of patients with severe respiratory distress. Scand J Infect Dis 24: 283–292
19. Schuller D, Spessert C, Fraser VJ, Goodenberger DM (1993). Herpes simplex virus from respiratory tract secretions: epidemiology, clinical characteristics, and outcome in immunocompromised and nonimmunocompromised hosts. Am J Med 94: 29–33
20. Byers RJ, Hasleton PS, Quigley A, et al (1996) Pulmonary herpes simplex in burns patients. Eur Respir J 9: 2313–2317
21. Cook CH, Yenchar JK, Kraner TO, Davies EA, Ferguson RM (1998) Occult herpes family viruses may increase mortality in critically ill surgical patients. Am J Surg 176: 357–360

VII

22. Cherr GS, Meredith JW, Chang M (2000) Herpes simplex virus pneumonia in trauma patients. J Trauma 49: 547–549
23. Cook CH, Martin LC, Yenchar JK, et al (2003) Occult herpes family viral infections are endemic in critically ill surgical patients. Crit Care Med 31: 1923–1929
24. Linssen CF, Jacobs JA, Stelma FF, et al (2008) Herpes simplex virus load in bronchoalveolar lavage fluid is related to poor outcome in critically ill patients. Intensive Care Med 34: 2202–2209
25. De Vos N, Van Hoovels L, Vankeerberghen A, et al (2009) Monitoring of herpes simplex virus in the lower respiratory tract of critically ill patients using real-time PCR: a prospective study. Clin Microbiol Infect 15: 358–363
26. Bouza E, Giannella MV, Torres P, et al (2011) Herpes simplex virus: A marker of severity in bacterial ventilator-associated pneumonia. J Crit Care 26: 432
27. Adler H, Beland JL, Del-Pan NC, et al (1997) Suppression of herpes simplex virus type 1 (HSV-1)-induced pneumonia in mice by inhibition of inducible nitric oxide synthase (iNOS, NOS2). J Exp Med 185: 1533–1540
28. Cook CH, Yenchar JK, Kraner TO, Davies EA, Ferguson RM (1998) Occult herpes family viruses may increase mortality in critically ill surgical patients. Am J Surg 176: 357–360
29. Tuxen DV, Wilson JW, Cade JF (1987) Prevention of lower respiratory herpes simplex virus infection with acyclovir in patients with the adult respiratory distress syndrome. Am Rev Respir Dis 136: 402–405
30. Limaye AP, Kirby KA, Rubenfeld GD, et al (2008) Cytomegalovirus reactivation in critically ill immunocompetent patients. JAMA 300: 413–422
31. Anderson LJ (1991) Major trends in nosocomial viral infections. Am J Med 91: 107S–111S
32. Kalil AC, Florescu DF (2009) Prevalence and mortality associated with cytomegalovirus infection in nonimmunosuppressed patients in the intensive care unit. Crit Care Med 37: 2350–2358
33. Papazian L, Fraisse A, Garbe L, et al (1996) Cytomegalovirus. An unexpected cause of ventilator-associated pneumonia. Anesthesiology 84: 280–287
34. Cook CH, Zhang Y, Sedmak DD, Martin LC, Jewell S, Ferguson RM (2006) Pulmonary cytomegalovirus reactivation causes pathology in immunocompetent mice. Crit Care Med 34: 842–849
35. Papazian L., Doddoli C, Chetaille B, et al (2007) A contributive result of open-lung biopsy improves survival in acute respiratory distress syndrome patients. Crit Care Med 35: 755–762
36. Raoult D, Audic S, Robert C, et al (2004) The 1.2-megabase genome sequence of Mimivirus. Science 306: 1344–1350
37. La Scola B, Marrie TJ, Auffray JP, Raoult D (2005) Mimivirus in pneumonia patients. Emerg Infect Dis 11: 449–452
38. Berger P, Papazian L, Drancourt M, La Scola B, Auffray JP, Raoult D (2006). Ameba-associated microorganisms and diagnosis of nosocomial pneumonia. Emerg Infect Dis 12: 248–255
39. Dare RK, Chittaganpitch M, Erdman DD (2008) Screening pneumonia patients for mimivirus. Emerg.Infect.Dis 14: 465–467
40. Vincent A, La Scola B, Forel JM, Pauly V, Raoult V, Papazian L (2009) Clinical significance of a positive serology for mimivirus in patients presenting a suspicion of ventilator-associated pneumonia. Crit Care Med 37: 111–118

VII

VIII Fungal Infections

Early Recognition of Invasive Candidiasis in the ICU

P.-E. Charles, R. Bruyere, and F. Dalle

Introduction

Invasive candidiasis, mainly due to *Candida albicans*, is a life-threatening complication encountered in intensive care units (ICUs) [1, 2]. *Candida* spp. is regularly
reported as the fourth most frequent microbial agent responsible for blood-borne
infections in ICU-acquired sepsis [3, 4]. Moreover, cumulative evidence supports
the fact that the incidence of invasive candidiasis is increasing. In addition, an
epidemiological shift, namely the emergence of non-*albicans* species against
which azoles are often less effective, has been reported over the past two decades
[5].

VIII

It is acknowledged that in most cases, the source of infection is the gut [1].
Thus, yeast growth within the intestinal lumen is the first step in the pathophysiological process that, in some cases, can lead to mucosal invasion and finally
blood stream infection.

Thanks to tremendous progress, new antifungal drugs, echinocandins, have
been developed so that safe, effective, broad-spectrum therapies are still available
[6, 7]. However, mortality rates remain high among patients with invasive candidiasis [8]. Besides the severity of the underlying disease of these patients, the fact
that antifungal treatments are frequently delayed is probably one of the main
causes of treatment failure [9]. This is because the commonly available diagnostic
tools are still not sufficiently reliable to provide an accurate and prompt diagnosis
of invasive candidiasis.

Two main questions arise from these observations: (i) How can patients with
the highest risk of invasive candidiasis patients be identified? (ii) What evidence
can justify the use of early antifungal drugs in this setting? In an attempt to
answer these issues, we have to make use of observational studies that assess risk
factors for invasive candidiasis, the few well-conducted clinical trials assessing
early antifungal therapy, and finally experts' guidelines.

How to Identify Patients With The Highest Risk of Invasive Candidiasis Among Critically Ill Patients?

A Few Words About the Pathophysiology of Invasive Candidiasis

Candida albicans is a commensal germ of the digestive tract [1]. Some conditions, such as exposure to antibiotics might favour colonization. The gut could
then become a putative source of yeasts, but additional circumstances are needed
to make *Candida* spp. a pathogen. The adhesion of yeast cells to the epithelial

J.-L. Vincent (ed.), *Annual Update in Intensive Care and Emergency Medicine 2012*
DOI 10.1007/978-3-642-25716-2 © Springer-Verlag Berlin Heidelberg 2012

surface is probably a very critical step [10]. Thereafter, *Candida* spp. has to cross the epithelial barrier. However, the underlying mechanisms are still unknown. It is hypothesized that the ability of *C. albicans* to form germ tubes allows it to go through epithelial cells and invade the gut mucosa [11, 12]. Another pathway could be intercellular spaces within the intestinal epithelia. Although these junctions are normally tight and almost impossible to penetrate, *Candida* spp. may be able to disrupt the junction to reach the deepest layers of the mucosa. Interestingly, although several virulence factors have been identified, it seems more likely that host factors play a major role during the pathogenesis of invasive candidiasis. One important conclusion that could be drawn from these experimental data is that it takes time for yeasts from the intestinal lumen to reach the blood compartment. In other words, yeast invasion precedes the positive blood culture. Although the time required is unknown, one can suppose that clinical as well as biological markers are present throughout this period. The challenge is therefore to recognize such early signs of a coming infection and to prescribe appropriate antifungal drugs.

Clinical Rules: Description, Relevance and Limitations

Several clinical rules have been established in an attempt to identify patients with an obvious risk of developing invasive candidiasis during their ICU stay. These rules were based on the assessment of the most relevant risk factors identified previously in large cohorts of critically ill patients. Thus, given the importance of invasive candidiasis from a pathophysiological point of view, in the early 1990s, Pittet et al. proposed a rule based on the assessment of fungal colonization density [13]. The so-called colonization index involves multiple sampling from the skin and mucosal surfaces. A threshold value of 0.5, meaning that at least half of the specimens was positive for *Candida* spp, predicted the risk of invasive candidiasis with 100 % sensitivity and 69 % specificity. The corrected colonization index takes into account only positive culture results (i.e., the number of strongly positive cultures divided by the number of all positive cultures), and shows even greater diagnostic accuracy since 100 % sensitivity and 100 % specificity were achieved using a threshold of 0.4. In addition, intense colonization was likely to precede the diagnosis of invasive candidiasis by 6 days. Although very attractive, Pittet's index raises several issues. First, from a practical point of view, the genuine colonization index cannot be assessed routinely in the ICU setting. This is because daily cultures are required as well as *Candida* spp. isolate genotyping since only isogenic strains from a given patient are considered for its calculation. Second, no studies have been conducted to demonstrate the external validity of the colonization index, that is to say the validation of its predictive value in a larger cohort of patients, as recommended before proposing any diagnostic tool. Such a validation study is, however, desirable given the findings in the so called 'inception' study in 29 high-risk surgical patients known to be colonized by *Candida* spp. according to a first screening. These patients accounted for only 5 % of all the admissions over the study period. Such patients should, therefore, be considered highly selected and not really representative of the general ICU population. On the basis of Pittet's findings, Piarroux et al. conducted a single-center study with a before-after design [14]. They showed that invasive candidiasis became very unlikely in their surgical ICU as soon as every patient was given fluconazole in accordance with the colonization index value. Interestingly, the patients included had undergone major abdominal surgery, and therefore resemble those included in the *princeps* study. However, the relevance of the index could be different in another population. We showed in a prospective study that a colonization index greater than 0.5 was a common finding in a 'medical' ICU since more than one third of the patients reached such a value, but none of them developed invasive candidiasis [15]. Moreover, the clinical relevance of the colonization index as a decision tool raised serious concerns after the publication of the EPCAN group study, since Leon et al. reported 72 % sensitivity and 47 % specificity for the colonization index in a cohort of more than 1000 critically ill patients from 36 distinct ICUs [16]. One can therefore conclude that *Candida* spp. colonization density cannot be the only predictor for invasive fungal disease in the ICU setting and that additional risk factors need to be assessed.

To this end, some authors have tested the predictive value of clinical rules including other risk factors. Ostrosky-Zeichner et al. proposed a rule based on the results from an observational study that included more than 2000 patients in the USA [17]. The independent risk factors identified (i.e., central venous catheter, dialysis, total parenteral nutrition, systemic antibiotic, surgery, pancreatitis, steroids and use of immunosuppressive agents) were included in a scoring system. This prediction rule exhibited 34 % sensitivity, 90 % specificity, a positive predictive value (PPV) of 1 % and a negative predictive value (NPV) of 97 %. Interestingly, fungal colonization was not assessed since it was not identified as an independent predictor in a previous study by the same group [18]. However, it is worth noting that only one single mycological sample was obtained in these patients, making any colonization density assessment unreliable. As a result, the clinical rule proposed by these authors exhibited very low PPV (i.e., 1 %) while the NPV reached 97 %. Playford et al. applied this rule to their own cohort of patients and obtained comparable results [19]. Interestingly, fungal colonization was assessed prospectively in these patients. Thus, they showed that using the previously described clinical rule generated a lot of false positive results. Moreover, including *Candida* spp. colonization as a risk factor led to an almost 10 % improvement in specificity. This illustrates the fact that invasive candidiasis is very unlikely in patients without apparent fungal colonization. Following on from these data, the EPCAN study group conducted a large cohort study to identify the most relevant risk factors for invasive candidiasis [20]. More than 1000 critically patients mainly from Spain were included. All consecutive patients free of prior fungal infection and without antifungal treatment were included as soon as they had spent at least 7 days in the ICU. Fungal colonization was assessed twice a week until death or discharge. This group found only four independent variables likely to predict the risk of invasive candidiasis: Severe sepsis, surgery, total parenteral nutrition (TPN) and multifocal colonization, defined as the presence of at least two samples from distinct body sites growing *Candida* spp. The "Candida score" construction was based on the respective statistical weight of each of the above-mentioned risk factors (severe sepsis: 2 points; surgery: 1 point; TPN: 1 point; multifocal colonization: 1 point). According to this first evaluation study, the accuracy of the Candida score was promising since sensitivity was 81 % and specificity was 74 % when a threshold of 2.5 points was used. A validation study was then conducted in another large cohort of critically ill patients admitted to the ICU for more than one week [16] (**Table 1**). The high NPV of the Candida score was emphasized since less than 3 % of the patients with a score less than 3 actually developed invasive candidiasis. However, the PPV was quite low (14 %)

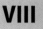

VIII

Table 1. Diagnostic accuracy of the Candida Score and the Colonization index according to validation study results [16].

	Candida Score ≥ 3 (95 % CI)	Colonization Index ≥ 0.5 (95 % CI)
Area under ROC curve	0.774 (0.715 – 0.832)	0.633 (0.557 – 0.709)
Sensitivity	77.6 (66.9 – 88.3)	72.4 (60.9 – 83.9)
Specificity	66.2 (63.0 – 69.4)	47.4 (44.0 – 50.8)
Predictive positive value	13.8 (10.0 – 17.5)	8.7 (6.2 – 11.3)
Predictive negative value	97.7 (96.4 – 98.9)	96.1 (94.2 – 98.0)
Relative risk for invasive candidiasis	5.98 (3.28 – 10.92)	2.24 (1.28 – 3.93)

ROC: receiver operating characteristic; CI: confidence interval

since sensitivity and specificity were 78 % and 66 %, respectively. Although better than fungal colonization alone as measured by the Pittet's index, the overall accuracy of the Candida score was disappointing since the area under the receiver operating characteristic (ROC) curve was 0.774, compared with 0.847 found in the first study.

Apart from the above-mentioned studies, other interesting data on high-risk surgical patients have been published. More than 20 years ago, Calandra et al. showed that abdominal surgery should not be considered an unequivocal risk factor for invasive candidiasis [21]. These authors showed that only patients with major surgery, especially those with anastomosis leakage and recurrent perforations, were the most likely to develop invasive candidiasis. Moreover, they showed that the presence of yeast in the peritoneal fluid had to be considered only if *Candida* spp. density was high and growing fast. More recently, other authors have proposed a clinical rule likely to predict the presence of *Candida* spp. within the peritoneal fluid of patients with gut perforation [22]. They showed that shock, upper gastrointestinal tract origin, female sex and exposure to antibiotics were independently associated with the risk of fungal peritonitis.

In conclusion, fungal colonization is considered a prerequisite for the development of invasive candidiasis. It therefore needs to be assessed in patients with suspected invasive candidiasis. The presence of multifocal *Candida* spp. colonization makes invasive candidiasis more likely, but other relevant risk factors should be thoroughly evaluated given the very poor PPV of colonization alone [23]. Several rules, including the Candida score calculation, have been reported so far. However, although helpful for the identification of patients with a very low risk of invasive candidiasis, such diagnosis strategies remain controversial given the unacceptably high rate of false positive results, which is likely to encourage useless if not harmful antifungal treatments. Additional markers of the disease are therefore urgently needed.

Biomarkers

As described above, whereas *Candida* spp. gut colonization is a critical step in the pathogenesis of invasive candidiasis, subsequent events are required to allow the yeast to reach the bloodstream. It is therefore challenging to identify patients who will actually develop invasive infection among those who are colonized.

Detecting circulating yeast is totally specific but may be unreliable if the current blood culture process is used, as the expected sensitivity is no more than

50 %, with a mean time to positivity of almost 2 days [24]. Using specific media for yeast could however enhance *Candida* spp. growth. Another approach relies on the detection of fungal DNA in the blood, since routine testing is already possible [25]. However, DNA extraction from the blood is still a concern, and as a result, false negative results are still possible. Another promising way to circumvent culture-based methods is to detect fungal outer membrane compounds, since convincing results have been obtained in immunosuppressed patients. We will focus on mannan and 1,3-ß-D-glucan. High positive and negative values have been reported with both markers in patients with prolonged neutropenia [26]. In addition, it has been shown that the detection of such biomarkers could precede candidemia by more than 1 week [27, 28]. One could, therefore, hypothesize that during the gut mucosa invasion process, fungal products reach the bloodstream before the yeast itself. However, no prospective studies have ascertained whether or not early detection of invasive candidiasis through biomarker assessment leads to earlier antifungal treatment and in turn improves the outcome. In addition, the above-mentioned studies used the EORTC (European Organisation for Research and Treatment of Cancer) diagnosis criteria, the relevance of which in the ICU setting is still unknown [29].

A few studies have addressed the question of 1,3-ß-D-glucan in critically ill non-neutropenic patients. Takesue et al. compared the positivity rate of the biomarker in a population of high-risk postoperative patients colonized with *Candida* spp. regarding the clinical response to empirical fluconazole therapy [30]. They showed that the number of colonized sites as well as the detection of a significant amount of 1,3-ß-D-glucan in serum was independently associated with an improvement under therapy. However, although fewer than 10 % of the fluconazole-responders exhibited a negative result, more than 50 % of the non-responders tested positive. Altogether, these data illustrate to what extent 1,3-ß-D-glucan lacks specificity in the ICU setting. Other observational studies have provided similar findings. Digby et al. showed that 1,3-ß-D-glucan was unable to differentiate between fungal and bacterial infections [31]. They also reported that *Candida* spp. colonization was likely to be associated with positive results regardless of the subsequent occurrence of invasive candidiasis. It is also worth noting that dialysis, albumin perfusion, antibiotics and surgical gauze are also likely to provide false positive results. In an attempt to increase the PPV of the test and to circumvent these issues, other authors applied a higher cut-off value (i.e., 80 instead of 20 pg/ml) [32]. As a result, they found a high number of false negative results. Finally, whether or not these biomarkers are of clinical interest in the ICU setting has yet to be demonstrated.

Systemic inflammation related biomarkers have proven useful for the early diagnosis of sepsis. Among them, procalcitonin (PCT) is one the most interesting. Unfortunately, our group has shown that PCT was of little value in patients with candidemia since only a mild elevation was detected as compared with bacteremia [33]. However, although weak, PCT increase is significantly greater during fungal infection than in patients with *Candida* spp. colonization alone [34].

Genetic Approach

More recent findings have raised comment and hopes. It has been shown that some genetic determinants could influence the ability of the host to become colonized or infected by *Candida* spp. Prior to these results, Bochud et al. reported that Toll-like receptor (TLR) 4 gene polymorphism was likely to worsen the prognosis of hematopoietic stem cell transplant recipients with pulmonary invasive aspergillosis [35]. Similarly, Plantinga et al. showed in similar patients that one variant of the dectin-1 gene was associated with the risk of developing both colonization and infection with *Candida* spp. [36]. Moreover, they showed *in vitro* that cells from these subjects were less responsive to yeast with respect to the release of inflammatory mediators, which could account for an increased susceptibility to these infections. Although data are not yet available in the ICU setting, one could imagine that screening for such polymorphisms on admission could be useful to stratify patients with regard to the risk of invasive candidiasis.

Conclusions

Predicting the risk of invasive candidiasis is challenging. Despite considerable knowledge of the clinical risk factors thanks to the results from several well-conducted large cohort studies, we are still unable to diagnose this life-threatening ICU-acquired infection in a reliable and timely manner. The detection of outer-membrane *Candida* spp. compounds could be a promising avenue, but the data published so far are disappointing. Other biomarkers are therefore required. Host factors should also be taken into account, and the genomic approach could therefore become a relevant way to improve risk assessment in critically ill patients.

VIII

What Evidence Supports the Use of Early Antifungal Drugs in this Setting?

As mentioned above, the earlier antifungal treatment is started, the better the prognosis. It has been shown that the mortality rate can increase from 15 % to 30 % if the time elapsed between the first positive blood culture and treatment exceeds 12 hours [9, 37]. Hence, because of the lack of reliable diagnostic tools, we are obliged to start antifungal drugs before evidence of infection is available.

Definitions: From Empirical Treatment to Prophylaxis

Essentially, antifungal administration should be considered in any patient with unexplained sepsis and risk factors for invasive candidiasis, including *Candida* spp. multifocal colonization, if no significant clinical improvement is achieved despite a 2-day course of broad spectrum antibiotics. This type of treatment is empirical. It has been proposed that patients should be treated earlier, that is as soon as they become intensively colonized with *Candida* spp. This type of treatment is pre-emptive therapy. Some high-risk patients may benefit from antifungal treatment at ICU admission if the risk of invasive candidiasis is too high. This type of treatment is prophylaxis.

Review and Limits of the Main Available Trials

Most of the available trials addressing the question of early antifungal therapy in critically ill patients were designed to evaluate prophylaxis. Inclusion criteria aimed at selecting a potentially high-risk population, because only patients with a prolonged ICU-stay and/or mechanical ventilation requirement were generally enrolled. Pelz et al. showed that fluconazole prophylaxis reduced the incidence of fungal invasive disease by one half in a single surgical ICU [38]. However, the definition of invasive disease raised some serious concerns since "presumed" and "suspected" infections (and not only proven) were also considered, representing 24 out of the 31 events. As a result, some patients with colonization rather than infection were falsely classified. Thus, despite a rate of invasive candidiasis exceeding 10 % in the study population, the length of stay was short and more than 85 % of the patients were discharged alive from the ICU, regardless of the randomization group. These data should, therefore, be taken very cautiously since mortality rates associated with invasive candidiasis are generally more than 30 %. Garbino et al. published an interesting trial on mechanically ventilated patients with an ICU length of stay exceeding 2 days [39]. In contrast to the previous study, the main endpoint was candidemia. These authors showed that fluconazole prophylaxis was likely to reduce the incidence of candidemia. Although underpowered, the authors failed to demonstrate any difference in mortality. In addition, the external validity of this single center study raised concerns since all the included patients underwent a selective digestive decontamination protocol, a condition likely to increase the risk of fungal disease. Thus, the candidemia rate reached 16 % in the control group, an unusual rate if prolonged mechanical ventilation was actually the only risk factor. The fact that *Candida* spp. colonization as assessed through Pittet's index calculation was obvious in most of the patients on inclusion could account for this, emphasizing the weight of this risk factor. In the already mentioned 'before-after' study published by Piarroux et al., it was shown that fluconazole prophylaxis could prevent invasive candidiasis in a selected population of postoperative patients with high levels of fungal colonization [14]. However, although statistically significant, the difference was not readily clinically relevant since the number of ICU-acquired candidemias (i.e., those which could really have been prevented by the intervention) decreased from 2.2 % to 0 %. In addition, the authors failed to demonstrate any survival benefit despite having included nearly 500 patients in each arm. We believe therefore that such a 'preemptive' strategy targets too many patients, leading to large numbers of antifungal treatments in order to avoid a very few episodes of invasive candidiasis.

Despite its small size (n = 49), an earlier study by Eggimann et al., showed that it was possible to select more accurately the patients who could really benefit from antifungal prophylaxis in the ICU [40]. Accordingly, the only patients with high-risk surgical condition (i.e., recurrent gut perforations, anastomose leakage, severe acute pancreatitis) were included and randomized to receive either fluconazole or placebo. As a result, a 30 % absolute risk reduction was achieved. It was however a single center study underpowered to demonstrate any decrease in mortality.

Apart from these studies, only one well conducted multicenter trial that evaluated empirical antifungal treatment in critically ill patients has been conducted [41] (**Table 2**). All patients with persistent fever despite broad-spectrum antibiotics were included. Schuster et al. randomized 270 ICU patients to either placebo or high-dose fluconazole in a double-blind fashion. The primary objective was to assess the clinical response to therapy using a composite endpoint. The response to treatment was defined as fever resolution in the absence of proven fungal infection, drug-related toxicity or introduction of a new antifungal drug. Around one third of the included patients in both arms were considered as responders given their favorable outcome according to the endpoint definition. However, the

Table 2. Main results from the multicenter randomized double-blind trial comparing fluconazole to placebo as empirical treatment of invasive candidiasis in the ICU. Success was defined as fever resolution in the absence of drug toxicity, proven invasive fungal disease or use of an alternative antifungal treatment [41].

Outcomes	Fluconazole recipients (n = 122)	Placebo recipients (n = 127)	Relative Risk	P value
Success	44 (36 %)	48 (38 %)	0.95 (0.69 – 1.32)	0.78
Failure	78 (64 %)	79 (62 %)	–	–

rate of invasive candidiasis was quite low in the placebo group (9 %) and probably even overestimated, since 5 of the 11 infected patients presented with candiduria. Consequently, one may consider that the risk of invasive fungal disease was too low in the study population, making any benefit from empirical fluconazole unlikely. Actually, less than half of the included patients exhibited multifocal *Candida* spp. colonization. However, such data emphasize to what extent empirical antifungal therapy administration should target a restrictive subset of critically ill patients.

Finally, the clinical trials described above have generally been single center studies underpowered for any survival assessment. Moreover, the patients included in the different studies have been different in terms of risk for fungal disease. Hence, various inclusion criteria have been used: Multifocal *Candida* spp. colonization, abdominal surgery or prolonged mechanical ventilation as some examples. In addition, although the incidence of invasive candidiasis is the main endpoint, the authors used various definitions of the disease. As a result, one cannot exclude that in some cases, patients with *Candida* spp. colonization were falsely considered as really infected. Since antifungal exposure is likely to reduce colonization density, such concerns may have led to an overestimation of the clinical benefit from prophylaxis.

However, despite the above mentioned serious methodological concerns, several meta-analyses have been performed [42, 43]. These analyses concluded that antifungal prophylaxis was likely to reduce the incidence of invasive fungal infection in the ICU and to a lesser extent to improve the outcome of high-risk critically ill patients. The authors acknowledged that a risk of invasive candidiasis of more than 15 % should be achieved in order to expect a benefit from early antifungal drug therapy [43]. They extrapolate from previous clinical trials results that the number needed to treat to prevent one invasive candidiasis episode was acceptable in such a high-risk subset of patients. However, it is worth noting that all these meta-analyses were published before publication of the study by Schuster et al. [41], the results of which may have led to different conclusions. In addition, none of those trials addressed the question of the risk of selection of azole-resistant *Candida* species. However, it is worth noting that these species, especially *C. glabrata*, are of growing importance in the ICU setting. As a result, fluconazole should not remain the first-intention drug when considering early antifungal therapy in a critically ill patient.

What Is the Place of Echinocandins?

Echinocandins are new antifungal drugs that have been available for about 10 years [7]. Caspofungin, anidulafungin and micafungin are the three licensed echinocandins. They all exhibit powerful fungicidal activity against most of the *Candida* spp., especially the non-*albicans* species known to develop resistance to azoles (i.e., *C. krusei* and *C. glabrata*). However, their minimal inhibitory concentrations against *C. parapsilosis* are higher, although actual clinical resistance has not yet been demonstrated. In addition, adverse effects are infrequent and only a few drug interactions have been described.

These drugs have been evaluated for the treatment of proven invasive candidiasis through several large and well conducted multicenter non-inferiority trials including non-neutropenic, mostly ICU patients. Caspofungin was compared to amphotericin B, and anidulafungin to fluconazole [44, 45]. In addition, micafungin was compared to caspofungin [46]. All these studies demonstrated at least the non-inferiority of the new drug. In addition, these studies provided data supporting to some extent the superiority of echinocandins compared to either amphotericin B (caspofungin) or fluconazole (anidulafungin). As a result, the most recent American guidelines recommend echinocandins as the first-choice drug in critically ill patients with proven invasive candidiasis (A-III) [47].

To the best of our knowledge, no published clinical trial has tested echinocandin in the early therapy of invasive candidiasis. Senn et al. performed an interesting study showing that if caspofungin was given as prophylaxis in some very high-risk surgical patients (i.e., recurrent perforations or anastomosis leakage), the risk of invasive fungal disease was 2 % compared to the 40 % rate reported previously in an historical cohort [48]. Although speculative, one could hypothesize that beyond the above mentioned methodological issues, more consistent data would have been obtained from previous trials if an echinocandin had been administered instead of fluconazole. Although promising, such findings must be confirmed by future randomized trials.

VIII

Current Guidelines

According to the most recent American guidelines, antifungal prophylaxis is not recommended in the ICU setting except in high-risk patients hospitalized in units where the incidence of invasive candidiasis is high (B-I) [47]. The recommended drug is fluconazole. In contrast, surprisingly, empirical treatment is recommended (B-III) for suspected invasive candidiasis in critically ill patients with unexplained fever and risk factors including multifocal fungal colonization, despite the lack of published evidence as reported above. However, the experts probably took into account the detrimental effect of any delay in antifungal administration. Another striking statement is that the echinocandins should be preferred to fluconazole in most critically ill patients, even if there are no consistent published data to support such recommendation. Given the high expected efficacy of these drugs and the poor prognosis generally associated with invasive fungal infection, it seems reasonable to promote echinocandins, while waiting for the results of ongoing clinical trials.

Conclusions

Early therapy of invasive fungal infection may be prophylactic, pre-emptive or empirical. Most published trials deal with prophylactic or pre-emptive therapies since differentiating these treatments remains difficult. Because of obvious methodological issues, the results from these studies should be taken cautiously. New trials are desirable and should aim at better selecting those patients who will really benefit from early antifungal therapy. Clinical practice needs to be improved in an attempt to: (i) treat early (if not prevent) *Candida* spp. invasive infection with the most efficient drug; (ii) avoid useless (if not deleterious) antifungal treatments.

Observational studies have shown that, in real life, antifungal administration to patients with invasive candidiasis is often delayed [49], but, on the other hand, antifungal drug consumption is increasing dramatically in the ICU, raising two major concerns: Increasing costs and the risk of emergence of resistant species [50]. Regarding the latter point, although controversial, it is worth noting that increased use of fluconazole may be responsible for a shift toward non-*albicans* species. Similarly, a relationship may exist between exposure to one echinocandin and the isolation of *C. parapsilosis* in patients with candidemia [51]. These aspects should be remembered every time one prescribes antifungal drugs.

VIII

Conclusion

Invasive candidiasis is a life-threatening infection in the ICU, management of which has improved over the past two decades. First, new efficient drugs have been developed: Fluconazole in the early 1990s, followed by echinocandins 10 years later. Simultaneously, our knowledge of fungal infection risk assessment has been enhanced by data obtained from large cohort studies. Obviously, *Candida* spp. colonization is considered as a prerequisite for infection but additional circumstances are clearly required prior to invasive disease development. However, apart from some specific high-risk surgical patients, we are still unable to reliably identify those patients who will actually benefit from early administration of antifungal agents. The development of biomarkers able to inform about the ongoing invasion process by *Candida* spp. is promising but has been disappointing. Knowledge of genetic host factors should be considered but cannot currently be implemented into every day practice.

Once suspected in a critically ill unstable patient, any *Candida* spp. infection should be treated with the most potent drug, namely an echinocandin, after samples from various body sites and blood cultures have been collected. If no evidence of infection is obtained within the next few days, there will still be time to withdraw the treatment, especially if another pathogen is recovered from blood culture as well as in the absence of multifocal *Candida* spp. colonization. However, improving early, reliable diagnosis of *Candida* spp. invasive infections is crucial: On the one hand to save lives and on the other hand to prevent any loss of efficacy of the available drugs, especially the most potent, namely echinocandins.

References

1. Eggimann P, Garbino J, Pittet D (2003) Epidemiology of Candida species infections in critically ill non-immunosuppressed patients. Lancet Infect Dis 3: 685–702
2. Falagas ME, Apostolou KE, Pappas VD (2006) Attributable mortality of candidemia: a systematic review of matched cohort and case-control studies. Eur J Clin Microbiol Infect Dis 25: 419–425
3. Kett DH, Azoulay E, Echeverria PM, et al (2011) Candida bloodstream infections in intensive care units: analysis of the extended prevalence of infection in intensive care unit study. Crit Care Med 39: 665–670
4. Wisplinghoff H, Bischoff T, Tallent SM, Seifert H, Wenzel RP, Edmond MB (2004) Nosocomial bloodstream infections in US hospitals: analysis of 24,179 cases from a prospective nationwide surveillance study. Clin Infect Dis 39: 309–317
5. Horn DL, Neofytos D, Anaissie EJ, et al (2009) Epidemiology and outcomes of candidemia in 2019 patients: Data from the Prospective Antifungal Therapy Alliance Registry. Clin Infect Dis 48: 1695–1703
6. Eggimann P, Garbino J, Pittet D (2003) Management of Candida species infections in critically ill patients. Lancet Infect Dis 3: 772–785
7. Sucher AJ, Chahine EB, Balcer HE (2009) Echinocandins: the newest class of antifungals. Ann Pharmacother 43: 1647–1657
8. Zaoutis TE, Argon J, Chu J, Berlin JA, Walsh TJ, Feudtner C (2005) The epidemiology and attributable outcomes of candidemia in adults and children hospitalized in the United States: a propensity analysis. Clin Infect Dis 41: 1232–1239
9. Garey KW, Rege M, Pai MP, et al (2006) Time to initiation of fluconazole therapy impacts mortality in patients with candidemia: a multi-institutional study. Clin Infect Dis 43: 25–31
10. Dalle F, Jouault T, Trinel PA, et al (2003) Beta-1,2- and alpha-1,2-linked oligomannosides mediate adherence of Candida albicans blastospores to human enterocytes in vitro. Infect Immun 71: 7061–7068
11. Bendel CM, Hess DJ, Garni RM, Henry-Stanley M, Wells CL (2003) Comparative virulence of Candida albicans yeast and filamentous forms in orally and intravenously inoculated mice. Crit Care Med 31: 501–507
12. Dalle F, Wachtler B, Coralie L, et al (2010) Cellular interactions of Candida albicans with human oral epithelial cells and enterocytes. Cell Microbiol 12: 248–271
13. Pittet D, Monod M, Suter PM, Frenk E, Auckenthaler R (1994) Candida colonization and subsequent infections in critically ill surgical patients. Ann Surg 220: 751–758
14. Piarroux R, Grenouillet F, Balvay P, et al (2004) Assessment of preemptive treatment to prevent severe candidiasis in critically ill surgical patients. Crit Care Med 32: 2443–2449
15. Charles PE, Dalle F, Aube H, et al (2005) Candida spp. colonization significance in critically ill medical patients: a prospective study. Intensive Care Med 31: 393–400
16. Leon C, Ruiz-Santana S, Saavedra P, et al (2009) Usefulness of the "Candida score" for discriminating between Candida colonization and invasive candidiasis in non-neutropenic critically ill patients: a prospective multicenter study. Crit Care Med 37: 1624–1633
17. Ostrosky-Zeichner L, Sable C, Sobel J, et al (2007) Multicenter retrospective development and validation of a clinical prediction rule for nosocomial invasive candidiasis in the intensive care setting. Eur J Clin Microbiol Infect Dis 26: 271–276
18. Blumberg HM, Jarvis WR, Soucie JM, et al (2001) Risk factors for candidal bloodstream infections in surgical intensive care unit patients: the NEMIS prospective multicenter study. The National Epidemiology of Mycosis Survey. Clin Infect Dis 33: 177–186
19. Playford EG, Lipman J, Kabir M, et al (2009) Assessment of clinical risk predictive rules for invasive candidiasis in a prospective multicentre cohort of ICU patients. Intensive Care Med 35: 2141–2145
20. Leon C, Ruiz-Santana S, Saavedra P, et al (2006) A bedside scoring system ("Candida score") for early antifungal treatment in nonneutropenic critically ill patients with Candida colonization. Crit Care Med 34: 730–737
21. Calandra T, Bille J, Schneider R, Mosimann F, Francioli P (1989) Clinical significance of Candida isolated from peritoneum in surgical patients. Lancet 2: 1437–1440

VIII

22. Dupont H, Bourichon A, Paugam-Burtz C, Desmonts JM (2003) Can yeast isolation in peritoneal fluid be predicted in intensive care unit patients with peritonitis? Crit Care Med 31: 752–757
23. Charles PE (2006) Multifocal Candida species colonization as a trigger for early antifungal therapy in critically ill patients: what about other risk factors for fungal infection? Crit Care Med 34: 913–914
24. Meyer MH, Letscher-Bru V, Jaulhac B, Waller J, Candolfi E (2004) Comparison of Mycosis IC/F and plus Aerobic/F media for diagnosis of fungemia by the bactec 9240 system. J Clin Microbiol 42: 773–777
25. Wahyuningsih R, Freisleben HJ, Sonntag HG, Schnitzler P (2000) Simple and rapid detection of Candida albicans DNA in serum by PCR for diagnosis of invasive candidiasis. J Clin Microbiol 38: 3016–3021
26. Senn L, Robinson JO, Schmidt S, et al (2008) 1,3-b-d-glucan antigenemia for early diagnosis of invasive fungal infections in neutropenic patients with acute leukemia. Clin Infect Dis 46: 878–885
27. Odabasi Z, Mattiuzzi G, Estey E, et al (2004) Beta-D-glucan as a diagnostic adjunct for invasive fungal infections: validation, cutoff development, and performance in patients with acute myelogenous leukemia and myelodysplastic syndrome. Clin Infect Dis 39: 199–205
28. Prella M, Bille J, Pugnale M, et al (2005) Early diagnosis of invasive candidiasis with mannan antigenemia and antimannan antibodies. Diagn Microbiol Infect Dis 51: 95–101
29. Ascioglu S, Rex JH, de Pauw B, et al (2002) Defining opportunistic invasive fungal infections in immunocompromised patients with cancer and hematopoietic stem cell transplants: an international consensus. Clin Infect Dis 34: 7–14
30. Takesue Y, Kakehashi M, Ohge H, et al (2004) Combined assessment of beta-D-glucan and degree of candida colonization before starting empiric therapy for candidiasis in surgical patients. World J Surg 28: 625–630
31. Digby J, Kalbfleisch JH, Glenn A, Larsen A, Browder W, Williams D (2003) Serum glucan levels are not specific for presence of fungal infections in intensive care unit patients. Clin Diagn Lab Immunol 10: 882–885
32. Alam FF, Mustafa AS, Khan ZU (2007) Comparative evaluation of (1, 3)-β-D-glucan, mannan and anti-mannan antibodies, and Candida species-specific snPCR in patients with candidemia. BMC Infect Dis 7: 103
33. Charles PE, Dalle F, Aho S, et al (2006) Serum procalcitonin measurement contribution to the early diagnosis of candidemia in critically ill patients. Intensive Care Med 32: 1577–1583
34. Charles PE, Castro C, Ruiz-Santana S, Leon C, Saavedra P, Martin E (2009) Serum procalcitonin levels in critically ill patients colonized with Candida spp: new clues for the early recognition of invasive candidiasis? Intensive Care Med 35: 2146–2150
35. Bochud PY, Chien JW, Marr KA, et al (2008) Toll-like receptor 4 polymorphisms and aspergillosis in stem-cell transplantation. N Engl J Med 359: 1766–1777
36. Plantinga TS, van der Velden WJ, Ferwerda B, et al (2009) Early stop polymorphism in human DECTIN-1 is associated with increased candida colonization in hematopoietic stem cell transplant recipients. Clin Infect Dis 49: 724–732
37. Morrell M, Fraser VJ, Kollef MH (2005) Delaying the empiric treatment of candida bloodstream infection until positive blood culture results are obtained: a potential risk factor for hospital mortality. Antimicrob Agents Chemother 49: 3640–3645
38. Pelz RK, Hendrix CW, Swoboda SM, et al (2001) Double-blind placebo-controlled trial of fluconazole to prevent candidal infections in critically ill surgical patients. Ann Surg 233: 542–548
39. Garbino J, Lew DP, Romand JA, Hugonnet S, Auckenthaler R, Pittet D (2002) Prevention of severe Candida infections in nonneutropenic, high-risk, critically ill patients: a randomized, double-blind, placebo-controlled trial in patients treated by selective digestive decontamination. Intensive Care Med 28: 1708–1717
40. Eggimann P, Francioli P, Bille J, et al (1999) Fluconazole prophylaxis prevents intraabdominal candidiasis in high-risk surgical patients. Crit Care Med 27: 1066–1072
41. Schuster MG, Edwards JE Jr, Sobel JD, et al (2008) Empirical fluconazole versus placebo for intensive care unit patients: a randomized trial. Ann Intern Med 149: 83–90

VIII

42. Vardakas KZ, Samonis G, Michalopoulos A, Soteriades ES, Falagas ME (2006) Antifungal prophylaxis with azoles in high-risk, surgical intensive care unit patients: a meta-analysis of randomized, placebo-controlled trials. Crit Care Med 34: 1216–1224
43. Playford EG, Webster AC, Sorrell TC, Craig JC (2006) Antifungal agents for preventing fungal infections in non-neutropenic critically ill and surgical patients: systematic review and meta-analysis of randomized clinical trials. J Antimicrob Chemother 57: 628–638
44. Reboli AC, Rotstein C, Pappas PG, et al (2007) Anidulafungin versus Fluconazole for Invasive Candidias. N Engl J Med 356: 2472–2482
45. Mora-Duarte J, Betts R, Rotstein C, et al (2002) Comparison of caspofungin and amphotericin b for invasive candidiasis. N Engl J Med 347: 2020–2029
46. Pappas PG, Rotstein CM, Betts RF, et al (2007) Micafungin versus caspofungin for treatment of candidemia and other forms of invasive candidiasis. Clin Infect Dis 45: 883–893
47. Pappas PG, Kauffman CA, Andes D, et al (2009) Clinical practice guidelines for the management of candidiasis: 2009 update by the Infectious Diseases Society of America. Clin Infect Dis 48: 503–535
48. Senn L, Eggimann P, Ksontini R, et al (2009) Caspofungin for prevention of intra-abdominal candidiasis in high-risk surgical patients. Intensive Care Med 35: 903–908
49. Bougnoux ME, Kac G, Aegerter P, d'Enfert C, Fagon JY, Group CS (2008) Candidemia and candiduria in critically ill patients admitted to intensive care units in France: incidence, molecular diversity, management and outcome. Intensive Care Med 34: 292–299
50. Marchetti O, Bille J, Fluckiger U, et al (2004) Epidemiology of candidemia in Swiss tertiary care hospitals: secular trends, 1991–2000. Clin Infect Dis 38: 311–320
51. Lortholary O, Desnos-Ollivier M, Sitbon K, Fontanet A, Bretagne S, Dromer F (2011) Recent exposure to caspofungin or fluconazole influences the epidemiology of candidemia: a prospective multicenter study involving 2,441 patients. Antimicrob Agents Chemother 55: 532–538

Management of Invasive Candidiasis in the Critically Ill

J. Garnacho-Montero, A. Díaz-Martín, and J.A. Márquez-Vácaro

Introduction

In the last few decades, fungi have become one of the most important and frequent opportunistic microorganisms involved in nosocomial infections in hospitalized patients. The most common organism implicated in fungal infections is the ubiquitous *Candida*, which is part of the human skin flora, mucosae, gastrointestinal tract, genital and urinary systems. Candidiasis encompasses diverse diseases that range from superficial infections of skin and mucosal membranes, to disseminated diseases with profound organ involvement. Deep-seated infections include candidemia, invasive candiadiasis, and peritonitis as well as other entities less frequently diagnosed in the critically ill patient [1].

However, in critically ill patients, *Candida* spp. are frequently isolated in non-sterile sites, which have a complex and controversial management. The mere isolation of *Candida* spp. in non-sterile sites does not always justify the administration of systemic antifungal therapy although it is important to bear in mind that it may indicate a disseminated candidiasis in certain situations [2].

Diagnosis of Invasive *Candida* Diseases

Diagnosis of candidemia is not problematic since it requires the isolation of *Candida* spp. in the blood [1]. *Candida* in a blood culture should never be viewed as a contaminant and should always prompt treatment initiation.

Conversely, the diagnosis of invasive non-candidemic candidiasis remains elusive in the majority of the patients. The problem is compounded by the absence of positive blood cultures in many patients with invasive disease. The definitive diagnosis requires histological demonstration of deep organ involvement with diffuse *Candida* microabscesses with a combined acute suppurative and granulomatous reaction. However, very frequently, the use of invasive diagnostic techniques for histopathological studies is not possible because of the underlying conditions of critically ill patients [3].

Candida spp. is isolated especially in secondary nosocomial peritonitis and in tertiary peritonitis. In the case of *Candida* peritonitis, diagnosis is made by a positive culture for *Candida* in the peritoneal fluid collected during operation or by percutaneous drainage. On the contrary, *Candida* positive samples in drainage fluid from postoperative patients are not diagnostic of Candida peritonitis but should be considered as colonization [2, 4].

J.-L. Vincent (ed.), *Annual Update in Intensive Care and Emergency Medicine 2012*
DOI 10.1007/978-3-642-25716-2 © Springer-Verlag Berlin Heidelberg 2012

Microbiology

Candida albicans continues to be the species that causes the largest number of cases of candidemia and is responsible for more than 50 % of all the isolates; it is followed, in order of frequency, by *C. parapsilosis*, *C. tropicalis* and *C. glabrata*. Other species, such as *C. krusei*, *C. lusitaniae*, *C. guilliermondii* and *C. dubliniensis*, are less frequent. In critically ill adult patients, the second most frequent species is *C. tropicalis*, followed by *C. glabrata*, since *C. parapsilopsis* is more frequent in pediatric patients [5, 6].

C. glabrata is responsible for approximately 15–20 % of the isolates although this rate seems to be higher (> 30 %) in the elderly population [7]. It seems that *C. glabrata* is very prone to being resistant to fluconazole, or at least needs a higher dose, which has serious implications for treatment [8]. Similarly, *C. krusei*, which generally affects severely immunocompromised patients, is intrinsically resistant to fluconazole [9].

Studies evaluating what effect prior use of fluconazole may have on infections caused by *Candida* non-*albicans* or by species potentially resistant to fluconazole (*C glabrata* or *C krusei*) have produced contradictory results [6, 10–14]. From a practical point of view, it is important to foresee when *Candida* infection may be caused by species with proven resistance to fluconazole. In a recent study including 226 patients with candidemia, exposure to fluconazole was not a variable associated with isolation of *Candida* non-*albicans* or potentially fluconazole-resistant yeast. Nevertheless, previous fluconazole exposure was an independent predictor associated with candidemia caused by fluconazole-resistant *Candida* spp. (OR 5.09; 95 % CI 1.66–15.6; p = 0.004) [15].

This information has been obtained predominantly in series of *Candida* bloodstream infections. Data in other forms of invasive candidiasis are scarce although distribution of species seems to be very similar [16, 17]. Similarly, the epidemiology of *Candida* peritonitis has been less frequently studied. *C. albicans* is the predominant species isolated in peritonitis and the rate of non-*albicans* species ranges from 17 to 43 % [18–20]. The routine use of fluconazole in the prophylaxis of high-risk surgical patients may potentially increase the colonization rate by fluconazole resistant species, although this hypothesis was not corroborated by a recent study [21]. *C. krusei* has seldom been reported as a cause of peritonitis.

Management of Patients With Invasive Disease

Candidemia

Empirical Therapy

Intravenous antifungal therapy must be initiated in all patients with candidemia without delay. However, management of positive cultures in blood specimens obtained through an intravascular catheter is a frequent dilemma, especially if the patient is afebrile when results are available. These positive results may be considered as contamination from skin flora on the catheter hub. However, considering the low toxicity of antifungal agents and the poor outcome of invasive disease, it is unwise, regardless of the source, to ignore the presence of *Candida* in a blood culture [22]. In contrast, a positive culture of the catheter tip in the absence of a positive blood culture does not necessarily imply that treatment is required [23].

VIII

Regarding choice of therapy, if the species of *Candida* is unknown, either fluconazole or an echinocandin is an appropriate initial therapy for most adult patients. Fluconazole is reserved for non-severely ill patients without recent exposure to azoles [1–4].

Current guidelines and opinion experts recommend the use of an echinocandin in hemodynamically unstable patients or in those with a history of recent fluconazole exposure [24–27]. However, the term 'hemodynamically unstable' is not clearly defined and patients without overt shock but with failure of another organ (severe sepsis criteria) should be initially treated with an echinocandin.

Three echinocandins are currently available: Caspofungin, micafungin, and anidulafungin. The mechanism of action is via inhibition of an enzyme, β-(1,3)-D-glucan synthase, which is necessary for the synthesis of an essential component of the cell wall of several fungi. Pharmacokinetic properties of the echinocandins are shown in **Table 1**. The echinocandins display fungicidal activity against *Candida* spp, including strains that are fluconazole-resistant [28]. The *in vitro* spectrum of activity is identical among the three echinocandins. However, minimum inhibitory concentrations (MIC) are somewhat lower for micafungin and anidulafungin than for caspofungin [29]. *C. parapsilosis* and *C. guilliermondii* have decreased susceptibilities to all three echinocandins but are generally susceptible (MIC < 2 μg/ml) [30]. Clinical transcendence of these *in vitro* data seems to be negligible (**Fig. 1**).

The main results of the randomized, double-blind, non-inferiority trials that have evaluated the efficacy and safety of echinocandins are summarized in **Table 2** [31–33]. Only one clinical trial has compared two echinocandins head to head in patients with invasive candidasis and the results showed that efficacy and safety were similar with two doses of micafungin (100 mg/d or 150 mg/d) or the conven-

VIII

Table 1. Pharmacokinetic properties of the three echinocandins

	Caspofungin	Micafungin	Anidulafungin
Absorption		Not orally absorbed. i.v. only	
Distribution		Extensive into the tissues. Minimal CNS and urinary penetration	
Metabolism	Spontaneous degradation, hydrolysis and N-acetylation	Arylsulfatase COMT hydroxylation	Spontaneous degradation
Protein Binding (%)	97	>99	85-90
Dose	70 mg i.v. on day 1, then 50 mg i.v. daily thereafter	Loading dose not required. 100 mg i.v. once daily	200 mg i.v. on day 1, then 100 mg i.v. daily thereafter
Dose adjustment in renal insufficiency		Not required. Not dialyzable. No adjustment in continuous renal replacement therapies	
Dose Adjustment with hepatic impairment	Child-Pugh 7-9 70 mg i.v. on day 1, then 35 mg i.v. daily thereafter CYP inducers 70 mg i.v. daily No experience with Child-Pugh > 9	None. No experience with Child-Pugh > 9	None. No experience with Child-Pugh > 9

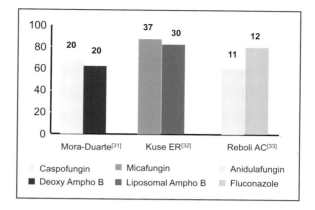

Fig. 1. Clinical cure rate in episodes of candidemia caused by *C. parapsilosis*

tional dose of caspofungin [34]. Nowadays, the three echinocandins can be considered interchangeable as therapy for invasive candidiasis in non-neutropenic patients [35]. Characteristics that differentiate the echinocandins include approved indications, requirement for a loading dose, and drug interaction profile. It is worth mentioning that critically ill patients comprise only a fraction of the general pool of patients enrolled in these trials, but secondary analyses in this subgroup of patients have been performed showing a lower efficacy of all antifungal drugs than in the entire cohort [36, 37].

Amphotericin B deoxycholate is considered obsolete in ICU patients because of its high toxicity. However, liposomal amphotericin B is also a valid alternative

Table 2. Comparison of the three randomized controlled trials designed to evaluate efficacy and safety of echinocandins

Author (ref)	Drug (number-of patients)	Response [%]	Mortality rate (%)	Commentary
Mora-Duarte et al [31]	Caspofungin (109)	73.4	34.2	In patients with study treatment for at least 5 days: favorable response in 80.7 % of patients in caspofungin arm compared with 64.9 % wth amphotericin B (difference, 15.4 %; 95 % CI, 1.1 – 29.7).
	Ampho B deoxyctolate (115)	61.7	30	
Kuse et al [32]	Micafungin (264)	89.6	40	
	Liposomal Ampho B (267)	89.5	40	
Reboli et al [33]	Anidulafungin (127)	75.6	22.8	Removing data from the site enrolling the largest number of patients: success rate was 73.2 % in the anidulafungin group and 61.1 % in the fluconazole group (difference, 12.1 %; 95 % CI, −1.1 to 25.3).
	Fluconazole (118)	60.2 (difference, 15.4 %; 95 % CI, 3.9 to 27.0).	31.4	

VIII

with a high efficacy similar to the echinocandins. Nevertheless, in two clinical trials, the rate of renal dysfunction and infusion-related reactions were significantly higher with liposomal amphotericin B than with an echinocandin [32, 38]. In contrast, voriconazole is not a first line agent. It was approved for the treatment of candidemia after it was compared with conventional amphotericin B/fluconazole in an open trial [39]. Nevertheless, its less predictable pharmacokinetics, frequent drug interactions, likely resistance in fluconazole-resistant *Candida* spp, and the recommendation not to use intravenously in renal failure (creatinine clearance < 30 ml/min) limit its use in critically ill patients [40].

Duration of therapy

Recommended duration of therapy for candidemia in non-neutropenic patients without metastatic complications is 2 weeks after documented clearance of *Candida* from the bloodstream and resolution of symptoms attributable to candidemia [24, 26].

An echocardiogram must be performed in all patients with recurrent candidemia to rule out endocarditis [1]. Fundoscopic evaluation for the presence of *Candida* endophthalmitis should be performed in patients with candidemia. This diagnosis has clear implications: Need for surgery, antifungal choice, and longer duration of treatment (at least four to six weeks). Treatments for *Candida* endophthalmitis have not been evaluated in well-designed clinical trials. Fluconazole and voriconazole achieve high concentrations in the vitreous humor. Liposomal amphotericin B at a dosage of 3–5 mg/kg daily is a valid option. Concentrations are very low with the three echinocnadins although case reports have communicated their utility, usually in combination with other antifungal drugs. For sight-threatening episodes, intravitreal injection of either amphotericin B or voriconazole should be used as adjunctive therapy [41, 42].

Directed therapy

Therapy can be modified based on susceptibility results. Hence, a change from the echinocandin empirically administered to fluconazole is recommended for patients whose clinical condition has improved, follow-up cultures have been negative for at least 48 hours, and candida isolates are susceptible to fluconazole [24, 25, 26]. The optimal duration of therapy before change to fluconazole is uncertain but it seems prudent to maintain the echinocandin for at least seven days, especially in critically ill patients with organ dysfunction. Obviously, these uncertainties warrant further research via randomized controlled trials or cohort studies.

Directed antifungal therapy can vary depending on the isolated species. Thus, for *C. parapsilosis*, the drugs of choice are fluconazole if the clinical condition is improving or liposomal amphotericin B in case of recurrent candidemia or in an unstable patient (persistence of severe sepsis or septic shock). *C. glabrata* should be treated with an echinocandin, with liposomal amphotericin B a valid alternative. De-escalation to fluconazole can be performed but always after verification of susceptibility to this azole. In candidemia caused by *C. lusitaniae* that appears to be less susceptible to amphotericin B, an echinocandin or fluconazole are suitable alternatives.

The use of antifungal associations for the treatment of candidemia is not recommended and should be considered only in selected cases with persistent candidemia after removal of the venous catheter, especially in neutropenic patients.

Management of the catheter

Conflicting data exist regarding the most appropriate time for catheter withdrawal, or the population of patients that will benefit most from such an intervention. Diverse studies have concluded that, in patients with *Candida* spp. bloodstream infection, early catheter removal is associated with a reduction in the death risk [43, 44], whereas others concluded that the timing of catheter withdrawal does not influence the outcome [45, 46]. Nevertheless, removal of all existing catheters is judicious as part of the correct management of a candidemia, especially in the critical care setting. *C. parapsilosis* is very frequently associated with catheters, especially if used for administration of total parenteral nutrition [47]. Therefore, catheter withdrawal is mandatory in episodes cause by this species.

Invasive Candidiasis

Candida colonization

The management of invasive candidiasis remains severely hampered by delays in diagnosis and the lack of reliable diagnostic methods for detection of tissue invasion by *Candida* spp. However, recovery of *Candida* spp. from multiple superficial sites has been identified as a risk factor for deeply invasive candidiasis [2, 15, 16].

Candida colonization is documented in nearly 60 % of non-neutropenic critically ill patients admitted to the ICU for more than 7 days. However, only 5 – 30 % of all colonized patients will develop invasive candidiasis [3]. Of note, patients with multifocal *Candida* colonization have a higher mortality than non-colonized patients or patients with unifocal colonization and a similar mortality to patients with demonstrated invasive *Candida* infection [48].

Furthermore, site of colonization may be of value to identify patients at high risk of invasive candidiasis. Thus, the risk of invasive candidiasis is significantly higher in patients with urinary or gastrointestinal colonization than when *Candida* spp. is isolated in other anatomic sites (skin, respiratory tract, oropharynx or stomach) [49]. In a surgical ICU, there was a statistically significant difference in the frequency of invasive candidiasis comparing patients with and without urinary (13.2 % versus 2.8 %), respiratory (8.0 % versus 1.2 %), and rectum/-ostomy (8.4 % versus 0 %) colonization. Moreover, patients with negative rectum/-ostomy cultures and patients with both negative urine and respiratory tract cultures did not develop invasive disease [50].

However, the unique presence of *Candida* colonization does not justify the use of systemic antifungal therapy [8]. In critically ill patients, there are many factors promoting colonization and subsequent infection, such as underlying diseases, presence of venous catheters, parenteral nutrition, use of broad-spectrum antibiotics, acute pancreatitis, abdominal surgery or intestinal leakages.

Clinical scores

Various diagnostic approaches have been proposed to identify patients at risk of invasive candidiasis because rigorous selection of high-risk patients is crucial to optimize the risk-benefit ratio of this therapy. Unselected ICU patients usually have an underlying risk of invasive candidiasis of 1 – 2 %.

The colonization index and the corrected colonization index were developed by Pittet and coworkers to predict the risk of invasive candidiasis in critically ill surgical patients [51]. A cut-off point ≥ 0.4 of the corrected colonization index

VIII

Table 3. Clinical indexes to predict risk of invasive candidiasis

	Study characteristics	Conditions required	Cut-off value	Sensitivity/ specificity	PPV/ NPV
Pittet's Colonization Index	Prospective study Surgical ICU patients	Ratio of the number of non-blood DBS colonized by *Candida* spp. to the total number of body sites cultured.	≥ 0.5	100 %/ 69 %	0.66/1
Pittet's Corrected Colonization Index	Prospective study Surgical ICU patients	Ratio of the numbers of DBS showing heavy growth$^{\Psi}$ to the total of DBS growing *Candida* spp.	≥ 0.4	100 %/ 100 %	1/1
Candida Score	At least 7 days at ICU No prior antifungal therapy Candidemia incidence 5.8 %	• Multifocal *Candida* colonization (1 point) • Surgery at admission (1 point) • Parenteral nutrition (1 point) • Severe sepsis (2 point)	≥ 3	77.6 %/ 66.2 %	0.138/ 0.977
Ostrosky-Zeichner Redefined Index	No prior antifungal therapy Immunocompetent IC incidence 3.7 %	≥ 4 days in ICU, plus: • MV ≥ 48h • Antibiotic use • Presence of CVC • And one of: – major surgery – pancreatitis – parenteral nutrition – renal replacement – immunosupresive therapy (corticoids included)	NA	50 %/ 83 %	0.10/ 0.97
Nebraska Medical Center (NMC) Rule	No prior antifungal therapy IC incidence 2.3 %	≥ 4 days in ICU, plus: • Broad spectrum antibiotic use (BSAbx) • Presence of CVC • Abdominal surgery • Corticosteroid therapy • Parenteral nutrition (TPN) • Mean pre-ICU LOS	2.45	84.1 %/ 60.2 %	0.047/ 0.994

DBS: distinct body sites; IC: invasive candidiasis; MV: mechanical ventilation; LOS: length of stay; TPN: total parenteral nutrition; PPV: positive predictive value; NPV: negative predictive value; $^{\Psi}$Heavy growth: large amount of *Candida* spp. in the semiquantitative culture (except for gastric juice and urine specimen), corresponding to ≥ 10^5 cfu/ml. NMC Rule: (1.537 x BSAbx*) + (0.873 x CVC*) + (0.922 x TPN*) + (0.402 x steroids§) + (0.879 x abdominal surgery) + (0.039 x pre-ICU LOS) where * = days 1 to 3 in ICU and § = days –7 to 3 in ICU

(CCI) is highly suggestive of invasive candidiasis although is a laborious tool for daily practice (**Table 3**).

In a prospective study involving 1,720 patients admitted to Spanish ICUs longer than one week, colonized patients were compared to those with a confirmed diagnosis of invasive fungal infection by *Candida* spp. Using a logistic regression model, a scoring system, termed Candida score, was obtained [48]. In a prospective study that included more than 1,000 critically patients, the same group validated this score that showed a higher sensitivity and specificity than the Pittet's colonization index [49] (**Table 3**).

In 2007, Ostrosky-Zeichner found that in intensive care patients, presence of a central venous catheter or broad-spectrum antibiotics in combination with at least two minor risk factors (**Table 3**) was predictive of invasive candidiasis [52]. More recently, in a retrospective matched case-control study, this prediction score was validated, giving a sensitivity of 73.9 with a specificity of 60.6 % yielding a high negative predictive value (NPV) of 99 % and a very low positive predictive value (PPV) of 4.2 % [53]. These authors also described a new prediction rule (Nebraska Medical Center rule) with a PPV of 0.047 and a NPV of 0.994 [53] (**Table 3**).

Procalcitonin

In critically ill patients with multifocal *Candida* colonization who develop invasive candidiasis, serum procalcitonin levels at day 7 are higher than in other patients, increasing the PPV of the Candida Score from 44.7 to 59.3 %, the NPV remaining high (88.9 %) [54].

Candida biomarkers

A number of methods based on the detection of *Candida* mannan, anti-mannan antibodies, *Candida albicans* germ-tube antibodies, and (1,3)-beta-D-glucan, have been used for the diagnosis of invasive candidiasis with conflicting results [55–57].

VIII

An assay to measure serum (1,3)-beta-D-glucan, derived from fungal cell walls, has been found to be a promising instrument for the early diagnosis of invasive candidiasis. In critically ill patients, (1,3)-beta-D-glucan was also an independent predictor of invasive candidiasis (OR 1.004, 95 % CI 1.0–1.007). Simultaneous use of the Candida score and the serum value of this biomarker can be of great help to differentiate colonization from true disseminated candidiasis [49]. In 57 surgical critically ill patients, sensitivity of a positive (1,3)-beta-D-glucan (cut-off point ≥ 80 pg/ml) for identifying invasive candidiasis was 87 %, with 73 % specificity. Importantly, although only three patients had proven invasive candidiasis, (1,3)-beta-D-glucan was detected in these patients 4 to 8 days prior to diagnosis [58]. (1,3)-beta-D-glucan can be detected in other fungal infections (caused by *Aspergillus, Fusarium, Scedosporium, Pneumocystis jiroveci*). In addition, false positive results have been reported in Gram-positive bacteremia, and in patients receiving hemodialysis or albumin, immunoglobulin and glucan-containing gauze [57, 59].

A new test based on detection, by indirect immunofluorescence assay, of antibodies against the surface of *C. albicans* germ tubes is now available. Surgery has been identified as the principal clinical factor associated with positive results in critically ill patients and results seem not to be altered by antifungal agents [60]. Detection of *C. albicans* germ tube antibody in patients with infections caused by non-*albicans* species may also be positive, although titers are lower than in candidiasis caused by *C. albicans*. Further studies are required to determine the role of this biomarker in distinguishing between colonization and infection and a possible drawback is that non-*albicans* species may not be recognized.

Management of invasive candidiasis

The clinician establishes the diagnosis of suspected invasive candidiasis based on clinical predictor scores and microbiological data. Colonization is crucial to the development of invasive candidiasis. Therefore, this diagnosis should be reserved for patients with multifocal colonization (or elevated serum (1,3)-beta-D-glucan) and risk factors included in the clinical indexes. As histological confirmation is not feasible in the great majority of critically ill patients, antifungal therapy should be started once this diagnostic test is performed. Delay of antifungal therapy increases mortality in patients with candidemia [61, 62], and, similarly, it is assumed that a delay in antifungal therapy will also be associated with a worse outcome in non-candidemic invasive candidiasis.

The number of patients with forms of invasive disease other than candidemia who have been included in clinical trials evaluating new antifungals agents is low, ranging from 7 to 19 % [31, 32, 33], impeding sub-analysis of these patients' data. Therefore, information obtained in candidemia has to be extrapolated to invasive candidiasis.

The therapeutic approach is similar to that previously described for candidemia. An echinocandin is preferred for patients with severe illness and/or recent azole exposure. In this case, selection of the antifungal therapy can be performed based on colonization culture data (susceptibility results).

Information about de-escalation therapy is not available in this clinical situation. Similarly, the optimal duration of therapy is unknown and negativization of blood culture cannot be used to monitor response as occurs in candidemia. Conversely, evolution of colonization cultures and/or sero-diagnostic tests can be used to guide length of therapy. It is assumed that course of antifungal therapy is longer in invasive candidiasis than in uncomplicated candidemia [63].

Candida Peritonitis

In a large cohort of patients with peritonitis, isolation of *Candida* from peritoneal samples was associated with worse fatality rates in nosocomial peritonitis, but not in community-acquired cases [64]. As for invasive candidiasis, few cases of *Candida* peritonitis have been included in clinical trials [20]. Dupont et al. identified four independent risk factors for yeast isolation in the peritoneal fluid of critically ill patients: Female gender, an upper gastrointestinal tract origin of the peritonitis, intraoperative cardiovascular failure, and previous antimicrobial therapy at least 48 h prior to the onset of peritonitis. This index was validated in a prospective cohort. The presence of at least three of these factors was associated with a sensitivity of 84 %, specificity of 50 %; positive and negative predictive values were 67 % and 72 %, respectively [65]. This approach can be helpful to initiate early antifungal therapy in the critical care setting.

An echinocandin is preferred in patients with severe sepsis or septic shock, in those previously exposed to an azole, or in infections caused by azole-resistant *Candida* species. Duration of therapy is not well established but should be continued for at least 2 – 3 weeks [4]. In a recent multicenter study, the median duration of antifungal treatment in patients with *Candida* peritonitis was 20 days for survivors [20].

Conclusion

Invasive candidiasis is a feared infection associated with high crude mortality (40–60 %). Moreover, delay in initiating antifungal treatment in critically ill patients is associated with a worse outcome. Therefore, use of early antifungal therapy in patients with a high suspicion of invasive candidiasis is justified. Recovery of *Candida* species from multiple superficial sites has been identified as a risk factor for deeply invasive candidiasis but its presence alone does not justify administration of antifungal agents. The use of clinical scores (especially the Candida score) and *Candida* biomarkers, such as (1,3)-beta-D-glucan, can help clinicians identify those patients who would benefit from early antifungal treatment. Regarding choice of treatment, either fluconazole or an echinocandin is an appropriate initial therapy for most patients with invasive candidiasis. Fluconazole is reserved for non-severely ill patients without recent exposure to azoles. An echinocandin is clearly recommended for hemodynamically unstable patients or those with previous fluconazole exposure.

References

1. Edwards JE (2010) Candida species. In: Mandell GR, Bennett JE, Dolin R (eds) Principles and Practice of Infectious Disease. Chrchill Livingstone Elsevier, Philadelphia, pp 3225–3240
2. Ostrosky-Zeichner L, Pappas PG (2006) Invasive candidiasis in the intensive care unit. Crit Care Med 34: 857–863
3. Eggimann P, Bille J, Marchetti O (2011) Diagnosis of invasive candidiasis in the ICU. Ann Intensive Care 1: 37
4. Blot SI, Vandewoude KH, De Waele JJ (2007) Candida peritonitis. Curr Opin Crit Care 13: 195–199
5. Peman J, Canton E, Gobernado M (2005) Epidemiology and antifungal susceptibilities of *Candida* species isolated from blood: results of a 2-year multicentre study in Spain. Eur J Clin Microbiol Infect Dis 24: 23–30
6. Almirante B, Rodriguez D, Park BJ, et al (2005). Epidemiology and predictors of mortality in cases of Candida bloodstream infection: results from population-based surveillance, Barcelona, Spain, from 2002 to 2003. J Clin Microbiol 43: 1829–1835
7. Pfaller MA, Messer SA, Hollis RJ, et al (2009) Variation in susceptibility of bloodstream isolates of Candida glabrata to fluconazole according to patient age and geographic location in the United States in 2001 to 2007. J Clin Microbiol 47: 3185–3190
8. Tumbarello M, Sanguinetti M, Trecarichi EM, et al (2008) Fungaemia caused by Candida glabrata with reduced susceptibility to fluconazole due to altered gene expression: risk factors, antifungal treatment and outcome. J Antimicrob Chemother 62: 1379–1385
9. Muñoz P, Sánchez-Somolinos M, Alcalá L, Rodríguez-Créixems M, Peláez T, Bouza E (2005) Candida krusei fungaemia: antifungal susceptibility and clinical presentation of an uncommon entity during 15 years in a single general hospital. J Antimicrob Chemother 55: 188–193
10. Playford EG, Marriott D, Nguyen Q, et al (2008) Candidemia in nonneutropenic critically ill patients: risk factors for non-albicans Candida spp. Crit Care Med 36: 2034–2039
11. Chow JK, Golan Y, Ruthazer R, et al (2008) Risk factors for albicans and non-albicans candidemia in the intensive care unit. Crit Care Med 36: 1993–1998
12. Davis SL, Vazquez JA, McKinnon PS (2007) Epidemiology, risk factors, and outcomes of Candida albicans versus non-albicans candidemia in nonneutropenic patients. Ann Pharmacother 41: 568–573
13. Lin MY, Carmeli Y, Zumsteg J, et al (2005) Prior antimicrobial therapy and risk for hospital- acquired Candida glabrata and Candida krusei fungemia: a case-case-control study. Antimicrob Agents Chemother 49: 4555–4560

VIII

14. Shorr AF, Lazarus DR, Sherner JH, et al (2007) Do clinical features allow for accurate prediction of fungal pathogenesis in bloodstream infections? Potential implications of the increasing prevalence of non-albicans candidemia. Crit Care Med 35: 1077–1083

15. Garnacho-Montero J, Díaz-Martín A, García-Cabrera E, et al (2010) Risk factors for fluconazole-resistant candidemia. Antimicrob Agents Chemother 54: 3149–3154

16. Eggimann P, Garbino J, Pittet D (2003) Epidemiology of *Candida* species infections in critically ill non-immunosuppressed patients. Lancet Infect Dis 3: 685–702

17. Leroy O, Gangneux JP, Montravers P, et al (2007) Epidemiology, management, and risk factors for death of invasive Candida infections in critical care: a multicenter, prospective, observational study in France (2005–2006). Crit Care Med 37: 1612–1618

18. Dupont H, Paugam-Burtz C, Muller-Serieys C, et al (2002) Predictive factors of mortality due to polymicrobial peritonitis with Candida isolation in peritoneal fluid in critically ill patients. Arch Surg 137: 1341–1347

19. Sandven P, Qvist H, Skovlund E, Giercksky KE (2002) Significance of Candida recovered from intraoperative specimens in patients with intraabdominal perforations. Crit Care Med 30: 541–547

20. Montravers P, Mira JP, Gangneux JP, Leroy O, Lortholary O (2011) A multicentre study of antifungal strategies and outcome of Candida spp. peritonitis in intensive-care units. Clin Microbiol Infect 17: 1061–1067

21. Magill SS, Swoboda SM, Shields CE, et al (2009) The epidemiology of Candida colonization and invasive candidiasis in a surgical intensive care unit where fluconazole prophylaxis is utilized: follow-up to a randomized clinical trial. Ann Surg 249: 657–665

22. Bennett JE (2006) Echinocandins for candidemia in adults without neutropenia. N Engl J Med 355: 1154–1159

23. Pérez-Parra A, Muñoz P, Guinea J, Martín-Rabadán P, Guembe M, Bouza E (2009) Is Candida colonization of central vascular catheters in non-candidemic, non-neutropenic patients an indication for antifungals? Intensive Care Med 35: 707–712

24. Pappas PG, Kauffman CA, Andes D, et al (2009) Clinical practice guidelines for the management of candidiasis: 2009 update by the Infectious Diseases Society of America. Clin Infect Dis 48: 503–535

25. De Rosa FG, Garazzino S, Pasero D, Di Perri G, Ranieri VM (2009) Invasive candidiasis and candidemia: new guidelines. Minerva Anestesiol 75: 453–458

26. Aguado JM, Ruiz-Camps I, Muñoz P, et al (2011) [Guidelines for the treatment of Invasive Candidiasis and other yeasts. Spanish Society of Infectious Diseases and Clinical Microbiology (SEIMC). 2010 Update.] Enferm Infecc Microbiol Clin 29: 345–361

27. Limper AH, Knox KS, Sarosi GA, et al (2011) An official american thoracic society statement: treatment of fungal infections in adult pulmonary and critical care patients. Am J Respir Crit Care Med 183: 96–128

28. Sucher AJ, Chahine EB, Balcer HE (2009) Echinocandins: the newest class of antifungals. Ann Pharmacother 43: 1647–1657

29. Cuenca-Estrella M, Gomez-Lopez A, Mellado E, Monzon A, Buitrago MJ, Rodriguez-Tudela JL (2009) Activity profile in vitro of micafungin against Spanish clinical isolates of common and emerging species of yeasts and molds. Antimicrob Agents Chemother 53: 2192–2195

30. Pfaller MA, Boyken L, Hollis RJ, et al (2008) In vitro susceptibility of invasive isolates of Candida spp. to anidulafungin, caspofungin, and micafungin: six years of global surveillance. J Clin Microbiol 46: 150–156

31. Mora-Duarte J, Betts R, Rotstein C, et al (2002) Comparison of caspofungin and amphotericin B for invasive candidiasis. N Engl J Med 347: 2020–2029

32. Kuse ER, Chetchotisakd P, da Cunha CA, et al (2007) Micafungin versus liposomal amphotericin B for candidaemia and invasive candidosis: a phase III randomised double-blind trial. Lancet 369: 1519–1527

33. Reboli AC, Rotstein C, Pappas PG, et al (2007) Anidulafungin versus fluconazole for invasive candidiasis. N Engl J Med 356: 2472–2482

34. Pappas PG, Rotstein CM, Betts RF, et al (2007) Micafungin versus caspofungin for treatment of candidemia and other forms of invasive candidiasis. Clin Infect Dis 45: 883–893

35. Garnacho-Montero J, Díaz-Martín A, Cayuela-Dominguez A (2008) Management of inva-

VIII

sive Candida infections in non-neutropenic critically ill patients: from prophylaxis to early therapy. Int J Antimicrob Agents 32 (Suppl 2): S137–141

36. DiNubile MJ, Lupinacci RJ, Strohmaier KM, Sable CA, Kartsonis NA (2007) Invasive candidiasis treated in the intensive care unit: observations from a randomized clinical trial. J Crit Care 22: 237–244

37. Dupont BF, Lortholary O, Ostrosky-Zeichner L, Stucker F, Yeldandi V (2009) Treatment of candidemia and invasive candidiasis in the intensive care unit: post hoc analysis of a randomized, controlled trial comparing micafungin and liposomal amphotericin B. Crit Care 13: R159

38. Walsh TJ, Teppler H, Donowitz GR, et al (2004) Caspofungin versus liposomal amphotericin B for empirical antifungal therapy in patients with persistent fever and neutropenia. N Engl J Med 351: 1391–1402

39. Kullberg BJ, Sobel JD, Ruhnke M, et al (2005) Voriconazole versus a regimen of amphotericin B followed by fluconazole for candidaemia in non-neutropenic patients: a randomised non-inferiority trial. Lancet 366: 1435–1442

40. Johnson LB, Kauffman CA (2003) Voriconazole: a new triazole antifungal agent. Clin Infect Dis 36: 630–637

41. Khan FA, Slain D, Khakoo RA (2007) Candida endophthalmitis: focus on current and future antifungal treatment options. Pharmacotherapy 27: 1711–1721

42. Riddell J 4th, Comer GM, Kauffman CA (2011) Treatment of endogenous fungal endophthalmitis: focus on new antifungal agents. Clin Infect Dis 52: 648–653

43. Rex JH, Bennett JE, Sugar AM, et al (1995) Intravascular catheter exchange and duration of candidemia. NIAID Mycoses Study Group and the Candidemia Study Group. Clin Infect Dis 21: 994–996

44. Liu CY, Huang LJ, Wang WS, et al (2009) Candidemia in cancer patients: impact of early removal of non-tunneled central venous catheters on outcome. J Infect 58: 154–160

45. Rodriguez D, Park BJ, Almirante B, et al (2007) Impact of early central venous catheter removal on outcome in patients with candidaemia. Clin Microbiol Infect 13: 788–793

46. Nucci M, Anaissie E, Betts RF, et al (2010) Early removal of central venous catheter in patients with candidemia does not improve outcome: analysis of 842 patients from 2 randomized clinical trials. Clin Infect Dis 51: 295–303

47. Almirante B, Rodríguez D, Cuenca-Estrella M, et al (2006) Epidemiology, risk factors, and prognosis of Candida parapsilosis bloodstream infections: case-control population-based surveillance study of patients in Barcelona, Spain, from 2002 to 2003. J Clin Microbiol 44: 1681–1685

48. León C, Ruiz-Santana S, Saavedra P, et al (2006) A bedside scoring system ("Candida score") for early antifungal treatment in nonneutropenic critically ill patients with Candida colonization. Crit Care Med 34: 730–737

49. León C, Ruiz-Santana S, Saavedra P, et al (2009) Usefulness of the "Candida score" for discriminating between Candida colonization and invasive candidiasis in non-neutropenic critically ill patients: a prospective multicenter study. Crit Care Med 37: 1624–1633

50. Magill SS, Swoboda SM, Johnson EA, et al (2006) The association between anatomic site of Candida colonization, invasive candidiasis, and mortality in critically ill surgical patients. Diagn Microbiol Infect Dis 55: 293–301

51. Pittet D, Monod M, Suter PM, Frenk E, Auckenthaler R (1994) Candida colonization and subsequent infections in critically ill surgical patients. Ann Surg 220: 751–758

52. Ostrosky-Zeichner L, Sable C, Sobel J, et al (2007) Multicenter retrospective development and validation of a clinical prediction rule for nosocomial invasive candidiasis in the intensive care setting. Eur J Clin Microbiol Infect Dis 26: 271–276

53. Hermsen ED, Zapapas MK, Maiefski M, Rupp ME, Freifeld AG, Kalil AC (2011) Validation and comparison of clinical prediction rules for invasive candidiasis in intensive care unit patients: a matched case-control study. Crit Care 15: R198

54. Charles PE, Castro C, Ruiz-Santana S, León C, Saavedra P, Martín E (2009) Serum procalcitonin levels in critically ill patients colonized with Candida spp: new clues for the early recognition of invasive candidiasis? Intensive Care Med 35: 2146–2150

55. Alam FF, Mustafa AS, Khan ZU (2007) Comparative evaluation of (1, 3)-beta-D-glucan, mannan and anti-mannan antibodies, and Candida species-specific snPCR in patients with candidemia. BMC Infect Dis 7: 103

VIII

56. Ostrosky-Zeichner L, Alexander BD, Kett DH, et al (2005) Multicenter clinical evaluation of the (133) -D-glucan assay as an aid to diagnosis of fungal infections in humans. Clin Infect Dis 41: 654–659

57. Pemán J, Zaragoza R (2010) Current diagnostic approaches to invasive candidiasis in critical care settings. Mycoses 53: 424–433

58. Mohr JF, Sims C, Paetznick V, et al (2011) Prospective survey of (1→3)-beta-D-glucan and its relationship to invasive candidiasis in the surgical intensive care unit setting. J Clin Microbiol 49: 58–61

59. Pickering JW, Sant HW, Bowles CA, Roberts WL, Woods GL (2005) Evaluation of a (1-> 3)-beta-D-glucan assay for diagnosis of invasive fungal infections. J Clin Microbiol 43: 5957–5962

60. Pemán J, Zaragoza R, Quindós G, et al (2011) Clinical factors associated with a Candida albicans germ tube antibody positive test in intensive care unit patients. BMC Infect Dis 11: 60

61. Morrell M, Fraser VJ, Kollef MH (2005) Delaying the empiric treatment of Candida bloodstream infection until obtaining positive blood culture results: A potential risk factor for hospital mortality. Antimicrob Agents Chemother 49: 3640–3645

62. Garey KW, Rege M, Pai MP (2006) Time to initiation of fluconazole therapy impacts mortality in patients with candidemia: A multicenter study. Clin Infect Dis 43: 25–31

63. De Rosa FG, Garazzino S, Pasero D, Di Perri G, Ranieri VM (2009) Invasive candidiasis and candidemia: new guidelines. Minerva Anestesiol 75: 453–458

64. Montravers P, Dupont H, Gauzit R, et al (2006) Candida as a risk factor for mortality in peritonitis. Crit Care Med 34: 646–652

65. Dupont H, Bourichon A, Paugam-Burtz C, Mantz J, Desmonts JM (2003) Can yeast isolation in peritoneal fluid be predicted in intensive care unit patients with peritonitis? Crit Care Med 31: 752–757

VIII

Use of Antifungal Drugs during Continuous Hemofiltration Therapies

P.M. Honoré, R. Jacobs, and H.D. Spapen

Introduction

Increased use of blood purification and continuous renal replacement therapies (CRRT) in critically ill patients and advances in these techniques have led to important questions being raised regarding the pharmacokinetics of antimicrobial, and especially antifungal, agents during these processes [1]. Clinicians may have doubts about the efficacy of prescribing antimicrobial regimens proposed for intermittent hemodialysis (IHD) in patients receiving CRRT. This concern is particularly true for antifungal agents for which differences in their pharmacokinetic behavior during IHD and CRRT may not only result in therapeutic failure but may also harm the patient.

Table 1. Characteristics of major antifungal agents including recommended dosages during continuous renal replacement therapy (CRRT)

Antifungal agent	Mechanism	Use	Adverse effects	Elimination	Dosages during CRRT
Lipid formulations of amphotericin B	Interacts with ergosterol in the fungal cell membrane	i.v.	Hepatic, renal and cardiovascular toxicity	Unaffected by CRRT	5 mg/kg/day
Fluconazole	Exhibits time-dependent activity	i.v. or oral	Hepatic toxicity	High elimination by CRRT	600 mg/12h
Voriconazole	Reduced ergosterol synthesis	i.v. or oral	Toxicity in AKI with IV use	Poor elimination of i.v. form by CRRT	Loading dose: 6 mg/kg Maintenance dose: 4 mg/kg/12h
Echinocandins	Inhibits β(1,3)-glucan synthesis	i.v.	Potential hepatic toxicity	Unaffected by CRRT	Anidulafungin: Loading dose: 200 mg Maintenance dose: 100 mg/day Caspofungin: Loading dose: 70 mg Maintenance dose: 50 mg/day

i.v.: intravenous

J.-L. Vincent (ed.), *Annual Update in Intensive Care and Emergency Medicine 2012*
DOI 10.1007/978-3-642-25716-2 © Springer-Verlag Berlin Heidelberg 2012

Dose recommendations can only be derived from pharmacological studies that specifically address antifungal therapy in critically ill patients under CRRT [2]. We, therefore, extensively searched the literature and collected, reviewed, and summarized all available pharmacological data on antifungal therapy in CRRT. Rather than discussing each antifungal drug in detail, we will focus only on the pharmacokinetic aspects of those drugs most relevant to the ICU environment, i.e., lipid formulations of amphotericin B (AMB), fluconazole, voriconazole and the echinocandins (**Table 1**). We use the retrieved information to propose guidelines that can be applied at the bedside.

Lipid Formulations of Amphotericin B

AMB is a broad-spectrum antifungal agent for intravenous use. It is available as AMB deoxycholate and as lipid-associated formulations, including AMB lipid complex (ABLC), liposomal AMB (L-AMB) and AMB colloidal dispersion (ABCD) [3]. AMB and its lipid derivatives exert their antifungal effect by interacting with ergosterol in the fungal cell membrane. Pores are formed through which intracellular contents leak, resulting in cell destruction [3]. The lipid formulations have been specifically developed to reduce infusion-related adverse effects and to decrease the unacceptably high hepatic, renal, and cardiovascular toxicity of AMB [4, 5]. Free AMB is insoluble in water at physiologic pH and, after dissociation from its lipid moiety, becomes more than 90 % bound to plasma proteins, mainly β-lipoproteins [6]. Because of unmeasurable free AMB plasma levels, the high antimycotic activity of lipid formulations of AMB is thought to be due to their potential accumulation at the site of infection [3, 7, 8]. Nevertheless, these drugs have remarkable differences in structure and in patterns of clearance and distribution volume. ABLC is a complex consisting of equimolar concentrations of AMB and lipids, forming ribbon-like structures with a length of 1600 to 11000 nm [7], whereas L-AMB consists of spherical liposomes of 45 to 80 nm in diameter containing roughly one AMB molecule for nine lipid molecules. ABCD forms disk-like structures of about 75 to 170 nm in diameter [7, 9]. According to recent studies, highest blood values are obtained during treatment with ABLC [10].

The pharmacokinetics of lipid AMB drugs, such as ABLC, has been studied in various clinical conditions [11]. Some investigators have also performed therapeutic drug monitoring in patients on CRRT treated with ABLC [12, 13]. It is recognized that continuous veno-venous hemofiltration (CVVH) creates a specific pharmacokinetic environment that influences appropriate dosing of ABLC in a general ICU clinical setting [12, 14]. However, data in ICU patients who receive lipid formulations while suffering from acute kidney injury (AKI) and/or receiving CRRT are disappointingly scarce [15, 16]. A recent study of L-AMB and ABCD infusion during CRRT showed that the pharmacokinetic behavior of ABCD but not of L-AMB was similar to ABLC [14]. In fact, plasma levels of L-AMB were found to exceed those of ABCD [14]. Because of their large size, filtration of the lipid formulations was negligible. In contrast, significant amounts of AMB were detected in the filtrate during ABLC therapy because ABLC was separated in the plasma into free AMB and its lipid moiety [14]. The plasma pharmacokinetics of liberated protein-bound AMB are probably similar for all lipid AMB drugs. Indeed, recent data suggest clinical equivalence of ABLC and L-AMB [17].

In conclusion, accumulation of ABLC has not so far been observed in AKI requiring CRRT and its elimination appears to be almost unaffected by CRRT. Plasma levels were found to be lower in critically ill patients as compared to other patient groups. Therefore, ICU patients may be more frequently under- than overdosed. Currently, a dose of 5 mg/kg/day can be safely recommended for all AMB lipid formulations in critically ill patients under CRRT. Importantly, no data are available in patients receiving CRRT at a dose of or exceeding 35 ml/kg/h [18].

Azoles

Azole antifungal agents are divided into imidazoles (ketoconazole, miconazole) and triazoles (fluconazole, itraconazole, voriconazole and posaconazole). They act primarily within the cell by inhibiting the enzyme C-14α demethylase, thus reducing ergosterol synthesis. The most relevant azoles for use in an ICU setting are fluconazole and voriconazole.

Fluconazole

Fluconazole is a fungistatic agent with excellent overall activity against common *Candida* species isolated from ICU patients. Fluconazole was shown to be less toxic and as effective as AMB in treating candidemia [19]. Despite being extensively used in the ICU, the adequate dose of fluconazole in patients receiving CRRT is still unknown. Current guidelines propose a once daily dose of 400 mg [19].

Fluconazole is pharmacokinetically classified as a drug that exhibits time-dependent activity [20]. Therefore, the adequacy of fluconazole treatment is determined by maintaining its plasma levels above the minimal inhibitory concentration (MIC) at the site of infection. Fluconazole is widely distributed throughout the body. Surprisingly, tissue concentrations (except for bone) are higher than plasma concentrations [21]. Most *Candida* strains are inhibited at a concentration of 6 µg/ml fluconazole [22] but for treating other fungi (e.g., *Cryptococcus neoformans*), concentrations above 10 µg/ml may be necessary [23]. Based on these findings, Yagasaki et al. decided to target fluconazole plasma trough concentrations above 10 µg/ml in patients on CRRT whilst administering a dose of either 400 mg every 12 h or 800 mg every 24 h [24]. In all but one patient, the dosing regimens did not reach the intended trough concentration. The pharmacokinetic characteristics of fluconazole did not significantly differ between the two dosing regimens. Elimination half-life (less than 10 hours) was markedly lower compared to that seen in normal volunteers (approximately 30 hours) [25]. These findings demonstrate that CRRT can efficiently remove fluconazole from the circulation and suggest that the currently proposed 400 mg dose of fluconazole clearly is not effective to maintain appropriate trough levels in CRRT-treated patients [24]. These results were corroborated by Kishino et al. [26] who reported a similar fluconazole elimination half-life below 10 hours in ICU patients under CRRT or less than one-third that of normal volunteers [25]. Finally, Bouman et al. [27] confirmed the effective high extracorporeal removal of fluconazole which exceeded the normal renal clearance and necessitated a higher daily maintenance dose. These authors hypothesized that in normal kidneys fluconazole is not only excreted but also in part reabsorbed. In line with the avail-

VIII

able data and, as long as hepatic function is or remains stable, we recommend a dose of fluconazole of 500–600 mg every 12 h in critically ill patients under CRRT in line with the findings of Yagasaki et al. [24].

Although poorly documented, ketoconazole [28], itraconazole [29], and posaconazole [30] probably do not require dose adjustment during CRRT since elimination is negligible. Admittedly, these azoles are not often used for acute treatment.

Voriconazole

Voriconazole has an extended activity spectrum against many *Candida* species, including fluconazole-resistant strains, and is considered to be the first-line treatment for invasive aspergillosis. Voriconazole is available for oral and intravenous use. Possible toxicity of intravenous voriconazole in the setting of AKI is linked to the solvent sulfobutylether-beta-cyclodextrin (SBECD), a cyclic oligosaccharide composed of 1,4-linked glucopyranose molecules that forms a truncated cone with a hydrophilic outer surface and a hydrophobic cavity [31, 32]. This structure leads to an inclusion complex carrying the lipophilic voriconazole in its center [33]. As such, use of intravenous voriconazole is strongly discouraged when creatinine clearance decreases below 50 ml/min. Oral voriconazole preparations do not contain SBECD and no dose reduction is required in patients with AKI. However, oral administration of antimicrobial agents is not preferred in the critically ill because of doubtful or erroneous digestive absorption [34]. SBECD appears to be well-tolerated in humans. In animals, however, repeated doses of SBECD produced vacuolization of epithelial cells in the urinary tract and activation of hepatic and pulmonary macrophages [35]. SBECD has a steady-state distribution volume approximating 0.2 l/kg of body weight, which is similar to the extracellular fluid volume in humans, and has only limited tissue penetration [36]. Ninety-five percent of SBECD is excreted by the kidneys at a clearance that is linearly correlated with creatinine clearance [37]. On the other hand, voriconazole is extensively metabolized via the hepatic cytochrome P-450 system with less than 2 % of the dose excreted unchanged in the urine [37]. The main metabolite, voriconazole-N-oxide, has only minimal antifungal activity, but its role in voriconazole-associated toxicity remains unclear. Voriconazole is poorly eliminated by IHD or CRRT and dose adjustments are, therefore, not mandatory [38, 39]. In contrast, SBECD is rapidly eliminated by IHD or CRRT [38, 39]. Despite being removed rapidly by hemodialysis with high-flux membranes, SBECD exposure is thought to remain significant because its elimination is only intermittently 'activated'. Lowering the dose of voriconazole to decrease SBECD exposure is not a valid option since it may jeopardize the desired antifungal effect. In view of the high severity of invasive fungal infections and the unreliable effect of oral voriconazole in critically ill patients with AKI, exposure to SBECD toxicity is generally accepted. CRRT may be an elegant solution to obviate the need to adapt the dose of intravenous voriconazole [39, 40]. We therefore suggest that 'classical' doses of intravenous voriconazole, regardless of the presence of SBECD, can be safely administered as long as AKI is controlled with CRRT [40, 41]. If IHD is used, the dose should be adapted. However, since this may result in less effective systemic drug exposure, close therapeutic drug monitoring is advised [41].

The recommended dose of voriconazole (6 mg/kg loading dose followed by a maintenance dose of 4 mg/kg every 12 hours) was found to be inadequate to achieve drug concentrations above 1 µg/ml over the entire dosing interval in some critically ill patients under CRRT [41]. This underlines the fact that more studies are warranted to define the most adequate and least toxic dosing regimen of voriconazole during CRRT [40, 41].

Echinocandins

Echinocandins represent the newest class of antifungal agents. Echinocandins are semi-synthetic cyclic lipopeptides which, by inhibiting β-(1,3)-glucan synthesis, cause disruption of the fungal cell wall and rapid cell death [42]. Currently, anidulafungin, caspofungin and micafungin are licensed for clinical use. Echinocandins have a broad-spectrum fungicidal effect, must be given intravenously, have very few drug interactions and a remarkably low adverse event rate [42]. They exhibit an extremely high protein binding rate (> 99 %) and might, therefore, not be affected by extracorporeal removal [43].

Anidulafungin pharmacokinetics during CRRT resemble those observed in healthy subjects and in adults infected by fungi. Therefore, the classical dosing regimen (200 mg loading dose on the first day, followed thereafter by 100 mg/day) remains the standard during CRRT [44]. The dose of caspofungin (70 mg loading dose followed by 50 mg/day) does not need to be adapted in renal failure. However, in patients with a body weight exceeding 80 kg, a maintenance dose of 70 mg/day is recommended [45]. At this dose, elimination of the drug by CRRT remains non-significant [45]. In animals with invasive candidiasis, a caspofungin dose up to 10 mg/kg has been administered without any significant renal elimination [46]. Caspofungin dose escalation up to 210 mg in healthy humans did not cause significant adverse effects and renal elimination was not increased [45]. Micafungin, in doses up to 150 mg twice daily, also did not result in any CRRT losses [47].

In conclusion, the available data on echinocandin pharmacokinetics during CRRT do not support any adaptation of the currently recommended doses in patients without AKI [44, 46, 47].

Conclusions and Recommendations for Antifungal Dosing during CRRT

The pharmacokinetic behavior of antifungal agents during CRRT in critically ill patients is still poorly understood. Elimination appears to be very different from one compound to another. Indeed, fluconazole is rapidly and effectively eliminated by CRRT, whereas the echinocandins, even at escalating doses, are not affected. The high elimination rate of fluconazole necessitates a dose increase (up to 600 mg twice daily) in patients on CRRT but care must be taken to avoid liver toxicity or unwarranted drug interactions. Lipid formulations of AMB in a dose of 5 mg/kg/day can still be recommended as the elimination of ABLC is unaffected by CRRT at a dose less than 35 ml/kg/h. Toxicity of the SBECD solvents during full-dose intravenous voriconazole treatment can be minimized by using CRRT as a standard blood purification method. However, the currently recommended voriconazole dose may still fail to achieve sufficiently high plasma drug concentrations over the entire dosing interval in some patients. The classical caspofungin

VIII

loading and maintenance doses, eventually adapted to the patient's weight, were not associated with any loss in the ultrafiltrate during CRRT; no increase in renal elimination was observed even for daily doses up to 210 mg. The sparse data available on anidulafungin and micafungin also confirm no loss of these agents in the ultrafiltrate and thus support the use of classically recommended doses during CRRT.

References

1. Heintz BH, Matzke GR, Dager WE (2009) Antimicrobial dosing concepts and recommendations for critically ill adult patients receiving continuous renal replacement therapy or intermittent hemodialysis. Pharmacotherapy 29: 562–577
2. Susla GM (2009) The impact of continuous renal replacement therapy on drug therapy. Clin Pharmacol Ther 86: 562–565
3. Wong-Beringer A, Jacobs RA, Guglielmo BJ (1998) Lipid formulations of amphotericin B: clinical efficacy and toxicities. Clin Infect Dis 27: 603–618
4. Hughes WT, Armstrong D, Bodey G, et al (2002) Guidelines for the use of antimicrobial agents in neutropenic patients with cancer. Clin Infect 34: 730–751
5. Walsh TJ, Finberg RW, Arndt C, et al (1999) Liposomal amphotericin B for empirical therapy in patients with persistent fever and neutropenia. National Institute of Allergy and Infectious Diseases Mycoses Study Group. N Engl J Med 340: 764–771
6. Ridente Y, Aubard J, Bolard J (1999) Absence in amphotericin B-spiked plasma of the free monomeric drug, as detected by SERS. FEBS Lett 446: 282–286
7. Adler-Moore JP, Proffitt RT (1993) Development, characterization, efficacy and mode of action of AmBisome, a unilamellar liposomal formulation of amphotericin B. J Liposome Res 3: 429–450
8. Wasan KM, Lopez-Berestein G (1996) Characteristics of lipid-based formulations that influence their biological behavior in the plasma of patients. Clin Infect Dis 23: 1126–1138
9. Boswell GW, Buell D, Bekersky I (1998) AmBisome (liposomal amphotericin B): a comparative review. J Clin Pharmacol 38: 583–559
10. Hiemenz JW, Walsh TJ (1996) Lipid formulations of amphotericin B:recent progress and future directions. Clin Infect Dis 22: S133–134
11. Diezi TA, Takemoto JK, Davies NM, Kwon GS (2011) Pharmacokinetics and nephrotoxicity of amphotericin B-incorporated poly(ethylene glycol)-block-poly(N-hexyl stearate l-aspartamide) micelles. J Pharm Sci 100: 2064–2070
12. Bellmann R, Egger P, Djanani A, Wiedermann CJ (2004) Pharmacokinetics of amphotericin B lipid complex in critically ill patients on continuous veno-venous haemofiltration. Int J Antimicrob Agents 23: 80–83
13. Humphreys H, Oliver DA, Winter R, Warnock DW (1994) Liposomal amphotericin B and continuous venous–venous haemofiltration. J Antimicrob Chemother 33: 1070–1071
14. Bellmann R, Egger P, Gritsch W, et al (2003) Amphotericin B lipid formulations in critically ill patients on continuous veno-venous haemofiltration. J Antimicrob Chemother 51: 671–681
15. Trotman RL, Williamson JC, Shoemaker DM, Salzer WL (2005) Antibiotic dosing in critically ill adult patients receiving continuous renal replacement therapy. Clin Infect Dis 15: 1159–1166
16. Muhl E (2005) Antimycotic drugs under continuous renal replacement therapy. Mycoses 48: 56–60
17. Fleming RV, Kantarjian HM, Husni R, et al (2001) Comparison of amphotericin B lipid complex (ABLC) vs. AmBisome in the treatment of suspected or documented fungal infections in patients with leukemia. Leuk Lymphoma 40: 511–520
18. Honore PM, Jacobs R,Joannes-Boyau O, et al (2011) Septic AKI in ICU patients. Diagnosis, pathophysiology, and treatment type, dosing, and timing: A comprehensive review of recent and future developments. Ann Intensive Care 1: 32

VIII

19. Rex JH, Bennett JE, Sugar AM, et al (1994) A randomized trial comparing fluconazole with amphotericin B for the treatment of candidemia in patients without neutropenia. N Engl J Med 331: 1325–1330

20. Klepser ME, Wolfe EJ, Jones RN, Nightingale CH, Pfaller MA (1997) Antifungal pharmacodynamic characteristics of fluconazole and amphoteri-cin B tested against Candida albicans. Antimicrob Agents Chemother 41: 1392–1395

21. Shrikhande S, Friess H, Issenegger C, et al (2000) Fluconazole penetration into the pancreas. Antimicrob Agents Chemother 44: 2569–2571

22. Hughes CE, Bennett RL, Tuna IC, Beggs WH (1988) Activities of fluconazole (UK 49:858) and ketoconazole against ketoconazole-susceptible and -resistant Candida albicans. Antimicrob Agents Chemother 32: 209–212

23. Fischman AJ, Alpert NM, Livnu E, et al (1993) Pharmacokinetics of F-labelled fluconazole in healthy human subjects by positron emission tomography. Antimicrob Agents Chemother 37: 1270–1277

24. Yagasaki K, Gando S, Matsuda N, et al (2003) Pharmacokinetics and the most suitable dosing regimen of fluconazole in critically ill patients receiving continuous hemodiafiltration. Intensive Care Med 29: 1844–1848

25. Debruyne D, Ryckelynck JP (1993) Clinical pharmacokinetics of fluconazole. Clin Pharmacokinet 24: 10–27

26. Kishino S, Koshinami Y, Hosoi T, et al (2001) Effective fluconazole therapy for liver transplant recipients during continuous hemodiafiltration. Ther Drug Monit 23: 4–8

27. Bouman CS, van Kan HJ, Koopmans RP, Korevaar JC, Schultz MJ, Vroom MB (2006) Discrepancies between observed and predicted continuous venovenous hemofiltration removal of antimicrobial agents in critically ill patients and the effects on dosing. Intensive Care Med 32: 2013–2019

28. Nakasato S, Shah GM, Morrissey RL, Winer RL (1983) Ketoconazole treatment of fungal infection in acute renal failure. Clin Exp Dial Apheresis 7: 191–196

29. Coronel B, Persat F, Dorez D, Moskovtchenko JF, Peins MA, Mercatello A (1994) Itraconazole concentrations during continuous haemodiafiltration. J Antimicrob Chemother 34: 448–449

30. Li Y, Theuretzbacher U, Clancy CJ, Nguyen MH, Derendorf H (2010) Pharmacokinetic/ pharmacodynamic profile of posaconazole. Clin Pharmacokinet 49: 379–96

31. Abel S, Allan R, Gandelman K, Tomaszewski K, Webb DJ, Wood ND (2008) Pharmacokinetics, safety and tolerance of voriconazole in renally impaired subjects: two prospective, multicentre, open-label, parallel-group volunteer studies. Clin Drug Investig 28: 409–420

32. Stella VJ, Rajewski VA (1997) Cyclodextrins: their future in drug formulation and delivery. Pharm Res 14: 556–567

33. Gage R, Venn RF, Bayliss MA, Edgington AM, Roffey SJ, Sorrell B (2000) Fluorescence determination of sulphobutylether-beta-cyclo-dextrin in human plasma by size exclusion chromatography with inclusion complex formation. J Pharm Biomed Anal 22: 773–780

34. Pea F, Pavan F, Furlanut M (2008) Clinical relevance of pharmacokinetics and pharmacodynamics in cardiac critical care patients. Clin Pharmacokinet 47: 449–462

35. Ghannoum M A, Kuhn DM (2002) Voriconazole–better chances for patients with invasive mycoses. Eur J Med Res 7: 242–256

36. von Mach MA, Burhenne J, Weilemann LS (2006) Accumulation of the solvent vehicle sulphobutylether beta cyclodextrin sodium in critically ill patients treated with intravenous voriconazole under renal replacement therapy. BMC Clin Pharmacol 6: 6

37. Karlsson MO, Lutsar I, Milligan PA (2009) Population pharmacokinetic analysis of voriconazole plasma concentration data from pediatric studies. Antimicrob Agents Chemother 53: 935–944

38. Hafner V, Czock D, Burhenne J, et al (2010) Pharmacokinetics of sulfobutylether-beta-cyclodextrin and voriconazole in patients with end-stage renal failure during treatment with two hemodialysis systems and hemodiafiltration. Antimicrob Agents Chemother 54: 2596–2602

39. Radej J, Krouzecky A, Stehlik P, et al (2011) Pharmacokinetic evaluation of voriconazole treatment in critically ill patients undergoing continuous venovenous hemofiltration. Ther Drug Monit 33: 393–397

40. Burkhardt O, Thon S, Burhenne J, Welte T, Kielstein JT (2010) Sulphobutylether-beta-cyclodextrin accumulation in critically ill patients with acute kidney injury treated with intravenous voriconazole under extended daily dialysis. Int J Antimicrob Agents 36: 93–94
41. Myrianthefs P, Markantonis SL, Evaggelopoulou P, et al (2010) Monitoring plasma voriconazole levels following intravenous administration in critically ill patients: an observational study. Int J Antimicrob Agents 35: 468–472
42. Kofla G, Ruhnke M (2011)Pharmacology and metabolism of anidulafungin, caspofungin and micafungin in the treatment of invasive candidosis: review of the literature. Eur J Med Res 28: 159–166
43. Bellmann R (2007) Clinical pharmacokinetics of systemically administered antimycotics. Curr Clin Pharmacol 2: 37–58
44. Leitner JM, Meyer B, Fuhrmann V, et al (2011). Multiple-dose pharmacokinetics of anidulafungin during continuous venovenous haemofiltration. J Antimicrob Chemother 66: 880–884
45. Migoya EM, Mistry GC, Stone JA, et al (2011) Safety and pharmacokinetics of higher doses of caspofungin in healthy adult participants. J Clin Pharmacol 51: 202–211
46. Wiederhold NP, Najvar LK, Bocanegra RA, et al (2011) Caspofungin dose escalation for invasive candidiasis due to resistant candida albicans. Antimicrob Agents Chemother 55: 3254–3260
47. Hirata K, Aoyama T, Matsumoto Y, et al (2007) Pharmacokinetics of antifungal agent micafungin in critically ill patients receiving continuous hemodialysis filtration. Yakugaku Zasshi 127: 897–901

VIII

IX Hemodynamic Optimization

Guytonian Approach to the Circulation

H.D. Aya, A. Rhodes, and M. Cecconi

Introduction

The cardiovascular system is highly complex and a good understanding of its physiology and pathophysiology is essential in order to diagnose and treat cardiovascular dynamics in critically ill patients. Much of what we know comes from the experiments and theories of Frank Starling and Guyton [1 – 4]. In this chapter we will review some of these aspects and present new technology that has the potential to monitor *in vivo* the Guytonian aspects of the circulation.

Frank Starling and Optimal Preload

IX

Starling [1, 2] stated in the so-called 'Law of the heart' that as the volume of blood that flows into the heart increases, the cardiac muscle responds by increasing the contractile strength. The more the cardiac muscle is stretched, the greater the contractile strength in the following systole and the greater volume is ejected. Preload, therefore, can be defined as the length of the sarcomere, or more precisely the tension within it, before contraction. This relationship between preload and stroke volume implies that stroke volume will increase together with preload, until there is a maximum stretching between actin and myosin. Before this point an increase in preload will lead to an increase in stroke volume, whereas after this

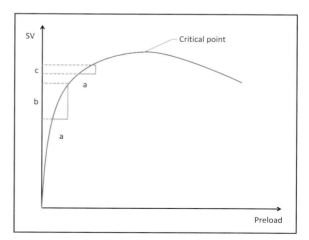

Fig. 1. Frank-Starling law of the heart: An increase in preload **a** will lead to an increase in stroke volume (SV) (**b** or **c**) until a critical point.

J.-L. Vincent (ed.), *Annual Update in Intensive Care and Emergency Medicine 2012*
DOI 10.1007/978-3-642-25716-2 © Springer-Verlag Berlin Heidelberg 2012

point any increase in preload will not have any effect on stroke volume and may actually be detrimental (**Fig. 1**).

Preload and Preload Responsiveness

It is not possible to directly measure preload in practice. Hence, trustable indicators of 'preload' and accurate predictors of 'volume responsiveness' have been the focus of research in critically ill patients in recent years. Several studies [5–13] over the last thirty years have investigated whether central venous pressure (CVP) and/or pulmonary artery occlusion or wedge pressure (PAOP) can be used as good markers of preload. No significant relationship has been found that would enable either to be used reliably in clinical practice. Kumar et al. [14] assessed the relationship between these pressure estimates of ventricular preload (PAOP and CVP) and end-diastolic ventricular volumes and stroke volume in healthy volunteers and again no significant correlation was found. Similar results were found with respect to changes in these variables following volume infusion. In the same way, Marik et al. [15] carried out a systematic review of the literature, including 24 studies and 803 patients, confirming no association between CVP and circulating blood volume and the inability of CVP or changes in CVP to predict the hemodynamic response to a fluid challenge.

In contrast with cardiac filling pressures, several studies have suggested that volumetric indicators such as intrathoracic blood volume index (ITBI) and global end-diastolic volume index (GEDVI) measured with transpulmonary thermodilution are superior in estimating cardiac preload [8, 16–19]. However, as the relationship between preload and stroke volume depends on ventricular contractility, the assessment of ventricular preload, as a static parameter, is not enough to predict a positive response to fluid therapy. These static parameters are more useful when their values are clearly low or high, but in the intermediate range, their yield is limited. Echocardiographic techniques have also been used to measure intracavitary dimensions and volumes. The end-diastolic area index (EDAI) and EDVI measured by 2D echo provides a better index of left-ventricular preload than PAOP [20]. Additionally, the changes in peak velocity (ΔVpeak) of aortic blood flow have been shown to be an accurate indicator of fluid responsiveness in patients with septic shock who are receiving mechanical ventilation [21]. The respiratory variation in inferior cava diameter (ΔD_{IVC}) in mechanically ventilated patients has also been reported as an accurate, simple and non-invasive parameter to investigate the pertinence of volume expansion [21, 22].

Part of the problem with indices of preload is that they aim to estimate an absolute value. The problem with this approach is that it does not provide information about the preload reserve of the patients. In practice, if a patient has preload reserve, then the stroke volume will go up in response to fluids. This concept is often referred to as 'fluid responsiveness'. Recently, dynamic indices have been investigated to see if they can predict fluid responsiveness. Marik and colleagues [23] carried out a systematic review to determine the ability of dynamic changes in arterial waveform-derived variables (pulse pressure variation [PPV], systolic pressure variation [SPV] and stroke volume variation [SVV]) to predict fluid responsiveness. Twenty-nine studies were included showing that dynamic changes in arterial waveform-derived variables measured during volume-controlled mechanical ventilation can predict volume responsiveness with a high

IX

degree of accuracy. These studies reported a diagnostic threshold of between 11 % and 13 % with a very high sensitivity and specificity. In this review, all the studies included in the analysis used a tidal volume (V_T) of 7 ml/kg or above. Recently, Zhang et al. [24] conducted a systematic review and meta-analysis of 23 studies investigating the diagnostic value of SVV in predicting fluid responsiveness. The odds ratio was 18.4 (95 % CI, 9.52–35.5), sensitivity was 0.81 and specificity 0.80. As the authors mentioned, these results were only validated in mechanically ventilated patients under controlled mode and V_T of more than 8 ml/kg.

Despite the good accuracy of waveform-derived variables, they cannot be used in patients with valvular heart disease, cardiac arrhythmia, intracardiac shunts, peripheral vascular disease, or decreased ejection fraction states. Moreover, the accuracy of these variables remains uncertain in patients under pressure-support ventilation or volume-controlled ventilation with a tidal volume of < 8 ml/kg [25]. In addition, the volume used for fluid challenge in these studies is quite variable, which may have some impact in some non-responsive cases and, importantly, none of these variables is a measure of the actual volemic state but only a predictor of the dynamic response of the ventricle if further volume is given [26].

Guytonian Model of Circulation

However, as pointed out by Guyton [27], it is not the heart itself that is the primary controller of cardiac output. Instead, the rate of blood flow to each tissue of the body is almost always accurately controlled by a combination of local signals in relation to, firstly, tissue needs (such as the availability of oxygen and other nutrients, the accumulation of carbon dioxide and other tissue waste products) and, secondly, sympathetic activity. Thus, cardiac output is finely controlled by the sum of all the local tissue flows, and the sum of all the local blood flows through all the individual tissue segments of the peripheral circulation is basically the venous return. Under steady conditions, the cardiac output and venous return are equivalent, and any parameter that determines venous return will, therefore, also determine cardiac output.

Following Guyton's argument, blood flow through a blood vessel is determined by two factors: Pressure difference, also called 'pressure gradient', along the vessel and the vascular resistance. This concept can be mathematically represented by the following formula, which is called Ohm's law:

$$F = \Delta P \: / \: R$$

in which F is blood flow, ΔP is the pressure difference (P1-P2) between two points of the vessel, and R is the resistance to venous return. Guyton himself pointed out that it is the *difference* in pressure between two points, not the absolute pressure in any point of the vessel that determines the rate of flow. In this way, the venous return is defined by three parameters: The mean systemic filling pressure, the right atrial pressure and the resistance to venous return. This can also be mathematically represented as follows:

$$VR = (Pms - RAP) \: / \: RVR$$

in which Pms is the mean systemic filling pressure, which is the degree of filling of the systemic circulation, RAP is the right atrial pressure, and RVR is the resistance to venous return.

The mean systemic filling pressure (Pms) is the pressure in the whole vascular system when the heart is stopped and there is no fluid motion, and was described by Bayliss and Starling [28] in a dog model of induced cardiac arrest. This concept may require further explanation: In static conditions, the volume to fill a distensible tube such as a tyre or a blood vessel with no pressure rise is called the 'unstressed' volume (V_o). Further volume additions imply necessarily a pressure rise (P) and an elastic distension of the wall of the tube which depends on the compliance (C) of the wall. This volume is the 'stressed' volume (V_e) and is related to the pressure in the next equation:

$$P = V_e / C$$

As it is reflected in this equation, the mean systemic pressure (Pms) depends totally on the stressed volume of the circulation (rather than the cardiac function per se – the heart by definition must have stopped for this pressure to be measured) and the compliance of the circulatory system. Therefore, if we could measure or estimate this variable, we could theoretically have a quantitative description of the volume state, independent of cardiac function.

Guyton [3] drew venous return curves (**Fig. 2**) in recently dead dogs with a pump replacing the heart and varying the right atrial pressure (RAP) by increasing or decreasing the minute capacity of the pump and, on the other side, the mean circulatory filling pressure by increasing or decreasing the total quantity of blood. These curves showed that for any given RAP, the greater the mean circulatory filling pressure, the greater the venous return; and importantly, under isovolumetric conditions, the greater the RAP, the lower is the venous return.

In another experiment, a healthy dog received a very large and rapidly administered transfusion of whole blood and the heart was stopped every two minutes by electrical fibrillation. The mean circulatory filling pressure was measured over a few seconds, and then the heart was defibrillated. Guyton measured RAP and cardiac output at the same time and traced a curve with the pressure gradient venous flow (Pms – RAP) against cardiac output (venous return) (**Fig. 3**). This curve illustrates that the venous return and cardiac output are approximately proportional to the pressure gradient of venous flow. The results of Guyton's experiments are still debated [29, 30], but have opened the way to a different understanding of cardiovascular regulation.

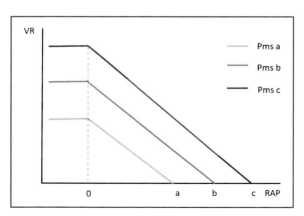

Fig. 2. Guyton's venous return curves representing the effect of isovolumetric variation of right atrial pressure (RAP) on venous return (VR) at different levels of mean circulatory filling pressure (Pms)

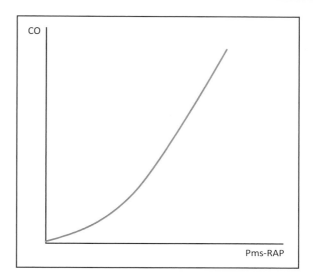

Fig. 3. Effect of the pressure gradient for venous return (mean systemic filling pressure [Pms] – right atrial pressure [RAP]) on cardiac output (CO).

The Mean Systemic Filling Pressure

The main problem in determining the pressure gradient for venous flow is that the Pms is not an easy variable to measure in patients with an intact circulation. Schipke et al. [31] performed a fibrillation–defibrillation sequence in 82 patients in order to measure the mean circulatory filling pressure over a duration of 13 ± 2 s. However, a true equilibrium pressure was not achieved, and the arterial–central venous blood pressure difference remained at 13.2 ± 6.2 mm Hg. This study suggested that Pms cannot be directly measured unless maintaining a time of cessation of flow of about 20 seconds, which is not ethically tolerable in human patients. Nonetheless, Guyton et al. [3] pointed out an important linear relationship between RAP and venous return, showing that the RAP corresponding to the zero-flow point in the curve reflects the Pms. This has been the base for many subsequent studies.

Pinsky [32] designed a model in animals with an intact circulation to construct venous return curves observing the relationship between instantaneous changes in right ventricular stroke volume and RAP during intermittent positive pressure breathing. The extrapolated Pms values were similar to the Pms measured during circulatory arrest. Other studies [33–35] have confirmed this linear relationship between venous return and CVP and derived Pms from the regression equation in animal models with an intact circulation. Maas and colleagues [36] applied the same rationale to study the effect of a 12-second inspiratory hold maneuver to three different steady-state levels on CVP and blood flow (cardiac output) measured via the pulse contour method during the last 3 seconds of the maneuver in mechanically ventilated postoperative cardiac patients. This interesting study again showed a linear relationship between CVP and cardiac output, and importantly, Pms could be estimated in intensive care patients with an intact circulation. Obviously this technique is only feasible in patients under volume-controlled ventilation and who have a regular pulse. Parkin and Wright [37] proposed an alternative approach describing a method for estimating a mean systemic filling pressure analog (Pmsa) using the mean blood pressure, the RAP, cardiac output and anthropometric data. In essence, they employed a mathematical algorithm to design a cardiovascular model that consists of a heart and a systemic circulation including compliant arterial and venous compartments and resistances to blood flow. The model uses real measured variables to adjust the model parameters, and then, the model heart is stopped, rather than stopping the patient's heart. This model is based on the following formula for estimating the analogous value, Pmsa:

$$Pmsa = 0.96RAP + 0.04MAP + cCO$$

where CO is cardiac output and c has the dimensions of resistance and is determined by patient anthropometrics (height, weight and age). The clinical validity of this approach was tested in 10 patients in acute renal failure receiving continuous venovenous hemofiltration (CVVH) [38]. Fluid replacement therapy was electro-mechanically controlled to a target value of Pmsa. In spite of some limitations of this study (the small sample of patients and some methodological aspects of the design of the study) this approach gives support for the idea of measuring Pmsa as a quantitative parameter of the volume state.

Efficiency of Heart Performance

IX

Parkin and Leaning [39] proposed, in addition, a model of reservoirs in order to explain the role of the heart in the circulation. Basically this model consist of four parts: (1) A large reservoir of fluid with a pressure P_D; (2) an exit pipe of resistance R and flow F through the base of the wall reservoir; (3) a small chamber of pressure head P_C; and within the chamber (4) a person throws buckets full of water back into the large reservoir (**Fig. 4**). The pipe fills the small chamber passively due to the pressure of the large reservoir and the person is careful to keep P_C low and constant; the bucketing output thus equals the flow F into the chamber where:

$$F = (P_D - P_C) / R$$

In this equation, P_D is analogous to Pms, P_C to the RAP, R to the resistance to venous return from RVR, F to the venous return and the performance of the per-

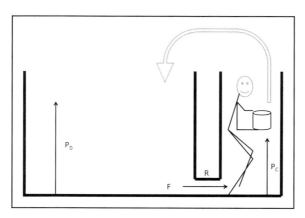

Fig. 4. The two reservoir model of circulation (see text for full explanation). P = pressure, R = resistance and F = flow

son throwing bucketfuls of water to the performance of the heart. If the person stops filling the bucket, P_C approaches P_D and the efficiency of the bucket thrower tends to zero. Conversely, vigorous bucketing causes P_C to approach zero and increases the efficiency of the bucket thrower. Thus, we can use the following dimensionless expression to describe the efficiency of the bucket thrower (E):

$$E = (P_D - P_C) / P_D = 1 - P_C / P_D$$

In the same way, the global pumping efficiency of the heart, E_H, is defined using the analog value of Pms, where

$$E_H = (Pmsa - RAP) / Pmsa = 1 - RAP/Pmsa$$

Therefore, if the heart stops, the RAP will approach Pmsa and E_H approaches zero, and if the cardiac output is increased, the RAP tends to zero and increases E_H. This relationship between cardiac output and RAP was already observed by Guyton when he pointed out that "right atrial pressure is not one of the primary determinants of cardiac output but, instead, is itself determined simultaneously along with cardiac output" [3]. This equation gives RAP a role of indicator of the relationship between volume state and cardiac function, rather than an indicator of preload or volume state [40].

The concepts sketched out above have been used in a new system (Navigator™, Applied Physiology, Pty Ltd, Sydney, Australia). This system uses the anthropometric data of the patient and hemodynamic variables from other monitors including RAP, MAP, cardiac output to calculate the values of heart performance (E_H) and Pmsa.

There is currently only one multicenter [41] clinical trial which has performed a clinical evaluation of this new system. It was a randomized controlled trial in 112 elective postoperative cardiac surgical patients. The Navigator™ system was used to attain and maintain physician-designated targets, and was compared with standard post-surgical care using a pulmonary artery catheter (PAC). The primary endpoint was a measure of the attainment and maintenance of MAP and cardiac output together in relation to the respective targets, called the average standardized distance (ASD). There was no significant difference between the groups with respect to this endpoint. Similarly, there was no difference with respect to postoperative rates of atrial fibrillation, adverse events and intensive care unit (ICU) or hospital lengths of stay. The authors concluded that guided therapy with the Navigator™ system was non-inferior to standard ICU therapy. However, none of the six centers in the study usually used protocol-guided hemodynamic care, and the use of fluids, inotropes or vasoactive drugs was totally based on clinician judgement, which makes the comparison somewhat unhelpful. Second, there were no predetermined targets and, what is more, target values in both groups could be altered at any time throughout the study period. In fact, 80 target changes of cardiac output or MAP were documented in the guidance group, compared with only 18 in the control group. Considering the objectives of the study and the main endpoint, this difference between interventions in each group brings into question the internal validity of the results. Finally, compliance with the guidance was not monitored, which means that the results in the guidance group were not necessarily a consequence of the monitor assistance.

IX

Conclusion

Absence of a quantitative estimation of the volume state has lead to a qualitative approach in terms of 'volume responsiveness'. However, as pointed out by other authors [39, 42], it is important to remember that volume responsiveness is not a pathological state. Numerous factors influence the response to a fluid challenge, such as venous compliance, ventricular compliance or ventricular dysfunction, volume administered, time of administration, and probably others [40, 43].

Thus, we have to admit that, in spite of the limitations mentioned above, a quantitative approach to the volume state based on the Guytonian concept of Pms, theoretically independent of cardiac function, has several possible applications in clinical practice. The mathematical approach of Parkin and colleagues will need more validation to see if it can be used in routine clinical practice. Importantly, it remains to be proven if the Pmsa or the E_H can guide cardiovascular therapy in critically ill patients in the near future. In this context, future studies are eagerly awaited.

References

1. Patterson SW, Piper H, Starling EH (1914) The regulation of the heart beat. J Physiol 48: 465–513
2. Patterson SW, Starling EH (1914) On the mechanical factors which determine the output of the ventricles. J Physiol 48: 357–379
3. Guyton AC (1955) Determination of cardiac output by equating venous return curves with cardiac response curves. Physiol Rev 35: 123–129
4. Guyton AC, Lindsey AW, Kaufmann BN (1955) Effect of mean circulatory filling pressure and other peripheral circulatory factors on cardiac output. Am J Physiol 180: 463–468
5. Calvin JE, Driedger AA, Sibbald WJ (1981) Does the pulmonary capillary wedge pressure predict left ventricular preload in critically ill patients? Crit Care Med 9: 437–443
6. Sakka SG, Reinhart K, Meier-Hellmann A (1999) Comparison of pulmonary artery and arterial thermodilution cardiac output in critically ill patients. Intensive Care Med 25: 843–846
7. Jardin F, Valtier B, Beauchet A, Dubourg O, Bourdarias JP (1994) Invasive monitoring combined with two-dimensional echocardiographic study in septic shock. Intensive Care Med 20: 550–554
8. Lichtwarck-Aschoff M, Zeravik J, Pfeiffer UJ (1992) Intrathoracic blood volume accurately reflects circulatory volume status in critically ill patients with mechanical ventilation. Intensive Care Med 18: 142–147
9. Hoeft A, Schorn B, Weyland A, et al (1994) Bedside assessment of intravascular volume status in patients undergoing coronary bypass surgery. Anesthesiology 81: 76–86
10. Buhre W, Weyland A, Schorn B, et al (1999) Changes in central venous pressure and pulmonary capillary wedge pressure do not indicate changes in right and left heart volume in patients undergoing coronary artery bypass surgery. Eur J Anaesthiol 16: 11–17
11. Tousignant CP, Walsh F, Mazer CD (2000) The use of transesophageal echocardiography for preload assessment in critically ill patients. Anesth Analg 90: 351–355
12. Calvin JE, Driedger AA, Sibbald WJ (1981) The hemodynamic effect of rapid fluid infusion in critically ill patients. Surgery 90: 61–76
13. Osman D, Ridel C, Ray P, et al (2007) Cardiac filling pressures are not appropriate to predict hemodynamic response to volume challenge. Crit Care Med 35: 64–68
14. Kumar A, Anel R, Bunnell E, et al (2004) Pulmonary artery occlusion pressure and central venous pressure fail to predict ventricular filling volume, cardiac performance, or the response to volume infusion in normal subjects. Crit Care Med 32: 691–699
15. Marik PE, Baram M, Vahid B (2008) Does central venous pressure predict fluid responsiveness? A systematic review of the literature and the tale of seven mares. Chest 134: 172–178

IX

16. Michard F, Alaya S, Zarka V, Bahloul M, Richard C, Teboul JL (2003) Global end-diastolic volume as an indicator of cardiac preload in patients with septic shock. Chest 124: 1900–1908

17. Wiesenack C, Prasser C, Keyl C, Rodig G (2001) Assessment of intrathoracic blood volume as an indicator of cardiac preload: single transpulmonary thermodilution technique versus assessment of pressure preload parameters derived from a pulmonary artery catheter. J Cardiothorac Vasc Anesth 15: 584–588

18. Reuter DA, Felbinger TW, Moerstedt K, et al (2002) Intrathoracic blood volume index measured by thermodilution for preload monitoring after cardiac surgery. J Cardiothorac Vasc Anesth 16: 191–195

19. Della Rocca G, Costa GM, Coccia C, Pompei L, Di Marco P, Pietropaoli P (2002) Preload index: pulmonary artery occlusion pressure versus intrathoracic blood volume monitoring during lung transplantation. Anesth Analg 95: 835–843

20. Thys DM, Hillel Z, Goldman ME, Mindich BP, Kaplan JA (1987) A comparison of hemodynamic indices derived by invasive monitoring and two-dimensional echocardiography. Anesthesiology 67: 630–634

21. Feissel M, Michard F, Mangin I, Ruyer O, Faller JP, Teboul JL (2001) Respiratory changes in aortic blood velocity as an indicator of fluid responsiveness in ventilated patients with septic shock. Chest 119: 867–873

22. Barbier C, Loubieres Y, Schmit C, et al (2004) Respiratory changes in inferior vena cava diameter are helpful in predicting fluid responsiveness in ventilated septic patients. Intensive Care Med 30: 1740–1746

23. Marik PE, Cavallazzi R, Vasu T, Hirani A (2009) Dynamic changes in arterial waveform derived variables and fluid responsiveness in mechanically ventilated patients: a systematic review of the literature. Crit Care Med 37: 2642–2647

24. Zhang Z, Lu B, Sheng X, Jin N (2011) Accuracy of stroke volume variation in predicting fluid responsiveness: a systematic review and meta-analysis. J Anesth 25: 904–916

25. De Backer D, Heenen S, Piagnerelli M, Koch M, Vincent JL (2005) Pulse pressure variations to predict fluid responsiveness: influence of tidal volume. Intensive Care Med 31: 517–523

26. Pinsky MR (2003) Rationale for cardiovascular monitoring. Curr Opin Crit Care 9: 222–224

27. Guyton AC (1971) Basic Human Physiology: Normal Function and Mechanisms of Disease. Saunders, Philadelphia

28. Bayliss WM, Starling EH (1894) Observations on venous pressures and their relationship to capillary pressures. J Physiol 16: 159–318

29. Magder S (2006) Point: the classical Guyton view that mean systemic pressure, right atrial pressure, and venous resistance govern venous return is/is not correct. J Appl Physiol 101: 1523–1525

30. Brengelmann GL (2006) Counterpoint: the classical Guyton view that mean systemic pressure, right atrial pressure, and venous resistance govern venous return is not correct. J Appl Physiol 101: 1525–1526

31. Schipke JD, Heusch G, Sanii AP, Gams E, Winter J (2003) Static filling pressure in patients during induced ventricular fibrillation. Am J Physiol Heart Circ Physiol 285: H2510–2515

32. Pinsky MR (1984) Instantaneous venous return curves in an intact canine preparation. J Appl Physiol 56: 765–771

33. Versprille A, Jansen JR (1985) Mean systemic filling pressure as a characteristic pressure for venous return. Pflugers Arch 405: 226–233

34. Den Hartog EA, Versprille A, Jansen JR (1994) Systemic filling pressure in intact circulation determined on basis of aortic vs. central venous pressure relationships. Am J Physiol 267: H2255–2258

35. Hiesmayr M, Jansen JR, Versprille A (1996) Effects of endotoxin infusion on mean systemic filling pressure and flow resistance to venous return. Pflugers Arch 431: 741–747

36. Maas JJ, Geerts BF, van den Berg PC, Pinsky MR, Jansen JR (2009) Assessment of venous return curve and mean systemic filling pressure in postoperative cardiac surgery patients. Crit Care Med 37: 912–918

37. Parkin WG, Wright CA (1991) Three dimensional closed loop control of the human circulation. Int J Clin Monit Comput 8: 35–42

IX

38. Parkin G, Wright C, Bellomo R, Boyce N (1994) Use of a mean systemic filling pressure analogue during the closed-loop control of fluid replacement in continuous hemodiafiltration. J Crit Care 9: 124–133
39. Parkin WG, Leaning MS (2008) Therapeutic control of the circulation. J Clin Monit Comput 22: 391–400
40. Cecconi M, Parsons AK, Rhodes A (2011) What is a fluid challenge? Curr Opin Crit Care 17: 290–295
41. Pellegrino VA, Mudaliar Y, Gopalakrishnan M, et al (2011) Computer based haemodynamic guidance system is effective and safe in management of postoperative cardiac surgery patients. Anaesth Intensive Care 39: 191–201
42. Jansen JR, Maas JJ, Pinsky MR (2010) Bedside assessment of mean systemic filling pressure. Curr Opin Crit Care 16: 231–236
43. Michard F, Teboul JL (2002) Predicting fluid responsiveness in ICU patients: a critical analysis of the evidence. Chest 121: 2000–2008

IX

Perioperative Hemodynamic Optimization: A Way to Individual Goals

J. Benes, R. Pradl, and I. Chytra

Introduction

Perioperative goal directed therapy (GDT) and hemodynamic optimization have been on the program of anesthesiology and intensive care meetings for almost 30 years. The idea that morbidity [1,2], incidence of infectious complications [3] and even short term [4] or long-term mortality [5] can be affected by improving hemodynamic status and oxygen delivery to organs at the time of surgical trauma is very attractive. Since 1988 when Shoemaker et al. published their study [6] much has changed in the approach to high-risk surgical patients, including less invasive therapies and new surgical methods. Hemodynamic monitoring options have also increased. But the problem of hemodynamic optimization has scarcely moved from the hypothetical level of controlled trials to every-day practice in many institutions. Although there is a strong movement towards adoption of this principle via national guidelines [7], the community of believers (mostly from the academic field) is opposed by the practicing 'infidels'. In a recently published survey among North American and European anesthesiologists, only 35 % of respondents used some cardiac output monitoring for high-risk surgical patients [8]. Lees et al. [9] named the following controversies as the major reasons for not-adopting GDT:

IX

- The right population (problem with defining the high-risk patient and surgery)
- The protocol itself (heterogeneity of goals, interventions and monitoring tools)
- Logistic reasons (economic and personal issues)

However, without elucidating the practical issues first, we will hardly be able to convince the staff of operating rooms and postoperative intensive care units (ICU) to accept GDT, or the hospital management to cover additional expenses.

Identifying and Monitoring the High-risk Population

Given the number of diagnostic tools and monitoring techniques available it is improbable that we will ever find one that is supreme over the others. As one size never fits all, individualization was introduced into the patient-monitor relationship using a stepwise approach guided by actual hemodynamic and laboratory markers and escalating the invasivity of the monitoring accordingly [10]. Kirov et al. further adapted this proposal to the surgical population, adding patient- and

J.-L. Vincent (ed.), *Annual Update in Intensive Care and Emergency Medicine 2012*
DOI 10.1007/978-3-642-25716-2 © Springer-Verlag Berlin Heidelberg 2012

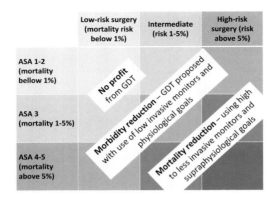

Fig. 1. Distribution of outcome benefits among different risk groups – a two dimensional scheme
ASA: American Society of Anesthesiologists' physical status classification;
GDT: goal-directed therapy.

surgery-related factors to constitute a two-dimensional decision scheme [11]. Defining high-risk by using the Boyd and Jackson assumption [12] (patients with a mortality risk of more than 5 % because of their health conditions or undergoing surgery associated with a 5 % risk of death) has one drawback. Patients with intermediate health-related risk under intermediate surgery-risk conditions can also reach the 'high-risk' threshold and should not be missed. By adapting this two-dimensional stratification not only is risk assessment possible, but the reasonable goals for therapy and predicted outcome benefit can also be estimated (**Fig. 1**). Brienza et al. [13] provided a meta-analysis of the influence of GDT on the risk of death according to control group mortality. They found that even though there was a mortality reduction in the overall population (30 studies, 4874 patients, odds ratio 0.54; 95 % confidence interval [CI] 0.38–0.77), the high-risk group (mortality > 10 %) had the risk further lowered (odds ratio 0.38; 95 % CI 0.25–0.57). The effect vanished in lower risk groups (5–10 % and < 5 %). However, even within these lower-mortality groups a reduction in organ and infectious complications was observed [1–3]. On the other hand, studies performed in patients with very low risk (ASA 1–3, peripheral surgery) showed no outcome benefit [14, 15]. The question still remains whether no benefit was proved, because these studies were underpowered to show reduction in rate of complications.

Defining the Goals

The quite extensive meta-analytical work performed in the last few years substitutes for the missing large multicenter study. There have been probably more than 34 different randomized trials published with about 5200 patients included. Their protocols differ substantially. **Table 1** lists 20 of the recent studies (published since the year 2002). Among these trials, 3 used a pulmonary artery catheter (PAC), 7 used esophageal Doppler devices, 1 a central venous catheter (CVC), and 9 studies used some sort of arterial pressure waveform analysis (2 of them in combination with the dilution technique). Three major groups of protocol goals could be distinguished: Supranormal oxygen delivery (DO_2) values (4 studies), maximization of the stroke volume (14 studies), and oxygen extraction targets (2 studies). In some trials, these goals overlapped [16, 17], in others the only target was normalization of the cardiac index [14, 18].

Table 1. Perioperative hemodynamic optimization studies (since 2002)

First author [ref]	Year	No. of patients	Timing of the intervention	Type of GDT	Intervention	Device
Bonazzi [40]	2002	100	B, D, A (48)	$DO_2I(600)$	F, I	PAC
Conway [41]	2002	57	D	SVMAX(FTc)	F	ED
Gan [42]	2002	100	D	SVMAX(FTc)	F	ED
Venn [43]	2002	59	D	SVMAX(FTc)	F	ED
Sandham [44]	2003	1994	B, D, A (24)	$DO_2I(550-600)$	F, I, CA	PAC
McKendry [45]	2004	179	A (4)	SVMAX	F, CA	ED
Pearse [17]	2005	122	A (8)	SVMAX; $DO_2I(600)$	F, I, CA	PWA
Wakeling [46]	2005	134	D	SVMAX(FTc)	F	ED
Lobo [23]	2006	50	B, D, A (24)	$DO_2I(600)$	F, I	PAC
Noblett [47]	2006	103	D	SVMAX(FTc)	F	ED
Donati [31]	2007	135	D, A (24)	O_2ER	F, I	CVC
Chytra [48]	2007	162	A (12)	SVMAX(FTc)	F	ED
Lopes [26]	2007	33	D	SVMAX(Dyn)	F	PWA
Goepfert [18]	2007	79	D, A (48)	CI(2,5)	F, CA	PWA
Kapoor [36]	2008	30	A (8)	SVMAX(Dyn); O_2ER; DO_2I (450-600)	F, I	PWA
Buettner [15]	2008	80	D	SVMAX(Dyn)	F, CA	PWA
Benes [49]	2010	120	D	SVMAX(Dyn)	F, I	PWA
Mayer [50]	2010	60	D	SVMAX(Dyn)	F, I, CA	PWA
Van der Linden [14]	2010	57	D	CI(2,5)	F, I	PWA
Cecconi [16]	2011	40	D, A (1)	SVMAX; $DO_2I(600)$	F, I	PWA

Timing of intervention: B – before operation, D – during surgery, A – postoperatively (length of treatment in hours); Type of GDT: DO_2I – oxygen delivery goal (target value), SVMAX – stroke volume maximization (parameter used), FTc – corrected flow time, Dyn – dynamic fluid responsiveness parameters, O_2ER – oxygen extraction or venous saturation goal, CI – cardiac index goal (target value); Intervention: F – fluids, I – inotropes, CA – other catecholamines; Device: PAC – pulmonary artery catheter, ED – esophageal Doppler, PWA – arterial pressure wave analysis, CVC – central venous catheter

IX

In 2002, a meta-analysis by Kern and Shoemaker of previous optimization efforts was published [19]. This work is an important milestone as it emphasized some important issues regarding hemodynamic optimization. First, the role of early treatment was stressed; optimization is only reasonable if started before organ dysfunction develops. The therapeutic effect of GDT appears to be related to microvascular flow improvement and local tissue DO_2 due to increased global parameters of DO_2 [20]. Local hemodynamic derangement, resulting in ischemia/reperfusion injury, ensuing inflammation, cell dysfunction and possible death, is the pathophysiological background of the hypoperfusion-induced injury. Increasing amounts of oxygen delivered to failed organs or dead cells is futile; there is a strong suspicion that this approach may even promote injury by increasing the production of reactive oxygen species (ROS) [21]. The second important information coming from this meta-analysis [19] was the disproportionate effect of supranormal values in the high and the low mortality groups. This lack of benefit in control groups with low mortality rates questioned the proposed 'supranormal' DO_2 values and hemodynamic status.

Shoemaker's Supranormal Values

In a large meta-analysis, Hamilton et al. cited 9 studies [4] in which a DO_2 index (DO_2I) of more than 600 ml/min/m^2 was used as the therapeutic goal. All of them showed either a morbidity or mortality benefit. The extent of postoperative higher-than-normal circulatory conditions was evaluated by Shoemaker et al. [6] and median values of survivors were proposed as goals of intervention for other high-risk patients as well. Originally, Shoemaker proposed a group of hemodynamic indices ($DO_2I > 600$ ml/min/m^2, oxygen uptake index [VO_2I] > 170 ml/min/m^2, cardiac index > 4.5 l/min/m^2), but as DO_2 is, from a physiology perspective, the most important index, the majority of subsequent studies only used DO_2I as the goal of therapy.

There are some hazards associated with the use of preset (and fixed) supranormal goals in every patient and every condition. When the median value is used, half of the survivors in Shoemaker's primary population did not reach supranormal values [6]. It is not clear whether these patients could not reach these goals due to inability to increase their cardiac performance or whether there was no physiological need. Nevertheless, pushing these patients with pharmacologic agents (fluids and inotropes) to reach these goals may pose unnecessary risks. In a study by Lobo et al. [22] a substantial percentage of the protocol group patients (58 %) were unable to reach the predefined goals although they received higher doses of dobutamine (19 ± 12 µg/kg/min vs. 9.6 ± 5.2 µg/kg/min in achievers) and more fluid (median value 6.5 vs. 4 l). Mortality of these protocol non-achievers was actually higher than that of those control patients who spontaneously achieved the predefined DO_2 goals. The values of oxygen consumption and extraction were higher in the protocol group than in the control group referring to possible negative influences of the interventions. In a study by Pearse et al. [17], 21 % of patients allocated to the protocol group did not reach the proposed goals of DO_2I of 600 ml/min/m^2. These non-achievers suffered from an increased incidence of cardiac morbidity: Six of them had severe tachycardia and one myocardial infarction. This emphasizes the risks of deliberate inotropic support. On the other hand, in another study performed by Lobo et al. [23] values of the mixed venous oxygen saturation (SvO_2) in the optimized group reached 83 – 86 %. These values are probably far higher than necessary. The number of patients who were unable to reach predefined supranormal targets or were possibly 'over-treated' is not negligible and there should be some mechanism integrated into our protocols to restrict the pursuit for fixed hemodynamic goals to a judicious level. The right question concerning DO_2 is probably not whether it is normal compared to some arbitrary value but whether it is adequate for the body's needs. When we decide to drive our goals and patients above physiological levels, we should be more 'supra-adequate' than 'supranormal'. To assess adequacy we need to look at the other (venous) side of the circulation.

Optimization of Position on the Frank-Starling Curve

Achieving stroke volume maximization is another concept of optimizing status in perioperative care. This approach was first proposed by Mythen and Webb [24] and subsequently by Sinclair et al. [25]. A great contribution to this change in perception of the optimization was the use of different monitoring techniques. Both these groups used esophageal Doppler instead of the PAC [24, 25], allowing them to use corrected flow time as a better predictor of fluid responsiveness to monitor the position of the patient on the Frank-Starling curve. The best heart performance under a given contractile state is reached by using consecutive fluid boluses to achieve initiation of the flat portion of the curve. Thereby the best-obtainable conditions are achieved, which are not normal, but still possible within physiological limits. Fluid loading could be guided either by change in the stroke volume observed after fluid challenge or by different fluid responsiveness parameters. Use of dynamic change in stroke volume instead of the exact value and/or predictors obtainable without hemodynamic measurements makes the concept very attractive and far reaching. There have been 14 studies published since 2002 (**Table 1**) that use stroke volume maximization as part of a protocol. Most of these trials showed a morbidity reduction. Esophageal Doppler (7 studies) and arterial pressure waveform analysis (5 studies) were used to assess hemodynamic status. In two studies, only fluid responsiveness predictors were used to drive the protocol without contribution of hemodynamic variables which were not considered [15] or even measured [26]. This low invasiveness and use of peripherally obtainable predictors poses on the other hand a certain risk. Corrected flow time was shown to be a better predictor of the positive reaction to fluid challenge than filling pressures [27], but its value is inversely proportional to systemic resistance. This could pose some limitations when used under anesthesia conditions with their vasodilatory potential. Arterial pressure wave analysis devices assess fluid responsiveness by so called dynamic predictors – variations of stroke volume or arterial pressure induced by ventilation. The limits of these parameters have been well described elsewhere [28]. The three most important are: The need for sedation, artificial ventilation and regular heart rhythm. Using the change in stroke volume (usually 10 %) is probably the safest way to reach the plateau of the Frank-Starling curve as it is applicable under many different conditions including spontaneous ventilation or vasoplegia. When the device being used is precise enough, the issue of accuracy is of lesser importance because relative changes are considered; this enables the use of non-calibrated monitors.

IX

The second limitation of use of stroke volume maximization is that it merely exploits the limits of the heart and that even optimal fluid loading may not increase DO_2 to satisfactory levels, especially in patients with advanced heart dysfunction. In the study by Pearse et al. [17], dopexamine infusion was ordered by the protocol to achieve a DO_2I of 600 ml/min/m^2 after the stroke volume was maximized. Such inotropic support was necessary in 55 of 62 patients (89 %). Cecconi et al. [16] described that 55 % of optimally loaded patients needed dobutamine infusion to reach the same target. Lobo et al. [23] compared the effect of fluids and inotropes versus fluids only on the ability to reach this DO_2 goal. They observed a high proportion of non-achievers in the fluid only group (28 % during anesthesia and 64 % during ICU stay) with consequent increase in pulmonary edema and heart failure incidence in this group. Both groups received similar amounts of fluids guided by pulmonary occlusion pressures, so the key difference was attributed to inotropic agents. The use of fluids only, and especially crystalloids, for optimization is also not without consequences. Under different pathological conditions, such as surgical trauma, dysfunction of vessel wall permeability and the glycocalyx layer occurs, increasing the extravascular fluid leak [29]. The resulting interstitial edema prolongs the diffusion distance for oxygen and thus deteriorates local cell DO_2. Hiltebrandt et al. observed a better oxygen tension in the perianastomotic tissue when colloids were used for intraoperative GDT and a steep deterioration when only crystalloids were infused [30]. The last issue to consider during stroke volume maximization is the change in loading conditions due to changes in vascular tone, or those induced by mechanical ventilation and positive end-expiratory pressure (PEEP). In most populations these limits have quite a small impact, but they can influence the approach in certain situations, for example reversible vasoparalysis during regional anesthesia [16]. Within the limits discussed above, stroke volume maximization is probably the

IX

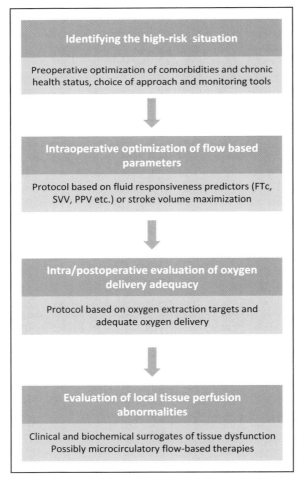

Fig. 2. Suggested 'four-step' algorithm for individualized goal-directed therapy in high risk surgical patients. FTc: corrected flow time, PPV: pulse pressure variation; SVV: stroke volume variation.

best way to start intraoperative fluid optimization, and may satisfy requirements in some patients with preserved functional limits. In patients with diminished cardiovascular performance, another supportive treatment would be necessary. Nevertheless, other steps must follow in both cases in order to evaluate the adequacy of the achieved global and local DO_2 (**Fig. 2**).

The Venous Side of the Circulation

Donati et al. [31] published a protocol based on use of the CVC and evaluated the surrogate marker of DO_2 adequacy – superior vena cava estimate of oxygen extraction (O_2ERe). They set the cut-off value for O_2ERe at 27 %, which equates to a central venous oxygen saturation ($ScvO_2$) of 72–73 % under normal oxygenation conditions. This cut-off is consistent with values proposed by other authors for the postoperative period [32, 33] and also for treatment of sepsis [34, 35]. The positive aspects of this study were its multicenter design and clear methodology including the protocol of the care. Two other studies have been published using venous saturation in the protocol. Kapoor et al. [36] used a goal of $ScvO_2$ > 70 % in the first 8 postoperative hours in cardiac surgery patients as the second step after adequate fluid loading. The proposed interventions were packed red blood cells (target hematocrit > 30 %) and dobutamine infusion. Polonen et al. [37] optimized cardiac surgery patients for 8 hours after admission to the ICU using SvO_2 > 70 % and serum lactate level < 2 mmol/l as targets. Also in this protocol, obtaining normal pulmonary artery occlusion pressure (PAOP, 12–18 mmHg) and hemoglobin levels preceded the proposed intervention with dobutamine. Oxygen extraction indices from the central vein or the pulmonary artery are a logical step to assess the effect of improved hemodynamic conditions. Their use in perioperative GDT has been proposed by many authors [32, 33], but some controversies need to be mentioned. First, there is a large disproportion between values obtained under general anesthesia and in conscious subjects. In a multicenter study on peri- and postoperative $ScvO_2$, values higher than 80 % were observed throughout surgery with a decrease after ICU admission. A similar pattern was observed by Pearse et al. [33]. There are many reasons for these findings, including decreased metabolism under general anesthesia and mechanical ventilation on one side, and pain, emergence from anesthesia and shivering due to intraoperative fall in body temperature on the other. Using the $ScvO_2$ as an estimate of SvO_2 is also not without consequence as values from the upper part of the body do not correlate with SvO_2 in various pathological states [38].

Another drawback of this optimization method lies in the possible frequency of measurement. Owing to recent development in cardiac output monitoring possibilities, we have become used to continuous measurement of hemodynamic indices. Under normal conditions, a blood sample is needed to obtain the SvO_2, which can limit the frequency of decisive points in optimization protocols. In the study by Polonen et al. [37], intermittent evaluation of goals was performed with a two-hour period between measurements. In following the protocol, there were only four decisive points which was not enough to adapt treatment. As a possible consequence, there was a large number of non-achievers (43 %) in the trial. Use of continuous measurement using some of the newer optical catheters may improve these results as well as applicability of this optimization goal, but the impact of these devices in the GDT trial setting has not yet been tested. In gen-

IX

eral, using oxygen extraction targets for optimization follows a more physiologic process which is adaptive to individual patient needs. In view of the steep increase in VO_2 in the early postoperative setting, this period is likely the golden hour for optimization (**Fig. 2**). One major disadvantage remains that the easily obtainable $ScvO_2$ is only an estimate of global body oxygen extraction and knowledge of the invasive SvO_2 does not exclude regional perfusion abnormalities.

Evaluating Possible Tissue Goals

As all of the described optimization goals are global hemodynamic parameters, the risk is that local tissue hypoperfusion will be missed. The interventions performed to achieve these goals make local tissue perfusion abnormalities unlikely, but they cannot be ruled out. There are few studies that have evaluated use of tissue oxygenation or perfusion goals to achieve an optimal hemodynamic state [39]. When considering local perfusion abnormalities, their probable localization has to be identified in order to monitor the affected tissue. Mythen et al. proposed the gastrointestinal tract (GIT) as one of the most affected organ systems and designed a GDT trial with a maximal stroke volume goal and gastric tonometry measurements [24]. The protocol group showed markedly reduced signs of gut hypoperfusion (higher pHi) and subsequent outcome improvement. In a porcine experiment, Hiltebrand and co-workers [30] demonstrated the beneficial effect of goal-directed colloid infusion compared with goal-directed crystalloid and restricted crystalloid infusion regimes on gut tissue perfusion. Finally, Jhanji et al. [20] observed marked improvement in sublingual microcirculatory flow and cutaneous tissue oxygen tension in the abdominal wall in patients optimized using colloids and dopexamine infusion during the ICU stay after major gastrointestinal tract surgery. These studies support the assumption that a 'local tissue perfusion' step is needed following fluid loading and after reaching global DO_2 adequacy (**Fig. 2**). However, none of the assessment techniques available today is easy enough to be clinically acceptable for establishing a GDT protocol. It is also unclear whether the interventions used to optimize the global circulation (mostly fluids and inotropes) are also effective at the local level. New 'tissue goals' could hasten our search for new interventions or for adaptation of old ones. Nevertheless, assessment of possible local hemodynamic abnormalities should be performed using standard clinical and biochemical markers (lactate, markers of organ injury). Diagnostic techniques, for example clearance of indocyanine-green, gastric mucosal tonometry, tissue oxygenation or microcirculatory visualization, could be of value but their routine use is still elusive.

Conclusion

The use of individual goals for perioperative hemodynamic optimization instead of arbitrary preset values should be encouraged. This approach utilizes the physiologic potential of each patient and hence minimizes the negative risks of GDT. Potentially compliance with the idea of hemodynamic optimization would also improve. Adequate position on the Frank-Starling curve using fluid loading and increasing DO_2 to reach adequate tissue oxygenation assessed by global extraction indices follow this principle of physiologic hemodynamic optimization.

Other goals including local microcirculatory or tissue perfusion parameters could add important information and help to guide our optimization efforts, but their evaluation as therapeutic targets is still lacking.

Acknowledgement: This work was supported by a research grant of the Czech Ministry of Education (MSM0021620819)

References

1. Giglio MT, Marucci M, Testini M, Brienza N (2009) Goal-directed haemodynamic therapy and gastrointestinal complications in major surgery: a meta-analysis of randomized controlled trials. Br J Anaesth 103: 637–646
2. Brienza N, Giglio MT, Marucci M, Fiore T (2009) Does perioperative hemodynamic optimization protect renal function in surgical patients? A meta-analytic study. Crit Care Med 37: 2079–2090
3. Dalfino L, Giglio MT, Puntillo F, Marucci M, Brienza N (2011) Haemodynamic goal-directed therapy and postoperative infections: earlier is better. a systematic review and meta-analysis. Crit Care 15: R154
4. Hamilton MA, Cecconi M, Rhodes A (2011) A systematic review and meta-analysis on the use of preemptive hemodynamic intervention to improve postoperative outcomes in moderate and high-risk surgical patients. Anesth Analg 112: 1392–1402
5. Rhodes A, Cecconi M, Hamilton M, et al (2010) Goal-directed therapy in high-risk surgical patients: a 15-year follow-up study. Intensive Care Med 36: 1327–1332
6. Shoemaker WC, Appel PL, Kram HB, Waxman K, Lee TS (1988) Prospective trial of supranormal values of survivors as therapeutic goals in high-risk surgical patients. Chest 94: 1176–1186
7. Powell-Tuck J, Gosling P, Lobo D, et al (2009) British consensus guidelines on intravenous fluid therapy for adult surgical patients (GIFTASUP). Available at http://www.renal.org/pages/media/download_gallery/GIFTASUP%20FINAL_05_01_09.pdf Accesed Nov 2011
8. Cannesson M, Pestel G, Ricks C, Hoeft A, Perel A (2011) Hemodynamic monitoring and management in patients undergoing high risk surgery: a survey among North American and European anesthesiologists. Crit Care 15: R197
9. Lees N, Hamilton M, Rhodes A (2009) Clinical review: Goal-directed therapy in high risk surgical patients. Crit Care 13: 231
10. Hofer CK, Cecconi M, Marx G, della Rocca G (2009) Minimally invasive haemodynamic monitoring. Eur J Anaesthesiol 26: 996–1002
11. Kirov MY, Kuzkov VV, Molnar Z (2010) Perioperative haemodynamic therapy. Curr Opin Crit Care 16: 384–392
12. Boyd O, Jackson N (2005) How is risk defined in high-risk surgical patient management? Crit Care 9: 390–396
13. Brienza N, Dalfino L, Giglio M (2011) Perioperative hemodynamic optimization. In: Vincent JL (ed) Annual Update in Intensive Care and Emergency Medicine. Springer, Heidelberg, pp 459–470
14. Van der Linden PJ, Dierick A, Wilmin S, Bellens B, De Hert SG (2010) A randomized controlled trial comparing an intraoperative goal-directed strategy with routine clinical practice in patients undergoing peripheral arterial surgery. Eur J Anaesthesiol 27: 788–793
15. Buettner M, Schummer W, Huettemann E, Schenke S, van Hout N, Sakka SG (2008) Influence of systolic-pressure-variation-guided intraoperative fluid management on organ function and oxygen transport. Br J Anaesth 101: 194–199
16. Cecconi M, Fasano N, Langiano N, et al (2011) Goal directed haemodynamic therapy during elective total hip arthroplasty under regional anaesthesia. Crit Care 15: R132
17. Pearse R, Dawson D, Fawcett J, Rhodes A, Grounds RM, Bennett ED (2005) Early goal-directed therapy after major surgery reduces complications and duration of hospital stay. A randomised, controlled trial [ISRCTN38797445]. Crit Care 9: R687–R693

IX

18. Goepfert MSG, Reuter DA, Akyol D, Lamm P, Kilger E, Goetz AE (2007) Goal-directed fluid management reduces vasopressor and catecholamine use in cardiac surgery patients. Intensive Care Med 33: 96–103

19. Kern J, Shoemaker W (2002) Meta-analysis of hemodynamic optimization in high-risk patients. Crit Care Med 30: 1686–1692

20. Jhanji S, Vivian-Smith A, Lucena-Amaro S, Watson D, Hinds C, Pearse R (2010) Haemodynamic optimisation improves tissue microvascular flow and oxygenation after major surgery: a randomised controlled trial. Crit Care 14: R151

21. Altemeier WA, Sinclair SE (2007) Hyperoxia in the intensive care unit: why more is not always better. Crit Care Med 13: 73–78

22. Lobo S, Salgado P, Castillo V, et al (2000) Effects of maximizing oxygen delivery on morbidity and mortality in high-risk surgical patients. Crit Care Med 28: 3396–3404

23. Lobo SM, Lobo FR, Polachini CA, et al (2006) Prospective, randomized trial comparing fluids and dobutamine optimization of oxygen delivery in high-risk surgical patients [ISRCTN42445141]. Crit Care 10: R72

24. Mythen M, Webb A (1995) Perioperative plasma volume expansion reduces the incidence of gut mucosal hypoperfusion during cardiac surgery. Arch Surg 130:423

25. Sinclair S, James S, Singer M (1997) Intraoperative intravascular volume optimisation and length of hospital stay after repair of proximal femoral fracture: randomised controlled trial. BMJ 315: 909–912

26. Lopes MR, Oliveira MA, Pereira V, Lemos I, Auler J, Michard F (2007) Goal-directed fluid management based on pulse pressure variation monitoring during high-risk surgery: a pilot randomized controlled trial. Crit Care 11: R100

27. Lee JH, Kim JT, Yoon SZ, et al (2007) Evaluation of corrected flow time in oesophageal Doppler as a predictor of fluid responsiveness. Br J Anaesth 99: 343–348

28. Marik PE, Cavallazzi R, Vasu T, Hirani A (2009) Dynamic changes in arterial waveform derived variables and fluid responsiveness in mechanically ventilated patients: a systematic review of the literature. Crit Care Med 37: 2642–2647

29. Chappell D, Jacob M, Hofmann-Kiefer K, Conzen P, Rehm M (2008) A rational approach to perioperative fluid management. Anesthesiology 109: 723–740

30. Hiltebrand LB, Kimberger O, Arnberger M, Brandt S, Kurz A, Sigurdsson GH (2009) Crystalloids versus colloids for goal-directed fluid therapy in major surgery. Crit Care 13: R40

31. Donati A, Loggi S, Preiser JC, et al (2007) Goal-directed intraoperative therapy reduces morbidity and length of hospital stay in high-risk surgical patients. Chest 132: 1817–1824

32. Collaborative Study Group on Perioperative ScvO2 Monitoring (2006) Multicentre study on peri- and postoperative central venous oxygen saturation in high-risk surgical patients. Crit Care Med 10: R158

33. Pearse R, Dawson D, Fawcett J, Rhodes A, Grounds RM, Bennett ED (2005) Changes in central venous saturation after major surgery, and association with outcome. Crit Care 9: R694-R699

34. Rivers E, Nguyen B, Havstad S, et al (2001) Early goal-directed therapy in the treatment of severe sepsis and septic shock. N Engl J Med 345: 1368–1377

35. Dellinger RP, Levy MM, Carlet JM, et al (2008) Surviving Sepsis Campaign: international guidelines for management of severe sepsis and septic shock: 2008. Crit Care Med 36: 296–327

36. Kapoor P, Kakani M, Chowdhury U, Choudhury M, Lakshmy R, Kiran U (2008): Early goal-directed therapy in moderate to high-risk cardiac surgery patients. Ann Card Anaesth 11: 27–34

37. Pölönen P, Ruokonen E, Hippeläinen M, Pöyhönen M, Takala J (2000) A prospective, randomized study of goal-oriented hemodynamic therapy in cardiac surgical patients. Anesth Analg 90: 1052–1059

38. Shepherd SJ, Pearse RM (2009) Role of central and mixed venous oxygen saturation measurement in perioperative care. Anesthesiology 111: 649–656

39. Turek Z, Sykora R, Matejovic M, Cerny V (2009) Anesthesia and the microcirculation. Semin Cardiothorac Vasc Anesth 13: 249–258

40. Bonazzi M, Gentile F, Biasi GM, et al (2002) Impact of perioperative haemodynamic monitoring on cardiac morbidity after major vascular surgery in low risk patients. A randomised pilot trial. Eur J Vasc Endovasc Surg 23: 445–451

IX

41. Conway D, Mayall R, Abdul-Latif M, Gilligan S, Tackaberry C (2002) Randomised controlled trial investigating the influence of intravenous fluid titration using oesophageal Doppler monitoring during bowel surgery. Anaesthesia 57: 845–845

42. Gan TJ, Soppitt A, Maroof M, et al (2002) Goal-directed intraoperative fluid administration reduces length of hospital stay after major surgery. Anesthesiology 97: 820–826

43. Venn R, Steele A, Richardson P, Poloniecki J, Grounds M, Newman P (2002) Randomized controlled trial to investigate influence of the fluid challenge on duration of hospital stay and perioperative morbidity in patients with hip fractures. Br J Anaesth 88: 65–71

44. Sandham JD, Hull RD, Brant RF, et al (2003) A randomized, controlled trial of the use of pulmonary-artery catheters in high-risk surgical patients. N Engl J Med 348: 5–14

45. McKendry M, McGloin H, Saberi D, Caudwell L, Brady AR, Singer M (2004) Randomised controlled trial assessing the impact of a nurse delivered, flow monitored protocol for optimisation of circulatory status after cardiac surgery. BMJ 329: 258

46. Wakeling HG, McFall MR, Jenkins CS, et al (2005) Intraoperative oesophageal Doppler guided fluid management shortens postoperative hospital stay after major bowel surgery. Br J Anaesth 95: 634–642

47. Noblett SE, Snowden CP, Shenton BK, Horgan AF (2006) Randomized clinical trial assessing the effect of Doppler-optimized fluid management on outcome after elective colorectal resection. Br J Surg 93: 1069–1076

48. Chytra I, Pradl R, Bosman R, Pelnár P, Kasal E, Zidková A (2007) Esophageal Doppler-guided fluid management decreases blood lactate levels in multiple-trauma patients: a randomized controlled trial. Crit Care 11: R24

49. Benes J, Chytra I, Altmann P, et al (2010) Intraoperative fluid optimization using stroke volume variation in high risk surgical patients: results of prospective randomized study. Crit Care 14: R118

50. Mayer J, Boldt J, Mengistu A, Rohm K, Suttner S (2010) Goal-directed intraoperative therapy based on autocalibrated arterial pressure waveform analysis reduces hospital stay in high-risk surgical patients: a randomized, controlled trial. Crit Care 14: R18

IX

Perioperative Goal-directed Therapy: Monitoring, Protocolized Care and Timing

M. Cecconi, C. Corredor, and A. Rhodes

Introduction

In the 1970s, Shoemaker observed that patients who survived high-risk surgical interventions had distinct hemodynamic patterns [1]. These included higher mean global oxygen delivery (DO_2), cardiac index (CI) and tissue oxygen demand (VO_2) than non-survivors. Shoemaker went on to develop the concept of perioperative optimization by using the survivors' patterns as therapeutic goals [2]. Amongst survivors, consistent 'supranormal' oxygen flow physiological values were noted of $DO_2 > 600$ ml/min/m², $VO_2 > 170$ ml/min/m² and CI > 4.5 l/min/m² [3]. Positive results in initial uncontrolled studies were corroborated by a controlled trial that used supranormal goals for hemodynamic optimization in the protocol group of high-risk surgical patients [4]. This protocol decreased mortality and spurred a wave of interest in perioperative goal directed therapy (GDT).

To understand these observations, it is necessary to review the physiology of how oxygen is delivered to and utilized by tissues. Global DO_2 is the product of cardiac output (CO) and arterial oxygen content (CaO_2) and is expressed by the equation:

$$DO_2 \text{ (ml/min)} = CO \text{ (l/min)} \times CaO_2 \times 10$$

Adequate DO_2 ensures that aerobic metabolism is maintained as the most efficient source of cellular energy. This energy is crucial for maintaining tissue structure and function [5]. The normal VO_2 at rest in healthy adults is 250–300 ml/min or 3.5 ml/kg, and is the amount required for basal metabolism. Exercise, sepsis, pain and anxiety can increase VO_2. Conversely, VO_2 is decreased by anesthesia and hypothermia. VO_2 can be calculated, using the modified Fick equation, as the product of the difference between CaO_2 and mixed venous blood oxygen content (CvO_2, in the pulmonary artery) and cardiac output (CO);

$$VO_2 = (CaO_2 - CvO_2) \times CO$$

The relationship between tissue VO_2 and DO_2 is known as the oxygen extraction ratio (O_2ER);

$$O_2ER = VO_2 / DO_2$$

DO_2 far exceeds the tissue VO_2 at rest and in health. A resting extraction ratio of 0.3 can increase to 0.8 during exercise in healthy individuals allowing for a 'supply-independent relationship' between DO_2 and VO_2. At a critical DO_2 point, however, VO_2 becomes 'supply-dependent'. Once critical DO_2 is reached, DO_2 is unable to support aerobic metabolism and lactic acidosis ensues [5]. Critical ill-

J.-L. Vincent (ed.), *Annual Update in Intensive Care and Emergency Medicine 2012*
DOI 10.1007/978-3-642-25716-2 © Springer-Verlag Berlin Heidelberg 2012

ness exhibits an abnormal relationship in which VO_2 becomes 'supply-dependent' even at levels above critical DO_2 [6]. Shoemaker and colleagues also used VO_2 values to identify a global state of impaired tissue oxygenation which occurred early in the postoperative period of the high-risk surgical patient. He described this as an 'oxygen deficit' or 'oxygen debt' and defined it as the difference between the pre-surgical normal VO_2 and the post-surgical insult VO_2. These investigators observed that the magnitude and duration of oxygen deficit in the postoperative period was strongly correlated with the subsequent appearance of organ failure and death [7].

The systemic inflammatory response that accompanies surgery increases requirements of the cardiovascular and respiratory systems to be able to deliver enough oxygen in the face of increased tissue demand. The consequences of not meeting these demands are a perpetuation of the inflammatory response, complement activation, cytokine release and endothelial dysfunction [8, 9]. An adequate partial pressure of oxygen is also crucial for neutrophil and macrophage bacterial killing mechanisms. Thus, low tissue oxygen has been linked to postoperative infections and impaired wound healing [10], translating into increased perioperative mortality and complications. Clinical criteria used to define 'high-risk' in perioperative GDT trials have a common denominator, which is the presence of a limited cardiovascular and respiratory reserve that is unable to meet the demands imposed by a variable degree of surgical stress [11]. It is, therefore, not surprising that the 'high-risk' group of patients account for more than 80 % of the deaths and postoperative complications related to surgery [12].

The impact of postoperative complications on long term survival after major surgery was highlighted by Khuri et al. [13]. In their work, data from the large National Surgical Quality Improvement Program (NSQIP) database was analyzed. They found that the occurrence of 30-day postoperative complications was the most important factor determining long-term survival after major surgery. The adverse effect of complications was independent of the patient's preoperative risk. They argue that the focus, therefore, should be on measures and processes to prevent the emergence of complications [13]. Similar findings have been presented for complications following pancreatic surgery and open aortic aneurysmectomy [14, 15].

Based on all these observations, attempts have been made over the last 30 years to increase DO_2 through hemodynamic manipulation, with the aim of improving outcomes of critically ill surgical patients. This is known as 'Goal-Directed Therapy' and encompasses all hemodynamic interventions aimed at ensuring adequate tissue perfusion and cellular oxygenation.

Outcome Evidence after Three Decades of Perioperative Goal-directed Therapy

Over the last three decades there have been a sizeable number of randomized controlled clinical trials (RCTs) and systematic reviews analyzing the impact of perioperative hemodynamic optimization strategies on mortality and morbidity of high-risk surgical patients. Meta-analyses and systematic reviews showed improved outcomes in different patient populations using different optimization techniques [16, 17]. A number of studies, however, found either no improved outcomes [18, 19], or even increased mortality rates [20] or complications in the optimized patient group [21].

The RCTs used in initial systematic reviews, differed in various aspects including the case mix of patients recruited (severity of surgical insult and comorbidity), thus affecting expected mortality; techniques and devices used to measure cardiac output; goals targeted (cardiac output, DO_2, stroke volume, etc); and methods used to achieve those goals (fluid plus inotropes or fluids alone). In addition there have been differences in methodological quality; some studies were not blinded and others had small population sizes limiting statistical power [22]. Recent systematic reviews have been undertaken using rigorous techniques for literature searching and data analysis. They have also addressed the impact of overall trial quality in the validity of the data produced.

In 2005, a meta-analysis of 30 RCTs, found that hemodynamic optimization techniques significantly decreased mortality when applied to perioperative patients without sepsis or multi-organ failure (RR 0.66, 95 % confidence interval [CI] 0.54 – 0.81). The authors conducted a formal methodological quality assessment and found wide variation in study quality. They also found that, in general, higher quality studies were less likely to report a significant reduction in mortality compared to lower quality studies. They concluded, however, that the reduction in mortality in high-risk surgical patients was not related to trial quality [22]. Hamilton et al., analyzed data from 29 RCTs involving 4805 moderate and high-risk surgical patients (overall mortality 7.6 %). They concluded that the use of the pre-emptive strategy of hemodynamic monitoring and associated therapy reduced surgical mortality (pooled OR 0.48, 95 % CI 0.33–0.70, p< 0.0002) and surgical complications (pooled OR 0.43, 95 % CI 0.35–0.55, p< 0.0001) [23]. Another recent systematic review of 32 clinical trials comprising 5056 high-risk surgical patients found that optimizing tissue perfusion in the perioperative period significantly reduced mortality (OR 0.67, 95 % CI 0.55–0.82, p < 0.001) and postoperative organ failure (OR 0.62, 95 % CI 0.55–0.70, p < 0.001) [24].

In addition, a number of recent systematic reviews and meta-analyses have focused on assessing the impact of GDT on specific postoperative complications. Postoperative kidney dysfunction is a significant cause of perioperative morbidity and mortality [25]. A meta-analytic study conducted by Brienza et al. found that the incidence of postoperative acute renal injury was significantly reduced in patients who received perioperative hemodynamic optimization compared with the control group (OR 0.64 p = 0.0007). Mortality was also significantly reduced in the treatment group (OR 0.50 p = 0.004) [26]. Giglio et al. found that patients undergoing major surgery benefitted from the protection that GDT provides to organs at risk of perioperative hypoperfusion, such as the bowel. Major gastrointestinal complications were significantly reduced by GDT when compared with a control group (OR 0.42; 95 % CI 0.27–0.65). These authors found no evidence, however, of GDT reducing the incidence of liver dysfunction [27]. Pneumonia, urinary tract infections and surgical site infections are leading causes of postoperative morbidity. They are particularly likely in the setting of high-risk surgical patients. Optimizing DO_2 using GDT protects patients against postoperative infections [28]. **Table 1** summarizes the findings of these systematic reviews and meta-analyses.

IX

Table 1. Summary of systematic reviews and meta-analyses on goal-directed therapy (GDT)

Author [ref]	Year	Focus	No of studies	No of patients	Mortality subgroup	Mortality effect	Type of Morbidity	Morbidity effect
Kern et al. [16]	2002	Mortality in high-risk surgery, trauma and septic patients if GDT is started before or after organ failure	21	NA	Mortality in all patients	difference ($\pm$ SD) -0.05 ($\pm$0.02) significant	NA	NA
			7	NA	Mortality with Control mortality > 20% after organ failure	difference ($\pm$ SD) - 0.01 ($\pm$ 0.06) non-significant	NA	NA
			7	NA	Mortality with Control mortality > 20% before organ failure	difference ($\pm$ SD) -0.23 ($\pm$ 0.07) significant	NA	NA
Poeze et al. [22]	2005	Mortality in perioperative and septic patients	30	5733	Mortality in all patients	0.61 (95 % CI 0.46 to 0.81) significant	NA	NA
			21	4,174	Perioperative studies and trauma	0.43 (95 % CI 0.28 to 0.66) significant	NA	NA
			10	1558	Septic shock or organ failure	0.85 (95 % CI 0.58 to 1.25)	NA	NA
Brienza et al. [26]	2009	Mortality and acute kidney injury	20	4220	Mortality in all patients	OR 0.50; CI 0.31–0.80; p = 0.004	Acute renal injury	OR 0.64; CI 0.50–0.83; p = 0.0007

NA: not available; CI: confidence interval; OR: odds ratio

IX

IX

Table 1. (*continued*)

Author [ref]	Year	Focus	No of studies	No of patients	Mortality subgroup	Mortality effect	Type of Morbidity	Morbidity effect
Giglio et al. [27]	2009	Gastrointestinal complications in major surgery	16	3410	NA	NA	Major gastrointestinal complications	OR, 0.42; 95 % CI, 0.27–0.65 significant
			16	3410	NA	NA	Minor gastrointestinal complications	OR, 0.29; 95 % CI, 0.17–0.50, significant
			16	3410	NA	NA	Hepatic injury	(OR, 0.54; 95 % CI, 0.19–1.55, not significant
Hamilton et al. [23]	2010	Mortality and morbidity in high-risk surgery	29	4805	Mortality in all patients	OR 0.48 (CI 0.33–0.70), p< 0.0002	All complications	OR 0.43 (0.35–0.55) p< 0.0001
Dalfino et al. [28]	2011	Infections in surgery in moderate to high-risk surgery	26	4188	NA	NA	All infections	OR 0.58, 95 % CI 0.46–0.74; p < 0.0001
			26	4188	NA	NA	Pneumonia	OR 0.71, 95 % CI 0.55–0.92; p = 0.009
			26	4188	NA	NA	Urinary tract Infection	0.44, 95 % CI 0.22–0.84; p = 0.02
Gurgel et al. [24]	2011	Mortality and organ dysfunction in high-risk surgery	32	5056	Mortality in all patients	0.67; 95 % CI: 0.55–0.82; p < 0.001	Organ dysfunction	0.62; 95 % CI: 0.55–0.70; p < 0.001

NA: not available; CI: confidence interval; OR: odds ratio

Earlier in this chapter, we highlighted the importance of postoperative complications as predictors of long term survival following major surgery. It is therefore logical to expect that preventing postoperative complications through the use of GDT would have an impact on long-term survival. Rhodes et al. assessed the long-term survival of patients enrolled in a previous RCT of GDT in high-risk surgical patients. They found that 15 years after the original study, long term survival was associated with three independent factors: Age (hazard ratio 1.04, 95 % CI 1.02–1.07, p< 0.0001), randomization to the GDT group (hazard ratio 0.61, 95 % CI 0.4–0.92, p = 0.02) and avoidance of significant postoperative cardiac complications (hazard ratio 3.78, 95 % CI 2.16–6.6, p = 0.007) [29]. The benefits conferred by GDT seem to be linked to various constant features appearing in all these studies, namely the use of cardiac output monitors, protocols guiding the clinical team and early initiation of GDT.

Cardiac Output Monitoring Devices and GDT

Clinical signs of hypovolemia are neither sensitive nor specific in the critically ill patient. When faced with hypovolemia, catecholamines and neural responses tend to maintain mean arterial pressure (MAP) even in the presence of decreasing blood flow [30]. Therefore, heart rate and pressure based measurements such as central venous pressure (CVP) and MAP bear little correlation with blood flow in critical illness and are poor predictors of survival [31]. Proof of this is that persistent tissue hypoxia can remain even when these parameters are normalized when used as end points of resuscitation [32]. Despite all this evidence, a recent survey by Cannesson et al. in USA and Europe has shown than 70 % of anesthesiologists still rely on these variables [33].

'Normal' values are 'abnormal' in the context of critical illness; survivors of major surgery and trauma have been found to be able to increase their DO_2 and VO_2 values to 'supranormal' values [34]. These observations were made possible by the inception of the pulmonary artery catheter (PAC) as the first bedside cardiac output monitoring system. Cardiac output and DO_2 monitoring have now become standard practice to ensure adequate tissue DO_2, and constitute the foundation of GDT. There are now many cardiac output monitors available for the clinician. As an indepth review of the technical aspects of all the different devices is beyond the scope of this chapter, emphasis is made on analyzing the available evidence behind the devices most commonly used in current GDT practice.

IX

The Pulmonary Artery Catheter

Despite the many cardiac output monitors currently available, cardiac output measurement by intermittent pulmonary artery thermodilution with the PAC remains the 'gold standard' against which other devices are compared. The conception of GDT is intimately linked to the PAC technology and they are sometimes considered synonymous. The initial observational studies that found 'supranormal' values of cardiac output and oxygen flow in survivors of critical illness used the PAC [35]. The PAC was also used in the pioneering prospective GDT trial by Shoemaker et al. in 1988 and in other early trials, such as that carried out by Boyd et al. in which GDT was associated with improved outcome [4, 36]. However, further studies using the PAC to guide hemodynamic optimization produced conflicting evidence with no improvement in outcome found with its use in trauma [37], sepsis [38] or critically ill patients [19]. There was, however, a reduction in morbidity and duration of hospital stay in cardiac surgical patients [39]. A meta-analysis of studies using the PAC conducted in 2002 by Kern and Shoemaker, found significantly lower mortality rates in high-risk elective surgical patients who were optimized at an early stage [16].

The uncertainty surrounding the benefits of GDT is also based on concerns arising from observational studies that linked PAC use to increased morbidity and mortality [40, 41]. Sandham et al. conducted a large RCT of the use of the PAC for GDT in high-risk surgical patients. They found neither mortality benefit nor evidence of any excess mortality linked to insertion of a PAC [21]. The apparent lack of evidence supporting the use of the PAC and the perceived associated risks, has led to a decline in enthusiasm to use this monitoring technique. Recent publications have, however, demonstrated that the use of PAC for certain groups of patients is associated with reductions in morbidity and mortality. In a meta-analysis of 29 randomized clinical trials evaluating the use of a pre-emptive hemodynamic intervention in high-risk surgical patients, Hamilton et al. found a statistically significant reduction in morbidity and mortality in studies using the PAC (OR 0.35; (0.19–0.65) p = 0.001) [23]. A systematic review of RCTs that used a hemodynamic protocol to maintain adequate tissue perfusion in the same group of patients found that monitoring cardiac output with a PAC and increasing oxygen transport and/or decreasing consumption also significantly reduced mortality [24].

In addition to cardiac output, the PAC can produce additional hemodynamic variables including mixed venous oxygen saturation (SvO_2), pulmonary artery pressures and conventional filling pressures. The PAC is, therefore, a valuable tool when monitoring of these variables is desirable or when other techniques fail to provide accurate cardiac output values.

Doppler Cardiac Output Monitoring

Estimation of cardiac output by esophageal Doppler monitoring devices is achieved by multiplying the cross sectional area of the aorta by the blood flow velocity measured in the descending aorta. Esophageal Doppler monitoring provides values for cardiac output, stroke volume and estimated systemic flow volume corrected time (FTc). Response to fluid loading in relation to stroke volume and FTc can be used to guide hemodynamic optimization (Cardio Q; Deltex Medical, Chichester UK). This non-invasive device has consistently demonstrated a reduction in complication rates and hospital length of stay when used for perioperative fluid optimization [42]. Hamilton et al. reported a reduction in postoperative complications in patients monitored using esophageal Doppler in their meta-analyisis of hemodynamic intervention trials in high-risk surgical patients (OR 0.41, 95 % CI 0.30–0.57) [23].

Despite the lack of multicenter prospective RCTs, the evidence base for outcome-benefit and cost-benefit is considered strong enough for the National Institute for Health and Clinical Excellence in the UK to recommend routine use of this device in high-risk surgical patients [43].

Pulse Contour Waveform Analysis

Arterial catheters are universally used for monitoring of the high-risk surgical patient during the perioperative period. Technologies that use the arterial waveform to derive cardiac output and stroke volume values have come to light in recent years as minimally invasive alternatives. The data provided by these techniques is continuous and allows the clinician to make decisions and apply interventions in real time.

The LiDCO™plus and LiDCO™ rapid systems (LiDCO Ltd, London, UK) use pulse power analysis techniques to track continuous changes in stroke volume. LiDCO™plus requires transpulmonary lithium dilution calibration for accurate cardiac output values and LiDCO™ rapid uses normograms for cardiac output estimation and does not require calibration. The PiCCOplus™ system (Pulsion Medical Systems AG, Munich, Germany) is a pulse contour analysis device that requires frequent transpulmonary thermodilution calibrations for cardiac output measurement. The Vigileo (Flotrac/Vigileo, Edwards Lifesciences, Irvine, CA, USA) system uses a specific arterial pressure transducer to characterize the pulse waveform. The data are analyzed together with patient demographics using an algorithm to provide an estimated stroke volume and cardiac output.

Both the LiDCO™plus and PiCCOplus™ monitors have been validated against the PAC and had a good degree of agreement when continuous and intermittent values of cardiac output were compared to those of the PAC [44]. Initial validation studies of the Vigileo system using earlier versions of the algorithm provided conflicting results. Subsequent modifications of the algorithm have shown improved perioperative performance [45]. The LiDCOplus™ system was used to measure cardiac output in an RCT in high-risk surgical patients using stroke volume optimization with colloid and dopexamine to achieve a DO_2 of > 600 ml/min/m^2. LiDCO-guided GDT was associated with reduced complications (p = 0.003) and length of hospital stay after major surgery (p = 0.001) [46].

A study in patients undergoing elective coronary artery bypass grafting (CABG) surgery used a PiCCO guided therapy algorithm protocol and compared these treated patients to a historical control group. Therapy guided by an algorithm based on global enddiastolic volume index (GEDVI) led to a shortened and reduced need for vasopressors, catecholamines, mechanical ventilation, and time patients stayed in the intensive care unit (ICU) [47]. Buettner et al. conducted a study in 80 elective major abdominal surgery patients comparing intraoperative fluid administration guided by systolic pressure variation monitored by PiCOO with standard care. They found no differences in organ perfusion and function, duration of mechanical ventilation, length of stay in the ICU or mortality between the groups [48].

The Flotrac/Vigileo system has been used to guide an intraoperative hemodynamic optimization protocol in high-risk patients undergoing major abdominal surgery. The use of the Flotrac/Vigileo-guided protocol reduced length of hospital stay and was associated with a lower incidence of complications compared to a standard management protocol (20 % vs 50 % p = 0.003) [49]. Cecconi et al. also incorporated the Flotrac/Vigileo system in a GDT protocol aiming to maximize stroke volume and target a DO_2 > 600 ml/min/m^2 in patients undergoing elective hip replacement. They reported a decreased number of minor postoperative complications in the protocol group compared to a control group that received standard care (100 % vs 75 %, p = 0.047) [50].

IX

Central Venous Oxygen Saturation and Oxygen Extraction Ratio

$ScvO_2$ can be easily measured by analyzing blood drawn from a central venous catheter (CVC) and has been used as a marker of the balance between global oxygen supply and demand [45]. A European multicenter study analyzed the association between peri- and postoperative $ScvO_2$ and outcome in high-risk surgical patients. This study found a relationship between a low ScvO2 perioperatively and an increased risk of postoperative complications in this group of patients [51].

In the light of the improved mortality outcomes reported by Rivers et al. in their early GDT (EGDT) trial for the treatment of septic shock, $ScvO_2$ has been used as a resuscitation endpoint in guidelines for treatment of patients with severe sepsis and septic shock [52, 53]. O_2ER can also be easily measured by drawing blood from arterial (SaO_2) and central venous catheters ($ScvO_2$) and putting the values into the equation:

$$O_2ER = SaO_2 - ScvO_2 / SaO_2.$$

Recently, investigators conducted a multicenter trial of 135 patients undergoing major abdominal surgery. The protocol group was managed with the goal to maintain an O_2ER of $< 27\%$ compared with standard targets of MAP > 80 mmHg and urinary output > 0.5 ml/kg/h in the control group. The authors found a reduction in length of stay (p< 0.05) and number of failing organs in the protocol group compared to the control group (p< 0.001). They found no difference in mortality [54].

The multiplicity of RCTs using an increasing array of cardiac output devices to guide perioperative GDT over the last few years called for a systematic review of the literature to appraise the impact of these technologies in outcomes. In their meta-analysis, Hamilton et al. conducted a subgroup analysis of morbidity and mortality outcomes for different monitoring devices when used to guide preemptive hemodynamic interventions in moderate and high-risk surgical patients. The PAC was alone in being associated with a statistically significant reduction in mortality (p $= 0.001$). Studies using esophageal Doppler, LiDCO™plus, FloTrac and CVP/arterial line demonstrated a significant reduction in the overall complication rate (OR 0.43, 95% CI 0.34–0.53) [23]. The complication rate was also reduced when O_2ER, pulse pressure variation, SvO_2 or lactate were used as a goals (OR 0.26, 95% CI 0.13–0.52) [23].

The evidence suggests that the use of cardiac output monitoring for hemodynamic interventions in the perioperative period is associated with better postoperative outcomes in moderate to high-risk patients. The choice of monitoring device will depend on a variety of factors: institutional (availability, level of experience, compatibility with existing devices); device related (invasiveness, technical limitations, validity & accuracy); and patient specific (arrhythmias, contraindications for insertion, type of operation, type of treatment protocol) [45]. The integrative approach to cardiac output monitoring proposed by Alhashemi et al. provides a logical framework for the use of different devices along the different stages of the clinical patient pathway. Device choices are made whilst balancing the invasiveness of the device with the need for more accurate hemodynamic variables and particular optimization protocol used [45].

IX

The Importance of Protocolized Care when Implementing Goal-directed Therapy

Perioperative hemodynamic optimization is carried out using patient specific physiological data to guide therapy aimed at achieving flow related goals. The variables required to calculate DO_2 are heart rate, stroke volume, SaO_2 and hemoglobin concentration. Different perioperative GDT trials have manipulated one or more of these physiological parameters in order to optimize tissue perfusion.

The first step in most GDT trials is usually stroke volume 'maximization' through administration of intravenous fluids titrated according to response. The objective is to attain the preload required for a near-maximal stroke volume or cardiac output in agreement with the Frank Starling law of the heart. This controlled technique is known as a 'fluid challenge' and serves two simultaneous purposes; it allows the clinician to administer fluids and at the same time test the preload reserve of the patient [55]. 'Stroke volume maximization' may be sufficient to achieve the desired flow goal. However, if the goal is not achieved, inotropes can be introduced in an attempt to further improve cardiac output and DO_2. Optimal oxygenation and hematocrit need to be maintained during the GDT process. Data from a recent meta-analysis suggest that the combination of fluid and inotropes is superior to fluids alone when expressed in terms of mortality reduction (OR 0.47, p = 0.002). When postoperative complications are considered, therapy with fluids plus inotropes (OR 0.47, 95 % CI 0.35–0.64) and with fluids alone (OR 0.38, 95 % CI 0.26–0.55) were both associated with improved outcomes [23].

The final step in GDT is achieving adequate DO_2. The parameters used as endpoints vary from trial to trial. Global DO_2 has historically been the most studied endpoint and was used in Shoemaker's prospective trial [4]. Various other indexes have also been used over the last few years e.g., O_2ER [54], FTc [56], SvO_2 [51], and lactate concentrations [39]. Recent data from a large hemodynamic optimization meta-analysis however suggested that only the use of DO_2 or cardiac index as endpoints conferred a statistically significant mortality reduction (p = 0.001) [23]. In addition, effects on mortality were more pronounced in studies using supranormal DO_2 resuscitation targets (p = 0.00001) [22, 23, 26]. Significant reductions in postoperative morbidity were observed when other targets, such as FTc/stroke volume (OR 0.41 95 % CI 0.28–0.58), pulse pressure variation (PPV), SvO_2 and lactate were used (OR 0.26, 95 % CI 0.13–0.52) [23]. Physiologically normal targets seem to be as effective as supranormal goals in terms of preventing complications, such as perioperative renal failure [26, 57].

Perioperative GDT trials have commonly used protocols or guidelines to direct implementation of therapy by investigators. There are crucial differences between the concepts of guidelines and protocols. Guidelines lack detail and only offer general guidance that require clinicians to fill in the many gaps. Protocols are detailed and, when used for complex clinical ICU problems, can generate patient-specific, evidence-based therapy instructions that can be carried out by different clinicians with almost no inter-clinician variability [58]. There is a strong body of evidence that suggests that the use of protocols in perioperative GDT is associated with improved outcomes. It remains important, however, for a clinician to be at the bedside and to ensure that the protocol is being followed in an appropriate fashion for each individual patient as important variances can and do occur.

The use of the PAC coupled with a hemodynamic optimization protocol has shown improved outcome benefits in multiple RCTs [4, 36, 39, 59, 60]. In contrast,

IX

there was no outcome benefit when the clinical management was left to the discretion of the treating physician following PAC insertion [61]. Similarly, no improved outcomes were found when only guidelines were followed [21]. Another example can be found in studies using minimally invasive devices. Takala et al. found no improvement in outcome when the FloTrac/Vigileo monitor was used early in addition to standard care in hemodynamically unstable ICU patients. This RCT did not use a protocol to guide therapy [62]. The use of the same device, in conjunction with an optimization protocol, has been associated with reduced postoperative complications [50, 63]. A recent systematic review of GDT that included 5056 high-risk surgical patients found a significant reduction in mortality rate ($p < 0.001$) and incidence of postoperative organ dysfunction ($p < 0.00001$) when a hemodynamic protocol was used to maintain tissue perfusion. Furthermore, additional mortality reduction benefits were found when the mortality rate was > 20 % in the control group [24].

Perioperative Goal-directed Therapy: Earlier is Better

Eighty percent of postoperative surgical deaths are from multi-organ failure [17]. High-risk surgical patients are particularly susceptible to develop organ dysfunction and account for most of the deaths and complications occurring after major surgery [3]. Organ dysfunction arises from persistent defects in DO_2 to the tissues that alter endothelial and cellular metabolism. If hypovolemia and impaired oxygen flow are not addressed early, mitochondrial damage ensues, and these effects become permanent [64, 65]. These defects accrue 'oxygen debt' in the tissues. The debt can be repaid in the early stages of the systemic inflammatory response syndrome (SIRS) that accompanies surgery, by optimizing oxygen flow. The repayment of oxygen debt is, however, time sensitive and once cellular and mitochondrial structures are permanently damaged attempts to improve oxygen flux are futile [66]. Some authors have demonstrated the presence of such permanent changes in the form of 'cytopathic hypoxia' in animal models of SIRS. Cytopathic hypoxia can be defined as an intrinsic derangement of the ability of the cells to use oxygen irrespective of adequate DO_2 [67].

These 'bench-side' observations have been corroborated at the 'bedside' by literature that reveals improved outcomes in patients in whom oxygen flow optimization interventions are started early in the disease process. Conversely, there is evidence suggesting that patients are insensitive to optimization techniques once organ failure develops. In septic patients, GDT was associated with important benefits in survival when started early in the emergency department [52]. When optimization protocols were applied late in the disease process, with organ dysfunction already established there were no survival benefits [19, 20]. Systematic reviews and meta-analyses of trials conducted in the era of the PAC reached similar conclusions. Early achievement of optimal oxygen flow goals in high-risk surgical and trauma patients before organ failure develops was associated with statistically significant mortality reductions [16, 17]. Kern and Shoemaker conducted a meta-analysis of 21 hemodynamic optimization RCTs trials in high-risk surgical, trauma and septic patients. They divided the studies into two groups: 'Early', 8 to 12 hours postoperatively or before organ failure developed; and 'late' or after the onset of organ failure. The authors found that in extremely high-risk patients (control mortalities group > 20 %), there was a 23 % mortality difference (p < 0.05) between the control and protocol groups with early optimization; however, patients optimized after the development of organ failure did not have significantly improved mortality [16].

Findings in a more recent meta-analysis studying GDT in surgical and critically ill patients have followed the same lines. The meta-analysis conducted by Poeze et al. found that the positive effect of hemodynamic optimization on outcomes was mostly due to the significant improvement in mortality in studies that included perioperative and trauma patients (relative risk [RR] 0.66, 95 % CI 0.54 to 0.81) compared to those that included septic patients (RR 0.92, 95 % CI 0.75 to 1.11). Peri-operative and trauma patients were less likely to have established organ dysfunction and benefited the most from hemodynamic optimization [22]. The meta-analysis conducted by Hamilton et al. included only RCTs that initiated hemodynamic interventions pre-emptively in the perioperative period. The perioperative period was defined as 24 hours preoperatively, intra-operatively or up to 24 hours after surgery. The authors did not analyze subgroups of patients according to the timing of hemodynamic intervention. They found that use of GDT pre-emptively yielded a significant reduction in mortality ($p = 0.0002$) and surgical complications ($p < 0.001$) compared to control groups [23].

Gut barrier failure because of hypoperfusion and bacterial translocation is linked to the development of infections and multi-organ failure in critically ill patients. A meta-analysis of 26 RCTs that included patients undergoing major surgery found that GDT initiated in the perioperative period significantly reduced the incidence of postoperative infections (pooled OR 0.44, 95 % CI 0.28–0.58; $p < 0.00001$). Only trials that initiated hemodynamic optimization "early" (within 8 hours of surgery) were included and those which included patients with already established sepsis and organ failure were excluded [28]. Similarly, a meta-analysis that found that GDT was associated with reduced postoperative acute renal injury and gastrointestinal complications excluded studies with patients undergoing late optimization or with established organ failure or sepsis [26, 27].

Conclusion

GDT can be defined as the early use of protocolized treatment guided by hemodynamic monitoring to optimize the status of high-risk surgical and septic patients. When the three features (monitoring, protocol and timing) are present, this appraoch has shown to improve patient outcome.

References

1. Shoemaker WC, Montgomery ES, Kaplan E, Elwyn DH (1973) Physiologic patterns in surviving and nonsurviving shock patients. Use of sequential cardiorespiratory variables in defining criteria for therapeutic goals and early warning of death. Arch Surg 106: 630–636
2. Shoemaker WC, Appel PL, Waxman K, Schwartz S, Chang P (1982) Clinical trial of survivors' cardiorespiratory patterns as therapeutic goals in critically ill postoperative patients. Crit Care Med 10: 398–403
3. Shoemaker WC, Appel PL, Kram HB (1993) Hemodynamic and oxygen transport responses in survivors and nonsurvivors of high-risk surgery. Crit Care Med 21: 977–990
4. Shoemaker WC, Appel PL, Kram HB, Waxman K, Lee TS (1988) Prospective trial of supranormal values of survivors as therapeutic goals in high-risk surgical patients. Chest 94: 1176–1186

IX

5. Connett RJ, Honig CR, Gayeski TE, Brooks GA (1990) Defining hypoxia: a systems view of VO2, glycolysis, energetics, and intracellular PO2. J Appl Physiol 68: 833–842
6. Leach RM, Treacher DF (1992) The pulmonary physician and critical care. 6. Oxygen transport: the relation between oxygen delivery and consumption. Thorax 47: 971–978
7. Shoemaker WC, Appel PL, Kram HB (1992) Role of oxygen debt in the development of organ failure sepsis, and death in high-risk surgical patients. Chest 102: 208–215
8. Karimova A, Pinsky DJ (2001) The endothelial response to oxygen deprivation: biology and clinical implications. Intensive Care Med 27: 19–31
9. Sibbald WJ, Fox G, Martin C (1991) Abnormalities of vascular reactivity in the sepsis syndrome. Chest 100 (3 Suppl): 155S–159S
10. Allen DB, Maguire JJ, Mahdavian M, et al (1997) Wound hypoxia and acidosis limit neutrophil bacterial killing mechanisms. Arch Surg 132: 991–996
11. Boyd O, Jackson N (2005) How is risk defined in high-risk surgical patient management? Crit Care 9: 390–396
12. Jhanji S, Thomas B, Ely A, Watson D, Hinds CJ, Pearse RM (2008) Mortality and utilisation of critical care resources amongst high-risk surgical patients in a large NHS trust. Anaesthesia 63: 695–700
13. Khuri SF, Henderson WG, DePalma RG, Mosca C, Healey NA, Kumbhani DJ (2005) Determinants of long-term survival after major surgery and the adverse effect of postoperative complications. Ann Surg 242: 326–341
14. Kamphues C, Bova R, Schricke D, et al (2012) Postoperative complications deteriorate long-term outcome in pancreatic cancer patients. Ann Surg Oncol (in press)
15. Nathan DP, Brinster CJ, Jackson BM, et al (2011) Predictors of decreased short- and long-term survival following open abdominal aortic aneurysm repair. J Vasc Surg 54: 1237–1243
16. Kern JW, Shoemaker WC (2002) Meta-analysis of hemodynamic optimization in high-risk patients. Crit Care Med 30: 1686–1692
17. Boyd O, Hayes M (1999) The oxygen trail: the goal. Br Med Bull 55: 125–139
18. Heyland DK, Cook DJ, King D, Kernerman P, Brun-Buisson C (1996) Maximizing oxygen delivery in critically ill patients: a methodologic appraisal of the evidence. Crit Care Med 24: 517–524
19. Gattinoni L, Brazzi L, Pelosi P, et al (1995) A trial of goal-oriented hemodynamic therapy in critically ill patients. SvO2 Collaborative Group. N Engl J Med 333: 1025–1032
20. Hayes MA, Timmins AC, Yau EH, Palazzo M, Hinds CJ, Watson D (1994) Elevation of systemic oxygen delivery in the treatment of critically ill patients. N Engl J Med 330: 1717–1722
21. Sandham JD, Hull RD, Brant RF, et al (2003) A randomized, controlled trial of the use of pulmonary-artery catheters in high-risk surgical patients. N Engl J Med 348: 5–14
22. Poeze M, Greve JW, Ramsay G (2005) Meta-analysis of hemodynamic optimization: relationship to methodological quality. Crit Care 9: R771–779
23. Hamilton MA, Cecconi M, Rhodes A (2011) A systematic review and meta-analysis on the use of preemptive hemodynamic intervention to improve postoperative outcomes in moderate and high-risk surgical patients. Anesth Analg 112: 1392–1402
24. Gurgel ST, do Nascimento P Jr (2011) Maintaining tissue perfusion in high-risk surgical patients: a systematic review of randomized clinical trials. Anesth Analg 112: 1384–1391
25. Jones DR, Lee HT (2008) Perioperative renal protection. Best Pract Res Clin Anaesthesiol 22: 193–208
26. Brienza N, Giglio MT, Marucci M, Fiore T (2009) Does perioperative hemodynamic optimization protect renal function in surgical patients? A meta-analytic study. Crit Care Med 37: 2079–2090
27. Giglio MT, Marucci M, Testini M, Brienza N (2009) Goal-directed haemodynamic therapy and gastrointestinal complications in major surgery: a meta-analysis of randomized controlled trials. Br J Anaesth 103: 637–646
28. Dalfino L, Giglio MT, Puntillo F, Marucci M, Brienza N (2011) Haemodynamic goal-directed therapy and postoperative infections: earlier is better. A systematic review and meta-analysis. Crit Care 15: R154
29. Rhodes A, Cecconi M, Hamilton M, et al (2010) Goal-directed therapy in high-risk surgical patients: a 15-year follow-up study. Intensive Care Med 36: 1327–1332

IX

30. Wo CC, Shoemaker WC, Appel PL, Bishop MH, Kram HB, Hardin E (1993) Unreliability of blood pressure and heart rate to evaluate cardiac output in emergency resuscitation and critical illness. Crit Care Med 21: 218–223

31. Shoemaker WC, Czer LS (1979) Evaluation of the biologic importance of various hemodynamic and oxygen transport variables: which variables should be monitored in postoperative shock? Crit Care Med 7: 424–431

32. Rady MY, Rivers EP, Nowak RM (1996) Resuscitation of the critically ill in the ED: responses of blood pressure, heart rate, shock index, central venous oxygen saturation, and lactate. Am J Emerg Med 14: 218–225

33. Cannesson M, Pestel G, Ricks C, Hoeft A, Perel A (2011) Hemodynamic monitoring and management in patients undergoing high risk surgery: a survey among North American and European anesthesiologists. Crit Care 15: R197

34. Bishop MH, Shoemaker WC, Appel PL, et al (1993) Relationship between supranormal circulatory values, time delays, and outcome in severely traumatized patients. Crit Care Med 21: 56–63

35. Bland RD, Shoemaker WC, Abraham E, Cobo JC (1985) Hemodynamic and oxygen transport patterns in surviving and nonsurviving postoperative patients. Crit Care Med 13: 85–90

36. Boyd O, Grounds RM, Bennett ED (1993) A randomized clinical trial of the effect of deliberate perioperative increase of oxygen delivery on mortality in high-risk surgical patients. JAMA 270: 2699–2707

37. Velmahos GC, Demetriades D, Shoemaker WC, et al (2000) Endpoints of resuscitation of critically injured patients: normal or supranormal? A prospective randomized trial. Ann Surg 232: 409–418

38. Tuchschmidt J, Fried J, Astiz M, Rackow E (1992) Elevation of cardiac output and oxygen delivery improves outcome in septic shock. Chest 102: 216–220

39. Polonen P, Ruokonen E, Hippelainen M, Poyhonen M, Takala J (2000) A prospective, randomized study of goal-oriented hemodynamic therapy in cardiac surgical patients. Anesth Analg 90: 1052–1059

40. Connors AF Jr, Speroff T, Dawson NV, et al (1996) The effectiveness of right heart catheterization in the initial care of critically ill patients. SUPPORT Investigators. JAMA 276: 889–897

41. Zion MM, Balkin J, Rosenmann D, et al (1990) Use of pulmonary artery catheters in patients with acute myocardial infarction. Analysis of experience in 5,841 patients in the SPRINT Registry. SPRINT Study Group. Chest 98: 1331–1335

42. Abbas SM, Hill AG (2008) Systematic review of the literature for the use of oesophageal Doppler monitor for fluid replacement in major abdominal surgery. Anaesthesia 63: 44–51

43. NICE (2011) MTG3 CardioQ-ODM (oesophageal Doppler monitor): guidance. www.nice.org.uk/guidance/MTG3. Accessed November 2011

44. Morgan P, Al-Subaie N, Rhodes A (2008) Minimally invasive cardiac output monitoring. Curr Opin Crit Care 14: 322–326

45. Alhashemi JA, Cecconi M, Hofer CK (2011) Cardiac output monitoring: an integrative perspective. Crit Care 15: 214

46. Pearse R, Dawson D, Fawcett J, Rhodes A, Grounds RM, Bennett ED (2005) Early goal-directed therapy after major surgery reduces complications and duration of hospital stay. A randomised, controlled trial [ISRCTN38797445]. Crit Care 9: R687–693

47. Goepfert MS, Reuter DA, Akyol D, Lamm P, Kilger E, Goetz AE (2007) Goal-directed fluid management reduces vasopressor and catecholamine use in cardiac surgery patients. Intensive Care Med 33: 96–103

48. Buettner M, Schummer W, Huettemann E, Schenke S, van Hout N, Sakka SG (2008) Influence of systolic-pressure-variation-guided intraoperative fluid management on organ function and oxygen transport. Br J Anaesth 101: 194–199

49. Mayer J, Boldt J, Mengistu AM, Rohm KD, Suttner S (2010) Goal-directed intraoperative therapy based on autocalibrated arterial pressure waveform analysis reduces hospital stay in high-risk surgical patients: a randomized, controlled trial. Crit Care 14: R18

50. Cecconi M, Fasano N, Langiano N, et al (2011) Goal-directed haemodynamic therapy during elective total hip arthroplasty under regional anaesthesia. Crit Care 15: R132

IX

51. Collaborative Study Group on Perioperative ScvO2 Monitoring (2006) Multicentre study on peri- and postoperative central venous oxygen saturation in high-risk surgical patients. Crit Care 10: R158
52. Rivers E, Nguyen B, Havstad S, et al (2001) Early goal-directed therapy in the treatment of severe sepsis and septic shock. N Engl J Med 345: 1368–1377
53. Dellinger RP, Levy MM, Carlet JM, et al (2008) Surviving Sepsis Campaign: international guidelines for management of severe sepsis and septic shock: 2008. Crit Care Med 36: 296–327
54. Donati A, Loggi S, Preiser JC, et al (2007) Goal-directed intraoperative therapy reduces morbidity and length of hospital stay in high-risk surgical patients. Chest 132: 1817–1824
55. Cecconi M, Parsons AK, Rhodes A (2011) What is a fluid challenge? Curr Opin Crit Care 17: 290–295
56. Noblett SE, Snowden CP, Shenton BK, Horgan AF (2006) Randomized clinical trial assessing the effect of Doppler-optimized fluid management on outcome after elective colorectal resection. Br J Surg 93: 1069–1076
57. Rhodes A, Cecconi M, Hamilton M, et al (2010) Goal-directed therapy in high-risk surgical patients: a 15-year follow-up study. Intensive Care Med 36: 1327–1332
58. Morris AH (2003) Treatment algorithms and protocolized care. Curr Opin Crit Care 9: 236–240
59. Wilson J, Woods I, Fawcett J, et al (1999) Reducing the risk of major elective surgery: randomised controlled trial of preoperative optimisation of oxygen delivery. BMJ 318: 1099–1103
60. Lobo SM, Lobo FR, Polachini CA, et al (2006) Prospective, randomized trial comparing fluids and dobutamine optimization of oxygen delivery in high-risk surgical patients [ISRCTN42445141]. Crit Care 10: R72
61. Harvey S, Harrison DA, Singer M, et al (2005) Assessment of the clinical effectiveness of pulmonary artery catheters in management of patients in intensive care (PAC-Man): a randomised controlled trial. Lancet 366: 472–477
62. Takala J, Ruokonen E, Tenhunen JJ, Parviainen I, Jakob SM (2011) Early non-invasive cardiac output monitoring in hemodynamically unstable intensive care patients: A multicenter randomized controlled trial. Crit Care 15: R148
63. Benes J, Chytra I, Altmann P, et al (2010) Intraoperative fluid optimization using stroke volume variation in high risk surgical patients: results of prospective randomized study. Crit Care 14: R118
64. Poeze M, Greve JW, Ramsay G (1999) Oxygen delivery in septic shock. Chest 116: 1145
65. Hollenberg SM, Cunnion RE (1994) Endothelial and vascular smooth muscle function in sepsis. J Crit Care 9: 262–280
66. Abid O, Akca S, Haji-Michael P, Vincent JL (2000) Strong vasopressor support may be futile in the intensive care unit patient with multiple organ failure. Crit Care Med 28: 947–949
67. Fink MP (2002) Bench-to-bedside review: Cytopathic hypoxia. Crit Care 6: 491–499

IX

Blood Lactate Levels: A Manual for Bedside Use

J. BAKKER and T.C. JANSEN

Introduction

In the first description of increased lactate levels in human beings [1], Joseph Scherer analyzed blood drawn from young women who had just died from what we now call septic shock. Since then increased levels and delayed clearance have been associated with many measures of morbidity and mortality [2, 3]. However, the source of increased lactate levels and/or the cause of its delayed clearance is not linked to one specific pathological process that, when positively influenced by therapy, will change lactate levels and improve outcome. Therefore, the clinical use of lactate levels to improve outcome of critically ill patients is subject to ongoing discussion. To use the complex signal of increased lactate levels and/or delayed clearance the clinician needs to understand the metabolism of lactate.

IX

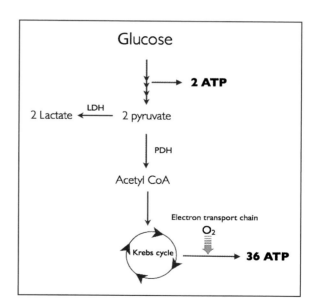

Fig. 1. Glucose metabolism.
LDH : lactate dehydrogenase;
PDH : pyruvate dehydrogenase

J.-L. Vincent (ed.), *Annual Update in Intensive Care and Emergency Medicine 2012*
DOI 10.1007/978-3-642-25716-2 © Springer-Verlag Berlin Heidelberg 2012

Normal Metabolism

Almost all cells in the human body can produce lactate from glucose exclusively mediated by the lactate dehydrogenase enzyme and lactate can thus be regarded as a key metabolite [4]. Normally, glucose is metabolized to pyruvate (**Fig. 1**), which, when entering the mitochondrial metabolic processes (Krebs cycle), produces (in the presence of oxygen) the large amount of ATP needed to maintain cell function. When excess pyruvate is present the conversion to lactate dominates. As erythrocytes have no mitochondria, lactate is the end product of glucose metabolism in these cells. In other cells, a lack of oxygen is an important cause of limited pyruvate metabolism, and thus lactate levels, by mass effect. In critically ill patients, this mechanism is the basis for using lactate levels to guide resuscitation with fluids and inotropes to improve tissue oxygenation and prevent the development of multiple organ failure [5]. Lactate is metabolized mainly in the liver (50 %) and kidneys (20 %), but (resting) muscle also metabolizes lactate. Therefore, in conditions of impaired liver perfusion and function, lactate levels can increase more significantly because of impaired clearance.

What is the Cause of Increased Lactate Levels?

The blood lactate level is the consequence of increased production and/or of impaired clearance.

Increased Production: The Hypoxic Pathway

In many experimental and some clinical studies the presence of a critical level of global/regional oxygen delivery (DO_2) has been identified [6, 7]. At DO_2 levels lower than this critical level, oxygen consumption (VO_2) is dependent on DO_2 (supply dependency). Both in experimental and clinical conditions, this phenomenon is associated with increased blood lactate levels in many disease states [7–12]. Moreover, in experimental conditions reversal of this supply dependency state is associated with normalization of blood lactate levels to baseline values [13] (**Fig. 2**). In clinical conditions, improvement in DO_2 in patients with increased lactate is associated with increased VO_2 [10]. In addition, the supply-dependent VO_2 phenomenon seems to be apparent in the early phase of critical illness and to resolve following adequate resuscitation associated with a normalization of lactate levels [8].

Increased Production: The Increased Metabolism Pathway

As lactate is a normal end-product of glucose metabolism increased glycolysis may thus exceed the capacity to metabolize pyruvate and, hence, increase lactate levels. In critically ill patients, and especially patients with sepsis, increased aerobic lactate production has been identified. In particular, the Na^+/K^+ pump, present in most cells, is a known producer of lactate in the presence of adequate oxygenation [14]. Epinephrine administration also results in increased glycolysis and a dose-dependent increase in lactate levels in human volunteers [15]. The presence of this mechanism has even been related to improved outcome in patients with clinical shock [16].

Fig. 2. Shock induced by cardiac tamponade. In this model cardiac tamponade resulted in a stepwise decrease in oxygen delivery (DO_2). The decrease in oxygen consumption (VO_2 – induction of shock) was associated with a significant rise in lactate levels. Following restoration of DO_2 (treatment) by release of intrapericardial pressure (dotted arrow lines) VO_2 increased and lactate levels returned to baseline values. Adapted from [13]

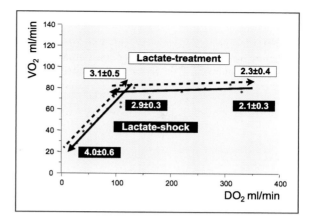

Many other causes of increased lactate levels not associated with inadequate tissue oxygenation have been identified although even in these cases increased lactate levels may be associated with a worse outcome [5].

Decreased Clearance

Although some have reported impaired clearance as a cause of increased lactate levels in patients with sepsis [17], others showed that in patients with septic and cardiogenic shock, lactate clearance was not the cause of increased lactate levels but rather lactate production [18]. Although in patients following cardiac surgery, lactate clearance is impaired [19] others have shown that in these circumstances inadequate tissue oxygenation may still be an important cause of increased lactate levels [20]. Although impaired liver perfusion and liver function may decrease lactate clearance the actual impact on clinical lactate levels is not straightforward [21, 22]. Nevertheless, abnormal lactate clearance has also been associated with outcome parameters in critically ill patients [23].

Summary

Although increased lactate levels do not necessarily imply inadequate oxygenation of tissues it seems reasonable to assume that in the early phase of shock, lactate production is increased due to impaired DO_2 to the tissues and that adequate treatment should result in normalization of lactate levels. Persistence of increased lactate levels in critically ill patients is associated with increased morbidity and mortality even in the presence of adequate tissue oxygenation [24].

What is the Initial Treatment of Patients Admitted with Increased Lactate Levels?

From the above summary of the causes of increased lactate levels it follows that initial treatment should be focused on improving tissue oxygenation. This can be accomplished in several ways (**Table 1**). As the transport of oxygen is a product of hemoglobin levels, arterial oxygen saturation and blood flow (cardiac output,

IX

Table 1. Optimizing tissue oxygenation

Category	Intervention
Oxygen demand	Treat pain, fear, tachypnea, high fever, delirium. Apply (non)invasive mechanical ventilation
Hemoglobin level	Infuse red blood cells to predefined minimum level
Arterial oxygen saturation	Increase FiO_2, optimize ventilation by use of PEEP, lung recruitment
Flow	Increase cardiac output by optimizing preload, improve regional/microcirculatory blood flow by limiting central venous pressure and/or use of vasodilators

FiO_2: inspired fraction of oxygen; PEEP: positive end-expiratory pressure

regional or microcirculatory perfusion) these are 3 important mechanisms to improve tissue DO_2. Also, one could decrease the oxygen demand to balance the delivery of oxygen to the demand for oxygen. Many of the interventions summarized in **Table 1** can be started at the same time. The tissues regulate the immediate delivery of oxygen to meet their oxygen demand by changing blood flow as we cannot change our hemoglobin level or arterial oxygen saturation rapidly and significantly. As blood flow can be increased by more then 100 % [25] when, for example, hemoglobin levels are decreasing this is a very important mechanism. Therefore, the initial treatment of patients with increased lactate levels targets improving tissue blood flow. This should first be accomplished by optimizing cardiac preload by fluid resuscitation that can effectively increase DO_2 and VO_2 [26]. Although optimal cardiac filling pressures have been advocated [27, 28], the use of a dynamic approach seems to be more physiology based [29]. When blood flow is still not optimal, it could be further increased by the use of inotropic agents [10]. Regional and microcirculatory blood flow can be optimized by use of inotropic agents and vasodilators [30–34]. Although the efficiency of improving tissue oxygenation by use of blood transfusion is unclear, this approach can optimize microcirculatory perfusion by increasing the number of perfused capillaries [35]. The optimal arterial oxygen saturation is unknown although high oxygen levels seem to be undesirable in critically ill patients [36–38].

In addition, an adequate perfusion pressure should accompany these interventions. Although the optimal perfusion pressure is not well defined, in general a mean arterial pressure (MAP) > 65 mmHg seems adequate in most patients and is thus recommended in international guidelines [28]. Norepinephrine has been shown to improve microcirculatory oxygenation, even in the early phase of septic shock [39] and seems to be superior to dopamine [40]. In specific patients (elderly, history of hypertension, brain injury, cardiac ischemia) a higher perfusion pressure may be necessary to maintain adequate organ perfusion.

An important question when optimizing tissue DO_2 to meet metabolic demands is: "when is delivery adequate?" Although a target of supranormal levels of DO_2 has been advocated for a long time this approach may be harmful in critically ill patients [41]. When tissues need more oxygen and delivery cannot be increased, the oxygen reserve present in the circulation is used. As in normal circumstances only 25 % of the amount of oxygen is used for consumption, a significant amount of oxygen returns unused to the right heart. In a condition in which this reserve is used, the venous oxygen saturation will decrease. Clinically the oxygen saturation in the superior vena cava ($ScvO_2$) is frequently measured and has been incorporated in treatment schedules that have resulted in improved outcomes in critically ill patients [42]. Although the use of $ScvO_2$ has some limitations, its trending seems to reflect the true mixed venous compartment (SvO_2) adequately [43]. Therefore general guidelines suggest maintaining $ScvO_2 > 70\%$ [28, 44].

What Decrease in Lactate Levels should be Aimed For?

This question is hard to answer as no studies have tried to solve this problem. Observational studies have shown that a small decrease (10 %) in the first six hours of treatment can discriminate survivors from non-survivors [3]. However, subsequent use of this clearance as a goal of therapy did not improve outcome over the use of $ScvO_2$ [45]. When we used a much higher clearance of lactate (20 % per two hours for the first 8 hours of treatment) together with a normal $ScvO_2$ as a goal of treatment in a randomized study, this strategy was associated with a significant decrease in mortality although ultimately the clearance of lactate was ± 5 % per hour in both groups [46]. We concluded from this study that lactate could help to optimize the balance between DO_2 and oxygen demand in the early phase of treatment in specific patients in whom lactate levels do not respond adequately to treatment. When using a target lactate clearance of 20 % per two hours, failure to meet this goal probably also served as a red flag to indicate suboptimal treatment or response to treatment.

IX

What to do When Lactate Levels do not Decrease Adequately?

When global DO_2 and oxygen demand have been optimized, inadequate regional/ microcirculatory perfusion could persist. This abnormality could be treated by the use of inotropes [30] and vasodilators [33]. In recent studies, we showed that impaired peripheral perfusion was associated with limited lactate clearance [47, 48] and, therefore, this condition could serve as a surrogate marker to optimize lactate clearance. Peripheral perfusion in septic shock can be optimized by improving perfusion pressure and global blood flow [39], by targeting coagulation abnormalities [49, 50] and with the use of vasodilators [34].

Conclusion

Lactate is a key metabolite in humans and although the interpretation of increased levels in critically ill patients is complex, the presence or persistence of increased lactate levels is associated with significant morbidity and mortality in these patients. As inadequate tissue oxygenation/perfusion is an important and significant cause of increased lactate levels, targeting optimal tissue oxygenation/ perfusion is an important goal in the first hours of treatment. Optimizing cardiac output and regional/microcirculatory flow by improving preload, use of inotropes and in some cases vasodilators and subsequently optimizing hemoglobin levels and arterial oxygen saturation, can improve the delivery of oxygen to the tissues.

Combined with reducing oxygen demand in the critically ill patient this approach may further optimize the balance between oxygen demand and oxygen supply. Using venous oxygen saturation and significant decreases in lactate levels as the goal of this initial treatment could optimize the chances of survival of critically ill patients.

References

1. Kompanje EJ, Jansen TC, van der Hoven B, Bakker J (2007) The first demonstration of lactic acid in human blood in shock by Johann Joseph Scherer (1814–1869) in January 1843. Intensive Care Med 33: 1967–1971
2. Bakker J, Gris P, Coffernils M, Kahn RJ, Vincent JL (1996) Serial blood lactate levels can predict the development of multiple organ failure following septic shock. Am J Surg 171: 221–226
3. Nguyen HB, Rivers EP, Knoblich BP, et al (2004) Early lactate clearance is associated with improved outcome in severe sepsis and septic shock. Crit Care Med 32: 1637–1642
4. Leverve XM, Mustafa I (2002) Lactate: A key metabolite in the intercellular metabolic interplay. Crit Care 6: 284–285
5. Jansen TC, van Bommel J, Bakker J (2009) Blood lactate monitoring in critically ill patients: a systematic health technology assessment. Crit Care Med 37: 2827–2839
6. Cain SM, Curtis SE (1991) Experimental models of pathologic oxygen supply dependency. Crit Care Med 19: 603–612
7. Ronco JJ, Fenwick JC, Tweeddale MG, et al (1993) Identification of the critical oxygen delivery for anaerobic metabolism in critically ill septic and nonseptic humans. JAMA 270: 1724–1730
8. Friedman G, De Backer D, Shahla M, Vincent JL (1998) Oxygen supply dependency can characterize septic shock. Intensive Care Med 24: 118–123
9. Bakker J, Vincent JL (1991) The oxygen supply dependency phenomenon is associated with increased blood lactate levels. J Crit Care 6: 152–159
10. Vincent JL, Roman A, De Backer D, Kahn RJ (1990) Oxygen uptake/supply dependency. Effects of short-term dobutamine infusion. Am Rev Respir Dis 142: 2–7
11. Cain SM (1965) Appearance of excess lactate in anesthetized dogs during anemic and hypoxic hypoxia. Am J Physiol 209: 604–608
12. Rixen D, Siegel JH (2005) Bench-to-bedside review: oxygen debt and its metabolic correlates as quantifiers of the severity of hemorrhagic and post-traumatic shock. Crit Care 9: 441–53
13. Zhang H, Spapen H, Benlabed M, Vincent JL (1993) Systemic oxygen extraction can be improved during repeated episodes of cardiac tamponade. J Crit Care 8: 93–99
14. Levy B, Gibot S, Franck P, Cravoisy A, Bollaert PE (2005) Relation between muscle Na+K+ ATPase activity and raised lactate concentrations in septic shock: a prospective study. Lancet 365: 871–875
15. Griffith FR Jr, Lockwood JE, Emery FE (1939) Adrenalin lactacidemia: proportionality with dose. Am J Physiol 127: 415–421
16. Wutrich Y, Barraud D, Conrad M, et al (2010) Early increase in arterial lactate concentration under epinephrine infusion is associated with a better prognosis during shock. Shock 34: 4–9
17. Levraut J, Ciebiera JP, Chave S, et al (1998) Mild hyperlactatemia in stable septic patients is due to impaired lactate clearance rather than overproduction. Am J Respir Crit Care Med 157: 1021–1026
18. Revelly JP, Tappy L, Martinez A, et al (2005) Lactate and glucose metabolism in severe sepsis and cardiogenic shock. Crit Care Med 33: 2235–2240
19. Mustafa I, Roth H, Hanafiah A, et al (2003) Effect of cardiopulmonary bypass on lactate metabolism. Intensive Care Med 29: 1279–1285
20. Ranucci M, De Toffol B, Isgro G, Romitti F, Conti D, Vicentini M (2006) Hyperlactatemia during cardiopulmonary bypass: determinants and impact on postoperative outcome. Critical Care 10: R167

IX

21. De Gasperi A, Mazza E, Corti A, et al (1997) Lactate blood levels in the perioperative period of orthotopic liver transplantation. Int J Clin Lab Res 27: 123–128

22. Joseph SE, Heaton N, Potter D, Pernet A, Umpleby MA, Amiel SA (2000) Renal glucose production compensates for the liver during the anhepatic phase of liver transplantation. Diabetes 49: 450–456

23. Levraut J, Ichai C, Petit I, Ciebiera JP, Perus O, Grimaud D (2003) Low exogenous lactate clearance as an early predictor of mortality in normolactatemic critically ill septic patients. Crit Care Med 31: 705–710

24. Jansen TC, van Bommel J, Woodward R, Mulder PG, Bakker J (2009) Association between blood lactate levels, Sequential Organ Failure Assessment subscores, and 28-day mortality during early and late intensive care unit stay: a retrospective observational study. Crit Care Med 37: 2369–2374

25. Weiskopf RB, Viele MK, Feiner J, et al (1998) Human cardiovascular and metabolic response to acute, severe isovolemic anemia. JAMA 279: 217–221

26. Kaufman BS, Rackow EC, Falk JL (1984) The relationship between oxygen delivery and consumption during fluid resuscitation of hypovolemic and septic shock. Chest 85: 336–340

27. Packman MI, Rackow EC (1983) Optimum left heart filling pressure during fluid resuscitation of patients with hypovolemic and septic shock. Crit Care Med 11: 165–169.

28. Dellinger RP, Levy MM, Carlet JM, et al (2008) Surviving Sepsis Campaign: international guidelines for management of severe sepsis and septic shock: 2008. Intensive Care Med 34: 17–60

29. Vincent JL, Weil MH (2006) Fluid challenge revisited. Crit Care Med 34: 1333–1337

30. De Backer D, Creteur J, Dubois MJ, et al (2006) The effects of dobutamine on microcirculatory alterations in patients with septic shock are independent of its systemic effects. Crit Care Med 34: 403–408

31. Creteur J, De Backer D, Vincent JL (1999) A dobutamine test can disclose hepatosplanchnic hypoperfusion in septic patients. Am J Respir Crit Care Med 160: 839–845

32. De Backer D, Berre J, Zhang H, Kahn RJ, Vincent JL (1993) Relationship between oxygen uptake and oxygen delivery in septic patients: effects of prostacyclin versus dobutamine. Crit Care Med 21: 1658–1664

33. Spronk PE, Ince C, Gardien MJ, Mathura KR, Oudemans-van Straaten HM, Zandstra DF (2002) Nitroglycerin in septic shock after intravascular volume resuscitation. Lancet 360: 1395–1396

34. den Uil CA, Caliskan K, Lagrand WK, et al (2009) Dose-dependent benefit of nitroglycerin on microcirculation of patients with severe heart failure. Intensive Care Med 35: 1893–1899

35. Sakr Y, Chierego M, Piagnerelli M, et al (2007) Microvascular response to red blood cell transfusion in patients with severe sepsis. Crit Care Med 35: 1639–1644

36. Cabello JB, Burls A, Emparanza JI, Bayliss S, Quinn T (2010) Oxygen therapy for acute myocardial infarction. Cochrane Database Syst Rev CD007160

37. de Jonge E, Peelen L, Keijzers PJ, et al (2008) Association between administered oxygen, arterial partial oxygen pressure and mortality in mechanically ventilated intensive care unit patients. Crit Care 12: R156

38. Reinhart K, Bloos F, Konig F, Bredle D, Hannemann L (1991) Reversible decrease of oxygen consumption by hyperoxia. Chest 99: 690–694

39. Hamzaoui O, Georger JF, Monnet X, et al (2010) Early administration of norepinephrine increases cardiac preload and cardiac output in septic patients with life-threatening hypotension. Crit Care 14: R142

40. De Backer D, Biston P, Devriendt J, et al (2010) Comparison of dopamine and norepinephrine in the treatment of shock. N Engl J Med 362: 779–789

41. Hayes MA, Yau EH, Timmins AC, Hinds CJ, Watson D (1993) Response of critically ill patients to treatment aimed at achieving supranormal oxygen delivery and consumption. Relationship to outcome. Chest 103: 886–895

42. Rivers E, Nguyen B, Havstad S, et al (2001) Early goal-directed therapy in the treatment of severe sepsis and septic shock. N Engl J Med 345: 1368–1377

43. Reinhart K, Rudolph T, Bredle DL, Hannemann L, Cain SM (1989) Comparison of central-

IX

venous to mixed-venous oxygen saturation during changes in oxygen supply/demand. Chest 95: 1216–1221

44. Pinsky MR, Vincent JL (2005) Let us use the pulmonary artery catheter correctly and only when we need it. Crit Care Med 33: 1119–1122

45. Jones AE, Shapiro NI, Trzeciak S, Arnold RC, Claremont HA, Kline JA (2010) Lactate clearance vs central venous oxygen saturation as goals of early sepsis therapy: a randomized clinical trial. JAMA 303: 739–746

46. Jansen TC, van Bommel J, Schoonderbeek FJ, et al (2010) Early lactate-guided therapy in intensive care unit patients: a multicenter, open-label, randomized controlled trial. Am J Respir Crit Care Med 182: 752–761

47. Lima A, Jansen TC, van Bommel J, Ince C, Bakker J (2009) The prognostic value of the subjective assessment of peripheral perfusion in critically ill patients. Crit Care Med 37: 934–938

48. Lima A, van Bommel J, Jansen TC, Ince C, Bakker J (2009) Low tissue oxygen saturation at the end of early goal-directed therapy is associated with worse outcome in critically ill patients. Crit Care 13 (Suppl 5): S13

49. Donati A, Romanelli M, Botticelli L, et al (2009) Recombinant activated protein C treatment improves tissue perfusion and oxygenation in septic patients measured by near-infrared spectroscopy. Crit Care 13 (Suppl 5): S12

50. Spronk PE, Rommes JH, Schaar C, Ince C (2006) Thrombolysis in fulminant purpura: observations on changes in microcirculatory perfusion during successful treatment. Thromb Haemost 95: 576–578

IX

X Fluids and Blood Transfusion

The Meaning of Fluid Responsiveness

R. Giraud, N. Siegenthaler, and K. Bendjelid

Introduction

The management of intravenous fluid infusion in intensive care unit (ICU) patients is complex and often corresponds to the clinical imperative for perfusion and tissue oxygenation [1]. This issue is important because it concerns a large proportion of ICU patients. Indeed, inappropriate volume restriction may cause low cardiac output and/or inappropriate use of vasopressive or inotropic drugs [2]. In contrast, adjusted volume restriction avoids excessive fluid infusion and related complications, which include pulmonary edema, microcirculatory dysfunction and organ failure [3, 4]. Excessive fluid resuscitation may also lead to electrolytic disorders such as hypernatremia and hyperchloremic acidosis [5] and/or coagulation impairments [6].

The understanding of this complex issue and the clinical application of fluid resuscitation involve the integration of different indices of volemia (preload and preload-dependent indices), of which the determinants are arterial and venous circulation, cardiac function, and their interaction with pulmonary mechanics [7, 8]. Ventricular preload indices (static indices) and preload-dependent indices (dynamic indices) can quantify the same hemodynamic status on quite distinct grounds [9]. In a specific hemodynamic status, each value of central venous pressure (CVP), pulmonary artery occlusion pressure (PAOP) or pulse pressure variation (PPV) is determined by the interaction between the two circulations (venous and arterial) and the heart-lung system [10]. Thus, coupling static indices (CVP and PAOP) and dynamic indices [PPV and systolic pressure variation [SPV]] could help to estimate the circulating blood volume and to predict fluid responsiveness [11]. However, in certain clinical situations, combining preload and preload-dependent indices does not facilitate the management of vascular filling in the ICU. This is particularly true in spontaneously breathing patients or mechanically ventilated patients under pressure support (triggering the ventilator), in whom PPV, for example, is not interpretable. In these cases, it is sometimes necessary to transitorily modify the patient's intravascular volume status by performing a passive leg raising maneuver, and to observe the effects on volemia, preload and cardiac output [12]. Here, we review the physiology of circulatory volume, how to optimize intravascular volume status, and the indices allowing prediction of fluid responsiveness.

X

J.-L. Vincent (ed.), *Annual Update in Intensive Care and Emergency Medicine 2012*
DOI 10.1007/978-3-642-25716-2 © Springer-Verlag Berlin Heidelberg 2012

Physiology of Circulatory Volume

The concept of preload dependence/independence describes the effect of fluid infusion on cardiac output. An increase in cardiac output of more than a clear percentage value (10–15 %) secondary to volume infusion defines the patient as a fluid responder [13]. Conversely, if cardiac output does not increase by more than the present percentage value (10–15 %) after volume expansion, the patient is defined as a non-responder. According to experimental studies, preload is defined by the myocardial fiber length before contraction [14]. However, in clinical practice, there is no consensus on the definition of ventricular preload. For each ventricle, the preload can be defined either as the ventricular dimension in diastole (diameter, area, and volume assessed principally by echocardiography), or as the loading conditions of the ventricle in diastole. The relationship between preload and stroke volume is called the Frank–Starling systolic function curve [14] .

The evaluation of preload-dependence and the use of various hemodynamic indices require knowledge of the physiological mechanisms involved in venous return [7, 15, 16]. Parameters which should be considered are: Stressed and unstressed venous volume, the pressure gradient generating venous return (mean systemic pressure minus CVP), cardiac function, and the effective arterial elastance [17] (**Fig. 1**). This systemic return corresponds to drainage by the cardiac pump of the blood volume from the peripheral venous bed towards the intrathoracic central vascular bed through large collapsible veins. When averaged over a period of time, systemic venous return and cardiac output are equal. The pressure gradient of venous return is the difference between the upstream driving pressure prevailing in the venous bed (mean circulatory filling pressure) and the downstream pressure of the venous return, represented by the intravascular right

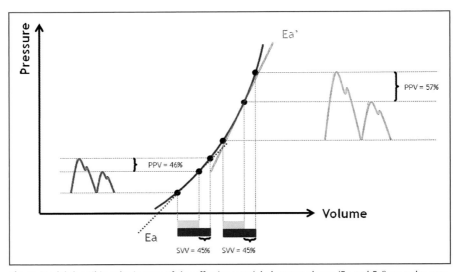

Fig. 1. Model describing the impact of the effective arterial elastance slopes (Ea and Ea′) on pulse pressure variation (PPV) values. For a same stroke volume variation (SVV) value = 45 %, PPVs vary from 46 to 57 %.

atrial pressure or CVP [7]. There is also a hemodynamically inactive blood volume that is necessary to maintain the vessels in an open shape, known as the unstressed volume. The ratio between stressed and unstressed volumes within the venous vascular bed depends upon venous tone and/or vasopressor treatment [2].

Volume expansion transiently increases circulating blood volume. Part of this volume may be lost in the case of capillary leakage, as observed in septic patients [18]. Extravascular distribution, which requires a period of equilibration, depends on the vascular permeability coefficient, the properties of the oncotic liquid, and the hydrostatic pressure. It is thus difficult to predict what fraction of the infused solution is contributing to the increase in intravascular volume or is recruited to the cardiac preload. This fraction varies according to time, vascular permeability and the clinical situation. Under stable conditions, an increase in stressed volume can be assessed by measuring the increase in cardiac pressure or ventricular volume [19]. However, stressed volume will increase venous return and cardiac preload only if vascular fillings increase the mean circulatory filling pressure to a greater extent than the CVP [20]. The present statement presupposes that all other determinants of venous return remain stable.

Several parameters can influence the determinants of the pressure gradient of venous return: the intra-abdominal pressure (in turn affected by abdominal compartment syndrome or positive pressure ventilation) [21], the variation of compliance and venous resistance associated with the use of vasoactive substances with venous tropism (e.g., nitroglycerin, norepinephrine), and the intrathoracic and cardiac functions [22]. These pathophysiological states can influence the pressure gradient of venous return, regardless of the stressed volume, and thus limit the effects of volume expansion.

For a given pressure gradient, the venous return generated can also be limited by the flow resistance (venous resistance). The vascular waterfall effect is an adaptive or pathological situation where venous return is impeded when intramural venous vessel pressure becomes lower than extramural pressure. Subsequently, as for example in the vena cava, the venous vessel collapses and flow is interrupted [21, 23]. This phenomenon could be an adaptive protection against an excessive increase in venous return, which would result in right ventricular overload. This is the case when there is an excessive decrease in CVP (during forced inspiration for example) occurring concomitantly with a high stressed volume [23]. In contrast, this mechanism may be harmful in the case of low stressed volume and a pathologically high extramural pressure (high abdominal pressure), where real preload dependence could occur following the collapse of the vena cava [21, 24]. In this case, the appropriate therapeutic approach may consist of not only increasing the circulating vascular volume, but also in reducing the extramural pressure, allowing the stressed volume to reach the cardiac chambers.

Venous Return During Mechanical Ventilation

Under positive pressure ventilation, intrathoracic pressure increases during inspiration. This increase in intrathoracic pressure is partially transmitted to the right atrium, thus reducing the mean circulatory filling pressure–CVP pressure gradient and inducing a decrease in venous return [25]. In a patient with balanced volume status, changes in intrathoracic pressure will have little effect on venous return. However, in cases of hypovolemia, the consequences will be significant.

The effect of positive pressure ventilation on venous return is the main determinant of dynamic indices [25]. The effect of intrathoracic pressure changes on CVP is also dependent on the transmission of this pressure to the abdominal compartment, and its consequences on the inferior vena cava (IVC) [21]. The IVC diameter is mainly determined by the transmural pressure of the vena cava [26], defined as the difference between intramural and extramural pressures. In addition, the impact of positive pressure ventilation on venous return is influenced by the stressed volume and venous compliance [26, 27].

Indications for Fluid Expansion

Four situations may indicate a need to investigate for preload-dependence:

- Systemic hypotension
- A low cardiac output
- Signs of tissue hypoperfusion (lactate, base excess, mixed venous oxygen saturation [SvO_2])
- A pathological but compensated medical state

In some cases, systemic blood pressure can be normalized by sympathetic stimulation, but this can be associated with inadequate tissue perfusion. In this situation, volume expansion may shift the cardiovascular system toward a new state of stability to reduce the often deleterious compensatory mechanisms, such as peripheral vasoconstriction and adrenergic stimulation.

X   On What Basis Should Volume Expansion Be Administered?

Static Indices

Although ventricular end-diastolic volume is a good preload marker [8], the relationship between ventricular volume and stroke volume is dependent on cardiac function [11]. For a determined ventricular preload (pressure, volume), preload-dependence can be estimated using the curve of cardiac function [28]. A normal ventricular volume associated with reduced cardiac function could correspond to a zone of preload-independence, while this same volume, in the presence of a hyper-contractile cardiac function, may be associated with a preload-dependent state (**Fig. 2**). Thus, the relationship linking ventricular preload and stroke volume cannot be addressed solely through knowledge of the degree of myocardial fiber stretch [29] (**Fig. 2**).

In clinical practice, in the absence of ventricular volume monitoring, the ventricular pressure measurement is used as a surrogate of preload (CVP, PAOP) [8]. This substitution is limited by two factors. First, the measured pressures represent a component of the transmural pressure; the intramural pressure does not take into account the extramural pressure, which may be important in many situations encountered in the ICU. Second, the relationship between diastolic volume and transmural pressure is determined by ventricular and pericardial elastance, both of which are difficult to assess [30]. Variations in extramural pressure, when measured at the bedside, can cause the intraluminal pressure to vary significantly without being translated into a change in preload [30]. Moreover, under positive pressure ventilation, the change in intrathoracic pressure depends upon the degree of pressure transmission (greater in the presence of increased lung com-

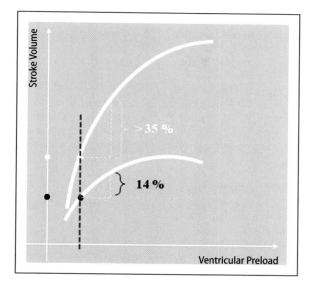

Fig. 2. Model highlighting that the relationship linking ventricular preload and changes in stroke volume (SV) following volume expansion cannot be addressed solely through the knowledge of the preload value. Example: For a same change in ventricular preload, SV increases by 14 % in a failing heart and by 35 % in a normal heart.

pliance). Taking into consideration the multiple pathophysiological concepts mentioned above, it is clear that static indices of cardiac preload cannot predict fluid responsiveness in critically ill patients, and cannot discriminate responders to volume expansion from non-responders [8].

Dynamic Indices

Over the last decade, pragmatic intensivists were more interested in the fluid responsiveness of the subject than in estimating the ventricular preload [31–34]. However, several authors have considered volume therapy in a different way [8, 19, 35, 36], based on the Frank–Starling relationship [14]. Their aim is to predict the response to volume expansion, which distinguishes patients whose cardiac output and blood pressure will increase (responders) from patients whose hemodynamic status is insensitive to volume infusion (non-responders), or in whom the infusion volume may be deleterious [3, 4].

Based on prospective physiological studies directed at understanding and treating circulatory failure, it became clear that assessing cardiac preload does not predict fluid responsiveness [9]. Static indices, based on the measurement of filling pressure, ventricular volumes and surfaces, were shown to be unreliable and of limited use [37] in patients with either spontaneous ventilation or positive pressure ventilation [8, 19, 35, 36]. In contrast, dynamic indices, based on estimation of preload dependence via a disturbance of the circulation by a mechanical breath, proved their utility and reliability for characterizing preload-dependence [8, 19, 35, 36]. These indices are based on heart-lung interactions under positive pressure ventilation in deeply sedated patients with regular heart rhythms, and are now increasingly used to estimate the need for volume expansion and to optimize circulatory status in critically ill patients [8, 35, 36].

Respiratory changes in systemic pulse pressure, stroke volume and systolic arterial pressure during mechanical ventilation reflect changes in left ventricular preload [35]. These variations in ventricular preload are due to changes in venous return, induced in turn by the cyclic variations of both pleural and transpulmonary pressures [28, 29]. Other dynamic indices, based on the variation of parameters not coupled to the systolic ejection period and stroke volume, have also demonstrated reliability in predicting fluid responsiveness [38–43].

The measurement of cardiac filling pressures and chamber volumes has little value as a predictor of fluid responsiveness. However, these measurements remain important, because they show that the fluid infusion has reached the heart and, therefore, that preload-dependence has been tested [19]. In the intensive care setting, the prevalence of patients presenting with significant capillary leakage (sepsis, acute pancreatitis, ischemia-reperfusion) is very high, and the volume required to load the heart may vary considerably. However, it should be kept in mind that basic conditions are necessary to enable the use of heart-lung interactions and derived dynamic indices. The heart rhythm has to be regular [8], tidal volume breathed through the respirator has to be more than 8 ml/kg [44, 45], and the patient should be deeply sedated and unable to trigger the ventilator [8, 44]. Apart from these specific cases, and in patients with spontaneous ventilation, passive leg raising appears to be the most robust method for predicting fluid responsiveness [12, 46, 47].

Passive Leg Raising

This maneuver mobilizes the blood from the legs and abdomen to the chest compartment and produces the hemodynamic effects of an autotransfusion [47]. The maximum increase in blood flow during this maneuver takes place within the first 20 seconds. Several studies have validated the passive leg raising maneuver as a predictor of fluid responsiveness in patients triggering the ventilator and in those with an arrhythmia [12, 46, 47]. This simple maneuver is easy to perform at the bedside, and can aid in judging whether or not fluid loading is indicated, in all critically ill patients.

Macrocirculation and Microcirculation

The final goal of hemodynamic management is to improve or maintain tissue perfusion. This functional perfusion is provided by the microvascular system. Concerning fluid infusion and after initial resuscitation in a stabilized situation, some considerations must be discussed: First, even if fluid infusion may improve microvascular perfusion, this effect seems to be independent (uncoupled) from the macro-hemodynamic parameters (hemodynamic indices or dynamic markers of preload responsiveness) [48]. Second, the effect of volume expansion on the microcirculation depends on the amount of fluid infused, a quantity which is very difficult to guess [49]. Finally, the effect of fluid infusion may be more effective in particular phases of the disease [48]. Consequently, these specificities of the microvascular response to fluid infusion further increase the complexity of assessing tissue fluid responsiveness. Indeed, vascular fluid responsiveness does not mean tissue fluid responsiveness.

Conclusion

The proposed techniques for monitoring fluid responsiveness should provide the clinician with reliable and reproducible information for deciding whether or not to administer volume expansion to a hypotensive patient, as well as information about how to administer volume expansion safely. Information collected through these indices may allow the intensivist to make more informed treatment decisions, to optimize the patient's hemodynamic status and possibly to improve their prognosis. The benefits of such an approach could result in the optimization of circulatory status, with improved peripheral tissue perfusion and consequent prevention of multiple organ dysfunctions. This reasoned approach, and the practical management of circulating blood volume in critically ill patients, should be based on the pathophysiology of venous return, heart–lung interactions and cardiac function.

References

1. Siegenthaler N, Giraud R, Piriou V, Romand JA, Bendjelid K (2010) Microcirculatory alterations in critically ill patients: pathophysiology, monitoring and treatments. Ann Fr Anesth Reanim 29: 135–144
2. Nouira S, Elatrous S, Dimassi S, et al (2005) Effects of norepinephrine on static and dynamic preload indicators in experimental hemorrhagic shock. Crit Care Med 33: 2339–2343
3. Arieff AI (1999) Fatal postoperative pulmonary edema: pathogenesis and literature review. Chest 115: 1371–1377
4. Boussat S, Jacques T, Levy B, et al (2002) Intravascular volume monitoring and extravascular lung water in septic patients with pulmonary edema. Intensive Care Med 28: 712–718
5. Mallie JP, Halperin ML (2001) A new concept to explain dysnatremia: the tonicity balance of entries and exits. Bull Acad Natl Med 185: 119–146
6. Fries D, Innerhofer P, Klingler A, et al (2002) The effect of the combined administration of colloids and lactated Ringer's solution on the coagulation system: an in vitro study using thrombelastograph coagulation analysis. Anesth Analg 94: 1280–1287
7. Bendjelid K (2005) Right atrial pressure: determinant or result of change in venous return? Chest 128: 3639–3640
8. Bendjelid K, Romand JA (2003) Fluid responsiveness in mechanically ventilated patients: a review of indices used in intensive care. Intensive Care Med 29: 352–360
9. Michard F, Reuter DA (2003) Assessing cardiac preload or fluid responsiveness? It depends on the question we want to answer. Intensive Care Med 29:1396
10. Tyberg JV (1992) Venous modulation of ventricular preload. Am Heart J 123: 1098–1104
11. Michard F (2005) Changes in arterial pressure during mechanical ventilation. Anesthesiology 103: 419–428
12. Monnet X, Rienzo M, Osman D, et al (2006) Passive leg raising predicts fluid responsiveness in the critically ill. Crit Care Med 34: 1402–1407
13. Stetz CW, Miller RG, Kelly GE, Raffin TA (1982) Reliability of the thermodilution method in the determination of cardiac output in clinical practice. Am Rev Respir Dis 126: 1001–1004
14. Starling E (1918) The Linacre Lecture On The Law Of The Heart Given At Cambridge, 1915. Longmans, Green and CO, London
15. Guyton AC, Lindsey AW, Abernathy B, Richardson T (1957) Venous return at various right atrial pressures and the normal venous return curve. Am J Physiol 189: 609–615
16. Levy MN (1979) The cardiac and vascular factors that determine systemic blood flow. Circ Res 44: 739–747
17. Giraud R, Siegenthaler N, Bendjelid K (2011) Pulse pressure variation, stroke volume variation and dynamic arterial elastance. Crit Care 15: 414

X

18. Levy MM, Fink MP, Marshall JC, et al (2003) 2001 SCCM/ESICM/ACCP/ATS/SIS International Sepsis Definitions Conference. Intensive Care Med 29: 530–538

19. Coudray A, Romand JA, Treggiari M, Bendjelid K (2005) Fluid responsiveness in spontaneously breathing patients: a review of indexes used in intensive care. Crit Care Med 33: 2757–2762

20. Guyton AC (1955) Determination of cardiac output by equating venous return curves with cardiac response curves. Physiol Rev 35: 123–129

21. Duperret S, Lhuillier F, Piriou V, et al (2007) Increased intra-abdominal pressure affects respiratory variations in arterial pressure in normovolaemic and hypovolaemic mechanically ventilated healthy pigs. Intensive Care Med 33: 163–171

22. Scharf SM, Caldini P, Ingram RH Jr (1977) Cardiovascular effects of increasing airway pressure in the dog. Am J Physiol 232: H35–43

23. Permutt S (1963) Hemodynamics of collapsible vessels with tone: the vascular waterfall. J Appl Physiol 18: 924–932

24. Vivien B, Marmion F, Roche S, et al (2006) An evaluation of transcutaneous carbon dioxide partial pressure monitoring during apnea testing in brain-dead patients. Anesthesiology 104: 701–707

25. Bendjelid K, Romand JA (2007) Cardiopulmonary interactions in patients under positive pressure ventilation. Ann Fr Anesth Reanim 26: 211–217

26. Takata M, Wise RA, Robotham JL (1990) Effects of abdominal pressure on venous return: abdominal vascular zone conditions. J Appl Physiol 69: 1961–1972

27. Bendjelid K, Romand JA, Walder B, Suter PM, Fournier G (2002) Correlation between measured inferior vena cava diameter and right atrial pressure depends on the echocardiographic method used in patients who are mechanically ventilated. J Am Soc Echocardiogr 15: 944–949

28. Feihl F, Broccard AF (2009) Interactions between respiration and systemic hemodynamics. Part I: basic concepts. Intensive Care Med 35: 45–54

29. Feihl F, Broccard AF (2009) Interactions between respiration and systemic hemodynamics. Part II: practical implications in critical care. Intensive Care Med 35: 198–205

30. Tyberg JV, Taichman GC, Smith ER, Douglas NW, Smiseth OA, Keon WJ (1986) The relationship between pericardial pressure and right atrial pressure: an intraoperative study. Circulation 73: 428–432

31. Horst HM, Obeid FN (1986) Hemodynamic response to fluid challenge: a means of assessing volume status in the critically ill. Henry Ford Hosp Med J 34: 90–94

32. Perel A (1998) Assessing fluid responsiveness by the systolic pressure variation in mechanically ventilated patients. Systolic pressure variation as a guide to fluid therapy in patients with sepsis-induced hypotension. Anesthesiology 89: 1309–1310

33. Perel A, Pizov R, Cotev S (1987) Systolic blood pressure variation is a sensitive indicator of hypovolemia in ventilated dogs subjected to graded hemorrhage. Anesthesiology 67: 498–502

34. Tavernier B, Makhotine O, Lebuffe G, Dupont J, Scherpereel P (1998) Systolic pressure variation as a guide to fluid therapy in patients with sepsis-induced hypotension. Anesthesiology 89: 1313–1321

35. Michard F, Teboul JL (2000) Using heart-lung interactions to assess fluid responsiveness during mechanical ventilation. Crit Care 4: 282–289

36. Michard F, Teboul JL (2002) Predicting fluid responsiveness in ICU patients: a critical analysis of the evidence. Chest 121: 2000–2008

37. Osman D, Ridel C, Ray P, et al (2007) Cardiac filling pressures are not appropriate to predict hemodynamic response to volume challenge. Crit Care Med 35: 64–68

38. Barbier C, Loubieres Y, Schmit C, et al (2004) Respiratory changes in inferior vena cava diameter are helpful in predicting fluid responsiveness in ventilated septic patients. Intensive Care Med 30: 1740–1746

39. Bendjelid K, Suter PM, Romand JA (2004) The respiratory change in preejection period: a new method to predict fluid responsiveness. J Appl Physiol 96: 337–342

40. Feissel M, Badie J, Merlani PG, Faller JP, Bendjelid K (2005) Pre-ejection period variations predict the fluid responsiveness of septic ventilated patients. Crit Care Med 33: 2534–2539

41. Feissel M, Michard F, Faller JP, Teboul JL (2004) The respiratory variation in inferior vena cava diameter as a guide to fluid therapy. Intensive Care Med 30: 1834–1837

42. Vieillard-Baron A, Chergui K, Rabiller A, et al (2004) Superior vena caval collapsibility as a gauge of volume status in ventilated septic patients. Intensive Care Med 30: 1734–1739

43. Vistisen ST, Struijk JJ, Larsson A (2009) Automated pre-ejection period variation indexed to tidal volume predicts fluid responsiveness after cardiac surgery. Acta Anaesthesiol Scand 53: 534–542

44. De Backer D, Heenen S, Piagnerelli M, Koch M, Vincent JL (2005) Pulse pressure variations to predict fluid responsiveness: influence of tidal volume. Intensive Care Med 31: 517–523

45. Szold A, Pizov R, Segal E, Perel A (1989) The effect of tidal volume and intravascular volume state on systolic pressure variation in ventilated dogs. Intensive Care Med 15: 368–371

46. Lamia B, Ochagavia A, Monnet X, Chemla D, Richard C, Teboul JL (2007) Echocardiographic prediction of volume responsiveness in critically ill patients with spontaneously breathing activity. Intensive Care Med 33: 1125–1132

47. Monnet X, Teboul JL (2008) Passive leg raising. Intensive Care Med 34: 659–663

48. Ospina-Tascon G, Neves AP, Occhipinti G, et al (2010) Effects of fluids on microvascular perfusion in patients with severe sepsis. Intensive Care Med 36: 949–955.

49. Pottecher J, Deruddre S, Teboul JL, et al (2010) Both passive leg raising and intravascular volume expansion improve sublingual microcirculatory perfusion in severe sepsis and septic shock patients. Intensive Care Med 36: 1867–1874

X

Respiratory Variation in the Perioperative and Critical Care Settings

R.H. Thiele, J. Raphael, and A.D. Shaw

Introduction

The American Society of Anesthesiologists' (ASA) Standards for Basic Anesthetic Monitoring recommend blood pressure monitoring every 5 minutes for all patients under general anesthesia. The selection of blood pressure as a standard monitoring tool is not based on physiologic rationale (indeed, physiologic studies suggest there is essentially no relationship between mean arterial pressure ([MAP] and global delivery of oxygen [DO_2] [1]) or evidence of improved outcomes.

The lack of data and questionable physiologic rationale behind pressure-based hemodynamic management has led to the development of alternative paradigms, collectively titled 'goal-directed therapy'. Over the last thirty years, investigators have incorporated a variety of goals into management algorithms, including maximization of global DO_2 [2], maintenance of mixed venous oxygen saturation (SvO_2) above a certain threshold [3], and optimization of stroke volume [4], all of which require use of additional, non-standard monitoring equipment.

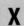

Respiratory variation, which attempts to quantify the likely increase in stroke volume following volume administration, has recently emerged as an attractive alternative to conventional goal-directed therapy targets. Its measurement is relatively simple (and intuitive) and theoretically does not require the use of additional monitoring equipment. While not a physiologic endpoint *per se*, respiratory variation tells the practitioner whether or not stroke volume is optimized given a particular set of loading conditions, allowing the practitioner to make rational decisions regarding fluid management.

Systemic Arterial Respiratory Variation

Historical Context

During normal spontaneous ventilation, systolic blood pressure decreases on inspiration, although typically not by more than 5 mmHg [5]. During constrictive conditions, such as pericardial tamponade, the right ventricular enlargement that normally occurs during negative-pressure inhalation impinges on the left ventricle, enhancing the decrease in blood pressure that accompanies inspiration [6]. In 1873, Adolf Kussmaul bestowed upon this phenomenon the unfortunate term "pulsus paradoxus"[7] (unfortunate because it is not paradoxical at all, it is simply an exaggeration of a normal physiologic phenomenon).

In 1966, Morgan et al. examined the effect of positive pressure ventilation on vena caval and aortic blood flow, stroke volume, and systemic blood pressure in

J.-L. Vincent (ed.), *Annual Update in Intensive Care and Emergency Medicine 2012*
DOI 10.1007/978-3-642-25716-2 © Springer-Verlag Berlin Heidelberg 2012

dogs during spontaneous and positive pressure ventilation (peak airway pressures ranged from 10–30 mmHg, I:E ratios ranged from 1:2 to 2:1). These authors found that initiation of positive pressure ventilation led to a decrease in venous return and, within two heartbeats, decreased aortic blood flow. Importantly, the extent of these changes was significantly related to peak airway pressures. [8]. In 1973, Massumi and colleagues described a series of conditions that could lead to "reversed pulsus paradoxus", in which inspiration led to an increase, rather than decrease in blood pressure (because this is the opposite of what normally occurs, it actually deserves the title "pulsus paradoxus". However, because the term "pulsus paradoxus" had been misused for at least half a century prior to their discovery [9], Massumi et al. had to resort to the more cumbersome and less appropriate title "reversed pulsus paradoxus" to describe their findings). Importantly, one of the conditions in which blood pressure might increase during inspiration was cardiac failure in the setting of positive pressure ventilation [10].

Based on Morgan and Massumi's work, Rick and Burke examined the arterial blood pressure and airway pressures in 65 critically ill patients undergoing positive pressure ventilation. In their study, 71 % of the patients who were thought to be hypovolemic had at least 10 mmHg of change in blood pressure with respiration (respiratory variation) [11]. In contrast, only 24 % of normovolemic patients had 10 mmHg of respiratory variation. Thus, Rick and Burke were the first to suggest that variations in blood pressure associated with positive pressure ventilation may be a means of assessing volume status. Subsequent experiments conducted by Perel and colleagues further elucidated the relationship between positive pressure ventilation, blood pressure variation, and volume status. This group made major contributions to the study of this new clinical variable, showing that respiratory variation was linearly and reliably related to graded hemorrhage in animal models (and could be reversed with fluid resuscitation) [12], that respiratory variation was related to tidal volumes [13], and that respiratory variation was inversely correlated with left ventricular end-diastolic volume (LVEDV) as determined by transesophageal echocardiography [14].

Of note, investigators have used different measurements to assess the impact of positive pressure ventilation on systemic blood pressure. The term 'respiratory variation' refers to any metric which seeks to quantitate the change in blood pressure that occurs with changes in intrathoracic pressure and is not limited to changes in systolic blood pressure. Commonly used metrics include systolic pressure variation (SPV, defined as the difference between maximal and minimal systolic pressure over the course of one respiratory cycle, i.e., $SP_{max} - SP_{min}$), SPV% (SPV as a percent of MAP), pulse pressure variation (PPV, defined as the difference between maximal and minimal pulse pressures over the course of one respiratory period), and PPV% (PPV as a percent of mean pulse pressure). Delta up (Δup) and delta down (Δdown) represent the change in maximal and minimal systolic pressures, respectively, with respect to a reference systolic pressure (SP_{ref}) measured at the beginning of an end-expiratory pause, although both have recently fallen out of favor. ΔPP is also commonly used, and is defined as $100 \times (PP_{max} - PP_{min})/[(PP_{max} + PP_{min})/2]$ [5].

Physiology: The Dynamic Approach to Volume Status

Although simply recognizing the existence of respiratory variation was a major discovery, the clinical utility of respiratory variation would have to await the next

X

major intellectual leap – from a static approach to the description of fluid status (i.e., measurement of central pressures or echocardiographic volumes) to a dynamic approach (correlation of respiratory variation to changes in hemodynamics that occur following fluid administration). To fully appreciate this approach, a more thorough understanding of the physiologic principles of respiratory variation is required. During application of a positive pressure breath, intrathoracic pressure is increased. The immediate result of this increase is a decrease in left ventricular afterload (because transmural pressure is transiently increased), an increase in right ventricular afterload (due to alveolar pressure increases), an increase in left ventricular preload (due to increased drainage of pulmonary venous blood), and a decrease in right ventricular preload. These four events result in a transient increase in left ventricular stroke volume and systemic blood pressure while at the same time decreasing right ventricular stroke volume.

Critically, the magnitude of this increase in left ventricular stroke volume depends on volume status. A left ventricle with adequate preload (i.e., on the flat portion of the Frank-Starling curve) will not respond to changes in preload, whether by positive pressure variation or any other means. On the other hand, a left ventricle with inadequate preload (i.e., on the steep portion of the Frank-Starling curve) will vigorously respond to changes in preload (see **Fig. 1**).

Of course, positive pressure ventilation is not identical to volume loading, and the benefits of positive pressure on the underloaded left ventricle are very short lived (one to two heart beats). Within seconds, the decrease in right ventricular preload and increase in right ventricular afterload manifest as a *decrease* in right ventricular stroke volume and thus a decrease in left ventricular preload. As

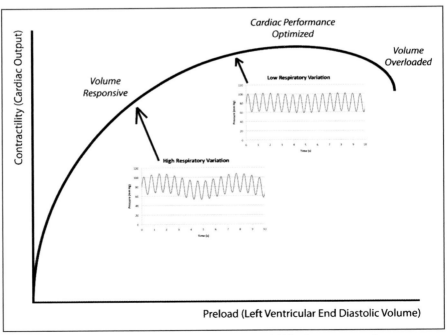

Fig. 1. influence of an idealized Frank-Starling curve on arterial blood pressure waveform

before, how the left ventricle responds to these changes depends on where it is on the Frank-Starling curve. Thus, positive pressure ventilation in some ways simulates a 'test dose' of volume, in that preload can be altered very transiently (for one or two heart beats) and the response subsequently analyzed. Readers interested in a more comprehensive explanation of the physiology behind this phenomena are referred to an excellent review by Michard [5], an important contributor to this field in his own right [15].

Clinical Studies and Validation

The logical extension of this reasoning is the hypothesis that patients who exhibit significant changes in systemic blood pressure during positive pressure ventilation will respond to volume expansion with an increase in cardiac output. Indeed, as of 2009 at least 27 studies (including over 600 patients) examining the relationship between SPV, PPV, and fluid responsiveness (i.e., change in cardiac output following fluid administration) had been published. Remarkably, the sum of all available data suggest that both PPV and SPV outperform central venous pressure (CVP), pulmonary artery occlusion pressure (PAOP), and echocardiographically-derived parameters in their abilities to predict fluid responsiveness [16, 17].

Subsequent to the review by Marik et al. [16], Cannesson and colleagues conducted a prospective, multicenter study comparing PPV to CVP and cardiac output in 413 patients undergoing general anesthesia and mechanical ventilation. The results of this study confirmed the findings of Marik et al., demonstrating clear superiority of PPV over CVP (areas under receiver operating characteristic curves [AUCs] 0.89 and 0.57, respectively) [18].

Limitations

X

Advocates of the dynamic approach to the assessment of volume status often overlook an important point regarding its predictive abilities: Because the Frank-Starling curve theoretically begins to decline after reaching its apex (whether or not this actually occurs in healthy humans is a matter of debate), and because the available techniques for measuring respiratory variation cannot discriminate between an *increase* in blood pressure and a *decrease* in blood pressure following a positive pressure breath, a slightly volume underloaded patient will have an identical arterial pressure tracing to a slightly volume overloaded patient. The only way to discriminate between slightly underloaded and overloaded patients is to change volume status and observe the response (an overloaded patient will respond to a fluid bolus with *increased* respiratory variation). Another limitation of this technology is the wide interindividual variability. Michard et al. demonstrated cardiac output changes ranging from 0 to 18 % in patients with a PPV of 10 % [15], and Cannesson et al. similarly showed changes in cardiac output ranging from -6 to 30 % in patients with a PPV of 10 % [18]. Thus, whereas the relationship between respiratory variation and volume responsiveness is statistically significant, on the individual level the range of possible hemodynamic outcomes following volume administration is wide.

Some of this interindividual variation may be attributable to interactions between the pulmonary and systemic vascular systems. Because fluid is generally administered into the systemic intravenous compartment, its ability to impact left ventricular function is dependent on the ability of the right ventricle to translocate incremental increases in volume into the pulmonic venous system. Patients with increased right ventricular afterload or decreased right ventricular function may not be able to effectively mobilize such increases in right ventricular preload. Indeed, recent animal [19] and human [20] studies have suggested that respiratory variation does not predict volume responsiveness in the setting of increased right ventricular afterload (and may actually be harmful), further lending credence to the admonition that volume responsiveness must be independently verified whenever possible.

Studies validating the utility of respiratory variation have generally been conducted in patients undergoing controlled mechanical ventilation using standardized tidal volumes and standardized fluid boluses. Often, subjects are arbitrarily labeled as either 'responders' or 'non-responders' based on whether or not cardiac index increases 15 % or more. In reality, a neat distinction does not exist – the data from both Michard et al. [15] and Cannesson et al. [18] show a clear, linear relationship between respiratory variation and changes in cardiac index. Lumping patients into arbitrary categories ('responders' or 'non-responders') is misleading because most patients respond to volume administration to some extent – the relevant question is "how much?"

Practitioners must be careful to take into account important physiological parameters that may deviate from the tightly-controlled values used by the validation studies. Changes in fluid volume, tidal volume, right heart function, and ventilation rate can all impact the predictive capabilities of these metrics. There are reports of successful use of respiratory variation in the setting of one lung ventilation [21]; however, the tidal volumes at which respiratory variation is meaningful are controversial [22, 23]. Multiple studies suggest that respiratory variation is not a reliable predictor of volume responsiveness in spontaneously ventilating patients [24, 25]. Not surprisingly, these metrics also appear to fail in the setting of open-chest procedures [26, 27].

Currently Available Means of Measurement

While the utility of respiratory variation is indisputable, and its connection with volume status was made in 1978 [11], the delay in the development of medical devices which quantitate this variable is regrettable. The first report of a real-time respiratory variation monitor came from Soncini et al., who connected an analog-to-digital converter to a personal computer running customized software, which displayed SPV [28]. In 2004, Aboy et al. developed an 'open source' algorithm for calculation of PPV [29], which Philips adopted into some of its Intellivue™ monitors (Philips Healthcare, Andover, MA, USA) [30]. General Electric (GE Healthcare, Little Chalfont, UK) has similarly begun to incorporate SPV and PPV into some of its newer monitors. Fortunately for clinicians and their patients, there are now at least ten pending US patent applications related to real-time assessment of fluid responsiveness.[7]

For practitioners interested in stand-alone devices, the PiCCO (Pulsion Medical Systems, Munich, Germany), LiDCO Rapid, and LiDCO+ (LiDCO, Cambridge, UK) devices are capable of estimating both stroke volume variation (SVV) and PPV and work independently of hemodynamic monitoring equipment. Similarly, the Flotrac (Edwards Lifesciences, Irvine, CA, USA) is also capable of measuring SVV (but does not measure PPV) [31]. From preliminary data, SVV appears comparable to PPV in its ability to predict volume responsiveness [31].

Alternative Measures of Respiratory Variation

Photoplethysmography

Several investigators have hypothesized that changes in the absorbance of red and infrared electromagnetic radiation (emitted by a pulse oximeter and referred to as the photoplethysmographic [PPG] waveform) may mimic changes in the arterial pressure tracing over short time intervals, concluding that the PPG tracing may offer an alternative measure for respiratory variation. Changes in PPG waveforms have been shown to correlate with fluid responsiveness in several studies [32–35], as well as predicting hypotension following the induction of general anesthesia [36]; however, when directly compared to PPV, PPG waveforms were not found to be a reliable surrogate for arterial pressure variation [37]. These seemingly confounding results may be partially explained by the apparent dependence of respiratory variation in the PPG waveform on waveform amplitude [38]. Masimo (Masimo Corporation, Irving, CA, USA) has developed a plethysmographic derivative of respiratory variation, the Pleth Variability Index (PVI^{TM}), currently the only commercially available device for estimating respiratory variation using the PPG waveform.

Echocardiography

Analysis of respiratory variation in arterial blood pressure or PPG waveforms assumes that changes in pressure (or light absorbance) are proportionate to changes in blood flow. Whether or not this is true has not been experimentally verified, thus measuring changes in blood *flow*, as opposed to *pressure*, may offer practitioners an attractive alternative and a potential means of improving upon this important concept. Several authors have analyzed changes in Doppler-based echocardiographic parameters that occur with respiration and found clinically significant correlations with volume responsiveness. Choi et al. compared respiratory variation in the peak velocity of aortic outflow (%V_{peak}, defined as the difference in maximal and minimal aortic outflow velocity [$V_{aortic\ outflow}$] throughout the respiratory cycle, divided by the average $V_{aortic\ outflow}$) using a transthoracic echocardiography probe in mechanically-ventilated children status-post ventricular septal defect (VSD) repair, finding a significant correlation with volume status (AUC 0.83 compared to 0.48 for CVP [39]. Similarly, Renner et al. compared PVI to transesophageal echocardiography-derived %V_{peak} and %VTI_{peak} (defined as the difference in maximal and minimal velocity time integral [VTI] throughout the respiratory cycle, divided by the average VTI) in infants with congenital heart disease post-induction but prior to surgical repair. The predictive abilities of PVI, %V_{peak}, and %VTI_{peak}, as assessed by the AUC, were 0.78, 0.92, and 0.84, respectively, suggesting that echocardiographic techniques may outperform peripherally-derived indices for the prediction of volume responsiveness [40]. Lamia et al. combined passive leg raising with VTI analysis in critically ill, spontaneously breathing patients, and using ROC analysis found that changes in VTI (AUC 0.96), but not in left ventricular end-diastolic area index (AUC 0.58) were predictive of fluid responsiveness [41].

In addition to the potential for increased accuracy and decreased intersubject variability, echocardiographically-derived indices offer the practitioner the ability to identify two clinical situations in which peripheral indices may be misleading (right heart failure and an optimal or over-distended left ventricular end-diastolic volume).

X

Future Techniques

Cannesson et al. explored the correlation between variation in the amplitude of the R-wave from an electrocardiogram (EKG) and PPV% (from an arterial blood pressure tracing) in patients undergoing general anesthesia, and found a significant correlation (r = 0.79, p < 0.01) [42]. The results of this study, which did not actually assess volume responsiveness, must be viewed as preliminary. Ma and Zhang measured respiratory variation in pulse wave transit time and noted a significant correlation with respiratory variation in the arterial blood pressure of healthy volunteers [43]. In an animal model of septic shock, Tang et al. noted a decrease in pulse transit time and an increase in respiratory variation in pulse transit time following endotoxin administration, presumably reflecting the simultaneous sympathetic nervous system activation and inflammation-mediated decreased in preload that accompanies sepsis [44]. Lastly, Maisch et al. utilized electrical impedance tomography (EIT, traditionally used to monitor ventilation) to estimate SVV in animal models, finding a significant correlation between estimated and measured stroke volume variation (r = 0.73; p < 0.001) [45].

Respiratory Variation and Goal-directed Therapy

Respiratory variation is unlike traditional goal-directed therapy targets in that it does not appear to be a rational physiologic end-point. Unlike DO_2, $ScvO_2$, and stroke volume, respiratory variation does not give the practitioner an indication of the amount or adequacy of DO_2. Instead, respiratory variation tells the practitioner whether, from a fluid management standpoint, stroke volume and DO_2 are optimized, i.e., whether there is any 'recruitable' stroke volume or whether increases in DO_2 will mandate either transfusion of red blood cells or initiation of ionotropic agents.

Indeed, the use of stroke volume monitoring, primarily via esophageal Doppler monitoring, has lead to a paradigm shift in fluid management: In this form of goal-directed therapy, fluid is not given arbitrarily but rather in order to ensure an adequate stroke volume is achieved. Meta-analyses have confirmed consistent and substantial benefits in terms of hospital length of stay, complications, overall cost, and in some cases, mortality [46, 47].

Knowledge of respiratory variation can guide the practitioner in making correct hemodynamic decisions with regards to well-validated physiologic end-points. Some investigators have hypothesized that optimization of stroke volume is a rational physiologic goal in and of itself, and studies utilizing respiratory variation as a physiologic end-point are starting to emerge.

Lopes et al. randomized 33 patients undergoing high-risk surgery to a control group (fluid management at the discretion at the anesthesiologist) or to an intervention group in which PPV was continuously monitored and maintained less than 10 %. The intervention resulted in increased intraoperative fluid administration, as well as statistically significant reductions in median hospital stay, duration of mechanical ventilation, and total complications [48]. Benes et al. [49] randomized 120 patients undergoing intra-abdominal surgery to routine intraoperative care versus management guided by SVV (in which SVV was kept below 10 %). As in the study by Lopes et al. [48], the SVV group received more intraoperative fluids. Lactate levels at the end of surgery were lower in the intervention group, and the perioperative complication rate was halved, although unlike in the study by Lopes et al., hospital stay between groups was not significantly different [49]. Forget et al. [50] randomized 82 patients undergoing major abdominal surgery to standard of care versus PVI-directed fluid management, in which PVI was maintained at < 13 % (and vasoactive drugs were administered to maintain MAPs in excess of 65 mmHg after fluid optimization). Unlike the results from the studies by Lopes et al. and Benes et al., the intervention group received less intravenous fluid. Still, lactate levels were significantly lower in the intervention group at all time points (both during surgery and 48 hours afterwards) [50].

Conclusion

Quantitative assessment of respiratory variation in the arterial blood pressure tracing is a well-validated, physiologically sound means of predicting the hemodynamic response to volume administration in mechanically ventilated patients. Although substantial interindividual variability remains, respiratory variation outperforms filling pressures and echocardiographically-derived volumetric measurements in the assessment of 'recruitable' stroke volume. Assessment of respiratory variation may be complicated in the settings of right heart failure, elevated pulmonary vascular resistance, and optimized left ventricular preload. The utility of respiratory variation in spontaneously ventilating patients, during one lung ventilation, and in open-chest procedures is less well established. Several completely noninvasive techniques for measuring respiratory variation are under development, with the most advanced being variation in the PPG waveform (PVI), the initial evaluations of which are, on the whole, promising. In the majority of clinical situations, respiratory variation can help guide those practitioners who implement goal-directed therapy by answering the critical question, "Should I administer volume or initiate ionotropic agents to achieve my hemodynamic goals?". Several small studies have suggested that maintaining respiratory variation of the arterial pressure or PPG waveforms under a pre-defined threshold may improve outcomes. However, until larger outcome-based studies are performed, respiratory variation should likely be used as an adjunct to a well-validated goal-directed therapy strategy (e.g., optimization of SV by esophageal Doppler monitoring) and not as an end-point in and of itself, although preliminary data are promising.

References

1. Barash PG (2006) Clinical Anesthesia, 5th ed.: Lippincott Williams and Wilkins, Philadelphia, p 303
2. Shoemaker WC, Appel PL, Kram HB, Waxman K, Lee TS (1988) Prospective trial of supranormal values of survivors as therapeutic goals in high-risk surgical patients. Chest 94: 1176–1186
3. Rivers E, Nguyen B, Havstad S, et al (2001) Early goal-directed therapy in the treatment of severe sepsis and septic shock. N Engl J Med 345: 1368–1377
4. Gan TJ, Soppitt A, Maroof M, et al (2002) Goal-directed intraoperative fluid administration reduces length of hospital stay after major surgery. Anesthesiology 97: 820–826
5. Michard F (2005) Changes in arterial pressure during mechanical ventilation. Anesthesiology 103: 419–428
6. Fauci A, Braunwald E, Kasper DL, et al (2008) Harrison's Principles of Internal Medicine. 17th ed. McGraw-Hill Professional, Columbus
7. Cannesson M, Aboy M, Hofer CK, Rehman M (2011) Pulse pressure variation: where are we today? J Clin Monit Comput 25: 45–56

8. Morgan BC, Martin WE, Hornbein TF, Crawford EW, Guntheroth WG.(1966) Hemodynamic effects of intermittent positive pressure respiration. Anesthesiology 27: 584–590
9. Katz L, Guauchat H (1924) Observation of pulsus paradoxus (with special reference to pericardial effusions). II. Experimental. Arch Intern Med 33: 371–393
10. Massumi RA, Mason DT, Vera Z, Zelis R, Otero J, Amsterdam EA (1973) Reversed pulsus paradoxus. N Engl J Med 289: 1272–1275
11. Rick JJ, Burke SS (1978) Respirator paradox. South Med J 71: 1376–1378
12. Perel A, Pizov R, Cotev S (1987) Systolic blood pressure variation is a sensitive indicator of hypovolemia in ventilated dogs subjected to graded hemorrhage. Anesthesiology 67: 498–502
13. Szold A, Pizov R, Segal E, Perel A (1989) The effect of tidal volume and intravascular volume state on systolic pressure variation in ventilated dogs. Intensive Care Med 15: 368–371
14. Preisman S, DiSegni E, Vered Z, Perel A (2002) Left ventricular preload and function during graded haemorrhage and retranfusion in pigs: analysis of arterial pressure waveform and correlation with echocardiography. Br J Anaesth 88: 716–718
15. Michard F, Boussat S, Chemla D, et al (2000) Relation between respiratory changes in arterial pulse pressure and fluid responsiveness in septic patients with acute circulatory failure. Am J Respir Crit Care Med 162: 134–138
16. Marik PE, Cavallazzi R, Vasu T, Hirani A (2009) Dynamic changes in arterial waveform derived variables and fluid responsiveness in mechanically ventilated patients: a systematic review of the literature. Crit Care Med 37: 2642–2647
17. Hofer CK, Muller SM, Furrer L, Klaghofer R, Genoni M, Zollinger A (2005) Stroke volume and pulse pressure variation for prediction of fluid responsiveness in patients undergoing off-pump coronary artery bypass grafting. Chest 128: 848–854
18. Cannesson M, Le Manach Y, Hofer CK, et al (2011) Assessing the diagnostic accuracy of pulse pressure variations for the prediction of fluid responsiveness: A "gray zone" approach. Anesthesiology 115: 231–241
19. Daudel F, Tuller D, Krahenbuhl S, Jakob SM, Takala J (2011) Pulse pressure variation and volume responsiveness during acutely increased pulmonary artery pressure: an experimental study. Crit Care 14: R122
20. Wyler von Ballmoos M, Takala J, Roeck M, et al (2011) Pulse-pressure variation and hemodynamic response in patients with elevated pulmonary artery pressure: a clinical study. Crit Care 14: R111
21. Suehiro K, Okutani R (2010) Stroke volume variation as a predictor of fluid responsiveness in patients undergoing one-lung ventilation. J Cardiothorac Vasc Anesth 24: 772–775
22. Lee JH, Jeon Y, Bahk JH, et al (2011) Pulse pressure variation as a predictor of fluid responsiveness during one-lung ventilation for lung surgery using thoracotomy: randomised controlled study. Eur J Anaesthesiol 28: 39–44
23. Suehiro K, Okutani R (2011) Influence of tidal volume for stroke volume variation to predict fluid responsiveness in patients undergoing one-lung ventilation. J Anesth 25: 777–780
24. Rooke GA, Schwid HA, Shapira Y (1995) The effect of graded hemorrhage and intravascular volume replacement on systolic pressure variation in humans during mechanical and spontaneous ventilation. Anesth Analg 80: 925–932
25. Heenen S, De Backer D, Vincent JL (2006) How can the response to volume expansion in patients with spontaneous respiratory movements be predicted? Crit Care 10: R102
26. Wyffels PA, Sergeant P, Wouters PF (2010) The value of pulse pressure and stroke volume variation as predictors of fluid responsiveness during open chest surgery. Anaesthesia 65: 704–709
27. de Waal EE, Rex S, Kruitwagen CL, Kalkman CJ, Buhre WF (2009) Dynamic preload indicators fail to predict fluid responsiveness in open-chest conditions. Crit Care Med 37: 510–515
28. Soncini M, Manfredi G, Redaelli A, et al (2002) A computerized method to measure systolic pressure variation (SPV) in mechanically ventilated patients. J Clin Monit Comput 17: 141–146
29. Aboy M, McNames J, Thong T, Phillips CR, Ellenby MS, Goldstein B (2004) A novel algorithm to estimate the pulse pressure variation index deltaPP. IEEE Trans Biomed Eng 51: 2198–203

X

30. McGee WT (2009) A simple physiologic algorithm for managing hemodynamics using stroke volume and stroke volume variation: physiologic optimization program. J Intensive Care Med 24: 352–360

31. Hofer CK, Senn A, Weibel L, Zollinger A (2008) Assessment of stroke volume variation for prediction of fluid responsiveness using the modified FloTrac and PiCCOplus system. Crit Care 12: R82

32. Cannesson M, Attof Y, Rosamel P, et al (2007) Respiratory variations in pulse oximetry plethysmographic waveform amplitude to predict fluid responsiveness in the operating room. Anesthesiology 106: 1105–1111

33. Cannesson M, Desebbe O, Rosamel P, et al (2008) Pleth variability index to monitor the respiratory variations in the pulse oximeter plethysmographic waveform amplitude and predict fluid responsiveness in the operating theatre. Br J Anaesth 101: 200–206

34. Keller G, Cassar E, Desebbe O, Lehot JJ, Cannesson M (2008) Ability of pleth variability index to detect hemodynamic changes induced by passive leg raising in spontaneously breathing volunteers. Crit Care 12: R37

35. Zimmermann M, Feibicke T, Keyl C, et al (2010) Accuracy of stroke volume variation compared with pleth variability index to predict fluid responsiveness in mechanically ventilated patients undergoing major surgery. Eur J Anaesthesiol 27: 555–61

36. Tsuchiya M, Yamada T, Asada A (2010) Pleth variability index predicts hypotension during anesthesia induction. Acta Anaesthesiol Scand 54: 596–602

37. Landsverk SA, Hoiseth LO, Kvandal P, Hisdal J, Skare O, Kirkeboen KA (2008) Poor agreement between respiratory variations in pulse oximetry photoplethysmographic waveform amplitude and pulse pressure in intensive care unit patients. Anesthesiology 109: 849–855

38. Broch O, Bein B, Gruenewald M, et al (2011) Accuracy of the pleth variability index to predict fluid responsiveness depends on the perfusion index. Acta Anaesthesiol Scand 55: 686–693

39. Choi DY, Kwak HJ, Park HY, Kim YB, Choi CH, Lee JY (2010) Respiratory variation in aortic blood flow velocity as a predictor of fluid responsiveness in children after repair of ventricular septal defect. Pediatr Cardiol 31: 1166–1170

40. Renner J, Broch O, Gruenewald M, et al (2011) Non-invasive prediction of fluid responsiveness in infants using pleth variability index. Anaesthesia 66: 582–589

41. Lamia B, Ochagavia A, Monnet X, Chemla D, Richard C, Teboul JL (2007) Echocardiographic prediction of volume responsiveness in critically ill patients with spontaneously breathing activity. Intensive Care Med 33: 1125–1132

42. Cannesson M, Keller G, Desebbe O, Lehot JJ (2010) Relations between respiratory changes in R-wave amplitude and arterial pulse pressure in mechanically ventilated patients. J Clin Monit Comput 24: 203–207

43. Ma HT, Zhang YT (2006) Spectral analysis of pulse transit time variability and its coherence with other cardiovascular variabilities. Conf Proc IEEE Eng Med Biol Soc 1: 6442–6445

44. Tang CH, Chan GS, Middleton PM, et al (2010) Pulse transit time variability analysis in an animal model of endotoxic shock. Conf Proc IEEE Eng Med Biol Soc 2010: 2849–2852

45. Maisch S, Bohm SH, Sola J, et al (2011) Heart-lung interactions measured by electrical impedance tomography. Crit Care Med 39: 2173–2176

46. Gurgel ST, do Nascimento P Jr (2011) Maintaining tissue perfusion in high-risk surgical patients: a systematic review of randomized clinical trials. Anesth Analg 112: 1384–1391

47. Hamilton MA, Cecconi M, Rhodes A (2011) A systematic review and meta-analysis on the use of preemptive hemodynamic intervention to improve postoperative outcomes in moderate and high-risk surgical patients. Anesth Analg 112: 1392–402

48. Lopes MR, Oliveira MA, Pereira VO, Lemos IP, Auler JO Jr, Michard F (2007) Goal-directed fluid management based on pulse pressure variation monitoring during high-risk surgery: a pilot randomized controlled trial. Crit Care 11: R100

49. Benes J, Chytra I, Altmann P, et al (2010) Intraoperative fluid optimization using stroke volume variation in high risk surgical patients: results of prospective randomized study. Crit Care 14: R118

50. Forget P, Lois F, de Kock M (2010) Goal-directed fluid management based on the pulse oximeter-derived pleth variability index reduces lactate levels and improves fluid management. Anesth Analg 111: 910–914

X

Fluid Resuscitation: Think Microcirculation

S. Tanaka, A. Harrois, and J. Duranteau

Introduction

The goal of fluid resuscitation in intensive care unit (ICU) patients is to restore effective tissue perfusion and oxygen delivery (DO_2). Fluid resuscitation must be started as a first-line treatment in the management of septic or hemorrhagic shock. Fluid administration should be titrated to clinical endpoints of perfusion (such as capillary refill and urine output) and also to macrocirculatory parameters of global perfusion. It is recommended that fluids should be given only if changes in preload result in significant changes in stroke volume. However, assessment of the adequacy of resuscitation requires attention to both the macro- and the microcirculation. Microcirculatory dysfunction is a central abnormality in septic and hemorragic shock and relationships between the macro- and microcirculations are complex. It is, therefore, impossible to predict the microvascular response after a positive fluid challenge in ICU patients without assessment of the microcirculation. However, techniques to monitor the microcirculation are not yet available for clinical practice.

Learning how fluid resuscitation impacts the microcirculation in the different vascular beds and how the emerging techniques assess the microcirculation are the first steps toward developing a fluid strategy that targets microcirculatory perfusion.

Titration of Fluid Resuscitation

The goal of fluid therapy in ICU patients is to preserve tissue oxygenation and metabolism. In patients with suspected hypovolemia, considering static measures of cardiac preload is unhelpful, and it is recommended that the circulation be challenged by performing maneuvers, such as passive leg raising (PLR) or end-expiratory occlusion, or fluid challenges to evaluate the patient's response and avoid development of pulmonary edema. The Surviving Sepsis Campaign guidelines recommend that early fluid resuscitation should consist of administration of repeated fluid challenges of $\geq$ 1,000 ml of crystalloids or 300 to 500 ml of colloids [1]. As stroke volume (and thus cardiac output) is related to cardiac preload according to the Frank-Starling relationship, an increase in stroke volume reveals preload dependency and proves the legitimacy of the volume expansion. When no increase in stroke volume is observed after fluid challenge, fluid administration should be stopped because stroke volume is no longer sensitive to preload increases (flat part of the Frank-Starling relationship).

J.-L. Vincent (ed.), *Annual Update in Intensive Care and Emergency Medicine 2012*
DOI 10.1007/978-3-642-25716-2 © Springer-Verlag Berlin Heidelberg 2012

However, a positive fluid challenge does not always mean that the patient needs fluid. Patients need fluids only when the fluid-induced increase in stroke volume is accompanied by an improvement in tissue perfusion. However, relationships between the macro- and microcirculations during resuscitation are complex. Indeed, different mechanisms are implicated in the regulation of microvascular and macrovascular perfusion and microcirculatory alterations in ICU patients may result from multiple factors, such as endothelial cell dysfunction, increased leukocyte adhesion, microthrombi, rheologic abnormalities, and functional shunting. A positive fluid challenge may improve the microcirculation and tissue oxygenation through an increase in microcirculatory blood flow, rheologic changes (decreased microvascular blood viscosity) or local vasodilation (shear stress). However, Sakr et al. [2] and Trzeciak et al. [3] reported persistent microcirculatory alterations in septic patients despite an improvement in cardiac output after fluid resuscitation. The microvascular fluid response was dissociated from the macrovascular response to fluids. This phenomenon was also noted by Ospina-Tascon et al. [4] in a recent study investigating the effect of fluid loading on the sublingual microcirculation during early (within 24 h after the diagnosis) or late (more than 48 h after the diagnosis) phases of septic shock with an improvement of the microcirculation during the early phase but not in the late phase. Once again, the microvascular response was dissociated from the macro-hemodynamic response to fluids. There was no relationship between changes in microvascular perfusion and initial arterial pressure or cardiac index changes during fluid administration. Despite an increase in stroke volume in the early or in the late phase, the microcirculation was only improved during the initial phase highlighting that the microcirculatory response to fluids varied over time. The authors suggested that fluid administration has a limited impact on tissue perfusion during the later stages of sepsis, even when cardiac output and arterial pressure may improve and that fluid resuscitation may thus be useless or even detrimental in later stages of sepsis. Pottecher et al. [5] investigated sublingual microcirculatory perfusion after fluid loading realized either by PLR but also by fluid expansion in severe sepsis and septic shock patients within the first 24 h of their admission to the ICU. All of the studied patients were preload-dependent, defined by respiratory variations in arterial pulse pressure (PPV) greater than 13 %. Both PLR and volume expansion improved sublingual microcirculatory perfusion. However, during fluid expansion the microcirculation was initially improved by the increase in cardiac output, but this improvement plateaued despite an additional increase in cardiac output. These results suggest that the microcirculation does not have the same dose response to fluid loading as the heart (**Fig. 1**). This was also very well illustrated by Jhanji et al. [6] in patients undergoing major gastrointestinal surgery. These authors tested the effects of central venous pressure (CVP) and stroke volume guided intravenous fluid on tissue microvascular flow (sublingual microscopy and laser Doppler flowmetry) and oxygenation (PtO_2, Clark electrode). Intravenous fluid therapy was guided by measurements of CVP or stroke volume. The main result was that microvascular flow remained constant in the stroke volume group but was altered in the CVP group despite more than 1,500 ml of fluid expansion.

The fact that independent determinants of microvascular flow can change the relationship between the macro- and microcirculations is true for all the circulatory beds. For example, in the renal microvascular bed, Legrand et al. [7] reported that improvement in renal microvascular perfusion was more pro-

X

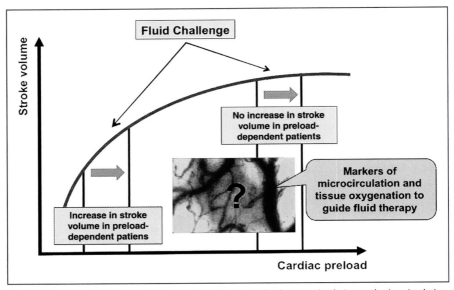

Fig. 1. Adequacy of fluid resuscitation requires attention to both macrocirculation and microcirculation. Microcirculatory dysfunction is a central abnormality in septic or hemorrhagic shock and relationships between the macro- and microcirculations are complex. Microcirculatory fluid response may be different to the macrovascular fluid response.

nounced when fluid resuscitation was performed immediately after lipopolysaccharide (LPS) administration in rats than when fluid resuscitation was delayed (i.e., 120 min), despite a similar restoration of renal blood flow. One of the determinants of this difference of response may be the fact that leukocyte infiltration in glomeruli was less in the early fluid resuscitation group compared to the late fluid administration group. A key point is that persistent alteration of renal microvascular oxygenation was observed in the two groups.

The challenge of fluid resuscitation is to improve the microcirculation and tissue oxygenation without inducing fluid overload. Thus, it is essential to have markers of microcirculation and tissue oxygenation to guide fluid therapy. The physician needs to know when fluid resuscitation cannot improve the microcirculation. He/she can then stop fluid administration to limit the risk of fluid overload, especially if the lung is injured, and consider other therapeutic strategies. It is obvious that fluid administration should be stopped when there is no fluid responsiveness, but the real target is the microcirculation and tissue oxygenation. However, which emerging techniques may be valuable in the future to evaluate the microcirculation at the bedside? There is a need to have quantifiable, validated, reproducible and practical techniques to evaluate the microcirculation in ICU patients.

Currently Available Techniques to Evaluate the Microcirculation at the Bedside

Orthogonal Polarization Spectral and Sidestream Darkfield Imaging Techniques

Orthogonal polarization spectral (OPS) and sidestream darkfield (SDF) imaging are two videomicroscopic imaging techniques that provide high contrast images of the microvasculature [8, 9]. These techniques can be used only on organs covered by a thin epithelial layer. These techniques have been validated against intravital videomicroscopy which is the goal standard for microvascular evaluation in experimental conditions. Both techniques are based on the principle that green light (530 nm) illuminates the depth of a tissue (up to 3 mm) and that the scattered green light is absorbed by hemoglobin of red blood cells (RBCs), independently of its oxygenation state. A key point to remember is the fact that only vessels containing RBCs are visualized. Several microvascular markers can be analyzed, including microvascular blood flow (microcirculatory flow index [MFI] and the proportion of perfused vessels; semiquantitative analysis), functional capillary density (FCD) and heterogeneity of perfusion. The reproducibility of this semiquantitative analysis is excellent, with intra- and interobserver variabilities within 5–10 %. This analysis requires time with off-line image processing and delayed evaluation of the image sequences. This point is crucial and limits the applicability of these technique at the bedside for titration of fluid resuscitation. However, it is very interesting to note that Arnold et al. [10] found that realtime point-of-care determination of MFI at the bedside has good agreement with conventional off-line analysis techniques in a heterogeneous patient population across a wide range of flow characteristics. This bedside point-of-care determination of the MFI was highly sensitive and specific for detecting impaired microvascular flow. In ICU patients, these techniques have been used to test the effects of fluid resuscitation mostly at the level of the sublingual microcirculation [5, 11, 12]. It can be argued that this region does not reflect other microvascular beds. But this remark is valid for all techniques which try to evaluate microcirculation in a specific vascular bed. Furthermore, it has been demonstrated that the severity and the time course of microcirculatory changes are similar in the sublingual and in the gut region during sepsis [13].

Near-Infrared Spectroscopy

Near-infrared spectroscopy (NIRS) is a continuous, non-invasive, bedside monitoring technique using the absorption of infrared light at two specific wavelengths (680 and 800 nm) by deoxyhemoglobin and oxyhemoglobin to define the saturation of hemoglobin in vessels of size < 1 mm located in the volume of tissue illuminated by the probe (StO_2). The depth of tissue measured is directly related to the distance between the illumination fibers and the detection fibers. The StO_2 is determined from the ratio oxyhemoglobin/(oxyhemoglobin + deoxyhemoglobin). In addition, from total light absorption, NIRS can provide two indices of the blood volume in the tissue crossed by near-infrared light: The total tissue hemoglobin (HbT) and the absolute tissue hemoglobin index (THI). StO_2 reflects arteriolar, capillary and venular oxygen saturations within the tissue sensed by the probe. Because in the muscle of healthy humans, the distribution of the blood volumes among microvessels is estimated to be 10, 20 and 70 % for the arteriolar, capillary and venular compartments, respectively [14], StO_2 measurements mostly represent venous hemoglobin oxygen saturation. StO_2 is not a direct measurement of microvascular blood flow, but an index of tissue oxygenation which is dependent on the balance between DO_2 and oxygen consumption (VO_2). This point is important because in septic shock, after the initial resuscitation phase, the values of StO_2 may be unchanged or slightly decreased despite alterations in the microcirculation. Indeed, even though microvascular blood flow is decreased in septic patients, a simultaneous decrease in VO_2 can lead to an unchanged StO_2. In addition, in these patients the StO_2 can, therefore, be normal or even increased when the venous blood compartment volume is relatively reduced and/or when arterio-venous shunting results in increased oxygen saturation of the venous blood.

The NIRS technique also allows the capacity of the microvascular bed to recruit microvessels in response to a hypoxic stimulus to be tested by performing a vascular occlusion test (VOT). The analysis, interpretation, and understanding of StO_2 measurements during VOT are still debated [15]. However, it is assumed that when the StO_2 recovery slope is reduced, the capacities of recruiting microvessels in response to a hypoxic stimulus are lower. Accordingly, Creteur et al. [16] showed that the StO_2 recovery slope was lower in septic patients and that the presence of this alteration in the first 24 h of sepsis and its persistence were associated with a worse outcome. Other studies have reported lower than normal StO_2 recovery slopes in patients with sepsis [17–19]. We may wonder whether the analysis of StO_2 during VOT could be useful to determine whether fluid resuscitation can result in recruitment of microvessels. Indeed, Georger et al. [20] reported that restoring mean arterial pressure (MAP) with norepinephrine improved the StO_2 recovery slope during severely hypotensive septic shock.

Tissue PCO_2

Several experimental and clinical studies have demonstrated that gastric mucosal (gastric tonometry) and sublingual PCO_2 are quantifiable, reproducible and practical techniques to assess microvascular blood flow during acute fluid resuscitation [21–24].

In stable respiratory condition, tissue PCO_2 reflects the balance between tissue production and its clearance by the local microcirculation. Among the factors determining tissue PCO_2 (arterial CO_2, regional blood flow, microvascular blood flow and tissue CO_2 production [aerobic and anaerobic]), microvascular blood flow is the major one. During hypoxic hypoxia, in which microvascular flow is preserved, the tissue PCO_2 should not increase because CO_2 is washed out by the microvascular blood flow [23, 25]. If the microvascular blood flow is altered, the CO_2 washes out from the tissue more slowly inducing accumulation of tissue CO_2. In septic patients, Creteur et al. [24] supported the concept that microvascular blood flow is the major factor determining tissue PCO_2, by reporting that the decrease in sublingual PCO_2 gap paralleled the increase in the proportion of well-perfused capillaries in each patient during dobutamine infusion.

Recently, the ear lobe cutaneous tissue CO_2 ($PcCO_2$) level has been evaluated as a reliable tool to investigate microcirculatory perfusion in ICU patients [26]. The differences between $PcCO_2$ and $PaCO_2$ ($PcCO_2$-$PaCO_2$), and between cutaneous $PcCO_2$ and end-tidal PCO_2 ($PcCO_2$-$etCO_2$) were evaluated during 36 hours in ICU patients. Twenty-four hours after ICU admission, a $PcCO_2$-$PaCO_2 > 16$ mmHg and a $PcCO_2$-$etCO_2$ > 26 mmHg was related to a poor outcome. $PcCO_2$-$PaCO_2$ and $PcCO_2$-$etCO_2$ variations during fluid challenge were inversely correlated with changes in skin microcirculatory blood flow (laser Doppler flowmetry) [26]. This non-invasive technique seems to be promising for futures studies.

Contrast Enhanced Ultrasonography

Recent progress in ultrasonography with microbubble contrast has allowed quantification of regional blood flow in real time at the bedside [27–29]. Contrast-enhanced ultrasonography (CEUS) is a non-invasive bedside technique based on the use of gas-filled microbubbles to assess microvascular tissue perfusion. With appropriate imaging modes and software, CEUS allows dynamic quantification of tissue flow in both the macro- and microvasculatures. This technique use microbubble contrast agents, which are composed of tiny bubbles of an injectable gas in a supporting shell. Microbubbles remain confined to the intravascular space because their size (1 to 6 µm) prevents them from diffusing through the endothelium. Changes in the shape of microbubbles with ultrasound waves result in the generation of nonlinear signals with a high echogenicity difference between the gas in the microbubbles and the soft tissue. This technique opens the way to evaluate the microcirculation in ICU patients at the bedside. Several authors have used these methods in various organs and tissues. For example, cerebral perfusion in dogs was assessed with CEUS at baseline and during hypercapnia and hypocapnia. Good correlation was found between cerebral microvascular blood volume derived from CEUS and cerebral blood flow measured by radiolabeled microspheres. Kishimoto et al. [30] reported that CEUS can be used for quantitatively evaluating changes induced by a therapeutic agent such as dopamine (2 mcg/min/kg) on renal cortical blood flow. Schwenger et al. [31] reported that determination of renal blood flow by CEUS had higher sensitivity (91 % vs. 82 %, p < 0.05), specificity (82 % vs. 64 %, p < 0.05) and accuracy (85 % vs. 73 %, p < 0.05) for the diagnosis of chronic allograft nephropathy than conventional Doppler ultrasonographic resistance indices. CEUS is a very exciting emerging technique which may be valuable for therapy guidance, especially for titration of fluid resuscitation. CEUS would be a helpful tool in the ICU to assess the microcirculation and the impact of therapeutic interventions on organ dysfunction, such as acute kidney injury.

Microdialysis

The microdialysis technique mimics the function of a blood capillary by positioning a thin dialysis tube in the tissue and can be used to analyze the chemical composition of the interstitial fluid. Microdialysis allows measurements of different molecules in the extracellular space. The concentration gradients between the interstitial fluid and the perfusate constitute the driving force for diffusion. The molecular weight of the molecules being sampled is limited by the pore size of the dialysis membrane (cut-off). The perfusate flows along the dialysis membrane slowly and at a constant speed, and the sample (dialysate) is collected and analyzed biochemically. The microdialysis technique has been used in most human tissues. Since microdialysis is an invasive technique, the tissue damage caused by the catheter and the possible complications are of special importance. These risks may be most obvious during intracerebral microdialysis. The brain is also the organ where we have most clinical experience [32, 33].

Glucose, pyruvate and lactate measurements provide information about the relative contributions of aerobic and anaerobic metabolism to bioenergetics. Increased lactate concentrations and elevation of the lactate/pyruvate ratio are robust and reliable indicators of increased anaerobic metabolism. In acute brain injury, several studies have shown that probes placed directly in contusions or infarcts reveal severe neurochemical alterations. Cerebral microdialysis provides substantial new information about the neurochemistry of the acutely injured brain and could be very useful in the future to prevent secondary neurological deterioration [33]. Alterations of metabolism during periods of intracranial hypertension have been associated with a reduction in brain glucose and elevation of the lactate/pyruvate ratio. Cerebral microdialysis has been used to guide cerebral perfusion pressure targets [34]. In patients with subarachnoid hemorrhage, an increased risk of metabolic alterations was noted at hemoglobin concentrations below 10 g/dl [35]. In septic shock, it has been reported that the lactate/pyruvate ratio may be increased [36].

Conclusion

The challenge of fluid resuscitation is to improve the microcirculation and tissue oxygenation without inducing fluid overload. Thus, it is essential to have markers of microcirculation and tissue oxygenation to guide fluid therapy. The physician needs to know when fluid resuscitation cannot improve the microcirculation. There is a need to have quantifiable, validated, reproducible and practical techniques to evaluate the microcirculation in ICU patients. Guiding fluid resuscitation with the use of emerging techniques will allow fluid strategies that target the microcirculatory perfusion in the future with the hope that this approach will decrease organ dysfunction.

References

1. Dellinger RP, Levy MM, Carlet JM, et al (2008) Surviving Sepsis Campaign: international guidelines for management of severe sepsis and septic shock: 2008. Crit Care Med 36: 296–327
2. Sakr Y, Dubois MJ, De Backer D, Creteur J, Vincent JL (2004) Persistent microcirculatory alterations are associated with organ failure and death in patients with septic shock. Crit Care Med 32: 1825–1831
3. Trzeciak S, Dellinger RP, Parrillo JE, et al (2007) Early microcirculatory perfusion derangements in patients with severe sepsis and septic shock: relationship to hemodynamics, oxygen transport, and survival. Ann Emerg Med 49: 88–98
4. Ospina-Tascon G, Neves AP, Occhipinti G, et al (2010) Effects of fluids on microvascular perfusion in patients with severe sepsis. Intensive Care Med 36: 949–955
5. Pottecher J, Deruddre S, Teboul JL, et al (2010) Both passive leg raising and intravascular volume expansion improve sublingual microcirculatory perfusion in severe sepsis and septic shock patients. Intensive Care Med 36: 1867–1874
6. Jhanji S, Vivian-Smith A, Lucena-Amaro S, Watson D, Hinds CJ, Pearse RM (2010) Haemodynamic optimisation improves tissue microvascular flow and oxygenation after major surgery: a randomised controlled trial. Crit Care 14: R151
7. Legrand M, Bezemer R, Kandil A, Demirci C, Payen D, Ince C (2011) The role of renal hypoperfusion in development of renal microcirculatory dysfunction in endotoxemic rats. Intensive Care Med 37: 1534–1542
8. Goedhart PT, Khalilzada M, Bezemer R, Merza J, Ince C (2007) Sidestream Dark Field

(SDF) imaging: a novel stroboscopic LED ring-based imaging modality for clinical assessment of the microcirculation. Opt Express 15: 15101–15114

9. De Backer D, Ospina-Tascon G, Salgado D, Favory R, Creteur J, Vincent J-L (2010) Monitoring the microcirculation in the critically ill patient: current methods and future approaches. Intensive Care Med 36: 1813–1825

10. Arnold RC, Parrillo JE, Dellinger RP, et al (2009) Point-of-care assessment of microvascular blood flow in critically ill patients. Intensive Care Med 35: 1761–1766

11. Ospina-Tascon G, Neves AP, Occhipinti G, et al (2010) Effects of fluids on microvascular perfusion in patients with severe sepsis. Intensive Care Med 36: 949–955

12. Dubin A, Pozo MO, Casabella CA, et al (2009) Comparison of 6 % hydroxyethyl starch 130/0.4 and saline solution for resuscitation of the microcirculation during the early goal-directed therapy of septic patients. J Crit Care 25: 659

13. Verdant CL, De Backer D, Bruhn A, et al (2009) Evaluation of sublingual and gut mucosal microcirculation in sepsis: A quantitative analysis. Crit Care Med 37: 2875–2881

14. Moens AL (2005) Flow-mediated vasodilation: A diagnostic instrument, or an experimental tool? Chest 127: 2254–2263

15. Bezemer R, Lima A, Myers D, et al (2009) Assessment of tissue oxygen saturation during a vascular occlusion test using near-infrared spectroscopy: the role of probe spacing and measurement site studied in healthy volunteers. Crit Care 13 (Suppl 5): S4

16. Creteur J, Carollo T, Soldati G, Büchele G, Backer D, Vincent J-L (2007) The prognostic value of muscle StO2 in septic patients. Intensive Care Med 33: 1549–1556

17. Doerschug KC, Delsing AS, Schmidt GA, Haynes WG (2007) Impairments in microvascular reactivity are related to organ failure in human sepsis. Am J Physiol Heart Circ Physiol 293: H1065–H1071

18. Leone M, Blidi S, Antonini F, et al (2009) Oxygen tissue saturation is lower in nonsurvivors than in survivors after early resuscitation of septic shock. Anesthesiology 111: 366–371

19. Skarda DE, Mulier KE, Myers DE, Taylor JH, Beilman GJ (2007) Dynamic near-infrared spectroscopy measurements in patients with severe sepsis. Shock 27: 348–353

20. Georger J-F, Hamzaoui O, Chaari A, Maizel J, Richard C, Teboul JL (2010) Restoring arterial pressure with norepinephrine improves muscle tissue oxygenation assessed by near-infrared spectroscopy in severely hypotensive septic patients. Intensive Care Med 36: 1882–1889

21. Duranteau J, Sitbon P, Teboul JL, et al (1999) Effects of epinephrine, norepinephrine, or the combination of norepinephrine and dobutamine on gastric mucosa in septic shock. Crit Care Med 27: 893–900

22. Jin X, Weil MH, Sun S, Tang W, Bisera J, Mason EJ (1998) Decreases in organ blood flows associated with increases in sublingual PCO2 during hemorrhagic shock. J Appl Physiol 85: 2360–2364

23. Dubin A, Murias G, Estenssoro E, et al (2002) Intramucosal-arterial PCO2 gap fails to reflect intestinal dysoxia in hypoxic hypoxia. Crit Care 6: 514–520

24. Creteur J, De Backer D, Sakr Y, Koch M, Vincent JL (2006) Sublingual capnometry tracks microcirculatory changes in septic patients. Intensive Care Med 32: 516–523

25. Vallet B, Teboul JL, Cain S, Curtis S (2000) Venoarterial CO(2) difference during regional ischemic or hypoxic hypoxia. J Appl Physiol 89: 1317–1321

26. Vallee F, Mateo J, Dubreuil G, et al (2010) Cutaneous ear lobe Pco at 37 degrees C to evaluate microperfusion in patients with septic shock. Chest 138: 1062–1070

27. Schneider A, Johnson L, Goodwin M, Schelleman A, Bellomo R (2011) Bench-to-bedside review: Contrast enhanced ultrasonography – a promising technique to assess renal perfusion in the ICU. Crit Care 15: 157

28. Schneider AG, Hofmann L, Wuerzner G, et al (2012) Renal perfusion evaluation with contrast-enhanced ultrasonography. Nephrol Dial Transplant (in press)

29. Larsen LPS (2010) Role of contrast enhanced ultrasonography in the assessment of hepatic metastases: A review. World J Hepatol 2: 8–15

30. Kishimoto N, Mori Y, Nishiue T, et al (2003) Renal blood flow measurement with contrast-enhanced harmonic ultrasonography: evaluation of dopamine-induced changes in renal cortical perfusion in humans. Clin Nephrol 59: 423–428

X

31. Schwenger V, Korosoglou G, Hinkel UP, et al (2006) Real-time contrast-enhanced sonography of renal transplant recipients predicts chronic allograft nephropathy. Am J Transplant 6: 609–615
32. Nordström CH (2009) Cerebral energy metabolism and microdialysis in neurocritical care. Childs Nerv Syst 26: 465–472
33. Rao GS, Durga P (2011) Changing trends in monitoring brain ischemia: from intracranial pressure to cerebral oximetry. Curr Opin Anaesthesiol 24: 487–494
34. Sarrafzadeh AS, Sakowitz OW, Callsen TA, Lanksch WR, Unterberg AW (2002) Detection of secondary insults by brain tissue pO2 and bedside microdialysis in severe head injury. Acta Neurochir Suppl 81: 319–321
35. Kurtz P, Schmidt JM, Claassen J, et al (2010) Anemia is associated with metabolic distress and brain tissue hypoxia after subarachnoid hemorrhage. Neurocrit Care 13: 10–16
36. Ellebaek Pedersen M, Qvist N, et al (2009) Peritoneal microdialysis. Early diagnosis of anastomotic leakage after low anterior resection for rectosigmoid cancer. Scand J Surg 98: 148–154

X

Human Albumin in the Management of Complications of Liver Cirrhosis

M. Bernardi, C. Maggioli, and G. Zaccherini

Introduction

Human serum albumin is the most abundant plasma protein, representing about 50 % of the total protein content (3.5–5 g/l). Albumin is a protein of 585 amino acids and molecular weight 66 kDa encoded by a gene on chromosome 4 and is exclusively synthesized by liver cells, which release it directly into the blood stream without storage. Under physiological conditions, only 20–30 % of hepatocytes are committed to the production of 9–12 g of albumin per day; therefore, the liver has a large functional reserve, so that it can increase the synthesis of this protein by 3–4 times, if necessary. The production of albumin is mainly regulated by the osmolarity and oncotic pressure of interstitial fluid in the liver extravascular space, but it is also induced by hormonal factors (insulin, cortisol and growth hormone) and inhibited by acute phase cytokines, such as interleukin (IL)-6 and tumor necrosis factor (TNF)-α [1].

Because serum albumin scarcely crosses the majority of capillaries, it remains in the blood stream and generates about 70 % of the plasma oncotic pressure. This feature is two-thirds because of a direct osmotic effect and one third because of the Gibbs-Donnan effect, as a result of the strong negative charges attracting positively charged molecules into the intravascular compartment. Albumin is, therefore, a main modulator of fluid distribution throughout body compartments [1].

The capacity of albumin to expand the plasma volume represents the pathophysiological background for the use of human albumin in many clinical conditions; nevertheless, its administration is often inappropriate, largely because of a common belief in its efficacy, whereas many indications are still under debate or have been disproved by evidence-based medicine. Indeed, the high cost, the theoretical risk of viral disease transmission, and the availability of cheaper alternatives should be carefully weighed when considering prescription of albumin [2]. At present, it is generally accepted that the administration of non-protein colloids and crystalloids represents the first-line treatment of resuscitation, and use of albumin in critically ill patients should be reserved for specific conditions, such as in patients with septic shock [3, 4]. Albumin administration is not recommended to correct hypoalbuminemia *per se* (i.e., not associated with hypovolemia) or for nutritional intervention [2, 5], but these indications are often disregarded in clinical practice. Albumin is also prescribed in certain specific conditions and diseases, such as kernicterus, plasmapheresis, and graft versus host disease [2], even though these indications are not supported by definite evidence.

Although the clinical use of albumin is mainly related to plasma volume expansion, albumin is more than a volume expander, having further biological

X

J.-L. Vincent (ed.), *Annual Update in Intensive Care and Emergency Medicine 2012*
DOI 10.1007/978-3-642-25716-2 © Springer-Verlag Berlin Heidelberg 2012

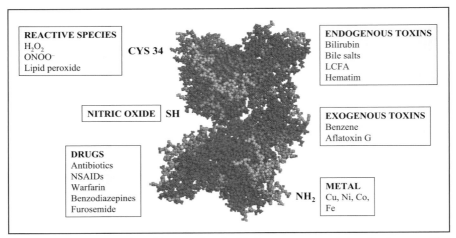

Fig. 1. Non-oncotic properties of human albumin: Binding, transport and detoxification capacities. H_2O_2: hydrogen peroxide; LCFA: long-chain fatty acids; ONOO⁻: peroxynitrite; NSAIDs: non-steroidal anti-inflammatory drugs; CYS: cysteine

properties: It binds and transports a variety of water-insoluble molecules, metals, and drugs, with implications for delivery and efficacy of drugs, including antibiotics, and for detoxification of endogenous and exogenous substances [5]. Furthermore, it constitutes the main circulating antioxidant in the body, being the major extracellular source of reduced sulfhydryl groups, potent scavengers of reactive oxygen species (ROS) (**Fig. 1**) [6].

Among the 35 cysteine residues of albumin, 34 are employed for intramolecular disulfide bonds, whereas cysteine 34 (Cys34) remains free. ROS react primarily with Cys34, leading to reversible, highly unstable derivatives: The sulfenic and sulfinic acids. The subsequent, final product of the reaction is the sulfonic acid-albumin complex. Oxidation alters the biological properties of albumin, which becomes more susceptible to proteinase digestion, undergoes faster degradation than the non-oxidized counterpart, and has reduced binding capacity to various substances, including bilirubin [6, 7]. In healthy adults, about 70–80 % of Cys34 contains a free sulfhydryl group (human mercaptalbumin); about 25 % forms a disulfide bond with small sulfhydryl compounds, such as cysteine, homocysteine or glutathione (human nonmercaptalbumin 1); and a small fraction is highly oxidized to sulfonic acid (human nonmercaptalbumin 2). In contrast, in chronic diseases, such as diabetes, renal failure, ischemic heart disease, and cancer, the oxidized form of albumin greatly increases, leading to an impairment of its biological activities [7]. Ischemia-modified albumin (IMA) has the capacity to bind cobalt and other metal ions, a property that contributes to the anti-oxidant activity of albumin by preventing these molecules from catalyzing pro-oxidative reactions. Increased IMA levels have been proposed as a mortality predictor in renal failure [8] and myocardial infarction [9].

Human Serum Albumin and Liver Cirrhosis

Patients with advanced cirrhosis almost always have hypoalbuminemia caused both by decreased synthesis by the hepatocytes and water and sodium retention that dilutes the content of albumin in the extracellular space. Other factors likely contribute to the development of hypoalbuminemia, including an increased transcapillary transport rate [10].

Oncotic Properties of Albumin in Cirrhosis

The therapeutic use of albumin in hepatology dates back to the 1960s when it was thought that hypoalbuminemia had a prominent role in the pathogenesis of ascites, because of alteration of the balance between the forces of Starling in the intrahepatic microcirculation. It was found that plasma albumin levels less than 3 g/l were almost constantly associated with the presence of ascites, which did not develop with plasma levels greater than 4 g/l [11]. Moreover, plasma oncotic pressure less than 20 mmHg significantly increased the probability of developing ascites in the presence of portal hypertension [10]. These findings may support supplementation with exogenous albumin in patients with ascites and hypoalbuminemia. However, the net flow of fluid from the vascular compartment to the interstitium is regulated by its transcapillary gradient rather than by its intravascular concentration alone. When the gradient between plasma and ascitic fluid oncotic pressure was taken into account, no correlation was found with the rate of ascites formation [12], indicating that hypoalbuminemia simply reflects a deterioration in liver synthetic function without playing a major, direct role in the pathogenesis of ascites formation.

From the 1990s better understanding of the cardiovascular alterations in patients with advanced cirrhosis led to a critical review of the clinical use of albumin. These patients typically have a hyperdynamic circulatory syndrome, characterized by a decrease in peripheral vascular resistance and a compensatory increase in cardiac output, which manifest at the clinical level with arterial hypotension, tachycardia and hyperkinetic arterial pulses. The primary cause of the hyperdynamic circulatory syndrome is arterial vasodilation, mainly localized in the splanchnic circulatory area, of sufficient magnitude to reduce the effective blood volume (i.e., the blood volume in the heart, lungs and central arterial tree that is sensed by arterial receptors). Arterial vasodilation in cirrhosis mainly results from the increased production of vasoactive substances, such as nitric oxide (NO), carbon monoxide, and endocannabinoids, which induce vasodilation and hamper the vascular response to vasoconstrictors. The ensuing effective hypovolemia evokes the compensatory activation of neuro-humoral systems, including the renin-angiotensin-aldosterone axis, sympathetic nervous system, and arginine-vasopressin, able to promote vasoconstriction and renal retention of sodium and water. As a result, from a functional point of view, patients with advanced cirrhosis are hypovolemic and exhibit cardiovascular hyporeactivity, even though their cardiac output is usually significantly elevated [13]. However, a decrease in cardiac output leading to an exacerbation of effective hypovolemia is observed in patients with severe disease, suggesting clinically relevant cardiac dysfunction in the more advanced stages of cirrhosis [13]. In addition to ascites, these cardiovascular alterations represent the pathophysiological background of several severe complications of cirrhosis, such as hepatorenal syndrome (HRS),

X

precipitated or not by spontaneous bacterial peritonitis (SBP), and post-paracentesis circulatory dysfunction (PPCD), which all share acute exacerbation of effective hypovolemia as the pathophysiological momentum.

Based on this background, preservation of central blood volume represents a major aim in the management of patients with advanced cirrhosis. Several controlled and/or randomized studies have shown that albumin administration is effective to prevent circulatory dysfunction after large-volume paracentesis [14] and renal failure after SBP [15], and to treat HRS when given together with vasocontrictors [16, 17]. Furthermore, it is currently believed that the capacity of albumin to expand the central blood volume in cirrhosis is superior to that of several other plasma-expanders [18]. In contrast, the chronic use of albumin to treat ascites is still debated, due to the lack of definitive scientific evidence supporting its clinical benefits. Thus, albumin is now given in patients with cirrhosis to expand effective volemia regardless of its plasma level.

Prevention of post-paracentesis circulatory dysfunction

Large-volume paracentesis is the treatment of choice for the management of patients with massive or refractory ascites. Although large-volume paracentesis is a safe procedure and the risk of local complications, such as hemorrhage or bowel perforation, is very low, it can favor the development of PPCD, which is characterized by the exacerbation of effective hypovolemia and is defined by an increase of more than 50 % in the basal plasma renin activity 4–6 days after paracentesis. PPCD predisposes to rapid re-accumulation of ascites, hyponatremia, renal failure, and shortened survival [19].

The occurrence of PPCD is significantly reduced when large-volume paracentesis is combined with infusion of albumin (8 g/l of ascites removed). Albumin was more effective than other plasma expanders (dextran-70 or polygeline) for the prevention of PPCD when more than 5 l of ascites were removed; however, the incidence of PPCD was similar when less than 5 l of ascites were tapped [18, 19]. Moreover, use of albumin after large-volume paracentesis compared with alternative but cheaper plasma expanders appears to be more cost-effective because albumin post-paracentesis is associated with fewer liver-related complications within the first month [20].

Despite these findings, the clinical value of albumin administration as an adjunct to large-volume paracentesis has been questioned because a survival benefit could not be shown in individual randomized trials. However, a meta-analysis that included all available randomized clinical trials comparing albumin with alternative treatments showed that albumin infusion significantly reduces the incidence of PPCD, hyponatremia and mortality, providing evidence-based support for the well-accepted clinical practice of infusing albumin as first choice in patients requiring large-volume paracentesis (Bernardi M, unpublished results).

Hepatorenal syndrome

HRS is defined as the occurrence of renal failure in patients with advanced liver disease without another identifiable cause of renal failure, and is usually classified into two types according to the definition of the International Ascites Club [21]. Type 1 HRS is a rapidly progressive acute renal failure diagnosed when the serum creatinine increases more than 100 % from baseline to a final level greater than 2.5 mg/dl within two weeks. It is usually precipitated by an acute insult often represented by a bacterial infection, although it may occur without any clear triggering event. Type 2 HRS is a relatively steady but moderate degree of functional renal failure with serum creatinine levels above 1.5 mg/dl. It is usually associated with refractory ascites and often hyponatremia. Patients with type 2 HRS may eventually develop type 1 HRS either spontaneously or following a precipitating event, such as SBP.

HRS can be seen as the final event of the hemodynamic disturbances characterizing advanced cirrhosis. The development of HRS is related to an extreme reduction in the effective arterial blood volume combined with a decrease in the mean arterial pressure (MAP). This condition results from either a marked vasodilatation mainly in the splanchnic arterial bed or an impairment of cardiac function as a result of cirrhotic cardiomyopathy. Thus, the cardiac output in patients with HRS may be low or normal (infrequently high), but always insufficient for the patient's needs [21]. Effective hypovolemia produces a very intense compensatory activation of the sympathetic nervous and renin-angiotensin-aldosterone systems which causes renal vasoconstriction and a shift in the renal autoregulatory curve, rendering renal blood flow much more sensitive to the negative effects of low MAP [22].

The prognosis of type 1 HRS is dismal with almost 90 % of patients dying without therapy within 2 weeks. In the last decade, combined therapy with vasoconstrictors and albumin has proved to be effective in reversing HRS in approximately half of the cases [22]. The rationale for this approach is to improve the markedly impaired circulatory function by causing vasoconstriction of the extremely dilated splanchnic vascular bed and by antagonizing effective hypovolemia so that MAP and renal perfusion can increase [22].

Terlipressin, a vasopressin analog, is the most studied vasoconstrictor and two multicenter randomized trials have demonstrated the efficacy of increasing doses of terlipressin in combination with albumin (1 g/kg or 100 g on day 1 followed by 20–40 g/day) (**Fig. 2**) [16, 17]. Albumin administration appears necessary to improve the efficacy of the vasoconstrictor as the rate of HRS reversal is significantly lower with terlipressin alone compared to combination therapy

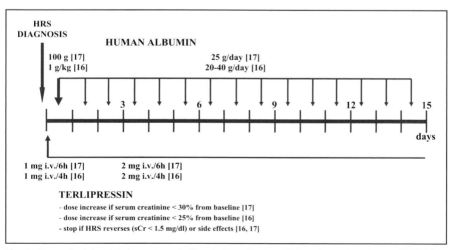

Fig. 2. Dose schedule of terlipressin and albumin in patients with hepatorenal syndrome (HRS) (data from [16, 17]). i.v.: intravenous

[23]. The most frequent side effects of treatment are cardiovascular or ischemic complications, which have been reported in more than 10 % of patients treated [24].

Vasoconstrictors other than vasopressin analogs that have been used in the management of type 1 HRS include norepinephrine and midodrine plus octreotide, both in combination with albumin. Although the number of patients enrolled in the studies evaluating these vasoconstrictors is quite small, their use appeared to improve renal function in a consistent number of patients with HRS [25, 26]. Finally, a systematic review of randomized studies using terlipressin as well as other vasoconstrictors, always in combination with albumin, has shown that treatment is associated with an improved short-term survival [24]. This result may be of paramount importance to keep patients waiting for liver transplantation alive until an organ becomes available [27].

Prevention of hepatorenal syndrome after spontaneous bacterial peritonitis

All patients with cirrhosis and ascites are at risk of developing a bacterial infection of the ascitic fluid, called SBP, which is diagnosed when the neutrophil count in ascitic fluid exceeds $250/mm^3$ as determined by microscopy [19]. SBP, even without septic shock, may precipitate circulatory dysfunction with severe liver failure, hepatic encephalopathy and type 1 HRS, causing the death of the patient in approximately 20 % of cases despite infection resolution with antibiotic treatment [19].

Administration of albumin at a dose of 1.5 g/kg body weight at diagnosis followed by 1 g/kg on day 3 significantly decreased the incidence of type 1 HRS from 30 % to 10 % and reduced mortality from 29 % to 10 % compared with cefotaxime alone in a randomized, controlled study in patients with SBP (**Fig. 3**) [15]. If the efficacy of albumin administration in patients with advanced disease, as witnessed by a serum bilirubin greater than 4 mg/dl and a serum creatinine greater than 1 mg/dl, appears to be undisputed, this is not the case for patients with

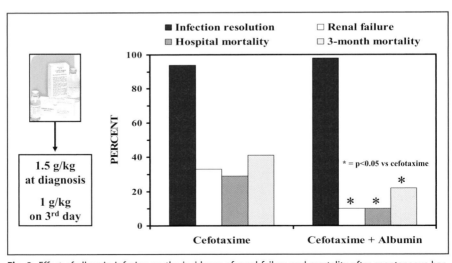

Fig. 3. Effect of albumin infusion on the incidence of renal failure and mortality after spontaneous bacterial peritonitis in patients with cirrhosis (data from [15]).

moderate liver failure and without renal dysfunction at diagnosis as they show a very low incidence of HRS precipitated by SBP [15]. At the same time, it is not established whether crystalloids or artificial colloids could replace albumin, although equivalent doses of hydroxyethyl starch (HES) have not been found to be as effective as albumin in preventing the circulatory dysfunction caused by SBP [28]. Interestingly, albumin infusion was able to prevent the increase in nitrate levels and to reduce the elevated plasma levels of Von Willebrand-related antigen observed in patients with SBP treated with HES [29]. This finding suggests an effect of albumin on endothelial function that appears to be related to the non-oncotic properties of this molecule rather than to its activity as plasma-expander.

Ascites

The chronic use of albumin to treat ascites is still debated, due to the lack of definitive scientific evidence supporting its clinical benefits. When human albumin became available, studies performed several decades ago failed to show clear usefulness of this substance in relieving ascites and preventing its recurrence; however, these investigations were uncontrolled and/or included a small number of patients [30]. Thus, treatment of cirrhotic ascites with diuretics and albumin has been practiced on anecdote and experience for many years. More than a decade ago, a controlled clinical trial in hospitalized patients with cirrhosis and ascites randomized to receive diuretics associated or not with low-doses of albumin (12.5 g/day) showed that treatment with diuretics plus albumin was overall more effective than diuretics alone in determining the disappearance of ascites and reducing the length of the hospital stay [31]. However, this result was only achieved in patients who received the initial dose of diuretics, whereas the difference in the treatment response was not statistically significant in those patients who required higher doses of diuretics or were refractory to diuretic treatment. Albumin administration at home also reduced the rate of ascites recurrence and readmission to the hospital due to ascites, but its prescription was very expensive and no effect on survival was observed [31]. More recently, the same research group showed, in an unblinded randomized trial, that long-term albumin administration is also able to increase patient survival and to reduce the risk of ascites recurrence [32].

No other controlled clinical trials have so far been performed to evaluate the effectiveness of prolonged albumin administration in the treatment of cirrhosis and ascites. Thus, the absence of confirmatory multicenter randomized studies, together with the high cost of human albumin, explains why albumin infusion is not usually included among the therapeutic options for difficult-to-treat ascites. A multicenter randomized clinical trial (NCT 01288794, www.clinicaltrials.gov) planning to enroll more than 400 patients is ongoing in Italy to cover this lack of information.

Non-Oncotic Properties of Albumin in Cirrhosis

In recent years, scientific interest into the non-oncotic properties of human serum albumin has progressively increased in the field of hepatology. Initial findings showed that patients with chronic liver disease have decreased amounts of circulating human nonmercaptalbumin (the 'good guy') and elevated levels of the oxidized form human nonmercaptalbumin 26 (the 'bad guy') [33, 34]. More recently, binding, transport, and detoxification capacities of albumin have been found to be severely impaired in cirrhotic patients, particularly in those with acute-on-chronic liver failure precipitated by bacterial infections [35]. As a result, endogenous and exogenous substances that are normally bound to albumin are free to react arbitrarily. The reduced detoxification capacity of albumin is especially important, as it suggests that the molecule cannot bind and remove waste products. Furthermore, IMA is significantly increased, suggesting an impaired metal chelation capacity that contributes to generate an environment of sustained oxidative stress by favoring radical formation through Fenton chemistry processes. Most important, the loss of albumin function and the increase in the IMA level were associated with poor survival [8, 9, 35].

From a clinical context, the non-oncotic properties of albumin have so far been exploited in extracorporeal albumin dialysis systems in patients with acute or acute-on-chronic liver failure. The two commercially available detoxification systems are the "Molecular Adsorbent Recirculating System" (MARS) and the "fractionated plasma separation and adsorption" (Prometheus), which are based on the association of a conventional dialysis membrane with a second dialysis circuit filled with a circulating 20 % albumin solution in the case of MARS or with a second filter containing albumin in the case of Prometheus. In addition to the positive consequences associated with the removal of toxic molecules, early studies of these systems showed a favorable impact on systemic hemodynamics likely due to the purification of substances involved in the pathogenesis of the hyperdynamic circulatory syndrome, such as NO, and the pro-inflammatory cytokines, TNF-α and IL-6 [36, 37]. Such systems, currently available only in specialized and transplant centers, have a potential therapeutic role in the following medical conditions: Acute fulminant liver failure, acute liver failure on chronic liver disease, primary dysfunction of the transplanted liver, liver failure after resection and intractable pruritus [37]. It has to be stressed, however, that the results of the first large-scale controlled trials that have employed either MARS or Prometheus in patients with cirrhosis and acute-on-chronic liver failure did not show a significant impact on major outcomes, such as survival [38, 39]. Likely, subgroups of patients who would actually benefit from these detoxification systems need to be identified, as suggested by the survival benefit observed in patients with severe cirrhosis (model for end-stage liver disease [MELD] score > 30) and HRS type 1 treated with the Prometheus system [39].

Conclusion

The use of human albumin in the setting of liver cirrhosis is supported by evidence arising from prospective randomized trials and meta-analyses. Albumin administration is, therefore widely accepted and recommended by current international guidelines for the prevention of PPCD and acute renal failure in patients with SBP, and the treatment of HRS as an adjunct to vasoconstrictors. All these complications share the common pathophysiological background of reduced effective volemia, mainly because of peripheral arterial vasodilation, and the rationale underlying the use of albumin is related to its activity as a plasma expander. However, it is likely that the beneficial effects of albumin are also linked to its non-oncotic properties, including binding capacity, antioxidant activity, and effects on capillary integrity. These effects represent the main fields

X

of current and future research, from which will likely arise further and more appropriate indications for albumin administration in patients with liver disease.

References

1. Quinlan GJ, Martin GS, Evans TW (2005) Albumin: biochemical properties and therapeutic potential. Hepatology 41: 1211–1219
2. Mirici-Cappa F, Caraceni P, Domenicali M, et al (2011) How albumin administration for cirrhosis impacts on hospital albumin consumption and expenditure. World J Gastroenterol 17: 3479–3486
3. Finfer S, Bellomo R, Boyce N, French J, Myburgh J, Norton R, SAFE Study Investigators (2004) A comparison of albumin and saline for fluid resuscitation in the intensive care unit. N Engl J Med 350: 2247–2256
4. Delaney AP, Dan A, McCaffrey J, Finfer S (2011) The role of albumin as a resuscitation fluid for patients with sepsis: a systematic review and meta-analysis. Crit Care Med 39: 386–391
5. Vincent JL (2009) Relevance of albumin in modern critical care medicine. Best Pract Res Clin Anaesthesiol 23: 183–191
6. Evans TW (2002) Review article: albumin as a drug. Biological effects of albumin unrelated to oncotic pressure. Aliment Pharmacol Ther 16: S6–S11
7. Oettl K, Stauber RE (2007) Physiological and pathological changes in the redox state of human serum albumin critically influence its binding properties. Br J Pharmacol 151: 580–590
8. Sharma R, Gaze DC, Pellerin D, et al (2006) Ischemia-modified albumin predicts mortality in ESRD. Am J Kidney Dis 47: 493–502
9. Van Belle E, Dallongeville J, Vicaut E, Degrandsart A, Baulac C, Montalescot G; OPERA Investigators (2010) Ischemia-modified albumin levels predict long-term outcome in patients with acute myocardial infarction. The French Nationwide OPERA study. Am Heart J 159: 570–576
10. Henricksen JH, Siemssen O, Krintel JJ, Malchow-Møller A, Bendtsen F, Ring-Larsen (2001) Dynamics of albumin in plasma and acitic fluid in patients with cirrhosis. J Hepatol 34: 53–60
11. Wood LJ, Colman J, Dudley FJ (1987) The relationship between portal pressure and plasma albumin in the development of cirrhotic ascites. J Gastroenterol Hepatol 2: 525–531
12. Rector WG Jr, Ibarra F, Openshaw K, Hoefs JC (1986) Ascites kinetics in cirrhosis: relationship to plasma-ascites hydrostatic-oncotic balance and intensity of renal sodium retention. J Lab Clin Med 107: 412–419
13. Møller S, Henriksen JH (2008) Cardiovascular complications of cirrhosis. 57: 268–278
14. Ginés P, Titó L, Arroyo V, et al (1998) Randomized comparative study of therapeutic paracentesis with and without intravenous albumin in cirrhosis. Gastroenterology 94: 1493–1502
15. Sort P, Navasa M, Arroyo V, et al (1999) Effect of intravenous albumin on renal impairment and mortality in patients with cirrhosis and spontaneous bacterial peritonitis. N Engl J Med 341: 403–409
16. Martín-Llahí M, Pépin MN, Guevara M, et al (2008) Terlipressin and albumin vs albumin in patients with cirrhosis and hepatorenal syndrome: a randomized study. Gastroenterology 134: 1352–1359
17. Sanyal AJ, Boyer T, Garcia-Tsao G, et al (2008) A randomized, prospective, double-blind, placebo-controlled trial of terlipressin for type 1 hepatorenal syndrome. Gastroenterology 134: 1360–1368
18. Ginès A, Fernandez-Esparrach G, Monescillo A, et al (1996) Randomized controlled trial comparing albumin, dextran-70 and polygelin in cirrhotic patients with ascites treated by paracentesis. Gastroenterology 111: 1002–1010
19. European Association for the Study of the Liver (2010) EASL clinical practice guidelines on the management of ascites, spontaneous bacterial peritonitis, and hepatorenal syndrome in cirrhosis J Hepatol 53: 397–417

X

20. Moreau R, Valla DC, Durand-Zaleski I, et al (2006) Comparison of outcome in patients with cirrhosis and ascites following treatment with albumin or a synthetic colloid: a randomised controlled pilot trail. Liver Int 26: 46–54
21. Salerno F, Gerbes A, Ginès P, Wong F, Arroyo V (2007) Diagnosis, prevention and treatment of hepatorenal syndrome in cirrhosis. Gut 56: 1310–1318
22. Ginès P, Schrier RW (2009) Renal failure in cirrhosis. N Engl J Med 361: 1279–1290
23. Ortega R, Gines P, Uriz J, et al (2002) Terlipressin therapy with and without albumin for patients with hepatorenal syndrome: results of prospective, non-randomized study. Hepatology 36: 941–948
24. Gluud LL, Christensen K, Christensen E, Krag A (2010) Systematic review of randomized trials on vasoconstrictor drugs for hepatorenal syndrome. Hepatology 51: 576–584
25. Angeli P, Volpin R, Gerunda G, et al (1999) Reversal of type 1 hepatorenal syndrome (HRS) with the combined administration of midodrine and octreotide. Hepatology 29: 1690–1697
26. Alessandria C, Ottobrelli A, Debernardi-Venon W, et al (2007) Noradrenalin vs terlipressin in patients with hepatorenal syndrome: a prospective, randomized, unblinded, pilot study. J Hepatol 47: 499–505
27. Caraceni P, Santi L, Mirici F, et al (2011) Long-term treatment of hepatorenal syndrome as a bridge to liver transplantation. Dig Liver Dis 43: 242–245
28. Sigal SH, Stanca CM, Fernandez J, Arroyo V, Navasa M (2007) Restricted use of albumin for spontaneous bacterial peritonitis. Gut 56: 597–599
29. Fernández J, Monteagudo J, Bargallo X, et al (2005) A randomized unblinded pilot study comparing albumin versus hydroxyethyl starch in spontaneous bacterial peritonitis. Hepatology 42: 627–634
30. Clermont RJ, Vlahevic ZR, Chalmers TC, Adham NF, Curtis GW, Morrosin RS (1967) Intravenous therapy of massive ascites in patients with cirrhosis. Long-term effects on survival and frequency of renal failure. Gastroenterology 53: 220–228
31. Gentilini P, Casini-Raggi V, Di Fiore G, et al (1999) Albumin improves the response to diuretics in patients with cirrhosis and ascites: results of a randomized, controlled trial. J Hepatol 30: 639–645
32. Romanelli RG, La Villa G, Barletta G, et al (2006) Long-term albumin infusion improves survival in patients with cirrhosis and ascites: an unblinded randomized trial. World J Gastroenterol 12: 1403–1407
33. Watanabe A, Matsuzaki S, Moriwaki H, Suzuki K, Nishiguchi S (2004) Problems in serum albumin measurement and clinical significance of albumin microheterogeneity in cirrhotics. Nutrition 20: 351–357
34. Oettl K, Stadlbauer V, Petter F, et al (2008) Oxidative damage of albumin in advanced liver disease. Biochim Biophys Acta 1782: 469–473
35. Jalan R, Schnurr K, Mookerjee RP, et al (2009) Alterations in the functional capacity of albumin in patients with decompensated cirrhosis is associated with increased mortality. Hepatology 50: 555–564
36. Oettl K, Stadlbauer V, Krisper P, Stauber RE (2009) Effect of extracorporeal liver support by molecular adsorbents recirculating system and Prometheus on redox state of albumin in acute-on-chronic liver failure. Ther Apher Dial 13: 431–436
37. Karvellas CJ, Gibney N, Kutsogiannis D, Wendon J, Bain VG (2007) Bench-to-bedside review: current evidence for extracorporeal albumin dialysis systems in liver failure. Crit Care 11: 215
38. Bañares R, Nevens F, Larsen FS, Jalan R, Albillos A, Dollinger M, Relief Study Group (2010) Extracorporeal liver support with the molecular adsorbent recirculating system (MARS) in patients with acute-on-chronic liver failure (AOCLF). The RELIEF Trial. J Hepatol 52: S459–S460
39. Rifai K, Kribben A, Gerken G, et al (2010) Extracorporeal liver support by fractionated plasma separation and adsorption (PROMETHEUS) in patients with acute-on-chronic liver failure (HELIOS Study): a prospective randomized controlled multicenter study. J Hepatol 52: S3 (abst)

X

The Ability of Red Blood Cell Transfusions to Reach the Microcirculation

K. Yuruk, R. Bezemer, and C. Ince

Introduction

The ultimate goal of red blood cell (RBC) transfusions in anemic patients is to provide oxygen-rich blood to the microcirculation to improve tissue oxygenation [1]. There is little evidence, however, that this is actually achieved in patients. RBCs undergo several biochemical and hemorheological changes during their storage. Several clinical studies have reported blood transfusion-related complications associated with the aging of blood, such as increased mortality, multiple organ failure, infections, and prolonged hospital length of stay. Other studies, in contrast, have not found differences in outcome following transfusion of fresh blood or aged blood. At present, the studies on transfusion medicine have been mainly focused on the role of the quality of the transfused blood. These changes are commonly referred to as storage lesions and are held responsible for many of the deleterious effects of RBC transfusions. The presence of leukocytes and their by-products in stored blood may be another factor affecting *in vivo* function of transfused blood. Taken together, these biochemical and hemorheological changes during RBC storage may adversely affect the ability of transfused RBCs to deliver oxygen-rich blood to the microcirculation [2, 3]. As the ultimate aim of RBC transfusions is to promote microcirculatory oxygen delivery (DO_2), the underlying disease should also be taken into consideration as this may interfere with the transfusion. In fact, in some disease states it has been shown that RBC transfusions may even have deleterious effects on the microcirculation [4, 5]. It seems that even though systemic hematocrit and hemoglobin levels rise following transfusion, the ability of transfused blood to actually reach the microcirculation and oxygenate the tissues may not be achieved [6]. In two clinical studies performed by our group, however, we demonstrated that RBC transfusions did promote microcirculatory perfusion and oxygenation in cardiac surgery patients [7] and anemic hematology out-patients [8]. However, in septic intensive care patients we too found a discrepancy in the macro- and microcirculatory response to RBC transfusions, because systemic hematocrit and hemoglobin levels rose, while the microcirculatory parameters did not [6, 9].

Most of the clinical and experimental studies performed have been focused on factors related to the impaired ability of transfused RBCs to improve the microcirculation in anemic patients, such as the additive solutions, the leukocyte content, and storage lesions. Yet, insight into the factors diminishing the efficacy of RBC transfusions is lacking because of the conflicting results of these studies. To date, little attention has been given to the potential role of the condition of the patients receiving the RBC transfusions (underlying disease, severity of disease,

J.-L. Vincent (ed.), *Annual Update in Intensive Care and Emergency Medicine 2012*
DOI 10.1007/978-3-642-25716-2 © Springer-Verlag Berlin Heidelberg 2012

degree of anemia, therapy being administered). In this chapter, we present a brief history of blood transfusion medicine and then evaluate studies investigating the efficacy of RBC transfusions, focusing on two main aspects: 1) The quality of the transfused blood and 2) the condition of the patient receiving the blood transfusion.

Historical Background

Long before William Harvey described the theory of the circulation of blood, transfusion of blood had been described on several occasions. The first known transfusion was performed on Pope Innocent VIII in 1490. The blood of three ten-year old boys (who died shortly after the procedure) was given into the veins of the sick pope [10]. The first documented animal-to-animal transfusion attempts were performed by Richard Lower and Jean-Baptiste Dennis in 1665. In 1667, Lower and Dennis each performed the first animal-to-human transfusions with sheep and lambs as donors. The next important step in transfusion medicine was taken by James Blundel, an English obstetrician who performed the first human-to-human transfusion in 1818. Between 1818 and 1829, Blundel performed 10 experiments using human blood, of which only 4 were successful. Until the 20th century, blood transfusion remained a risky treatment due to fatal hemolytic transfusion reactions and coagulation of donor blood. The discovery of ABO blood groups by Karl Landsteiner in 1901 and sodium citrate as an anticoagulant storage solution by Richard Lewisohn in 1915 had a major impact on transfusion medicine. Later, the introduction of the rhesus (Rh) blood group system by Karl Landsteiner and Alexander Wiener in 1940 was a huge step forwards. Both world wars also stimulated transfusion medicine and opened new research into colloid or plasma resuscitation. The past three decades have mainly been focused on improvement in the quality of stored blood.

Quality of the Transfused Blood
Biochemical and Hemorheological Studies

RBCs undergo several biochemical and hemorheological changes during their storage [11]. These changes are commonly referred to as the storage lesion and are held responsible for many of the deleterious effects of RBC transfusion. The biochemical changes include a decrease in 2,3-diphosphoglycerate (2,3 DPG) and ATP levels [12], a decrease in membrane sialic acid [13], RBC membrane lipid peroxidation [14], a loss of intrinsic RBC membrane proteins [15], a loss of cellular antioxidant capability [16], a decrease in pH [17], an increase in free hemoglobin as a result of hemolysis [18], and a decrease in S-nitrosohemoglobin concentrations [19]. Furthermore, the hemorheological properties of the RBCs are altered in terms of reduced deformability [20, 21] and increased aggregability and adhesiveness to vascular endothelial cells [22]. In a very elegant study by Donadee et al., storage of human RBCs resulted in the accumulation of cell-free and microparticle-encapsulated hemoglobin, which scavenges the vasodilator nitric oxide (NO) approximately a thousand times faster than intact erythrocytes [18]. In line, the authors showed that cell-free and microparticle-encapsulated hemoglobin is a highly potent vasoconstrictor *in vivo* and that even the infusion of the plasma from stored RBC units produced significant vasoconstriction in the rat due to storage-related hemolysis.

Taken together, these biochemical and hemorheological changes during RBC storage may adversely affect the ability of transfused RBCs to deliver oxygen-rich blood to the microcirculation. The biochemical changes, and especially the depleted 2,3-DPG levels, increase the hemoglobin oxygen affinity in stored RBCs which leads to impaired oxygen offloading in the tissues. It has been shown, however, that the 2,3-DPG levels recover within 72 hours after transfusion *in vivo* [23]. In a recent experimental study by our group, we showed that the storage-related decline in RBC ATP levels, which is responsible for the worsening of RBC viability during storage, could be reverted by treatment of cells with a rejuvenation solution. This method was, in addition to restoring ATP levels, also successful in restoring the ability of the stored RBCs to transport oxygen to the renal microcirculation of anemic rats [24]. Finally, the altered hemorheological properties of stored RBCs in terms of increased stiffness, aggregability, and adhesiveness may severely impair the ability of transfused cells to enter the microcirculation [2].

Leukocyte Studies

Leukocytes and their by-products in stored blood may be another confounding factor affecting the *in vivo* efficacy of transfused blood. It is generally thought that the cytokines, enzymes, and inflammatory mediators derived from leukocytes during blood storage may worsen storage lesion and cause transfusion-related immunomodulation. Leukoreduction is performed to reduce some of the negative immunosuppressive effects of blood transfusions and to mitigate RBC storage lesions [25, 26]. However, there are conflicting data in the literature regarding the clinical impact of transfusion of non-leukoreduced blood. Anniss and Sparrow examined endothelial RBC adherence and compared non-leukodepleted blood, buffy-coat-poor blood, and leukodepleted blood and demonstrated that leukodepleted blood showed significantly lower adhesiveness to vascular endothelial cells, an effect which would be beneficial for the microvascular perfusion of transfused blood [27]. Consistent with the idea that leukoreduction provides a better quality stored blood, van de Watering et al. reported increased survival rates in cardiac surgery patients receiving leukoreduced RBC units compared to patients transfused with buffy-coat-removed packed RBCs units [28]. In addition, Netzer et al. reported an association between leukoreduced RBC transfusion and decreased mortality rates [29]. In contrast, a randomized prospective study in 2780 patients receiving either leukoreduced or non-leukoreduced RBC units showed no beneficial effect of leukoreduction on clinical outcome, including mortality, length of intensive care unit (ICU) stay, and readmission rate [30]. Nathens et al., moreover, randomized 268 of 1864 trauma patients to receive leukoreduced or non-leukoreduced RBC units and demonstrated no difference in mortality or morbidity [31].

Experimental Studies

Several experimental studies have shown that transfusion of fresh RBCs is more effective at improving the microcirculation in anemic animals compared to transfusion of aged RBCs. Van Bommel et al. showed that transfusion of rat blood stored for four weeks was not as effective in improving intestinal microcirculatory

X

oxygenation following hemorrhage as compared to fresh rat blood [20]. No such differences were observed in the changes in venous saturation levels which responded equally well to both RBC solutions. The authors furthermore showed that the type of preservation solution used to store the RBCs could significantly affect the RBC rheological properties and consequently the efficacy of RBC transfusion with respect to improving microvascular oxygenation. Tsai et al. showed that transfusion of stored RBCs resulted in significantly malperfused and underoxygenated skin microvasculature in severely hemodiluted hamsters [32]. This effect was not detectable at the systemic level, underscoring the importance of studying the effects of RBC transfusions at the microcirculatory level. It must be noted, however, that the blood was hamster blood stored for 28 days, which may correspond to much older human blood than is conventionally used (e.g. [33]) and, in addition, the blood was not leukodepleted so the results of this study should be evaluated with care. Raat et al., in pursue of a more clinically relevant model, developed a rat model that tolerated transfusion of human RBCs [12]. The authors measured intestinal microcirculatory oxygenation and tested whether transfused human RBCs functionally transport oxygen to the rat microcirculation. It was shown that at low hematocrit, the oxygen-delivering capacity of human RBCs stored for 5–6 weeks was significantly reduced compared to the capacity of fresh human RBCs and human RBCs stored for 2–3 weeks.

Clinical Studies

Several clinical studies have reported blood transfusion-related complications associated with the aging of blood, such as increased mortality [34, 35], multiple organ failure [36], infections [37], and prolonged hospital length of stay [38]. Other studies, in contrast, have not found differences in outcome following transfusion of fresh or aged blood [39–42]. The clinical studies that identified complications associated with aging of blood are listed in **Table 1** and the clinical studies that did not are listed in **Table 2**.

Table 1. Clinical studies that identified complications associated with aging of blood.

First author [ref]	Year of publication	Patients	Complication(s) associated with transfusion of aged blood
Marik [4]	1993	23 septic patients	gastric PCO_2
Purdy [34]	1997	31 septic ICU patients	mortality
Vamvakas [37]	1999	416 cardiac surgery patients	postoperative pneumonia
Zallen [36]	1999	63 trauma patients	multiple organ failure
Offner [38]	2002	61 trauma patients	prolonged ICU length of stay major infections
Weinberg [43]	2008	1813 trauma patients	mortality renal failure pneumonia
Koch [35]	2008	6002 cardiac surgery patients	mortality postoperative complications

Table 2. Clinical studies that did not identify complications associated with aging of blood.

First author [ref]	Year of publication	Patients	Tested outcome parameters
Vamvakas [39]	2000	268 cardiac surgery patients	ICU length of stay post-operative pneumonia
Walsh [40]	2004	22 septic shock patients	gastric tissue oxygenation
Murrell [41]	2005	275 trauma patients	mortality
Van de Watering [42]	2006	2732 cardiac surgery patients	mortality ICU length of stay
Yuruk	unpublished data	20 hematology outpatients	microvascular density microvascular oxygenation

In septic ICU patients, Purdy et al. reported that the 19 who died received more and older RBCs compared to the 12 surviving patients [34]. Vamvakas et al. demonstrated in a retrospective cohort study in 416 cardiac surgery patients that transfusion of aged RBC units was associated with an increased risk of postoperative pneumonia [37]. Zallen et al. retrospectively reviewed a database of trauma patients who had received 6–20 units of RBCs in the first 12 hours after admission to the trauma center and found that 23 of 63 patients who developed multiple organ failure had received RBCs that had been stored for more than a month [36]. Offner et al. [38] reported a trauma cohort of 61 patients who received 6–20 units of RBCs in the first 12 hours after admission (same institute and study design as that of Zallen et al. [36]). In this second study, it was found that transfusion of RBCs stored for more than two weeks was associated with an increased risk of major infections and longer stay in the ICU [38]. However, in contrast to the first study, no association was found between the age of the transfused blood and the occurrence of multiple organ failure or mortality. Weinberg et al. [43] retrospectively examined the role of the age of transfused blood with respect to mortality in 1813 trauma patients. Trauma patients were considered eligible for analysis when receiving more than 1 unit of packed RBCs within the first 24 hours after admission. The authors showed that larger transfusion volumes of blood, irrespective of storage age, were associated with increased risk of mortality. This was, moreover, shown to be potentiated by the aging of blood. However, for patients transfused with smaller blood volumes, blood age had no effect on mortality [43]. In a large retrospective study, Koch et al. reviewed the outcome of cardiac surgery patients who received either RBCs stored for 14 days or less (2872 patients) or RBCs stored for more than 14 days (3130 patients). The authors found that patients who were given older units had higher rates of in-hospital and out-hospital mortality. Furthermore, patients who had been transfused with aged RBCs had a significantly higher risk of postoperative complications [35]. These results, however, should be interpreted with caution since these authors attributed their results to storage length while about half of the transfused blood was nonleukodepleted and, in addition, the length of storage tolerated in the US is considerably longer than that allowed in Europe.

In contrast to the studies described above, other studies have found no link between duration of RBC storage and clinical outcome of the recipient. Vamvakas et al., previously reporting that transfusion of aged RBC units was associated with

X

an increased risk of postoperative pneumonia, in a subsequent retrospective study in 268 consecutive cardiac surgery patients receiving RBC transfusion found no relationship between length of ICU and hospital stays and the age of the transfused blood [39]. In a randomized prospective clinical trial by Walsh et al., 22 patients with septic shock were randomized to receive transfusion of RBCs stored for longer than 20 days (12 patients) or transfusion of RBCs stored for less than 5 days (10 patients). The authors found no differences in outcome between the two groups [40]. Murrell et al. performed a retrospective cohort study including 275 patients in a trauma center. They found no relationship between the age of the RBC units and the mortality rate of studied patients. However, ICU length of stay was longer in those receiving older RBC units [41]. Van de Watering et al. performed a large retrospective review consisting of 2732 patients who underwent cardiac surgery and received non-leukoreduced RBC units. The multivariate analysis demonstrated no independent effect of storage duration of RBC units on survival or length of ICU stay [42]. The above studies all need to be interpreted with care because the transfusion conditions are often no longer applied in modern transfusion practice, at least in Europe. That is why the recent study by Sakr et al. is of significance. These authors retrospectively analyzed the results of 5925 patients in a surgical ICU and found that higher hemoglobin concentrations and blood transfusion were independently associated with a lower risk of in-hospital death in patients admitted to the ICU after non-cardiovascular surgery, in patients with higher severity scores, and in patients with severe sepsis. This was noted to be the case especially in patients aged from 66 to 80 years [6].

With the aim of studying the effects of storage duration on the ability of RBC transfusions to reach the microcirculation, our group performed a prospective randomized pilot clinical study. Twenty anemic hematology outpatients were randomized to receive transfusion of leukodepleted RBCs in saline-adenine-glucose-mannitol (SAGM) stored for less than one week (n = 10) or transfusion of leukodepleted RBCs in SAGM stored for 3–4 weeks (n = 10). We were able to show a parallel increase in both systemic hemoglobin and hematocrit values and microvascular perfused vessel density and oxygen saturation with differences between the two groups (Yuruk et al., unpublished data).

Condition of the Patient Receiving Blood Transfusion

Underlying Disease

At present, studies on transfusion medicine have been mainly focused on the role of the quality of the transfused blood. As the ultimate aim of RBC transfusions is to promote microcirculatory DO_2, the underlying disease should also be taken into consideration as this may interfere with the efficacy of transfusion. For example, in some disease states, such as sepsis, blood transfusion has been shown to be ineffective in improving the microcirculation possibly due to altered rheological, coagulation, and inflammation factors already present in the host circulation in combination with microvascular obstruction and shunting often seen in septic patients [2, 4].

Only a few studies have investigated the direct effects of RBC transfusions on the microcirculation [7, 8, 44–46] and only three studies have shown a beneficial effect of RBC transfusions on the microcirculation, of which one was in adults undergoing cardiac surgery [7], one in hematological outpatients [8], and one in

Table 3. Clinical studies on the effects of blood transfusion on the microcirculation.

First author [ref]	Year of publication	Patients	Effect on microcirculation
Genzel-Boroviczény [46]	2004	13 preterm infants	Increased skin functional capillary density 2 hours and 24 hours after transfusion.
Sakr [44]	2007	35 severely septic patients	No changes in the sublingual microcirculation after transfusion; however, the microcirculation improved after transfusion in patients with depressed baseline values.
Creteur [45]	2009	44 intensive care patients (18 patients with sepsis)	No changes in muscle tissue oxygenation, oxygen consumption, and microvascular reactivity after transfusion; however, oxygen consumption and microvascular reactivity improved after transfusion in patients with depressed baseline values.
Yuruk [7]	2011	24 cardiac surgery patients	Increased sublingual microcirculatory density and tissue oxygenation after transfusion.
Yuruk [8]	2011	20 hematology outpatients	Increased sublingual and muscle tissue oxygenation after transfusion.

anemic preterm infants [46]. The contrasting results (**Table 3**) of these studies might be explained by the studied patient populations as the studies showing no effect of RBC transfusions were carried out in (septic) ICU patients [44, 45], in which the microcirculation is significantly impaired with endothelial dysfunction and abnormal endogenous RBCs [47, 48]. These depressed microcirculatory conditions are much less prevalent in surgical patients [7], hematological outpatients [8], and preterm infants [46], possibly explaining the discrepancy between these studies.

Sakr et al. studied the sublingual microcirculation in 35 septic patients using orthogonal polarization spectral (OPS) imaging. They performed the measurements just before RBC unit transfusion and one hour after transfusion of one or two leukoreduced RBC units with a mean age of 24 days. They found that although mean arterial pressure (MAP) and DO_2 increased following RBC transfusion, oxygen uptake and microcirculatory parameters did not. It must be noted, however, that there was interindividual variability with an increase in sublingual capillary perfusion in patients with depressed perfusion at baseline and a decrease in perfusion in patients with normal baseline perfusion [44]. Creteur et al. obtained similar results studying muscle oxygenation, oxygen consumption, and microvascular reactivity using near-infrared spectroscopy (NIRS) in ICU patients receiving one leukoreduced RBC unit with a mean age of 18 days [45]. In contrast, Genzel-Boroviczény et al. observed an increased functional capillary density in the skin 2 hours and 24 hours after transfusion of 9.3–14.2 ml of packed RBCs per kg body weight (age of packed RBCs unknown) in pediatric patients [46]. In line with the study by Genzel-Boroviczény et al., our group demonstrated increased sublingual microcirculatory density and tissue oxygenation after transfusion of one to three RBCs units with a mean age of 18 days in cardiac surgery patients [7] and increased sublingual and muscle tissue oxygenation after transfusion of two or three RBCs units with a mean age of 21 days in hematology outpatients [8]. In these studies, we have been able to verify that transfused blood is effective in improving oxygen transport to the tissue by promoting RBC delivery to the microcirculation and we also identified the mechanism by which this is accomplished: i.e., not by increasing microcirculatory flow velocity but rather by filling empty capillaries, by which the oxygen diffusion distances to the tissue cells is reduced. In an attempt to confirm the findings by Sakr et al. and Creteur et al., we have recently conducted a pilot study testing the ability of RBC transfusions to improve microcirculatory density as studied using sidestream dark field (SDF) imaging and oxygenation as studied using NIRS in adult septic patients [9] and critically ill pediatric patients, both groups with severely disturbed microcirculations.

Conclusion

The ultimate aim of blood transfusion is to provide oxygen-rich RBCs to the microcirculation to improve DO_2 to the tissue cells that is required for maintaining organ function. However, only a few clinical studies have actually evaluated the effects of blood transfusions at the microcirculatory level. Therefore, the ability of blood transfusions to improve microcirculatory DO_2 should be addressed in larger clinical trials. As several studies have shown that the septic microcirculation is resistant to blood transfusion, new maneuvers to increase the efficacy of blood transfusions in septic patients should be investigated. However, first it is important to gain understanding of the mechanisms responsible for the resistance of the septic microcirculation to blood transfusion. With this knowledge, adjunct therapies can be developed to optimize the efficacy of blood transfusion for septic (and non-septic) patients to achieve improved oxygen transport to the tissues.

Acknowledgement: KY and RB were in part supported by the Landsteiner Foundation for Blood Transfusion Research (grant 1365) and in part by the Dutch Kidney Foundation (grant 1103).

X

References

1. Hébert PC, Wells G, Tweeddale M, et al (1997) Does transfusion practice affect mortality in critically ill patients? Transfusion Requirements in Critical Care (TRICC) Investigators and the Canadian Critical Care Trials Group. Am J Respir Crit Care Med 155: 1618–1623
2. Almac E, Ince C (2007) The impact of storage on red cell function in blood transfusion. Best Pract Res Clin Anaesthesiol 21: 195–208
3. Raat NJH, Ince C (2007) Oxygenating the microcirculation: the perspective from blood transfusion and blood storage. Vox Sanguin 93: 12–18
4. Marik PE, Sibbald WJ (1993) Effect of stored-blood transfusion on oxygen delivery in patients with sepsis. JAMA 269: 3024–3029.
5. Fernandes CJ Jr, Akamine N, De Marco FV, De Souza JA, Lagudis S, Knobel E (2001) Red blood cell transfusion does not increase oxygen consumption in critically ill septic patients. Crit Care 5: 362–367
6. Sakr Y, Lobo S, Knuepfer S, et al (2010) Anemia and blood transfusion in a surgical intensive care unit. Crit Care 14: R92
7. Yuruk K, Almac E, Bezemer R, Goedhart P, de Mol B, Ince C (2011) Blood transfusions recruit the microcirculation during cardiac surgery. Transfusion 51: 961–967
8. Yuruk K, Bartels SA, Milstein DM, Bezemer R, Biemond BJ, Ince C (2012) Red blood cell transfusions and tissue oxygenation in anemic hematology outpatients. Transfusion (in press)

9. Ayhan B, Yuruk K, Bakker J, de Mol BAJM, Ince C (2010) Blood transfusions recruit the microcirculation in on-pump cardiac surgery patients, but not in septic patients. Intensive Care Med 36 (Suppl S) 0489 (abst)

10. Starr D (2002) Blood – An Epic History of Medicine and Commerce. Perennial, New York

11. Hess JR (2010) Red cell changes during storage. Transfus Apher Sci 43: 51–59

12. Raat NJ, Verhoeven AJ, Mik EG, et al (2005) The effect of storage time of human red cells on intestinal microcirculatory oxygenation in a rat isovolemic exchange model. Crit Care Med 33: 39–45

13. Bratosin D, Leszczynski S, Sartiaux C, et al (2001) Improved storage of erythrocytes by prior leukodepletion: flow cytometric evaluation of stored erythrocytes. Cytometry 46: 351–356

14. Knight JA, Voorhees RP, Martin L, Anstall H (1992) Lipid peroxidation in stored red cells. Transfusion 32: 354–357

15. Messana I, Ferroni L, Misiti F, et al (2000) Blood bank conditions and RBCs: the progressive loss of metabolic modulation. Transfusion 40: 353–360

16. Racek J, Herynková R, Holecek V, Jerábek Z, Sláma V (1997) Influence of antioxidants on the quality of stored blood. Vox Sang 72: 16–19

17. Högman CF (1998) Preparation and preservation of red cells. Vox Sang 74 (Suppl 2): 177–187

18. Donadee C, Raat NJ, Kanias T, et al (2011) Nitric oxide scavenging by red blood cell microparticles and cell-free hemoglobin as a mechanism for the red cell storage lesion. Circulation 124: 465–476

19. Reynolds JD, Ahearn GS, Angelo M, Zhang J, Cobb F, Stamler JS (2007) S-nitrosohemoglobin deficiency: a mechanism for loss of physiological activity in banked blood. Proc Natl Acad Sci USA 104: 17058–17062

20. van Bommel J, de Korte D, Lind A, et al (2001) The effect of the transfusion of stored RBCs on intestinal microvascular oxygenation in the rat. Transfusion 41: 1515–1523

21. Berezina TL, Zaets SB, Morgan C, et al (2002) Influence of storage on red blood cell rheological properties. J Surg Res 102: 6–12

22. Luk CS, Gray-Statchuk LA, Cepinkas G, Chin-Yee IH (2003) WBC reduction reduces storage-associated RBC adhesion to human vascular endothelial cells under conditions of continuous flow in vitro. Transfusion 43: 151–156

23. Heaton A, Keegan T, Holme S (1989) In vivo regeneration of red cell 2,3-diphosphoglycerate following transfusion of DPG-depleted AS-1, AS-3 and CPDA-1 red cells. Br J Haematol 71: 131–136

24. Raat NJ, Hilarius PM, Johannes T, de Korte D, Ince C, Verhoeven AJ (2009) Rejuvenation of stored human red blood cells reverses the renal microvascular oxygenation deficit in an isovolemic transfusion model in rats. Transfusion 49: 427–424

25. Hébert PC, Fergusson D, Blajchman MA, et al (2003) Clinical outcomes following institution of the Canadian universal leukoreduction program for red blood cell transfusions. JAMA 289: 1941–1949

26. Shapiro MJ (2004) To filter blood or universal leukoreduction: what is the answer? Crit Care 8 (Suppl) 2: S27–S30

27. Anniss AM, Sparrow RL (2006) Storage duration and white blood cell content of red blood cell (RBC) products increases adhesion of stored RBCs to endothelium under flow conditions. Transfusion 46: 1561–1567

28. van de Watering LM, Hermans J, Houbiers JG, et al (1998) Beneficial effects of leukocyte depletion of transfused blood on postoperative complications in patients undergoing cardiac surgery: a randomized clinical trial. Circulation 97: 562–568

29. Netzer G, Shah CV, Iwashyna TJ, et al (2007) Association of RBC transfusion with mortality in patients with acute lung injury. Chest 132: 1116–1123

30. Dzik WH, Anderson JK, O'Neill EM, Assmann SF, Kalish LA, Stowell CP (2002) A prospective, randomized clinical trial of universal WBC reduction. Transfusion 42: 1114–1122

31. Nathens AB, Nester TA, Rubenfeld GD, Nirula R, Gernsheimer TB (2006) The effects of leukoreduced blood transfusion on infection risk following injury: a randomized controlled trial. Shock 26: 342–347

32. Tsai AG, Cabrales P, Intaglietta M (2004) Microvascular perfusion upon exchange transfu-

X

sion with stored red blood cells in normovolemic anemic conditions. Transfusion 44: 1626–1634

33. d'Almeida MS, Jagger J, Duggan M, White M, Ellis C, Chin- Yee IH (2000) A comparison of biochemical and functional alterations of rat and human erythrocytes stored in CPDA-1 for 29 days: implications for animal models of transfusion. Transfus Med 10: 291–303

34. Purdy FR, Tweeddale MG, Merrick PM (1997) Association of mortality with age of blood transfused in septic ICU patients. Can J Anaesth 44: 1256–1261

35. Koch CG, Li L, Sessler DI, et al (2008) Duration of red-cell storage and complications after cardiac surgery. N Engl J Med 358: 1229–1239

36. Zallen G, Offner PJ, Moore EE, (1999) Age of transfused blood is an independent risk factor for postinjury multiple organ failure. Am J Surg 178: 570–572.

37. Vamvakas EC, Carven JH (1999) Transfusion and postoperative pneumonia in coronary artery bypass graft surgery: effect of the length of storage of transfused red cells. Transfusion 39: 701–710

38. Offner PJ, Moore EE, Biffl WL, Johnson JL, Silliman CC (2002) Increased rate of infection associated with transfusion of old blood after severe injury. Arch Surg 137: 711–716

39. Vamvakas EC, Carven JH (2000) Length of storage of transfused red cells and postoperative morbidity in patients undergoing coronary artery bypass graft surgery. Transfusion 40: 101–109

40. Walsh TS, McArdle F, McLellan SA, et al (2004) Does the storage time of transfused red blood cells influence regional or global indexes of tissue oxygenation in anemic critically ill patients? Crit Care Med 32: 364–371

41. Murrell Z, Haukoos JS, Putnam B, Klein SR (2005) The effect of older blood on mortality, need for ICU care, and the length of ICU stay after major trauma. Am Surg 71: 781–785

42. van de Watering L, Lorinser J, Versteegh M, Westendord R, Brand A (2006) Effects of storage time of red blood cell transfusions on the prognosis of coronary artery bypass graft patients. Transfusion 46: 1712–1718

43. Weinberg JA, McGwin G Jr, Griffin RL, et al (2008) Age of transfused blood: an independent predictor of mortality despite universal leukoreduction. J Trauma 65: 279–282

44. Sakr Y, Chierego M, Piagnerelli M, et al (2007) Microvascular response to red blood cell transfusion in patients with severe sepsis. Crit Care Med 35: 1639–1644

45. Creteur J, Neves AP, Vincent JL (2009) Near-infrared spectroscopy technique to evaluate the effects of red blood cell transfusion on tissue oxygenation. Crit Care 13 (Suppl 5): S11

46. Genzel-Boroviczény O, Christ F, Glas V (2004) Blood transfusion increases functional capillary density in the skin of anemic preterm infants. Pediatr Res 56: 751–755

47. Ince C (2005) The microcirculation is the motor of sepsis. Crit Care 9 (Suppl 4): S13–S19.

48. Ait-Oufella H, Maury E, Lehoux S, Guidet B, Offenstadt G (2010) The endothelium: physiological functions and role in microcirculatory failure during severe sepsis. Intensive Care Med 36: 1286–1298

X

Transfusion-related Pulmonary Complications

A.D. Goldberg, L. Clifford, and D.J. Kor

Background

Physicians have long recognized, though incompletely understood, the respiratory symptoms their patients may manifest after receiving a blood product transfusion [1, 2]. Today, two distinct pulmonary transfusion reactions are recognized as the likely etiology. Although both share a similar clinical phenotype of pulmonary edema and hypoxemic respiratory insufficiency, each have different management schemes and preventative strategies [3–6]. One reaction, called transfusion-related acute lung injury (TRALI) is a life-threatening complication marked by acute inflammation and injury to the pulmonary parenchyma and vasculature with resultant alveolar flooding. The second, transfusion-associated circulatory overload (TACO) results from the compensatory capacity of the cardiovascular system being overwhelmed by an increase in intravascular volume. This overloaded state manifests as respiratory distress from hydrostatic pulmonary edema.

In a time when it is estimated that nearly 1 of every 2 patients admitted to an intensive care unit (ICU) will receive at least one allogenic blood product [7], a comprehensive understanding of these two pulmonary transfusion reactions is needed more than ever. TRALI has become the leading cause of transfusion-related morbidity and mortality in the world [8, 9]. Likewise in 2010, the U.S. Food and Drug Administration (FDA) noted that TACO was the second leading cause of transfusion-related mortality, accounting for 20 % of all transfusion-related fatalities [8]. In this chapter, we review the epidemiology, pathophysiology, clinical management and future directions of research for TRALI and TACO. We will also describe the diagnostic tools available to the clinician faced with the challenge of differentiating between the two.

Transfusion-related Acute Lung Injury

Epidemiology

Although initially described decades ago [2, 10], uniform diagnostic criteria for TRALI were only established following a Consensus Conference in Toronto, Canada in 2004 [11]. These recommendations (**Box 1**) have since gained broad endorsement, facilitating efforts to better understand TRALI epidemiology and pathophysiology. Recent estimates suggest that TRALI occurs at a rate of 0.02 % – 0.05 % per component transfused and in 0.04 % – 0.16 % of patients transfused, making it substantially more common than both hemolytic transfusion reactions and transfusion-mediated microbial infections [8]. However, because of reliance

J.-L. Vincent (ed.), *Annual Update in Intensive Care and Emergency Medicine 2012*
DOI 10.1007/978-3-642-25716-2 © Springer-Verlag Berlin Heidelberg 2012

Box 1. TRALI Consensus Criteria [11]

ALI:	a) Acute onset
	b) Hypoxemia
	i. PaO$_2$/FiO$_2$ $\leq$300 or SpO$_2$ < 90 % on room air (or other clinical evidence of hypoxemia)
	c) Bilateral infiltrates on frontal chest radiograph
	d) No evidence of left atrial hypertension (i.e circulatory overload)
Plus:	e) No pre-existing ALI before transfusion
	f) During or within 6 hours of transfusion
	g) Bearing no temporal relationship to an alternative risk factor for ALI

on passive reporting rather than active surveillance, as well as persistent problems with poor syndrome recognition, these estimates likely fall short. Indeed, in 2002, Kopko et al. found that only 13.4 % of cases with symptoms suggestive of TRALI on *post hoc* analysis were reported as possible transfusion reactions [12]. Furthermore, a recent prospective cohort study, using the 2004 consensus criteria, noted an 8 % incidence of TRALI in a tertiary care ICU setting [4]. Although the ICU represents a higher-risk subgroup of transfusion recipients, these findings support the fact that TRALI is far more common than previously believed.

Although it is recognized that all blood products are associated with TRALI, those containing higher volumes of plasma (e.g., whole blood, fresh frozen plasma [FFP], plasma stored within 24 hours, and apheresis platelets) have consistently carried the greatest risk [4]. The American Red Cross recently reported per component risks of fatality from probable TRALI [13]. This report confirms a higher TRALI-related fatality rate with FFP (4.93 deaths per 106 components) and single-donor apheresis platelets (3.12 per 106 components), when compared to red blood cells (RBCs, 0.40 deaths per 106 components) and random donor platelet products (0.46 deaths per 106 components). Most implicated units contained greater than 50 ml of plasma [14].

Importantly, robust data from hemovigilance programs worldwide have suggested a decreased incidence of TRALI reactions [3, 9]. Notably, this reduction has not been consistent across all blood component therapies. This was exemplified by the American Red Cross, who recently reported a significant decrease in TRALI cases due to plasma from 2006 to 2008 [15], without a significant decrease in cases associated with RBCs. Several other agencies have subsequently supported these findings [3]. This discrepancy among various blood products is believed to be largely because of changes in donor procurement strategies aimed at minimizing donation from allo-immunized donors: For example, male-only donation policies for components containing high plasma volumes, suspensions of buffy coat platelet pools in male-only plasma, and increased use of whole-blood derived platelet products. Many centers have also incorporated anti-human leukocyte antigen (HLA) testing into their donor screening strategies. [16]

In 2003, TRALI emerged as the leading cause of transfusion-related death reported to the FDA [8, 9]. Today, despite the recent fall in TRALI cases, it remains the leading cause of transfusion-related mortality in the United States [8]. In the fiscal year of 2010, 18 TRALI-related fatalities were reported to the FDA. This nearly equals the total number of all other transfusion-related deaths in that year (n = 22). Notably, however, with appropriate supportive care, most cases of TRALI will recover. Generally, recovery is quite rapid, with most TRALI patients showing evidence of both clinical and radiographic resolution within

48–96 hours of syndrome onset [14]. However, approximately 20 % of TRALI cases exhibit refractory hypoxemia, and these patients have been suggested to have a higher mortality rate of 6 % – 14 % [14].

Pathophysiology

Although the pathogenesis of TRALI remains incompletely understood, antibodies found in donor plasma that are directed at HLAs or human neutrophil antigens (HNA) in the recipient have been implicated in 65–90 % of cases [17]. In this scenario, donor anti-HLA/anti-HNA antibodies are believed to interact with cognate antigens on the recipient leukocytes and/or pulmonary endothelial cells (anti-HLA antibodies only) [18]. This process results in leukocyte activation and aggregation within the pulmonary microcirculation. The subsequent neutrophil respiratory burst, along with concomitant compliment activation, activates and injures endothelial cells resulting in capillary leak, alveolar flooding, and the full acute lung injury (ALI) phenotype. Importantly, although some antibodies appear capable of inciting a TRALI episode independently, by inducing both neutrophil priming and activation (referred to as leukoagglutinins), others appear to require an initial neutrophil priming event such as surgery or a concomitant infection [18]. A number of antibodies capable of producing this cascade of events have been described, including HLA class I, HLA class II, and neutrophil-specific antibodies. Of these, the anti-HNA-3a antibody has been noted to be a high-frequency antibody, which appears to be associated with severe TRALI reactions [18]. Indeed, anti-HNA-3a is one class of antibodies believed capable of both neutrophil priming and activation.

Importantly, a sizable proportion of TRALI reactions appear not to be antibody mediated. For example, donor antibodies have been reported absent in greater than 15 % of documented TRALI reactions [19]. In addition, a number of

X

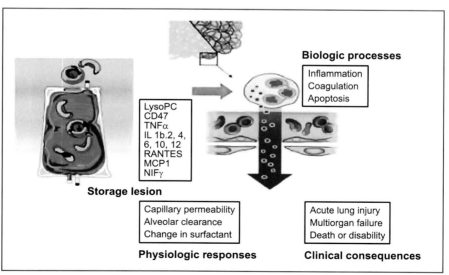

Fig. 1. Putative biologic and physiologic consequences of storage lesion. TNF: tumor necrosis factor; IL: interleukin; RANTES: Regulated upon Activation, Normal T-cell Expressed, and Secreted; MCP: monocyte chemoattractant protein; IFN: interferon;

TRALI cases have been identified in which the recipient did not possess a matching cognate antigen [20]. These inconsistencies have generated interest in a second non-antibody-mediated mechanism for TRALI which has been termed the "two-hit" model [21]. As with the antibody-mediated mechanism, this model generally describes a neutrophil priming event such as trauma, surgery or a concomitant infection [4, 21]. This priming event results in adhesion and sequestration of neutrophils to activated pulmonary endothelium. In the case of TRALI, the second event that leads to neutrophil activation is postulated to be the infusion of biologically active triggering substances that accumulate within cellular blood products during storage [18]. Although a variety of soluble biologic response modifiers such as bioactive lipids and soluble CD40 ligand, have been implicated as potential TRALI triggers, the true causal agents underlying this second hit remain under investigation (**Fig. 1**) [19, 22]. Whatever the true activating agents may be, the respiratory burst of activated neutrophils ultimately leads to capillary injury, alveolar edema and inflammatory pulmonary edema.

Management

Initial evaluation
If TRALI is suspected, the transfusion should be immediately discontinued. The event should be reported to the blood bank and a transfusion reaction work-up initiated. The implicated blood component should be returned to the blood bank to aid in the transfusion reaction evaluation [11].

Supportive therapies
At present, the mainstay of TRALI management is supportive care with the supplementation of oxygen to correct hypoxemia being the cornerstone of therapy [11]. Previous reports suggest that nearly 70 % of patients will also require ventilatory assistance. Approximately 20 % of TRALI cases have been reported to result in persistent hypoxemia and are often associated with systemic hypoperfusion and acute respiratory distress syndrome (ARDS) [14, 23]. As expected, these cases may require more aggressive concomitant therapies.

Mechanical ventilation
Although there have been no systematic evaluations detailing the optimal ventilator management of patients with TRALI, we would agree with previous recommendations that it would be prudent to adopt evidence-based practices from the histopathologically similar ALI [5, 24]. Specifically, we would endorse the use of low-tidal volume ventilation (≤ 6 ml per kg of ideal body weight) while maintaining the inspiratory plateau pressures at ≤ 30 cmH$_2$O [25].

The use of positive-end expiratory pressure (PEEP) levels in mechanically ventilated patients with ALI remains a matter of debate [26]. As such, we cannot provide any firm recommendations on the management of PEEP for patients with TRALI.

Management of intravascular volume status
Patients with TRALI are often hypovolemic and hypotensive. Therefore, the initial goal of hemodynamic management is to ensure adequate end-organ perfusion. This may be achieved with fluid resuscitation, vasoactive support, or a combination of the two. Diuretic therapy may result in hypotension and should be used with caution in the early phases of a TRALI reaction [27]. Importantly, conserva-

X

tive fluid management in patients with the more general syndrome of ALI has been shown to improve outcomes. The ARDS-Network Fluid and Catheter Treatment Trial (FACTT) demonstrated an increase in the number of ventilator-free days (14.6 ± 0.5 vs. 12.1 ± 0.5) and ICU-free days (13.4 ± 0.4 vs. 11.2 ± 0.4) for patients with lung injury who received an aggressive diuretic regimen [28]. Whether or not these findings generalize to patients with TRALI remains unclear, and it should be emphasized that diuresis was not attempted in patients who were hypotensive in the FACTT trial [28]. However, for patients with sustained hypoxemia and hemodynamic stability, diuretic therapy may be a reasonable intervention.

Corticosteroids

Despite a strong biologic rationale, the role of corticosteroid therapy in ALI remains a matter of debate [29, 30]. Early investigations of high-dose corticosteroid therapy failed to identify a beneficial effect and indeed suggested the potential for harm [31]. Subsequent investigations evaluating lower-dose protocols have yielded mixed results [29, 30]. Notably, the largest randomized clinical trial evaluating corticosteroids in the treatment of ALI performed to date suggests the potential for harm when initiating therapy more than 14 days after syndrome onset [30]. Aside from case reports, no well-designed studies to evaluate steroids in TRALI exist. Therefore, in the face of conflicting and inconclusive data, we cannot advocate the use of corticosteroids in the setting of TRALI. Moreover, we would advise against the use of corticosteroid therapy when the lung injury is fully established and has been present for more than 14 days.

HMG-CoA reductase inhibitors

HMG-CoA reductase inhibitors (statins) have anti-inflammatory, immunomodulatory and antioxidant characteristics and have been shown to attenuate inflammation and ameliorate injury in animal models of ALI [32]. As such, statin therapy may have a role in TRALI prevention and/or treatment as well. In an initial observational study evaluating the role of statins in patients with established ALI, we were not able to confirm a lung protective effect with statin therapy [33]. In contrast, O'Neal and colleagues reported reduced rates of ALI in patients receiving statin medications [34]. To help clarify this potential association, the ARDS-Network is currently enrolling patients into a multicenter randomized clinical trial. Until these results become available, we believe it would be premature to suggest statin therapy for the treatment and/or prevention of TRALI.

Management of the Donor

All blood products given during the 6-hour period preceding the first clinical manifestation of TRALI are considered to be associated with the TRALI reaction [11]. When TRALI is suspected, the remaining products from each associated donor unit should be returned to the blood bank for antibody testing, specifically anti-HLA and anti-HNA. If antibodies are identified, their specificity to the recipient's antigens must be determined. A donor is considered to be implicated in the TRALI reaction if either specificity between donor antibody and recipient antigen is found or if there is a positive cross-match [5, 11]. In the interest of the safety of future transfusion recipients, all implicated donors should be permanently deferred from future apheresis and whole blood donation. If they are not deferred indefinitely, their RBCs should be washed before transfusions and the plasma should be fractionated, with no platelets manufactured [5, 11]. In addition, because HNA-3a is a high-frequency antigen and the chance of a reaction with a future recipient is high, some blood centers have instituted a policy of indefinite deferral for any donor who expresses the anti-HNA-3a antibody [35].

Prevention

As with most conditions, preventive strategies will likely have a far greater influence on reducing the impact of TRALI than will improved treatments for the syndrome [3, 4, 16]. Until recently, deferral of implicated blood donors was the primary prevention strategy. However, recent advances in the understanding of TRALI pathogenesis have led to important new donor procurement strategies. Specifically, the association of donor antibodies with TRALI pathogenesis has stimulated efforts to reduce the transfer of these TRALI-related antibodies to transfusion recipients. Examples of these efforts include the deferral of female plasma donors, avoidance of apheresis platelet donation from multiparous donors, suspension of buffy coat platelet pools in male-only plasma and increased utilization of whole-blood derived platelet products [3]. Of note, female donor plasma is still used for fractionation and the production of plasma derivatives. Substantial evidence supports these changes in donor procurement strategies [4] and multiple hemovigilance reports have subsequently confirmed a fall in the number of TRALI cases following their implementation [3, 8]. As an additional TRALI prevention strategy, many blood centers have also begun to utilize HLA/HNA antibody testing for plateletpheresis donors [16].

Future Directions

Evidence-based transfusion practices

The adoption of more conservative, evidence-based transfusion practices is the most effective way to reduce transfusion reactions, such as TRALI. To this end, the literature suggests that we have substantial opportunities for improvement. Recently, it was estimated that approximately 40 % of patients in the ICU will receive an RBC transfusion [7]. Notably, the average pre-transfusion hemoglobin was 8.5 g/dl. These data arise in the setting of a growing body of literature which suggests either no benefit, or worse yet, the potential for harm with more aggressive RBC transfusion practices [36].

Aggressive transfusion practices have also been documented with other blood components, and it has been suggested that up to 25–30 % of plasma transfusions are administered without evidence-based support [37]. Moreover, although evidence would suggest minimal risk for bleeding in patients with platelet counts greater than 50×10^9/l, a recent observational study has shown an average pre-transfusion platelet count in excess of 84×10^9/l in patients undergoing non-cardiac surgery and 102×10^9/l in those undergoing cardiopulmonary bypass [38].

Blood donation procurement strategies

In addition to the blood procurement strategies mentioned above, practices such as leukoreduction, RBC storage duration and RBC washing have also been suggested to potentially reduce the risk of TRALI. Blumberg and colleagues have recently reported a decreased incidence of TRALI following the introduction of universal leukoreduction [39]. However, no such effect was noted by Watkins and colleagues [40]. Studies evaluating the relation of RBC storage duration to TRALI are similarly conflicted. Whereas the concentration of many immunologically active substances is known to increase during the storage of cellular blood products [19, 41], the clinical implications of these effects are unclear. Likewise, clinical studies evaluating the potential impact of an RBC storage lesion have yielded mixed results [42, 43].

A third proposed intervention for reducing the risk of TRALI is the washing of RBCs and platelets prior to transfusion [39, 44, 45]. In support of this intervention, Biffl et al. have shown the ability to remove biologically active lipids by washing the RBCs with saline [45]. However, additional resource requirements as well as a 15 % loss of hemoglobin and the short outdate of washed units remain barriers to the implementation of RBC washing [44].

Alternatives to blood component therapies

Increasingly, we are finding potential alternatives to traditional blood component therapies (e.g., RBC substitutes, prothrombin complex concentrates (PCC), fibrinogen concentrates, activated factor VII). Proposed benefits of these agents include more rapid replacement of deficient coagulation factor content, a low volume of administration, and reduced risk for viral transmission [46]. Additionally, there is a notable absence of anti-HLA/anti-HNA antibodies with these strategies [47]. As a result, the theoretical risk for TRALI, at least from the pathophysiologic mechanisms currently described, are believed minimal. However, while a reduced risk of TRALI may be one potential benefit of these novel therapies, the net sum of the risk/benefit profile requires additional study.

Transfusion-associated Circulatory Overload

Epidemiology

X

A major barrier in TACO-related research has been the lack of a uniform definition. Historically, TACO has been broadly characterized by acute respiratory distress, tachycardia and hypertension following blood product administration [46]. Although this clinical presentation appears relatively clear, there is a common misconception that TACO is an easy diagnosis to make. In fact, multiple lines of evidence suggests that TACO is frequently missed entirely or, alternatively, misdiagnosed as TRALI or congestive heart failure (CHF) [49].

The difficulty in identifying cases of TACO has been one reason why only a small number of investigations have attempted to define its incidence. In a recent prospective cohort study, Li and colleagues reported that 51 of 901 (6 %) patients transfused in a tertiary ICU setting developed TACO [50]. In comparison, previous publications have reported a TACO incidence ranging from < 1 % [51] to 11 % [52]. This variability in incidence is also influenced by factors, such as case ascertainment strategies (e.g., passive reporting vs. active surveillance) and unique characteristics of a study population (e.g., ICU versus all transfusion recipients). In addition, many biovigilance networks have only recently tracked TACO cases, including the FDA, which began tracking TACO as a unique clinical syndrome in 2005 [53].

In the context of inconsistent case definitions, poor clinical recognition and inconsistent reporting, the true incidence of TACO is likely best represented by the upper limits of the reported range. This hypothesis was recently confirmed by Finlay et al. in a retrospective cohort study [54]. Using computer-assisted algorithms to facilitate the identification of potential TRALI and TACO cases, it was noted that 12 % of confirmed TACO cases had previously gone unrecognized and unreported [54].

The incidence of TACO also appears dependent on the location of the transfusion. Specifically, TACO appears more common in patients who are transfused in an ICU setting as compared to an unmonitored ward [49]. A higher prevalence of associated risk factors and comorbid conditions of ICU patients, such as advanced age, cardiovascular and renal disease, may partially explain the different rates of TACO within the hospital [36]. In addition, ICU populations more frequently require high volumes and rates of blood product administration, both known risk factors for developing the complication [50].

As with the incidence rates for TACO, reported rates of TACO-related mortality also vary. In 2002, the French hemovigilance system reported a TACO case-fatality rate of 3.6 % [55]. More recent studies suggest mortality rates as high as 5–15 % [8]. In 2010, the United Kingdom's Serious Hazards of Transfusion (SHOT) committee reported TACO to be the most common cause of transfusion-related death [9]. In contrast, a nested case-control study by Li et al. failed to identify a significant association between TACO and mortality when comparing ICU patients with TACO to matched and transfused ICU controls [56]. Specifically, the authors failed to identify an increased risk of mortality at hospital discharge, 1- and 2-year follow-up. Clearly, additional studies are needed to more accurately define the attributable mortality of TACO.

Whereas the relationship between TACO and mortality remains somewhat unsettled, the impact of TACO on patient morbidity appears clear. Numerous investigations have associated TACO with an increased length of ICU and hospital stay [8] and up to 21 % of TACO cases have been categorized as 'life threatening' [53] using a commonly utilized 4-level severity score [57]. Recently, the SHOT committee reported that 13 out of 15 TACO cases in the United Kingdom (UK) resulted in ICU admission.

To improve the recognition of TACO cases and to address the need for a uniform definition, the Center for Disease Control (CDC), National Healthcare Safety Network Manual on Transfusion Biovigilance has recently outlined their recommendations for adjudicating TACO diagnoses (**Box 2**) [58]. Specifically, the definition requires that at least 3 of these variables are present within 6 h of transfusion. In the future, improved TACO recognition and case reporting will further detail the morbidity and mortality associated with this important transfusion reaction.

Box 2. National Healthcare Safety Network Diagnostic Criteria for TACO [58]

New onset or exacerbation of ≥ 3 of the following within 6 hours of transfusion:
Acute respiratory distress
Radiographic evidence of pulmonary edema
Evidence of left heart failure
Evidence of elevated central venous pressure (CVP)
Evidence of positive fluid balance
Elevated B-type naturietic peptide (BNP)

Pathophysiology and Risk Factors

In keeping with Starling's Law, increased left ventricular (LV) end-diastolic volume generally results in improved LV performance. However, markedly hypervolemic states or compromised LV function can lead to over-distention, elevated left atrial filling pressures, alveolar flooding and hypoxemia [43]. Although simplified, this is the general mechanism for the development of pulmonary edema in patients with CHF. Likewise, when administered in high volumes and/or at high infusion rates [50], transfusion therapies can exceed the compensatory capacity of the left ventricle. In this context, the resultant clinical phenotype within 6 h of blood product administration is termed TACO.

As noted, both large volume and high transfusion rates are risk factors for TACO [50]. It is important to note, however, that TACO can also occur in the setting of low-volume transfusion. Indeed, a number of reports have described patients developing TACO after a single unit of RBC transfusion [53]. It is hypothesized that in such cases the recipient was simply more susceptible to circulatory overload due to pre-existing cardiac dysfunction or a hypervolemic state [50].

Alternatively, volume overload may not be the sole mechanism underlying TACO pathophysiology. Indeed, two potential alternative mechanisms for TACO pathogenesis have been described. In the first scenario, it is hypothesized that defective nitric oxide (NO) metabolism in stored RBCs may result in post-transfusion NO trapping in the microcirculation [59]. The resultant increase in vascular resistance may, in turn, precipitate LV dysfunction and ultimately lead to hydrostatic pulmonary edema (TACO). A second alternative theory regarding TACO pathogenesis builds on the previously described associations between inflammatory mediators and exacerbations of CHF [39, 60]. In support of this potential mechanism, Blumberg et al. noted a dramatic fall in the incidence of TACO following the introduction of universal pre-storage leukoreduction of their RBCs [39].

Further to this, additional risk factors for the development of TACO include the extremes of age (< 3 yrs or > 60 yrs), severe chronic anemia and plasma transfusion for the reversal of oral anticoagulant therapy [43]. It should be emphasized that while the syndrome appears to disproportionately affect the extremes of age, no age group is exempt, and clinicians should maintain a high index of suspicion for TACO in all patients. In this context, the Quebec hemovigilance study noted that 9 % of TACO cases occurred in transfusion recipients who were < 50 yrs of age, 15 % in those < 60 yrs and approximately 7 % occurred in those aged 18–49 yrs [61]. Chronic anemia is believed to be a risk factor for TACO because of an associated hyperdynamic state and the relative intolerance of the cardiovascular system to acute increases in circulating blood volume. Plasma transfusion for the reversal of oral anticoagulant therapy is presumed to be related to TACO because of the large volume of plasma required to achieve the desired endpoints (frequently greater than 1–2 l).

Management

If a TACO reaction is believed present, the first course of action is to discontinue the transfusion. Subsequent TACO management strategies are similar to the treatment principles employed for hydrostatic pulmonary edema resulting from CHF.

At present, the cornerstones of such therapies include oxygen supplementation, ventilator support when needed [62, 63], and efforts to induce a negative fluid balance when feasible. As the hemodynamic response in most TACO episodes is one of hypertension, the administration of intravenous diuretics to enhance urine output and foster negative fluid balance is generally recommended [62, 63]. Non-invasive ventilation with continuous positive airway pressure (CPAP) has been shown to reduce the need for endotracheal intubation as well as mortality in patients with acute hypoxemic respiratory insufficiency resulting from heart failure [64]. As such, we would recommend consideration of this technique in TACO cases as well, provided the subjects remain hemodynamically stable. When ventilatory support is required, lung protective ventilation strategies should be employed (see discussion on TRALI management). Importantly, the suspected transfusion reaction should be reported to the Blood Bank in order to facilitate a thorough evaluation and appropriate reporting of the adverse transfusion-related event.

Prevention

As with TRALI prevention, the avoidance of unnecessary transfusions through the use of conservative, evidence-based transfusion practices is expected to have the most meaningful impact on TACO prevention. When transfusion is deemed necessary, efforts to determine the recipient's risk for TACO (e.g., assessing for evidence of cardiopulmonary disease or pre-existing fluid overload) are warranted. For those determined to be 'high-risk', total volume and rate of transfusion should be minimized. Unfortunately, evidence guiding clinicians as to what constitutes a safe volume or rate of transfusion is limited. Generally, the American Association of Blood Banks (AABB) recommends a transfusion rate of 150–300 ml/h. For patients with known cardiac dysfunction, a reduced rate of 1 ml/kg/h is recommended [6]. However, in clinical practice this may be technically challenging, particularly in patients with active bleeding [65]. Additionally, the use of low-volume alternatives to current blood component therapies may mitigate risk of TACO in the future. Although mechanistically attractive, such alternatives require more thorough testing before receiving broad endorsement. A third potential prevention strategy is the prophylactic use of diuretics in those determined to be at high-risk of developing TACO. Although many clinicians are currently applying this potentially preventative measure to high-risk transfusion recipients, it should be emphasized that this strategy remains untested, and the associated risks (e.g., hypotension, electrolyte imbalance and cardiac arrhythmias) remain poorly defined.

Future Directions

Improved understanding of TACO epidemiology

As discussed above, surprisingly little work has been done to improve our understanding of TACO epidemiology. Indeed, substantial knowledge gaps remain in understanding the risk factors, incidence, clinical circumstances, and attributable burden of TACO. The adoption of a common definition for TACO will be fundamental to progress. In this regard, we would endorse the definitions put forth by the CDC, National Healthcare Safety Network Manual on Transfusion Biovigilance [58].

Predicting risk of TACO

Because no single factor can accurately assess a transfusion recipient's risk of developing TACO, a combination of risk factors is necessary to provide adequate predictive value. In this light, the lack of accurate TACO prediction models, particularly our inability to identify high-risk patients, is precluding the provision of best transfusion practices. As such, we believe the development and validation of an accurate TACO risk prediction model is an important goal for future research.

Improved understanding of TACO pathophysiology

Improved understanding of TACO pathophysiology will ultimately assist in improved prevention and treatment strategies. To this end, multiple novel mechanisms for TACO pathogenesis have been recently described and warrant further study. We continue to explore our recent findings noting an association between RBC transfusion, elevated systemic vascular resistance and subsequent development of hypoxemia (TACO). As discussed above, Blumberg et al. noted an impressive 83 % reduction in the incidence of TACO cases following the implementation of universal pre-storage leukoreduction for RBCs [39]. It is perhaps most interesting to note that when RBCs (n = 28,120) and platelets (n = 69,325) were washed and leukoreduced, there were no reported cases of TRALI or TACO over the 14-year evaluation interval. These findings would suggest a potential role for soluble biologic response modifiers in TACO pathogenesis and provides another hypothesis for research [60].

Differentiating Between TRALI and TACO

Accurately identifying a transfusion-related pulmonary complication is important, as it can influence therapeutic considerations and assist blood centers with component safety and donor management strategies [66]. However, differentiating between TACO and TRALI can often be quite challenging, particularly in the critically ill. This difficulty is largely the result of similar clinical phenotypes, with the differentiation of hydrostatic (TACO) and non-hydrostatic (TRALI) edema being mostly dependent on the assessment of volume status. In addition to the aforementioned challenges, it is possible for the conditions to co-exist as well.

X

Clinical Signs

Although no clinical sign can confirm the presence or absence of a specific pulmonary transfusion reaction, distinct clinical features have been associated with each syndrome (**Table 1**) [66]. TACO classically presents with evidence of volume overload and respiratory symptoms generally improve with diuresis. CHF is a known risk factor for the development of TACO, and findings such as jugular venous distention, normal to elevated systemic blood pressures and an S3 gallop on auscultation are frequently found on physical examination. Although elevated pulmonary artery occlusion pressures (PAOP > 18 mmHg) are common in patients with hydrostatic pulmonary edema, it is important to recognize that they do not effectively exclude TRALI. This point was emphasized in the recent ARDS Network sponsored FACTT trial, where a full 29 % of patients determined to have non-hydrostatic pulmonary edema (ALI) had a PAOP of > 18 mmHg [67].

Table 1. Characteristic features of transfusion-related pulmonary complications [66]

Feature	TRALI	TACO
Body temperature	Fever may be present	Unchanged
Blood pressure	Hypotension	Hypertension
Respiratory symptoms	Acute dyspnea	Acute dyspnea
Neck veins	Unchanged	May be distended
Auscultation	Rales	Rales and S3 may be present
Chest radiograph	Diffuse bilateral infiltrates	Diffuse bilateral infiltrates
Ejection fraction	Normal or decreased	Decreased
PAOP	Most often 180 mmHg or less	> 180 mmHg
Pulmonary edema fluid	Exudate	Transudate
Fluid balance	Positive, neutral or negative	Positive
Response to diuretics	No change or deterioration	Significant improvement
White cell count	Transient leukopenia	Unchanged
BNP	< 250 pg/ml	> 1200 pg/ml
Leukocyte antibodies	Present +/- cognate antigens	May or may not be present

PAOP: pulmonary artery occlusion pressure; BNP: B-type natriuretic peptide

Regarding TRALI, patients often present with fever, hypovolemia and associated hypotension, although frank distributive shock is uncommon [66].

Imaging

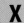

Chest radiography, particularly in the absence of objective measurements such as vascular pedicle width and the cardiothoracic ratio [68], is generally of little value in determining intravascular volume status. When these measurements are present, they have been reported to improve the estimation of an individual's volume status and hence the likely classification of lung edema (hydrostatic vs non-hydrostatic) [68]. Specifically, the presence of a vascular pedicle width > 70 mm and a cardiothoracic ratio > 0.55 have been shown to improve from 56 % to 70 % the accuracy of predicting a PAOP > 18 mmHg [68]. Echocardiographic measurements of cardiac dysfunction may also be useful. LV dysfunction (ejection fraction < 45 % – a marker of systolic dysfunction) or a ratio of mitral peak inflow velocity of early filling to early diastolic mitral annular velocity (E/e') > 15 (a marker of elevated left atrial filling pressures and diastolic dysfunction), have been identified as predictors for TACO and may assist in differentiating TACO from TRALI [50]. However, as with elevated PAOP, the presence of these criteria does not effectively exclude a TRALI diagnosis. Rather, they are an additional element to consider when attempting to differentiate these two transfusion-related respiratory complications.

Laboratory Testing

B-type natriuretic peptide (BNP)

Increased wall tension of the myocardium results in increased production and release of BNP in cardiac myocytes. When combined with clinical information, the measurement of BNP has been useful in establishing the diagnosis of volume overloaded states, such as acute decompensated CHF [69]. As the current understanding of TACO is based on a similar mechanism of ventricular overload, it has been hypothesized that BNP levels may have diagnostic utility when differentiating TACO and TRALI. The potential utility of BNP was supported by Zhou et al. [70] who noted that a > 50 % increase in BNP following transfusion had a sensitivity and specificity of 81 % and 89 %, respectively, for making a diagnosis of TACO. A subsequent case-control investigation found the accuracy of post-transfusion N-terminal pro-BNP (NT-proBNP) for making a diagnosis of TACO to be 87.5 % [71]. Neither of the above mentioned investigations, however, used BNP or NT-proBNP to differentiate TACO from TRALI. Rather, the evaluated control group did not experience a transfusion-related pulmonary complication. Therefore, while elevated levels of BNP and/or NT-proBNP have been associated with the diagnosis of TACO, the ability of these biomarkers to assist in differentiating TACO from TRALI was not tested. To address this limitation, a recent prospective cohort investigation was performed by Li and colleagues [72]. Contrasting with prior publications, the results of this study suggest that BNP and NT-pro-BNP have limited diagnostic value when attempting to distinguish TACO from TRALI. In part, this lack of discrimination may result from the multitude of factors (e.g., age, sex, concomitant medications, sepsis, renal failure) that can affect natriuretic peptide levels [72].

It should be noted that whereas elevated levels of BNP and/or NT-proBNP are of unclear diagnostic utility when attempting to differentiate TACO from TRALI, normal levels may prove more useful. Specifically, when measured near the onset of symptoms, BNP values < 250 pg/ml have been shown to reliably exclude heart failure as the sole explanation for acute pulmonary edema [73]. In such circumstances, TRALI becomes the more likely diagnosis.

Leukopenia

Whether the result of an immune-mediated reaction between donor antibodies and recipient HLA/HNA antigens, or the infusion of activating substances in a sensitized host, leukocyte activation and sequestration within the lungs are central to TRALI pathogenesis [74]. Not surprisingly, therefore, TRALI reactions have been associated with reports of transient leukopenia [75]. In a look back investigation by Fadeyi et al., 75 % (9/12) of patients who sustained a transfusion reaction developed leukopenia compared to 34.6 % (9/26) of patients who did not (p< 0.05) [75]. Church et al. described a TRALI case in which leukopenia developed prior to the onset of pulmonary edema and the development of respiratory insufficiency [76]. These findings highlight the potential utility of serial white blood cell (WBC) counts for patients in whom a TRALI reaction is suspected [76]. Importantly, however, TRALI cases have not always been associated with a decrease in WBC count, and transfusion recipients may experience a decrease in WBC count with no associated respiratory compromise [76]. Therefore, while a transient leukopenia may suggest a potential TRALI reaction, it cannot effectively rule in or out TRALI. Of note, TACO has not been associated with a characteristic change in the WBC count.

Fluid to serum ratio

As the nature of the pulmonary edema in TACO and TRALI is believed to be hydrostatic and inflammatory, respectively, the pulmonary fluid to serum protein ratio may assist in determining the etiology of pulmonary edema following blood transfusion. Specifically, a pulmonary fluid to serum protein ratio ≤ 0.65 has been suggested to identify a transudative process, supporting the diagnosis of hydrostatic pulmonary edema (TACO) [77]. In contrast, a ratio ≥ 0.75 is suggested to be consistent with non-hydrostatic permeability edema (TRALI) [77]. Although conceptually straightforward, significant limitations have prevented the broad endorsement of this test when attempting to correctly diagnose transfusion-related pulmonary complications. Perhaps the greatest of these limitations is the test's limited feasibility in patients who are not mechanically ventilated. Additionally, alveolar epithelial cells actively resorb protein rich fluid in cases of inflammatory pulmonary edema. Therefore, the ratio becomes much less reliable if taken > 1 hour after symptom onset [78].

Antibody testing

Although important for donor management, anti-HLA/HNA antibody testing has a limited role when differentiating TRALI from TACO in the acute setting. In part, this is because the finding of anti-HLA antibodies in an associated donor may be incidental, as 9 %-20 % of all female donors have been shown to express anti-HLA antibodies [11, 79]. In addition, anti-HLA/HNA antibodies to a recipient's antigen with high specificity confirm the diagnosis of TRALI. Therefore, while testing may not facilitate the differentiation of TACO and TRALI in the acute setting, it should still be pursued in circumstances in which TRALI is considered a potential etiology for respiratory compromise.

Although consensus definitions for TRALI require the absence of left atrial hypertension and/or circulatory overload, we acknowledge that TRALI and TACO may co-exist. Indeed, the findings of Rana et al. suggest that up to one third of patients with ALI have concomitant acute or chronic cardiac dysfunction [73]. Moreover, 25 % of patients with ALI have demonstrated components of hydrostatic pulmonary edema [5]. If after clinical evaluation it appears that a transfusion reaction may have components of both TRALI and TACO, it is recommended that the case be classified as TRALI. Such cases should be reported to the blood center in order to trigger the appropriate evaluations and antibody testing [5, 11].

Conclusion

The transfusion-related pulmonary complications, TRALI and TACO, remain the leading causes of transfusion-related morbidity and mortality. Although first described nearly 60 years ago, effective pharmacologic and therapeutic interventions for patients with TRALI are scarce, and management relies primarily on supportive care. A future consensus definition of TACO will likely improve disease recognition, surveillance and pathophysiologic understanding. Importantly, the implementation of conservative, evidence-based transfusion practices may have the greatest effect in mitigating the impact of both TRALI and TACO. Efforts to reduce the number of high-plasma containing transfusions from potentially alloimmunized donors (e.g., multiparous females) have also proved effective in reducing the adverse consequences of TRALI. Continued efforts toward improving the diagnostic accuracy of post-transfusion respiratory symptoms should lead to better management strategies.

References

1. Tung CL, Bien WN, Ch'u YC, Wang SH, Ma WS (1937) Chin Med J 52: 479
2. Barnard RD (1951) Indiscriminate transfusion: a critique of case reports illustrating hypersensitivity reactions. N Y State J Med 51: 2399–2402
3. Lin Y, Saw CL, Hannach B, Goldman M (2012) Transfusion-related acute lung injury prevention measures and their impact at Canadian Blood Services. Transfusion (in press)
4. Gajic O, Rana R, Winters JL, et al (2007) Transfusion-related acute lung injury in the critically ill, prospective nested case-control study. Am J Respir Crit Care Med 176: 886–891
5. Kleinman SH, Popovsky MA (2008) TRALI: Mechanisms, Management, and Prevention, 1st Ed edn. American Association of Blood Banks Press, Bethesda
6. Gresens CJ, Holland PV (2001) Blood Safety and Surveillance. Marcel Dekker Inc, New York
7. Napolitano LM, Kurek S, Luchette FA (2009) Clinical practice guideline: red blood cell transfusion in adult trauma and critical care. Crit Care Med 37: 3124–3157
8. Fatalities Reported to FDA Following Blood Collection and Transfusion: Annual Summary for Fiscal Year 2010. Available at: http://www.fda.gov/BiologicsBloodVaccines/SafetyAvailability/ReportaProblem/TransfusionDonationFatalities/ucm254802.htm Accessed November 2011
9. SHOT Steering Group (2010) Serious Hazards of Transfusion Annual Report 2010 Summary Available at: http://www.shotuk.org/wp-content/uploads/2011/07/SHOT-2010-Summary1.pdf Accessed November 2011
10. Popovsky MA, Abel MD, Moore SB (1983) Transfusion-related acute lung injury associated with passive transfer of antileukocyte antibodies. Am Rev Respir Dis 128: 185–189
11. Kleinman S, Caulfield T, Chan P, et al (2004) Toward an understanding of transfusion-related acute lung injury: statement of a consensus panel. Transfusion 44: 1774–1789
12. Kopko PM, Marshall CS, MacKenzie MR, Holland PV, Popovsky MA (2002) Transfusion-related acute lung injury: report of a clinical look-back investigation. JAMA 287: 1968–1971
13. Eder AF, Herron R, Strupp A, et al (2007) Transfusion-related acute lung injury surveillance (2003–2005) and the potential impact of the selective use of plasma from male donors in the American Red Cross. Transfusion 47: 599–607
14. Goldman M, Webert KE, Arnold DM, Freedman J, Hannon J, Blajchman MA (2005) Proceedings of a consensus conference: towards an understanding of TRALI. Transfus Med Rev 19: 2–31
15. Eder AF, Herron RM, Jr., Strupp A, et al (2010) Effective reduction of transfusion-related acute lung injury risk with male-predominant plasma strategy in the American Red Cross (2006–2008). Transfusion 50: 1732–1742
16. Kleinman S, Grossman B, Kopko P (2010) A national survey of transfusion-related acute lung injury risk reduction policies for platelets and plasma in the United States. Transfusion 50: 1312–1321
17. Brown CJ, Navarrete CV (2011) Clinical relevance of the HLA system in blood transfusion. Vox Sang 101: 93–105
18. Bux J, Sachs UJ (2007) The pathogenesis of transfusion-related acute lung injury (TRALI). Br J Haematol 136: 788–799
19. Silliman CC, Moore EE, Kelher MR, Khan SY, Gellar L, Elzi DJ (2011) Identification of lipids that accumulate during the routine storage of prestorage leukoreduced red blood cells and cause acute lung injury. Transfusion 51: 2549–2554
20. Kopko PM, Paglieroni TG, Popovsky MA, Muto KN, MacKenzie MR, Holland PV (2003) TRALI: correlation of antigen-antibody and monocyte activation in donor-recipient pairs. Transfusion 43: 177–184
21. Silliman CC (2006) The two-event model of transfusion-related acute lung injury. Crit Care Med 34 (5 Suppl): S124–131
22. Kor DJ, Van Buskirk CM, Gajic O (2009) Red blood cell storage lesion. Bosn J Basic Med Sci 9 (Suppl 1): 21–27
23. Popovsky MA, Moore SB (1985) Diagnostic and pathogenetic considerations in transfusion-related acute lung injury. Transfusion 25: 573–577

24. Gajic O, Moore SB (2005) Transfusion-related acute lung injury. Mayo Clin Proc 80: 766–770
25. The Acute Respiratory Distress Syndrome Network (2000) Ventilation with lower tidal volumes as compared with traditional tidal volumes for acute lung injury and the acute respiratory distress syndrome. N Engl J Med 342: 1301–1308
26. Briel M, Meade M, Mercat A, et al (2010) Higher vs lower positive end-expiratory pressure in patients with acute lung injury and acute respiratory distress syndrome: systematic review and meta-analysis. JAMA 303: 865–873
27. Jawa RS, Anillo S, Kulaylat MN (2008) Transfusion-related acute lung injury. J Intensive Care Med 23: 109–121
28. Wiedemann HP, Wheeler AP, Bernard GR, et al (2006) Comparison of two fluid-management strategies in acute lung injury. N Engl J Med 354: 2564–2575
29. Steinberg KP, Hudson LD, Goodman RB, et al (2006) Efficacy and safety of corticosteroids for persistent acute respiratory distress syndrome. N Engl J Med 354: 1671–1684
30. Meduri GU, Headley AS, Golden E, et al (1998) Effect of prolonged methylprednisolone therapy in unresolving acute respiratory distress syndrome: a randomized controlled trial. JAMA 280: 159–165
31. Weigelt JA, Norcross JF, Borman KR, Snyder WH 3rd (1985) Early steroid therapy for respiratory failure. Arch Surg 120: 536–540
32. Jacobson JR, Barnard JW, Grigoryev DN, Ma SF, Tuder RM, Garcia JG (2005) Simvastatin attenuates vascular leak and inflammation in murine inflammatory lung injury. Am J Physiol Lung Cell Mol Physiol 288: L1026–1032
33. Kor DJ, Iscimen R, Yilmaz M, Brown MJ, Brown DR, Gajic O (2009) Statin administration did not influence the progression of lung injury or associated organ failures in a cohort of patients with acute lung injury. Intensive Care Med 35: 1039–1046
34. O'Neal HRJ, Koyama T, Koehler EAS (2011) Prehospital statin and aspirin use and the prevalence of severe sepsis and acute lung injury/acute respiratory distress syndrome. . Crit Care Med 39: 1343–1350
35. Su L, Kamel H (2007) How do we investigate and manage donors associated with a suspected case of transfusion-related acute lung injury. Transfusion 47: 1118–1124
36. Hébert PC, Wells G, Blajchman MA (1999) A multicenter, randomized, controlled clinical trial of transfusion requirements in critical care. Transfusion Requirements in Critical Care Investigators. N Engl J Med 340: 409–417
37. Wilson K, MacDougall L, Fergusson D, Graham I, Tinmouth A, Hebert PC (2002) The effectiveness of interventions to reduce physician's levels of inappropriate transfusion: what can be learned from a systematic review of the literature. Transfusion 42: 1224–1229
38. Cameron B, Rock G, Olberg B, Neurath D (2007) Evaluation of platelet transfusion triggers in a tertiary-care hospital. Transfusion 47: 206–211
39. Blumberg N, Heal JM, Gettings KF, et al (2010) An association between decreased cardiopulmonary complications (transfusion-related acute lung injury and transfusion-associated circulatory overload) and implementation of universal leukoreduction of blood transfusions. Transfusion 50: 2738–2744
40. Watkins TR, Rubenfeld GD, Martin TR, et al (2008) Effects of leukoreduced blood on acute lung injury after trauma: a randomized controlled trial. Crit Care Med 36: 1493–1499
41. Silliman CC, Clay KL, Thurman GW, Johnson CA, Ambruso DR (1994) Partial characterization of lipids that develop during the routine storage of blood and prime the neutrophil NADPH oxidase. J Lab Clin Med 124: 684–694
42. Koch CG, Li L, Sessler DI et al (2008) Duration of red-cell storage and complications after cardiac surgery. N Engl J Med 358: 1229–1239
43. Vamvakas EC, Blajchman MA (2010) Blood still kills: six strategies to further reduce allogenic blood transfusion-related mortality. Transfus Med Rev 24: 77–124
44. Silliman CC, Moore EE, Johnson JL, Gonzalez RJ, Biffl WL (2004) Transfusion of the injured patient: proceed with caution. Shock 21: 291–299
45. Biffl WL, Moore EE, Offner PJ, Ciesla DJ, Gonzalez RJ, Silliman CC (2001) Plasma from aged stored red blood cells delays neutrophil apoptosis and primes for cytotoxicity: abrogation by poststorage washing but not prestorage leukoreduction. J Trauma 50: 426–431

X

46. Preston FE, Laidlaw ST, Sampson B, Kitchen S (2002) Rapid reversal of oral anticoagulation with warfarin by a prothrombin complex concentrate (Beriplex): efficacy and safety in 42 patients. Br J Haematol 116: 619–624

47. Baker RI, Coughlin PB, Gallus AS, Harper PL, Salem HH, Wood EM (2004) Warfarin reversal: consensus guidelines, on behalf of the Australasian Society of Thrombosis and Haemostasis. Med J Aust 181: 492–497

48. Roback JD, Combs MR, Grossman BJ, Hillyer CD (2008) Technical Manual 16th edn. American Association of Blood Banks, Bethesda

49. Narick C, Triulzi DJ, Yazer MH (2011) Transfusion-associated circulatory overload after plasma transfusion. Transfusion (in press)

50. Li G, Rachmale S, Kojicic M (2011) Incidence and transfusion risk factors for transfusion-associated circulatory overload among medical intensive care unit patients. Transfusion 51: 338–343

51. Audet AM, Andrzejewski C, Popovsky MA (1998) Red blood cell transfusion practices in patients undergoing orthopedic surgery: a multi-institutional analysis. Orthopedics 21: 851–858

52. Rana RM, Rana SM, Fernandez ERM, Khan SAM, Gajic OM (2005) Transfusion related pulmonary edema in the intensive care unit (ICU). Chest 128 (Suppl):130s (abst)

53. Popovsky MA (2010) The Emily Cooley Lecture 2009: To breathe or not to breathe – that is the question. Pulmonary consequences of transfusion. Transfusion 50: 2057–2062

54. Finlay HE, Cassoria L, Feiner J, Toy P (2005) Designing and testing a computer-based screening system for transfusion-related acute lung injury. Am J Clin Path 124: 601–609

55. David B (2002) Haemovigilance: A comparison of three national systems. Proceedings of the 27th Congress of the International Society of Blood Transfusion: August 24–29th 2002, Vancouver (abst)

56. Li GM, Kojicic MM, Reriani MKM, et al (2010) Long-term survival & quality of life after transfusion-associated pulmonary edema in critically ill medical patients. Chest 137: 783–789

57. Whitaker BI. Reporting TACO and TRALI: Using the New National Hemovigilance Protocol to Categorize Transfusion Adverse Reactions. Available at: http://www.aabb.org/programs/biovigilance/us/Documents/reportingtralitaco.pdf Accessed November 2011

58. Center for Disease Control (2010) National Healthcare Safety Network Manual – Biovigilance Component Protocol. In: Transfusion Associated Circulatory Overload. Center for Disease Control, Altanta

59. Singel DJ, Stamler JS (2005) Chemical physiology of blood flow regulation by red blood cells: the role of nitric oxide and S-nitrosohemoglobin. Annu Rev Physiol 67: 99–145

60. Celis R, Torre-Martinez G, Torre-Amione G (2008) Evidence for activation of immune system in heart failure: is there a role for anti-inflammatory therapy? Curr Opin Cardiol 3: 254–260

61. Robillard P, Itaj NK, Chapdelaine A (2008) Increasing incidence of transfusion-associated circulatory overload reported to the Quebec Hemovigilance System 2000–2006. Transfusion 48:204A (abst)

62. Nieminen MS, Bohm M, Cowie MR, et al (2005) Executive summary of the guidelines on the diagnosis and treatment of acute heart failure – The Task Force on Acute Heart Failure of the European Society of Cardiology. Eur Heart J 26: 384–416

63. Jessup M, Abraham WT, Casey DE, et al (2009) 2009 Focused Update: ACCF/AHA Guidelines for the Diagnosis and Management of Heart Failure in Adults: A Report of the American College of Cardiology Foundation/American Heart Association Task Force on Practice Guidelines: Developed in Collaboration With the International Society for Heart and Lung Transplantation. Circulation 119: 1977–2016

64. Winck JC, Azevedo LF, Costa-Pereira A, Antonelli M, Wyatt JC (2006) Efficacy and safety of non-invasive ventilation in the treatment of acute cardiogenic pulmonary edema--a systematic review and meta-analysis. Crit Care 10:R69

65. Popovsky MA (2007) Transfusion Reactions, 3rd edn. AABB Press, Bethesda

66. Skeate RC, Eastlund T (2007) Distinguishing between transfusion related acute lung injury and transfusion associated circulatory overload. Curr Opin Haematol 14: 682–687

67. Wheeler AP, Bernard GR, Thompson BT et al (2006) Pulmonary-artery versus central venous catheter to guide treatment of acute lung injury. National Heart, Lung, and Blood

X

Institute Acute Respiratory Distress Syndrome (ARDS) Clinical Trials Network. N Engl J Med 354: 2213–2224

68. Ely EW, Smith AC, Chiles C, et al (2001) Radiologic determination of intravascular volume status using portable, digital chest radiography: a prospective investigation in 100 patients. Crit Care Med 8: 1502–1512

69. Maisel AS, Krishnaswamy P, Nowak RM et al (2002) Rapid measurement of B-type natriuretic peptide in the emergency diagnosis of heart failure. N Engl J Med, 347(3):161–167.

70. Zhou I, Giacherio D, Cooling L, Davenport RD (2005) Use of B-natriuretic peptide as a diagnostic marker of the differential diagnosis of transfusion-associated circulatory overload. Transfusion 45: 1056–1063

71. Tobain AAR (2008) N-Terminal pro-brain natriuretic peptide is a useful diagnostic marker for transfusion-associated circulatory overload. Transfusion 48: 1143–1150.

72. Li G, Daniels CE, Kojicic M (2009) The accuracy of naturietic peptides (brain naturietic peptids and N-terminal pro-brain naturietic) in differentiation between transfusion-related acute lung injury and transfusion-related circulatory overload in the critically ill. Transfusion 49: 13–20

73. Rana R, Vlahakis NE, Daniels CE, et al (2006) B-type natriuretic peptide in the assessment of acute lung injury and cardiogenic pulmonary edema. Crit Care Med 34: 1941–1946

74. Gilliss BM, Looney MR (2011) Experimental models of transfusion-related acute lung injury. Transfus Med Rev 25: 1–11

75. Fadeyi EA, De Los Angeles Muniz M, Wayne AS, Klein HG, Leitman SF, Stroncek DF (2007) The transfusion of neutrophil-specific antibodies causes leukopenia and a broad spectrum of pulmonary reactions. Transfusion 47: 545–550

76. Church GD, Price C, Sanchez R, Looney MR (2006) Transfusion-related acute lung injury in the paediatric patient: Two case reports and a review of the literature. Transfus Med 16: 343–348

77. Fein A, Grossman RF, Jones JG, et al (1979) The value of edema fluid protein measurement in patients with pulmonary edema. Am J Med 67: 32–38

78. Gajic O, Gropper MA, Hubmayr RD (2006) Pulmonary edema after transfusion: How to differentiate transfusion-associated circulatory overload from transfusion-related acute lung injury. Crit Care Med 34 (Suppl 5): s109–s113

79. Payne R (1962) The development and persistence of leukoagglutinins in parous women. Blood 19: 411–424

X

XI Pulmonary Edema

Confounders in the Diagnosis of Pulmonary Edema in Surgical Patients

F.Y. Lui, G. Luckianow, and L.J. Kaplan

Introduction

A host of clinical conditions may be accompanied by an increase in extravascular lung water (EVLW), and may have a cardiogenic or non-cardiogenic etiology [1, 2]. Regardless of the inciting cause, the increased tissue water (and electrolyte) component is often identifiable on clinical examination and supported by confirmatory radiographic analysis [3–5]. When the edema component is severe, clinical signs and symptoms are readily apparent and include, but are not limited to, an increased work of breathing (including accessory muscle use), rales, hypoxemia, hypercarbia, respiratory (and often metabolic) acidosis, as well as frothy, thin sputum that can be aspirated after placing an endotracheal tube for mechanical ventilatory support [6]. Medical patients are often diagnosed with pulmonary edema during an exacerbation of a pre-existing comorbidity such as myocardial ischemia, chronic obstructive pulmonary disease (COPD), acute-on-chronic renal insufficiency, as well as after early goal-directed therapy-based resuscitation for severe pneumonia.

In contrast, this constellation is not the predominant pattern for patients in whom the diagnosis of pulmonary edema is made after surgical illness or injury. Instead, the surgical patient may not demonstrate the typical signs and symptoms, but instead may have their diagnosis initially made on the basis of total body salt and water excess coupled with an abnormal chest radiograph. The factors that confound the accuracy of rendering a diagnosis of pulmonary edema in this patient population form the subject of this chapter. A clinical case will be a platform from which to explore many of these confounders.

XI

Case Presentation

A 68 year-old woman is admitted, 2 years after a successful cadaveric renal transplant, with pneumonia (**Fig. 1**) and acute renal failure that is believed to be due to acute tubular necrosis (ATN). She is hypoxemic and requires oral endotracheal intubation to manage her work of breathing, CO_2 clearance and oxygenation while she undergoes plasma volume expansion. She is placed on mechanical ventilation using assist control/volume cycled ventilation (AC/VCV) at a rate of 12, tidal volume (V_T) 650 ml, inspired oxygen fraction (FiO_2) 0.6, positive end-expiratory pressure (PEEP) 10 with a flow rate of 40 l/min on a decelerating waveform generating a peak airway pressure (Paw_{peak}) of 32 cmH$_2$O, Paw_{mean} 14 cmH$_2$O pressure, and minute ventilation (V_E) = 7.8 l/min. A post-intubation arterial

J.-L. Vincent (ed.), *Annual Update in Intensive Care and Emergency Medicine 2012*
DOI 10.1007/978-3-642-25716-2 © Springer-Verlag Berlin Heidelberg 2012

blood gas (ABG) was 7.32/38/74 (pH/PCO$_2$ [mmHg]/PO$_2$$_{mm}$Hg). She received 3000 ml of crystalloid and one unit of packed red blood cells (RBCs) over the next 3 hours; a subsequent ABG was 7.38/48/62, but the PO$_2$ now reflected 100 % O$_2$. The falling A-a gradient prompted a repeat chest x-ray (CXR) (**Fig. 2**) that was read as worsened pulmonary edema and the primary service marshaled the resources to initiate continuous renal replacement therapy (CRRT). However, the patient had cool extremities and a narrow pulse pressure; a bedside 2-D echocardiogram revealed a hyperdynamic and relatively empty left ventricle.

Instead of diuresis, she received 2000 ml of colloid (6 % hydroxyethyl starch [HES] in a balanced salt solution) and an additional 3000 ml of crystalloid (1/2 normal saline solution + 75 meq/l NaHCO$_3$) while she was started on a low-dose norepinephrine infusion to support her mean arterial pressure (MAP) in the setting of pulmonary sepsis. Her ventilator mode was changed from AC/VCV to airway pressure release ventilation (APRV) with settings of P$_{high}$ 30, P$_{low}$ 2, T$_{high}$ 7.0 sec, and T$_{low}$ 0.7 sec. As the FiO$_2$ requirement decreased, a repeat CXR was

XI

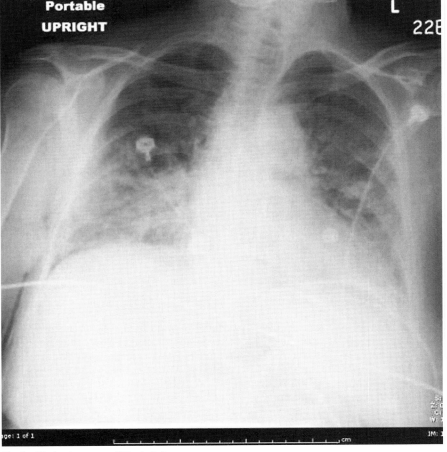

Fig. 1. AP chest x-ray on ICU admission

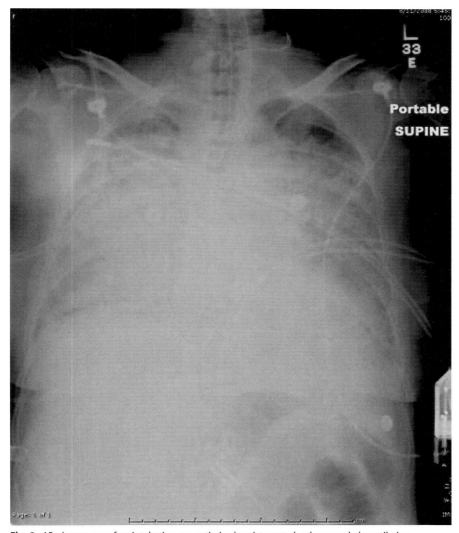

Fig. 2. AP chest x-ray after intubation on optimized assist control volume cycled ventilation

XI

obtained (**Fig. 3**), which demonstrated resolution of the "pulmonary edema" and markedly improved alveolar recruitment. A concomitant ABG returned as 7.45/ 38/245 on an FiO_2 of 0.4.

This case highlights several important principles that inform the clinician with regard to the accuracy of the diagnosis of 'pulmonary edema'. First, clinical examination is of greater importance than radiographic evidence with regard to volume status. Second, alveolar under-recruitment may mimic pulmonary edema by creating vascular crowding, and an increased radiodensity on frontal CXR. Third, diagnosis may be changed by altering the ventilator mode and enabling secretion clearance by hydration of the mucociliary blanket and reengaging the

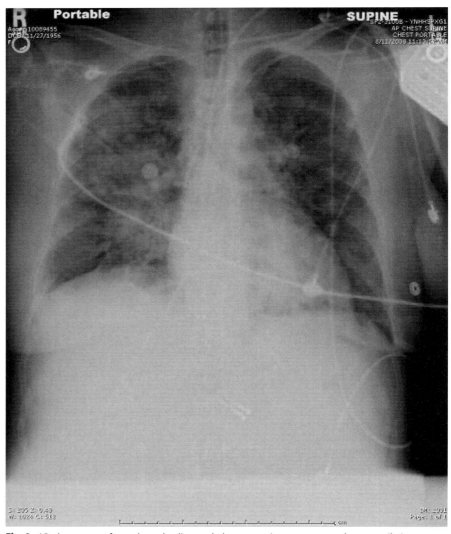

Fig. 3. AP chest x-ray after volume loading and change to airway pressure release ventilation

mucociliary elevator mechanism. Fourth, serial assessment regarding the efficacy of therapy is critical in titrating therapy to a physiologic endpoint. With these points in mind, let us explore what factors after surgical illness or injury may create the confounders that may mimic pulmonary edema.

Diagnosing Pulmonary Edema

Accurate diagnosis of pulmonary edema is facilitated by the synthesis of a thorough clinical history, a detailed physical examination, and the appropriate and timely use of laboratory tests and radiographic evaluation. As with other working diagnoses, inconsistencies between data elements should prompt reconsideration to include an alternate diagnosis. In a related fashion, known alterations in physiology that stem from a known process should alter the pre-test probability that a patient has a specific diagnosis. It is the latter principle that we will apply when examining confounders of the diagnosis of pulmonary edema in surgical patients. A brief review of the common criteria utilized in diagnosing pulmonary edema is in order and provides a frame of reference [7].

Diagnostic Elements for Pulmonary Edema

Elements supportive of the diagnosis of pulmonary edema are presented in **Table 1**. When the diagnosis of pulmonary edema is entertained and it is unclear if it is of cardiogenic or non-cardiogenic etiology, additional testing such as transthoracic or transesophageal echocardiography may be helpful to analyze chamber size and contractility [8, 9]. Of course, pulmonary artery catheterization may be useful to evaluate the pulmonary artery occlusion pressure (PAOP) to rule in or out left atrial hypertension and determine whether the edema is related to volume overload. Other techniques such as transthoracic bioimpedance to determine EVLW content may be useful, but often not uniformly so [10, 11]. Relatedly, identifying large changes in pulse pressure variation (PPV) during a straight-leg raise test in a spontaneously breathing patient, indicative of volume depletion, would guide one away from diagnosing pulmonary edema [12]. Nonetheless, surgical patients demonstrate physiology that is perturbed in manners that may impact the diagnostic accuracy of the reviewed elements when taken in isolation or a variety of montages that drive the clinician towards or away from the diagnosis of pulmonary edema.

Table 1. Data elements supportive of the diagnosis of pulmonary edema

XI

History	Physical Examination	Lab	Radiography
Coronary artery disease	Rales	Elevated BNP	Cardiomegaly (CXR)
Valvular disease	Crackles	Elevated creatinine	Pleural effusion(s) (CXR)
Pulmonary HTN	Edema	Acute anemia	Interstitial edema (CXR)
Renal failure	S3	Hyponatremia	Cephalization (CXR)
MI	JVD	Acute kidney injury	Enlarged pulmonary hila (CXR)
COPD	Cool extremities	Acute renal failure	Dilated chambers (ECHO)
Volume loading	Decreased capillary refill	Hypoalbuminemia	Acute valvular regurgitation (ECHO)

HTN: hypertension; JVD: jugular venous distension; CXR: chest x-ray; ECHO: echocardiogram (transthoracic or transesophageal); MI: myocardial infarction; S3: third heart sound; COPD: chronic obstructive pulmonary disease
Note: these elements are supportive but not individually diagnostic of pulmonary edema of cardiogenic or non-cardiogenic cause.

Postoperative Perturbations of Known Physiology

Abdominal or thoracic surgery reduces thoracic volume as a reflection of pain-induced thoracic splinting. As a result, atelectasis ensues and engenders several important changes in pulmonary physiology, cardiac performance, and thoracic radiology [13, 14]. Because of reduced inspiratory effort, alveolar collapse occurs as critical closing volume and pressure are exceeded. The atelectic alveolar units create local hypoxia. The locally reduced oxygen is a potent signal for physiologically adaptive shunting away from unventilated alveoli. This downstream event is termed hypoxic pulmonary vasoconstriction, and is well described in a variety of clinical conditions [15, 16]. However, the vasoconstriction has a number of maladaptive consequences.

As the pulmonary arteriolar tree total cross-sectional diameter is reduced, the space available for right-sided cardiac output is also reduced. This volume mismatch leads to a relative increase in pulmonary artery pressure, and proportionately reduced right ventricular (RV) performance. Consequently, RV ejection fraction declines, and RV end-diastolic pressure increases. This in turn leads to an increase in right atrial pressure and the measured central venous pressure (CVP) as well as a pressure related decrease in venous return. Furthermore, any acidosis will induce pulmonary artery vasoconstriction [15, 16]. Surgical patients often receive large volumes of crystalloid solutions for pre-, intra-, and often postoperative resuscitation [17]. Therefore, such patients are expected to demonstrate hyperchloremic metabolic acidosis as well as pulmonary artery vasoconstriction even without the added impact of atelectasis [17]. Thus, surgical patients have at least two pulmonary vasoconstricting influences that may work in synergy to reduce pulmonary arterial blood flow, and reduce right-sided cardiac performance. Hence, one may detect and erroneously interpret a CVP reading as consistent with volume excess when a patient actually demonstrates volume-recruitable cardiac performance.

Since venous return and left-sided cardiac output are identical, systemic flow may also reduce when there is significant hypoxic pulmonary vasoconstriction. Systemic hypotension may result when atelectasis is so severe that the dead space (V_D) to V_T ratio (V_D/V_T) exceeds 0.7 and acute respiratory failure ensues as a result of an unsupportable work of breathing. Such acute respiratory failure may be misinterpreted as volume overload when the CVP reading is high and the patient is hypoxic.

Radiographic abnormalities also reflect the above process. As a result of reduced alveolar gas volume, the imaged pulmonary parenchyma appears reduced in size, and more radiodense. Vascular crowding is common, and the pulmonary hila appear more prominent. Since there is relative pulmonary artery hypertension, the heart may appear enlarged due to an increase in right-sided chamber volume and size. Additionally, visceral edema that follows in the wake of surgery for injury, peritonitis, intestinal obstruction, or mesenteric ischemia may similarly elevate the diaphragm and exacerbate parechymal volume loss due to atelectasis [18]. Similarly, intraperitoneal packing that is utilized in damage control surgery for near-exsanguinating injury or emergency general surgery may directly elevate one or both hemi-diaphragms [19]. Moreover, intra-abdominal and sub-diaphragmatic irritation or purulence may engender a sympathetic pleural effusion or one or both sides, further compressing the pulmonary parenchyma, and adding to the cascade of cardiopulmonary compromise outlined above [20].

Pulmonary contusions after blunt or penetrating injury may also lead to radiodensities, capillary leak and EVLW that may be read as pulmonary edema on chest radiography [21, 22]. When thoracic injury requires surgical therapy, direct lung manipulation, as well as single lung ventilation with subsequent reinflation may demonstrate findings consistent with pulmonary edema. Of course, such patients have also typically required large volume resuscitation (> 10 l of crystalloid) within the first 24 hours after injury. Despite the radiographic appearance, such patients are often intravascularly depleted and benefit from additional volume resuscitation.

One unanticipated consequence of massive injury and resuscitation is the thoracic equivalent of the abdominal compartment syndrome – the thoracic compartment syndrome [23, 24]. It is likely that this syndrome is under-diagnosed in the critically ill as there is no safe, rapid, and repeatedly accurate means to measure intrathoracic pressure in mechanically ventilated patients. Thus far, the syndrome has been identified in patients whose thoracic cages have already been opened for injury or cardiac surgery, and that cannot be closed because of geometric constraints, or hemodynamic compromise upon attempted closure. Imaging in these patients will appear similarly radiodense with cephalization and pleural effusions as a result of capillary leak and not intravascular volume overload.

A unique condition that establishes excessive alveolar fluid in a euvolemic or even hypovolemic surgical patient is negative pressure pulmonary edema. This edema stems from a different physiology than primary pump failure or intravascular volume overload. Instead, this condition occurs principally in young healthy patients with normal muscle mass and endurance who have undergone an operation utilizing general anesthesia and endotracheal intubation. If the patient is extubated and tries to forcefully inhale against a closed glottis, they are capable of generating substantial negative intrathoracic and endoalveolar pressure. As a result, there is a pressure gradient that draws capillary fluid into the alveoli leading to alveolar flooding. Chest radiography supports these findings, and the patient does demonstrate hypoxia. Supportive care with mechanical ventilation, enhanced PEEP to reverse the pressure gradient and improve functional residual capacity with or without diuresis rapidly resolves this condition. Non-invasive ventilation may be unsafe as it does not address the underlying problem of a closed or nearly closed glottis [25, 26].

XI

Potential Consequences of Inappropriate Volume Reduction Therapy

Regardless of the modality selected, when intravascular volume reduction therapy is undertaken and not required the patient may suffer unintended consequences. Diuretic therapy (targeting the loop of Henle or other aspects of the renal tubular system) is the most common modality undertaken for volume reduction therapy in hospitalized patients by comparison to osmotic diuretics, hemodialysis (intermittent or continuous), or gastrointestinal track catharsis. Therefore, it is likely that the majority of the time no deleterious effects occur and the most common consequence is a lack of response to the administered diuretic. However, if a patient does respond to diuretic therapy that is not required, intravascular and then interstitial volume loss may ensue. In such circumstances, dessication of pulmonary mucus may occur, crippling the mucociliary elevator mechanism, and leading to secretion retention. In the presence of an indwelling endotracheal tube and the attendant biofilm, such secretion inspissation encourages atelectasis and is likely related to subsequent invasive pulmonary infection [27, 28].

As many surgical patients suffer hypoperfusion related to anesthesia, blood loss, sepsis, and capillary leak after injury, they are at high risk of ATN leading to acute kidney injury or acute renal failure. As creatinine increases and urine flow falls, diuretic therapy is often undertaken to 'ease volume management' [29]. However, oliguria may be a protective mechanism to reduce renal work and manage oxygen utilization related to solute and water clearance after injury. Pharmacologically driving such work may exert a negative influence of subsequent renal recovery. Such a hypothesis is supported by at least one study utilizing a propensity scoring system, and calls into question this time-honored, but not evidence-based common practice [30]. It is further recognized that renal injury or failure may be tracked using the RIFLE criteria (Risk, Injury, Failure, Loss and End-stage disease). Moreover, the worst RIFLE category that one reaches during hospitalization strongly correlates with mortality [31]. The influence of diuretic therapy on progression through RIFLE stages remains unclear at present, but additional renal hypoperfusion events would plausibly relate to worsened parencyhmal injury and reduced performance. Thus, one should be mindful of the potential deleterious and unintended potential consequences on outcome when prescribing diuretic therapy.

Conclusion

The diagnosis of pulmonary edema remains a clinical one; however, surgical patients may present with unique challenges that mislead the clinician to the diagnosis of 'pulmonary edema'. The primary pathophysiology of the presenting surgical disease, the younger patient population, and the prevalence of confounding factors, such as alveolar under-recruitment, may make the diagnosis more difficult. For these patients, an aggressive search for an underlying cause of pulmonary edema needs to be sought to justify the diagnosis. Use of APRV or other re-recruitment techniques may aid in elucidating the pulmonary pathophysiology and may be sufficient treatment for respiratory failure without the use of diuretic therapy. In fact, many patients with a radiographic diagnosis of pulmonary edema may have volume recruitable performance. Additional data derived from the increasingly liberal application of echocardiography, PPV and, in selected patients, the pulmonary artery catheter, may help identify postoperative patients who may benefit from intravascular volume reduction. It is a rare surgical patient who requires diuretic therapy early in their postoperative course. Alternative explanations for the clinical condition should be sought prior to the application of volume reduction therapies.

References

1. Ware, LB, Matthay, MA (2005) Clinical practice: Acute pulmonary edema. N Engl J Med 353: 2788–2796
2. Martin GS, Eaton S, Mealer M, Moss M (2005) Extravascular lung water in patients with severe sepsis: a prospective cohort study. Crit Care 9: R74-R82
3. Cotter G, Metra M, Milo-Cotter O, Dittrich HC, Gheorghiade M (2008) Fluid overload in acute heart failure – redistribution and other mechanisms beyond fluid accumulation. Eur J Heart Fail 10: 165–169.
4. Collins SP, Lindsell CJ, Storrow AB, Abraham WT, ADHERE Scientific Advisory Committee, Investigators and Study Group (2006) Prevalence of negative chest radiography results in the emergency department patient with decompensated heart failure. Ann Emerg Med 47: 13–18

XI

5. Mahdyoon H, Klein R. Eyler W, Lakier JB, Chakko SC, Gheorghiade M (1989) Radiographic pulmonary congestion in end-stage congestive heart failure. Am J Cardiol 63: 625–627
6. Parissis JT, Nikolaou M, Mebazaa A, et al. (2010) Acute pulmonary oedema: clinical characteristics, prognostic factors, and in-hospital management. Eur J Heart Fail 12: 1193–1202
7. Robin ED, Cross Ce, Zelis R (1973) Pulmonary edema. N Eng J Med 288: 292–304
8. Copetti R, Soldati G, Copetti P (2008) Chest sonography: a useful tool to differentiate acute cardiogenic pulmonary edema from acute respiratory distress syndrome. Cardiovasc Ultrasound 6: 16
9. Wallace DJ, Esper S, Gunn SR, Stone MB (2010) Ultrasonographic lung appearance of transfusion-related acute lung injury. Resuscitation 81: 632–633
10. Milzman D, Napoli A, Hogan C, Zlidenny A. Janchar T (2009) Thoracic impedance vs chest radiograph to diagnose acute pulmonary edema in the ED. Am J Emerg Med 27: 770–775
11. Abraham WT (2007) Intrathoracic impedance monitoring for early detection of impending heart failure decompensation. Congest Heart Fail 13: 113–115
12. Mannet X, Riwnzo M, Osman D, et al (2006) Passive leg raising predicts fluid responsiveness in the critically ill. Crit Care Med 34: 1402–1407
13. Fan E, Wilcox ME, Brower RG, et al (2008) Recruitment maneuvers for acute lung injury: a systematic review. Am J Respir Crit Care Med 178: 1156–1163
14. Santiago VR, Rzezinski AF, Nardelli LM, et al (2010) Recruitment maneuver in experimental acute lung injury: the role of alveolar collapse and edema. Crit Care Med 38: 2207–2214
15. Aaronson PI, Robertson TP, Ward JP (2002) Endothelium-derived mediators and hypoxic pulmonary vasoconstriction. Respir Physiol Neurobiol 132: 107–120
16. Aaronson PI, Robertson TP, Knock GA, et al (2006) Hypoxic pulmonary vasoconstriction: mechanisms and controversies. J Physiol 570: 53–58
17. Kaplan LJ, Cheung NH-T, Maerz LL, et al (2009) A physicochemical approach to acid-base balance in critically ill trauma patients minimizes errors and reduces inappropriate plasma volume expansion. J Trauma 66: 1045–1051
18. Lui F, Sangosanya A, Kaplan LJ (2007) Abdominal compartment syndrome: clinical aspects and monitoring. Crit Care Clin 23: 415–433
19. Waibel BH, Rotondo MF (2010) Damage control in trauma and abdominal sepsis. Crit Care Med 38 (9 Suppl): S421–430
20. Light RW (1985) Exudative pleural effusions secondary to gastrointestinal diseases. Clin Chest Med 6: 103–111
21. Whelan DB, Byrick RJ, Mazer CD, et al (2010) Posttraumatic lung injury after pulmonary contusion and fat embolism: factors determining abnormal gas exchange. J Trauma 69: 512–518
22. Cohn SM, Dubose JJ (2010) Pulmonary contusion: an update on recent advances in clinical management. World J Surg 34: 1959–1970
23. Kaplan LJ, Trooskin SZ, Santora TA (1996) Thoracic compartment syndrome. J Trauma 40: 291–293
24. Rizzo AG, Sample GA (2003) Thoracic compartment syndrome secondary to a thoracic procedure: a case report. Chest 124: 1164–1168
25. Krodel DJ, Bittner EA, Abdulnour R, Brown R, Eikermann M (2010) Case scenario: acute postoperative negative pressure pulmonary edema. Anesthesiology 113: 200–207
26. Udeshi A, Cantie SM, Pierre E (2010) Postobstructive pulmonary edema. J Crit Care 25: 538.e1–5
27. Kollef MH, Afessa B, Anzueto A, et al (2008) Silver-coated endotracheal tubes and incidence of ventilator-associated pneumonia: the NASCENT randomized trial. JAMA 300: 805–813
28. Lorente L, Blot S, Rello J (2010) New issues and controversies in the prevention of ventilator-associated pneumonia. Am J Respir Crit Care Med 182: 870–876
29. Macedo E, Bouchard J, Soroko SH, et al (2010) Program to Improve Care in Acute Renal Disease Study. Fluid accumulation, recognition and staging of acute kidney injury in critically-ill patients. Crit Care 14: R82

XI

30. Mehta RL, Pascual MT, Soroko S, Chertow GM, PICARD Study Group (2002) Diuretics, mortality and nonrecovery of renal function in acute renal failure. JAMA 288: 2547–2553
31. Hoste EA, Clermont G, Kersten A, et al (2006) RIFLE criteria for acute kidney injury are associated with hospital mortality in critically ill patients: a cohort analysis. Crit Care 10: R73

Neurogenic Pulmonary Edema

D.L. Davison, M. Terek, and L.S. Chawla

Introduction

Neurogenic pulmonary edema (NPE) is a clinical syndrome characterized by the acute onset of pulmonary edema following a significant central nervous system (CNS) insult. The etiology is thought to be a surge of catecholamines that results in cardiopulmonary dysfunction. A myriad of CNS events, including spinal cord injury, subarachnoid hemorrhage (SAH), traumatic brain injury (TBI), intracranial hemorrhage, status epilepticus, meningitis, and subdural hemorrhage, have been associated with this syndrome [1–5]. Although NPE was identified over 100 years ago, it is still underappreciated in the clinical arena. Its sporadic and relatively unpredictable nature and a lack of etiologic-specific diagnostic markers and treatment modalities may in part be responsible for its poor recognition at the bedside. In this manuscript, we will review the anatomical origin of NPE, outline the various possible pathophysiologic mechanisms responsible for its development, and propose a clinical framework for the classification of NPE.

Historical Background

The syndrome of NPE has been recognized for over a century. In 1903, Harvey Williams Cushing, described the connection between CNS injury and hemodynamic dysfunction [6]; and, in 1908, W. T. Shanahan reported 11 cases of acute pulmonary edema as a complication of epileptic seizures [7]. Francois Moutier described the sudden onset of pulmonary edema among soldiers shot in the head in World War I [8]. Similar reports exist of observed alveolar edema and hemorrhage in the lungs of 17 soldiers dying after isolated bullet head wounds in the Vietnam War [1].

Epidemiology

Because much of the clinical information on NPE has been derived from case reports and autopsy series, the true incidence of NPE is unknown and is likely under-reported. Any acute CNS insult, including spinal cord trauma, can result in pulmonary edema. In patients with SAH, reports of NPE incidence range from 2 % to 42.9 % [3, 9, 10]. Clinically, the likelihood of developing NPE following SAH correlates with increasing age, delay to surgery, vertebral artery origin, and the severity of clinical and radiographic presentation (e.g., Hunt-Hess and Fischer

J.-L. Vincent (ed.), *Annual Update in Intensive Care and Emergency Medicine 2012*
DOI 10.1007/978-3-642-25716-2 © Springer-Verlag Berlin Heidelberg 2012

grades) [10, 11]. Patients with SAH who develop NPE have a higher mortality rate, nearing 10 % [3]. In patients with TBI, the incidence of NPE has been estimated to be up to 20 % [12]. Rogers et al. examined a large autopsy and inpatient database on patients with acute head injury in an effort to better characterize NPE in this patient population. The authors found that the incidence of NPE in patients with TBI who died at the scene was 32 %. Among the TBI patients who died within 96 hours, the incidence of NPE rose to 50 % [2]. There was a direct correlation between decreasing cerebral perfusion pressure (CPP) and reduced PaO_2/FiO_2 ratios in the TBI patients [2]. NPE in patients who suffer seizures is rare; however, up to 80 to 100 % of epileptics who die unexpectedly of seizures are also found to have NPE [13]. In other series, close to one-third of patients with status epilepticus also developed NPE [14]. Other conditions, including aqueductal glioma, multiple sclerosis, medication overdose, arteriovenous malformations, meningitis/encephalitis and spinal cord infarction, have been reported and linked to the formation of NPE [5, 15–17].

Pathophysiology

The pathophysiology linking the neurologic, cardiac, and pulmonary conditions in NPE has been subject to debate and controversy since the recognition of NPE as a clinical entity. A common thread among all case descriptions of NPE is the severity and acuity of the precipitating CNS event. Neurologic conditions that cause abrupt, rapid, and extreme elevation in intracranial pressure (ICP) appear to be at greatest risk of being associated with NPE [18, 19]. Elevated ICP levels correlate with increased levels of extravascular lung water (EVLW) and NPE [2, 20]. The abrupt increase in ICP leading to neuronal compression, ischemia or damage is believed to give rise to an intense activation of the sympathetic nervous system and the release of catecholamines [2, 21]. This fundamental role of catecholamines is supported by the fact that the blockade of sympathetic activity in animal models via intrathecal lidocaine, phentolamine infusion, or pretreatment with phenoxybenzamine mitigates the pathologic neuro-pulmonary process [22, 23] (**Table 1**). In addition to pharmacologic intervention, anatomical interruption of the nervous system pathway (e.g., spinal cord transection) has also been shown to protect against the formation of NPE (**Table 1**). In one animal model, NPE was prevented by removal of one lung followed by reimplantation. This was in contrast to the pulmonary edema that developed in the innervated intrinsic lung [24]. In a human example, NPE has been reported in soldiers who died suddenly after gunshot wounds to the head. The soldiers with concomitant cervical spinal cord injury (and presumably severed neuronal connection) did not have evidence of pulmonary edema on post-mortem exam [1]. Pulmonary edema has also been reported in patients with pheochromocytoma, presumably from catecholamine surge [25].

Anatomical Origin of NPE

Although the exact source of sympathetic outflow has not been identified, certain centers in the brain have been implicated. These 'NPE trigger zones' include the hypothalamus and the medulla, specifically area A1, A5, nuclei of solitary tract

Table 1. Animal studies assessing possible therapeutic interventions for neurogenic pulmonary edema (NPE)

Intervention	Animal model	Study design/results
Alpha Blockade		
Phentolamine (1 mg/kg)	Rats	Prevented pulmonary edema after induced injury to anterior hypothalamus [23]
Phenoxybenzamine (3 mg/kg)	Dogs	Prevented pulmonary artery and systemic pressure increase after CSF pressure was increased from 100 to 200 mmHg [22]
Phenoxybenzamine (1.5 mg/kg)	Dogs	Prevented increases in pulmonary perfusion pressure and PVR and associated increases in lung water, Qs/Qt, VD, and hypoxemia induced by ICP elevation [50]
Phentolamine (2 mg/kg)	Sheep	Prevented the expected increase in permeability and lymph flow after CNS insult [38]
Beta Blockade		
Propranolol (0.5 mg/kg)	Dogs	Pulmonary artery and systemic pressure unchanged with use of beta blocker after CSF pressure was increased from 100 to 200 mmHg [22]
Propranolol (1.5 mg/kg)	Dogs	Pretreatment with beta blocker attenuated the increase in PVR during elevation in ICP but did not prevent increases in lung water, Qs/Qt, VD, and hypoxemia [50]
Sympathetic Outflow Denervation		
Bilateral thoracic sympa-thectomy	Dogs & Rabbits	Sympathectomy prior to induced CNS insult did not prevent pulmonary pressure elevation [35]
Spinal cord transection	Monkeys	NPE prevented by sympathetic denervation [18]
Cholinergic Influence		
Vagotomy	Dogs & Rabbits	Vagotomy did not prevent increases in pulmonary vascular pressures [35]
Vagotomy	Monkeys	Vagotomy did not prevent NPE [18]
Other		
Methylprednisone (40 mg/kg)	Rats	Prevented aconitine induced NPE and systemic HTN [51]
Hypovolemia	Rats	Lowering pulmonary blood volume by phlebotomy prevented aconitine induced NPE [51]
Naloxone	Sheep	Induced NPE could be prevented by opiate antagonism, suggesting a role for endorphins [45]

CSF: cerebrospinal fluid; PVR: pulmonary vascular resistance; CNS: central nervous system; VD: dead space; Qs/Qt: pulmonary shunt

XI

and the area postrema [5]. Area A1 is located in the ventrolateral aspect of the medulla and is composed of catecholamine neurons which project into the hypothalamus [5]. The neurons from area A5, located in the upper portion of the medulla, project into the preganglionic centers for spinal cord sympathetic outflow [5]. Injury to Area A1 or disruption of the efferent pathway between A5 and the cervical cord has been shown to result in the formation of pulmonary edema [26]. Stimulation of area A5 also causes increases in systemic blood pressure [27].

The nuclei of solitary tract and the area postrema of the medulla have also been linked to the formation of NPE. These areas are related to respiratory regulation and receive input from the carotid sinus. In animal models, bilateral irritation of the nuclei solitary tract causes severe hypertension and NPE [23]. Unilateral stimulation of the area postrema also results in profound hemodynamic changes, including increased cardiac output, peripheral vascular resistance, and hypertension [5]. Finally, NPE was shown to develop after lesions were induced in the hypothalamus of laboratory animals [28]. In a case series of 22 patients suffering from NPE, 11 of the patients had significant radiographic abnormalities in the hypothalamus. The presence of hypothalamic lesions among these NPE patients conferred a worse prognosis [29].

Pathogenesis

It is the prevailing view that the autonomic response to elevated ICP plays an important role in the pathogenesis of NPE. However, what occurs mechanistically at the level of the pulmonary vascular endothelium remains enigmatic and theoretical. Several clinicopathologic paradigms have been proposed to explain the clinical syndrome of NPE: 1) Neuro-cardiac; 2) Neuro-hemodynamic; 3) "blast theory"; and 4) pulmonary venule adrenergic hypersensitivity.

Neuro-cardiac NPE

Whereas NPE has traditionally been described as a 'non-cardiogenic' form of pulmonary edema, there is evidence that, in at least a subset of patients, neurologic insult leads to *direct* myocardial injury and the development of pulmonary edema. Takotsubo's cardiomyopathy is a reversible condition characterized by depressed cardiac contractility following a neurologically 'stressful' event. The transiently diminished lusitropy, diastolic dysfunction, and global hypokinesis of the Takotsubo heart can render these patients susceptible to cardiogenic pulmonary edema [30]. Connor was one of the first investigators to describe the myocytolysis and contraction-band necrosis on myocardial biopsies of neurosurgical patients with pulmonary edema [31]. Since this original report, several cases of cardiac injury associated with pulmonary edema following a CNS event have been described. In a retrospective analysis, patients with no previous cardiac history developed acute onset of pulmonary edema in association with a SAH. The patients all demonstrated segmental wall motion abnormalities on echocardiogram, mildly elevated cardiac enzymes, electrocardiogram (EKG) abnormalities, and elevated pulmonary artery occlusion pressures (PAOPs). These patients were noted to have focal myocardial necrosis, yet had no evidence of infarction and had normal coronary arteries [32]. Similar descriptions of reversible cardiac dysfunction have been reported among patients with TBI and NPE [30].

As with all forms of NPE, massive sympathetic discharge following CNS insult is thought to be the precipitating factor. More specifically, in this subset of patients with 'neuro-cardiac' NPE, it is catecholamines that induce *direct* myocyte injury. This is supported by the fact that the wall motion abnormalities seen on echocardiogram in patients with neurogenic stunned myocardium follow a pattern of sympathetic nerve innervation [33]. Similarly, myocardial lesions have

XI

been shown in patients with pheochromocytoma, supporting the role of catecholamine surge in the pathogenesis of stunned myocardium [34].

Neuro-hemodynamic NPE

Unlike the *direct* toxic effects to the myocardium as detailed above, the 'neuro-hemodynamic' theory posits that ventricular compliance is *indirectly* altered by the abrupt increases in systemic and pulmonary pressures following CNS injury. In the original studies by Sarnoff and Sarnoff, substantial increases in aortic and pulmonary pressures were observed following the injection of thrombin into the intracisterna magna of dogs and rabbits [35]. The authors noted that following the sympathetic surge, the left ventricle had reached its work-failure threshold and failed to effectively pump against the systemic pressures. A translocation of blood flow from the highly resistant systemic circulation to the low resistance pulmonary circuit subsequently ensued, leading to a hydrostatic form of pulmonary edema. The increased sizes of the left atrium and pulmonary veins in the animals were well documented in this study, and the authors subsequently coined the term "neuro-hemodynamic pulmonary edema" [35]. Several other animal models have documented large elevations in left atrial, systemic and pulmonary pressures associated with NPE [18, 22, 36]. One study induced graded levels of ICP in chimpanzees. All of the animals developed systemic hypertension, but only those with a marked increase in left atrial pressure and a decrease in cardiac output developed pulmonary edema [18].

Blast Theory

The neuro-cardiac and neuro-hemodynamic theories outlined above both suggest that alterations in hydrostatic and Starling forces are central to the formation of pulmonary edema following CNS injury. Although hydrostatic pressures may play a role in the pathogenesis, this mechanism alone cannot explain the presence of red blood cells (RBCs) and protein observed in the alveolar fluid in many NPE subjects [37, 38]. The exudative properties of the pulmonary fluid imply that alterations in vascular permeability play a role in the pathogenesis of NPE. In order to explain the presence of both hydrostatic factors and vascular leak, Theodore and Robin introduced the "blast theory" of NPE [39]. Similar to the neuro-hemodynamic model, the "blast theory" posits that the severe abrupt increases in systemic and pulmonary pressures following the catecholamine surge result in a net shift of blood volume from the systemic circulation to the low resistance pulmonary circulation. This increase in pulmonary venous pressure leads to the development of transudative pulmonary edema. The "blast theory" further posits that the acute rise in capillary pressure induces a degree of barotrauma capable of damaging the capillary-alveolar membrane. The structural damage to the pulmonary endothelium ultimately leads to vascular leak and persistent protein-rich pulmonary edema [39]. The pulmonary edema according to the "blast theory" is thus the result of two mechanisms which act synergistically: A high-pressure hydrostatic influence and pulmonary endothelial injury. Several pre-clinical models support this mechanism [40, 41]. Maron showed that barotrauma and vascular permeability occurred when pulmonary pressures exceeded 70 torr following CNS injury in dogs [40]. In another study, EVLW was observed when pulmonary artery pressures reached 25 torr or greater in rabbits [41]. The authors concluded

XI

that some degree of pulmonary hypertension is required for the development of pulmonary edema, and that the degree of permeability is "pressure dependent" [41].

Theodore and Robin in the "blast theory" acknowledged that it is rare to document elevated systemic and pulmonary pressures in human cases of NPE. According to their theory, this can be explained by the fact that the sympathetic surge and subsequent hemodynamic instability occurs at the time of the inciting event when hemodynamic monitoring is rare [39]. During the later stages of NPE, systemic and pulmonary pressures can return to normal, whereas the endothelial injury and vascular leak may persist [39]. A few case reports have been able to document this sequence of events in human subjects, lending credence to the "blast theory". One case study described a patient who had hemodynamic monitoring at the time of a seizure that led to NPE. Within minutes of the seizure, marked increases in systemic, pulmonary and pulmonary artery occlusion pressures were recorded. The hemodynamics quickly normalized and two hours later, pulmonary edema developed, which was determined to be high in protein content [37]. In another case report of a patient with an intracranial hemorrhage, extreme increases in systemic and mean pulmonary pressures (410/200 mmHg and 48 mmHg, respectively) lasted 4 minutes. This was followed by a dramatic decrease in the patient's oxygen levels. The patient's pulmonary edema did not clear on radiograph for 72 hours following the last episode of transient systemic and pulmonary hypertension. The authors concluded that persistent vascular leak was the basis for these findings [42].

Pulmonary Venule Adrenergic Hypersensitivity

Many reports of NPE fail to consistently demonstrate the hypertensive surges and changes in left atrial pressures as described in the theories above. This suggests that systemic hypertension and its effect on cardiac contractility may not always contribute to the development of NPE. An alternative hypothesis is that the massive sympathetic discharge following CNS injury *directly* affects the pulmonary vascular bed, and that the edema develops regardless of any systemic changes. We refer to this as the 'pulmonary venule adrenergic hypersensitivity' theory. This concept of neurally induced changes to endothelial integrity is made plausible by the fact that pulmonary vascular beds contain α- and β-adrenergic receptors [43]. In a well designed study by McClellan et al. [44], CNS injury and elevated ICP was induced in dogs by cisternal saline infusion. Autonomic activation following the CNS insult was evidenced by an increase in systemic and pulmonary vascular pressures. The pulmonary edema developed in the dogs and was proven to be exudative in content. When the same degree of pulmonary hypertension and increased left atrial pressure was induced with a left atrial balloon in the control group, pulmonary edema did not develop. The authors concluded that neurologic insult resulted in acute lung injury (ALI), which could not be explained by hemodynamic changes, but rather by *direct* neurological influences on the pulmonary endothelium [44]. In other studies of intracranial lesions induced in sheep, pulmonary edema developed despite normal or only mildly increased left atrial and systemic pressures [38, 45]. In one of these studies, α-adrenergic blockade prevented the formation of pulmonary edema with little systemic effect, further supporting the role of *direct* adrenergic influence [38]. In human examples, continuous cardiac monitoring during the development of NPE in patients with SAH and brain tumor resection failed to demonstrate preceding hemodynamic changes [46–48]. These findings suggest that isolated pulmonary venoconstriction or endothelial disruption following CNS injury may be responsible for the formation of pulmonary edema [47, 48].

Clinical Characteristics

Two distinct clinical forms of NPE have been described. The *early* form of NPE is most common and is characterized by the development of symptoms within minutes to hours following neurologic injury. In contrast, the *delayed* form develops 12 to 24 hours after the CNS insult [5]. The abrupt nature of respiratory distress is an impressive feature of NPE. Typically, the patient becomes acutely dyspneic, tachypneic, and hypoxic within minutes. Pink, frothy sputum is commonly seen and bilateral crackles and rales are appreciated on auscultation. Sympathetic hyperactivity is common and the patient may be febrile, tachycardic, and hypertensive, and leukocytosis may occur. Chest radiograph will reveal bilateral hyperdense infiltrates consistent with acute respiratory distress syndrome (ARDS) [5]. Symptoms often spontaneously resolve within 24 to 48 hours; however, in patients with ongoing brain injury and elevated ICP, the NPE often persists.

Differential Diagnosis

Because alternative conditions are common, NPE is a difficult diagnosis to establish. The diagnosis of 'pure' NPE is a diagnosis of exclusion and, by traditional definition, requires documentation of non-cardiogenic pulmonary edema in the setting of neurological injury. Aggressive fluid hydration is frequently administered to neurologically injured patients. Large volume resuscitation is especially common in SAH patients suspected of having vasospasm, thus rendering these patients at risk for volume overload and pulmonary edema [9]. Aspiration pneumonia is also common among CNS injured patients and must be excluded. Aspiration pneumonia differs from NPE by the presence of clinical clues (vomiting, gastric contents in the oropharynx, witnessed aspiration) and the distribution of alveolar disease in dependent portions of the lungs. In contrast, NPE is characterized by a frothy, often blood-tinged sputum and more centrally distributed alveolar disease on radiograph [5].

XI

Previous Treatment in Humans

Although numerous case reports have described the various precipitating CNS insults and clinical scenarios associated with NPE, few studies have identified specific treatment modalities for this condition. The management of NPE to date has largely focused on treating the underlying neurologic condition in order to quell the sympathetic discharge responsible for causing the lung injury. Treatment efforts to reduce ICP, including decompression and clot evacuation, osmotic diuretics, anti-epileptics, tumor resection, and steroids have all been associated with improvements in oxygenation [3, 16, 28]. Pharmacological intervention, specifically anti-α-adrenergic agents, which potentially interrupt the vicious cycle of hemodynamic instability and subsequent respiratory failure, has shown promise in animal models. However, there are few reports documenting its use in humans. In one case report, a patient with TBI developed sudden onset of bilateral infiltrates and hypoxia in the setting of elevated blood pressures, sinus tachycardia and normal central venous pressure (CVP). This patient was successfully treated with the α-blocking agent, chlorpromazine, as evidenced by rapid improvement in oxygenation and hemodynamics; catecholamine levels were not measured in this report [49].

Proposed Clinical Framework, Diagnostic Criteria, and Management of NPE

NPE is an exotic form of pulmonary edema and can be considered a form of ARDS per the consensus definition. While all cases of NPE follow a CNS event and likely originate from sympathetic activation, downstream effects on the cardiopulmonary system vary. Some patients may have direct myocardial injury resulting in left ventricular failure and pulmonary edema. Others develop pulmonary edema from a non-cardiogenic mechanism as described in the pulmonary venule hypersensitivity models. Differentiating between 'cardiogenic involvement' and 'non-cardiogenic' mechanisms is essential in the clinical realm, as there are clear therapeutic implications. In order for this clinical entity to be effectively studied and treated, a definition that captures a subset of patients with NPE who may benefit from sympathetic interference would be helpful. We, therefore, propose the following diagnostic criteria for this subset of NPE: 1) Bilateral infiltrates; 2) PaO_2/FiO_2 ratio < 200; 3) no evidence of left atrial hypertension; 4) presence of CNS injury (severe enough to have caused significantly increased ICP); 5) absence of other common causes of acute respiratory distress or ARDS (e.g., aspiration, massive blood transfusion, sepsis). For those patients who meet the above NPE criteria, measurement of serum catecholamines may be helpful. In those patients in whom blood pressure permits, a trial of an α-adrenergic blocking agent, such as phentolamine, can be considered.

XI

Conclusion

Despite decades of scientific experiments and case descriptions, the diagnosis and management of NPE remains controversial and challenging. Although this syndrome has been described for over a millennium, it remains underdiagnosed and underappreciated. The exact pathophysiology of NPE is still debated and the wide variety of clinical situations in which it occurs can obfuscate diagnosis. The sudden development of hypoxemic respiratory failure following a catastrophic CNS event, which cannot be attributed to other causes of ARDS, is the only universally agreed upon characteristic of NPE. A common denominator in all cases of NPE is likely a surge in endogenous serum catecholamines that may result in changes in cardiopulmonary hemodynamics and Starling forces. It appears that the specific clinical manifestations of this surge may vary depending on the individual circumstance. In some patients, cardiac dysfunction may predominate; in others, capillary leak is the primary manifestation. These patterns have obvious implications for the diagnosis and treatment of individual cases, including cardiac evaluation, fluid management, and choice of inotropic or vasoactive substances such as α-adrenergic blockade.

References

1. Simmons RL, Heisterkamp CA 3rd, Collins JA, Genslar S, Martin AM Jr (1969) Respiratory insufficiency in combat casualties. 3. Arterial hypoxemia after wounding. Ann Surg 1: 45–52
2. Rogers FB, Shackford SR, Trevisani GT, Davis JW, Mackersie RC, Hoyt DB (1995) Neurogenic pulmonary edema in fatal and nonfatal head injuries. J Trauma 5: 860–866
3. Fontes RB, Aguiar PH, Zanetti MV, Andrade F, Mandel M, Teixeira MJ (2003) Acute neurogenic pulmonary edema: case reports and literature review. J Neurosurg Anesthesiol 2: 144–150
4. Kaufman HH, Timberlake G, Voelker J, Pait TG (1993) Medical complications of head injury. Med Clin North Am 1: 43–60
5. Colice GL (1985) Neurogenic pulmonary edema. Clin Chest Med 3: 473–489
6. Cushing H (1902) I. On the avoidance of shock in major amputations by cocainization of large nerve-trunks preliminary to their division. With observations on blood-pressure changes in surgical cases. Ann Surg 3: 321–345
7. Shanahan W (1908) Acute pulmonary edema as a complication of epileptic seizures. NY Med J 54–56
8. Moutier F (1918) Hypertension et mort par oedeme pulmo aigu chez les blesses cranio-encephaliques. Presse Med 108–109
9. Friedman JA, Pichelmann MA, Piepgras DG, et al (2003) Pulmonary complications of aneurysmal subarachnoid hemorrhage. Neurosurgery 5: 1025–1031
10. Solenski NJ, Haley EC, Jr., Kassell NF, et al (1995) Medical complications of aneurysmal subarachnoid hemorrhage: a report of the multicenter, cooperative aneurysm study. Participants of the Multicenter Cooperative Aneurysm Study. Crit Care Med 6: 1007–1017
11. Ochiai H, Yamakawa Y, Kubota E (2001) Deformation of the ventrolateral medulla oblongata by subarachnoid hemorrhage from ruptured vertebral artery aneurysms causes neurogenic pulmonary edema. Neurol Med Chir (Tokyo) 11: 529–534
12. Bratton SL, Davis RL (1997) Acute lung injury in isolated traumatic brain injury. Neurosurgery 4: 707–712
13. Wayne SL, O'Donovan CA, McCall WV, Link K (1997) Postictal neurogenic pulmonary edema: experience from an ECT model. Convuls Ther 3: 181–184
14. Simon RP (1993) Neurogenic pulmonary edema. Neurol Clin 2: 309–323
15. Gentiloni N, Schiavino D, Della Corte F, Ricci E, Colosimo C (1992) Neurogenic pulmonary edema: a presenting symptom in multiple sclerosis. Ital J Neurol Sci 5: 435–438
16. Phanthumchinda K, Khaoroptham S, Kongratananan N, Rasmeechan S (1988) Neurogenic pulmonary edema associated with spinal cord infarction from arteriovenous malformation. J Med Assoc Thai 3: 150–153
17. Wagle VG, Hall A, Voytek T, Silberstein H, Uphoff DF (1990) Aqueductal (pencil) glioma presenting as neurogenic pulmonary edema: a case report. Surg Neurol 6: 435–438
18. Ducker TB, Simmons RL (1968) Increased intracranial pressure and pulmonary edema. 2. The hemodynamic response of dogs and monkeys to increased intracranial pressure. J Neurosurg 2: 118–123
19. Kosnik EJ, Paul SE, Rossel CW, Sayers MP (1977) Central neurogenic pulmonary edema: with a review of its pathogenesis and treatment. Childs Brain 1: 37–47
20. Gupta YK, Chugh A, Kacker V, Mehta VS, Tandon PN (1998) Development of neurogenic pulmonary edema at different grades of intracranial pressure in cats. Indian J Physiol Pharmacol 1: 71–80
21. Demling R, Riessen R (1990) Pulmonary dysfunction after cerebral injury. Crit Care Med 7: 768–774
22. Brashear RE, Ross JC (1970) Hemodynamic effects of elevated cerebrospinal fluid pressure: alterations with adrenergic blockade. J Clin Invest 7: 1324–1333
23. Nathan MA, Reis DJ (1975) Fulminating arterial hypertension with pulmonary edema from release of adrenomedullary catecholamines after lesions of the anterior hypothalamus in the rat. Circ Res 2: 226–235
24. Sugg WL, Craver WD, Webb WR, Ecker RR (1969) Pressure changes in the dog lung secondary to hemorrhagic shock: protective effect of pulmonary reimplantation. Ann Surg 4: 592–598

XI

25. de Leeuw PW, Waltman FL, Birkenhager WH (1986) Noncardiogenic pulmonary edema as the sole manifestation of pheochromocytoma. Hypertension 9: 810–812

26. Blessing WW, West MJ, Chalmers J (1981) Hypertension, bradycardia, and pulmonary edema in the conscious rabbit after brainstem lesions coinciding with the A1 group of catecholamine neurons. Circ Res 4: 949–958

27. Loewy AD, McKellar S (1980) The neuroanatomical basis of central cardiovascular control. Fed Proc 8: 2495–2503

28. Brown RH, Jr., Beyerl BD, Iseke R, Lavyne MH (1986) Medulla oblongata edema associated with neurogenic pulmonary edema. Case report. J Neurosurg 3: 494–500

29. Imai K (2003) Radiographical investigations of organic lesions of the hypothalamus in patients suffering from neurogenic pulmonary edema due to serious intracranial diseases: relationship between radiographical findings and outcome of patients suffering from neurogenic pulmonary edema. No Shinkei Geka 7: 757–765

30. Bahloul M, Chaari AN, Kallel H, et al (2006) Neurogenic pulmonary edema due to traumatic brain injury: evidence of cardiac dysfunction. Am J Crit Care 5: 462–470

31. Connor RC (1969) Myocardial damage secondary to brain lesions. Am Heart J 2: 145–148

32. Mayer SA, Lin J, Homma S, et al (1999) Myocardial injury and left ventricular performance after subarachnoid hemorrhage. Stroke 4: 780–786

33. Zaroff JG, Rordorf GA, Ogilvy CS, Picard MH (2000) Regional patterns of left ventricular systolic dysfunction after subarachnoid hemorrhage: evidence for neurally mediated cardiac injury. J Am Soc Echocardiogr 8: 774–779

34. Di Pasquale G, Andreoli A, Lusa AM, et al (1998) Cardiologic complications of subarachnoid hemorrhage. J Neurosurg Sci 1 (Suppl 1):33–36

35. Sarnoff SJ, Sarnoff LC (1952) Neurohemodynamics of pulmonary edema. II. The role of sympathetic pathways in the elevation of pulmonary and stemic vascular pressures following the intracisternal injection of fibrin. Circulation 1: 51–62

36. Minnear FL, Kite C, Hill LA, van der Zee H (1987) Endothelial injury and pulmonary congestion characterize neurogenic pulmonary edema in rabbits. J Appl Physiol 1: 335–341

37. Carlson RW, Schaeffer RC, Jr., Michaels SG, Weil MH (1979) Pulmonary edema following intracranial hemorrhage. Chest 6: 731–734

38. van der Zee H, Malik AB, Lee BC, Hakim TS (1980) Lung fluid and protein exchange during intracranial hypertension and role of sympathetic mechanisms. J Appl Physiol 2: 273–280

39. Theodore J, Robin ED (1976) Speculations on neurogenic pulmonary edema (NPE). Am Rev Respir Dis 4: 405–411

40. Maron MB (1989) Effect of elevated vascular pressure transients on protein permeability in the lung. J Appl Physiol 1: 305–310

41. Bosso FJ, Lang SA, Maron MB (1990) Role of hemodynamics and vagus nerves in development of fibrin-induced pulmonary edema. J Appl Physiol 6: 2227–2232

42. Wray NP, Nicotra MB (1978) Pathogenesis of neurogenic pulmonary edema. Am Rev Respir Dis 4: 783–786

43. Richardson JB (1987) Innervation of the pulmonary circulation: An overview. In: Will JA (ed) The Pulmonary Circulation in Health and Disease. Academic Press, Orlando, pp 9–14

44. McClellan MD, Dauber IM, Weil JV (1989) Elevated intracranial pressure increases pulmonary vascular permeability to protein. J Appl Physiol 3: 1185–1191

45. Peterson BT, Ross JC, Brigham KL (1983) Effect of naloxone on the pulmonary vascular responses to graded levels of intracranial hypertension in anesthetized sheep. Am Rev Respir Dis 6: 1024–1029

46. Keegan MT, Lanier WL (1999) Pulmonary edema after resection of a fourth ventricle tumor: possible evidence for a medulla-mediated mechanism. Mayo Clin Proc 3: 264–268

47. Fein A, Grossman RF, Jones JG, et al (1979) The value of edema fluid protein measurement in patients with pulmonary edema. Am J Med 1: 32–38

48. Fein IA, Rackow EC (1982) Neurogenic pulmonary edema. Chest 3: 318–320

49. Wohns RN, Tamas L, Pierce KR, Howe JF (1985) Chlorpromazine treatment for neurogenic pulmonary edema. Crit Care Med 3: 210–211

50. Malik AB (1985) Mechanisms of neurogenic pulmonary edema. Circ Res 1: 1–18

51. Minnear FL, Connell RS (1982) Prevention of aconitine-induced neurogenic pulmonary edema (NPE) with hypovolemia or methylprednisolone. J Trauma 2: 121–128

XI

XII Emergencies

Pre-hospital Resuscitative Interventions: Elemental or Detrimental?

M.J. Lippmann, G.A. Salazar, and P.E. Pepe

Introduction

Emergency prehospital resuscitative medical care, as we have come to know it in recent years, had many of its roots in the 1960s and 1970s when several intrepid physicians ventured into the out-of-hospital setting and published their experiences with lifesaving approaches to managing patients with acute coronary syndromes and, most specifically, cardiopulmonary arrest due to out-of-hospital ventricular dysrhythmias [1–5]. Although physician-staffed ambulance services and out-of-hospital emergency medical care responses had been in place for more than a century in many venues worldwide, this modern iteration of emergency medical rescue was highlighted by scientific documentation of lifesaving outcomes in the early years of development [1–3]. In turn, this reportable success prompted widespread adoption of emergency medical services (EMS) systems of care across the globe [6].

At the same time, the development of contemporary EMS was also remarkable in some locales for the development of formal training and community-wide deployment of non-physician personnel who could provide both basic and even advanced (procedurally-invasive) care interventions [2–6]. Such interventions, which, traditionally, had been provided in the in-hospital setting, ranged from basic spinal immobilization and extremity splinting to more advanced electrocardiographic (EKG) interpretation, defibrillation attempts and so-called 'invasive' procedures such as intravenous (i.v.) cannulation, needle decompression of the chest, and endotracheal intubation. Particularly in the arena of out-of-hospital cardiac arrest, early data supported the notion that 'the earlier the intervention, the better the results' [3, 4]. For example, published studies showed a distinct correlation between the response interval for emergency care responders and eventual survival to hospital discharge for patients who had sudden out-of-hospital ventricular fibrillation (VF)-related cardiac arrest [4]. Although, in retrospect, the most important factors may have been early, aggressive, uninterrupted chest compressions and rapid delivery of defibrillatory countershocks, those early out-of-hospital emergency care practitioners (**Fig. 1**) were also providing endotracheal intubation, i.v. administration of cardiac anti-arrhythmic medications and β-adrenergic drugs and vasopressor infusions [2–4, 7, 8]. It was, therefore, assumed that all of these interventions were providing a beneficial effect.

Over time, many other prehospital care interventions were adopted for a plethora of emergency medical conditions, ranging from i.v. fluid resuscitation for presumed hemorrhage and infusions of benzodiazepines for persistent seizures to subcutaneous administration of epinephrine for anaphylaxis and i.v. diuretics for

XII

J.-L. Vincent (ed.), *Annual Update in Intensive Care and Emergency Medicine 2012*
DOI 10.1007/978-3-642-25716-2 © Springer-Verlag Berlin Heidelberg 2012

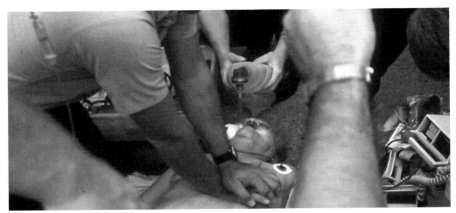

Fig. 1. Prehospital care interventions may be either effective or deleterious, depending on circumstances. Early (1970s) experience with prehospital resuscitative interventions provided on-scene by specially-trained out-of-hospital emergency medical responders proved to be dramatically life-saving in several clinical care scenarios. Subsequent scientific scrutiny also demonstrated that many interventions shown to be helpful for certain conditions, may also be detrimental in other circumstances, especially in the absence of expert medical oversight and appropriate delineation of treatment application (photo by Dr. Paul Pepe).

pulmonary edema. In the United States and several other countries, it was physician-trained, physician-supervised paramedics who generally provided the interventions [2–6]. In other venues, such as Europe and Asia, specialized physicians were assigned to the prehospital arena for the more critical emergencies. As a result, many of the interventions that physicians provided in the in-hospital setting were transitioned to the 'field' with the same presumption that they were both beneficial and necessary. In retrospect, however, and for a myriad of reasons ranging from EMS system design and evolving understanding of the physiology and timing of certain interventions, many of those prehospital procedures have not only been found to be relatively ineffective, but actually detrimental under various circumstances [8–13].

In the following discussion, choosing a few representative examples, some of the historical and current resuscitative interventions that have been delivered in the prehospital arena will be reviewed and analyzed as being 'elemental' or 'detrimental'. In essence, many of these interventions can be both helpful and harmful, but, to quote Oscar Wilde, "the truth is rarely pure and never simple" (from: The Importance of Being Earnest, 1895, Act I). The following review is one attempt to provide some perspectives on this important concept.

Prehospital Interventions for Trauma

Post-trauma Fluid Resuscitation

Following a series of elegant experimental models of severe hemorrhage in the 1950s and 1960s, scientists and clinicians alike adopted the concept that infusions of isotonic crystalloid were an important therapeutic intervention to restore intravascular volume loss [14, 15]. With the intuitive presumption that the earlier the intervention could be provided, the better the outcome would be, the evolution of EMS provided a mechanisms to deliver expedient infusion of i.v. fluids in the out-of-hospital setting, either on-scene or enroute to definitive surgical care, for patients with presumed or confirmed hemorrhage. In turn, by the 1990s, pre-hospital fluid resuscitation had become established as a mainstream intervention for trauma patients who had significant bleeding or suspected internal hemorrhage [16].

In recent years, however, there has been growing evidence that rapid fluid resuscitation prior to the control of hemorrhage, may be detrimental, and particularly in the case of penetrating injuries in which a distinct intrathoracic or intraabdominal vascular injury is likely to be involved [9, 17–23]. Experimental research in numerous models supports the concept that when fluid infusions are provided before bleeding has been controlled they will lead to a hydraulic increase in bleeding, disruption of early soft clot formation and even dilute coagulation factors [17–20, 22, 23].

Existing clinical research findings, although limited, have also supported this concept of not treating hypotension during uncontrollable hemorrhage and the evolving concept of 'damage control resuscitation', particularly in the absence of severe traumatic head injury [25, 26]. For example, a large, prospective, controlled clinical trial of fluid resuscitation for post-injury hypotension, compared immediate prehospital i.v. fluid resuscitation to fluid resuscitation that was deferred until arrival in the operating room (OR) [9]. Specifically, patients presenting with systolic blood pressure (SBP) < 90 mmHg following thoraco-abdominal gunshot or stab wounds were provided with either liberal lactated Ringer's fluid resuscitation preoperatively or no fluid resuscitation until arrival in the OR. The results demonstrated that patients in the preoperative fluid resuscitation group had a higher mortality rate and a higher rate of postoperative complications compared with patients in the delayed resuscitation group [9]. A second prospective randomized clinical trial involved both penetrating *and* blunt trauma patients [21]. Those with SBP < 90 mmHg were randomized to a fluid resuscitation strategy targeted to a lower than normal SBP (80 mmHg) or to conventional care (SBP > 100 mmHg). Mortality was identical (4/55 patients in each group) but there were fewer complications and a shorter duration of hemorrhage in the low-pressure group [21].

Accordingly, in this approach to trauma resuscitation, if the bleeding is easily controlled (such as a hemorrhaging vascular injury in an extremity, then fluids can be infused once mechanical hemostasis (e.g., tourniquet, direct pressure, clamping) is achieved. However, if the bleeding is uncontrollable in the prehospital setting, such as an intra-abdominal hemorrhage, there is now a strong precaution that this preoperative (pre-surgical) intervention may be harmful, particularly if provided overzealously or too early in the course of resuscitative care. Traditionally, the management strategy had been to return patients with system arterial hypotension to a more 'normotensive' state. However, with the evolving paradigm, a low systemic arterial blood pressure is generally tolerated until the time of surgical intervention unless palpable pulses are lost and the patient has become unresponsive [25–27].

Nevertheless, studies have not fully addressed the more complicated issue of blunt trauma involving severe traumatic brain injury (TBI), often characterized by numerous sites of hemorrhage and substantially greater direct tissue injury overall and greater extravascular sequestration of free fluid. Blunt trauma is more

XII

likely to include some degree of TBI, which is thought to be exquisitely sensitive to episodes of hypotension [28]. In such cases, the rationale for i.v. fluid infusions is much stronger and they continue to be recommended by many practitioners for such circumstances [27]. However, some would also argue that the observation of hypotension may simply be a surrogate variable for a more severely injured patient [25, 26]. Patients with polytrauma can also have distinct vascular injuries that are subject to some of the same concerns held for those with penetrating injuries. Creation of a secondary bleed following fluid infusions may also worsen the outcome, even with severe head injuries [20]. Controlled experimental evidence supports the notion that if there is concurrent on-going uncontrolled hemorrhage, early infusions of i.v. fluids are still detrimental in head injury, especially early and aggressive bolus doses [20]. One theory is that early fluid resuscitation in the prehospital stage of therapy may dislodge early soft clot formation before a more stable fibrinous clot has a chance to form [20]. This construct is consistent with the notion that soft clots may not tolerate higher pressures until fibrin deposition occurs, a process thought to occur about a half-hour into the clotting process. Therefore, future research initiatives should not only stratify patients with blunt trauma and those with severe head injury, but also the timing and rate of fluid infusions.

With respect to fluid type, it has been argued that early colloid infusion or even hypertonic saline infusions may be a better choice of fluid in the prehospital arena considering that they may be associated with smaller volumes of fluid [17, 24, 29]. Also, products such as hypertonic saline may have anti-inflammatory properties [26, 29]. This attribute may be advantageous in severe polytrauma, a process that can be associated with massive soft tissue injury and subsequent massive inflammatory response. However, to date, data have not fully documented an outcome difference with the use of hypertonic saline, including a recent major multicenter trial of hypertonic saline sponsored by the U.S. National Institutes of Health [29].

Although perhaps an over-simplified interpretation of the data, the evolving evidence is leaning away from early prehospital fluid resuscitation, unless bleeding can be readily controlled [23, 25–27]. Likewise, similar considerations would also apply to non-traumatic internal hemorrhage threats, such as aortic disruption or active gastrointestinal bleeding. Nevertheless, studies have also suggested that blood or fluid administration may be of value in patients with 'severe circulatory compromise' (i.e., mean systemic arterial blood pressure [MAP] < 40 mmHg). Patients with such a degree of hypotension typically present without a measurable SBP and are usually unconscious [9, 18, 19, 27]. Considering the grim outlook for these patients (airway obstruction, tension pneumothorax, cardiac tamponade, single vessel hemorrhage), rapid fluid infusion might be empirically reasonable [27]. In practice, the few survivors of prehospital loss of pulse are limited to those patients with anatomically discrete injuries (airway, aorta, heart) for whom rapid resuscitation is combined with equally rapid control of the underlying etiology [30, 31].

Post-trauma Airway and Ventilatory Management

While endotracheal intubation is considered the 'gold standard' definitive airway, several studies, including a controlled clinical trial in a pediatric population, have now suggested a detrimental effect or, at least, no significant advantage to prehospital endotracheal intubation [32–34]. In the controlled (33.5 month) trial of 830 children (age 12 years or younger), neurological outcomes were not significantly different for 92 of 404 (23 %) children receiving bag-valve-mask (BVM) devices versus 85 of 416 (20 %) receiving prehospital endotracheal intubation [34]. In another case-control study of severely head injured patients receiving endotracheal intubation facilitated by rapid sequence induction (RSI), outcomes were worse for patients receiving the procedure versus those with similar injuries not receiving it [33]. Also, in deference to other studies indicating a survival advantage to prehospital endotracheal intubation in post-trauma circulatory arrest, endotracheal intubation has been associated with increased mortality in other studies [30–32]. In view of these studies, one could even argue that there is no strong support for endotracheal intubation in terms of survival advantage, despite the intuitive value of performing it in critically ill and injured patients [12]. However, the problem may not be the endotracheal tube in itself, but the way in which it is used, including prehospital practitioners being facile at placement and the ensuing techniques of ventilatory support once endotracheal intubation has been performed [12, 13, 26, 30].

Most trauma patients do not require invasive airway management, but the most severely injured patients, those with very profound hemorrhagic states or obtunding TBI, are classic candidates [16, 33]. Endotracheal intubation would be provided not only to ensure adequate oxygenation and ventilation (carbon dioxide elimination), but also to protect the airway from rapid edema formation or aspiration of blood or gastric contents. In that sense, endotracheal intubation traditionally has been part of the clinical portfolio for prehospital care personnel [12]. However, although endotracheal intubation may be considered the definitive airway, in view of the aforementioned studies, it has become a controversial topic in recent years, particularly with the universal proliferation of advanced life support personnel (paramedics).

The number of paramedics in an EMS agency may affect skills performance [12]. The skill of endotracheal intubation requires not only proper initial training, but also multiple opportunities to provide the intervention to retain the skill, especially in the uncontrolled circumstances encountered in the prehospital setting where multiple challenges abound, such as bright ambient light, awkward positioning, hypopharyngeal blood and vomitus and portability of only rudimentary equipment. The original EMS systems were staffed by a core team of skilled physicians or a core cadre of paramedics who were focused on the relatively smaller group of critically ill patients [2,3]. In turn, skills utilization was frequent and, accordingly, endotracheal intubation performance was quite strong and routinely successful [12]. However, in the U.S. and other locales, a popular philosophy evolved in the 1970s that more paramedics in a system would provide trauma victims closer proximity to advanced prehospital care. As a result, there was also a resulting dilution of skills utilization. With a larger pool of advanced providers who must compete for the opportunity to attempt endotracheal intubation in the relatively small number of patients who require the procedure, skills experience is much less frequent and has led to less expedient or common occurrence of failed intubation [12, 34–36]. Thus, with evolving data demonstrating this phenomenon of skills-based failure to intubate successfully, there has been a growing sentiment among EMS system medical directors in the U.S. and other similar paramedic-based systems of care that endotracheal intubation is a relatively deleterious intervention in the prehospital setting. This has become particularly

XII

weighted when considering the relative risks of paralytics and sedative drugs to facilitate endotracheal intubation in the TBI patient and concomitant delays if endotracheal intubation is not performed rapidly and adeptly [12, 33, 34, 37]. With recent development of alternative airways such as the laryngeal airway mask, King airway and Combitube, the pressure to perform endotracheal intubation has lessened more than ever.

Even when prehospital practitioners are facile at endotracheal intubation and achieve successful tube placement, endotracheal intubation may actually lead to more harm if the practitioners' ventilatory practices are improper. In many venues, prehospital providers have been demonstrated to overzealously ventilate the patient once an endotracheal tube has been placed [12, 13]. Overzealous, or even relatively controlled ventilation (tidal volume and rate) with positive pressure breaths, can have a profound deleterious effect, especially in the bleeding patient who has experienced significant intravascular volume loss [13, 26]. Although relatively infrequent positive pressure breaths can maintain adequate oxygenation and ventilation in such fragile patients and even correlate with improved outcomes, even 'normal' rates of ventilation can be relatively harmful and likely lethal in extremis conditions [13, 30]. Therefore, endotracheal intubation may often be an appropriate intervention in the prehospital setting, but it can also be detrimental if the system is not designed to enhance skills for the practitioners and if they are not controlling the delivery of positive pressure ventilation [13, 31–37].

Prehospital Interventions for Cardiopulmonary Resuscitation

Defibrillation, Rescue Breathing and Basic Cardiopulmonary Resuscitation (CPR)

As previously discussed, considerable advances in lifesaving have been documented in terms of out-of-hospital interventions for cardiac arrest, particularly in terms of rapid on-scene defibrillation [2–5,7]. For example, a study was conducted at the airports in Chicago (USA) to evaluate the value of placing automated external defibrillator (AED) devices in public settings for use by bystanders, including those with no duty to act [7]. That investigation not only confirmed the safety and facile use of this prehospital intervention and that bystanders, without duty to act, would retrieve and operate it very rapidly, but it also demonstrated a profound lifesaving effect. In the first year of study alone, all persons collapsing in the ticket counter and gate areas with cardiac arrest were found to have VF and every single person survived, neurologically-intact [7]. Moreover, in contrast to traditional EMS experiences following paramedic defibrillation in which survivors often remain in coma for several hours (or even days) following resuscitation, almost every one of these survivors was waking prior to arrival of traditional EMS responders. In turn, this scenario diminished the need for critical care interventions, such as mechanical ventilation and other related interventions, thus diminishing the immediate requirement for high-end critical care resources. This noteworthy publication demonstrated a compelling principle that 'the earlier the intervention, the better the results'. It not only confirmed the corollary that a 'gram of the right prehospital care will save a kilogram of ICU care', but it also documented the remarkable potential for reversibility of one of the most common causes of death worldwide. Clearly, this prehospital intervention was shown to be both 'elemental' and resource-sparing at the same time. Similar experiences, in terms of eliminating the need for endotracheal intubation and mechanical ventilation, have been found with the prehospital application of continuous positive airway pressure (CPAP) for persons with congestive heart failure and acute onset of pulmonary edema formation.

Unfortunately, many other longstanding interventions applied in the prehospital setting for cardiac arrest may now be seen as being detrimental, particularly the traditional approaches to rescue breathing. The classic triad of 'ABC' (airway, breathing, circulation) has been emphasized for nearly three decades in numerous textbooks of resuscitative management, but, over the past decade, the 'breathing' component has been re-appraised [10, 13]. Current consensus guidelines have supported a renewed focus on minimally interrupted chest compressions and de-emphasized rescuer ventilation altogether [38, 39]. The concept here is to maintain the key determinant for return of spontaneous circulation (ROSC), namely adequate coronary artery perfusion pressure, without interruption [38–40]. Current studies show that when hands come off the chest (i.e., when chest compressions are interrupted in order to give rescue breathes, change rescuers, assess for a pulse or whatever), coronary perfusion pressure rapidly falls off, and it takes many seconds to build up the pressure head again [40]. Accordingly, if one stops for too long an interval (and too often) to provide rescue breaths, pulse assessments or delivery of a shock, the average coronary perfusion pressure calculated over a minute is dramatically diminished and, thus, resuscitation efforts become incompatible with ROSC [38–40]. On the other hand, if the compressions are maintained without interruption, a reasonable minute coronary perfusion pressure may be maintained, increasing the chances of ROSC and ultimate survival with intact neurological status.

Based on intuitive thinking, one might worry about desaturation of the arterial bloodstream without intermittent rescue breaths. However, under the conditions of markedly slow circulation during CPR attempts, the arterial bloodstream can stay fairly well-saturated for a few minutes, such as in the case of a sudden VF cardiac death [10, 39, 41]. With the obvious caveat of cardiac arrest presumably attributable to a respiratory compromise or a rapidly failing heart (with evolving cardiac shock and/or pulmonary edema), sudden circulatory arrest due to unexpected onset of VF should be associated with fully saturated arterial red blood cells (RBCs) at the time of onset of the sudden collapse [10, 39, 41]. Still, even if RBC desaturation did begin to occur, some investigators would argue that continuous delivery of even low content oxygen and lower oxygen tensions (relatively desaturated RBCs) is much more important in terms of achieving ROSC than a markedly interrupted flow of RBCs, even if 100 % saturated [38, 41]. Recent studies, although not yet confirmed with a gold standard controlled clinical trial, provide compelling evidence that providing minimally-interrupted chest compressions without rescue breathing, even after EMS arrival, affords significant survival advantages [38].

At the same time, as in the case of trauma patients, positive pressure ventilation, regardless of the inspired oxygen fraction carries its own detrimental effects on circulation [13]. Again, overzealous ventilation in a low-flow (e.g., CPR in this case) can be very deleterious [12, 13]. Even if the patient achieves ROSC, overzealous ventilation can mask pulses, impede or reverse the resuscitative effort [13, 42]. Some studies have documented that paramedics and other prehospital care responders have delivered overzealous ventilation, even when specifically trained to provide much slower rates [33, 42]. Also, as noted in the case of trauma resus-

XII

citation, less experienced providers may interrupt chest compressions too much in their attempts to place the tube in the trachea when they are less than facile. In turn, many resuscitative guidelines thus recommend that endotracheal intubation be deferred in the early stages of cardiac resuscitation [38]. Despite the concerns, however, endotracheal intubation is still the gold standard for airway control and protection, let alone controlled ventilatory procedures. One could still argue that (at some point in the resuscitation), endotracheal intubation is still the definitive airway and thus 'elemental' in prehospital resuscitation (as indicated). Nevertheless, prolonged attempts by less experienced care providers and/or overzealous ventilation following endotracheal intubation in the 'heat of action' may also be quite detrimental [12, 13, 33, 42].

The Quality of CPR and CPR Adjuncts

Although it is now clear that getting back to the basics of performing minimally interrupted CPR (chest compressions) is a paramount focus in restoring spontaneous circulation (and ultimate long-term survival with intact neurological status), one must also focus on the quality of the CPR [39, 41, 43–45]. Studies over the last decade have not only determined that chest compressions were interrupted too often but that there also is frequent inadequacy of the depth and rate of compressions as well as improper performance of basic CPR that does not allow enough thoracic recoil to occur [43–45]. At the same time, there also is evolving evidence to suggest that compressions can be delivered too fast. Even with well-performed CPR, if the rate of compressions is excessive, this may be associated with diminished survival chances. Once again, a critical (elemental) prehospital intervention, if not taught appropriately or implemented properly, can be systematically detrimental [5, 6, 13, 33, 36].

This concern leads to a renewed focus on adjuncts that might improve blood flow even further [46–50]. Many devices have already been approved for use by governmental product regulators, including the U.S. Food and Drug Administration (FDA), for use in cardiac arrest, even prior to definitive clinical trials [46–48]. One of these devices, the impedance threshold device (ITD), had been supported by compelling evidence both in the laboratory and clinical environment, but the results of a recent multicenter, controlled clinical trial did not support such a conclusion [48]. Still, the ITD was not found to be harmful and in another study, in which the ITD was combined with an active compression-decompression device (ACD), there was a demonstrable life-saving effect [49]. Whether this positive effect was due to the ITD and ACD combined or the ACD alone is not clear [46, 48–50].

As another example, the so-called "AutoPulse" device has been extremely impressive in terms of preliminary experience, but mixed results (including both positive and negative effects) in clinical trials and its attendant costs have hindered its widespread acceptance [46, 47]. Similarly, the so-called LUCAS and LifeStat devices have held great promise, but most clinicians and researchers are awaiting more confirmatory trials [46]. These recent findings do reflect some of the reasons why it is difficult to definitively conclude on the value of some interventions and, in turn, justify their use and cost. Often there are unrecognized detrimental confounding variables that may mask the actual effectiveness of a resuscitative intervention, even when the 'definitive' multicenter trial appears to be well-designed [13].

XII

Interestingly, however, if these devices do dramatically improve flow, then, physiologically, it may be incumbent upon rescuers to provide an increased number of intermittent rescue breaths given the concept that 'ventilation should match perfusion'. If perfusion (flow) is extremely low, there is a lesser need for matching ventilation, but if flow is high, there may be a greater need for ventilation [13, 41]. Again, these are the kinds of considerations that must be entertained as new interventions are considered for use in the prehospital emergency care and resuscitative arena.

Conclusion

Over the past four decades, many resuscitative interventions have been adopted for a plethora of emergency medical conditions occurring in the out-of-hospital setting. Many of those resuscitative interventions are now specifically provided on-scene in that 'prehospital' clinical arena and, in some cases, they have been demonstrated to be profoundly life-saving, markedly diminishing both morbidity and mortality. Moreover, in many cases, data have indicated that the earlier the intervention is provided, the better the results will be. Furthermore, they indicate that a small degree of properly-applied prehospital care will obviate a tremendous amount of in-hospital care requirements and concomitant advanced-level ICU resource utilization. However, it has also been demonstrated that certain early interventions that may be helpful in one set of circumstances, may actually be detrimental in other scenarios, even among similar-appearing conditions. Likewise, some procedures that have been correlated with good outcomes may also be very harmful if not implemented in the right setting or if they are used improperly. Concomitantly, some prehospital resuscitative interventions that actually may be truly-effective lifesaving modalities, may not be demonstrated as being advantageous because of some unrecognized confounding variables that may mask the positive effect of those modalities during clinical trials.

References

1. Pantridge JF, Geddes JF (1967) A mobile intensive-care unit in the management of myocardial infarction. Lancet 2: 271–273
2. Cobb LA, Alvarez H, Copass MK (1976) A rapid response system for out-of-hospital cardiac emergencies. Med Clin North Am 60: 283–290
3. McManus WF, Tresch DD, Darin JC (1977) An effective prehospital emergency system. J Trauma 17: 304–310
4. Eisenberg M, Bergner L, Hallstrom A (1979) Paramedic programs and out-of-hospital cardiac arrest: I. Factors associated with successful resuscitation. Am J Public Health 69: 30–38
5. Pepe PE, Mattox KL, Duke JH (1993) Effect of full-time specialized physician supervision on the success of a large, urban emergency medical services system. Crit Care Med 21: 1279–1286
6. Pepe PE, Copass MK, Fowler RL, Racht EM (2009) Medical direction of emergency medical services systems. In: Cone DC, Fowler R, O'Connor RE (eds) Emergency Medical Services: Clinical Practice and Systems Oversight. Kendall-Hunt Publications, Dubuque, IA, pp 22–52
7. Caffrey SL, Willoughby PJ, Pepe, PE, Becker LB (2002) Public use of automated defibrillators. N Engl J Med 347: 1242–1247
8. Olasveengen TM, Sunde K, Brunborg C, et al (2009) Intravenous drug administration during out-of-hospital cardiac arrest. JAMA 302: 2222–2229

XII

9. Bickell WH, Wall MJ, Pepe PE, et al (1994) Immediate versus delayed fluid resuscitation for hypotensive patients with penetrating torso injuries. N Engl J Med 331: 1105–1109
10. Becker LB, Berg RA, Pepe PE, et al (1997) A reappraisal of mouth-to-mouth ventilation during bystander-initiated cardiopulmonary resuscitation. Resuscitation 35: 189–201
11. Pepe PE, Fowler R, Roppolo L, Wigginton J 2004) Re-appraising the concept of immediate defibrillatory attempts for out-of-hospital ventricular fibrillation. Crit Care 8: 41–45
12. Wigginton JG, Benitez FL, Pepe PE (2005) Endotracheal intubation in the field: caution needed. Hospital Medicine 66: 91–94
13. Roppolo LP, Wigginton JG, Pepe PE (2004). Emergency ventilatory management as a detrimental factor in resuscitation practices and clinical research efforts. In: Vincent JL (ed) Yearbook of Intensive Care and Emergency Medicine, Springer-Verlag, Heidelberg, pp 139–151
14. Wiggers C (1950) Physiology of Shock. Commonwealth Fund, New York, USA, pp 121–146
15. Shires T, Coln D, Carrico CJ, et al (1964) Fluid therapy in hemorrhagic shock. Arch Surg 88: 688–693
16. American College of Surgeons Committee on Trauma Chapter 3: Shock (1997) In: Advanced Trauma Life Support Program for Physicians Instructor Manual. Publication of the American College of Surgeons, Chicago, pp 97–146
17. Bickell WH, Bruttig SP, Millnamow GA, et al (1991) The detrimental effects of intravenous crystalloid after aortotomy in swine. Surgery 110: 529–536
18. Capone A, Safar P, Stezoski W, et al (1995) Improved outcome with fluid restriction in treatment of uncontrolled hemorrhagic shock. J Am Coll Surg 180: 49–56
19. Stern SA, Wang X, Mertz M, et al (2001) Under-resuscitation of near-lethal uncontrolled hemorrhage: effects on mortality and end-organ function at 72 hours. Shock 15: 16–23
20. Stern SA, Zink BJ, Mertz M, Wang Z, Dronen SC (2000) Effect of initially limited resuscitation in a combined model of fluid-percussion brain injury and severe uncontrolled hemorrhagic shock. J Neurosurg 93: 305–314
21. Dutton RP, Mackenzie CF, Scalea T (2002) Hypotensive resuscitation during active hemorrhage: impact on in-hospital mortality. J Trauma 52: 1141–1146
22. Owens TM, Watson WC, Prough DS, et al (1995) Limiting initial resuscitation of uncontrolled hemorrhage reduces internal bleeding and subsequent volume requirements. J Trauma 39: 200–207
23. Mapstone J, Roberts I, Evans P (2003) Fluid resuscitation strategies: a systematic review of animal trials J Trauma 55: 571–589
24. Rafie AD, Rath PA, Michell MW, et al (2004) Hypotensive resuscitation of multiple hemorrhages using crystalloid and colloids. Shock 22: 262–269
25. Holcomb JB, Jenkins D, Rhee P, et al (2007) Damage control resuscitation: directly addressing the early coagulopathy of trauma. J Trauma 62: 307–310
26. Roppolo LP, Wigginton JG, Pepe PE (2011) Advances in resuscitative trauma care. Minerva Anestesiologica 77: 993–1002
27. Pepe PE, Mosesso VN Jr, Falk JL (2002) Prehospital fluid resuscitation of the patient with major trauma. Prehosp Emerg Care 6: 81–91
28. Chesnut RM, Marshall LF, Klauber MR, et al (1993) The role of secondary brain injury in determining outcome from severe head injury J Trauma 34: 216–222
29. Bulger EM, May S, Brasel K, et al (2010) Out-of-hospital hypertonic resuscitation following severe traumatic brain injury: a randomized controlled trial JAMA 304: 1455–1464
30. Pepe PE, Swor RA, Ornato JP, et al (2001) Resuscitation in the out-of-hospital setting: medical futility criteria for on-scene pronouncement of death. Prehosp Emerg Care 5: 79–87
31. Durham LA, Richardson RJ, Wall MJ, Pepe PE, Mattox KL (1992) Emergency center thoracotomy: Impact of prehospital resuscitation. J Trauma 32: 775–779
32. Eckstein M, Chan L, Schneir A, Palmer R (2000) The effect of prehospital advanced life support on outcomes of major trauma patients. J Trauma 48: 643–648
33. Davis DP, Hoyt DB, Ochs M, et al (2003) The effect of paramedic rapid sequence intubation on outcome in patients with severe traumatic brain injury. J Trauma 54: 444–453
34. Gausche M, Lewis RJ, Stratton S, et al (2000) Effect of out-of-hospital pediatric endotracheal intubation on survival and neurological outcome. JAMA 283: 783–790

XII

35. Stout J, Pepe PE, Mosesso VN (2000) All-advanced life support vs. tiered-response ambulance systems. Prehosp Emerg Care 4: 1–6

36. Persse DE, Key CB, Bradley RN, Miller CC, Dhingra A (2003) Cardiac arrest survival as a function of ambulance deployment strategy in a large urban emergency medical services system. Resuscitation 59: 97–104

37. Wang HE, Peitzman AB, Cassidy LD, et al (2004) Out-of-hospital endotracheal intubation and outcome after traumatic brain injury. Ann Emerg Med 44: 439–450

38. Bobrow BJ, Clark LL, Ewy GA, et al (2008) Minimally interrupted cardiac resuscitation by emergency medical services for out-of-hospital cardiac arrest. JAMA 299: 1158–1165

39. Sayre MR, Berg RA, Cave DM, Page RL, Potts J, White RD (2008) Hands-only (compression-only) cardiopulmonary resuscitation: a call to action for bystander response to adults who experience out-of-hospital sudden cardiac arrest. Circulation 117: 2162–2167

40. Koster RW (2003) Limiting 'hands-off' periods during resuscitation. Resuscitation 58: 275–276

41. Roppolo LP, Pepe PE, Bobrow BJ (2010) The role of gasping in resuscitation. In: Vincent JL (ed) The Yearbook of Intensive Care and Emergency Medicine. Springer-Verlag, Heidelberg, pp 83–95

42. Aufderheide TP, Sigurdsson G, Pirrallo RG, et al (2004) Hyperventilation-induced hypotension during cardiopulmonary resuscitation. Circulation 109: 1960–1965

43. Wik L, Kramer-Johansen J, Myklebust H, et al (2005) Quality of cardiopulmonary resuscitation during out-of-hospital cardiac arrest. JAMA 293: 299–304

44. Abella BS, Alvarado JP, Myklebust H, et al (2005) Quality of cardiopulmonary resuscitation after in-hospital cardiac arrest. JAMA 293: 305–310

45. Aufderheide TP, Pirallo RG, Yannopoulos D, et al (2005) Incomplete chest wall compressions: a clinical evaluation of CPR performance by EMS personnel and assessment of alternate manual chest compression-decompression techniques. Resuscitation 64: 353–362

46. Wigginton JL, Miller AH, Benitez FL, et al (2005) Mechanical devices for cardiopulmonary resuscitation. Curr Opin Crit Care 11: 219–223.

47. Hallstrom A, Rea TD, Sayre MR, Christenson J, et al (2006) Manual chest compression vs. use of an automated chest compression device during resuscitation following out-of-hospital cardiac arrest: a randomized trial. JAMA 295: 2620–2628

48. Aufderheide TP, Nichol G, Rea TD, et al (2011) A trial of an impedance threshold device in out-of-hospital cardiac arrest. N Engl J Med 365: 798–806

49. Aufderheide TP, Frascone RJ, Wayne MA, et al (2011) Standard cardiopulmonary resuscitation versus active compression-decompression cardiopulmonary resuscitation with augmentation of negative intrathoracic pressure for out-of-hospital cardiac arrest: a randomised trial. Lancet 377: 301–311

50. Plaisance P, Lurie KG, Vicaut E, et al (1999) A comparison of standard cardiopulmonary resuscitation and active compression-decompression resuscitation for out-of-hospital cardiac arrest. N Engl J Med 341: 569–575

XII

Afferent Limb of Rapid Response System Activation

J. Moore, M. Hravnak, and M.R. Pinsky

Introduction

Fundamental to the implementation of a functional rapid response system for the treatment of hospitalized patients is the identification of instability by the bedside caregivers who must activate the alert. This afferent limb of the rapid response system has the primary goal of crisis detection and is, therefore, the essential first element of effective rapid response system operations. More specifically, its purpose is the early recognition of 'emergent unmet patient needs', defined as mismatches between the care a patient is receiving and the care that patient immediately requires [1]. The afferent limb has the unique challenge of moving from its inception point, characterized by the clinical surveillance of all hospital inpatients during their admission, to its distinct endpoint of efferent limb activation of a rescue response for specific patients at specific times during their hospital stay. It may even be speculated that the inability for any trial to demonstrate that the application of a rapid response system definitively decreases mortality [2] may lie with failures to adequately monitor patients for instability, recognize instability once it occurs, and decide to make the call to escalate care – all components of the rapid response system afferent arm. In order to meet this challenge to safely and effectively rescue unstable patients, those wishing to design and maintain a timely, effective and efficient afferent limb of a rapid response system must address three components. These components are: 1) A set of objective and quantifiable criteria for triggering activation of the efferent limb that are both sensitive and specific for true instability; 2) human and technological monitoring or tracking of patients so as to detect when triggering criteria are met; and 3) a communication mechanism by which the efferent limb is activated. Below, we discuss these three components, review current barriers that threaten the proper functioning of the afferent limb and identify new and developing ways of overcoming these barriers.

Triggering Criteria

In order for a rapid response system to successfully identify a patient crisis, a set of clinical 'triggering' or 'crisis' criteria must be established. The rationale for instituting such criteria is based on the observation that most patients have quantifiable clinical antecedents that demonstrate cardiopulmonary instability prior to full cardiac arrest [3]. These criteria are generally objective in nature; however subjective clinical assessments, including staff concern or worry, are also used

J.-L. Vincent (ed.), *Annual Update in Intensive Care and Emergency Medicine 2012*
DOI 10.1007/978-3-642-25716-2 © Springer-Verlag Berlin Heidelberg 2012

Box 1. Bedside trigger criteria for rapid response system activation

Respiratory
- Rate < 8 or > 36/min
- New onset difficulty breathing
- Pulse oximeter (SpO_2) < 85 % for more than 5 minutes (unless patient is known to have chronic hypoxemia)
- New requirement for > 50 % oxygen to keep SpO_2 > 85 %

Heart Rate
- < 40 or > 140/min with new symptoms; or any rate > 160/min

Blood Pressure
- Systolic blood pressure < 80 OR > 200 mmHg or diastolic blood pressure > 110 mmHg with symptoms (neurologic change, chest pain, difficulty breathing)

Acute Neurological Change
- Acute loss of consciousness
- New onset lethargy or difficulty walking
- Sudden collapse,
- Seizure (outside of seizure monitoring unit)
- Sudden loss of movement (or weakness) of face, arm or leg

Other
- More than 1 STAT PAGE required to assemble team needed to respond to a crisis
- patient complaint of (cardiac) chest pain, (unresponsive to nitroglycerine, or MD unavailable)
- Skin color change (of patient or extremity): Pale, dusky, gray or blue
- Unexplained agitation more than 10 minutes
- Suicide attempt
- Uncontrolled bleeding
- Bleeding into airway
- Naloxone use without immediate response
- Large acute blood loss
- Crash cart must be used for rapid delivery of medications

within the afferent limb to complement objective data. Ideally, triggering criteria can be used by any hospital personnel, including nurses, physicians, and other clinical or non-clinical hospital staff. Hospital-wide acceptance and use of these criteria eliminates the need for additional calls to senior physicians to make emergent treatment or triage decisions and reduces the adverse consequences of erroneous interpretation of patient data. Overall, these criteria serve to eliminate unnecessary delays in efferent arm activation. **Box 1** lists the rapid response system activation criteria for one medical system, although the general structure of this list is common to all rapid response system criteria.

Objective criteria used in triggering systems use data obtained from the vital signs of heart rate, blood pressure, respiratory rate, and peripheral oxygen saturation by pulse oximetry, and some also use temperature, urine output and reduced consciousness, and at times temperature. Triggering criteria are often developed based upon existing risk-prediction of single trigger models [4]. Well known risk-prediction models such as Acute Physiology and Chronic Health Evaluation (APACHE) and Simplified Acute Physiology Score (SAPS) are poorly suited for routine use in the afferent limb of a rapid response system because they are difficult to use quickly at the bedside for dynamic vital sign changes, and they are only designed for risk prediction upon admission. The more recently devel-

XII

oped Modified Early Warning Score (MEWS) is a well validated model that has only five clinical variables, but assigns a weighted score for each variable with respect to degree of departure from 'normal', which are then added to develop a single composite score with a threshold for triggering a call. MEWS has been shown to predict an increased risk of death [5], but although superior to other risk-prediction models for the purpose of efferent limb activation, the MEWS model still requires clinical staff to utilize the model and calculate the score for a given patient. This process takes a significant amount of time and is not always practical on a busy hospital ward, and has been associated with low utilization rates [6]. 'Single trigger' activation systems, although not as sensitive and specific in risk-prediction, have the advantage of requiring only one unaltered or manipulated criterion to quickly initiate a rapid response system response [3]. However, accepting subjective clinical judgment is also considered an appropriate indication for efferent limb activation, and may empower staff to call for help sooner, improve staff morale, and be an effective complement to objective data. Efferent limb activation often leads to improvements in patient care even if the response team ultimately determines that no emergent patient need exists.

There is debate regarding which vital sign numeric thresholds, be they a part of single-parameter or aggregated early warning scores, are 'best' at identifying patients at risk of deterioration, because they have generally evolved based primarily upon expert clinical opinion. [4, 7, 8, 9]. Additionally, these thresholds are based on their statistical likelihood association with a retrospectively evaluated untoward event, such as prediction of death or requirement for ICU admission, and do not accommodate those patients who were unstable but rescued prior to the negative event.

Recently, Tarrassenko et al. [10] used a different approach to develop an early warning system simply based on the statistical properties of vital signs in hospitalized patients, irrespective of a later instability state. They utilized data from 863 acutely ill patients with 64,622 hours of continuously acquired vital sign data acquired from bedside monitors to develop normalized histograms (unit area under the curve) and cumulative distribution functions for each of four vital signs: Heart rate, respiratory rate, peripheral oxygen saturation by pulse oximetry, and systolic blood pressure (SBP). From these curves and distributions they determined distribution centiles, and an alerting system based on these centiles. For example, an Early Warning Score of 3 is associated with vital signs of which the distances from the mean of the distribution are between the 99th and 100th centiles, a score of 2 for values between the 95th and 99th centiles, a score of 1 for values between the $90 - 95^{th}$ centiles, and normal or a zero score for values below the 90th centile. The scoring system then aggregates the centile-based scores of each of the four vital sign parameters to develop a single aggregated score to serve as the trigger. Such a system has the advantage of identifying departure from normality at the present time, and not based on the likelihood of a future event. However, this centile-based early warning score has yet to be tested.

Combining demographic variables with dynamic physiologic variables must also be explored in the development of triggering systems. For example, age [11] and the number of pre-existing comorbid conditions have both been shown to be positively associated with instability prediction. Thus taking these 'static' characteristics into account [12] when evaluating the dynamic clinical condition may also be helpful in developing improved prediction models.

Recent advancements in monitoring technology may result in changes in the development of trigger criteria and in the afferent limb itself. Electronic integrated monitoring systems, such as the Visensia® system, are being actively studied to determine their utility within the afferent limb. In addition to alerting the clinician to patient abnormalities meeting response arm trigger criteria, these systems can also alert the clinician to more complex abnormalities of multiple clinical variables that indicate developing physiologic instability. These multivariable abnormalities often present in patterns and may exist without any one variable meeting current efferent arm trigger thresholds. Ultimately, these systems may result in a paradigm shift in developing trigger criteria.

Human and Technological Monitoring

The most complex aspect of the afferent arm involves monitoring of the large number of hospital inpatients and the data associated with them. The term 'technological monitoring' refers to our use of technology to view and record patient data, while 'human monitoring' refers to the cognitive process that is central to interpretation of patient data and abnormality detection. Hospital areas using current monitoring systems have many advantages over those areas without monitoring capability. On these monitored floors, nurses have completed additional training to be able to recognize abnormalities on the monitor more easily. Along with junior physicians and medical trainees, these nurses serve as the front-line caregivers for their patients, and they are often the first to identify clinical deterioration. The monitoring systems themselves non-invasively measure and record vital signs individually and then display these variables on one screen. Alarms alert the clinical staff of any variable that is outside a pre-determined range, improving nursing efficiency by allowing the staff to track vital sign abnormalities without being constantly at the bedside. Significant abnormalities can be recognized quickly and easily by the clinical staff in this way, and when used in the setting of an existing set of trigger criteria, the efferent arm of the rapid response system can subsequently be activated.

Although current systems have many advantages, there are several limitations as well. Technological limitations often stem from problems with patient identification, monitor accuracy, and system oversight. It is difficult to determine which patients benefit from continuous monitoring and which do not, since there are no data for any specific outcome that differentiate between the two groups. In addition, shortages of monitored hospital beds and qualified nursing resources limit the number of patients who can receive monitored care. Artifacts occur on the monitor frequently and typically arise from various system, staff, and patient related sources including removal of monitoring devices or faulty monitor hardware. The large number of false alarms caused by artifact can lower the sense of urgency felt at the bedside by the clinical staff and can ultimately worsen response time to such alerts. Alarms may also inappropriately call attention if alarm limits are set tighter than need be for true clinical concern. This over-alerting of staff engenders a state of 'alarm fatigue', which desensitizes them to true instability events and impairs patient safety [13, 14]. Proper human oversight of monitored data is another difficulty with the current system. Patient data displays may not always be positioned so that they can be readily seen by bedside nurses. Such information is often forwarded to a central site where there are no dedicated

XII

personnel responsible for data interpretation. Nurse-to-patient ratios in monitored areas may be no different from the high ratios on unmonitored floors, and additional responsibilities taken on by nurse caregivers may prevent prompt evaluation of monitor alarms.

Hravnak et al. [15] examined the ability of bedside nurses trained in rapid response system activation to identify and activate the rapid response system using traditional bedside non-invasive monitoring and routine periodic visual inspection in a medical-surgical step-down unit. These authors collected data on all 323 patients monitored on that unit over a 6-week interval. In this prospective blinded observational study, three aspects of the step-down patient population were demonstrated. First, most (approximately 75 %) of the patients in a monitored step-down unit were stable for the duration of their unit stay. Second, patients who were unstable were so only for very short intervals, and many bouts of severe cardiorespiratory insufficiency occurred without bedside nursing staff being aware. Lastly, the instability that developed rarely manifested as acute collapse, but rather as a progressive deterioration and then recovery such that unstable patients had episodes of stability interspaced with cardiovascular crisis. Since instability occurs only infrequently and often is bordered by periods of relative stability, direct intermittent patient observation is a highly inefficient and insensitive means by which to detect existing or developing cardiorespiratory insufficiency. These findings underscore the problems faced in afferent limb activation based on existing monitoring approaches.

One final technological limitation that is addressed less often is the inability of monitoring systems to assess more than one clinical variable at a time. These systems are designed to measure several vital signs individually. Monitors will alarm when a particular vital sign reaches a critical value, but they do not have the capability to synthesize these data to evaluate multiple variables as a single group. It is possible, therefore, for several variables to worsen without setting off a monitor alarm as long as no individual variable meets alarm criteria. This approach will miss patients with more gradual or subtle cardiovascular deterioration and may ultimately delay appropriate patient care.

XII

Integrated Monitoring Systems

The development of electronic integrated monitoring systems with the ability to synthesize patient data into a single marker of physiologic instability may reduce the time for deteriorating patients to be identified and treated. The Visensia system is one such system that is designed to detect these patterns using non-invasive monitoring devices and synthesizing physiologic data from patients to develop a single neural-networked score called the Visensia Index (VSI). Studies have shown that a VSI of ≥ 3 represents patient deterioration and that a VSI elevation precedes cardiorespiratory instability by as much as 6 hours in some patients [15, 16]. Although the effect on overall patient outcome is still unknown, the Visensia integrated monitoring systems provides an earlier and more sensitive detection of clinical instability compared to current systems and may be able to reduce efferent limb activation failures. In addition to being more sensitive, integrated monitoring systems are less subject to the high false-alarm rate seen with single channel monitoring. Using an integrated monitoring system may, therefore, reduce the number of false-alarms, be more specific for true instability, and allow nurses to be more efficient with their work. Over time, this could result in decreased hospital expense for hospital staffing outside the intensive care unit (ICU).

Using the initial medical-surgical step-down unit patient cohort as a 'calibration' training set, Hravnak et al. recalibrated the Visensia integrated monitoring system [17]. This recalibration resulted in the best receiver-operator characteristics curve with a VSI of > 3.2 representing cardiorespiratory insufficiency. They then trained the nursing staff to immediately respond to a VSI alarm (audible) representing a VSI > 3.2 and if the cause of cardiorespiratory insufficiency was not immediately correctable, to activate the integrated monitoring system. The investigators then prospectively studied the impact of this integrated monitoring system on patient cardiorespiratory instability over the next 8 weeks [17]. They defined any monitored parameters even transiently beyond local cardiorespiratory instability as concern triggers (heart rate < 40 or > 140 beats/min, respiratory rate < 8 or > 36 breaths/min, SBP < 80 or > 200 mmHg, diastolic BP [DBP] > 110 mmHg, SpO_2 < 85 %) and labeled then "INSTABILITYmin". "INSTABILITYall" was the number of times an alert was made even if the cause of the alert was a lost vital sign signal or poor signal quality. The difference between INSTABILITYall and INSTABILITYmin reflected 'false alarms' because of technical artifacts. INSTABILITYmin that was further judged as both persistent and serious defined "INSTABILITYfull". The authors then compared these directly measured physiological estimates of cardiorespiratory insufficiency to the integrated monitoring system alerts, referred to as INDEX. INDEX alert states were defined as INDEXmin and INDEXfull using the same classification. The calibration and intervention admission numbers (323 vs. 308) and monitoring hours (18,258 vs. 18,314) were similar. INDEXmin and INDEXfull correlated significantly with INSTABILITYmin and INSTABILITYfull (r = 0.713 and r = 0.815, respectively, p < 0.0001). INDEXmin occurred before INSTABILITYmin in 80 % of cases (mean advance time 9.4 ± 9.2 minutes). The calibration and intervention admission numbers were similarly likely to develop INSTABILITYmin (35 % vs. 33 %), but INSTABILITYmin duration/admission decreased from the calibration periods to the intervention interval (p = 0.018). INSTABILITYfull episodes/admission (p = 0.03), number of false alarms and INSTABILITYfull duration/admission (p = 0.05) decreased in the intervention period (**Fig. 1**).

XII

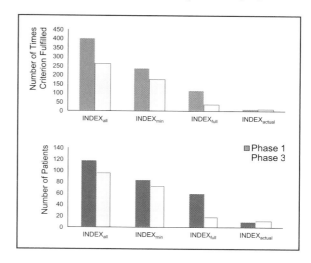

Fig. 1. Comparison of the number of times criterion for instability were fulfilled in which patients were across the thresholds of instability-concern criteria for each phase (upper panel), and the number of patients who were across the thresholds (lower panel). Data from [17]

Another aspect of monitoring is the degree to which caregivers become desensitized to the alarms and spend less time insuring that the signals that are used to define instability are accurately recorded. In essence, this effect can be considered the false alarm rate. To address this issue directly we also quantified both the total number of alerts made by the integrated monitoring system as compared to the INDEXmin values. **Figure 1** summarizes the effect of the integrated monitoring system on the number of false alarms as the difference between INSTABILITYall and INSTABILITYmin. Bedside nurses were educated about the integrated monitoring system as part of system implementation. Once they understood that the quality of the non-invasive monitoring signals was needed to drive the integrated monitoring system, the number and duration of false alarm signals decreased by 40 and 58 %, respectively. Furthermore, although the number of INDEXmin also decreased the real changes were in both the duration of time patients were in INDEXmin states and the amount and time that they were in INDEXfull. These data, although from a single study, strongly support the conclusion that our integrated monitoring system INDEX correlated significantly with cardiorespiratory instability-concern criterion, usually occurred before overt instability, and when coupled with nursing alert was associated with decreased cardiorespiratory instability-concern criterion in step-down unit patients.

The Human Aspect of Monitoring

The human aspect of monitoring involves many of the cognitive skills used in patient triage. Most importantly, these skills include the interpretation of patient data and the recognition of patterns within that data that suggest instability. An expert panel of critical care medicine experts described three models of triage in 1999 [18]. The "priority model" differentiates between patients who will benefit from ICU care and patients who will not; the "diagnosis model" lists particular diseases that require ICU management; and the "objective parameters model" lists a series of criteria indicating clinical deterioration. Although there are no data explicitly describing how triage is performed by experts, it is reasonable to say that experts in patient triage are able to recognize patterns within the clinical data of a given patient. More specifically, triage experts can use any or all of the described models to put objective patient data into context allowing for a more accurate assessment of illness severity and need for urgent care. Conversely, it is more difficult for triage novices, such as newly hired nurses, junior physicians, and medical trainees, to switch between models because they often lack the knowledge and the experience to do so. As a result, triage novices take more time to make complex clinical judgments and are more likely to make judgment errors. Criteria from the objective parameters model are particularly useful as efferent arm trigger criteria because of their measurable and specific nature and the fact that they can easily be employed by triage novices at the bedside. Interestingly, an electronic integrated monitoring system could serve to detect patterns in the clinical data of a patient much like a triage expert would. Errors in clinical judgment could be avoided and patient care expedited through integrated monitoring system use. Unfortunately, the current system typically places people with the least knowledge and experience at the bedside as primary caregivers.

The process of identification and characterization of physiologic instability by triage novices is where the technological and human aspects of monitoring intersect. When an alarm sounds, the primary caregiver must determine whether the alarm is truly reflective of patient status (not artifact) and then decide if the abnormality is clinically relevant. If the abnormality is significant, one of three scenarios generally occurs. First, the patient is in obvious distress or a monitored variable is abnormal enough to result in efferent limb activation. Next, the patient does not meet efferent limb trigger criteria but clearly needs further attention. The last and most troubling scenario is that the abnormality is not recognized as significant and the patient continues to deteriorate. In the latter two circumstances, technological innovations and an expanded role for clinical protocols may reduce unnecessary patient deterioration.

Clinical protocols are known to improve patient care in various areas of medicine. Expanding the role of similar protocols in patients with developing cardiorespiratory instability may expedite the delivery of appropriate care. Patients who trigger a monitor alarm but do not meet crisis criteria usually depend on the bedside caregiver, most generally a nurse, to determine the urgency of the situation. This task is often difficult for triage novices since it requires putting objective data into the context of the patient's disease. Clinical protocols addressing this situation may include an order set to obtain additional clinical information or suggest consultation with a triage expert. Such protocols may work most efficiently in conjunction with an electronic integrated monitoring system. Integrated monitoring systems may also prevent adverse events as a result of reducing false alarms and being a more sensitive way to detect physiologic instability. Since multiple-channel monitoring is more resistant to false alarms, caregivers at the bedside are more likely to maintain a sense of urgency for a given alert. The increased sensitivity of these systems may also result in improved recognition of instability and earlier initiation of proper care.

Communication Mechanism of Efferent Limb Activation

The final component of the afferent limb is the specific mechanism by which the efferent arm is activated. The structure of this mechanism must be immediately available and easy to use for all hospital personnel. For a mature rapid response system, the triggering apparatus may be a specific phone number, pager, or overhead call system. Notification is also accomplished by pager, overhead call, or a combination of these two methods. Developing a hospital culture that encourages activation of the rapid response system is difficult and often takes time to achieve. Barriers to efferent limb activation include lack of empowerment for bedside clinical staff including nurses and trainee doctors, lack of knowledge regarding outcome benefits for rapid response systems, and resistance to change by those clinicians practicing according to traditional norms [1]. The results of the Medical Emergency Response and Intervention Trial (MERIT) indicated that even within medical emergency team (MET) hospitals, only 30 % of patient events meeting trigger criteria resulted in MET activation [19]. It is important to reduce the burden on the caller to one call only with the established notification apparatus taking over from that point. Eliminating negative feedback and maximizing positive feedback by either verbal or written means will allow hospital staff to be more comfortable with efferent limb activation. There are many notable examples in which a well-developed response team giving appropriate positive feedback has demonstrated the benefits of rapid response systems to clinical staff in nursing units around the entire hospital system. Maintenance of this culture

XII

may be achieved by continued positive reinforcement for people activating the response team. Reminder immersion using pocket cards, phone stickers, and computer screen savers will also encourage continued use of the system. Ultimately, the goal is to have a self-propagating culture whereby the senior staff teaches the junior staff about the merits of the rapid response system and how to activate the efferent limb.

The afferent limb is given the task of the surveillance of hospital inpatients, and then challenged with the identification of patients developing even the most subtle signs of clinical decline. Although the current state of inpatient monitoring is vastly more developed than it once was, there remain many barriers to the detection of cardiopulmonary instability. Encouraging hospital employees to accept the rapid response system as a critical aspect of patient care and empowering them to become conscientious elements of the afferent limb are important steps that can be taken now to improve our crisis detection ability. Innovative tools, such as the Visensia® integrated monitoring system, with its low incidence of false positive alerts and new clinical protocols that prompt nurses to activate rapid response system activation using objective data may enhance our ability to identify and treat deteriorating patients earlier and more efficiently in the very near future.

Acknowledgement: This work was supported in part by NIH grant HL67181–06

References

1. Devita MA, Bellomo R, Hillman K, et al (2006) Findings of the First Consensus Conference on Medical Emergency Teams. Crit Care Med 34: 2463–2478
2. Jones DA, DeVita MA, Bellomo R (2011) Rapid-response teams. N Engl J Med 365: 139–146
3. Hillman K, Parr M, Flabouris A, Bishop G, Stewart A (2001) Redefining in-hospital resuscitation: The concept of the medical emergency team. Resuscitation 48: 105–110
4. Smith GB, Prytherch DR, Schmidt PE, Featherstone PI, Higgins B. (2008) A review and performance evaluation of single-parameter "track-and-trigger" systems. Resuscitation 79: 11–21
5. Subbe CP, Kruger M Rutherford P, Gemmel L (2001) Validation of a modified early warning score in medical admissions. Q J Med 2001 94: 521–526
6. Ludikhuize J, DeJonge E, Goosens A (2011) Measuring adherence among nurses one year after training in applying the Modified Early Warning Score and Situation-Background-Assessment-Recommendation instruments. Resuscitation 82: 1428–1433
7. Gao H, McDonnell A, Harrison DA, et al (2007) Systematic review and evaluation of track and trigger warning systems for identifying at-risk patients in the ward. Intensive Care Med 33: 667–679
8. Cuthbertson BH, Boroujerdi M, McKie L, Aucott L, Prescott G (2007) Can physiological variables and early warning scoring systems allow early detection of the deteriorating surgical patient? Crit Care Med 35: 402–409
9. Cuthbertson BH, Smith GB (2007) A warning on early-warning scores! Br J Anaesth 98: 704–706
10. Tarrassenko L, Clifton DA, Pinsky M, Hravnak M, Woods JR, Watkinson PJ (2011) Centile-based early warning scores derived from statistical distributions of vital signs. Resuscitation 82: 1013–1018
11. Smith GB, Prytherch DR, Schmidt PE, et al (2008) Should age be included as a component of track and trigger systems used to identify sick adult patients? Resuscitation 78: 109–115
12. Yousef K, Pinsky MR, DeVita MA, Sereika S, Hravnak M (2011) Demographic and clinical predictors of cardiorespiratory instability in a step-down unit: pilot study. Am J Crit Care (in press)

XII

13. Borowski M, Görges M, Fried R, Such O, Wrede C, Imhoff M (2011) Medical device alarms. Biomed Tech (Berl) 56: 73–83
14. Graham KC, Cvach M (2010) Monitor alarm fatigue: standardizing use of physiological monitors and decreasing nuisance alarms. Am J Crit Care 19: 28–34
15. Hravnak M, Edwards L, Clontz A, Valenta C, Devita MA, Pinsky MR (2008) Defining the incidence of cardiorespiratory instability in patients in step-down units using an electronic integrated monitoring system. Arch Intern Med 168: 1300–1308
16. Tarassenko L, Hann A, Young D (2006) Integrated Monitoring and Analysis for Early Warning of Patient Deterioration. Br J Anaesth 97: 64–68
17. Hravnak M, DeVita MA, Clontz A, Edwards L, Valenta C, Pinsky MR (2011) Cardiorespiratory instability before and after implementing an integrated monitoring system. Crit Care Med 39: 65–72
18. Task Force of the American College of Critical Care Medicine and the Society of Critical Care Medicine (1999) Guidelines for intensive care unit admission, discharge, and triage. Crit Care Med 27: 633–638
19. Hillman K, Chen J, Cretikos M, et al (2005) Introduction of the Medical Emergency Team (MET) system: A cluster-randomized controlled trial. Lancet 365: 2091–2097

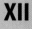

XII

Bradykinin-mediated Angioedema

B. Floccard, E. Hautin, and B. Allaouchiche

Introduction

Angioedema is a clinical syndrome characterized by transient and recurrent episodes of subcutaneous or mucosal edema that are referred to as attacks. These episodes of swelling can affect the skin, airways or digestive tract. Depending on the location, the attacks can be severe and potentially life-threatening [1]. This syndrome, which has various causes, is associated with excessive levels of bradykinin and is not an allergic reaction [2]. Although misunderstood and rare, this disease can be encountered by any intensive care unit (ICU) physician [3]. Reports from international consensus conferences have been published and specific molecules have been developed in recent years for the treatment of acute attacks [4, 5]. The aim of this article is to present the current protocols used for the emergency management of acute attacks. Pediatric cases will not be discussed because of the lack of new studies [6, 7]. Additionally, short-term prophylaxis to protect against attacks during a procedure or personal event (e.g., endoscopy, dental care, surgery and stressful everyday events) will not be discussed here [4, 5].

XII Bradykinin-Dependent Angioedema: A Clinical Syndrome, a Mediator and Multiple Causes

A Clinical Syndrome

The clinical picture of angioedema is characterized by recurrent episodes of white, soft, deforming, circumscribed, non-pruritic edema. The edema develops slowly over a period up to 36 hours, resolves spontaneously within 2 to 3 days and does not cause residual effects [8, 9]. The presence of such an episode of edema is called an attack. The clinical signs result from the topography of the edema, as these can be either isolated or in combination and can affect the skin of the torso, face, genitalia and limbs as well as the mucous membranes of the airways or the digestive tract (**Fig. 1**). About 75 % of patients will have attacks localized to the neck, face, tongue or respiratory tract, which result in voice alteration, dysphagia or a lump sensation in the throat [3, 10–12]. The mean interval between onset and maximum development of laryngeal edema is 8.3 hours [12]. About 93 % of patients will have abdominal attacks that are associated with edema of the intestinal wall (i.e., abdominal pain, diarrhea, vomiting, pseudo-obstructive syndrome, ascites and peritoneal effusion) and can result in unnecessary surgery (14 to 37 % of patients) (**Fig. 2**) [8, 10, 13–15]. In 50 % of cases,

J.-L. Vincent (ed.), *Annual Update in Intensive Care and Emergency Medicine 2012*
DOI 10.1007/978-3-642-25716-2 © Springer-Verlag Berlin Heidelberg 2012

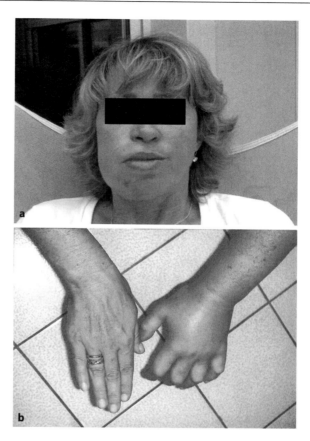

Fig. 1. Swelling in patient with hereditary angioedema. Facial attack and asymmetric swelling of the hand. From [50] with permission.

XII

patients are able to identify a trigger for their attack, such as trauma (even slight), dental care (dental extraction, scaling), stress (exams/tests), infection (urinary tract, sinusitis, dental) or hormonal changes (pills, pregnancy, menstruation) [8]. Tooth extractions without prophylaxis were followed by facial swelling and risk of laryngeal edema in 21.5 % of patients [16].

Some attacks are severe due to the localization of the swelling and may become life-threatening [6, 8]. In the absence of specific treatment, the mortality rate is 25 to 30 % [1, 8]. Therefore, all attacks localized to the neck, face, tongue, lips, pharynx or larynx must be considered severe. Even in the absence of signs of respiratory distress, these attacks should be regarded as severe because their prognosis is unpredictable; death has been found to occur within 20 minutes or several hours as a result of laryngeal edema and acute asphyxiation [11, 12]. Abdominal attacks with pain rated > 5 on the visual analog scale (VAS) are considered severe because of the risk of hypovolemic shock as a result of plasma leakage [8, 13].

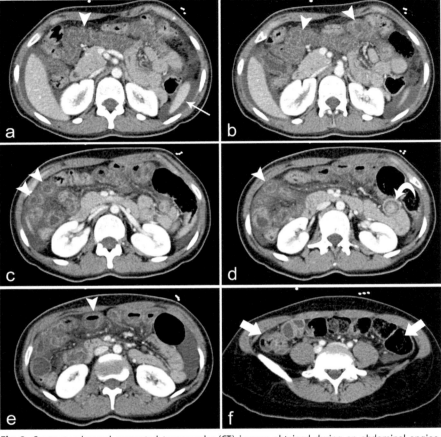

Fig. 2. Contrast-enhanced computed tomography (CT) images obtained during an abdominal angioedema attack, showing peritoneal fluid (**Fig. 2a**, thin arrow) and thickening and edema of the ileum wall (**Fig. 2a**-e, arrowheads). The jejunum was normal (**Fig. 2c**-d, arrows). At the jejuno-ileal junction, a target-like image corresponding to an intussusception was visible (**Fig. 2d**, curved arrow). The colon was normal (**Fig. 2f**, large arrow). From [15] with permission.

Bradykinin, a Mediator

Bradykinin is the key mediator of angioedema attacks. It is released following the activation of a cascade of proteases in the kallikrein-kinin pathway, which is activated by factor XII [8]. Vascular stress activates excessive contact-activated coagulation and leads to the release of large amounts of bradykinin [17]. Bradykinin will bind to specific B_2 vascular receptors, which then open intercellular junctions causing an increase in vascular permeability, plasma leakage and edema (**Fig. 3**) [18–21]. Bradykinin B_1 receptors also seem to be involved [22]. Bradykinin is degraded by three enzymes, with kininase activity: These consist of angiotensin-converting enzyme (ACE), aminopeptidase P and carboxypeptidase enzymes. Bradykinin levels can be increased by increases in kininogenase activity (i.e., the

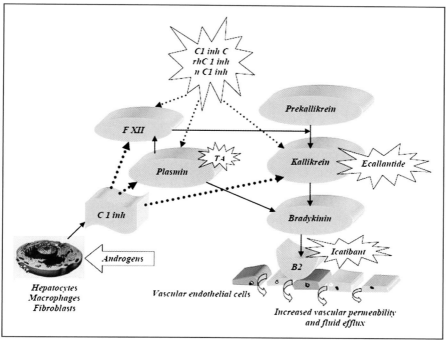

Fig. 3. Pathophysiological model of bradykinin-mediated angioedema and targets of treatments. The solid arrows represent an activation mechanism. The dotted arrows represent a mechanism of inhibition. Treatments inhibiting physiological pathways are represented as white stars. Therapeutic agents acting through activation of a physiological pathway are represented by a white arrow. C1 inh: C1 inhibitor physiological; F XII: factor XII; C1 inh C: C1 inhibitor concentrate; rhC1 inh: recombinant C1 inhibitor concentrate; n C1 inh: nanofiltered C1 inhibitor concentrate; TA: Tranexamic acid; B2: endothelial vascular receptor. From [21] with permission.

XII

proteolytic activities of Hageman factor, plasmin and kallikrein) or by a decrease in kininase activity [18, 23].

Multiple Causes

Typically, there are two types of angioedema: Hereditary angioedema and acquired angioedema, and the prevalence of both forms of the disease is low (estimated between 1:10,000 and 1:50,000 for hereditary angioedema; undetermined for acquired angioedema) [1, 24, 25].

Angioedema can be classified according to the presence or absence of C1 inhibitor deficiency (**Fig. 4**). The C1 inhibitor is the main regulator of the kallikrein-kinin pathway and regulates the activation of kallikrein, plasmin, factor Xa and XIIa, proteins involved in fibrinolysis and the contact phase of coagulation [1, 8, 18, 19, 26]. Quantitative (type I hereditary angioedema) or qualitative (type II hereditary angioedema) C1 inhibitor deficiency results in an excess of bradykinin [1]. A recently described type III hereditary angioedema exists, in which increased activity of kininogenase is associated with increased factor XII activity,

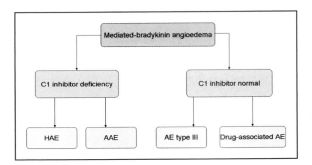

Fig. 4. Pathophysiological classification of mediated-bradykinin angioedema (AE). HAE: hereditary angiodema; AAE: acquired angioedema

and this leads to the excessive release of bradykinin. For type III hereditary angioedema, C1 inhibitor levels are normal, but function mutations in the factor XII gene, which may or may not be influenced by estrogen, have been described for some patients [4, 27, 28]. Acquired forms of the disease have also been described, and these are thought to be due to increased activity of kininogenase in response to a hyper-consumption of the C1 inhibitor (type I acquired angioedema) or a neutralization of the C1 inhibitor by C1 inhibitor antibodies (type II acquired angioedema). These forms are often associated with lymphoproliferative disorders or autoimmune diseases that may appear several years after the initial episode [25, 29]. Drug-induced acquired angioedema associated with kinase abnormalities has been reported. The drugs involved (ACE inhibitors, angiotensin receptor blockers [ARBs] and ACE inhibitors plus gliptins in combination) block the kinase that degrades bradykinin, which reduces its catabolism and thus increases its activity [30, 31]. Therefore, ACE inhibitors expose patients to a 0.5 – 1 % risk for angioedema, which can become severe and localize to the face or larynx [32, 33]. Because of the widespread use of ACE inhibitors, this etiology has dramatically increased over the past 20 years. Familial forms of the disease that target kinases have also been described [25].

Emergency Diagnosis

Two emergency situations are possible depending on whether the diagnosis has already been established:

- A patient whose diagnosis had not been established. This is the most difficult situation and is encountered in emergency departments. The diagnosis can be made by answering the following three questions [1, 19]:
  - First, is this an angioedema? This question must be asked when faced with a localized, transient, non-inflammatory and recurrent edema.
  - Second, is this a non-histaminergic angioedema? For these cases, there is no associated rash or itching, and the swelling will last for a few days. In particular, treatments with corticosteroids and anti-histamines are ineffective for cases of non-histaminergic angioedema.
  - Is this a bradykinin-induced angioedema? These types of angioedema are often associated with a gastrointestinal disorder. Family history reports similar episodes of edema or patient medication use (ACE inhibitors, ARBs).

XII

At this stage, the diagnosis is strictly clinical; no laboratory tests are available for emergency cases [21].

- A patient whose diagnosis has already been established. The patient should carry a wallet card that explains his/her illness and two doses of a specific treatment [4, 5].

Specific Treatments Available

Currently, several specific treatments are available, but a guideline for proper treatment has not been established. In fact, the results of numerous phase III clinical studies for these specific treatments cannot be directly compared because different treatment protocols were used. Above all, no study has compared the effectiveness of the available treatment options [5, 34]. Furthermore, the availability of different treatments and patient access to them differ by country [34, 35]. Updated information is available at the website of the hereditary angioedema international community (www.haei.org).

Randomized studies have been designed for patients with type I or type II hereditary angioedema. For the other clinical situations (type III hereditary angioedema, acquired and drug-induced angioedema), only clinical cases been published documenting the use of C1 inhibitor concentrate or icatibant outside of the authorized indications.

C1 Inhibitor Concentrate

C1 inhibitor concentrate (Berinert®, CSL Bering) is obtained by plasma fractionation after several stages of viral inactivation and pasteurization. Sites of action are presented in **Figure 3**. Various studies have reported the effectiveness of C1 inhibitor concentrate for all types of angioedema [36–39]. Two early, randomized, double-blind studies using fixed doses for patients with hereditary angioedema demonstrated symptom relief, and 95 % of patients were responsive to treatment within 4 hours [4]. Another randomized, double-blind, multicenter study compared two doses of C1 inhibitor concentrate to placebo in patients with hereditary angioedema (International Multicenter Prospective Angioedema C1-inhibitor Trial [IMPACT] 1) [40]. In this study, only the 20 U/kg dose led to a more rapid improvement in symptoms. An open follow-up study confirmed these results and demonstrated good long-term effectiveness (IMPACT 2) [41]. No viral transmission has been described using this concentrate, and the tolerance to treatment is good [36, 37]. Rare cases of anaphylaxis have been reported. In acquired angioedema, clinical cases have been reported that have occasionally required increased dosages [25].

C1 inhibitor concentrate is available in 500-U vials, the standard dose is 20 U/kg, and it is administered by rapid intravenous injection after reconstitution. The efficacy of this treatment is manifest within 30 minutes, and the half-life varies with the consumption of the C1 inhibitor (but can be up to 40 hours). In the absence of any improvement, it is possible to administer a repeated dose of 500 to 1000 U after 2 hours. The shelf life is 30 months at a temperature less than 25 °C. Depending on the frequency and severity of the attacks, it may be necessary to provide the patient with an emergency supply at home [5]. This product has been approved for treatment attacks in patients with hereditary angioedema in Europe, the United States and Australia [35].

XII

Icatibant

Icatibant (Firazyr®, Shire HGT) is a synthetic antagonist of the bradykinin B_2 receptor and blocks edema formation (**Fig. 3**). An uncontrolled pilot study demonstrated the efficacy and rapid action of icatibant and found reduced serum concentrations of bradykinin following treatment [42]. Two randomized, double-blind, multicenter studies compared icatibant to either placebo (For Angioedema Subcutaneous Treatment [FAST] 1) or tranexamic acid (FAST 2) in patients with hereditary angioedema [43]. Symptoms improved faster after icatibant treatment, and the duration of the attacks was shorter. In 90 % of cases, a single injection was sufficient. Patient self-administration was also assessed. For type III hereditary angioedema and acquired angioedema, and particularly for the drug-induced types, clinical cases have reported improvement following icatibant treatment.

This treatment is presented in a pre-filled 3-ml syringe containing 30 mg of icatibant. The dose is 30 mg subcutaneously. The injection can be repeated at 6-hour intervals (up to three injections per day). Its bioavailability is excellent, its efficacy is evident within 20 to 30 minutes, and its half-life is 2 hours. Shelf life is 24 months at room temperature. Adverse effects mainly consist of pain at the injection site. There have been no studies in children or pregnant women. Because of its ease of use and good tolerance, it is recommended that patients have this drug available at home and be trained for self-administration [5]. This product is approved to treat attacks in patients with hereditary angioedema and is approved for self-administration in Europe and the United States [35].

Recombinant C1 Inhibitor

Recombinant C1 inhibitor (Rhucin®/Ruconest™, Pharming) is analogous to human C1 inhibitor and is obtained from the milk of transgenic rabbits. Studies using two different doses have documented the efficacy safety of recombinant C1 inhibitor for the treatment of acute hereditary angioedema attacks [44]. Because of its unique glycosylation pattern, its half-life is approximately 3 hours. This drug is available in 2100 U vials, and the dose is 50 U/kg administered intravenously after reconstitution. Prior to treatment and also either once a year or after 10 uses, the absence of IgE antibodies directed against rabbit epithelium should be confirmed. Type I and II hypersensitivity reactions have been described and the production of neutralizing antibodies may occur. This product is not self-administered by patients, and it can only be used in emergency situations for patients who have tested negative for IgE rabbit epithelium antibodies. Recombinant C1 inhibitor is approved to treat attacks in patients with hereditary angioedema in Europe [35].

Nanofiltered C1 Inhibitor Concentrate

Two randomized studies have evaluated the effectiveness of a fixed dose of nanofiltered C1 inhibitor concentrate (Cinryze®, from ViroPharma, Cetor®, from Sanquin) over that of placebo for the treatment of attacks or as a crossover treatment for prophylaxis [45]. In the first study, the median time for the onset of efficacy was 2 hours versus 4 hours with the placebo, but 70 % of patients required a second injection. In the second study, the numbers of attacks and the level of the severity and duration of attacks decreased significantly after treatment [45]. There have been no studies that have compared different doses, and rare allergic reactions have been described. The dose for this drug is 1000 U, which is administered by slow intravenous injection after reconstitution for the treatment of attacks or as a prophylaxis. This product is approved in Europe for the treatment and prophylaxis of hereditary angioedema in adults and children and in the United States for the prophylaxis of acute hereditary angioedema attacks [35].

Ecallantide

Ecallantide (Kalbitor®, Dyax) is a specific recombinant kallikrein inhibitor (**Fig. 3**). Several randomized studies have demonstrated its rapidity of action, efficacy and safety [46]. Anaphylactic reactions and antibody production have been described, and the half-life of this drug is approximately 2 hours. Ecallantide is available in 1 ml vials containing 10 mg of ecallantide and is to be kept cool and in the dark. The dose is 30 mg subcutaneously. It is not recommended for self infusion at this time because of a small risk of anaphylaxis. It is approved in the United States but not in Europe [35].

Emergency Treatment of Acute Attacks

Severe attacks must be identified because their prognosis is unpredictable, and laryngeal edema or hypovolemic shock may cause a life-threatening situation. A severe attack is defined as any face or ENT localization or the presence of abdominal attack with VAS scores > 5. All patients experiencing a major attack should be hospitalized and treated with a specific drug [5, 21]. Corticosteroids and antihistamines are ineffective for the emergency treatment of acute attacks [1, 5].

Treatment of Severe Attacks

Specific treatment
A specific treatment should be initiated as early as possible [5]. Phase III studies have recommended the use of C1 inhibitor concentrate, icatibant, recombinant C1 inhibitor, nanofiltered C1 inhibitor or ecallantide for the treatment of severe hereditary angioedema attacks [5]. No studies concerning the superiority or inferiority of the relative actions of these molecules exist, and a guideline for the selection of these treatments has not yet been defined. Phase IV studies and international consensus conferences are needed [5]. In practice, the choice should be based on the local availability of the treatments and should reflect the national consensus of each country, depending on local customs [5].

XII

Treatment of laryngeal edema
Laryngeal edema is the complication that is primarily responsible for disease severity.

- Specific treatments. In open-phase studies, the effectiveness of C1 inhibitor concentrate, icatibant, nanofiltered C1 inhibitor and ecallantide has been examined for resolving laryngeal edema [43, 45–47]. Only the recombinant C1 inhibitor was not evaluated for this condition. Symptoms began to improve within approximately 15 to 30 minutes, and each of these treatments resulted in symptom improvement.

- Intubation. Intubation can become very difficult because of distortion and swelling of the upper airway. This technique should be performed by an experienced physician [1, 5, 19]. To avoid complications, intubation should be considered during the early stages of progressive laryngeal edema [5]. Intubations using a fiberscope may be affected by the presence of edema [48]. If these fail, it is necessary to perform a cricothyroidotomy, which can also be difficult or impossible as a result of the edema [3]. Occasionally, surgical tracheotomy is the only remaining option for treatment.
- Inhaled epinephrine. Clinical reports have suggested a moderate and transient efficacy for inhaled epinephrine, when provided during the early stages of edema. Due to the pathophysiology of angioedema and the questionable effectiveness of this treatment, the use of aerosolized epinephrine should not delay the initiation of other specific treatments [4].

Other treatments

- Fresh-frozen plasma (FFP). The administration of FFP provides the patient with the C1 inhibitor of the donor. Clinical case reports have been the only studies to demonstrate the effectiveness of FFP. This treatment has also been shown to worsen edema attacks [1, 4]. Indeed, FFP contains contact-activated coagulation proteins, which can produce additional bradykinin and thus worsen the attack. Additionally, the risk of exposure to transmissible diseases (e.g., non-enveloped viruses and prions) is present, as it is with any blood component. Currently, the use of FFP is strongly discouraged in countries where specific molecular treatment options are available [5].
- Analgesics. Although attacks are not usually painful, patients may experience significant pain if the swelling affects points of support, especially in the abdominal area, and these conditions may lead to a surgical emergency. Any class of analgesic, antiemetic or antispasmodic may be used for these cases [1, 3, 5].
- Fluid therapy. During an abdominal attack, the patient may experience a major collapse, secondary to fluid sequestration in the gastrointestinal tract and the abdominal cavity. For these situations, crystalloids and colloids can be used, but dextrans should be excluded [1, 3, 5].

XII

Treatment of Moderate Attacks

Specific treatments

All available treatment options can be used for the treatment of moderate attacks [5]. However, the high price of these treatments raises questions about the real benefit in terms of public health (i.e., lost work days, social life, quality of life, etc.) [49]. For all cases, the aim should be to reduce the morbidity of the disease and to enable patients to live as normally as possible, with the same approach as for hemophilia [5]. Health education programs should be developed to empower the patient, and self-administration studies for C1 inhibitor concentrate and icatibant have been conducted [5].

Tranexamic acid

This is an antifibrinolytic agent that controls the formation of plasmin and effectively 'saves' the C1 inhibitor and reduces the excessive synthesis of bradykinin (**Fig. 3**). Two early, controlled studies confirmed its effectiveness, and this treatment is more effective when started early. The adverse effects of treatment with tranexamic acid include nausea, faintness and dizziness. It is available in tablets or injectable ampoules, and the dose is 1 – 2 g per 6 h for 48 hours [4].

Conclusion

Angioedema is a disease that any ICU physician could encounter. Bradykinin-mediated angioedema should be evoked in cases of recurrent and transitory edema. Severe attacks must be identified. All patients with severe attacks should benefit from early treatment with a specific molecule. Without these treatments, life-threatening situations may arise. The availability of these treatments varies by country, and there is currently no consensus as to the optimal choice of a specific treatment.

It is important to encourage the patient to carry two doses of any specific treatment for emergency treatment. Self-administration of the product should be the goal. The rarity of this disease and the characteristics of the specific drugs (i.e., their retention periods, modes of delivery, prices and methods for reimbursement) should encourage hospitals to make strategic choices regarding the creation of an emergency supply of drugs or an institute-wide protocol for the rapid transfer of patients to specialized centers for treatment.

References

1. Zuraw BL (2008) Clinical practice. Hereditary angioedema. N Engl J Med 359: 1027 – 1036
2. Kaplan AP, Greaves MW (2005) Angioedema. J Am Acad Dermatol 53: 373 – 388
3. Levy JH, Freiberger DJ, Roback J (2010) Hereditary angioedema: current and emerging treatment options. Anesth Analg 110: 1271 – 1280
4. Bowen T, Cicardi M, Farkas H, Bork K, et al (2010) 2010 International consensus algorithm for the diagnosis, therapy and management of hereditary angioedema. Allergy Asthma Clin Immunol 6: 24
5. Bowen T (2011) Hereditary angioedema: beyond international consensus – circa December 2010 – The Canadian Society of Allergy and Clinical Immunology Dr. David McCourtie Lecture. Allergy Asthma Clin Immunol 7: 1
6. Farkas H, Varga L, Szeplaki G, Visy B, Harmat G, Bowen T (2007) Management of hereditary angioedema in pediatric patients. Pediatrics 120: e713 – 722
7. Farkas H (2010) Pediatric hereditary angioedema due to C1-inhibitor deficiency. Allergy Asthma Clin Immunol 6: 18
8. Agostoni A, Aygoren-Pursun E, Binkley KE, et al (2004) Hereditary and acquired angioedema: problems and progress: proceedings of the third C1 esterase inhibitor deficiency workshop and beyond. J Allergy Clin Immunol 114: S51 – 131
9. Zuraw BL (2008) Hereditary angiodema: a current state-of-the-art review, IV: short- and long-term treatment of hereditary angioedema: out with the old and in with the new? Ann Allergy Asthma Immunol 100: S13 – 18
10. Agostoni A, Cicardi M (1992) Hereditary and acquired C1-inhibitor deficiency: biological and clinical characteristics in 235 patients. Medicine 71: 206 – 215
11. Bork K, Siedlecki K, Bosch S, Schopf RE, Kreuz W (2000) Asphyxiation by laryngeal edema in patients with hereditary angioedema. Mayo Clinic proceedings 75: 349 – 354
12. Bork K, Hardt J, Schicketanz KH, Ressel N (2003) Clinical studies of sudden upper airway

XII

obstruction in patients with hereditary angioedema due to C1 esterase inhibitor deficiency. Arch Intern Med 163: 1229–1235

13. Bork K, Staubach P, Eckardt AJ, Hardt J (2006) Symptoms, course, and complications of abdominal attacks in hereditary angioedema due to C1 inhibitor deficiency. Am J Gastroenterol 101: 619–627

14. Nzeako UC (2010) Diagnosis and management of angioedema with abdominal involvement: a gastroenterology perspective. World J Gastroenterol 16: 4913–4921

15. Guichon C, Floccard B, Coppere B, et al (2011) One hypovolaemic shock...two kinin pathway abnormalities. Intensive Care Med 37: 1227–1228

16. Bork K, Hardt J, Staubach-Renz P, Witzke G (2011) Risk of laryngeal edema and facial swellings after tooth extraction in patients with hereditary angioedema with and without prophylaxis with C1 inhibitor concentrate: a retrospective study. Oral Surg Oral Med Oral Pathol Oral Radiol Endod 112: 58–64

17. Maurer M, Bader M, Bas M, et al (2011) New topics in bradykinin research. Allergy Aug 66: 1397–1406

18. Davis AE 3rd (2005) The pathophysiology of hereditary angioedema. Clin Immunol 114: 3–9

19. Bas M, Adams V, Suvorava T, Niehues T, Hoffmann TK, Kojda G (2007) Nonallergic angioedema: role of bradykinin. Allergy 62: 842–856

20. Kaplan A (2011) Bradykinin and the pathogenesis of hereditary angiodema. World Allergy Organiz J 4: 73–75

21. Floccard B, Crozon J, Rimmele T, et al (2011) Management of bradykinin-mediated angioedema. Ann Fr Anesth Reanim 30: 578–588

22. Bossi F, Fischetti F, Regoli D, et al (2009) Novel pathogenic mechanism and therapeutic approaches to angioedema associated with C1 inhibitor deficiency. J Allergy Clin Immunol 124: 1303–1310

23. Cugno M, Nussberger J, Cicardi M, Agostoni A (2003) Bradykinin and the pathophysiology of angioedema. Int Immunopharmacol 3: 311–317

24. Cicardi M, Zanichelli A (2010) Angioedema due to C1 inhibitor deficiency in 2010. Intern Emerg Med 5: 481–486

25. Cicardi M, Zanichelli A (2010) Acquired angioedema. Allergy Asthma Clin Immunol 6: 14

26. Davis AE, 3rd, Lu F, Mejia P (2010) C1 inhibitor, a multi-functional serine protease inhibitor. Thromb Haemost 104: 886–893

27. Bork K, Wulff K, Hardt J, Witzke G, Staubach P (2009) Hereditary angioedema caused by missense mutations in the factor XII gene: clinical features, trigger factors, and therapy. J Allergy Clinical Immunol 124: 129–134

28. Bouillet L (2010) Hereditary angioedema in women. Allergy Asthma Clin Immunol 6: 17

29. Cugno M, Castelli R, Cicardi M (2008) Angioedema due to acquired C1-inhibitor deficiency: a bridging condition between autoimmunity and lymphoproliferation. Autoimmunity Rev 8: 156–159

30. Brown NJ, Byiers S, Carr D, Maldonado M, Warner BA (2009) Dipeptidyl peptidase-IV inhibitor use associated with increased risk of ACE inhibitor-associated angioedema. Hypertension 54: 516–523

31. Hoover T, Lippmann M, Grouzmann E, Marceau F, Herscu P (2010) Angiotensin converting enzyme inhibitor induced angio-oedema: a review of the pathophysiology and risk factors. Clin Exp Allergy 40: 50–61

32. Miller DR, Oliveria SA, Berlowitz DR, Fincke BG, Stang P, Lillienfeld DE (2008) Angioedema incidence in US veterans initiating angiotensin-converting enzyme inhibitors. Hypertension 51: 1624–1630

33. Tai S, Mascaro M, Goldstein NA (2010) Angioedema: a review of 367 episodes presenting to three tertiary care hospitals. Ann Otol, Rhinol Laryngol 119: 836–841

34. Morgan BP (2010) Hereditary angioedema-therapies Old and new. N Engl J Med 363: 581–583

35. Blankart CR, Stargardt T, Schreyogg J (2011) Availability of and access to orphan drugs: an international comparison of pharmaceutical treatments for pulmonary arterial hypertension, Fabry disease, hereditary angioedema and chronic myeloid leukaemia. PharmacoEconomics 29: 63–82

XII

36. De Serres J, Groner A, Lindner J (2003) Safety and efficacy of pasteurized C1 inhibitor concentrate (Berinert P) in hereditary angioedema: a review. Transfus Apher Sci 29: 247–254

37. Longhurst HJ (2005) Emergency treatment of acute attacks in hereditary angioedema due to C1 inhibitor deficiency: what is the evidence? Int J Clin Pract 59: 594–599

38. Farkas H, Jakab L, Temesszentandrasi G, et al (2007) Hereditary angioedema: a decade of human C1-inhibitor concentrate therapy. J Allergy Clin Immunol 120: 941–947

39. Cicardi M, Zingale L, Zanichelli A, Deliliers DL (2007) Established and new treatments for hereditary angioedema: An update. Mol Immunol 44: 3858–3861

40. Craig TJ, Levy RJ, Wasserman RL, et al (2009) Efficacy of human C1 esterase inhibitor concentrate compared with placebo in acute hereditary angioedema attacks. J Allergy Clin Immunol 124: 801–808

41. Craig TJ, Bewtra AK, Bahna SL, et al (2011) C1 esterase inhibitor concentrate in 1085 Hereditary Angioedema attacks – final results of the I.M.P.A.C.T.2 study. Allergy 66: 1604–1611

42. Bork K, Frank J, Grundt B, Schlattmann P, Nussberger J, Kreuz W (2007) Treatment of acute edema attacks in hereditary angioedema with a bradykinin receptor-2 antagonist (Icatibant). J Allergy Clin Immunol 119: 1497–1503

43. Cicardi M, Banerji A, Bracho F, et al (2010) Icatibant, a new bradykinin-receptor antagonist, in hereditary angioedema. N Engl J Med 363: 532–541

44. Longhurst H (2008) Rhucin, a recombinant C1 inhibitor for the treatment of hereditary angioedema and cerebral ischemia. Curr Opin Investig Drugs 9: 310–323

45. Zuraw BL, Busse PJ, White M, et al (2010) Nanofiltered c1 inhibitor concentrate for treatment of hereditary angioedema. N Engl J Med 363: 513–522

46. Cicardi M, Levy RJ, McNeil DL, et al (2010) Ecallantide for the treatment of acute attacks in hereditary angioedema. N Engl J Med 363: 523–531

47. Craig TJ, Wasserman RL, Levy RJ, et al (2010) prospective study of rapid relief provided by C1 esterase inhibitor in emergency treatment of acute laryngeal attacks in hereditary angioedema. J Clin Immunol 30: 823–829

48. Jensen NF, Weiler JM (1998) C1 esterase inhibitor deficiency, airway compromise, and anesthesia. Anesth Analg 87: 480–488

49. Wilson DA, Bork K, Shea EP, Rentz AM, Blaustein MB, Pullman WE (2010) Economic costs associated with acute attacks and long-term management of hereditary angioedema. Ann Allergy Asthma Immunol 104: 314–320

50. Floccard B, Crozon J, Coppere B, Bouillet L, Allaouchiche B (2010) Angio-oedème à bradykinine. In: Leone M (ed) Maladies Rares en Réanimation. Springer, Paris, pp 236–274

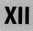

XIII Cardiac Arrest

Controlled Oxygenation after Cardiac Arrest

C.E. Hommers and J.P. Nolan

Introduction

Sudden cardiac arrest is the most common lethal manifestation of cardiovascular disease. Even when successfully resuscitated and admitted to the intensive care unit (ICU), the majority of patients do not survive [1]. This disappointingly low survival rate has resulted in a shift of focus from interventions that improve success of cardiopulmonary resuscitation (CPR) to factors that may modify outcome favorably after return of spontaneous circulation (ROSC) [2]. Whilst early restoration of blood flow to ischemic tissues is essential to halt progression of cellular damage, it is now clear that reperfusion initiates a complex series of reactions that paradoxically injure tissues. This global ischemia/reperfusion response is responsible for the post-cardiac arrest syndrome observed in survivors of cardiac arrest [3]. The brain is particularly vulnerable to ischemia/reperfusion and post-cardiac arrest brain injury is the most common cause of death and disability [4]. The recent success of therapeutic hypothermia has emphasized that the course of reperfusion injury can be mitigated and as such the search for other interventions that may further attenuate injury and improve outcome has focused recently on the high concentrations of oxygen administered routinely during CPR and for prolonged periods after ROSC.

Progress in understanding the pathophysiology of ischemia/reperfusion injury over the last 30 years has strongly implicated oxidative stress and mitochondrial dysfunction in the development of acute brain injury [5, 6]. Formation of reactive oxygen species (ROS) and reactive nitrogen species (RNS) are integral to this process. Several of these ROS are produced at low levels during normal physiological conditions and are scavenged by endogenous antioxidant systems. Following ischemia/reperfusion, a burst of ROS occurs, many combining to produce even more potent oxidant molecules, which overwhelm the endogenous scavenging mechanisms. A series of complex harmful effects can ensue, including direct protein nitration and oxidative damage to membrane lipids, proteins, RNA and DNA. In addition to the loss of cellular integrity, ROS can block mitochondrial respiration. This complex interplay combines with other pathogenic mechanisms including excitotoxicity, glutamate-mediated intracellular calcium overload and inflammation culminating in lethal cell injury, necrosis, apoptosis and the phenomenon of delayed neuronal death [7].

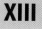

During cardiac arrest, the brain tissue oxygen tension ($PbtO_2$) falls rapidly to zero. However, at the onset of reperfusion there is commonly a hyperemic phase whereby tissue oxygenation becomes supranormal [8, 9]. Administering 100 % oxygen during this phase dramatically increases the PO_2 gradient between the

J.-L. Vincent (ed.), *Annual Update in Intensive Care and Emergency Medicine 2012*
DOI 10.1007/978-3-642-25716-2 © Springer-Verlag Berlin Heidelberg 2012

capillary bed and cell, exposing tissues to abnormally high PO_2. It is postulated that exposing ischemic brain tissue to significant hyperoxemia during this period of heightened vulnerability exacerbates the formation of ROS and hence post-ischemic oxidative injury and cellular death.

Concerns about the use of 100 % oxygen are not new. The hypothesis that oxygen is toxic by generation of oxygen free radicals has been around since the 1950s [10]. Detrimental effects of high-inspired concentrations of oxygen in neonatal resuscitation are well described [11], although clearly immature anti-oxidant defenses and the presence of fetal hemoglobin may alter the balance of potential risks. In adults, damaging pulmonary and circulatory consequences of prolonged exposure to 100 % oxygen are also well established. The lack of demonstrated benefit and distinct possibility of harm has brought into question the routine use of oxygen in many clinical contexts, including acute myocardial ischemia [12] and stroke [13].

Whereas it is intuitive to avoid too little oxygen and the inherent risks of hypoxemia, there is growing experimental and emerging clinical data that the indiscriminate use of unnecessarily high concentrations of oxygen may contribute to worse outcomes after cardiac arrest [14]. Many of the major international advisory organizations now advocate controlled re-oxygenation following ROSC. The International Liaison Committee on Resuscitation suggests avoidance of unnecessary arterial hyperoxemia, proposing a target of 94–96 % oxygen saturation [3]; similar guidance has been issued by the European Resuscitation Council [15], American Heart Association [2] and the British Thoracic Society [16].

The primary aim of this review is to systematically evaluate the current evidence for advocating controlled re-oxygenation in the setting of cardiac arrest. Supporting evidence from other forms of clinical ischemia/reperfusion injury will also be reviewed and discussed.

Animal Data

Most of the evidence on the effect of hyperoxemia after cardiac arrest is based on animal experimentation. Small and large animals have been studied extensively over the last 20 years in a variety of cardiac arrest models (Tables 1, 2 and 3). The most clinically relevant to adult cardiac arrest is the ventricular fibrillation (VF) arrest model whereby VF is induced for 8–10 min, usually by direct electrical stimulation of the heart, followed by open-chest CPR. A global cerebral ischemia model has also been commonly studied with occlusion of the carotid arteries bilaterally (10–30 min) with or without systemic hypotension induced either by atrial balloon inflation or temporary exsanguination. Finally, asphyxia induced by paralysis and ventilator disconnection has been examined and may be particularly useful for modeling non-cardiac and pediatric arrests. The majority of these models extend the oxygenation strategy throughout resuscitation as well as the post-ROSC period. Most consider the effects of hyperoxemia within the first 60 min of reperfusion but the duration studied ranges from 10 min to 6 h.

XIII

Table 1. Animal studies with cardiac arrest model demonstrating detrimental effect of hyperoxaemic resuscitation

Author, date [ref]	Study design	Number and characteristics of study population	Model	Oxygenation strategy compared	Outcomes reported for hyperoxia
Marsala 1992 [17]	Prospective controlled	13 adult dogs	15 min VF arrest	21 % vs 100 % During CPR and 1 h post-ROSC PaO_2 87 ± 13 vs 440 ± 37	↑ neuronal degeneration in 4 brain regions
Zwemer 1994 [28]	Prospective	27 adult male dogs	9 min VF arrest	21 % vs 100 % vs 100 % + antioxidant pre-treatment Pre-arrest, during CPR and 1 h post-ROSC	↑ NDS at 12 and 24 h Hyperoxia > normoxia > pretreated Attenuated by antioxidant pre-treatment
Liu 1998 [18]	Prospective	18 female dogs	10 min VF arrest	21 % vs 100 % During CPR and 1 h post-ROSC PaO_2 83 ± 4 vs 454 ± 34	↑ oxidized brain lipids Worse neurological outcome (NDS) at 24 h ↑ brain tissue lactate at 2 h
Richards 2006 [19]	Prospective controlled	?24 female dogs	10 min VF arrest	21 % vs 100 % During CPR and 1 h post-ROSC PaO_2 89 ± 4 vs 467 ± 30	↓ PDHC activity ↑ 3NT immunoreactivity Hippocamus but not cortex
Balan 2006 [25]	Prospective randomized	17 female dogs	10 min VF arrest	Oximetry guided O_2 (94–96 %) vs 100 % 1 h post-ROSC (100 % during CPR) PaO_2 94 ± 4 vs 564 ± 36	↑ NDS at 24 h ↑ Hippocampal CA1 neuronal injury at 24 h
Vereczki 2006 [20]	Prospective randomized	12 female dogs	10 min VF arrest	21 % v 100 % During CPR and 1 h post-ROSC PaO_2 76 ± 2 vs 384 ± 68	↓ PDHC immunostaining by 90 % at 2 h ↑ Protein nitration x2–3 at 2 h ↑ Hippocampal neuronal death at 24 h
Richards 2007 [21]	Prospective	20 female dogs	10 min VF arrest	21–30 % vs 100 % During CPR and 1 h post-ROSC ^{13}C glucose infusion PaO_2 96 ± 23 v 506 ± 63	↑ unmetabolized ^{13}C glucose ↓ incorporation ^{13}C into glutamate at 2h post-ROSC Hippocampus but not cortex
Brucken 2010 [26]	Retrospective	15 pigs	8 min VF arrest	100 % 10 min v 60 min (100 % during CPR) PaO_2 442 ± 140	↑ histopathological change hippocampus at 5 days Trend to worse neurological outcome (NDS and neurocognitive testing)

NDS: neurological deficit score; PDHC: pyruvate dehydrogenase complex; 3NT: 3-nitrityrosine; VF: ventricular fibrillation; CPR: cardiopulmonary resuscitation; ROSC: return of spontaneous circulation; PaO_2 in mmHg

XIII

Table 2. Animal studies with global cerebral ischemia model demonstrating detrimental effect of hyperoxemic resuscitation

Author, date [ref]	Study design	Number and characteristics of study population	Model	Oxygenation strategy compared	Outcomes reported for hyperoxia
Mickel 1987 [22]	Prospective controlled	28 male gerbils	15 min GCI (bilateral carotid occlusion)	21 % v 100 % 3 or 6 h post reperfusion	↑ pentane production (measured up to 180 min post reperfusion) x3 mortality at 14 days (p< 0.001)
Feng 1998 [23]	Prospective	?40 rats	20 or 30 min GCI (4 vessel occlusion)	15 % v 30 % v 100 % 10 min → 30 % or 100 % for rest of 4 h reperfusion	↑ tissue and mitochondrial hyperoxygenation Delayed recovery evoked potentials if worse insult Trend to slower extracellular K+ activity
Douzinas 2001 [31]	Prospective randomized controlled	28 male pigs	10 min GCI and systemic ischemia (carotid occlusion, RA balloon, apnea → MAP 15–35)	12 % v 100 % During CPR and 10 min post-ROSC PaO$_2$ 37 ± 5 v 446 ± 110	Worse neurological outcome (OPC) at 0, 8 and 24 h ↑ markers lipid peroxidation at 1 h Trend to slower lactate metabolism
Douzinas 2001 [29]	Prospective randomized	16 male pigs	10 min GCI and systemic ischemia (carotid occlusion, RA balloon, apnea → MAP 15–35)	PaO$_2$ 35 v > 300 mmHg During CPR and 10 min post-ROSC	↑ neuronal degeneration at 24 h Worse neurological outcome (OPC) at 0, 8 and 24 h
Hazelton 2010 [27]	Prospective randomized controlled	30 rats	10 min GCI and systemic ischemia (Carotid occlusion and withdrawal blood to MAP 31–35)	21 % v 100 % 1 h post reperfusion PaO$_2$ 86 ± 3 v 486 ± 22	↑ Hippocampal CA1 neuronal death at 7 and 30 days Trend to ↑ behavioural deficits at 23–30 days
Walson 2011 [24]	Prospective randomized controlled	50 rats (day 16–18 post natal)	9 min asphyxial arrest Pediatric model	21 % v 100 % v 100 % + antioxidant During CPR and I h post-ROSC PaO$_2$ 66 ± 6 v 397 ± 110	↓ reduced glutathione and ↑ superoxide dismutase activity at 6 h ↑ protein nitration and lipid peroxidation at 72 h in hippocampus Prevented by antioxidant treatment

RA: right atrial; MAP: mean arterial pressure; OPC: overall performance category; CPR: cardiopulmonary resuscitation; ROSC: return of spontaneous circulation; GCI: global cerebral ischemia; PaO$_2$ in mmHg

XIII

Table 3. Animal studies demonstrating neutral effect of hyperoxemic resuscitation

Author, date [ref]	Study design	Number and characteristics of study population	Model utilized	Oxygenation strategy compared	Outcomes reported for hyperoxia
Zwemer 1995 [32]	Prospective	17 adult male dogs	9 min VF arrest (electrical stimulation)	8.5 % vs 12 % vs 21 % During CPR and 15 min post-ROSC PaO$_2$ 26 ± 3 v 33 ± 4 vs 61 ± 17 mmHg	Hypoxia trend to: ↑ NDS at 24 h ↓ survival at 24 h No difference in markers of oxidant injury
Lipinski 1998 [30]	Prospective	22 male rats	8 min asphyxial arrest	21 % vs 100 % During CPR and 1 hour after ROSC	No difference in survival, NDS or hippocampal neuronal injury at 24, 48 or 72 h

CPR: cardiopulmonary resuscitation; ROSC: return of spontaneous circulation; NDS: neurological deficit score; VF: ventricular fibrillation

Evidence of Benefit For Controlled Re-Oxygenation

Neurochemical measures of oxidative stress and cellular dysfunction

Eight studies encompassing all types of model in both large and small animals demonstrated significantly raised biomarkers of oxidative stress and impaired cerebral energy metabolism when animals were exposed to 100 % oxygen early post-ROSC when compared with room air [17–24]. Increases in brain lipid per-oxidation, protein nitration, an oxidized shift in tissue redox state, reduced gluta-thione and increased superoxide dismutase activity have all been reported. Even exposure to short periods of post-reperfusion hyperoxemia, for as little as 10 min [23], increases oxidative injury, with mitochondrial hyperoxidation persisting long after PaO$_2$ and tissue hyperoxidation have normalized. A recent study of pediatric asphyxial cardiac arrest demonstrated prevention of some of these effects by using air or antioxidant treatment [24].

Contrary to the belief that supplying oxygen to ischemic tissues promotes aer-obic metabolism, early exposure to hyperoxemia has been associated with reduced activity of the pyruvate dehydrogenase complex, a key mitochondrial metabolic enzyme and the sole bridge between aerobic and anaerobic metabolism [19, 20], inhibition of glucose metabolism to aerobic energy metabolites (using C^{13} labeling) [21] and increased brain lactate levels [18].

XIII

Neuronal damage

One of the earliest animal studies [17] reported in 1992 a statistically significant increase in the proportion of neuronal degeneration identified histologically in four brain regions in a canine model of potassium chloride (KCl)-induced VF car-diac arrest resuscitated and reperfused with an FiO$_2$ of 1.0 for 60 min. Subsequent studies have used more sophisticated techniques to quantitatively assess histolog-ical changes and have focused on the selectively vulnerable neurons of the hippo-campal region. Increased neuronal injury and death, particularly in the CA1 region of the hippocampus, has been demonstrated at 12 h, 24 h and more recently up to 5, 7 and 30 days after early hyperoxemic reperfusion [20, 25–27].

Neurological outcome

The first animal study to demonstrate a harmful effect on functional outcome of early post-reperfusion exposure to 100 % oxygen was published in 1994 [28]. Dogs resuscitated from 9 min VF arrest and ventilated with FiO_2 1.0 for 60 min had statistically worse neurological deficit scores (NDS) at 12 and 24 h post-ROSC compared with those ventilated with room air. In proof of concept, this effect was attenuated by antioxidant pre-treatment. Four other studies have subsequently corroborated these findings at a 24 h reperfusion interval using VF and global cerebral ischemia models [18, 20, 25, 29]. Sustained effects on functional outcome beyond the first 24 h have not, however, been conclusively demonstrated. Two recent studies have reported longer-term follow up and outcome. One compared ventilation with FiO_2 1.0 for either 10 or 60 min following 8 min VF cardiac arrest in pigs [26]; at 5 days post-ROSC more prolonged exposure to hyperoxemia was associated with significantly more necrotic striatal brain damage and perivascular inflammation. However, a trend towards improved recovery in both NDS and neurocognitive testing failed to reach statistical significance. Design limitations, including small numbers, retrospective data collection and the 10 min exposure to hyperoxia in the control group, all confound interpretation. Hazelton et al. [27] recently attempted to again address the issue of whether avoiding hyperoxemic reperfusion could provide long-term protection. Using a rat model of 10 min global cerebral ischemia ventilated with either 21 % or 100 % O_2 after reperfusion, animals were followed up for 30 days. Whereas a significant difference in neuronal death was identified, no clear clinical effects were demonstrated; there were subtle neurobehavioral changes only. Variations in the type of model probably contributed to these findings, with a longer duration of ischemia necessary to generate significant differences in neurological impairment compared with the no-flow VF model.

Clearly, there are major limitations in extrapolating the results of these heterogeneous animal studies to clinical practice and it is worth dwelling on the most clinically relevant publication [25]. This was the first study to specifically consider post-ROSC oxygenation and still the only pre-clinical study to titrate post resuscitation oxygen therapy using pulse oximetry. To model current clinical practice accurately, dogs were resuscitated after 10 min VF arrest with 100 % oxygen. Immediately post-ROSC, the animals were randomized to receive 60 min ventilation with either FiO_2 1.0 or FiO_2 titrated to arterial oxygen saturations using pulse oximetry (SpO_2) of 94–96 %. Titrated oxygenation resulted in significant improvements in both neurological outcome and hippocampal CA1 neuronal injury at 24 h.

Mortality

To date, only one animal study has demonstrated a survival effect of an early post-reperfusion oxygenation strategy. In 1987, the earliest study of global cerebral ischemia [22] reported a three-fold increase in mortality in gerbils exposed to 15 min ischemia and either 3 or 6 h exposure to 100 % O_2 compared with room air post-reperfusion. The longer ischemic time and prolonged exposure to a hyperoxic environment may account for the dramatic findings. No subsequent studies have been adequately designed or powered to detect a mortality difference.

XIII

Studies neutral to the effect of hyperoxaemia

Of studies specially designed to consider hyperoxemic reperfusion, only one failed to find any differences in outcome [30]. Using an asphyxial model of cardiac arrest in rats ventilated with either 21 % or 100 % oxygen for 60 min post-ROSC, no differences in histological or clinical outcome were demonstrated at 24, 48 or 72 h. Given that asphyxial models generally produce worse functional deficits and neuronal damage compared with the no-flow VF model, demonstrating differential treatment effects is likely to be more difficult.

Evidence of Adverse Effects Using Controlled Re-oxygenation

No published experimental study to date has demonstrated any detrimental effects of resuscitating animals with titrated oxygen or room air. Given that normoxic resuscitation, in experimental cardiac arrest at least, is undoubtedly superior to hyperoxic reperfusion, a number of investigators have gone on to consider whether hypoxic reperfusion may confer additional benefit. In a porcine model of global cerebral ischemia, one group reported that hypoxemic conditions (FiO_2 of 0.12 or a PaO_2 target of 35 mmHg) produced improvements in markers of lipid oxidation, and functional and histological outcome compared with hyperoxemia ($PaO_2 > 300$ mmHg) [29, 31]. However, when compared with room air, Zwemer et al. [32] demonstrated that an $FiO_2 < 0.21$ during CPR and for 15 min post-ROSC tended to worsen neurological outcome and survival. The obvious and inherent concern of promoting normoxic resuscitation is that of inadvertently precipitating hypoxia.

Human Data

Until recently, the only human study that had been conducted was a small, randomized controlled, pilot study of 28 patients resuscitated from witnessed out-of-hospital cardiac arrest [33]. Patients were ventilated with either 30 % or 100 % oxygen for 60 min post-ROSC with continuous pulse oximetry and oxygen titration to maintain $SpO_2 > 94$ %. Most patients maintained acceptable arterial oxygenation with 30 % oxygen although the FiO_2 had to be increased in 5 of 14 patients. The use of 100 % oxygen was associated with a numerically increased concentration of neuron specific enolase (NSE) and S-100 at 24 and 48 h. This effect reached statistical significance only in an *a priori* subgroup analysis of patients not treated with therapeutic hypothermia (only for NSE at 24 h). As NSE is an established marker of neuronal injury, this result suggests that hypothermic conditions may protect against hyperoxygenation-generated reperfusion injury. This trial was underpowered to make any assessment of outcome or survival and was designed more as a feasibility study with a view to a larger randomized controlled trial (RCT).

XIII

Two large retrospective cohort database analyses have subsequently been published, one using the Project IMPACT database in the United States (US) [34] and the second, the Australian and New Zealand Adult Patient Database (ANZ-APD) [35]. Using data generated from a critical care database in 120 US hospitals, the first of these studies demonstrated a possible association between post-resuscitation hyperoxemia and poor clinical outcome [34]. Of the 6326 patients included in the study, 1156 (18 %) were hyperoxemic, defined as $PaO_2 > 300$ mmHg within 24 h of arriving in the ICU, 3999 (63 %) were hypoxemic with a $PaO_2 < 60$ mmHg or PaO_2/FiO_2 (P/F) ratio < 300, and 1171 (19 %) were normoxemic. In-hospital mortality was 63 % in the hyperoxemic group, significantly higher than the 57 % mortality in the hypoxic group and 45 % mortality in the normoxemic group (p< 0.001). Hyperoxemia was also associated with a lower likelihood of independent functional status at hospital discharge. After controlling for a predefined set of confounders in a multivariate analysis, hyperoxemia remained an independent predictor of in-hospital mortality (odds ratio [OR] 1.8; 95 % confidence interval [CI] 1.2–2.2).

Significant methodological limitations of the study were acknowledged. The observational retrospective data collection raises the possibility of residual confounding factors existing even after risk adjustment. The lack of information on the temporal relationship of hyperoxemia to admission and paucity of outcome data limits the ability to interpret any relationship between hyperoxemia and survival or the effect of extracerebral deleterious consequences of hyperoxemia. There were also, inexplicably, 2410 patients excluded for lack of blood gas analysis within the first 24 hours after admission, the effect of which is unquantified and may well represent significant selection bias.

A secondary analysis of these data was published in 2011 [36]. This time, the hypoxemic group ($PaO_2 < 60$ or P/F ratio < 200) was excluded and data from the remaining 4459 patients were analyzed with PaO_2 as a continuous variable in the multivariate analysis. Aiming to define better the relationship between PaO_2 and outcome, the authors found a dose-dependent association with mortality and independent status at hospital discharge. For every 100 mmHg rise in PaO_2, mortality increased by 24 % (OR 1.24; 95 % CI 1.18–1.24). Whereas this finding may have implications for future clinical trial design, the discussed limitations still apply, particularly the risk that FiO_2 represents an unmeasured surrogate marker of illness severity.

The second, Australasian study, generated data from 12,108 patients from across 125 ICUs [35]. Specifically configured to facilitate direct comparisons with the US study, definitions were maintained. Fewer patients, 1285 (10.6 %), were found to be hyperoxemic, 1919 (15.9 %) were normoxemic and 8904 (73.5 %) hypoxemic. An additional 'isolated hypoxemic' group (1168 or 9.7 %) was included in an attempt to separate out low PaO_2 effects from those of low P/F ratios. The primary outcome of in-hospital mortality was 59 % in the hyperoxemic group, significantly higher than the 47 % mortality with normoxemia (p < 0.0001) but not higher than the hypoxemic group with a mortality of 60 %. It was, however, the isolated hypoxemia group that had the highest mortality (70 %) and lowest rate of discharge to home (19 %). After multivariate analysis similar to that used in the US study, hyperoxemia had an OR for death of 1.5 (95 % CI 1.3–1.8). Additional modeling, which importantly included illness severity using an APACHE-based model, decreased the OR to 1.2 (95 % CI 1.1–1.6). After further evaluation using a Cox proportional hazards ratio combined with sensitivity analysis, timing period matching, adjustment for discharge to home and FiO_2, hyperoxemia was no longer independently associated with mortality. Isolated hypoxemia, however, remained an independent risk factor. The Australians concluded that hyperoxemia is relatively uncommon and that there is 'no robust or consistently reproducible relationship with mortality' and cautioned against policies of deliberately reducing FiO_2 due to the risks of precipitating the well-established adverse effects of hypoxemia [35].

Although undoubtedly rigorously conducted with multifaceted assessments and a larger, more complete data set (only 5.4 % were excluded) than the US

XIII

study, there are a number of important differences between these two studies that are worth highlighting. First, the US study used the first blood gas at an unspecified time during the first 24 h of admission whereas the ANZ study chose the worst blood gas in the first 24 h. When considering the effect of hyperoxemia, neither could be considered ideal, accepting that both situations are likely to bias towards the null hypothesis. Although an attempt was made in the ANZ study to correlate the worst blood gas with the mean PaO_2 in the first 24–48 h, it remains likely that a significant proportion of patients exposed to hyperoxemia were not identified in either study. Moreover, duration and timing of exposure, which may be critical to the adverse effects of hyperoxemia, cannot be considered.

Second, although most baseline characteristics were comparable, a marked difference in lowest median body temperature was noted (ANZ 34.9 °C, US 36 °C). As speculated, this presumably represents a far higher uptake of therapeutic hypothermia in Australasia and is more representative of current clinical practice. It was also postulated to explain the 50 % increase in favorable outcome seen in the ANZ study (65 % discharged home verses only 44 % in the US). It may, however, also provide an explanation for the difference in primary outcome. Hypothermia is known to mitigate reperfusion injury, as also suggested by the NSE result in the study by Kuisma et al [33], and this would feasibly reduce the magnitude of effect of hyperoxemia on mortality.

Discussion

Experimental data undoubtedly prove that early exposure to high-inspired concentrations of oxygen following cardiac arrest and ROSC increases oxidative stress and delayed neuronal cell death in healthy animals. These effects seems to correlate well with detrimental effects on short-term neurological function at 24 h. Although suggested, it remains far from clear whether these findings translate into any significant effect on longer-term outcome.

Human studies offer little to clarify the situation at present. There are no human data that consider direct measures of oxidative stress or neuronal damage after cardiac arrest. Outcome effects are based on limited, low quality, contradictory data from several retrospective observational studies and a single underpowered RCT. Whether the dose-dependent increase in mortality with PaO_2 observed by the US EMShockNet [36] investigators represents administration of higher FiO_2 in sicker patients and hence hyperoxemia is merely a marker of illness severity or whether significant methodological and population-based factors, such as blood gas selection and use of therapeutic hypothermia, account for the contradictory results remains to be determined. Only definitive well-designed prospective controlled trials can prove whether hyperoxemia is truly an independent risk factor for mortality and functional status at hospital discharge post cardiac arrest.

XIII

Is A Controlled Re-oxygenation Strategy Safe?

There is no evidence from the pre-clinical data that post-arrest ventilation with room air in healthy animals is detrimental. The pilot study by Kuisma et al. [33] demonstrated that using 30 % oxygen immediately post-ROSC was insufficient to maintain $SpO_2 > 94$ % in 36 % of patients following out of hospital VF arrest. Clearly, fear of hyperoxemia post-arrest should not lead to indiscriminate decreases in FiO_2 that risk precipitating hypoxemia, which is undoubtedly bad for the injured brain. The rapid but stepwise reduction in FiO_2 successfully used by Balan et al. [25] in a canine VF arrest model would present the safest and most logical approach, assuming adequate and reliable monitoring.

When and For How Long Is Exposure to Hyperoxemia Detrimental?

Most animal data suggest that exposure to hyperoxemia in the first 60 min after ROSC results in harm, but even periods as short as 10 min have been associated with adverse outcomes. One group found no difference in survival with exposure of between 3 and 6 h [22]. Interestingly, a study in 2003 [37] reported that hyperbaric oxygen initiated 1 h after reperfusion in a canine VF arrest model actually improved clinical and histological outcome compared with oxygen targeted to a PaO_2 80–100 mmHg. It seems likely, therefore, that the very early post-reperfusion period, within 60 min, is the critical time period. The relative risks and benefits of later and more prolonged exposure remain uncertain.

What Level of Hyperoxemia Is Detrimental and How Does Arterial Oxygenation Relate To Tissue Oxygenation?

Although the beneficial effects of air and detrimental effects of 100 % O_2 may be established in resuscitating healthy animals, extrapolating this to survivors of cardiac arrest, who are often elderly with multiple co-morbidities, is very difficult. The EMShockNet study [36] suggested a progressive graded effect of hyperoxemia rather than a threshold effect. It seems that defining safe limits of hyperoxia and hypoxia is fraught with difficulty. Oxygen has a complex biological role that we are only just beginning to understand. Oxygen-sensing mechanisms have evolved to enable the body to adapt and survive hypoxic insults [38], but individual and disease-related responses to both low and supernormal PO_2 will vary. There is no simple test to measure the therapeutic adequacy of O_2 therapy and we know PaO_2 is not necessarily a good reflection of tissue PO_2. At a cellular level, PO_2 will be affected not only by arterial O_2 content (CaO_2) but PO_2 gradient, diffusion distance and blood flow. In health, 100 % oxygen is known to cause vasoconstriction of key vascular beds. The marginal increase in CaO_2 conferred by 100 % oxygen is offset by a variable reduction in perfusion which can result in a paradoxical decrease in oxygen delivery [39].

XIII

How Do Hypothermia and Hyperoxemia Interact?

One of the proposed mechanisms of improved outcome with therapeutic hypothermia post-cardiac arrest includes suppression of free radical formation and the oxidative stress associated with reperfusion [3]. Animal studies evaluating the effect of hyperoxemia post-ROSC have considered only normothermic models. Differences between the US and ANZ studies may suggest that hypothermia negates the detrimental effect of exposure to high-inspired concentration of oxygen. Further studies are needed to establish an independent effect over and above hypothermia.

How Does The Effect Of Hyperoxemia On Other Organ Systems Affect Outcome?

It is important to emphasize that the summarized experimental data consider the effects of hyperoxemic reperfusion on ischemic brain injury in otherwise healthy animals. Clearly, this is very different to the clinical situation in human cardiac arrests. Post-cardiac arrest syndrome constitutes not only brain injury but also myocardial dysfunction, a systemic ischemia/reperfusion response and the persistent precipitating pathology [3]. Hyperoxemia may well have effects on each of these processes and on global end-organ function.

The best studied of these areas is the myocardial effect of oxygen, worth considering here as cardiac arrest in adults frequently occurs in the context of an acute coronary syndrome or myocardial infarction (MI). Hyperoxia causes an 8–29 % reduction in coronary blood flow associated with a significant increase in coronary vascular resistance and reduced myocardial oxygen consumption in healthy subjects and in patients with cardiac disease [40]. As early as the 1950s, it was reported that supplemental oxygen failed to improve electrocardiogram (EKG) and clinical symptoms in MI patients [41] and in 1976 a double-blinded RCT [42] of oxygen therapy in uncomplicated MI found that high-flow oxygen was associated with greater rise in serum aspartate aminotransferase and a non-significant tripling of mortality compared with air. Although these findings need to be interpreted with caution in the context of current clinical practice, a recent systematic review concluded, on the basis of the limited evidence, that routine use of supplemental oxygen may result in greater infarct size and a possible increased risk of mortality [43]. A Cochrane review in 2010 [44] concluded that the evidence is suggestive of harm but lacks power and neither supports nor refutes the routine use of oxygen. The British Thoracic Society guideline for emergency oxygen use recommends that oxygen should be given to patients with acute myocardial ischemia only if they are hypoxemic and to aim for a saturation range of 94–98 % [16]. This guideline was echoed by the National Institute for Health and Clinical Excellence (NICE) and endorsed by several other societies. Plans for a further RCT (the Air Verses Oxygen In myocarDial Infarction (AVIOD) study) are underway in Australia (ClinicalTrials.gov NCT01272713). The maintenance of normoxemia post-cardiac arrest may logically, therefore, have beneficial effects for myocardial function particularly in an age of early coronary revascularization.

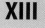

Evidence From Other Areas Of Clinical Practice Where Ischemia/Reperfusion Injury Occurs

The most robust clinical data demonstrating an adverse effect of 100 % relates to neonatal resuscitation. Even brief exposure to hyperoxemia after birth has been shown to trigger elevation in markers of oxidative stress, which persists to 28 days of life [45]. The consequences for growth and development are not entirely understood. However, several meta-analyses looking at over 2000 newborn infants have reported a 30 % reduction in mortality when resuscitation was carried out with 21 % instead of 100 % oxygen (number needed to treat = 20) [11, 46]. This has had a significant effect on practice with the recommendation that newborns are now resuscitated with room air initially [47]. Few data exist with respect to pediatric cardiac arrests. A recent experimental study is the first to suggest that a similar effect may occur in older children [24].

Acute ischemic stroke is another controversial area. After much early interest in hyperbaric oxygen (HBO), which failed to translate into any clear clinical benefit in a recent systematic review [48], subsequent focus has been on the more clinically feasible normobaric oxygen therapy (NBO). Current guidelines advocate routine administration of supplemental oxygen in the first 6 hours after acute ischemic stroke [49]. Preclinical data utilizing both transient and permanent models of stoke generally support a beneficial effect of NBO on pathological, neuroimaging and neurobehavioral outcomes [13]. Clinical data are limited to several small pilot studies and one controlled trial. One group has demonstrated transient improvement in clinical features and magnetic resonance imaging (MRI) parameters of ischemia when supplemental oxygen is administered within 12 hours of stroke onset [50]; however, there were no significant differences in outcome at 3 months. A second clinical study by the same group reported reduced lactate and preserved N-acetyl-aspartate values using magnetic resonance spectroscopy [51]. The authors concluded that NBO improves aerobic metabolism after stoke. A final feasibility study found a trend to reduced mortality, complications and hospital length of stay when FiO_2 0.4 was administered within 48 h to patients with severe middle cerebral artery (MCA) strokes [52]. None of these studies were adequately powered for outcome because few (between 6 and 17) patients were included. The only large study published to date was a quasi-randomized controlled trial involving 550 acute stroke patients who received either supplemental oxygen or room air for 24 h [53]. Overall 1-year mortality was no different; however, in a subgroup of patients with mild-moderate stroke, mortality was increased significantly (OR 0.45; 95 % CI 0.23 – 0.9) in the supplemental oxygen group. Major methodological flaws in the study limit interpretation of these results.

Explanation for these disparate findings may lie in the pathophysiology of acute ischemic stroke. Although the mechanisms of reperfusion injury, oxidative stress and neuroinflammation are similar to those of global cerebral ischemia, the pattern of injury is very different. Acute ischemic stroke consists of an ischemic core of irreversibly damaged tissue and an ischemic penumbra of potentially salvageable tissue [54]. The rationale for oxygen therapy in stroke assumes that improving oxygen availability to these impaired but viable brain cells is beneficial. Timing of supplemental oxygen therapy is likely to be key to its therapeutic benefit. Starting early after the onset of symptoms to salvage ischemic tissue and extending the therapeutic window for additional treatments (e.g., thrombolysis) are generally accepted benefits. What remains to be clarified is whether oxygen should be continued after reperfusion. A recent study of transient MCA occlusion in rodents delineated two distinct phases in acute ischemic stroke [55]. During occlusion, 100 % oxygen significantly attenuated the size of the stroke lesion and corrected the penumbral tissue PO_2, whereas identical treatment initiated immediately after reperfusion exacerbated the lesion volume. Given that spontaneous reperfusion is reported to occur in 53 % of stroke patients sometime during the first 7 days [56] and that many of the published clinical trials failed to control for time periods of treatment overlapping with thrombolytic therapy and reperfusion, the reported mixed outcomes are not surprising. A large prospective trial was underway in the US but was terminated early because of an imbalance in deaths favoring the control arm, reportedly not attributed to the treatment (ClinicalTrials.gov NCT00414726).

Concerns about excessive exposure to high-inspired concentrations of oxygen have been raised in numerous other settings including traumatic brain injury

XIII

(TBI) [57], ventilator-induced lung injury (VILI) [58] and even the general ICU patient population. In a retrospective database review of 50 Dutch ICUs [59] looking at 36,307 consecutive admissions, high FiO_2 and both high and low PaO_2 in the first 24 hours were all found to be independently associated with in-hospital mortality. FiO_2 had a linear relationship and PaO_2 had a U-shaped relationship with mortality. Reflecting the US EMShockNet study [34] in cardiac arrest, it remains to be seen whether this association is causal or reflects unmeasured differences in disease severity.

Conclusion

Preclinical and limited clinical evidence suggest that hyperoxemia may be associated with worse outcomes after cardiac arrest. However, the data are universally of low quality and consideration must, therefore, be given to the relative risks and benefits. Given the potential for harm, the lack of proven benefit in favor of hyperoxemia and the relative ease of titrating inspired oxygen concentration to maintain adequate arterial oxygen saturation, it seems reasonable to advocate a controlled re-oxygenation strategy provided adequate and reliable monitoring is available to guard against hypoxemia. As also suggested by the available evidence, this strategy is likely to be most effective if initiated as early as possible after ROSC which will have inherent implications for early and pre-hospital delivery of care.

Supplemental oxygen is ubiquitous in clinical practice, so embedded that it has become accepted as safe and appropriate management. On the premise of 'first do no harm', the burden of proof should be to establish whether hyperoxemia is safe after ROSC and in many other acute care settings. A definitive prospective clinical trial is warranted to establish both the efficacy and safety of controlled re-oxygenation post-cardiac arrest.

References

1. Nolan JP, Soar J (2010) Postresuscitation care: entering a new era. Curr Opin Crit Care 16: 216–222
2. Peberdy MA, Callaway CW, Neumar RW, et al (2010) Part 9: Post-cardiac arrest care: 2010 American Heart Association Guidelines for Cardiopulmonary Resuscitation and Emergency Cardiovascular Care. Circulation 122: S768–786
3. Nolan JP, Neumar RW, Adrie C, et al (2008) Post-cardiac arrest syndrome: epidemiology, pathophysiology, treatment, and prognostication. A Scientific Statement from the International Liaison Committee on Resuscitation; the American Heart Association Emergency Cardiovascular Care Committee; the Council on Cardiovascular Surgery and Anesthesia; the Council on Cardiopulmonary, Perioperative, and Critical Care; the Council on Clinical Cardiology; the Council on Stroke. Resuscitation 79: 350–379
4. Laver S, Farrow C, Turner D, Nolan J (2004) Mode of death after admission to an intensive care unit following cardiac arrest. Intensive Care Med 30: 2126–2128
5. Lewen A, Matz P, Chan PH (2000) Free radical pathways in CNS injury. J Neurotrauma 17: 871–890
6. Fiskum G, Danilov CA, Mehrabian Z, et al (2008) Postischemic oxidative stress promotes mitochondrial metabolic failure in neurons and astrocytes. Ann NY Acad Sci 1147: 129–138
7. Nakka VP, Gusain A, Mehta SL, Raghubir R (2008) Molecular mechanisms of apoptosis in cerebral ischemia: multiple neuroprotective opportunities. Mol Neurobiol 37: 7–38

XIII

8. Wolbarsht ML, Fridovich I (1989) Hyperoxia during reperfusion is a factor in reperfusion injury. Free Radic Biol Med 6: 61–62

9. Imberti R, Bellinzona G, Riccardi F, Pagani M, Langer M (2003) Cerebral perfusion pressure and cerebral tissue oxygen tension in a patient during cardiopulmonary resuscitation. Intensive Care Med 29: 1016–1019

10. Gerschman R, Gilbert DL, Nye SW, Dwyer P, Fenn WO (1954) Oxygen poisoning and x-irradiation: a mechanism in common. Science 119: 623–626

11. Davis PG, Tan A, O'Donnell CPF, Schulze A (2004) Resuscitation of newborn infants with 100 % oxygen or air: a systematic review and meta-analysis. Lancet 364: 1329–1333

12. Conti CR (2011) Is hyperoxic ventilation important to treat acute coronary syndromes such as myocardial infarction? Clin Cardiol 34: 132–133

13. Michalski D, Hartig W, Schneider D, Hobohm C (2011) Use of normobaric and hyperbaric oxygen in acute focal cerebral ischemia – a preclinical and clinical review. Acta Neurol Scand 123: 85–97

14. Neumar RW (2011) Optimal oxygenation during and after cardiopulmonary resuscitation. Curr Opin Crit Care 17: 236–240

15. Nolan JP, Soar J, Zideman DA, et al (2010) European Resuscitation Council Guidelines for Resuscitation 2010 Section 1. Executive summary. Resuscitation 81: 1219–1276

16. O'Driscoll BR, Howard LS, Davison AG (2008) BTS guideline for emergency oxygen use in adult patients. Thorax 63 (Suppl) 6: vi1–68

17. Marsala J, Marsala M, Vanicky I, Galik J, Orendacova J (1992) Post cardiac arrest hyperoxic resuscitation enhances neuronal vulnerability of the respiratory rhythm generator and some brainstem and spinal cord neuronal pools in the dog. Neurosci Lett 146: 121–124

18. Liu Y, Rosenthal RE, Haywood Y, Miljkovic-Lolic M, Vanderhoek JY, Fiskum G (1998) Normoxic ventilation after cardiac arrest reduces oxidation of brain lipids and improves neurological outcome. Stroke 29: 1679–1686

19. Richards EM, Rosenthal RE, Kristian T, Fiskum G (2006) Postischemic hyperoxia reduces hippocampal pyruvate dehydrogenase activity. Free Radic Biol Med 40: 1960–1970

20. Vereczki V, Martin E, Rosenthal RE, Hof PR, Hoffman GE, Fiskum G (2006) Normoxic resuscitation after cardiac arrest protects against hippocampal oxidative stress, metabolic dysfunction, and neuronal death. J Cereb Blood Flow Metab 26: 821–835

21. Richards EM, Fiskum G, Rosenthal RE, Hopkins I, Mckenna MC (2007) Hyperoxic reperfusion after global ischemia decreases hippocampal energy metabolism. Stroke 38: 1578–1584

22. Mickel HS, Vaishnav YN, Kempski O, von Lubitz D, Weiss JF, Feuerstein G (1987) Breathing 100 % oxygen after global brain ischemia in Mongolian Gerbils results in increased lipid peroxidation and increased mortality. Stroke 18: 426–430

23. Feng ZC, Sick TJ, Rosenthal M (1998) Oxygen sensitivity of mitochondrial redox status and evoked potential recovery early during reperfusion in post-ischemic rat brain. Resuscitation 37: 33–41

24. Walson KH, Tang M, Glumac A, et al (2011) Normoxic versus hyperoxic resuscitation in pediatric asphyxial cardiac arrest: effects on oxidative stress. Crit Care Med 39: 335–343

25. Balan IS, Fiskum G, Hazelton J, Cotto-Cumba C, Rosenthal RE (2006) Oximetry-guided reoxygenation improves neurological outcome after experimental cardiac arrest. Stroke 37: 3008–3013

26. Brucken A, Kaab AB, Kottmann K, et al (2010) Reducing the duration of 100 % oxygen ventilation in the early reperfusion period after cardiopulmonary resuscitation decreases striatal brain damage. Resuscitation 81: 1698–1703

27. Hazelton JL, Balan I, Elmer GI, et al (2010) Hyperoxic reperfusion after global cerebral ischemia promotes inflammation and long-term hippocampal neuronal death. J Neurotrauma 27: 753–762

28. Zwemer CF, Whitesall SE, D'Alecy LG (1994) Cardiopulmonary-cerebral resuscitation with 100 % oxygen exacerbates neurological dysfunction following nine minutes of normothermic cardiac arrest in dogs. Resuscitation 27: 159–170

29. Douzinas EE, Patsouris E, Kypriades EM, et al (2001) Hypoxaemic reperfusion ameliorates the histopathological changes in the pig brain after a severe global cerebral ischaemic insult. Intensive Care Med 27: 905–910

XIII

30. Lipinski CA, Hicks SD, Callaway CW (1999) Normoxic ventilation during resuscitation and outcome from asphyxial cardiac arrest in rats. Resuscitation 42: 221–229
31. Douzinas EE, Andrianakis I, Pitaridis MT, et al (2001) The effect of hypoxemic reperfusion on cerebral protection after a severe global ischemic brain insult. Intensive Care Med 27: 269–275
32. Zwemer CF, Whitesall SE, D'Alecy LG (1995) Hypoxic cardiopulmonary-cerebral resuscitation fails to improve neurological outcome following cardiac arrest in dogs. Resuscitation 29: 225–236
33. Kuisma M, Boyd J, Voipio V, Alaspää A, Roine RO, Rosenberg P (2006) Comparison of 30 and the 100 % inspired oxygen concentrations during early post-resuscitation period: a randomised controlled pilot study. Resuscitation 69: 199–206
34. Kilgannon JH, Jones AE, Shapiro NI, et al (2010) Association Between arterial hyperoxia following resuscitation from cardiac arrest and in-hospital mortality. JAMA 303: 2165–2171
35. Bellomo R, Bailey M, Eastwood GM, et al (2011) Arterial hyperoxia and in-hospital mortality after resuscitation from cardiac arrest. Crit Care 15: R90
36. Kilgannon JH, Jones AE, Parrillo JE, et al (2011) Relationship between supranormal oxygen tension and outcome after resuscitation from cardiac arrest. Circulation 123: 2717–2722
37. Rosenthal RE, Silbergleit R, Hof PR, Haywood Y, Fiskum G (2003) Hyperbaric oxygen reduces neuronal death and improves neurological outcome after canine cardiac arrest. Stroke 34: 1311–1316
38. Eltzschig HK, Carmeliet P (2011) Hypoxia and inflammation. N Engl J Med 364: 656–665
39. Iscoe S, Beasley R, Fisher JA (2011) Supplementary oxygen for nonhypoxemic patients: O2 much of a good thing? Crit Care 15: 305
40. Farquhar H, Weatherall M, Wijesinghe M, et al (2009) Systematic review of studies of the effect of hyperoxia on coronary blood flow. Am Heart J 158: 371–377
41. Bourassa MG, Campeau L, Bois MA, Rico O (1969) The effects of inhalation of 100 percent oxygen on myocardial lactate metabolism in coronary heart disease. Am J Cardiol 24: 172–177
42. Rawles JM, Kenmure AC, (1976) Controlled trial of oxygen in uncomplicated myocardial infarction. BMJ 1: 1121–1123
43. Wijesinghe M, Perrin K, Ranchord A, Simmonds M, Weatherall M, Beasley R (2009) Routine use of oxygen in the treatment of myocardial infarction: systematic review. Heart 95: 198–202
44. Cabello JB, Burls A, Emparanza JI, Bayliss S, Quinn T (2010) Oxygen therapy for acute myocardial infarction. Cochrane Database Syst Rev 6: CD007160
45. Vento M, Asensi M, Sastre J, Garcia-Sala F, Pallardo FV, Vina J (2001) Resuscitation with room air instead of 100 % oxygen prevents oxidative stress in moderately asphyxiated term neonates. Pediatrics 107: 642–647
46. Saugstad OD, Ramji S, Soll RF, Vento M (2008) Resuscitation of newborn infants with 21 % or 100 % oxygen: an updated systematic review and meta-analysis. Neonatology 94: 176–182
47. Saugstad OD (2007) Optimal oxygenation at birth and in the neonatal period. Neonatology 91: 319–322
48. Bennett MH, Wasiak J, Schnabel A, Kranke P, French C (2005) Hyperbaric oxygen therapy for acute ischaemic stroke. Cochrane Database Syst Rev CD004954
49. Adams HP Jr, del Zoppo G, Alberts MJ, et al (2007) Guidelines for the early management of adults with ischemic stroke: a guideline from the American Heart Association/American Stroke Association Stroke Council, Clinical Cardiology Council, Cardiovascular Radiology and Intervention Council, and the Atherosclerotic Peripheral Vascular Disease and Quality of Care Outcomes in Research Interdisciplinary Working Groups: The American Academy of Neurology affirms the value of this guideline as an educational tool for neurologists. Circulation 115: e478–534
50. Singhal AB, Benner T, Roccatagliata L, et al (2005) A pilot study of normobaric oxygen therapy in acute ischemic stroke. Stroke 36: 797–802
51. Singhal AB, Ratai E, Benner T, et al (2007) Magnetic resonance spectroscopy study of oxygen therapy in ischemic stroke. Stroke 38: 2851–2854

52. Chiu EH, Liu CS, Tan TY, Chang KC (2006) Venturi mask adjuvant oxygen therapy in severe acute ischemic stroke. Arch Neurol 63: 741–744
53. Ronning OM, Guldvog B (1999) Should stroke victims routinely receive supplemental oxygen? A quasi-randomized controlled trial. Stroke 30: 2033–2037
54. Singhal AB, Lo EH, Dalkara T, Moskowitz MA (2005) Advances in stroke neuroprotection: hyperoxia and beyond. Neuroimaging Clin N Am 15: 697–720
55. Rink C, Roy S, Khan M, Ananth P, Kuppusamy P, Sen CK, Khanna S (2010) Oxygen-sensitive outcomes and gene expression in acute ischemic stroke. J Cereb Blood Flow Metab 30: 1275–1287
56. Rha JH, Saver JL (2007) The impact of recanalization on ischemic stroke outcome: a meta-analysis. Stroke 38: 967–973
57. Diringer MN (2008) Hyperoxia: good or bad for the injured brain? Current Opinion in Critical Care 14: 167–171
58. Altemeier WA, Sinclair SE (2007) Hyperoxia in the intensive care unit: why more is not always better. Curr Opin Crit Care 13: 73–78
59. de Jonge E, Peelen L, Keijzers PJ, et al (2008) Association between administered oxygen, arterial partial oxygen pressure and mortality in mechanically ventilated intensive care unit patients. Crit Care 12: R156

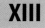

Is There Still a Place for Vasopressors in the Treatment of Cardiac Arrest?

C. Sandroni, F. Cavallaro, and M. Antonelli

Introduction

Around 300,000 people in the United States experience an out-of-hospital cardiac arrest each year, and less than 10 % of them survive to hospital discharge [1]. Survival is only slightly better for in-hospital cardiac arrest [2]. While provision of basic measures like bystander cardiopulmonary resuscitation (CPR) or early defibrillation is consistently associated with better survival [3], the benefit of advanced life support (ALS) measures, such as ventilation with advanced airway and administration of drugs, has not been clearly demonstrated [4].

Among drugs, after the recent removal of atropine from ALS protocols [5], and considering that antiarrhythmics are recommended only for the minority of cardiac arrest patients with persistent ventricular fibrillation/ventricular tachycardia (VF/VT), the mainstay of drug therapy for cardiac arrest is represented by vasopressors, namely epinephrine or vasopressin.

Rationale for the Use of Vasopressors in Cardiac Arrest

During cardiovascular collapse following cardiac arrest, flow to vital organs decreases to zero. CPR partially restores this blood flow, but cardiac output remains low, about 20 % of its normal value. The blood flow to the heart is driven by the coronary perfusion pressure, defined as the difference between the aortic diastolic pressure and the right atrial pressure. The importance of maintaining an adequate coronary perfusion pressure during CPR has been highlighted in animal and human studies. Kern et al. [6] showed that a coronary perfusion pressure < 20 mmHg measured after 20 minutes of CPR was associated with poor survival in dogs with VF. Brown et al. [7] found a positive association between myocardial blood flow and defibrillation rates in a swine model of VF. These results were confirmed in adult cardiac arrest patients by Paradis and colleagues [8], who found that initial and maximal coronary perfusion pressure values were significantly higher in patients who attained recovery of spontaneous circulation (ROSC) versus those with no ROSC. No patient whose coronary perfusion pressure was below 15 mmHg was resuscitated.

Vasopressor drugs increase coronary perfusion pressure by increasing aortic diastolic pressure and also increase systemic vascular resistance (SVR), diverting blood flow from peripheral to vital organs. Animal studies [6, 7] have demonstrated that epinephrine increases both myocardial and cerebral blood flow during CPR, and facilitates ROSC.

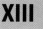

XIII

J.-L. Vincent (ed.), *Annual Update in Intensive Care and Emergency Medicine 2012*
DOI 10.1007/978-3-642-25716-2 © Springer-Verlag Berlin Heidelberg 2012

Epinephrine

Epinephrine has been the standard vasopressor in cardiac arrest for more than 30 years. The current European Resuscitation Council (ERC) guidelines for ALS [5] recommend epinephrine at a dose of 1 mg to be administered as soon as possible in patients with asystole or pulseless electrical activity, or after three unsuccessful defibrillation shocks in those with VF/VT. Similar recommendations are made by the American Heart Association (AHA) [9]. During CPR, epinephrine should be repeated every 3 to 5 minutes, because of its short half-life.

The pharmacological effects of epinephrine are mediated by the α and β adrenergic receptors. The α-receptors mediate mainly vasoconstriction, while β-receptors are responsible for stimulating effects on the heart (β_1) along with vaso-dilatation in some vascular beds (β_2) [10]. The vasoconstrictor α effect represents the scope of the administration of epinephrine during CPR, whereas cardiac stimulation from β effects is not beneficial in this context, because the heart is not contracting and cardiac output depends essentially on chest compression. In fact, β effects increase myocardial oxygen consumption and may cause an imbalance between oxygen demand and supply in the heart tissue. In an animal model, Ditchey and Lindenfeld [11] demonstrated that the administration of intravenous epinephrine during CPR significantly increased not only left ventricular (LV) coronary blood flow but also myocardial lactate concentration. β-adrenergic inotropic and chronotropic actions of epinephrine are mediated by calcium channel opening and calcium influx into the heart cells [12]. However, calcium ions are also intracellular mediators of ischemic damage [13].

There is evidence that the β_1 effects of epinephrine worsen post-resuscitation myocardial dysfunction. This effect consists of a transient reduction in myocardial performance from pre-arrest levels, which is commonly observed after ROSC [14]. In a study by Laurent et al. [15], post-resuscitation myocardial dysfunction occurred in 73/165 (44 %) patients resuscitated from out of-hospital cardiac arrest. Persistent dysfunction was associated with early death from multiorgan failure. In an experimental model of cardiac arrest and resuscitation, Tang et al. [16] demonstrated that post-resuscitation myocardial dysfunction was more severe in animals treated with epinephrine than in those treated with the α-agonist, phenylephrine, or with a combination of epinephrine and the β_1-blocker, esmolol, thus suggesting that β_1 stimulation has a role in determining this phenomenon.

Recent experimental evidence shows that, despite an increase in cerebral perfusion pressure, epinephrine can reduce cerebral tissue perfusion. In a pig model of cardiac arrest, Ristagno et al. [17] measured the cerebral microcirculatory blood flow, using orthogonal polarization spectral (OPS) imaging, and the cerebral cortical CO_2 and O_2 tensions (PbO_2 and $PbCO_2$) during and after CPR. Animals were randomized to either epinephrine or a combination of epinephrine with α_1- and β-receptor blockade (prazosin + propranolol) or a combination of epinephrine with α_2 and β receptor blockade (yohimbine + propranolol). Results showed that administration of epinephrine alone was associated with a significant reduction in post-resuscitation cerebral microcirculation and PbO_2, and with a significant increase in $PbCO_2$. The phenomenon was reduced after combined α_1 and β blockade but persisted after α_2 plus β blockade. The authors attributed this effect of epinephrine to small-vessel constriction, probably mediated by activation of the α_1 receptor subtype on cerebral and pial arterioles.

Vasopressin

Vasopressin is an endogenous nonapeptide that is synthesized by neurons of the supraoptic and paraventricular nuclei of the hypothalamus and is released in the posterior part of the pituitary gland. In normal conditions, vasopressin is released in response to decreased blood volume or increased plasma osmolality. Three types of vasopressin receptors have been identified: V1, V2 and V3. Whereas the V2 receptors mediate water reabsorption and V3 mediate the effects of vasopressin on central nervous system, the V1 receptors mediate cardiovascular effects, consisting of skin, skeletal muscle and splanchnic blood vessel vasoconstriction.

Vasopressin has been proposed as an alternative to epinephrine in cardiac arrest, based on the finding that its levels were significantly higher in successfully resuscitated patients than in patients who died [18]. In comparison with epinephrine, vasopressin has several advantages: First, its V1-mediated effects increase arterial peripheral resistance without causing direct myocardial stimulation. Moreover, it has a longer half-life (10 – 20 minutes vs. 3 – 5 minutes) and is more resistant to acidosis [19].

A series of animal studies were conducted on vasopressin during CPR. These studies consistently demonstrated that vasopressin doses between 0.4 and 0.8 U/kg led to a significantly higher coronary perfusion pressure and myocardial blood flow than epinephrine and were associated with a higher percentage of successfully resuscitated animals [20 – 23]. However, adverse cardiovascular effects from vasopressin have been described as well. They are related to the persistent vasoconstriction and increased myocardial afterload induced by this drug. In an observational study on patients with cirrhosis who received intravenous vasopressin during portacaval shunt operation [24], 13 of 52 patients developed signs of myocardial ischemia requiring treatment with vasodilators. In a pig model of prolonged VF [25], vasopressin was associated with significantly higher SVR and blood pressure after ROSC but also with a significantly lower cardiac index and contractility when compared with epinephrine, although survival at 24 h was not affected.

Epinephrine versus Vasopressin: Results of Clinical Trials

XIII

A series of clinical trials comparing vasopressin with epinephrine was conducted between 1997 and 2009 (**Table 1**). In a first small randomized trial on 40 prehospital patients who had not responded to three consecutive defibrillation shocks, the administration of 40 IU of vasopressin versus 1 mg of epinephrine was associated with a 50 % increase in survival to hospital admission and to a 66 % increase of survival at 24 hours [26]. However, a subsequent randomized placebo-controlled trial on 200 adult in-hospital patients comparing the same doses as in the previous study did not confirm those results [27]. In fact, 40 (39 %) patients in the vasopressin group versus 34 (35 %) patients in the epinephrine group survived 1 hour (p = 0.66; 95 % confidence interval [CI] for absolute increase in survival: -10.9 % to 17.0 %) whereas 12 (12 %) versus 13 (14 %) patients, respectively, survived to hospital discharge (p = 0.67; 95 % CI -11.8 % to 7.8 %). In this study, vasopressin and epinephrine were randomized only at the first bolus, and epinephrine was given as subsequent boluses to all patients. This single and early

Table 1. Summary of the characteristics of the clinical trials that have compared vasopressin with epinephrine in cardiac arrest

Author, year [ref]	Setting	Number of enrolled patients	Intervention	Mean time to first vasopressin bolus, min
Lindner, 1997 [26]	OHCA	40	Vasopressin 40 IU followed by epinephrine	13.9
Stiell, 2001 [27]	IHCA	200	Vasopressin 40 IU followed by epinephrine	6.7
Wenzel, 2004 [29]	OHCA	1186	Vasopressin 40 IU for up to 2 cycles, followed by epinephrine	17.5
Gueugniaud, 2008 [30]	OHCA	2894	Vasopressin 40 IU plus epinephrine for up to 2 cycles, followed by epinephrine	21.4
Mentzelopoulos, 2009 [31]	IHCA	100	Vasopressin 20 IU plus epinephrine for up to 5 cycles, plus methylprednisolone 40 mg (once only)	< 5

Treatment in the control group was epinephrine in all studies. IHCA: in-hospital cardiac arrest; OHCA: out-of-hospital cardiac arrest; IU: International Units.

administration of vasopressin has been criticized because, according to animal studies, vasopressin appears to be more beneficial in conditions of severe acidosis and, therefore, at a later phase of resuscitation [28].

A subsequent randomized controlled trial [29] enrolled 1186 out-of-hospital cardiac arrest patients to receive either 40 IU of vasopressin or 1 mg of epinephrine during two consecutive ALS cycles, followed by additional boluses of epinephrine if needed. The study demonstrated no significant differences in outcome between the two groups, except for the subgroup of patients with asystole, in whom survival to both hospital admission and hospital discharge were significantly higher with vasopressin (76/262 [29.0 %] vs. 54/266 [20.3 %]; p = 0.02 and 2/257 [4.7 %] vs. 4/262 [1.5 %] p = 0.04, respectively); however, the number of patients who survived to discharge in that group was negligible. In a post-hoc analysis of patients with prolonged cardiac arrest in whom additional doses of epinephrine were needed, vasopressin was associated with higher survival both to admission and to discharge, although patients who were given vasopressin had higher rates of poor neurological outcome (10/20 [50 %] vs. 1/5 [20 %]). Again, the effect was particularly evident in patients with asystole. Being the results of a post-hoc analysis, these data lack statistical power and are subject to bias.

To investigate the potential synergistic effects of vasopressin plus epinephrine, a larger, multicenter placebo-controlled study was carried out on 2894 out-of-hospital cardiac arrest patients who were randomized to receive either 1 mg of epinephrine plus 40 IU of vasopressin or epinephrine alone. In both groups, additional epinephrine was given if needed [30]. Unfortunately, the study did not show any differences between the two interventions in terms of ROSC (28.6 % vs. 29.5 %; relative risk, 1.01; 95 % CI 0.97 to 1.06), survival to hospital admission (20.7 % vs. 21.3 %; relative risk of death, 1.01; 95 % CI 0.97 to 1.05), or survival to hospital discharge (1.7 % vs. 2.3 %; relative risk, 1.01; 95 % CI 1.00 to 1.02). The

XIII

rates of good neurological recovery were also similar in the two groups. The study included a high percentage of patients with asystole (82.4 %), which made it very suitable for investigating the possible benefit of vasopressin in that specific group suggested by the previous study.

In a recent single center placebo-controlled trial [31], 100 consecutive patients with in-hospital cardiac arrest were randomized to receive either 1 mg epinephrine or epinephrine plus 20 IU vasopressin per resuscitation cycle for the first five cycles, followed by additional epinephrine if needed. Based on the results of previous observational studies which documented low cortisol levels in patients resuscitated from cardiac arrest, the intervention group received 40 mg methylprednisolone sodium succinate during the first resuscitation cycle. In addition, resuscitated patients with clinical signs of shock in the study group were treated with hydrocortisone sodium succinate at a dose of 300 mg/day for a maximum of seven days. Results showed that the experimental group had significantly higher rates of ROSC (39/48 [81 %] vs. 27/52 [52 %]; p = .003) and survival to hospital discharge 9/48 [19 %] vs. 2/52 [4 %]; p = .02). In 31 patients an arterial line was in place when cardiac arrest occurred; among those patients, systolic, diastolic and mean arterial blood pressures were significantly higher in the intervention group both during CPR and after ROSC. Moreover, vasopressor use during follow-up was significantly lower in the intervention group (p = .002).

The above study was undertaken in the hospital environment, where several patients had venous access in place (36 % of cardiac arrests occurred in the intensive care unit [ICU] or in the operating room [OR]) and response times were relatively short [32]. For this reason, the administration of the study drug occurred in less than 5 minutes, much earlier than in other trials. Another feature was the high dosage of vasopressin (mean 73.3 [± 30.1] IU, range 20–100 IU) administered to the intervention group. Unfortunately, because of the study design, the effects of vasopressin and those of steroids could not be analyzed separately.

A very recent meta-analysis [33] summarized the results of clinical trials on vasopressin for cardiac arrest. It included 4475 patients from six randomized controlled trials published between 1997 and 2009. In all trials, vasopressin was compared with epinephrine. The authors carried out subgroup analyses according to the initial cardiac rhythm and time from collapse to drug administration. Results showed that vasopressin did not improve overall rates of ROSC, long-term survival, or favorable neurological outcome. In the subgroup of patients with asystole in whom the time to drug administration was shorter than 20 minutes, vasopressin was associated with a significantly higher rate of both ROSC and long-term survival (OR 1.70 [95 % CI 1.17–2.47], p = 0.005, and OR 2.84 [95 % CI 1.19–6.79], p = 0.02, respectively). However, this subgroup included only 27 patients (20 in the vasopressin group and 7 in the control group) from three different trials. No data on favorable neurological outcome are available for this subgroup. In contrast to what has been hypothesized by other authors [28] these results seem to suggest that the effects of vasopressin are more beneficial when it is administered early.

XIII

Based on the neutral results of clinical trials, the 2010 Guidelines for Adult Advanced Cardiovascular Life Support of the AHA [9] recommended vasopressin as an alternative to the first or the second dose of epinephrine, at a dose of 40 IU via either intravenous or intraosseous routes. Arginine vasopressin is not or is scarcely available in some European Countries. The ERC 2010 Guidelines for Resuscitation did not make any specific recommendation on vasopressin and refer uniquely to epinephrine as the standard vasopressor drug for cardiac arrest [5].

Drugs versus no Drugs

During recent years, the limited evidence in favor of ALS measures and the evidence of possible harm from epinephrine in the post-resuscitation phase have raised concern as to whether drugs should be used at all during cardiac arrest. To address this point, a trial was conducted by Olasveengen et al. in Norway and its results published on 2009 [34]. In this study, 851 patients were randomized to receive ALS with or without intravenous drug administration. In the no-drug group, venous access and drugs were only allowed 5 minutes after ROSC (**Table 2**). To assess a possible interference from venous access, which is a time-consuming procedure that could divert focus from good-quality resuscitation, CPR quality was monitored using transthoracic impedance. Measures of CPR quality, such as time without compressions, CPR pauses before defibrillation shocks, compression rate and ventilation rate, were calculated. A special characteristic of this trial was that resuscitation was performed according to a local protocol that included three minutes of CPR both before defibrillation and between subsequent shocks in patients with VF (instead of no CPR before defibrillation and two minutes of CPR between subsequent shocks, as in the standard ALS Guidelines).

Results showed that survival to hospital discharge did not differ significantly between the groups, despite a small trend in favor of the drug group (10.5 % vs. 9.2 %, OR 1.16 [95 %CI 0.74 – 1.82], p = .61). Patients in the drug group had significantly higher rates of ROSC (40 % vs. 25 %, OR 1.99 [95 %CI 1.48 – 2.67], p.001), and had longer CPR attempts, during which a higher number of defibrillation shocks were given. There were no differences in the causes of ICU deaths, most of which (69.5 %) were due to brain damage, and no differences in neurological outcome between the two groups were observed. The results of the Olasveengen study [34] suggest that in adults with out-of-hospital cardiac arrest, the administration of drugs does not improve any relevant outcomes, except short-term survival. However, the study was not specifically focused on vasopressors. Epinephrine was administered in 79 % of patients in the drug group but its specific clinical effect could not be assessed separately. Moreover, the intervention could not be blinded for obvious reasons.

A very recent single center, randomized, double-blind, placebo-controlled trial by Jacobs et al. [35] was specifically designed to assess the effects of administration of epinephrine on survival from cardiac arrest (**Table 2**). The study included 534 adult patients (out of the planned 4426) with out-of-hospital cardiac arrest from any cause who were randomized to receive either epinephrine 1 mg or placebo. No other drug was used during ALS. Study drug and placebo were administered at the same time intervals recommended in the ALS guidelines and were repeated up to a maximum of 10 times. Patients in VF/VT who responded early to defibrillation were not randomized.

The results of the study showed that, after adjustment for confounding variables, patients in the epinephrine group had a significantly higher likelihood of achieving ROSC (23.5 % vs. 8.4 %; OR 3.5 [95 % CI 2.1 – 6.0]) and more than twice the odds of surviving to hospital discharge, although the difference was not sig-

Table 2. Methodological features and results of recent clinical trials comparing advanced life support treatment with or without drugs.

Author, year [ref]	Study design	Actual/ planned sample size (%)	Treatment in the intervention group	Treatment in the control group	Controlled for CPR quality	Causes of death documented	Survival (%) ROSC	Survival (%) Discharge
Olas-veengen, 2009 [34]	Random-ized, open-label	851/900 (94.6 %)	Epineph-rine, amio-darone, atropine	No drug or venous access up to 5 minutes after ROSC	Yes	Yes	26.1	9.9
Jacobs, 2011 [35]	Random-ized, dou-ble-blind placebo-controlled	534/4426 (12.1 %)	Epineph-rine	Intravenous placebo	No	No	16.1	3.0

ROSC: recovery of spontaneous circulation. CPR: cardiopulmonary resuscitation.

nificant (4.0 % vs. 1.9 %; OR 2.1 [0.7 – 6.3]). The study was largely underpowered, having recruited only 12 % of the planned sample. This was mainly due to ethical concerns, which prevented four of the five ambulance services that had been initially involved from continuing the study. Funding restrictions and final expiry of the study drug were additional issues. The trial confirmed that ALS drugs, especially vasopressors, significantly increase ROSC rates in adults with out-of-hospital cardiac arrest. There was also a clear trend towards an increased survival to hospital discharge. The main limitation of the trial was the limited sample size, because of its failure to achieve full patient recruitment. Another limitation was that the study did not control for CPR quality, although its placebo-controlled design probably prevented imbalances in CPR quality among the study groups.

Vasopressors for Cardiac Arrest: Benefit or Harm?

XIII

Results of recent clinical trials indicate that use of vasopressors during cardiac arrest increases the rate of successful resuscitation, and this effect is somewhat expected since they increase organ perfusion during CPR. However, there is no definite evidence that vasopressors increase either survival to discharge or neurological prognosis. There are three possible explanations for this:

- A first explanation could be that vasopressors restore spontaneous circulation in patients who are simply 'too ill to survive' and who die as soon as the temporary effect of resuscitation maneuvers and drugs has finished. This would confirm the results of the observational Ontario Prehospital Advanced Life Support (OPALS) study [4], which showed no improvement of survival to discharge when ALS was added to basic life support in an emergency medical system. In this case, vasopressors would just provide futile cardiac resuscitation to patients destined to die shortly afterwards from irreversible organ damage.

- However, it is also possible that patients resuscitated because of the extra benefit of vasopressors are potentially salvageable with the improvement or better implementation of post-resuscitation care. Most patients who die in the ICU after having been resuscitated from cardiac arrest do so from neurological causes [34, 36]. Mild therapeutic hypothermia can reduce postanoxic brain damage and improve survival to hospital discharge and neurological outcome after cardiac arrest [37, 38]. However, recent surveys showed that implementation of mild therapeutic hypothermia in many ICUs in the Western world is still incomplete [39, 40]. Rigorous application of post-resuscitation bundles [41] and triage of resuscitated patients towards specialized cardiac arrest centers where optimal post-resuscitation care is provided [42] represent possible resources to improve prognosis of resuscitated patients in the near future.
- A third explanation could be that vasopressors increase the success rate of cardiac resuscitation because they improve coronary perfusion but also reduce the chances of survival for many resuscitated patients because of their side effects, such as increased post-resuscitation myocardial dysfunction or decreased cerebral microcirculation. However, in the Olasveengen trial [34], distribution of the causes of death was similar in the group that received vasopressors and in the group that received no drug. A second potential indirect harmful effect of vasopressors could be their interference with the resuscitation process, introducing delays in CPR for drug preparation and intravenous access, and diverting team resources from more important tasks. However, the Olasveengen trial did not demonstrate any delay or deterioration in CPR quality in the drug versus no-drug groups.

Conclusion

The role of vasopressors during resuscitation from cardiac arrest needs to be further investigated. In experimental models, vasopressors increase diastolic blood pressure and blood flow to vital organs during CPR and facilitate resuscitation but also have detrimental effects on post-resuscitation myocardial performance and cerebral circulation. Two recent controlled trials in out-of-hospital cardiac arrest patients demonstrated that administration of epinephrine and other drugs was associated with a significant increase in short-term survival but not in survival to hospital discharge. In one of those trials, patients in the epinephrine group had more than twice the odds of surviving to hospital discharge than those who received placebo, but the difference did not reach statistical significance, possibly because of inadequate sample size. Future placebo-controlled trials on larger populations are needed to assess more clearly the association between epinephrine and survival to hospital discharge. Clinical studies are also needed to investigate the occurrence of side effects from vasopressors in humans after resuscitation and their possible influence on hospital survival. At present, epinephrine is the most widely used vasopressor in advanced life support. To date, no advantage from the use of vasopressin rather than epinephrine in any of the relevant outcomes from cardiac arrest has been identified in clinical studies.

References

1. McNally B, Robb R, Mehta M, et al (2011) Out-of-Hospital Cardiac Arrest Surveillance --- Cardiac Arrest Registry to Enhance Survival (CARES), United States, October 1, 2005-- December 31, 2010. MMWR Surveill Summ 60: 1 – 19
2. Sandroni C, Nolan J, Cavallaro F, Antonelli M (2007) In-hospital cardiac arrest: incidence, prognosis and possible measures to improve survival. Intensive Care Med 33: 237 – 245
3. Sasson C, Rogers MA, Dahl J, Kellermann AL (2010). Predictors of survival from out-of-hospital cardiac arrest: a systematic review and meta-analysis. Circ Cardiovasc Qual Outcomes 3: 63 – 81
4. Stiell IG, Wells GA, Field B, et al (2004) Advanced cardiac life support in out-of-hospital cardiac arrest. N Engl J Med 351: 647 – 656
5. Deakin CD, Nolan JP, Soar J, et al (2010) European Resuscitation Council Guidelines for Resuscitation 2010 Section 4. Adult advanced life support. Resuscitation 81: 1305 – 1352
6. Kern KB, Ewy GA, Voorhees WD, Babbs CF, Tacker WA (1988) Myocardial perfusion pressure: a predictor of 24-hour survival during prolonged cardiac arrest in dogs. Resuscitation 16: 241 – 250
7. Brown CG, Katz SE, Werman HA, Luu T, Davis EA, Hamlin RL (1987) The effect of epinephrine versus methoxamine on regional myocardial blood flow and defibrillation rates following a prolonged cardiorespiratory arrest in a swine model. Am J Emerg Med 5: 362 – 369
8. Paradis NA, Martin GB, Rivers EP, et al (1990) Coronary perfusion pressure and the return of spontaneous circulation in human cardiopulmonary resuscitation. JAMA 263: 1106 – 1113
9. Neumar RW, Otto CW, Link MS, et al (2010) Part 8: adult advanced cardiovascular life support: 2010 American Heart Association Guidelines for Cardiopulmonary Resuscitation and Emergency Cardiovascular Care. Circulation 122: S729 – 767
10. Schumann HJ (1983) What role do alpha- and beta-adrenoceptors play in the regulation of the heart? Eur Heart J 4 (Suppl A): 55 – 60
11. Ditchey RV, Lindenfeld J (1988) Failure of epinephrine to improve the balance between myocardial oxygen supply and demand during closed-chest resuscitation in dogs. Circulation 78: 382 – 389
12. Brown AM, Birnbaumer L (1988) Direct G protein gating of ion channels. Am J Physiol 254: H401 – 410
13. Meissner A, Morgan JP (1995) Contractile dysfunction and abnormal Ca2+ modulation during postischemic reperfusion in rat heart. Am J Physiol 268: H100 – 111
14. Gonzalez MM, Berg RA, Nadkarni VM, et al (2008) Left ventricular systolic function and outcome after in-hospital cardiac arrest. Circulation 117: 1864 – 1872
15. Laurent I, Monchi M, Chiche JD, et al (2002) Reversible myocardial dysfunction in survivors of out-of-hospital cardiac arrest. J Am Coll Cardiol 40: 2110 – 2116
16. Tang W, Weil MH, Sun S, Noc M, Yang L, Gazmuri RJ (1995) Epinephrine increases the severity of postresuscitation myocardial dysfunction. Circulation 92: 3089 – 3093
17. Ristagno G, Tang W, Huang L, et al (2009) Epinephrine reduces cerebral perfusion during cardiopulmonary resuscitation. Crit Care Med 37: 1408 – 1415
18. Lindner KH, Strohmenger HU, Ensinger H, Hetzel WD, Ahnefeld FW, Georgieff M (1992) Stress hormone response during and after cardiopulmonary resuscitation. Anesthesiology 77: 662 – 668
19. Zhong JQ, Dorian P (2005) Epinephrine and vasopressin during cardiopulmonary resuscitation. Resuscitation 66: 263 – 269
20. Krismer AC, Lindner KH, Wenzel V, et al (2001) The effects of endogenous and exogenous vasopressin during experimental cardiopulmonary resuscitation. Anesth Analg 92: 1499 – 1504
21. Lindner KH, Prengel AW, Pfenninger EG, et al (1995) Vasopressin improves vital organ blood flow during closed-chest cardiopulmonary resuscitation in pigs. Circulation 91: 215 – 221
22. Wenzel V, Lindner KH, Krismer AC, Miller EA, Voelckel WG, Lingnau W (1999) Repeated administration of vasopressin but not epinephrine maintains coronary perfusion pressure

XIII

after early and late administration during prolonged cardiopulmonary resuscitation in pigs. Circulation 99: 1379–1384

23. Wenzel V, Lindner KH, Prengel AW, et al (1999) Vasopressin improves vital organ blood flow after prolonged cardiac arrest with postcountershock pulseless electrical activity in pigs. Crit Care Med 27: 486–492

24. Sirinek KR, Adcock DK, Levine BA (1989) Simultaneous infusion of nitroglycerin and nitroprusside to offset adverse effects of vasopressin during portosystemic shunting. Am J Surg 157: 33–37

25. Prengel AW, Lindner KH, Keller A, Lurie KG (1996) Cardiovascular function during the postresuscitation phase after cardiac arrest in pigs: a comparison of epinephrine versus vasopressin. Crit Care Med 24: 2014–2019

26. Lindner KH, Dirks B, Strohmenger HU, Prengel AW, Lindner IM, Lurie KG (1997) Randomised comparison of epinephrine and vasopressin in patients with out-of-hospital ventricular fibrillation. Lancet 349: 535–537

27. Stiell IG, Hebert PC, Wells GA, et al (2001) Vasopressin versus epinephrine for inhospital cardiac arrest: a randomised controlled trial. Lancet 358: 105–109

28. Wenzel V, Lindner KH (2001) Vasopressin and epinephrine for cardiac arrest. Lancet 358: 2080–2081

29. Wenzel V, Krismer AC, Arntz HR, Sitter H, Stadlbauer KH, Lindner KH (2004) A comparison of vasopressin and epinephrine for out-of-hospital cardiopulmonary resuscitation. N Engl J Med 350: 105–113

30. Gueugniaud PY, David JS, Chanzy E, et al (2008) Vasopressin and epinephrine vs. epinephrine alone in cardiopulmonary resuscitation. N Engl J Med 359: 21–30

31. Mentzelopoulos SD, Zakynthinos SG, Tzoufi M, et al (2009) Vasopressin, epinephrine, and corticosteroids for in-hospital cardiac arrest. Arch Intern Med 169: 15–24

32. Sandroni C, Cavallaro F, Ferro G, et al (2003) A survey of the in-hospital response to cardiac arrest on general wards in the hospitals of Rome. Resuscitation 56: 41–47

33. Mentzelopoulos SD, Zakynthinos SG, Siempos I, Malachias S, Ulmer H, Wenzel V (2011) Vasopressin for cardiac arrest: Meta-analysis of randomized controlled trials. Resuscitation 83: 32–39

34. Olasveengen TM, Sunde K, Brunborg C, Thowsen J, Steen PA, Wik L (2009) Intravenous drug administration during out-of-hospital cardiac arrest: a randomized trial. JAMA 302: 2222–2229

35. Jacobs IG, Finn JC, Jelinek GA, Oxer HF, Thompson PL (2011) Effect of adrenaline on survival in out-of-hospital cardiac arrest: A randomised double-blind placebo-controlled trial. Resuscitation 82: 1138–1143

36. Laver S, Farrow C, Turner D, Nolan J (2004) Mode of death after admission to an intensive care unit following cardiac arrest. Intensive Care Med 30: 2126–2128

37. Bernard SA, Gray TW, Buist MD, et al (2002) Treatment of comatose survivors of out-of-hospital cardiac arrest with induced hypothermia. N Engl J Med 346: 557–563

38. The Hypothermia After Cardiac Arrest Study Group (2002) Mild therapeutic hypothermia to improve the neurologic outcome after cardiac arrest. N Engl J Med 346: 549–556

39. Merchant RM, Soar J, Skrifvars MB, et al (2006) Therapeutic hypothermia utilization among physicians after resuscitation from cardiac arrest. Crit Care Med 34: 1935–1940

40. Binks AC, Murphy RE, Prout RE, et al (2010) Therapeutic hypothermia after cardiac arrest – implementation in UK intensive care units. Anaesthesia 65: 260–265

41. Stub D, Bernard S, Duffy SJ, Kaye DM (2011) Post cardiac arrest syndrome: a review of therapeutic strategies. Circulation 123: 1428–1435

42. Soar J, Packham S (2010) Cardiac arrest centres make sense. Resuscitation 81: 507–508

Cerebral Blood Flow after Cardiac Arrest

L.L.A. Bisschops, C.W.E. Hoedemaekers, and J.G. van der Hoeven

Introduction

Patients resuscitated from a cardiac arrest have a high (in-hospital) mortality rate between 50–90 %. Although in the past few decades more patients have a return of spontaneous circulation (ROSC), overall prognosis has not substantially improved [1] and only a minority of patients survive with a favorable neurological recovery [2]. In 1972, Negovsky described the 'post-resuscitation syndrome', a constellation of pathophysiological processes occurring after ROSC. In 2008, the International Liaison Committee on Resuscitation (ILCOR) proposed a new term: The post-cardiac arrest syndrome [3]. Growing understanding of the post-cardiac arrest syndrome has contributed to the development of new therapeutic strategies. For example, mild therapeutic hypothermia was effective in improving neurological outcome after cardiac arrest in two randomized controlled trials [4, 5]. These results were recently confirmed in a retrospective, multicenter observational study showing that the implementation of mild therapeutic hypothermia in Dutch intensive care units (ICUs) was associated with a 20 % relative reduction in hospital mortality [6].

Post-cardiac Arrest Syndrome

The post-cardiac arrest syndrome is usually divided into 4 phases: (1) Immediate post-arrest phase (0–20 minutes after ROSC); (2) early post-arrest phase (period between 20 minutes and 6 to 12 hours after ROSC) when interventions are probably most effective; (3) intermediate post-arrest phase (period between 6 to 12 hours to 72 hours after ROSC) when injury pathways are still active; and finally (4) the recovery phase (> 72 hours after ROSC).

XIII

Pathophysiological Processes after ROSC

Instead of denominating the different phases of the post-cardiac arrest syndrome, describing its underlying pathophysiology is probably more informative. The post-cardiac arrest syndrome is a unique and complex combination of different processes including: (a) post-cardiac arrest brain injury; (b) post-cardiac arrest myocardial dysfunction; (c) systemic ischemia/reperfusion injury; and (d) persistent precipitating pathology such as acute myocardial infarction, pulmonary disease, thromboembolic disease, central nervous system (CNS) disease, hypovolemia, infection (sepsis) or toxicological factors.

J.-L. Vincent (ed.), *Annual Update in Intensive Care and Emergency Medicine 2012*
DOI 10.1007/978-3-642-25716-2 © Springer-Verlag Berlin Heidelberg 2012

In patients admitted to the ICU, brain injury is the leading cause of death in 68 % of patients after out-of-hospital cardiac arrest and in 23 % after in-hospital cardiac arrest [7]. The amount of brain damage is mainly determined by the period of primary cerebral ischemia. Of all the different body tissues, the brain is the most vulnerable for ischemia, with irreversible tissue damage occurring within minutes. The mechanisms leading to superimposed secondary neurological damage are complex and the result of cerebral perfusion failure due to impaired cerebrovascular autoregulation, cerebral edema and post ischemic neurodegeneration. In animal experiments cerebral blood flow (CBF) after cardiac arrest is characterized by 4 consecutive phases: (I) No-reflow; (II) global hyperemia, (III) delayed global hypoperfusion, and (IV) return to normal, increased or decreased CBF [8]. Different cell death pathways (neuronal necrosis and apoptosis) are mediated by various injury cascades [9]. Because many of the injury cascades develop over a period of hours to days, this implies a potential neuroprotective therapeutic window.

It is important to recognize myocardial dysfunction shortly after ROSC because it may contribute to a further decrease in CBF and to the development of multiple organ failure. Global myocardial dysfunction is usually transient and full recovery within days is common. During cardiopulmonary resuscitation (CPR), oxygen delivery (DO_2) and removal of metabolites is insufficient. Whole body ischemia/reperfusion injury with associated oxygen debt leads to activation of coagulation and several inflammatory pathways, which may result in multiple organ failure (MOF). Specific treatment of the precipitating cause is necessary and preferably happens in concordance with the treatment of the post-cardiac arrest syndrome, directed to brain preservation and optimization of CBF.

Cerebral Blood Flow

Although the brain is only about 2 % of the total body weight, it receives 15 % of the cardiac output. Under normal circumstances, regulation of the CBF is under direction of the brain itself, and is controlled through three different mechanisms changing cerebrovascular resistance: (1) Metabolic activity; (2) pressure autoregulation; and (3) cerebrovascular reactivity. Although perivascular adrenergic nerves richly supply the cerebral circulation, the importance of neural regulation of the cerebral circulation remains controversial [10, 11].

Cerebral Blood Flow after Cardiac Arrest

The amount of brain damage after cardiac arrest strongly depends on the recovery of the cerebral circulation. Understanding the pathophysiology and temporal pattern of cerebral perfusion is essential. Unfortunately, human studies are rare and the bulk of our present knowledge is obtained from animal studies. ROSC does not automatically restore normal cerebral circulation. Animal experiments demonstrate that the course of CBF after cardiac arrest is abnormal for several days. CBF with normotensive reperfusion after ROSC apparently progresses through 4 different stages.

Multifocal No-reflow

When blood flow to the brain is interrupted for more than a few minutes, vascular changes occur which interfere with the re-establishment of normal CBF. This has been referred to as the 'no-reflow phenomenon'. First described by Ames et al. post-ischemic perfusion defects increased in number and size with the duration of global ischemia [12]. Kågström et al. showed that areas of no-reflow appeared after 10 minutes of ischemia, were more extensive after 15 minutes, and occupied a major part of the brain after 30 minutes [13]. Several authors confirmed these data in different animal models. The threshold duration of ischemia for the manifestation of no-reflow is approximately 7 minutes of complete ischemia and is close to the ischemic threshold of irreversible brain damage [14].

Different mechanisms may contribute to the multifocal no-reflow: (1) Red blood cell (RBC) aggregation resulting in increased blood viscosity. However, the role of blood viscosity in the no-reflow phenomenon remains disputed, because hypothermia attenuates multifocal no-reflow, while increasing blood viscosity; (2) narrowing and occlusion of vascular lumina due to ischemia-induced swelling of perivascular glia and endothelial cells. A decrease in ATP levels may result in failure of active transport processes, resulting in movement of salts and water from plasma into perivascular cells; (3) cerebrovascular resistance increases during ischemia because of an increase in extracellular potassium concentration which depolarizes vascular smooth muscle cell membranes; (4) leukocyte adhesion; (5) intravascular coagulation [15]; (6) post-cardiac arrest hypotension, occurring in a high proportion of cardiac arrest survivors on admission to the ICU [16]. If autoregulation is disturbed, severe hypotension leads to decreased and insufficient perfusion pressure of the brain.

Transient Global Hyperemia (Vasoparalysis)

This next phase (15–30 minutes) is characterized by transient global vasoparalysis and 'reactive' hyperemia, which can co-exist with the no-reflow phase [17]. Since the no-reflow is heterogeneous, post-ischemic reactive hyperemia is heterogeneous as well. Measurement of global CBF after ischemia may therefore reveal normal or even increased flow rates, although focal areas of no-reflow are still present. The vasoparalysis is attributed to tissue acidosis and does not respond to changes in blood pressure or carbon dioxide. After ROSC, the viscosity of streaming blood declines. As a result of brain swelling, which already starts to develop in the no-reflow phase, and the following hyperemia, intracranial pressure (ICP) may increase sharply but usually normalizes before the next hypoperfusion phase starts.

XIII

Delayed (Protracted) Global Hypoperfusion

The severity of the protracted global hypoperfusion phase is independent of the duration of ischemia. In contrast, the timing of the hypoperfusion phase correlates with the duration of ischemia: The longer the ischemia, the later the onset of hypoperfusion. Based on various lines of evidence, the underlying pathophysiology appears to indicate a functional disturbance because of an increased arterio-arteriolar vascular tone. During the delayed hypoperfusion phase, CBF is characterized by an (inhomogeneous) decrease to about 50 % or less [18]. In cardiac arrest patients treated with normothermia, cerebrovascular resistance was initially high and gradually decreased during the first 24 hours [19]. This may be explained by an imbalance between local production of vasoconstrictors and vasodilators such as endothelin-1 and nitric oxide (NO). Another possible factor contributing to hypoperfusion is platelet and leukocyte adhesion triggered by morphological changes of the vascular lumen or by increased expression of adhesion molecules.

An abnormal coupling between CBF and brain metabolism is controversial. Several studies conclude that the ratio of CBF to cerebral metabolic rate of oxygen ($CMRO_2$) is normal [20]. Other studies indicate uncoupling (increase in $CMRO_2$ while CBF decreases) aggravating ischemia [21].

Normal, Low or Increased Cerebral Blood Flow

Finally, after 20–24 hours, CBF either returns to normal values, remains low (with low global oxygen uptake/coma) or increases. Secondary hyperemia may be a sign of severe postanoxic cerebral impairment or brain death [22].

Treatment Strategies in the ICU to Improve Cerebral Blood Flow

Treatment in the ICU is directed towards limiting the pathophysiological changes and creating an optimal environment for cerebral recovery. Prevention of secondary brain damage is a major concern. International guidelines on CPR recommend maintaining normotension, normoglycemia and normocapnia. However, so far it has been insufficiently clarified whether 'normal' is also ideal for the injured brain and if supraphysiological parameters should be pursued.

Arterial Blood Pressure

Many cardiac arrest patients face hypotension, dysrhythmias, and low cardiac output [23]. Nevertheless the effect of inotropes and vasopressors on survival has not been studied in clinical trials. No data are available from prospective clinical studies to determine the optimal blood pressure after ROSC. Normally, CBF is relatively constant when cerebral perfusion pressure (CPP = mean arterial pressure [MAP] – ICP) varies between 50–150 mmHg. Most (normothermic) cardiac arrest survivors show abnormal or absent cerebral pressure autoregulation [24]. Animal studies suggest that increasing MAP is important to improve outcome by mitigating both no-reflow and delayed hypoperfusion. A good outcome after cardiac arrest has been reported in studies in which the target MAP was as low as 65–75 mmHg or as high as 90–100 mmHg [25]. Hypertension (MAP > 100 mmHg) in the first 5 minutes after ROSC did not improve neurological recovery, but a higher MAP in the first 2 hours after ROSC showed a positive correlation with neurological outcome in a retrospective evaluation of 136 patients. Sasser and Safar examined the data from 1,234 cardiac arrest patients who survived at least 12 hours. After controlling for age, sex, arrest time, CPR time and pre-existing diseases, higher systolic arterial pressures at 1–2 min, 5 min, 10 min, 20 min, and 60 min were associated with CPC 1 or 2 (good outcome) [26]. In a prospective observational study we showed that a higher MAP (80–90 mmHg) may enhance the protective effects of hypothermia on cerebrovascular autoregulation

XIII

[27]. Although the optimal blood pressure in humans is still unknown, a MAP ≥ 65 mmHg is considered a reasonable goal by most.

It is debated whether sympathetic activity also influences CBF and cerebral oxygenation. If sympathetic influence on CBF exists, this could be important in the management of hypotensive patients. Without α-adrenergic influence on CBF, a low MAP can be increased to the cerebral autoregulation range by α-adrenergic receptor agonists to secure CBF and cerebral oxygenation. If CBF is influenced by cerebral α-adrenergic stimulation, CBF and cerebral oxygenation may decline while MAP increases. The direct effects of norepinephrine on CBF in cardiac arrest survivors are unknown and probably also depend on the metabolic activity of the brain, the integrity of the blood brain barrier and the level of autoregulation.

Cardiac Output

Impaired autoregulation is thought to play an important role in the relationship between cardiac output and CBF. However, no human study has investigated this relationship. In severely head injured patients no correlation existed between changes in cardiac output and changes in CBF, regardless of the status of autoregulation. According to Poiseuille's law, flow is the quotient of perfusion pressure and vascular resistance, without cardiac output fitting in this equation. At controlled levels of $PaCO_2$ moderate hypovolemia that did not change MAP, significantly decreased cardiac output and CBF in normal cats. The effect of cardiac output on CBF in cardiac arrest patients needs further studies. Central venous oxygen saturation ($ScvO_2$) is frequently used as a substitute for an adequate cardiac output. Although post-cardiac arrest care guidelines suggest an ideal target for $ScvO_2 \geq 70$ %, there are no human data available to support this.

Volume Expansion

As a result of ischemia/reperfusion injury, volume expansion is indicated in most cardiac arrest patients. Prospective clinical trials to assess the effects of early goal directed therapy as studied in sepsis or postoperative patients are not available for post-cardiac arrest patients. Animal data indicate that volume expansion with hypertonic solutions may have a beneficial effect on CBF when given during CPR by preventing post-ischemic hemoconcentration. Cerebral no-reflow after 15 minutes of cardiac arrest was significantly reduced by small volume hypertonic solutions in cats [28]. Krep et al. [29] demonstrated that infusion of hypertonic solutions during CPR preserved total and regional CBF and prevented post-cardiac arrest delayed cerebral hypoperfusion. Improvement may be due to the rapid volume expansion or to osmotic dehydration reversing endothelial swelling and augmenting reoxygenation. Cell shrinkage also reduces ICP and, therefore, improves CPP. Finally, hypertonic solutions reduce leukocyte adherence, which is another potential contributing factor to the delayed hypoperfusion phase.

XIII

Hematocrit/viscosity

The relationship between perfusion pressure and blood flow is partly determined by blood viscosity. Viscosity decreases as the shear rate, determined by blood flow velocity and vessel diameter, increases. The rheological properties of blood depend on hematocrit and plasma constituents. Blood cells increase viscosity whereas (colloidal) plasma expanders decrease blood viscosity. Viscosity also increases as temperature decreases. Hemodilution increases CBF in both normal and ischemic brain. It is debated whether CBF improves after hemodilution because of a diminished oxygen content with ensuing vasodilation or due to a decrease in blood viscosity. However, in the ischemic brain, local coupling of CBF to oxygen demand may be disrupted and the importance of blood viscosity probably increases [30]. The optimal hematocrit in cardiac arrest patients is still unknown.

Carbon Dioxide

Hypocapnic alkalosis shifts the oxyhemoglobin dissociation curve leftwards and reduces cerebral oxygen supply. Furthermore, cerebral vessels are very sensitive to changes in CO_2. Decreases in CO_2 result in marked cerebral vasoconstriction with a subsequent decrease of CBF. Hypercapnia preferentially dilates the smaller arterioles, but the vasoconstrictor effect of hypocapnia is size-independent. Changes in hydrogen ion concentration of the extracellular fluid in the vicinity of the cerebral blood vessels exert their effect directly on cerebral vascular smooth muscle cells [31]. Molecular CO_2 and the bicarbonate ion do not have inherent vasoactivity unless a change in pH is allowed to occur. The effect of changes in CO_2 depends on the prevailing bicarbonate ion concentration in the cerebrospinal fluid and extracellular fluid, since the blood brain barrier is freely permeable to CO_2 but impermeable to bicarbonate ions.

Hypocapnia-induced brain ischemia may also occur as a result of increased neuronal excitability. Increased neuronal excitability may worsen brain injury by an augmented cerebral oxygen demand and raised production of cytotoxic excitatory amino acids. Although hypocapnia-induced cerebral vasoconstriction has a beneficial effect on ICP, it is generally outweighed by the effects of a reduced oxygen supply.

One form of hypocapnic alkalosis is rarely discussed. During CPR, a critical reduction in pulmonary blood flow results in dissociation between central venous blood (high $PcvCO_2$ and low pH) and arterial blood (low $PaCO_2$ and high pH). This condition is referred to as pseudorespiratory alkalosis [32] and potentially results in severe cerebral vasoconstriction. After ROSC, cardiac arrest patients are generally treated with mild therapeutic hypothermia. Under normothermic conditions, cerebrovascular reactivity to changes in arterial PCO_2 is preserved [19]. We demonstrated intact CO_2 reactivity during a 24 h period of mild therapeutic hypothermia in comatose patients after cardiac arrest. Hypocapnia and hypercapnia were induced by adjusting mechanical ventilator settings. The mean change in mean flow velocity in the middle cerebral artery (MFV_{MCA}) as a parameter of CBF was 3.6 ± 2.9 %/mmHg. Hypoventilation resulted in a 4.4 ± 3.5 %/mmHg increase in MFV_{MCA} and hyperventilation resulted in a 2.8 ± 2.2 %/mmHg decrease in MFV_{MCA} (**Fig. 1**) [27]. Falkenbach et al. observed a high incidence of unintentional, iatrogenic hypo- and hypercapnia with marked delays in correction in cardiac arrest patients treated with mild therapeutic hypothermia. These studies emphasize the importance of strict control of mechanical ventilation in cardiac arrest survivors [33].

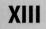

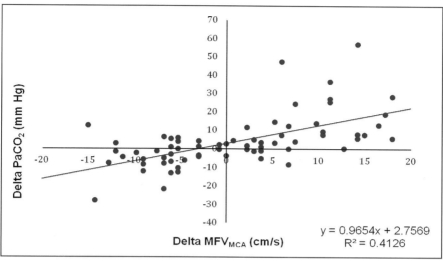

Fig. 1. Correlation between the change in $PaCO_2$ and mean flow velocity in the middle cerebral artery (MFV_{MCA}). From [27] with permission

Hypoxia/Hyperoxia

In contrast to CO_2, CBF is relatively insensitive to changes in PaO_2. A measurable increase in CBF is only found with a decrease in PaO_2 to < 55 mmHg. In normal rabbits, hypoxic hypoxia and hemodilution resulted in a similar increase in CBF as arterial oxygen content fell. In ischemic rabbits, hemodilution resulted in a progressive increase in CBF in both ischemic and non-ischemic brain regions. With hypoxic hypoxia, however, CBF in the ischemic region showed no increase or even a slight decrease. Therefore, blood flow augmentation by hemodilution in ischemic brain is probably related to a direct hemorheologic effect rather than the resulting hypoxemia. During ischemia the cerebral vessels are probably maximally dilated, and only perfusion pressure and viscosity influence CBF.

According to the current ILCOR consensus statement, unnecessary arterial hyperoxia should be avoided, especially during the initial post-cardiac arrest period. This advice is based on the growing preclinical evidence suggesting that hyperoxia in the early stages of reperfusion causes excessive oxidative stress. Balan et al. concluded that, in dogs, graded reoxygenation with oximetry guidance in order to reduce postresuscitative hyperoxia resulted in less neurological injury [34]. A recent study by Bellomo et al. found no evidence for an increase in cerebral damage with higher PaO_2 levels in humans [35]. The effects of hyperoxia on CBF in humans after cardiac arrest have not been studied. Although most evidence up to now suggests a detrimental effect of post-cardiac arrest hyperoxia, fear of hyperoxia should not lead to an indiscriminate decrease in inspired oxygen levels. Hypoxemia is certainly bad for the damaged brain.

Pharmacological Treatment

Theoretically, post-ischemic hypoperfusion can be improved by reducing vascular tone. Animal data show that the administration of vasodilators, anti-serotonergic agents and α-adrenergic blockers resulted in a decrease in cerebral vascular tone. However, peripheral vasodilation induces a decrease in CPP with a resultant net unchanged effect on CBF. Administration of calcium antagonists and endothelin antagonists also led to controversial results. Pre- and post-arrest anti-thrombotic therapy with plasminogen activator and heparin showed a strong reduction in cerebral no-reflow in animal studies [36]. Clinical trials have been disappointing thus far.

Hypothermia

Nowadays, mild therapeutic hypothermia is considered the standard of care in most cardiac arrest patients. However, mild therapeutic hypothermia reduces cardiac output and blood pressure and may reduce CBF. We measured low mean flow velocities in the middle cerebral artery in 10 cardiac arrest patients during mild hypothermia (**Fig. 2**). Despite low CBF, the cerebral oxygen extraction remained normal (**Fig. 3**). This suggests decreased metabolic activity with preserved metabolic coupling [27]. Royl et al. measured preserved neurovascular coupling in rats without a temperature threshold below which neurovascular coupling was impaired or lost [37].

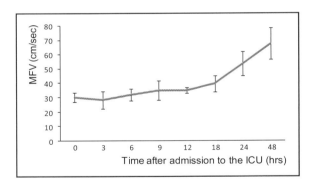

Fig. 2. Mean flow velocity in the middle cerebral artery as measured by transcranial Doppler. Values expressed as mean ± SD. MFV: mean flow velocity in the middle cerebral artery. From [27] with permission

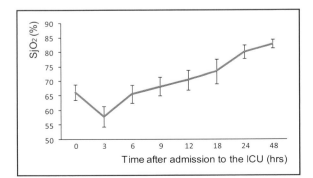

Fig. 3. Jugular bulb oxygen saturation (SjO$_2$). Values are expressed as mean ± SD. From [27] with permission

Blood viscosity increases when blood temperature decreases. However, the increase in viscosity is observed mostly at a temperature below 15 °C. This is congruent with the finding that hypothermia reduces the development of no-reflow in dogs, despite a potential increase in viscosity. In a model with a fixed vessel diameter with laminar flow the linear relationship between flow velocity and blood flow was not affected by hypothermia, underlining that measuring CBF by transcranial Doppler (TCD) is appropriate. The influence of mild therapeutic hypothermia on viscosity-induced changes in CBF appears to be negligible.

Monitoring Cerebral Blood Flow in the ICU

Translation of experimental ischemia-related research to clinical practice is complicated. The complex imaging methods used for research are of limited value in observing and improving CBF in cardiac arrest patients admitted to an ICU. Positron-emission tomography (PET) and magnetic resonance imaging (MRI) are widely used for imaging cerebral ischemia and blood flow. However, for obvious practical reasons these methods suffer from limited relevance in monitoring the ICU patient. In accordance with experimental data which demonstrate that raised ICP is limited to the short hyperemic phase, monitoring ICP in humans demonstrated no sustained increase in ICP during the first 24 hours [38]. Microdialysis is able to show ischemia-induced neurochemical changes after cardiac arrest and during rewarming and could potentially play a role in the guidance of rewarming in those patients not receiving anticoagulant therapy.

Near-infrared spectroscopy (NIRS) is a non-invasive optical technique that calculates oxygen saturation in the arteriovenous capillary beds. NIRS of the brain reflects mostly cerebral venous saturation. The critical level of NIRS at which neurological complication occurs has not been established. So far the utilization of NIRS has not been studied in cardiac arrest patients treated with mild therapeutic hypothermia. In patients undergoing deep hypothermic circulatory arrest NIRS does not closely correlate with jugular venous bulb saturation (SjO_2).

SjO_2 sampling is an invasive technique that allows measurement of the mixed venous saturation of the brain. It provides useful information on the global balance of cerebral oxygen demand and supply. A decrease in SjO_2 points towards a mismatch between oxygen demand and supply that may be amenable to several therapeutic measures. For example, hypocapnia leads to a decrease in SjO_2 and should result in a change in mechanical ventilator settings. Finally, serial TCD examinations may suggest a change in CBF and guide therapy.

XIII

Conclusion

The severity of brain damage after cardiac arrest strongly depends on the recovery of the cerebral circulation. ROSC does not automatically restore normal CBF. Understanding of the pathophysiology of cerebral perfusion is essential. The protracted abnormal level of CBF implies a neuroprotective therapeutic window. Treatment in the ICU is directed towards limiting these pathophysiological changes and creating an optimal environment for cerebral recovery. International guidelines on CPR recommend maintaining normotension, normoglycemia and normocapnia. Unfortunately, optimal blood pressure, amount of CBF, hemoglobin level, PaO_2 and $PaCO_2$ are still unknown.

References

1. Eckstein M, Stratton SJ, Chan LS (2005) Cardiac Arrest Resuscitation Evaluation in Los Angeles: CARE-LA. Ann Emerg Med 45: 504–509
2. Holzer M, Bernard SA, Hachimi-Idrissi S, Roine RO, Sterz F, Mullner M (2005) Hypothermia for neuroprotection after cardiac arrest: systematic review and individual patient data meta-analysis. Crit Care Med 33: 414–418
3. Neumar RW, Nolan JP, Adrie C, et al (2008) Post-cardiac arrest syndrome: epidemiology, pathophysiology, treatment, and prognostication. A consensus statement from the International Liaison Committee on Resuscitation (American Heart Association, Australian and New Zealand Council on Resuscitation, European Resuscitation Council, Heart and Stroke Foundation of Canada, InterAmerican Heart Foundation, Resuscitation Council of Asia, and the Resuscitation Council of Southern Africa); the American Heart Association Emergency Cardiovascular Care Committee; the Council on Cardiovascular Surgery and Anesthesia; the Council on Cardiopulmonary, Perioperative, and Critical Care; the Council on Clinical Cardiology; and the Stroke Council. Circulation 118: 2452–2483
4. HACA-study group (2002) Mild therapeutic hypothermia to improve the neurologic outcome after cardiac arrest. N Engl J Med 346: 549–556
5. Bernard SA, Gray TW, Buist MD, et al (2002) Treatment of comatose survivors of out-of-hospital cardiac arrest with induced hypothermia. N Engl J Med 346: 557–563
6. van der Wal G, Brinkman S, Bisschops LL, et al (2011) Influence of mild therapeutic hypothermia after cardiac arrest on hospital mortality. Crit Care Med 39: 84–88
7. Laver S, Farrow C, Turner D, Nolan J (2004) Mode of death after admission to an intensive care unit following cardiac arrest. Intensive Care Med 30: 2126–2128
8. Safar P (1993) Cerebral resuscitation after cardiac arrest: research initiatives and future directions. Ann Emerg Med 22: 324–349
9. Martin LJ, Al-Abdulla NA, Brambrink AM, Kirsch JR, Sieber FE, Portera-Cailliau C (1988) Neurodegeneration in excitotoxicity, global cerebral ischemia, and target deprivation: A perspective on the contributions of apoptosis and necrosis. Brain Res Bull 46: 281–309
10. van Lieshout JJ, Secher NH (2008) Point:Counterpoint: Sympathetic activity does/does not influence cerebral blood flow. Point: Sympathetic activity does influence cerebral blood flow. J Appl Physiol 105: 1364–1366
11. Edvinsson L (2008) Comments on Point:Counterpoint: Sympathetic activity does/does not influence cerebral blood flow. Sympathetic nerves influence the cerebral circulation. J Appl Physiol 105: 1370–1371
12. Ames A, III, Wright RL, Kowada M, Thurston JM, Majno G (1968) Cerebral ischemia. II. The no-reflow phenomenon. Am J Pathol 52: 437–453
13. Kagstrom E, Smith ML, Siesjo BK (1983) Local cerebral blood flow in the recovery period following complete cerebral ischemia in the rat. J Cereb Blood Flow Metab 3: 170–182
14. Hossmann KA (1997) Reperfusion of the brain after global ischemia: hemodynamic disturbances. Shock 8: 95–101
15. Bottiger BW, Motsch J, Bohrer H, et al (1995) Activation of blood coagulation after cardiac arrest is not balanced adequately by activation of endogenous fibrinolysis. Circulation 92: 2572–2578
16. Trzeciak S, Jones AE, Kilgannon JH, et al (2009) Significance of arterial hypotension after resuscitation from cardiac arrest. Crit Care Med 37: 2895–2903
17. Snyder JV, Nemoto EM, Carroll RG, Safar P (1975) Global ischemia in dogs: intracranial pressures, brain blood flow and metabolism. Stroke 6: 21–27
18. Safar P, Stezoski W, Nemoto EM (1976) Amelioration of brain damage after 12 minutes' cardiac arrest in dogs. Arch Neurol 33: 91–95
19. Buunk G, van der Hoeven JG, Meinders AE (1997) Cerebrovascular reactivity in comatose patients resuscitated from a cardiac arrest. Stroke 28: 1569–1573
20. Beckstead JE, Tweed WA, Lee J, MacKeen WL (1978) Cerebral blood flow and metabolism in man following cardiac arrest. Stroke 9: 569–573

21. Nemoto EM, Hossmann KA, Cooper HK (1981) Post-ischemic hypermetabolism in cat brain. Stroke 12: 666–676
22. Cohan SL, Mun SK, Petite J, et al (1989) Cerebral blood flow in humans following resuscitation from cardiac arrest. Stroke 20: 761–765
23. Peberdy MA, Callaway CW, Neumar RW, et al (2010) Part 9: post-cardiac arrest care: 2010 American Heart Association Guidelines for Cardiopulmonary Resuscitation and Emergency Cardiovascular Care. Circulation 122 (18 Suppl 3): S768-S786
24. Sundgreen C, Larsen FS, Herzog TM, Knudsen GM, Boesgaard S, Aldershvile J (2001) Autoregulation of cerebral blood flow in patients resuscitated from cardiac arrest. Stroke 32: 128–132
25. Rincon F (2010) Preserved cerebral coupling and cerebrovascular reactivity after cardiac arrest: lessons learned in the era of therapeutic hypothermia. Crit Care Med 38: 1603–1605
26. Sasser HC, Safar P (1999) Arterial hypertension after cardiac arrest is associated with good cerebral outcome in patients. Crit Care Med 27: A29 (abst)
27. Bisschops LL, Hoedemaekers CW, Simons KS, van der Hoeven JG (2010) Preserved metabolic coupling and cerebrovascular reactivity during mild hypothermia after cardiac arrest. Crit Care Med 38: 1542–1547
28. Fischer M, Hossmann KA (1996) Volume expansion during cardiopulmonary resuscitation reduces cerebral no-reflow. Resuscitation 32: 227–240
29. Krep H, Breil M, Sinn D, Hagendorff A, Hoeft A, Fischer M (2004) Effects of hypertonic versus isotonic infusion therapy on regional cerebral blood flow after experimental cardiac arrest cardiopulmonary resuscitation in pigs. Resuscitation 63: 73–83
30. Korosue K, Heros RC (1992) Mechanism of cerebral blood flow augmentation by hemodilution in rabbits. Stroke 23: 1487–1492
31. Wahl M, Deetjen P, Thurau K, Ingvar DH, Lassen NA (1970) Micropuncture evaluation of the importance of perivascular pH for the arteriolar diameter on the brain surface. Pflugers Arch 316: 152–163
32. Adrogue HJ, Madias NE (1998) Management of life-threatening acid-base disorders. Second of two parts. N Engl J Med 338: 107–111
33. Falkenbach P, Kamarainen A, Makela A, et al (2009) Incidence of iatrogenic dyscarbia during mild therapeutic hypothermia after successful resuscitation from out-of-hospital cardiac arrest. Resuscitation 80: 990–993
34. Balan IS, Fiskum G, Hazelton J, Cotto-Cumba C, Rosenthal RE (2006) Oximetry-guided reoxygenation improves neurological outcome after experimental cardiac arrest. Stroke 37: 3008–3013
35. Bellomo R, Bailey M, Eastwood GM, et al (2011) Arterial hyperoxia and in-hospital mortality after resuscitation from cardiac arrest. Crit Care 15: R90
36. Fischer M, Bottiger BW, Popov-Cenic S, Hossmann KA (1996) Thrombolysis using plasminogen activator and heparin reduces cerebral no-reflow after resuscitation from cardiac arrest: an experimental study in the cat. Intensive Care Med 22: 1214–1223
37. Royl G, Fuchtemeier M, Leithner C, et al (2008) Hypothermia effects on neurovascular coupling and cerebral metabolic rate of oxygen. Neuroimage 40: 1523–1532
38. Nordmark J, Rubertsson S, Mortberg E, Nilsson P, Enblad P (2009) Intracerebral monitoring in comatose patients treated with hypothermia after a cardiac arrest. Acta Anaesthesiol Scand 53: 289–298

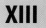

Post-resuscitation Care: What's Most Important for a Good Outcome?

P. Meybohm, J.-T. Graesner, and B. Bein

Introduction

Optimization of survival after cardiac arrest is achieved ideally by strengthening all four links of the chain of survival. Recently, developments in post-resuscitation care have had a particularly positive impact on outcome. The following chapter aims to provide some answers to the question, "Which post-resuscitation treatment yields best results with respect to outcome?"

Approximately one-third of patients admitted to an intensive care unit (ICU) after cardiac arrest survive to hospital discharge [1], but there is considerable variation in post-resuscitation care and patient outcome among different hospitals [2]. Sustained global ischemia during cardiac arrest and the subsequent reperfusion injury that starts immediately with cardiopulmonary resuscitation (CPR) result in the so-called post-cardiac arrest syndrome [3], which includes:

- brain injury
- myocardial dysfunction
- the systemic ischemia/reperfusion response, and
- the persistent precipitating pathology

Interventions that optimize neurological and myocardial recovery after successful CPR will be most likely to influence the chance of long-term survival.

Targeted Temperature Management

Based on two clinical studies reporting a better long-term neurological outcome [4, 5], mild therapeutic hypothermia at 32–34 °C for 12–24 hours is currently a mainstay of post-cardiac arrest care and is recommended in patients following initial successful CPR but remaining comatose [6]. It should be emphasized that both these studies also showed an improvement in overall survival among those treated with mild hypothermia. A decrease in post-cardiac arrest neurological deaths may account for this outcome benefit, but a decrease in post-cardiac arrest myocardial dysfunction and subsequent cardiac deaths could also have contributed. Several experimental studies have addressed the positive effects of mild hypothermia on post-cardiac arrest myocardial dysfunction [7, 8]. Jacobshagen et al. [9] investigated the influence of mild hypothermia on hemodynamic variables in resuscitated patients. These authors were able to progressively decrease the epinephrine dose as mild hypothermia progressed.

J.-L. Vincent (ed.), *Annual Update in Intensive Care and Emergency Medicine 2012*
DOI 10.1007/978-3-642-25716-2 © Springer-Verlag Berlin Heidelberg 2012

Use of mild hypothermia is accepted to treat comatose survivors of out-of-hospital ventricular fibrillation/ventricular tachycardia (VF/VT) cardiac arrest. In survivors of cardiac arrest from non-shockable rhythms, however, the use of mild hypothermia is more controversial [10]. A recent analysis by the German Resuscitation Registry Study Group [11] found that mild hypothermia was associated with increased 24 h-survival (adjusted OR 8.24 [95 % CI 4.24–16.0]). Interestingly, these favorable effects were observed irrespective of the initial electrocardiogram (EKG) rhythm: 24 h-survival rate was 92 % in patients with shockable and 90 % in those with an initial non-shockable rhythm. With respect to neurological recovery, regression analysis further revealed that mild hypothermia was an independent factor for good neurological outcome at hospital discharge (adjusted OR 2.13 [95 % CI 1.17–3.90]). In contrast, recent data from a large French cardiac arrest registry did not show any benefit of mild hypothermia in patients with non-shockable rhythms [12]. Mild hypothermia was associated with good neurological outcome in patients with VF/VT (adjusted OR 1.90 [95 % CI 1.18–3.06]) but not in the pulseless electrical activity (PEA)/asystole group (adjusted OR 0.71 [95 % CI 0.37 – 1.36]).

It is conceivable that the reduction in hyperthermia, rather than the use of mild hypothermia, may be the key factor that improves neurological recovery after successful resuscitation. No studies have yet compared mild hypothermia with strict normothermia. The recently launched 'Target Temperature Management After Cardiac Arrest' trial, which compares temperature management at 33 °C with 36 °C, may provide some answers (NCT01020916).

In terms of the optimal time for initiation of cooling, clinical trials have not yet shown that a shorter time elapsed before initiating hypothermia improves outcome. Ultimately, cooling during cardiac arrest may provide the most effective neuroprotection, a strategy that has been investigated with the use of intranasal evaporative cooling [13].

Adverse events, such as aspiration, myocardial dysfunction and hemodynamic instability, are common in the post-cardiac arrest period but the extent, if any, to which these adverse events are aggravated by mild hypothermia, is controversial. In a recent review, it was suggested that hypothermia may not increase complications at all [10]. On the basis of these data derived from a few randomized clinical trials, the rate of pneumonia/sepsis was 50/300 (17 %) in the hypothermia group versus 36/285 (13 %) in the control group. However, recent studies have documented much higher rates of infection in post-cardiac arrest patients. A registry-based study of out-of-hospital cardiac arrest patients who were treated with mild hypothermia in 22 hospitals in Europe and the United States documented the diagnosis 'pneumonia/sepsis' in 52 % of patients [14]. Infectious complications were more common in those patients admitted to an ICU after cardiac arrest and treated with mild hypothermia compared with those who were not cooled (69 versus 59 %, p = 0.03) [15].

Because the term 'therapeutic' implies a favorable effect that has not yet been demonstrated to be true in all circumstances, it has very recently been recommended that the term 'targeted temperature management' be used instead of 'therapeutic hypothermia' [16].

XIII

Coronary Reperfusion Therapy

In non-cardiac arrest patients with acute myocardial ischemia, early reperfusion by either percutaneous coronary intervention (PCI) or pharmacological thrombolysis is currently considered the treatment of first choice and is strongly recommended [17, 18]. Because the underlying causes of out-of-hospital cardiac arrest are mostly cardiac arrhythmia and acute myocardial ischemia subsequent to coronary artery occlusion [19–21], therapeutic coronary reperfusion strategies may be equally appropriate in cardiac arrest patients. Some years ago, however, an international multicenter study of 1050 cardiac arrest patients failed to demonstrate any benefit for systemic thrombolysis [22]. In contrast, in a selected group of cardiac arrest patients, primary PCI had a good success rate and reasonably good results in terms of short and longer term survival. In 25 patients with ST elevation myocardial infarction (STEMI) after out-of-hospital cardiac arrest, in-hospital and 1 year survivals without severe neurological disability were 68 % and 64 %, respectively [23]. Gorjup and colleagues [24] also reported that cardiac arrest patients with acute myocardial infarction benefited from primary PCI such that their outcome was comparable to that of non-cardiac arrest patients. Interestingly, immediate PCI may also be beneficial in cardiac arrest patients without any ST-segment elevation. A recent multivariate analysis of the 'Parisian Region Out of hospital Cardiac ArresT' (PROCAT) registry that included 435 patients with no obvious extracardiac cause of arrest, revealed that successful coronary angioplasty was an independent predictive factor of survival, regardless of the post-resuscitation EKG pattern (adjusted OR 2.06 [95 % CI 1.16–3.66]) [12]. In addition, at least one significant coronary artery lesion was detected in 96 % of patients with ST-segment elevation, but also in 58 % of patients without any ST-segment elevation. Under these circumstances, the early post-resuscitation 12-lead EKG may be less reliable for predicting acute coronary occlusion than it is in patients who do not have a cardiac arrest. Also, the high incidence of coronary lesions within the PROCAT study cohort highlights that acute coronary syndrome and out-of-hospital cardiac arrest are very closely linked. Coronary plaque rupture or erosion, fragmentation, and embolization of thrombus were identified as factors able to trigger pre-hospital cardiac arrest.

Within the German Resuscitation Registry [11], PCI was an independent predictor of an increased chance of 24 h-survival and good neurological outcome at hospital discharge. The proportion of patients with cerebral performance category 1 or 2 at hospital discharge increased from 10 % to 54 % if PCI was performed within 24 h after return of spontaneous circulation (ROSC). Even in the subgroup of patients with an initial non-shockable rhythm, 24 h-survival interestingly increased from 56 % to 88 % if PCI was performed. Thus, patients with poorer baseline conditions (initial non-shockable rhythm) may also benefit from coronary intervention. Based on these data it is reasonable that all survivors of cardiac arrest from a likely cardiac cause, regardless of the EKG pattern, should be considered for urgent coronary angiography and PCI.

To go even further, a standardized post-resuscitation care bundle including a liberal decision for urgent coronary intervention should be offered to most out-of-hospital cardiac arrest patients with successful resuscitation and hospital admission [25]. It should be noted that a typical history of coronary artery disease or EKG changes typical of STEMI was absent in up to 57 % of cardiac arrest patients, in whom coronary angiography revealed pathological findings with

XIII

therapeutic options [26, 27]. Clinical symptoms, such as chest pain, or risk factors are also often lacking in the setting of out-of-hospital cardiac arrest.

Hemodynamic Optimization

There is ample evidence that goal-directed therapy (GDT) may improve outcomes both in surgical patients and in patients in the early stage of sepsis [28–30]. Despite this, GDT algorithms have not yet gained widespread use in daily clinical routine. In a recent report on 15,002 subjects presenting with sepsis from 165 different sites in Europe, the USA and South America, compliance with recommended bundles from the Surviving Sepsis Campaign and hospital mortality were analyzed [31]. Compliance with the entire resuscitation bundle increased from 10.9 % in the first site quarter to 31.3 % by the end of 2 years and unadjusted hospital mortality decreased significantly from 37 % to 30.8 %. However, according to these data, approximately 70 % of patients were still not being treated according to current recommendations at the end of 2008.

It has been suggested that post-resuscitation disease and systemic inflammatory response syndrome (SIRS)/sepsis show many similarities, among those the pronounced inflammation that happens after the initial hit [32]. In this respect, GDT seems to be a logical approach to treat post-cardiac arrest patients. In a recent meta-analysis, however, Jones and co-workers were unable to identify a single trial that tested the efficacy of GDT in the post-resuscitation period [33]. Gaieski et al. reported on their experience with an algorithm based on mean arterial pressure (MAP), central venous pressure (CVP) and central venous oxygen saturation (ScvO$_2$) [34]. These authors found no difference compared to historic controls with respect to mortality or other important endpoints on an intention-to-treat basis, but those patients who completed the algorithm driven therapy successfully had lower mortality rates. However, the studied patient sample was small and the study was merely a feasibility trial rather than a conclusive study. Also, since therapeutic hypothermia was simultaneously rolled out in the authors' institution, it was impossible to discern the relative contributions of the GDT protocol and hypothermia on outcome.

It remains elusive, therefore, whether the proposed algorithm (based on MAP, CVP and ScvO$_2$) is suitable for post-cardiac arrest patients or whether other variables, such as cardiac index, pulse pressure or stroke volume variation (PPV, SVV) may be more appropriate. Since adequate tissue oxygenation is key to survival and outcome, ScvO$_2$ as a variable reflecting global oxygen supply/demand balance may be a reasonable part of a GDT algorithm. However, use of ScvO$_2$ for therapy guidance has been questioned during sepsis because there is a pronounced and sustained increase in ScvO$_2$ due to microvascular shunting [35, 36]. An alternative approach that has been successfully used for optimization of surgical patients is based upon analysis of fluid responsiveness by PPV [37]. On the other hand, our group has recently shown that functional hemodynamic monitoring by PPV is limited in the immediate post-resuscitation period, probably due to impaired left ventricular function after global ischemia [38]. In this respect, echocardiography-derived evaluation of fluid responsiveness may be advantageous. Fluid responsiveness was correctly assessed with high sensitivity and acceptable specificity by echocardiography naïve physicians who were shown a left ventricular two chamber view obtained in pigs during the immediate post-resuscitation

XIII

period [39]. This finding could qualify echocardiography for implementation into treatment protocols, but further research on this issue is urgently needed.

Blood Glucose Management

As an integral part of the post-resuscitation care bundle, control and therapy of blood glucose and electrolyte derangements is recommended. The optimal adjustment of blood glucose in critically ill patients has been the subject of several recent large scale trials but remains controversial. Recommendations with respect to insulin and glucose management derived from the The Diabetes Mellitus Insulin-Glucose Infusion in Acute Myocardial Infarction (DIGAMI) I-study in patients after acute myocardial infarction were not confirmed by the subsequent DIGAMI II trial [40, 41].

Blood glucose derangements after successful resuscitation following cardiac arrest are common in diabetic and non-diabetic patients and and are closely correlated to the duration of CPR. Beiser and co-workers analyzed the national registry on CPR (NRCPR) and reported on changes of blood glucose in patients after in-hospital cardiac arrest. In diabetic patients, blood glucose values up to 307 mg/dl and in non-diabetic patients up to 239 mg/dl were observed [42]. Worse outcomes were reported for diabetic patients with blood glucose levels above 240 mg/dl and for non-diabetic patients with levels below 70 mg/dl. The only randomized trial available to date in patients after successful CPR studied the influence of a strict (blood glucose between 72–108 mg/dl) versus a moderate therapeutic approach (blood glucose between 108–144 mg/dl) [43]. Whereas this study did not find an improved survival in patients receiving strict blood glucose management, patients in the moderately adjusted group had increased neuron specific enolase (NSE) levels, as a marker of possible cerebral damage. As a key determinant for defining a reasonable target range these authors identified pre-existing diabetes, which must be determined upon initiation of blood glucose management. Losert et al. studied the impact of blood glucose variability during the first 24 hours after ROSC on neurologic outcome after 6 months in a multicenter trial on 234 patients [44]. There was no difference between patients who received strict (blood glucose between 67–115 mg/dl) or moderate (blood glucose between 116–143 mg/dl) glucose control.

Recent trials in critically ill patients, such as the NICE-SUGAR study, reported a detrimental effect of strict (blood glucose between 108–144 mg/dl) compared with more moderate blood glucose control (blood glucose < 180 mg/dl) [45]. The 2005 guideline recommendation for strict glucose control (between 72–108 mg/dl) was modified in 2010 in favor of a more liberal regimen (blood glucose < 180 mg/dl) [6]. Although the upper limit of acceptable blood glucose is still under debate, expert consensus agrees on prevention of hypoglycemia, which is associated with poor outcomes in critically ill patients in general and also in patients after successful CPR. Unfortunately, studies published so far largely differ with respect to study design, time schedule for blood glucose determination and treatment, and do not adequately account for possible confounders that may have influenced neurologic outcome.

Seizures

The therapeutic bundles mentioned above also comment on the prevention and therapy of seizures [6]. Myoclonus, which may represent a diagnostic challenge, was also classified as requiring treatment. Both conditions may occur in up to 15 % of patients after successful resuscitation [46]. Specifically, in comatose survivors after CPR, seizures can be observed in up to 40 % of patients, a number that is further increased by shivering during therapeutic hypothermia [47]. Since seizures and myoclonus are associated with increased oxygen consumption, current guidelines suggest a prompt and targeted intervention to control them. Unfortunately there are no controlled trials on the therapy of seizures after successful CPR. Preventive administration of anticonvulsant drugs cannot be recommended at present because of the lack of evidence.

Oxygenation after Successful CPR

High inspired oxygen concentration may aggravate an existing neuronal deficit by generation of free oxygen radicals [48]. In 1994, Zwemer and colleagues reported on possible negative sequelae of high inspiratory oxygen concentrations in terms of neurologic dysfunction, in a study on 27 dogs [49]. Brücken et al. retrospectively analyzed the effect of 100 % oxygen during early reperfusion after successful resuscitation in 15 pigs and found increased brain necrosis and perivascular inflammation in the striatum [50]. Analyses of large patient registries have also pointed to a correlation between ventilation with high oxygen concentration during the immediate post-resuscitation period and an increased proportion of patients with poor neurological outcome [51]. Although the exact mechanism by which high oxygen contributes to tissue damage is still unresolved, an increasing oxidative mitochondrial stress level may be involved, which may have deleterious effects on the brain in the vulnerable time period directly after ROSC [52]. In a first small study in humans, Kuisma and coworkers [53] described the effects of either 30 % or 100 % inspired oxygen on outcome. With an FiO_2 of 0.3, acceptable arterial oxygen content was achieved in most patients, whereas in patients who had received a FiO_2 of 1.0 an increasing NSE concentration was observed after 24 h. Based on these and similar findings current International Liaison Committee on Resuscitation (ILCOR) recommendations were changed and at present recommend an arterial oxygen saturation of 94 %-96 %. Since complex interactions of oxygen and hypothermia are conceivable at the cellular level, future randomized trials are necessary to address the question of optimal oxygen concentration after CPR. Both the time period in which the brain is most susceptible for high oxygen concentrations and the cumulative time on high oxygen leading to brain damage need to be more clearly specified. Optimal ventilator support at present is challenging, since both hyperoxia and hypoxia should be avoided.

XIII

Post-resuscitation Care Bundle

Wolfrum et al. previously reported that mild hypothermia in combination with primary PCI was feasible and safe in patients resuscitated from out-of-hospital cardiac arrest following acute myocardial infarction [21]. In our previous registry analysis [11] we found 73 patients who received both mild hypothermia and PCI, irrespective of first EKG findings; 49 % of these patients were discharged from the hospital with good neurological outcome compared to 11 % of patients without any therapeutic procedure. Using logistic regression analysis including all patients (n = 584), only PCI was independently associated with an increased chance of good neurological outcome (adjusted OR 5.66 [95 % CI 3.54 – 9.03]), but not mild hypothermia (adjusted OR 1.27 [95 % CI 0.79 – 2.03]). These data are in agreement with most of the recent studies demonstrating either a trend or significant benefit for mild hypothermia [53]. Very importantly, most of the published data did not undergo adjustment for multiple independent predictors, thus interpretation and comparison with other results is difficult. We are not aware of any randomized controlled study investigating the combination of mild hypothermia with coronary intervention. However, a few small clinical studies including historical control groups, and case reports have recently indicated that the combination may be feasible and may indeed be associated with benefits for the individual patient [21, 25, 54, 55].

Taking a step backward, Sunde et al. previously demonstrated that a standardized post-resuscitation care bundle focusing on vital organ function including target temperature management, liberal decision for urgent coronary intervention, and control of hemodynamics, blood glucose, ventilation and seizures was most beneficial compared to a historical control group [25].

Conclusion

Post-resuscitation care is still a challenge for intensivists. **Box 1** shows the key elements of a post-resuscitation care bundle protocol. Although therapeutic hypothermia is an accepted mainstay of therapy after cardiac arrest, treatment of the underlying cause (mostly cardiac ischemia) may be even more important with respect to outcome. Several other issues, such as hemodynamic optimization, blood glucose control and adequate oxygenation, may also have an important impact on outcome, but data on these subjects are sparse. Further studies are urgently needed to more clearly define optimal therapeutic bundles for the treatment of survivors after cardiac arrest.

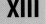

Box 1. Post-resuscitation care bundle protocol

* Target temperature management (32 – 34 C for 12 – 24 hours)
* Treatment of underlying cause (coronary reperfusion therapy)
* Adjuvant therapies
    - Hemodynamic optimization (goal directed therapy)
    - Blood glucose management (< 180 mg/dl)
    - Prevention and therapy of seizures
    - Prevention of hyperoxygenation (SpO$_2$ 94 – 96 %)

References

1. Nolan JP, Laver SR, Welch CA, Harrison DA, Gupta V, Rowan K (2007) Outcome following admission to UK intensive care units after cardiac arrest: a secondary analysis of the ICNARC Case Mix Programme Database. Anaesthesia 62: 1207–1216
2. Carr BG, Kahn JM, Merchant RM, Kramer AA, Neumar RW (2009) Inter-hospital variability in post-cardiac arrest mortality. Resuscitation 80: 30–34
3. Neumar RW, Nolan JP, Adrie C, et al (2008) Post-cardiac arrest syndrome: epidemiology, pathophysiology, treatment, and prognostication. A consensus statement from the International Liaison Committee on Resuscitation (American Heart Association, Australian and New Zealand Council on Resuscitation, European Resuscitation Council, Heart and Stroke Foundation of Canada, InterAmerican Heart Foundation, Resuscitation Council of Asia, and the Resuscitation Council of Southern Africa); the American Heart Association Emergency Cardiovascular Care Committee; the Council on Cardiovascular Surgery and Anesthesia; the Council on Cardiopulmonary, Perioperative, and Critical Care; the Council on Clinical Cardiology; and the Stroke Council. Circulation 118: 2452–2483
4. HACA (2002) Mild therapeutic hypothermia to improve the neurologic outcome after cardiac arrest. N Engl J Med 346: 549–556
5. Bernard SA, Gray TW, Buist MD, et al (2002) Treatment of comatose survivors of out-of-hospital cardiac arrest with induced hypothermia. N Engl J Med 346: 557–563
6. Peberdy MA, Callaway CW, Neumar RW, et al (2010) Part 9: post-cardiac arrest care: 2010 American Heart Association Guidelines for Cardiopulmonary Resuscitation and Emergency Cardiovascular Care. Circulation 122 (18 Suppl 3): S768–786
7. Hsu CY, Huang CH, Chang WT, et al (2009) Cardioprotective effect of therapeutic hypothermia for postresuscitation myocardial dysfunction. Shock 32: 210–216
8. Meybohm P, Gruenewald M, Albrecht M, et al (2009) Hypothermia and postconditioning after cardiopulmonary resuscitation reduce cardiac dysfunction by modulating inflammation, apoptosis and remodeling. PLoS One 4: e7588
9. Jacobshagen C, Pelster T, Pax A, et al (2010) Effects of mild hypothermia on hemodynamics in cardiac arrest survivors and isolated failing human myocardium. Clin Res Cardiol 99: 267–276
10. Holzer M (2010) Targeted temperature management for comatose survivors of cardiac arrest. N Engl J Med 363: 1256–1264
11. Grasner JT, Meybohm P, Caliebe A, et al (2011) Postresuscitation care with mild therapeutic hypothermia and coronary intervention after out-of-hospital cardiopulmonary resuscitation: a prospective registry analysis. Crit Care 15: R61
12. Dumas F, Cariou A, Manzo-Silberman S, et al (2010) Immediate percutaneous coronary intervention is associated with better survival after out-of-hospital cardiac arrest: insights from the PROCAT (Parisian Region Out of hospital Cardiac ArresT) registry. Circ Cardiovasc Interv 3: 200–207
13. Castren M, Nordberg P, Svensson L, et al (2010) Intra-arrest transnasal evaporative cooling: a randomized, prehospital, multicenter study (PRINCE: Pre-ROSC IntraNasal Cooling Effectiveness). Circulation 122: 729–736
14. Nielsen N, Sunde K, Hovdenes J, et al (2011) Adverse events and their relation to mortality in out-of-hospital cardiac arrest patients treated with therapeutic hypothermia. Crit Care Med 39: 57–64
15. Mongardon N, Perbet S, Lemiale V, et al (2011) Infectious complications in out-of-hospital cardiac arrest patients in the therapeutic hypothermia era. Crit Care Med 39: 1359–1364
16. Nunnally ME, Jaeschke R, Bellingan GJ, et al (2011) Targeted temperature management in critical care: a report and recommendations from five professional societies. Crit Care Med 39: 1113–1125
17. Boden WE, Gupta V (2008) Reperfusion strategies in acute ST-segment elevation myocardial infarction. Curr Opin Cardiol 23: 613–619
18. Antman EM, Anbe DT, Armstrong PW, et al (2004) ACC/AHA guidelines for the management of patients with ST-elevation myocardial infarction--executive summary: a report of the American College of Cardiology/American Heart Association Task Force on Practice

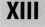

Guidelines (Writing Committee to Revise the 1999 Guidelines for the Management of Patients With Acute Myocardial Infarction). Circulation 110: 588–636

19. Pell JP, Sirel JM, Marsden AK, Ford I, Walker NL, Cobbe SM (2003) Presentation, management, and outcome of out of hospital cardiopulmonary arrest: comparison by underlying aetiology. Heart 89: 839–842

20. Böttiger BW, Grabner C, Bauer H, et al (1999) Long term outcome after out-of-hospital cardiac arrest with physician staffed emergency medical services: the Utstein style applied to a midsized urban/suburban area. Heart 82: 674–679

21. Wolfrum S, Pierau C, Radke PW, Schunkert H, Kurowski V (2008) Mild therapeutic hypothermia in patients after out-of-hospital cardiac arrest due to acute ST-segment elevation myocardial infarction undergoing immediate percutaneous coronary intervention. Crit Care Med 36: 1780–1786

22. Böttiger BW, Arntz HR, Chamberlain DA, et al (2008) Thrombolysis during resuscitation for out-of-hospital cardiac arrest. N Engl J Med 359: 2651–2662

23. Marcusohn E, Roguin A, Sebbag A, et al (2007) Primary percutaneous coronary intervention after out-of-hospital cardiac arrest: patients and outcomes. Isr Med Assoc J 9: 257–259

24. Gorjup V, Radsel P, Kocjancic ST, Erzen D, Noc M (2007) Acute ST-elevation myocardial infarction after successful cardiopulmonary resuscitation. Resuscitation 72: 379–385

25. Sunde K, Pytte M, Jacobsen D, et al (2007) Implementation of a standardised treatment protocol for post resuscitation care after out-of-hospital cardiac arrest. Resuscitation 73: 29–39

26. Spaulding CM, Joly LM, Rosenberg A, et al (1997) Immediate coronary angiography in survivors of out-of-hospital cardiac arrest. N Engl J Med 336: 1629–1633

27. Reynolds JC, Callaway CW, El Khoudary SR, Moore CG, Alvarez RJ, Rittenberger JC (2009) Coronary angiography predicts improved outcome following cardiac arrest: propensity-adjusted analysis. J Intensive Care Med 24: 179–186

28. Dalfino L, Giglio MT, Puntillo F, Marucci M, Brienza N (2011) Haemodynamic goal-directed therapy and postoperative infections: earlier is better. a systematic review and meta-analysis. Crit Care 15: R154

29. Lees N, Hamilton M, Rhodes A (2009) Clinical review: Goal-directed therapy in high risk surgical patients. Crit Care 13: 231

30. Rivers E, Nguyen B, Havstad S, et al (2001) Early goal-directed therapy in the treatment of severe sepsis and septic shock. N Engl J Med 345: 1368–1377

31. Levy MM, Dellinger RP, Townsend SR, et al (2010) The Surviving Sepsis Campaign: results of an international guideline-based performance improvement program targeting severe sepsis. Crit Care Med, 38: 367–374

32. Adrie C, Adib-Conquy M, Laurent I, et al (2002) Successful cardiopulmonary resuscitation after cardiac arrest as a "sepsis-like" syndrome. Circulation 106: 562–568

33. Jones AE, Shapiro NI, Kilgannon JH, Trzeciak S (2008) Goal-directed hemodynamic optimization in the post-cardiac arrest syndrome: a systematic review. Resuscitation 77: 26–29

34. Gaieski DF, Band RA, Abella BS, et al (2009) Early goal-directed hemodynamic optimization combined with therapeutic hypothermia in comatose survivors of out-of-hospital cardiac arrest. Resuscitation 80: 418–424

35. Pope JV, Jones AE, Gaieski DF, Arnold RC, Trzeciak S, Shapiro NI (2011) Multicenter study of central venous oxygen saturation (ScvO(2)) as a predictor of mortality in patients with sepsis. Ann Emerg Med 55: 40–46

36. Perel A (2008) Bench-to-bedside review: the initial hemodynamic resuscitation of the septic patient according to Surviving Sepsis Campaign guidelines--does one size fit all? Crit Care 12: 223

37. Lopes MR, Oliveira MA, Pereira VO, Lemos IP, Auler JO Jr, Michard F (2007) Goal-directed fluid management based on pulse pressure variation monitoring during high-risk surgery: a pilot randomized controlled trial. Crit Care 11: R100

38. Gruenewald M, Meybohm P, Koerner S, et al (2011) Dynamic and volumetric variables of fluid responsiveness fail during immediate postresuscitation period. Crit Care Med 39: 1953–1959

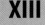

39. Gruenewald M, Meybohm P, Broch O, et al (2011) Visual evaluation of left ventricular performance predicts volume responsiveness early after resuscitation from cardiac arrest. Resuscitation 82: 1553–1557
40. Malmberg K, Norhammar A, Ryden L (2001) Insulin treatment post myocardial infarction: the DIGAMI study. Adv Exp Med Biol 498: 279–284
41. Malmberg K, Ryden L, Wedel H, et al (2005) Intense metabolic control by means of insulin in patients with diabetes mellitus and acute myocardial infarction (DIGAMI 2): effects on mortality and morbidity. Eur Heart J 26: 650–661
42. Beiser DG, Carr GE, Edelson DP, Peberdy MA, Hoek TL (2009) Derangements in blood glucose following initial resuscitation from in-hospital cardiac arrest: a report from the national registry of cardiopulmonary resuscitation. Resuscitation 80: 624–630
43. Oksanen T, Pettila V, Hynynen M, Varpula T (2007) Therapeutic hypothermia after cardiac arrest: implementation and outcome in Finnish intensive care units. Acta Anaesthesiol Scand 51: 866–871
44. Losert H, Sterz F, Roine RO, et al (2008) Strict normoglycaemic blood glucose levels in the therapeutic management of patients within 12h after cardiac arrest might not be necessary. Resuscitation 76: 214–220
45. Finfer S, Chittock DR, Su SY, et al (2009): Intensive versus conventional glucose control in critically ill patients. N Engl J Med 360: 1283–1297
46. Lu-Emerson C, Khot S (2010) Neurological sequelae of hypoxic-ischemic brain injury. NeuroRehabilitation 26: 35–45
47. Krumholz A, Stern BJ, Weiss HD (1988) Outcome from coma after cardiopulmonary resuscitation: relation to seizures and myoclonus. Neurology 38: 401–405
48. Becker LB (2004) New concepts in reactive oxygen species and cardiovascular reperfusion physiology. Cardiovasc Res 61: 461–470
49. Zwemer CF, Whitesall SE, D'Alecy LG (1994) Cardiopulmonary-cerebral resuscitation with 100 % oxygen exacerbates neurological dysfunction following nine minutes of normothermic cardiac arrest in dogs. Resuscitation 27: 159–170
50. Brücken A, Kaab AB, Kottmann K, et al (2010) Reducing the duration of 100 % oxygen ventilation in the early reperfusion period after cardiopulmonary resuscitation decreases striatal brain damage. Resuscitation 81: 1698–1703
51. Kilgannon JH, Jones AE, Shapiro NI, et al (2011) Association between arterial hyperoxia following resuscitation from cardiac arrest and in-hospital mortality. JAMA 303: 2165–2171
52. Cataldi A (2011) Cell responses to oxidative stressors. Current pharmaceutical design, 16: 1387–1395
53. Kuisma M, Boyd J, Voipio V, Alaspää A, Roine RO, Rosenberg P (2006) Comparison of 30 and the 100% inspired oxygen concentrations during early post-resuscitation period: a randomised controlled pilot study. Resuscitation 69: 199–206
54. Nielsen N, Hovdenes J, Nilsson F, et al (2009) Outcome, timing and adverse events in therapeutic hypothermia after out-of-hospital cardiac arrest. Acta Anaesthesiol Scand 53: 926–934
55. Hovdenes J, Laake JH, Aaberge L, Haugaa H, Bugge JF (2007) Therapeutic hypothermia after out-of-hospital cardiac arrest: experiences with patients treated with percutaneous coronary intervention and cardiogenic shock. Acta Anaesthesiol Scand 51: 137–142

XIV Pathogenesis of AKI

Role of Leukocytes in the Pathogenesis of Acute Kidney Injury

G.R. Kinsey and M.D. Okusa

Introduction

Acute kidney injury (AKI) is a significant cause of morbidity and mortality in hospitalized patients, especially those who are critically ill. The mortality rate in patients with severe AKI requiring renal replacement therapy (RRT) can exceed 50 % [1]. Numerous factors contribute to the development of AKI, including reductions in renal blood flow, actions of nephrotoxic drugs, cellular injury/death of proximal tubule epithelial cells, pro-inflammatory responses of renal endothelial cells, influx and activation of inflammatory leukocytes that further reduces renal blood flow through vascular congestion and promotes and extends injury to kidney parenchymal cells [2, 3]. The immune response in AKI involves cells of both the innate and adaptive immune systems. Although numerous studies have demonstrated the detrimental role of many different types of immune cells, recent reports have uncovered a protective and possibly therapeutic role of other immune cells in AKI. Studies in animal models of AKI have revealed that innate immune cells, such as neutrophils, macrophages, dendritic cells, natural killer (NK) cells and natural killer T (NKT) cells, and adaptive CD4$^+$ T cells promote renal injury. Indeed, renal inflammation is a common feature of human AKI [4] and detailed analyses of biopsy samples from patients with AKI demonstrated the presence of mononuclear leukocytes (some CD3$^+$ T cells) and neutrophils [5]. In contrast, CD4$^+$FoxP3$^+$ regulatory T cells (Tregs) can protect the kidney from ischemic and nephrotoxic injury in animal models. Understanding the immune mechanisms of renal injury and protection should yield new approaches to prevention and treatment of AKI. This review will summarize current knowledge on the role of the immune system in the pathogenesis of AKI.

Detrimental Actions of Pro-inflammatory Leukocytes

Neutrophils

Polymorphonuclear cells (PMNs or neutrophils) are critical mediators of innate immunity. They respond rapidly (within minutes) to invading pathogens and to sites of tissue damage. Neutrophils clear invading pathogens by phagocytosis or by releasing toxic granules containing proteases and other enzymes and reactive oxygen species (ROS). For this reason, neutrophil degranulation can lead to damage of host cells in the inflamed tissue. In several mouse models of AKI (e.g., ischemia/reperfusion injury and cisplatin-induced kidney injury), neutrophil accumulation in the injured kidney is a consistent and early finding [6–8] and

J.-L. Vincent (ed.), *Annual Update in Intensive Care and Emergency Medicine 2012*
DOI 10.1007/978-3-642-25716-2 © Springer-Verlag Berlin Heidelberg 2012

depletion of neutrophils [6] or prevention of neutrophil trafficking to the kidney [9] reduces kidney injury. In addition to releasing granules, neutrophils have been shown to produce the pro-inflammatory cytokines, interferon (IFN)-γ and interleukin (IL)-17, and the chemokine CXCL1, in the injured kidney [7, 9]. These findings demonstrate the involvement of neutrophils in the pathogenesis of kidney injury in the commonly used murine model of ischemia/reperfusion-induced AKI. Studies in some other species have reported a lack of significant neutrophil accumulation and no benefit after neutrophil depletion; however, these results may be related to differences in experimental models and limitations to methods for neutrophil depletion (see [10] and references therein).

Macrophages

Macrophages are phagocytic cells that arise from monocytes in the blood. Macrophage numbers increase early in the injured kidney (within 1 hour of reperfusion in an ischemia/reperfusion model [11]), and this infiltration is mediated by CCR2 and CX3CR1 signaling pathways [12, 13]. These macrophages have a distinct 'inflamed' F4/80^{low}Ly6C^{high}GR-1$^+$CX3CR1^{low} phenotype [12]. Depletion of macrophages, using liposomal clodronate, prior to kidney ischemia/reperfusion injury, reduced renal injury and adoptive transfer of macrophages reconstituted AKI [14]. Although macrophage infiltration is observed in cisplatin-induced experimental AKI, blockade of macrophage trafficking to the kidney did not prevent renal injury [15]. Analysis of post-ischemic kidney infiltrating macrophages by flow cytometry demonstrated that they are significant producers of many pro-inflammatory cytokines, including IL-6 and tumor necrosis factor (TNF)-α [12]. Another study identified IL-6 expression in renal outer medulla macrophages by *in situ* hybridization 4 hours after ischemia/reperfusion injury and IL-6 deficient mice are protected from kidney ischemia/reperfusion injury [16]. Recently, different types of macrophages have been described that either promote or inhibit inflammation, M1 and M2 macrophages, respectively [17]. New experimental evidence has demonstrated that once recruited to the post-ischemic kidney, macrophages display an M1 pro-inflammatory phenotype, but several days later those same macrophages change to an M2 phenotype and are vital in the repair process of the kidney [18].

Natural Killer Cells

NK cells are similar to lymphocytes of the adaptive immune system but lack a T cell receptor. Their activation is governed by signals received from activating and inhibitory receptors on their cell surface. The ligands for these NK cell receptors are expressed on target cells and are regulated by cell stress such as viral infection. During experimental AKI, the proximal tubule epithelial cells (TECs) upregulate the expression of an NK cell activating ligand, Rae-1, which promotes TEC killing by activating the NKG2D receptor on NK cells [19]. The NK cells utilize perforins to kill the TECs in this model and their numbers in the kidney are elevated as early as 4 h after ischemic insult [19].

Dendritic Cells

Dendritic cells classified by the expression of CD11c$^+$ are the most abundant leukocyte subset in the normal mouse kidney [20] suggesting an important role in renal immunity and inflammation. Upon stimulation, dendritic cells transform to a mature phenotype characterized by high levels of class II major histocompatibility complex (MHC class II) and co-stimulatory molecules with low phagocytic capacity. Mature dendritic cells are ideally suited to activate conventional T cells. Dendritic cells migrate to the renal draining lymph nodes after ischemia/reperfusion injury and induce T cell proliferation suggesting that kidney dendritic cells are vital to the adaptive immune response to ischemia/reperfusion injury [21]. Dendritic cells are also important in the innate immune response through several mechanisms. These include releasing pro-inflammatory factors, interacting with NKT cells via the co-stimulatory molecule, CD40, and presenting glycolipid to NKT cells via the CD1d molecule. Dong et al. demonstrated that after ischemia/reperfusion injury, renal dendritic cells produce the pro-inflammatory cytokines/chemokines, TNF, IL-6, monocyte chemotactic protein (MCP)-1 and RANTES (Regulated on Activation, Normal T Expressed and Secreted), and depletion of dendritic cells prior to ischemia/reperfusion injury significantly reduced the kidney levels of TNF produced after ischemia/reperfusion injury [22]. IL-12 and IL-23 are mainly produced from activated dendritic cells and their downstream cytokines, IFN-γ and IL-17, promote macrophage activation and neutrophil recruitment and amplify the immune response following ischemic kidney injury [9]. The use of a genetically-engineered mouse in which the promoter for the mainly dendritic cell-specific surface protein, CD11c, drives expression of the human diphtheria toxin receptor (CD11c-DTR mouse) has facilitated understanding of the role of renal dendritic cells in experimental AKI. Recent studies have demonstrated that dendritic cells can promote or prevent injury to the kidney depending on the stimulus. For example, depletion of dendritic cells prior to ischemia/reperfusion injury reduces subsequent reperfusion injury and renal dysfunction [11]. On the other hand, depletion of dendritic cells prior to cisplatin exposure resulted in worse renal dysfunction and inflammation [8]. These findings suggest that dendritic cells play an important role in orchestrating the immune response during AKI; additional studies are needed to understand what determines whether dendritic cells promote or inhibit kidney inflammation as this information may translate into new therapeutic strategies.

Lymphocytes

T and B cells are the major effector cells of the adaptive immune system. Recognition of antigens, presented by antigen-presenting cells, in the presence of sufficient co-stimulation, causes expansion and activation of T cells with a T-cell receptor specific for that antigen. B cells recognize soluble antigens through cell surface immunoglobulin type receptors. T cell contribution to the pathogenesis of kidney ischemia/reperfusion injury has been established in different mouse models lacking certain types of lymphocytes. In mice which lack CD4 and CD8 T cells (nu/nu mice), kidney injury and dysfunction were significantly reduced compared to wild-type controls after ischemia/reperfusion injury and cisplatin induced injury [23, 24]. Reconstitution of nu/nu mice with CD4+ T cells alone but not with CD8+ T cells alone restored kidney injury after ischemia/reperfusion injury [23] and mice lacking CD8 or CD4 T cells alone suffered less kidney dysfunction after cisplatin administration [24]. To investigate the requirement of antigen-dependent CD4 T cell activation in ischemia/reperfusion injury, Satpute et al. reconstituted nu/nu mice with either polyclonal CD4 T cells (with a diverse array of T-cell receptor specificities) or CD4 T cells from the DO11.10 mouse which nearly all express the same T-cell receptor, specific for a chicken ovalbumin peptide [25]. Whereas polyclonal T cells reconstituted injury in the T cell deficient mice, DO11.10 T cells did not, unless their cognate antigen was co-administered with the T cells [25]. These results suggest that antigen specific activation of CD4 T cells is important for early (within 24 h) AKI.

The results of B cell deficiency in mouse models of AKI are not consistent. Mice lacking T and B cells (RAG-1 KO) were protected in some studies [26, 27] and in others had similar injury to wild-type mice [28, 29]. Deficiency of B cells alone in mu MT mice conferred protection against ischemia/reperfusion injury in one study [30] but resulted in more severe renal dysfunction after ischemia/reperfusion injury in another [31]. Therefore, more studies are needed to determine the role of B cells in AKI.

Natural Killer T Cells

NKT cells are a unique subset of T lymphocytes with surface receptors and functional properties shared with conventional T cells and NK cells. Invariant or Type I NKT cells express a conserved T-cell receptor (Vα14/Jα18 and Vβ8.2,Vβ2 or Vβ7) together with the NK cell marker, NK1.1. In contrast to conventional T cells, this invariant NKT cell T-cell receptor does not recognize peptide antigens presented by MHC-class I or II; it recognizes glycolipids in the context of the class I-like molecule, CD1d. One of the most important functions of NKT cells is their ability to rapidly produce large amounts of cytokines, including Th1-type (IFN-γ, TNF) and Th2-type (IL-4, IL-13) at the same time. The rapid response by NKT cells following activation can amplify and regulate the function of dendritic cells, Tregs, NK and B cells, as well as conventional T cells. The number of IFN-γ producing type I NKT cells in the kidney is significantly increased by 3 hours of reperfusion after ischemic insult [7] and NKT cells were observed in kidneys of patients with acute tubular necrosis (ATN) [32]. Blockade of NKT cell activation with the anti-CD1d mAb, NKT cell depletion with an anti-NK1.1 monoclonal antibody in wild-type mice, or use of type I NKT cell-deficient mice (Jα18$^{-/-}$) inhibited the accumulation of IFN-γ producing neutrophils after IRI and prevented AKI [7]. Type II NKT cells are not restricted to an invariant T-cell receptor but still recognize glycolipids, such as sulfatide. In a recent study by Yang et al. sulfatide-activated Type II NKT cells migrated to the injured kidney and protected mice from ischemia/reperfusion injury [32]. Taken together these studies suggest that different types of NKT cells may play divergent roles in AKI.

Protective Actions of Regulatory T Cells

Tregs make up an indispensible counter-balance to the pro-inflammatory cells of the immune system. This aspect is illustrated in patients with immunodysregulation, polyendocrinopathy, enteropathy, x-linked (IPEX) syndrome and scurfy mice which both have devastating autoimmunity caused by a lack of functional Tregs [33]. Numerous types of Tregs have been described in the literature, but the most abundant are CD4$^+$ T cells, which express CD25, and the Treg-specific transcription factor, FoxP3. FoxP3 suppresses the expression of pro-inflammatory genes and promotes the anti-inflammatory phenotype of Tregs [34]. The main mechanisms of suppression employed by Tregs include production of anti-inflammatory cytokines, such as IL-10 and transforming-growth factor (TGF)-β, generation of extracellular adenosine, direct contact-mediated inhibition of dendtritic cells through cell surface molecules such as lymphocyte activation gene (LAG)-3 and cytotoxic T-lymphocyte antigen (CTLA)-4 and several others [35, 36]. Based on the important contribution of the pro-inflammatory immune cells to AKI discussed above we hypothesized that Tregs would serve to protect the kidney from inflammation and injury. To test this hypothesis, Tregs were partially depleted from naïve wild-type mice prior to a short ischemic insult that was not severe enough to induce kidney dysfunction in control mice [37]. Reduction in numbers of Tregs predisposed mice to tubular necrosis, renal inflammation and loss of function [37]. In other studies, Treg depletion prior to more severe ischemia also worsened renal injury measured at 72 h of reperfusion [38]. These results suggest that enhancement of Treg numbers or function may be an effective preventative therapy for AKI. Indeed, adoptive transfer of isolated Tregs, by i.v. injection prior to ischemia/reperfusion injury [37, 39] or cisplatin administration [40] protected mice from kidney injury. This protection was associated with a reduction in infiltrating innate immune cells and pro-inflammatory gene expression in the kidney [37, 39, 40]. In the ischemia/reperfusion injury model, IL-10-deficient Tregs were unable to offer any protection [37], suggesting that IL-10 production is an important mechanism for Treg-mediated protection from kidney injury. Two other methods of protecting the kidney, ischemic preconditioning [39, 41] and use of FTY720 [42], have been shown to be partially dependent on the presence of Tregs.

In addition to prevention of injury, Tregs also promote the recovery of kidney function after ischemia/reperfusion injury [43]. This effect was demonstrated by depleting Tregs after ischemic injury, which caused reduced renal repair and increased mortality; on the other hand, adoptive transfer of Tregs 24 h after ischemic insult accelerated the recovery of renal function in mice [43]. The effects on kidney recovery did not appear to be mediated through effects on infiltrating innate immune cells, but were associated with increased tubular epithelial cell proliferation and reduced cytokine production from infiltrating T cells [43]. This study is important since it is difficult to detect renal injury in a timely manner and this suggests that manipulations to enhance Treg numbers or function can have beneficial effects after injury has occurred.

Recently, a clinical trial was conducted to determine the safety and feasibility of *ex vivo* expansion of human Tregs for adoptive transfer into patients [44]. The authors demonstrated that it is possible to expand Tregs *in vitro* and then infuse up to 3 million Tregs/kg to patients, with no adverse effects observed [44]. Although this trial was conducted in the study of a different disease model, it demonstrates that Treg cells themselves may be a novel therapeutic strategy in humans for many diseases, including AKI.

XIV

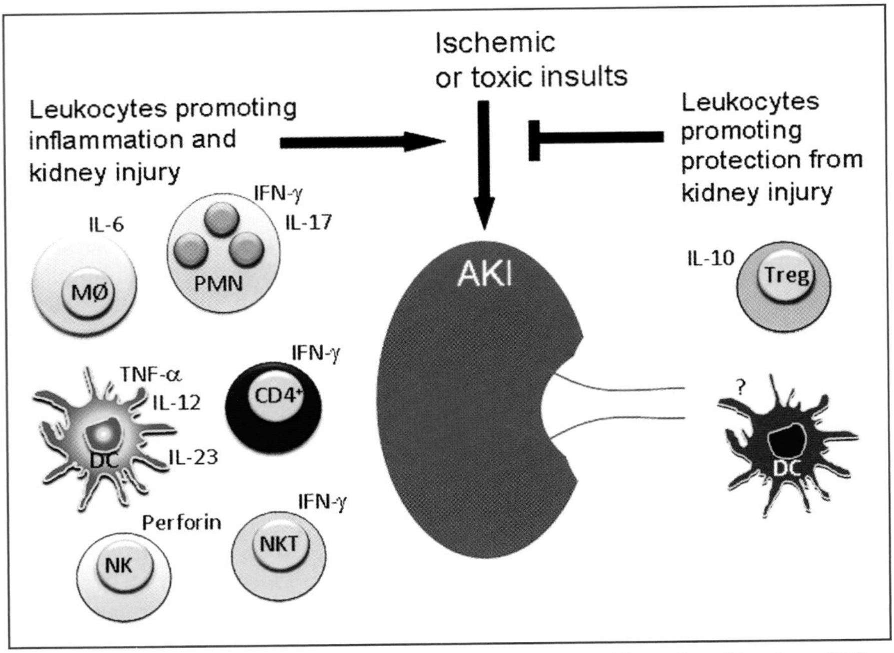

Fig. 1. Toxic or ischemic insults initiate inflammation in the kidney which consists of interferon (IFN)-γ- and interleukin (IL)-17-producing neutrophils (PMN), IL-6-producing macrophages (MØ), dendritic cells (DC) which produce tumor necrosis factor (TNF)-α, IL-12 and IL-23, IFN-γ-producing CD4+ T cells, invariant type I natural killer T (NKT) cells and natural killer (NK) cells which kill renal tubule epithelial cells in a perforin-dependent manner. On the other hand toxic and ischemic injuries are prevented by regulatory T cells (Tregs) which produce IL-10, and in cisplatin-induced nephrotoxicity DCs protect the kidney by an unknown mechanism.

Conclusion

The immune response to kidney damage during AKI is an important contributor to the prolonged lack of renal function and progression of kidney injury. This response is complex, involving numerous pro-inflammatory leukocytes which employ diverse effector mechanisms inside the kidney (**Fig. 1**). The response also involves an anti-inflammatory arm that protects the kidney from sub-threshold insults, which is mediated by Tregs and possibly dendritic cells in some conditions (**Fig. 1**). In the future, it may be possible to prevent AKI or treat existing AKI by inhibiting the pro-inflammatory immune response to kidney injury and/ or promoting the anti-inflammatory response through drugs or maneuvers that enhance Treg action or by direct administration of Tregs themselves.

XIV

References

1. Murugan R, Kellum JA (2011) Acute kidney injury: what's the prognosis? Nat Rev Nephrol 7: 209–217
2. Kinsey GR, Okusa MD (2011) Pathogenesis of acute kidney injury: foundation for clinical practice. Am J Kidney Dis 58: 291–301

3. Schrier RW, Wang W, Poole B, Mitra A (2004) Acute renal failure: definitions, diagnosis, pathogenesis, and therapy. J Clin Invest 114: 5–14
4. Solez K, Morel-Maroger L, Sraer JD (1979) The morphology of "acute tubular necrosis" in man: analysis of 57 renal biopsies and a comparison with the glycerol model. Medicine (Baltimore) 58: 362–376
5. Friedewald JJ, Rabb H (2004) Inflammatory cells in ischemic acute renal failure. Kidney Int 66: 486–491
6. Kelly KJ, Williams WW Jr, Colvin RB, et al (1996) Intercellular adhesion molecule-1-deficient mice are protected against ischemic renal injury. J Clin Invest 97: 1056–1063
7. Li L, Huang L, Sung SS, et al (2007) NKT cell activation mediates neutrophil IFN-gamma production and renal ischemia-reperfusion injury. J Immunol 178: 5899–5911
8. Tadagavadi RK, Reeves WB (2010) Renal dendritic cells ameliorate nephrotoxic acute kidney injury. J Am Soc Nephrol 21: 53–63
9. Li L, Huang L, Vergis AL, et al (2010) IL-17 produced by neutrophils regulates IFN-gamma-mediated neutrophil migration in mouse kidney ischemia-reperfusion injury. J Clin Invest 120: 331–342
10. Bolisetty S, Agarwal A (2009) Neutrophils in acute kidney injury: not neutral any more. Kidney Int 75: 674–676
11. Li L, Okusa MD (2010) Macrophages, dendritic cells, and kidney ischemia-reperfusion injury. Semin Nephrol 30: 268–277
12. Li L, Huang L, Sung S, et al (2008) The chemokine receptors CCR2 and CX3CR1 mediate monocyte/macrophage trafficking in kidney ischemia-reperfusion injury. Kidney Int 74: 1526–1537
13. Oh DJ, Dursun B, He Z, et al (2008) Fractalkine receptor (CX3CR1) inhibition is protective against ischemic acute renal failure in mice. Am J Physiol Renal Physiol 294: F264–271
14. Day YJ, Huang L, Ye H, Linden J, Okusa MD (2005) Renal ischemia-reperfusion injury and adenosine 2A receptor-mediated tissue protection: role of macrophages. Am J Physiol Renal Physiol 288: F722–731
15. Lu LH, Oh DJ, Dursun B, et al (2008) Increased macrophage infiltration and fractalkine expression in cisplatin-induced acute renal failure in mice. J Pharmacol Exp Ther 324: 1111–1117
16. Kielar ML, John R, Bennett M, et al (2005) Maladaptive role of IL-6 in ischemic acute renal failure. J Am Soc Nephrol 16: 3315–3325
17. Martinez FO, Sica A, Mantovani A, Locati M (2008) Macrophage activation and polarization. Front Biosci 13: 453–461
18. Lee S, Huen S, Nishio H, et al (2011) Distinct macrophage phenotypes contribute to kidney injury and repair. J Am Soc Nephrol 22: 317–326
19. Zhang ZX, Wang S, Huang X, et al (2008) NK cells induce apoptosis in tubular epithelial cells and contribute to renal ischemia-reperfusion injury. J Immunol 181: 7489–7498
20. Soos TJ, Sims TN, Barisoni L, et al (2006) CX3CR1+ interstitial dendritic cells form a contiguous network throughout the entire kidney. Kidney Int 70: 591–596
21. Dong X, Swaminathan S, Bachman LA, Croatt AJ, Nath KA, Griffin MD (2005) Antigen presentation by dendritic cells in renal lymph nodes is linked to systemic and local injury to the kidney. Kidney Int 68: 1096–1108
22. Dong X, Swaminathan S, Bachman LA, Croatt AJ, Nath KA, Griffin MD (2007) Resident dendritic cells are the predominant TNF-secreting cell in early renal ischemia-reperfusion injury. Kidney Int 71: 619–628
23. Burne MJ, Daniels F, El Ghandour A, et al (2001) Identification of the CD4(+) T cell as a major pathogenic factor in ischemic acute renal failure. J Clin Invest 108: 1283–1290
24. Liu M, Chien C, Burne-Taney M, et al (2006) A pathophysiologic role for T lymphocytes in murine acute cisplatin nephrotoxicity. J Am Soc Nephrol 17: 765–774
25. Satpute SR, Park JM, Jang HR, et al (2009) The role for T cell repertoire/antigen-specific interactions in experimental kidney ischemia reperfusion injury. J Immunol. 183: 984–992
26. Bajwa A, Jo SK, Ye H, et al (2010) Activation of sphingosine-1-phosphate 1 receptor in the proximal tubule protects against ischemia-reperfusion injury. J Am Soc Nephrol 21: 955–965

27. Day YJ, Huang L, Ye H, Li L, Linden J, Okusa MD (2006) Renal ischemia-reperfusion injury and adenosine 2A receptor-mediated tissue protection: the role of CD4+ T cells and IFN-gamma. J Immunol 176: 3108–3114
28. Burne-Taney MJ, Yokota-Ikeda N, Rabb H (2005) Effects of combined T- and B-cell deficiency on murine ischemia reperfusion injury. Am J Transplant 5: 1186–1193
29. Park P, Haas M, Cunningham PN, Bao L, Alexander JJ, Quigg RJ (2002) Injury in renal ischemia-reperfusion is independent from immunoglobulins and T lymphocytes. Am J Physiol Renal Physiol 282: F352–357
30. Burne-Taney MJ, Ascon DB, Daniels F, Racusen L, Baldwin W, Rabb H (2003) B cell deficiency confers protection from renal ischemia reperfusion injury. J Immunol 171: 3210–3215
31. Renner B, Strassheim D, Amura CR, et al (2010) B cell subsets contribute to renal injury and renal protection after ischemia/reperfusion. J Immunol 185: 4393–4000
32. Yang SH, Lee JP, Jang HR, et al (2011) Sulfatide-reactive natural killer T cells abrogate ischemia-reperfusion injury. J Am Soc Nephrol 22: 1305–3514
33. Wildin RS, Freitas A (2005) IPEX and FOXP3: clinical and research perspectives. J Autoimmun 25 (Suppl): 56–62
34. Fontenot JD, Gavin MA, Rudensky AY (2003) Foxp3 programs the development and function of CD4+CD25+ regulatory T cells. Nat Immunol 4: 330–336
35. Sakaguchi S, Wing K, Onishi Y, Prieto-Martin P, Yamaguchi T (2009) Regulatory T cells: how do they suppress immune responses? Int Immunol 10: 1105–1111
36. Vignali DA, Collison LW, Workman CJ (2008) How regulatory T cells work. Nat Rev Immunol 8: 523–532
37. Kinsey GR, Sharma R, Huang L, et al (2009) Regulatory T cells suppress innate immunity in kidney ischemia-reperfusion injury. J Am Soc Nephrol 20: 1744–1753
38. Monteiro RMM, Camara NOS, Rodrigues MM, et al (2009) A role for regulatory T cells in renal acute kidney injury. Transplant Immunol 21: 50–55
39. Kinsey GR, Huang L, Vergis AL, Li L, Okusa MD (2010) Regulatory T cells contribute to the protective effect of ischemic preconditioning in the kidney. Kidney Int 77: 771–780
40. Lee H, Nho D, Chung HS, Shin MK, Kim SH, Bae H (2010) CD4+CD25+ regulatory T cells attenuate cisplatin-induced nephrotoxicity in mice. Kidney Int 78: 1100–1109
41. Cho WY, Choi HM, Lee SY, Kim MG, Kim HK, Jo SK (2010) The role of Tregs and CD11c(+) macrophages/dendritic cells in ischemic preconditioning of the kidney. Kidney Int 78: 981–992
42. Kim MG, Lee SY, Ko YS, et al (2011) CD4+ CD25+ regulatory T cells partially mediate the beneficial effects of FTY720, a sphingosine-1-phosphate analogue, during ischaemia/reperfusion-induced acute kidney injury. Nephrol Dial Transplant 26: 111–124
43. Gandolfo MT, Jang HR, Bagnasco SM, et al (2009) Foxp3(+) regulatory T cells participate in repair of ischemic acute kidney injury. Kidney Int 76: 717–729
44. Brunstein CG, Miller JS, Cao Q, et al (2011) Infusion of ex vivo expanded T regulatory cells in adults transplanted with umbilical cord blood: safety profile and detection kinetics. Blood 117: 1061–1070

XIV

Worsening Renal Function during Decompensated Heart Failure: The Cardio-abdomino-renal Syndrome

F.H. Verbrugge, W. Mullens, and M. Malbrain

Introduction

The syndrome of heart failure is characterized by complex hemodynamic alterations with the hallmark being elevated filling pressures leading to symptoms of congestion. The pathophysiology of the interactions between heart and kidney is still insufficiently elucidated and in the setting of acute decompensated heart failure, coexisting renal insufficiency often complicates the treatment course. Historically, poor forward flow, i.e., low cardiac output, has been considered the culprit mechanism of acute decompensated heart failure, but growing evidence has emphasized the importance of venous congestion, not only for the progression of heart failure, but also for the development of worsening renal function during its treatment course. A potential role of the abdomen, through coexisting elevated intra-abdominal pressure (IAP), has recently been proposed. Therefore, the traditional perception of worsening renal function secondary to hypoperfusion of the kidneys through low-flow states has been challenged by the actual hemodynamics present, characterized by congestion and elevated IAP, leading to the concept of 'congestive kidney failure' or 'cardio-abdomino-renal syndrome'. This review will discuss the contemporary pathophysiological insights into the role of systemic venous congestion and elevated IAP in acute decompensated heart failure and its repercussions on the heart, kidneys and abdominal compartment. Current and future treatment strategies, aiming to relieve congestion while preserving renal function, will also be discussed.

Definition and Epidemiology

XIV

The definition 'cardiorenal syndrome' has been used to describe a wide range of clinical conditions implying concomitant impairment of cardiac and renal function. A more strict definition of cardiorenal syndrome is the extreme of cardiorenal dysregulation whereby therapy to relieve congestive symptoms of heart failure is limited by further decline in renal function. A more pragmatic approach is to define 'worsening renal function' as a 0.3–0.5 mg/dl rise in serum creatinine or a decrease in glomerular filtration rate (GFR) of 9–15 ml/min during hospitalization for acute decompensated heart failure [1, 2]. This definition has been used in most clinical outcome studies as worsening renal function occurs in 30 % of patients admitted for heart failure regardless of whether there is depressed or preserved systolic function. Worsening renal function typically occurs early, within days of hospitalization, suggesting a direct causative effect of the hemody-

J.-L. Vincent (ed.), *Annual Update in Intensive Care and Emergency Medicine 2012*
DOI 10.1007/978-3-642-25716-2 © Springer-Verlag Berlin Heidelberg 2012

namic alterations that occur while treatment for acute decompensated heart failure is initiated [3]. Worsening renal function is associated with a longer length of hospital stay and is a strong independent predictor of adverse outcomes [4–6]. Pre-existing renal dysfunction is one of the strongest risk factors for the development of worsening renal function, as it determines the 'intrinsic reserve' available for the kidneys [7].

Altered Hemodynamics in the Pathophysiology of Heart Failure and Worsening Renal Function

The exact pathophysiological mechanisms responsible for worsening renal function are multifactorial and not well defined. An overall imbalance in interactions between the failing heart, kidneys, abdominal compartment, neurohormonal system and inflammatory response, has been implicated. Traditionally, worsening renal function complicating the treatment of acute decompensated heart failure has been attributed to hypoperfusion of the kidney due to low-output failure, so-called 'pre-renal hypoperfusion' [4, 8]. Clinically, this is rarely the case. Autoregulation mechanisms in the kidneys will counteract the reduced renal blood flow through a compensatory increase in filtration fraction, which preserves glomerular filtration. It is only in very severe systolic heart failure, leading to an extremely high renal vascular resistance (through activation of the neurohormonal axis), that renal blood flow and the GFR will fall markedly without further increase in filtration fraction [8]. In addition, two observations from the Acute Decompensated Heart Failure National Registry (ADHERE) cast further doubt on the hypothesis of pre-renal hypoperfusion. First, worsening renal function is equally common among patients with preserved rather than reduced systolic function [9]. Second, most patients with acute decompensated heart failure have a normal or elevated blood pressure and many of them develop worsening renal function [10]. Thus, while diminished renal blood flow may still contribute to worsening renal function, it is important to recognize that other hemodynamic factors, including venous congestion, elevated IAP and right ventricular function, are at least equally important.

Systemic Venous Congestion

Pathophysiology

XIV

Systemic venous congestion, manifesting as elevated jugular venous pressure and often leading to anasarc edema is the hallmark feature of the heart failure syndrome. Patients presenting with acute decompensated heart failure are much more likely to have symptoms of congestion than of low-output heart failure [10]. As a result, it is recognized that the presence of low cardiac output in acute decompensated heart failure can only explain part of the pathophysiology. The failing heart tries to balance 'preload' and 'afterload' to compensate for impaired contractility. This results in stimulation of baroreceptors and the juxtaglomerular apparatus, leading to orthosympathetic activation, activation of the renin-angiotensin-aldosterone system, release of arginine vasopressin and stimulation of thirst [11]. Therefore, heart failure patients have a strong tendency to retain water and salt, leading to systemic venous congestion. Although this cardiocentric idea of congestion is indicative of a lack of compensatory reserve, it does not explain why some cases of low-output heart failure present without congestion or the occurrence of flash pulmonary edema that is often secondary to vascular redistribution and precedes any form of systemic congestion.

Systemic venous congestion is an important treatment target, and its relief or prevention is often considered as treatment success. At the same time, it is vital to emphasize that systemic venous congestion is not specific for heart failure, because it occurs in various states of end-stage organ dysfunction, such as cirrhosis and nephropathy. Importantly, intracardiac pressures rise about 5 days preceding hospitalization for acute decompensated heart failure, reflecting a state of systemic venous congestion and probably also increased vasoconstriction of the venous capacitance beds [12]. Moreover, systemic venous congestion itself can promote the progression of heart failure (**Fig. 1**). First, an increase in volume overload exacerbates myocardial remodeling. Second, dilation of the left ventricle worsens functional mitral regurgitation, providing a substrate for atrial fibrillation, a common trigger for acute decompensated heart failure. Third, activation of the venous endothelium occurs in acute decompensated heart failure, contributing to a pro-inflammatory and vasoconstrictive environment, with increased oxidative stress [13].

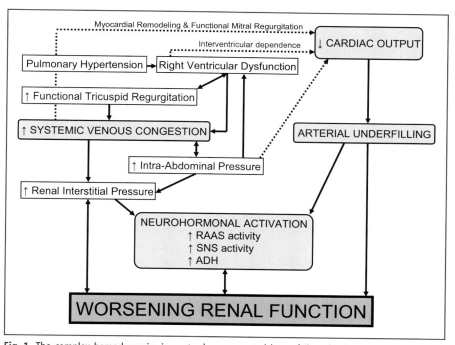

Fig. 1. The complex hemodynamics in acute decompensated heart failure, leading to worsening renal function. RAAS: renin-angiotensin-aldosterone system; SNS: sympathic nervous system; ADH: antidiuretic hormone

XIV

A paradigm shift to the concept of 'congestive kidney failure'

The concept that elevated venous pressure is transmitted back to the renal veins and kidneys leading to 'congestive kidney failure' is supported by a substantial (and largely forgotten) amount of older animal literature. Already in 1931, Winton described the detrimental influence of acute venous pressure increase on renal function in an *ex vivo* canine kidney model [14]. This effect seemed to be reversible, as release of renal vein compression immediately improved urine output and the GFR.

Recently, a resurgence of interest in the role of venous congestion in the development of worsening renal function complicating the treatment of acute decompensated heart failure has arisen [15–17]. In a study of 145 patients admitted with advanced decompensated low-output heart failure states, central venous pressure (CVP) was the only hemodynamic parameter related to the occurrence of worsening renal function, whereas cardiac index was not [17]. This correlation was even more evident in patients with pulmonary hypertension and in those with low renal blood flow [15, 16]. The exact pathophysiological mechanisms for this relation remain speculative (**Fig. 1**). Because the kidney is an encapsulated organ, congestion of the venules surrounding the renal tubules might obliterate their lumen until the hydrostatic pressure of the ultrafiltrate exceeds that in the veins, leading to worsening renal function [14]. Backwards transmission of the CVP via the renal veins, may be another explanation. Importantly, intrarenal and systemic angiotensin II concentrations increase with increasing renal venous pressure, which will further reduce the GFR [18, 19].

Elevated Intra-abdominal Pressure

Definitions

The compliance of the abdominal wall normally prevents an increase in IAP as the abdominal girth increases. Depending on body mass index (BMI) and body position, a normal IAP for a healthy adult is considered to be 5–7 mmHg [20]. However, once a critical volume is reached, compliance falls abruptly. Further distension leads to a rapidly augmenting IAP and results in organ dysfunction [21, 22]. Intra-abdominal hypertension (IAH) is arbitrarily defined as an IAP ≥ 12 mmHg, whereas abdominal compartment syndrome (ACS) is defined as a sustained increase in IAP ≥ 20 mmHg in the presence of new organ dysfunction [20].

Hemodynamic effects of increased intra-abdominal pressure

Cardiac function can be distilled into three essential components: Preload, afterload and contractility. Elevated IAP negatively impacts upon all three of these interrelated components (**Fig. 2**) [23].

Decreased preload: It has been demonstrated that an IAP of only 10 mmHg can significantly reduce inferior vena cava blood flow and cardiac preload. Reduced venous return has the immediate effect of decreasing cardiac output through decreased stroke volume by the Frank-Starling relationship. In patients with IAH, multiple mechanisms are responsible for the reduced cardiac preload. First, an increased intrathoracic pressure, as the result of an upwards movement of the diaphragm because of increased IAP, decreases blood flow through the inferior vena cava and limits venous return. Second, when IAP increases, the upwards deviation of the diaphragm narrows the inferior vena cava as it passes through the dia-

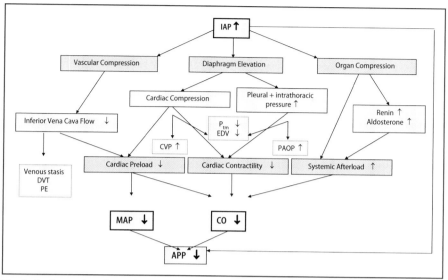

Fig. 2. Cardiovascular effects of elevated intra-abdominal pressure. APP: abdominal perfusion pressure; CO: cardiac output; CVP: central venous pressure; DVT: deep vein thrombosis; EDV: end-diastolic volume; IAP: intra-abdominal pressure; MAP: mean arterial pressure; PAOP: pulmonary artery occlusion pressure; PE: pulmonary embolism; P_{tm}: transmural pressure

phragm (through altered anatomy of the diaphragmatic crura), which impedes proper venous return and has a profound effect on cardiac preload [24]. Importantly, the impact of an elevated IAP is not limited to the abdominal compartment as it may result in elevated pulmonary artery, central venous, and pulmonary artery occlusion pressure (PAOP) readings from the pulmonary artery catheter (PAC), which makes preload assessment difficult. Furthermore, measured intravascular pressures are not always reflective of intravascular volumes, which can lead to inappropriate diuretic therapy that increases the risk of worsening renal function. These changing hemodynamics may occur with an IAP as low as 10 mmHg [25]. This effect may explain why effective venous return is decreased in patients with acute decompensated heart failure even though venous pressure is increased.

Decreased contractility: Diaphragmatic elevation and increased intrathoracic pressure also have marked effects on cardiac contractility. Traditionally, the right ventricle has been considered to be solely a conduit for delivering blood to the lungs and left ventricle. Compression of the pulmonary parenchyma increases pulmonary vascular resistance and right ventricular afterload. The right ventricle responds with dilation and increased myocardial oxygen demand [26]. Through the mechanism of interventricular dependence, the dilated failing right ventricle also impedes left ventricular function. Reduced left ventricular output may contribute to the development of systemic hypotension, worsening right coronary artery blood flow and leading to ischemia, which further compromises right ventricular contractility. This effect ultimately culminates in further activation of the neurohormonal axis, triggering systemic venous congestion which in turn leads to further augmentation of IAP, creating a vicious cycle which further compromises the already-impaired left ventricle (**Figs. 1** and **2**).

XIV

Increased afterload: Elevated IAP can cause increased systemic vascular resistance in two ways. First, through direct compressive effects on the aorta and systemic vasculature, and second (and more commonly) as compensation for the reduced venous return and falling stroke volume. As a result of this physiologic compensation, mean arterial pressure (MAP) typically remains stable in the early stages of IAH, despite reductions in venous return and cardiac output. This increasing afterload may be poorly tolerated by patients with marginal cardiac contractility or inadequate intravascular volume.

Renal effects of increased intra-abdominal pressure

Elevated IAP significantly decreases renal venous and arterial blood flow, leading to renal dysfunction and failure. Oliguria develops at an IAP of 15 mmHg and anuria at 30 mmHg in the presence of normovolemia, and even lower levels of IAP are implicated in patients with hypovolemia [27]. Abdominal or kidney perfusion pressure is defined as MAP minus IAP [20]. Therefore, theoretically, decreased kidney perfusion can be prevented by either decreasing IAP or increasing MAP. The filtration gradient (FG) is possibly a more appropriate parameter to explain acute kidney injury (AKI) associated with IAH. It is defined as the glomerular filtration pressure minus the proximal tubular pressure, which in conditions of IAH can be simplified as follows: FG = MAP − 2xIAP. Thus, changes in IAP have a greater impact on renal function and urine production than do changes in MAP. It should, therefore, not be surprising that decreased renal function, as evidenced by the development of oliguria, is one of the first visible signs of IAH.

Right Ventricular Function

The goal of the right ventricle is to generate flow into the highly compliant, low-resistant pulmonary circulation, while maintaining the lowest possible pressures in the right heart cavities to optimize venous return. In addition, the right ventricle is important for adequate filling of the left ventricle. Right ventricular systolic dysfunction is widely accepted as a strong and independent predictor of adverse outcomes in patients with heart failure [28, 29]. In patients with advanced heart failure, it even more closely predicts exercise capacity and survival than does left ventricular function [28]. Amelioration of right ventricular function in response to intensive medical treatment for acute decompensated heart failure portends a better long-term prognosis [30].

XIV

Remarkably, echocardiographic signs of right ventricular dysfunction at the moment of acute decompensated heart failure characterize the subgroup with the greatest improvement in renal function after medical treatment for acute decompensated heart failure [31]. This suggests the importance of systemic venous congestion secondary to right ventricular failure in the development of worsening renal function. Indeed, right ventricular dilation induces tricuspid regurgitation leading to reduced left ventricular preload and worsening systemic venous congestion. These patients often respond very well to decongestive therapies, resulting in an improvement in renal function [30, 31].

Defining the Cardio-abdomino-renal Syndrome

Only recently, it was shown that IAP is often raised in patients with acute decompensated heart failure. In a study of 40 patients hospitalized for acute decompensated heart failure, more than 50 % presented with raised IAP, mostly with minimal or no abdominal complaints [32]. Interestingly, ascites was only found in a small subset of cases, so the presence of raised IAP in acute decompensated heart failure is probably due to visceral (tissue) edema as a result of progressive whole-body fluid accumulation or systemic congestion [32, 33].

Elevated IAP seems to correlate with more impaired renal function in patients presenting with acute decompensated heart failure and reduction of IAP after tailored medical therapy is associated with improvement in renal function [32]. Furthermore, in the subgroup of patients in which intensive medical treatment fails to reduce IAP, mechanical fluid removal with either paracentesis in case of ascites or ultrafiltration might be effective at reducing IAP and subsequently ameliorating renal function [33].

Notably, although organ dysfunction has only been described in the literature when IAP exceeds 12 mmHg, patients with acute decompensated heart failure may already develop worsening renal function with a much lower IAP [32]. This suggests that the underlying reserve of the kidneys to counteract an increased IAP is limited in this setting. It is also vital to emphasize that although the degree of renal dysfunction is probably correlated with the degree of elevated IAP, there can be a wide range of IAPs in relation to serum creatinine levels at presentation [32]. Although we can only speculate why this discrepancy exists, it is clear that other mechanisms, including coexisting systemic congestion, pre-existing renal insufficiency, and drugs used during the treatment of acute decompensated heart failure, probably play a role.

Because of the central role that IAP plays in cardiovascular and renal hemodynamics in critically ill patients, we believe that it may present the missing link between the heart and the kidney. Therefore, we would like to coin the term "cardio-abdomino-renal syndrome".

Therapeutic Strategies to Relieve Congestion in Acute Decompensated Heart Failure

Water and Salt Restriction

Because of their stimulated neurohormonal axis, heart failure patients have a tendency to retain sodium and water. A daily salt intake above 3 g typically increases the need for diuretics, which further augments neurohormonal stimulation and reduces the GFR [34, 35]. Water restriction is often difficult to achieve in the presence of thirst. Plasma osmolarity is normally tightly regulated by the thirst center in the brain. Preventing hyperosmolarity through limitation of the salt intake and adequate control of glycemia suppresses thirst and facilitates water restriction.

XIV

Diuretic Therapy

Loop diuretics are among the most widely prescribed drugs in the treatment of acute decompensated heart failure [9]. A recent, large, double-blind, randomized clinical trial could not prove a benefit for high versus low dosing or administration with bolus versus continuous infusions, although a trend towards worse renal function was seen in the high dose group [36].

There are several potential mechanisms by which diuretics could worsen heart failure progression and increase the risk of worsening renal function. First, diuretics further stimulate the neurohormonal axis which is implicated in the progression of heart failure. Second, diuretics can cause marked electrolyte abnormalities, such as potassium and magnesium depletion, as well as metabolic alkalosis, possibly resulting in lethal arrhythmias. Third, intravascular underfilling can occur if diuresis exceeds the plasma refilling time, which is about 3–4 ml/kg/h. This effect causes decreased renal blood flow and often provokes a significant decrease in GFR. Nevertheless, recent data suggest that in cases of clear hypervolemia, achieving hemoconcentration through extensive use of diuretic therapy – despite transient worsening renal function – may be associated with a better prognosis [37]. This finding suggests that transient worsening of renal function may be acceptable if it allows a complete decongestive state to be achieved. This suggestion is again in line with ADHERE data, which clearly documented that more than half the patients admitted with signs of congestion during acute decompensated heart failure, do not lose weight during hospitalization [9].

Remarkably, data from the Evaluation Study of Congestive Heart Failure and Pulmonary Artery Catheterization Effectiveness (ESCAPE) trial demonstrated that worsening renal function did not occur when diuretic therapy was tailored to invasively measured filling pressures. In contrast, worsening renal function occured more frequently when therapy was guided by clinical judgment alone [38]. Overall, however, the ESCAPE trial did not reveal a benefit on mortality or rehospitalization frequency of routine PAC placement to guide therapy for patients with acute decompensated heart failure [39]. These seemingly contradicting observations are an illustration of the heterogeneity of the heart failure population that impedes the development of good randomized clinical trials.

Vasodilator Therapy

Most patients presenting with acute decompensated heart failure have normal or elevated blood pressures [10]. In these cases, especially when cardiac output is impaired, unloading the heart with vasodilator therapy is beneficial and often leads to enhanced diuresis, without or with significantly less diuretic therapy. Sodium nitroprusside has been used for years in the treatment of acute decompensated heart failure with excellent results. A recent study emphasized its safety and efficacy in a population with low-output states, pointing to possibly favorable long-term outcomes [40]. Recent observations raise questions about our current management strategy for acute decompensated heart failure, which has been traditionally focused on enhancing the cardiac index (often through inotropic agents) instead of lowering filling pressures.

Novel Renal-preserving Treatments

A variety of novel agents is under investigation for the treatment of systemic and/or pulmonary venous congestion in the setting of acute decompensated heart failure. These therapies all aim to relieve congestion with preservation of renal function. However, nesiritide, vasopressin receptor antagonists and the adenosine A1

XIV

receptor antagonist, rolofylline, have all failed to fulfill their promise in the latest clinical trials [41 – 43].

Ultrafiltration

Whereas diuretics (and vasopressin receptor antagonists) promote diuresis of *hypo*tonic urine, mechanical removal of fluid through ultrafiltration removes *iso*tonic fluid. Thus, while diuretic-induced diuresis and ultrafiltration might (temporarily) both reduce total body water, only ultrafiltration adequately removes salt. Moreover, because isotonic plasma is eliminated, electrolyte abnormalities are most often avoided.

A device that permits ultrafiltration through peripheral access, thereby being less invasive, minimizing hemodynamic effects and having the theoretical advantage of being able to be performed on a regular nursing floor, has been available for more than 5 years. A pilot study in congested heart failure patients showed 90 % ultrafiltration success during a single 8 h session, achieving a total net fluid removal of 4650 ml per patient, without the need for a central venous line [44]. Consequently, the Ultrafiltration versus Intravenous Diuretics for Patients Hospitalized for Acute Decompensated Heart Failure (UNLOAD) trial was designed to compare intravenous diuretics with ultrafiltration for the treatment of patients with ≥ 2 signs of hypervolemia [45]. Two hundred patients (mean age 63 years; 63 % men) were randomized to ultrafiltration or intravenous diuretics. Weight and net fluid loss were greater in the ultrafiltration group. Whereas symptom relieve was comparable in both groups, there was a significant reduction in subsequent rehospitalization for heart failure favoring the ultrafiltration group [45]. Other outcomes of UNLOAD are presented in **Table 1**. Remarkably, the improved outcome was achieved even though a trend towards worsening renal function was noted in the ultrafiltration group. One could, therefore, speculate that the underlying pathophysiology of worsening renal function, more than its occurrence, seems to have prognostic impact. Thus, worsening renal function should not be used as a single prognostic parameter when evaluating the effects of future decongestive therapies.

Ultrafiltration remains the only fluid removal strategy which has been shown to improve outcomes in randomized clinical trials of patients with acute decompensated heart failure. However, invasiveness and costs still hamper a widespread strategy of early ultrafiltration. Efforts are being made to develop a hemofilter for continuous ambulatory ultrafiltration and a prototype exists with promising results [46]. A possible advantage is that such a device makes slower fluid

XIV

Table 1. Important outcome parameters from the UNLOAD trial [45]

	Ultrafiltration group mean (standard error mean)	Diuretics group mean (standard error mean)	p-value
Weight loss at 48 h (kg)	5.0 (3.1)	3.1 (3.5)	0.001
Net fluid loss at 48 h (l)	4.6	3.3	0.001
Re-hospitalization for heart failure at 90 days	0.22 (0.54)	0.46 (0.76)	0,022
Re-hospitalization days per patient at 90 days	1.4 (4.2)	3.8 (8.5)	0.022
Serum potassium < 3.5 meq/l (%)	1	12	0.018
Episodes of hypotension	4	3	NS

removal possible, so that refilling from the extravascular compartment can be maintained.

Decreasing IAP

The World Society on Abdominal Compartment Syndrome (WSACS, www.wsacs.org) has recently published recommendations for the treatment of IAH and ACS focused on improvement of abdominal wall compliance, evacuation of intraluminal contents, evacuation of free abdominal fluid, correction of capillary leak and fluid balance and maintaining abdominal perfusion pressure above 60 mmHg [47]. All these interventions may help in cardio-abdomino-renal syndrome.

Conclusion

Acute decompensated heart failure is a state of altered hemodynamics. Systemic venous congestion and elevated IAP are characteristic findings for this syndrome and together with right heart failure may contribute to worsening renal function and further organ dysfunction with profound negative impact on long-term prognosis. The concept of 'congestive kidney injury' has gained attention and the term "cardio-abdomino-renal syndrome" is coined here for the first time. Because the kidney is an encapsulated organ, augmented venous pressure increases renal interstitial pressure, upregulating further the neurohormonal axis with detrimental effects on heart failure progression. Right ventricular dysfunction and functional tricuspid regurgitation play an important role in the development of systemic venous congestion. Although a lot of research has focused on new ways to relieve congestion to preserve renal function, IAP seems to play a key role and ultrafiltration is the only fluid removal strategy that has been shown to improve outcomes in a randomized clinical trial of patients with acute decompensated heart failure.

References

1. Damman K, Navis G, Voors AA, et al (2007) Worsening renal function and prognosis in heart failure: systematic review and meta-analysis. J Card Fail 13: 599–608
2. Gottlieb SS, Abraham W, Butler J, et al (2002) The prognostic importance of different definitions of worsening renal function in congestive heart failure. J Card Fail 8: 136–141
3. Krumholz HM, Chen YT, Vaccarino V, et al (2000) Correlates and impact on outcomes of worsening renal function in patients > or =65 years of age with heart failure. Am J Cardiol 85: 1110–1113
4. Forman DE, Butler J, Wang Y, et al (2004) Incidence, predictors at admission, and impact of worsening renal function among patients hospitalized with heart failure. J Am Coll Cardiol 43: 61–67
5. Hillege HL, Girbes AR, de Kam PJ, et al (2000) Renal function, neurohormonal activation, and survival in patients with chronic heart failure. Circulation 102: 203–210
6. Cowie MR, Komajda M, Murray-Thomas T, Underwood J, Ticho B (2006) Prevalence and impact of worsening renal function in patients hospitalized with decompensated heart failure: results of the prospective outcomes study in heart failure (POSH). Eur Heart J 27: 1216–1222
7. Heywood JT, Fonarow GC, Costanzo MR, Mathur VS, Wigneswaran JR, Wynne J (2007) High prevalence of renal dysfunction and its impact on outcome in 118,465 patients hospi-

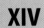

talized with acute decompensated heart failure: a report from the ADHERE database. J Card Fail 13: 422–430

8. Ljungman S, Laragh JH, Cody RJ (1990) Role of the kidney in congestive heart failure. Relationship of cardiac index to kidney function. Drugs 39 (Suppl 4): 10–21

9. Yancy CW, Lopatin M, Stevenson LW, De Marco T, Fonarow GC (2006) Clinical presentation, management, and in-hospital outcomes of patients admitted with acute decompensated Heart Failure with preserved systolic function: a report from the Acute Decompensated Heart Failure National Registry (ADHERE) Database. J Am Coll Cardiol 47: 76–84

10. Adams KF Jr, Fonarow GC, Emerman CL, et al (2005) Characteristics and outcomes of patients hospitalized for heart failure in the United States: rationale, design, and preliminary observations from the first 100,000 cases in the Acute Decompensated Heart Failure National Registry (ADHERE). Am Heart J 149: 209–216

11. Schrier RW, Abraham WT (1999) Hormones and hemodynamics in heart failure. N Engl J Med 341: 577–585

12. Adamson PB, Magalski A, Braunschweig F, et al (2003) Ongoing right ventricular hemodynamics in heart failure: clinical value of measurements derived from an implantable monitoring system. J Am Coll Cardiol 41: 565–571

13. Colombo PC, Banchs JE, Celaj S, et al (2005) Endothelial cell activation in patients with decompensated heart failure. Circulation 111: 58–62

14. Winton FR (1931) The influence of venous pressure on the isolated mammalian kidney. J Physiol 72: 49–61

15. Damman K, Navis G, Smilde TD, et al (2007) Decreased cardiac output, venous congestion and the association with renal impairment in patients with cardiac dysfunction. Eur J Heart Fail 9: 872–878

16. Damman K, van Deursen VM, Navis G, Voors AA, van Veldhuisen DJ, Hillege HL (2009) Increased central venous pressure is associated with impaired renal function and mortality in a broad spectrum of patients with cardiovascular disease. J Am Coll Cardiol 53: 582–588

17. Mullens W, Abrahams Z, Francis GS, et al (2009) Importance of venous congestion for worsening of renal function in advanced decompensated heart failure. J Am Coll Cardiol 53: 589–596

18. Fiksen-Olsen MJ, Strick DM, Hawley H, Romero JC (1992) Renal effects of angiotensin II inhibition during increases in renal venous pressure. Hypertension 19: II137–II141

19. Kastner PR, Hall JE, Guyton AC (1982) Renal hemodynamic responses to increased renal venous pressure: role of angiotensin II. Am J Physiol 243: F260–F264

20. Malbrain ML, Cheatham ML, Kirkpatrick A, et al (2006) Results from the International Conference of Experts on Intra-abdominal Hypertension and Abdominal Compartment Syndrome. I. Definitions. Intensive Care Med 32: 1722–1732

21. Doty JM, Saggi BH, Blocher CR, et al (2000) Effects of increased renal parenchymal pressure on renal function. J Trauma 48: 874–877

22. Malbrain ML, Chiumello D, Pelosi P, et al (2005) Incidence and prognosis of intraabdominal hypertension in a mixed population of critically ill patients: a multiple-center epidemiological study. Crit Care Med 33: 315–322

23. Cheatham ML, Malbrain ML (2007) Cardiovascular implications of abdominal compartment syndrome. Acta Clin Belg Suppl 98–112

24. Schein M, Wittmann DH, Aprahamian CC, Condon RE (1995) The abdominal compartment syndrome: the physiological and clinical consequences of elevated intra-abdominal pressure. J Am Coll Surg 180: 745–753

25. Diamant M, Benumof JL, Saidman LJ (1978) Hemodynamics of increased intra-abdominal pressure: Interaction with hypovolemia and halothane anesthesia. Anesthesiology 48: 23–27

26. Eddy AC, Rice CL, Anardi DM (1988) Right ventricular dysfunction in multiple trauma victims. Am J Surg 155: 712–715

27. De Laet I, Malbrain ML, Jadoul JL, Rogiers P, Sugrue M (2007) Renal implications of increased intra-abdominal pressure: are the kidneys the canary for abdominal hypertension? Acta Clin Belg Suppl 119–130

28. Di Salvo TG, Mathier M, Semigran MJ, Dec GW (1995) Preserved right ventricular ejec-

XIV

tion fraction predicts exercise capacity and survival in advanced heart failure. J Am Coll Cardiol 25: 1143–1153

29. Ghio S, Gavazzi A, Campana C, et al (2001) Independent and additive prognostic value of right ventricular systolic function and pulmonary artery pressure in patients with chronic heart failure. J Am Coll Cardiol 37: 183–188

30. Verhaert D, Mullens W, Borowski A, et al (2010) Right ventricular response to intensive medical therapy in advanced decompensated heart failure. Circ Heart Fail 3: 340–346

31. Testani JM, Khera AV, St John Sutton MG, et al (2010) Effect of right ventricular function and venous congestion on cardiorenal interactions during the treatment of decompensated heart failure. Am J Cardiol 105: 511–516

32. Mullens W, Abrahams Z, Skouri HN, et al (2008) Elevated intra-abdominal pressure in acute decompensated heart failure: a potential contributor to worsening renal function? J Am Coll Cardiol 51: 300–306

33. Mullens W, Abrahams Z, Francis GS, Taylor DO, Starling RC, Tang WH (2008) Prompt reduction in intra-abdominal pressure following large-volume mechanical fluid removal improves renal insufficiency in refractory decompensated heart failure. J Card Fail 14: 508–514

34. Bayliss J, Norell M, Canepa-Anson R, Sutton G, Poole-Wilson P (1987) Untreated heart failure: clinical and neuroendocrine effects of introducing diuretics. Br Heart J 57: 17–22

35. Gottlieb SS, Brater DC, Thomas I, et al (2002) BG9719 (CVT-124), an A1 adenosine receptor antagonist, protects against the decline in renal function observed with diuretic therapy. Circulation 105: 1348–1353

36. Felker GM, Lee KL, Bull DA, et al (2011) Diuretic strategies in patients with acute decompensated heart failure. N Engl J Med 364: 797–805

37. Testani JM, Chen J, McCauley BD, Kimmel SE, Shannon RP (2010) Potential effects of aggressive decongestion during the treatment of decompensated heart failure on renal function and survival. Circulation 122: 265–272

38. Nohria A, Hasselblad V, Stebbins A, et al (2008) Cardiorenal interactions: insights from the ESCAPE trial. J Am Coll Cardiol 51: 1268–1274

39. Binanay C, Califf RM, Hasselblad V, et al (2005) Evaluation study of congestive heart failure and pulmonary artery catheterization effectiveness: the ESCAPE trial. JAMA 294: 1625–1633

40. Mullens W, Abrahams Z, Francis GS, et al (2008) Sodium nitroprusside for advanced low-output heart failure. J Am Coll Cardiol 52: 200–207

41. O'Connor CM, Starling RC, Hernandez AF, et al (2011) Effect of nesiritide in patients with acute decompensated heart failure. N Engl J Med 365: 32–43

42. Konstam MA, Gheorghiade M, Burnett JC Jr, et al (2007) Effects of oral tolvaptan in patients hospitalized for worsening heart failure: the EVEREST Outcome Trial. JAMA 297: 1319–1331

43. Massie BM, O'Connor CM, Metra M, et al (2010) Rolofylline, an adenosine A1-receptor antagonist, in acute heart failure. N Engl J Med 363: 1419–1428

44. Bart BA, Boyle A, Bank AJ, et al (2005) Ultrafiltration versus usual care for hospitalized patients with heart failure: the Relief for Acutely Fluid-Overloaded Patients With Decompensated Congestive Heart Failure (RAPID-CHF) trial. J Am Coll Cardiol 46: 2043–2046

45. Costanzo MR, Guglin ME, Saltzberg MT, et al (2007) Ultrafiltration versus intravenous diuretics for patients hospitalized for acute decompensated heart failure. J Am Coll Cardiol 49: 675–683

46. Gura V, Ronco C, Nalesso F, et al (2008) A wearable hemofilter for continuous ambulatory ultrafiltration. Kidney Int 73: 497–502

47. Cheatham ML, Malbrain ML, Kirkpatrick A, et al (2007) Results from the International Conference of Experts on Intra-abdominal Hypertension and Abdominal Compartment Syndrome. II. Recommendations. Intensive Care Med 33: 951–962

XIV

XV Diagnosis of AKI

Subclinical Damage in Acute Kidney Injury: A Novel Paradigm

S.M. Bagshaw and M. Haase

Introduction

Acute kidney injury (AKI) remains a challenging clinical problem for clinicians caring for critically ill patients. Its occurrence in the critically ill is remarkably common, frequently iatrogenic, and it consistently predicts an increase in the complexity and intensity of care. Moreover, AKI appears to consistently have a negative impact on both short and long-term survival and recovery of kidney function, along with greatly intensifying health resource utilization [1, 2]. Accordingly, there has been considerable effort to better understand the pathophysiology and improve the outcomes associated with the development of AKI.

Defining Acute Kidney Injury

The term AKI broadly defines a wide spectrum of abrupt changes to kidney function, encompassing mild elevations in serum creatinine (sCr) to overt anuric kidney failure requiring support with renal replacement therapy (RRT). Traditionally, inferences on the epidemiologic burden of AKI have been imprecise due to the lack of agreement on an acceptable standardized definition. However, in 2004, the Acute Dialysis Quality Initiative (ADQI) proposed the consensus-driven RIFLE (Risk Injury Failure Loss End-stage) classification scheme [3]. The RIFLE criteria define three grades of AKI severity (Risk, Injury and Failure) based on detected changes to sCr from a known baseline and to urine output, along with two clinical outcomes (Loss, End-stage). Since this publication, AKI has largely been defined according to these criteria (or the proposed modifications presented by the AKI Network [AKIN]) [4].

These consensus criteria represent the current diagnostic paradigm in AKI and have clearly been a monumental advance in the field [5]. However, the RIFLE (and AKIN) criteria are imperfect and not without significant shortcomings. For example, the use of sCr, which is a poor surrogate marker of changes to glomerular filtration rate (GFR), is immensely problematic. sCR can require hours and/or days to accumulate and achieve steady state following acute declines in GFR (and may only show significant increases after loss of > 50 % of GFR). The volume of distribution of sCr can be inconsistent and heavily modified by age, sex, muscle mass, drugs, critical illness and fluid resuscitation [6]. Finally, experimental data have shown that the expression of creatinine from muscle may be suppressed in septic states [7]. Consequently, this current diagnostic paradigm for AKI, utilizing sCr as the principal marker, is highly prone to not only delayed detection but

XV

J.-L. Vincent (ed.), *Annual Update in Intensive Care and Emergency Medicine 2012*
DOI 10.1007/978-3-642-25716-2 © Springer-Verlag Berlin Heidelberg 2012

also missed episodes of important declines in GFR. In addition, and perhaps more importantly, this diagnostic paradigm does not allow the segregation of aspects of genuine 'damage', in terms of the type, timing of onset, evolution and/or recovery phases, from actual decrements in GFR. This is clearly inadequate when the timely diagnosis of AKI among critically ill patients is such a clinical priority given the prognostic consequences associated with overt kidney failure.

Novel Biomarkers of Kidney Injury

Numerous promising novel kidney injury-specific biomarkers have recently been discovered, characterized, validated, and are increasingly available in clinical practice for the early detection and diagnosis of AKI. Importantly, these novel biomarkers are better capable of detecting real-time 'injury' to renal tubular epithelial tissue and provide considerable 'lead-time' for potential overt AKI when compared with AKI diagnosed by conventional measures such as sCr [8].

Neutrophil gelatinase-associated lipocalin (NGAL) is one such promising biomarker. NGAL is a 25 kDa polypeptide that is rapidly upregulated in renal tubular epithelial tissue in response to distal nephron injury [9]. The protein by-product of this gene upregulation, NGAL, is easily measured in the urine and plasma, where its concentration increases in a dose-dependent relationship with the severity and duration of acute tubular injury [10, 11]. A number of observational studies have suggested that NGAL is a sensitive biomarker for anticipating (in advance by 24–48 hours) the occurrence of conventionally-diagnosed AKI (i.e., sCr-based criteria) [12–14]. In addition, NGAL has shown value for discriminating established AKI from milder forms of AKI, such as pre-renal states, that are rapidly reversible [8, 15]. Moreover, NGAL may provide important prognostic information on the risk of worsening AKI, need for RRT and mortality [10, 11]. Although encouraging, these findings have not been universally consistent [16, 17]. Interestingly though, it has been speculated that the observed uncertainty on the performance of NGAL, in particular in critically ill patients, may be more specifically related to the use of a suboptimal surrogate marker (i.e., sCr) as the diagnostic gold standard for AKI [18].

Detection of Subclinical Kidney Injury

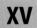

This observation that sCr may be suboptimal is perhaps best illustrated by patients who have been exposed to a kidney 'injury' stimulus, such as cardiopulmonary bypass (CPB) or contrast media, and who clearly develop detectable increases in kidney injury-specific biomarkers, such as NGAL, yet do not develop concomitant increases in sCr to fulfill conventional consensus definitions for AKI [12]. Such patients thus have detectable kidney 'injury' with preserved kidney 'function', and could be best described as having a syndrome of 'subclinical' AKI. This is a prime example of how these novel kidney-injury specific biomarkers are adding new information to our understanding of the pathophysiology and perhaps the short- and long-term clinical course of patients who develop this syndrome. Is there increased risk for worsening/future AKI or accelerated development of chronic kidney disease or progression to end-stage kidney disease or increased susceptibility to other adverse events? What do we know about this subgroup with apparent subclinical AKI?

Recently, in a pooled analysis of prospective observational studies, we evaluated the hypothesis that detectable elevations in urine and/or plasma NGAL, in the absence of detectable changes in sCr fulfilling the conventional diagnosis of AKI, would identify a unique cohort of patients with 'subclinical AKI' whose risk of adverse events and clinical course would be more complicated and whose prognosis would be negatively modified [11]. We performed a pooled analysis of aggregate data from 10 studies, including 2322 patients, which evaluated the significance of NGAL for the early diagnosis of AKI. The patients were classified into four discreet groups for analysis: NGAL(-)/sCr(-), NGAL(+)/sCr(-), NGAL(-)/sCr(+), and NGAL(+)/sCr(+). In total, 19.2 % (n = 445) of these patients were classified as having 'subclinical AKI' defined as NGAL(+)/sCr(-) (**Table 1**). The identification of this subgroup by NGAL only would have resulted in an additional 43 % of patients being diagnosed with AKI, rather than being missed and classified as non-AKI by sCr-criteria alone. More importantly, this subclinical AKI subgroup had significantly higher use of RRT, higher mortality, and long durations of stay in the intensive care unit (ICU) and hospital, when compared with the NGAL(-)/sCr(-) subgroup. This finding was consistent regardless of whether NGAL was measured from the urine or plasma. These observations strongly support the hypothesis of the existence of a clinically important state of subclinical 'injury' detectable only by injury-specific biomarkers, such as NGAL, that occurs without significant loss to GFR and which is completely missed by our current diagnostic paradigm for AKI [11].

Moreover, the biologic plausibility of this hypothesis is further supported by studies that evaluated the urine sediment for detection of renal tubular 'injury'. Examination of the urine sediment, a long-standing practice in nephrology, may represent an additional ideal surrogate for 'structural' damage to renal tubular epithelial tissue. It is also plausible that assessment of the urine sediment may provide 'lead-time', analogous to kidney-injury biomarkers, for the early diagnosis of AKI prior to detectable increases in sCr. Likewise, urine sediment evaluation may provide additional information about prognosis, specifically about the severity of injury and/or its expected clinical course [19–22]. Perazella and colleagues recently reported the results of two prospective observational studies assessing the diagnostic significance of a novel urine microscopy score (UMS) in non-ICU hospitalized patients with AKI to predict the occurrence of a composite of 'worsening AKI', defined as an increase in AKIN stage, need for RRT and/or

Table 1. Summary of outcomes stratified by aggregate subgroups of neutrophil gelatinase-associated lipocalin (NGAL) and serum creatinine (sCr) [11].

	NGAL(-)/sCr(-)	NGAL(+)/sCr(-)	NGAL(-)/sCr(+)	NGAL(+)/sCr(+)
n, %	1296 (55.8)	445 (19.2)	107 (4.6)	474 (20.4)
peak NGAL§ (ng/mL)	59 (20–97)	213 (117–1124)	69 (21–118)	354 (208–1888)
RRT (n, %)	2 (0.015)	11 (2.5)	8 (7.5)	38 (8.0)
Composite¶ (n, %)	63 (4.9)	69 (15.5)	10 (9.3)	84 (17.7)
ICU stay§ (days)	4.2 (2.2–6.4)	7.1 (5.4–10.3)	6.5 (3.0–11.7)	9.0 (8.0–14.0)
Hospital stay§ (days)	8.8 (7.7–19.0)	17 (8.4–24.2)	17.8 (5.1–26.4)	21.9 (15.8–29.9)

§ Median (IQR); ¶ Composite = RRT or death.

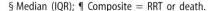

hospital death [21, 22]. In this study, a higher UMS, suggestive of greater detectable 'structural' tubular damage, was closely correlated with an increased adjusted-risk for worsening AKI.

More recently, we reported our findings of a prospective observational study examining the urine microscopy profile in a cohort of critically ill patients with AKI and its association with urine/plasma NGAL, worsening AKI, need for RRT initiation and hospital mortality [23]. We found that a higher UMS, implying a greater degree of 'structural' renal tubular damage, correlated significantly with higher urine NGAL (this correlation was less robust for plasma NGAL) and was associated with higher adjusted odds of worsening AKI, defined as a progression in AKI to a higher RIFLE category or need for RRT. Interestingly, this study also demonstrated that commonly used urine biochemical indices (e.g., fractional excretion of sodium, fractional excretion of urea) correlated poorly with UMS and failed to reliably discriminate whether patients would develop worsening AKI. In fact, a significant proportion of those patients with an elevated UMS had relatively preserved 'global' tubular function when expressed as a capacity to generate a fractional excretion of sodium $< 1\,\%$. This is an important observation and would suggest the association between true 'structural' tubular damage, detected by either NGAL or urine microscopy, and tubular function is more complex than appreciated. Traditionally, patients fulfilling the conventional RIFLE definition for AKI and having evidence of preserved tubular function (i.e., fractional excretion of sodium $< 1\,\%$) would be classified as having 'functional' AKI (i.e., pre-renal azotemia). However, this was before the era of the availability of injury-specific biomarkers. Clearly, this premise can now be challenged by observations suggesting that 'structural' tubular damage, independent of detectable declines in tubular function and/or glomerular filtration, conveys an increased risk for a more complicated clinical course and worse outcome [11, 23]. Moreover, these data further support the hypothesis of the existence of a syndrome of subclinical AKI, again characterized by detectable 'structural' tubular injury but relative preservation of global kidney function.

The Next Phase

The implication of these observations, and the next logical step, would be to integrate these measures of 'structural' injury (e.g., NGAL, urine microscopy) into the next iteration of a consensus definition for AKI so as to ensure this novel subgroup with subclinical AKI is appropriately identified and captured (**Fig. 1**). This approach would certainly translate into an improvement in the diagnostic performance of current consensus criteria, but also have far reaching implications not only for diagnostics, but also for risk identification, monitoring for toxicity and, importantly, risk modification, by providing an earlier window of opportunity for therapeutic interventions that may limit ongoing injury, promote renal repair, and improve the outcomes of a cohort of patients who have traditionally fared poorly.

XV

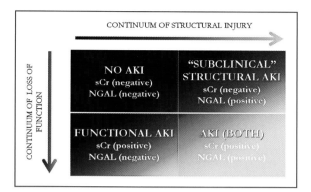

Fig. 1. Novel framework for acute kidney injury (AKI), integrating the concept of 'subclinical' AKI and kidney-injury specific biomarkers and conventional measures of kidney function. NGAL: neutrophil gelatinase-associated lipocalin; sCr: serum creatinine

References

1. Ishani A, Xue JL, Himmelfarb J, et al (2009) Acute kidney injury increases risk of ESRD among elderly. J Am Soc Nephrol 20: 223–228
2. Wald R, Quinn RR, Luo J, et al (2009) Chronic dialysis and death among survivors of acute kidney injury requiring dialysis. JAMA 302: 1179–1185
3. Bellomo R, Ronco C, Kellum JA, Mehta RL, Palevsky P (2004) Acute renal failure – definition, outcome measures, animal models, fluid therapy and information technology needs: the Second International Consensus Conference of the Acute Dialysis Quality Initiative (ADQI) Group. Crit Care 8: R204–212
4. Mehta RL, Kellum JA, Shah SV, et al (2007) Acute Kidney Injury Network: report of an initiative to improve outcomes in acute kidney injury. Crit Care 11: R31
5. Ricci Z, Cruz D, Ronco C (2008) The RIFLE criteria and mortality in acute kidney injury: A systematic review. Kidney Int 73: 538–546
6. Macedo E, Bouchard J, Soroko SH, et al (2010) Fluid accumulation, recognition and staging of acute kidney injury in critically-ill patients. Crit Care 14: R82
7. Doi K, Yuen PS, Eisner C, et al (2009) Reduced production of creatinine limits its use as marker of kidney injury in sepsis. J Am Soc Nephrol 20: 1217–1221
8. Paragas N, Qiu A, Zhang Q, et al (2011) The Ngal reporter mouse detects the response of the kidney to injury in real time. Nat Med 17: 216–222
9. Mishra J, Dent C, Tarabishi R, et al (2005) Neutrophil gelatinase-associated lipocalin (NGAL) as a biomarker for acute renal injury after cardiac surgery. Lancet 365: 1231–1238
10. Haase M, Bellomo R, Devarajan P, Schlattmann P, Haase-Fielitz A (2009) Accuracy of neutrophil gelatinase-associated lipocalin (NGAL) in diagnosis and prognosis in acute kidney injury: a systematic review and meta-analysis. Am J Kidney Dis 54: 1012–1024
11. Haase M, Devarajan P, Haase-Fielitz A, et al (2011) The outcome of neutrophil gelatinase-associated lipocalin-positive subclinical acute kidney injury: a multicenter pooled analysis of prospective studies. J Am Coll Cardiol 57: 1752–1761
12. Bennett M, Dent CL, Ma Q, et al (2008) Urine NGAL predicts severity of acute kidney injury after cardiac surgery: a prospective study. Clin J Am Soc Nephrol 3: 665–673
13. Cruz DN, de Cal M, Garzotto F, et al (2010) Plasma neutrophil gelatinase-associated lipocalin is an early biomarker for acute kidney injury in an adult ICU population. Intensive Care Med 36: 444–451
14. Zappitelli M, Washburn KK, Arikan AA, et al (2007) Urine neutrophil gelatinase-associated lipocalin is an early marker of acute kidney injury in critically ill children: a prospective cohort study. Crit Care 11: R84
15. Nickolas TL, O'Rourke MJ, Yang J, et al (2008) Sensitivity and specificity of a single emergency department measurement of urinary neutrophil gelatinase-associated lipocalin for diagnosing acute kidney injury. Ann Intern Med 148: 810–819

XV

16. Siew ED, Ware LB, Gebretsadik T, et al (2009) Urine neutrophil gelatinase-associated lipocalin moderately predicts acute kidney injury in critically ill adults. J Am Soc Nephrol 20: 1823–1832

17. Wagener G, Gubitosa G, Wang S, Borregaard N, Kim M, Lee HT (2008) Urinary neutrophil gelatinase-associated lipocalin and acute kidney injury after cardiac surgery. Am J Kidney Dis 52: 425–433

18. Haase-Fielitz A, Bellomo R, Devarajan P, et al (2009) Novel and conventional serum biomarkers predicting acute kidney injury in adult cardiac surgery--a prospective cohort study. Crit Care Med 37: 553–560

19. Chawla LS, Dommu A, Berger A, Shih S, Patel SS (2008) Urinary sediment cast scoring index for acute kidney injury: a pilot study. Nephron Clin Pract 110: c145–150

20. Marcussen N, Schumann J, Campbell P, Kjellstrand C (1995) Cytodiagnostic urinalysis is very useful in the differential diagnosis of acute renal failure and can predict the severity. Ren Fail 17: 721–729

21. Perazella MA, Coca SG, Hall IE, Iyanam U, Koraishy M, Parikh CR (2010) Urine microscopy is associated with severity and worsening of acute kidney injury in hospitalized patients. Clin J Am Soc Nephrol 5: 402–408

22. Perazella MA, Coca SG, Kanbay M, Brewster UC, Parikh CR (2008) Diagnostic value of urine microscopy for differential diagnosis of acute kidney injury in hospitalized patients. Clin J Am Soc Nephrol 3: 1615–1619

23. Bagshaw SM, Haase M, Haase-Fielitz A, Bennett M, Devarajan P, Bellomo R (2012) A prospective evaluation of urine microscopy in septic and non-septic acute kidney injury. Nephrol Dial Transplant (in press)

A Troponin for the Kidney: Not There Yet

L.G. FORNI, M. OSTERMANN, and B.J. PHILIPS

> *"If a lot of cures are suggested for a disease,*
> *it means that the disease is incurable."*
> Anton Pavlovich Chekhov, The Cherry Orchard, 1904

Introduction

The reclassification of the syndrome formerly known as "acute renal failure" as "acute kidney injury" (AKI) has generated considerable interest since the initial publication of the RIFLE (Risk Injury Failure Loss End-stage) criteria and subsequent modifications by the AKI Network (AKIN) [1, 2]. This interest is reflected in the number of publications citing AKI which has increased from less than 60 in 2004 to over 700 in 2010. The genesis of this 'rebranding' stems from the desire to have robust criteria to enable research questions to be answered, coupled with the realization that even relatively small changes in serum creatinine (sCr) translate into a significantly poorer outcome for patients. It is this observation that has stimulated such international interest in the 'AKI Epidemic'.

The definition of AKI is based on two parameters: The urine output or the sCr (or the derived glomerular filtration rate [GFR]) and an inherent problem with such definitions is in the utility of using serum creatinine (sCr) as the 'gold standard' [3]. The formation of creatinine is relatively constant under most conditions outside the intensive care unit (ICU) and yet it is being targeted as a marker of an acute metabolic disturbance. Furthermore, creatinine kinetics are such that acute injury, as heralded by a rise in sCr, is not diagnosed until 24–48 hours post initial insult and factors such as comparing creatinine measurements obtained from different laboratories, biological and nutritional variation and enhanced tubular secretion of creatinine confound the diagnosis further. It follows that any attempts to either prevent AKI in patient populations or indeed identify patients at risk are thwarted by the fact that the variable used to define it, creatinine, is such an imprecise tool. Hence, there has been much interest in the pursuit of a quantifiable indicator which will allow for the early detection of AKI. Understandably, this has been earmarked as an area of considerable research interest, driven, in part, by the clinical models of care based on other biomarkers with cardiac troponins being the best known examples.

The cardiac troponins I (cTnI) and T (cTnT) are cardiac regulatory proteins controlling the calcium-mediated interaction of actin and myosin. Cardiac troponin is now the preferred marker for the diagnosis of myocardial infarction as well as risk stratification given its highly sensitive features that aid in the detection of myocardial cell damage [4]. However, the clinical application of cardiac troponin must be taken in context with available clinical information and electrocardiographic (EKG) changes. Therefore, if one employs troponin testing indiscriminately in patients with a low pretest probability of myocardial thrombotic disease then any positive predictor value of the test will be decreased. Indeed, elevated

J.-L. Vincent (ed.), *Annual Update in Intensive Care and Emergency Medicine 2012*
DOI 10.1007/978-3-642-25716-2 © Springer-Verlag Berlin Heidelberg 2012

troponin levels have been described in a wide range of conditions ranging from subarachnoid hemorrhage to extreme exercise as is seen in marathon runners and are also often elevated in our ICU population [5]. Perhaps crucially, following acute myocardial infarction there is a delay in troponin rise but definitive reperfusion treatment following an ST elevation infarct should not be delayed until the troponin level has risen! Perhaps the same could apply to our patients at risk of AKI in whom best practice should not be delayed until there is an elevation in creatinine or indeed biomarker levels.

Biomarkers

What defines a good biomarker? Clearly the sensitivity and specificity together with the time course of a biomarker's profile are critical in determining its use in any disease process. However, more importantly, the utility of a biomarker depends on the purpose it is expected to fulfill and the current view is that an ideal biomarker for AKI should fulfill the following criteria [6, 7]:

i)   It should distinguish pre-renal AKI from apoptotic and necrotic injury
ii) It should be specific for renal injury in the presence of concomitant injury involving other organs
iii) It should allow timing of the onset or stage of injury
iv) It should predict outcome
v)   It should act as a surrogate end-point useful for clinical interventional studies

Therefore, in order to be accepted as a useful biomarker, these criteria should, if possible, be fulfilled. Ultimately the acid test for any biomarker(s) of AKI is whether it performs in the clinical arena, facilitating early identification of patients and hopefully improving outcomes through timely interventions.

Potential Candidate Molecules

To date, the search for biomarkers for AKI have followed animal studies and involve candidates in both plasma and urine. **Table 1** outlines the array of biomarkers for AKI described to-date with **Figure 1** outlining the anatomical site within the kidney where elevations in each biomarker are thought to imply renal damage. There have been numerous studies on biomarkers for AKI which have spawned several review articles; however, comparison of studies is hampered by factors such as variation in what is deemed of diagnostic significance as well as the heterogeneity of study populations.

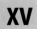

Studies in Cardiothoracic Patients

In 2005, the first clinical validation of neutrophil gelatinase-associated lipocalin (NGAL) as a potential biomarker was published describing the predictive value of urinary (uNGAL) for AKI in children undergoing cardiothoracic surgery. Seventy-one children undergoing cardiopulmonary bypass (CPB) were studied of whom 28 % developed AKI as defined by an increase in baseline sCr by 50 %. The results were encouraging with multivariate analysis demonstrating that the 2-hour post-CPB uNGAL value was the most powerful independent predictor of AKI with an

Table 1. Acute kidney injury (AKI) biomarkers

AKI biomarker	Production/origin	Handling by the kidney	Sample sources	Detection time after renal injury	Confounding factors
Neutrophil gelatinase-associated lipocalin (NGAL)	25 kDa glycoprotein produced by epithelial tissues throughout the body	plasma NGAL excreted via glomerular filtration and undergoes complete reabsorption in healthy tubular cells. NGAL is also produced in distal tubular segments	plasma and urine	2–4 hours post AKI	sepsis malignancy chronic kidney disease systemic lupus erythematosus
Cystatin C (CysC)	13 kDa cysteine protease inhibitor produced by all nucleated human cells and released into plasma	glomerular filtration and reabsorbed and catabolized by proximal tubular cells; no tubular secretion (generally not detectable in urine)	plasma; only detectable in urine after tubular injury	12–24 hours post renal injury	systemic inflammation malignancy thyroid disorders glucocorticoid deficiency excess smoking
Interleukin-18 (IL-18)	18 kDa pro-inflammatory cytokine	released from proximal tubule following injury	plasma and urine	12–24 hours after renal injury	systemic inflammation sepsis heart failure
Kidney injury molecule-1 (KIM-1)	transmembrane glycoprotein produced by proximal tubular cells after ischaemic or nephrotoxic injury; no systemic source	present in urine after ischaemic or nephrotoxic damage of proximal tubular cells	urine	12–24 hours after renal injury	renal cell carcinoma chronic proteinuria chronic kidney disease
Liver-type fatty acid-binding protein (L-FABP)	14 kDa intracellular lipid chaperone produced in liver, intestine, pancreas, lung, nervous system, stomach and kidneys	freely filtered in glomeruli and reabsorbed in proximal tubular cells; increased urinary excretion after tubular cell damage	plasma and urine	1 hour after ischemic tubular injury	chronic kidney disease polycystic kidney disease
N-acetyl-β-D-glucosaminidase (NAG)	> 130 kDa lysosomal enzyme; produced in many cells including proximal and distal tubules	too large to undergo glomerular filtration; urinary elevations imply tubular origin	plasma and urine	12 hours	

XV

Table 1. (continued)

AKI biomarker	Production/origin	Handling by the kidney	Sample sources	Detection time after renal injury	Confounding factors
α/π glutathione S-transferase (GST)	47–51 kDa cytoplasmic enzyme produced in proximal tubule (α GST) and distal tubule (π GST)	limited glomerular filtration; increased urinary levels following tubular injury	urine	12 hours	
Alanine aminopeptidase (AAP) Alkaline phosphatase (ALP) γ-glutamyl transpeptidase (γ-GT)	enzymes located on the brush border villi of the proximal tubular cells	released into urine after tubular injury	urine	?	
α1-microglobulin	31 kDa low molecular weight plasma protein; produced in liver	freely filtered in glomeruli and reabsorbed in proximal tubular cells	plasma and urine; detection in urine consistent with tubular injury	?	
β2-microglobulin	12 kDa low molecular weight plasma protein	freely filtered and significant tubular uptake (fractional excretion into urine 2 %)			
Hepcidin	low molecular peptide hormone predominantly produced in hepatocytes; some production in kidney, heart and brain		urine and plasma	Preliminary studies have shown an inverse association between degree of urinary hepcidin rise and risk of AKI ("negative" biomarker)	systemic inflammation

XV

Fig. 1. Acute kidney injury (AKI) biomarkers as indicators of site of renal injury
NGAL: neutrophil gelatinase-associated lipocalin; NAG: N-acetyl-β-D-glucosaminidase; α-GST: α glutathione S-transferase; π-GST: π glutathione S-transferase; KIM-1: kidney injury molecule–1; IL-18: interleukin 18; RBP: retinol binding protein; L-FABP: Liver-type fatty acid binding protein. I = glomerulus; II = proximal convoluted tubule; III = proximal tubule; IV = loop of Henle; V = distal tubule; VI = distal convoluted tubule; VII = collecting duct

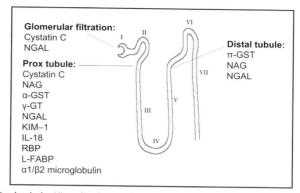

area under the receiving operating curve (AUROC) of 0.998 and a sensitivity of 1.0 [8,9]. Clearly this was extremely encouraging in terms of a potential early marker of AKI and led to several subsequent studies in both the pediatric and adult populations, principally because these patients represent a reasonably homogenous group for investigation with a well-defined risk for AKI allowing investigation before, during, and after insult, in this case CPB. Despite these advantages, results for the various potential biomarkers have been mixed and subsequent studies have been less favorable, especially in adults and less homogenous groups. **Table 2** out-

Table 2. Major clinical studies employing neutrophil gelatinase-associated lipocalin (NGAL) as a biomarker of acute kidney injury (AKI) biomarkers in adult patients

Clinical Setting	References
Prediction of AKI:	
• Post-cardiopulmonary bypass surgery	14–16, 19, 20, 22, 34–38
• After contrast exposure	39, 40
• In sepsis	41, 42
• Trauma patients	38
• In critically ill adult patients	30, 43, 44
• In delayed graft function after renal transplantation	45
Prediction of outcome:	
• Duration/severity of AKI and length of stay in ICU	15, 19
• Adverse outcomes in patients with AKI	46
• Need for RRT	15, 16, 28, 29, 32, 35–37
• Mortality in patients on RRT	47
Differentiation between transient and sustained AKI in adults on admission to ICU	31
Differentiation between "pre-renal" and intrinsic AKI	48
Prediction of severity of AKI and need for RRT in patients in the emergency department	32, 49
Prediction of decreased GFR in patients with chronic kidney disease	50

RRT: renal replacement therapy; ICU: intensive care unit; GFR: glomerular filtration rate

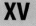

lines the major studies employing NGAL highlighting the different groups that have been examined. As can be seen, NGAL has been applied to a variety of situations many of which are not comparable in terms of renal insult.

In a study of 311 children undergoing surgery for congenital cardiac disease an AUROC of 0.71 was reported for the prediction of AKI by uNGAL [10]. The first urine sample obtained after surgery was investigated and a 4.1 fold increased risk of severe AKI observed. Of 1217 adults undergoing cardiac surgery (90 % on bypass), AKI developed in 60 patients [defined as either the requirement for renal replacement therapy [RRT] or a 2-fold increase in creatinine (RIFLE Injury)] [11]. Urine interleukin (IL)-18, uNGAL and plasma NGAL (pNGAL) were measured 0–6 h after surgery with AUROC values obtained of 0.74, 0.67 and 0.7, respectively. In comparison, the initial sCr had an area under the curve (AUC) of 0.72 for predicting AKI [11]. The addition of a clinical model composed of risk factors for AKI improved the performance of all the biomarkers to 0.75. These results are in keeping with a further study of 876 patients post-coronary bypass surgery which reported similar AUROC values for the predictive value of NGAL and emphasized the limited value of NGAL in these circumstances [12]. Further confounders in terms of NGAL performance include pre-existing renal function. Studies on 426 adult patients undergoing cardiac surgery stratified the group according to the pre-existing estimated glomerular filtration rate (eGFR). Urinary NGAL performed best for patients with eGFR 90–120 ml/min (AUC 0.88) but for patients with eGFR > 120 ml/min or < 30 ml/min, the predictive value of NGAL for AKI was very poor (AUC 0.27 and 0.34 respectively) [13].

Cystatin C (CysC), measured in either serum or urine has been investigated in patients undergoing cardiac surgery with variable results [14–16]. This variation is apparent when comparing studies in which CysC has been reported to be a reasonable discriminator for the development of AKI (AUROC 0.7) and other studies which are less encouraging (AUROC 0.5) [14, 16]. An alternative method is to adopt a less indiscriminant approach and attempt to identify patients at risk of AKI before cardiac surgery, which may provide opportunity for modifying management to avoid AKI. For example, Shlipak et al. investigated the role of pre-operative serum CysC in the prediction of AKI [17]. Results suggested that CysC was superior in predicting the development of AKI compared with conventional approaches, such as sCr or creatinine-derived eGFR. However, the effect observed was marginal and further studies in children failed to demonstrate a relationship between pre-operative CysC and AKI [18].

Given the array of insults that may befall the kidney in our patients, an alternative may be to examine a panel of biomarkers, which was performed in a study of 103 patients [14]. The candidate molecules included kidney injury molecule 1 (KIM-1), N-acetyl-β-D-glucosaminidase (NAG), IL-18, uNGAL, CysC and α-1 microglobulin. In this study, the AUROC for uNGAL was 0.55 and for urinary CysC, 0.66, with KIM-1 being the only biomarker found to predict postoperative AKI with an AUROC of 0.78. However, this result improved significantly to 0.88 with incorporation of a clinical score. No single biomarker has yet emerged as an ideal predictor of AKI and considerable efforts have been directed at improving performance by the panel approach [11, 14, 19–24]. The main difficulty in interpreting these studies is that the results are inconsistent. To date, no single biomarker can be recommended, in isolation, to predict AKI after CPB surgery. It may be that in the future, combinations of biomarkers may improve

XV

performance regarding prediction of AKI risk. However, one must not forget that tried and tested robust clinical scores are also available and should not be dismissed.

Studies in Non-cardiac Patients

Clearly efforts to validate the role of biomarkers for AKI have so far focused predominantly on cardiac patients for the reasons described above. However, a few studies have been performed in patients undergoing solid organ transplantation. In keeping with cardiothoracic surgery, orthotopic liver transplantation (OLT) carries a significant risk of postoperative AKI with estimates as high as 60 %. Postoperative AKI is also an independent risk factor for mortality during the first year after transplantation and significantly reduces graft survival. Initial studies performed on liver transplant patients suggested that plasma and uNGAL may have some predictive ability in terms of AKI and a recent study does show promise. Wagener and colleagues report the results from a large prospective cohort study of 92 patients undergoing OLT at a single center between 2008 and 2010 in whom uNGAL was measured [25]. Transplantation occurred for a variety of reasons and importantly no patient required RRT preoperatively with 'normal' serum creatinine (88+/-56 μmol/l). uNGAL was measured prior to surgery, after reperfusion of the liver graft and then at timed intervals thereafter. uNGAL/urine creatinine ratios were calculated and AKI defined by the RIFLE criteria. Interestingly uNGAL increased immediately after reperfusion with a peak at 3 hours and those who developed post-transplant AKI had elevated levels at 3 and 18 h after reperfusion with an AUROC of 0.800 (95 % CI: 0.732–0.869) reported at 3 hours although at 18 hours the discriminatory power was less impressive (AUROC 0.636). Plasma NGAL (pNGAL) was not measured in this study. As pointed out, the uNGAL/urine creatinine ratio was calculated. This ratio 'compensates' for possible urinary dilution or concentration which is yet another confounder in terms of intepretation. Correction for urinary creatinine implies steady state production of urinary creatinine during AKI development, which is a considerable flaw and plagues the literature with regard to uNGAL reporting. What is clear, however, is that studies which do normalize for urine creatinine in general show slightly higher AUROC values and increased statistical significance. In earlier studies, pNGAL outperformed uNGAL in similar patient groups; however, the incidence of anuria was significantly higher [26]. This study found that a combination of APACHE score and NGAL was predictive of AKI. Similarly, cadaveric renal transplant recipients have been studied. Ninety-one patients underwent serial measurements of uNGAL, IL-18, and KIM-1 [27]. The cohort was described as having slow, delayed or immediate graft function and uNGAL and IL-18 were superior to decrease in creatinine in predicting need for dialysis at one week when measured on the first postoperative day.

XV

Studies in ICU Patients

AKI in critically ill patients is often multifactorial with no clear indication of the exact etiology and time of onset. The role of NGAL in this heterogenous population has been explored with particular focus on early diagnosis of AKI, differentiation between transient and sustained AKI, need for RRT and prediction of death. Cruz et al. measured pNGAL in 301 heterogeneous ICU patients and showed that pNGAL allowed a diagnosis of AKI up to 48 hours prior to RIFLE criteria with an AUROC of 0.78 at this timepoint as well as an AUROC of 0.82 to predict RRT [28]. In another study involving 88 patients, a single pNGAL measurement on admission to the ICU predicted the onset of AKI 48 hours before AKI as per the RIFLE criteria [29]. Despite an impressive AUROC of 0.92, it should be noted that patients with a history of chronic kidney disease were excluded. Endre et al. evaluated six urinary biomarkers (NGAL, KIM-1, IL-18, alkaline phosphatase, γ-glutamyltransptidase and CysC) prospectively in 529 patients on admission to ICU [30]. No biomarker had an AUROC above 0.7 for the prediction of AKI, RRT or mortality. The differentiation between transient and sustained AKI can be difficult in ICU patients. In a study involving 510 critically ill patients, de Geus et al. confirmed that serial uNGAL results were superior to pNGAL and CysC in differentiating between transient and sustained AKI on admission to the ICU [31]. However, the article also showed that adding uNGAL to a model with clinical parameters improved the prediction model only marginally, i.e., the AUROC increased only from 0.79 to 0.82. Although pNGAL has also been shown to predict the need for RRT in ICU patients, in the absence of an interventional study it is difficult to make any recommendations on how to act on a raised pNGAL level [28, 29].

Studies in Emergency/specific Patient Groups

A potentially exciting role for biomarkers of early AKI could be the stratification of patients at risk presenting as acute emergencies rather than to the ICU. Recently, several studies have addressed this issue using NGAL. A study on over 600 patients presenting to an emergency department demonstrated that 30 patients with AKI at presentation had significantly elevated uNGAL levels [32]. Using multiple logistic regression, uNGAL was predictive of clinical outcomes including need for ICU admission bot the use of NGAL as a predictor of AKI was not determined. Shapiro and colleagues attempted to address this by measuring pNGAL in emergency patients with suspected sepsis [33]. This cohort was deemed at higher risk for AKI as defined by a sCr level of > 0.5 mg/dl during the 72 hours post-admission. Using a cut-off of > 150 ng/ml, pNGAL demonstrated 81 % sensitivity for predicting RIFLE Risk increasing to 93 % at RIFLE Injury. However, specificity was poor at 51 % (95 % CI 47 – 55 %), although these results do show promise.

Pitfalls

The studies described above show that in most circumstances the application of biomarkers is not of sufficient specificity to enable them to be used routinely as a 'screen' or diagnostic aid in assessing AKI. Indeed, the most basic of measurements in our patients, urine output, has been shown to be of utility in assessing risk of AKI, and in preoperative assessment of cardiothoracic patients the addition of NGAL measurements to a validated clinical score only improved the AUROC from 0.84 to 0.85.

Why is this the case when animal work, and indeed pediatric work, seemed to show such promise? Perhaps the fault lies not with the biomarkers but the concept of AKI itself. The application of an acronym to a constellation of signs does not confer disease or indeed pathophysiological status upon it. Our patients in the ICU are exposed to a wide ranging array of insults. Sepsis, hypotension, contrast, antibiotics, nephrotoxins, the list goes on. Indeed the causes of AKI in the ICU are also numerous and although sepsis is probably the major contributor there are a variety of potential culprits. Furthermore, most animals do not suffer from the typical co-morbidities that are seen in humans with AKI, in particular diabetes, chronic kidney disease, and proteinuria. Therefore is it surprising that no one biomarker has to-date proved its worth? The animal work and indeed early human studies were in select populations with a timed insult and as such bear little relation to the majority of patients with AKI that populate our ICUs. Expectation that any single biomarker will have universal application is probably naïve. The kidney is not the heart. Perhaps, more importantly, AKI is not myocardial infarction. Although AKI has been described as 'renal angina' the situation is much more complex than that.

Finally, studies to date have concentrated on the diagnosis of AKI and the early prediction of outcome. None of the putative biomarkers has been used to track the course of AKI or even define the severity of injury. There are no well defined 'treatments' of AKI and absolutely no evidence that biomarkers can be used to measure the efficacy of an intervention. Until we define AKI or its many versions in terms of the pathology occurring, we are unlikely to find highly specific markers.

Conclusion

The current literature contains numerous publications on the possible clinical applications of biomarkers to enable the early identification of AKI in high risk groups. Despite early promise, no one biomarker has proved itself to be of universal application in identifying AKI in ICU patients. Early studies used a variety of platforms for biomarker assay (particularly NGAL) and were in relatively well-defined patient groups with a known renal insult. In the ICU, patients (and their kidneys!) are exposed to a heterogeneity of insults. So far, we have focused on determining the relationship between changes in creatinine compared to changes in the concentrations of new biomarkers and how much they agree or disagree, rather than exploring new methods to explore their full relationship. Despite the large number of different studies describing new 'biomarkers of tubular injury', there is a lack of data examining the relationship with tubular function including its concentrating or diluting ability, electrolyte reabsorption and novel imaging techniques. Perhaps herein lies part of the problem. Our quest for a new marker of AKI has become almost all encompassing, whereas a different approach may be to utilize these fingerprints as a way to understand the pathophysiology at a tubular and, indeed, cellular level.

XV

It is of no great surprise that we are still searching for the 'renal troponin'. This does not mean that the search for an early marker of kidney damage should cease, rather the search should be broadened and perhaps the way forward is the application of a panel of biomarkers to cover the range of insults the kidney is exposed to, combined with more sophisticated analyses of renal function to determine what these new biomarkers are truly telling us, and coupled with an intervention. This approach is certainly gaining popularity. If as intensivists and nephrologists we do find the holy grail(s) this will herald an exciting time in critical care nephrology. All we will be left with then, is trying to determine the best treatment to prevent AKI, unless of course, Chekhov was right.

References

1. Bellomo R, Ronco C, Kellum JA, et al (2004) The ADQI workgroup: Acute renal failure – definition, outcome measures, animal models, fluid therapy and information technology needs: the Second International Consensus Conference of the Acute Dialysis Quality Initiative (ADQI) Group. Crit Care 8: R204-R212
2. Mehta RL, Kellum JA, Shah SV, et al (2007) Acute kidney injury network: report of an initiative to improve outcomes in acute kidney injury. Crit Care 11: R31
3. Waikar SS, Betensky RA, Bonventre JV (2009) Creatinine as the gold standard for kidney injury biomarker studies? Nephrol Dial Transplant 24: 3263–3265
4. Katus HA, Remppis A, Scheffold T, et al (1991) Intracellular compartmentation of cardiac troponin T and its release kinetics in patients with reperfused and nonreperfused myocardial infarction. Am J Cardiol 67: 1360–1367
5. Thygesen K, Alpert JS, White HD, Joint ESC/ACCF/AHA/WHF Task Force for the Redefinition of Myocardial Infarction (2007) Universal definition of myocardial infarction. Eur Heart J 28: 2525–2538
6. Bouman CS, Forni LG, Joannidis M (2010) Biomarkers and acute kidney injury: dining with the Fisher King? Intensive Care Med 36: 381–384
7. Soni SS, Ronco C, Katz N, et al (2009) Early Diagnosis of Acute Kidney Injury: The Promise of Novel Biomarkers. Blood Purif 28: 165–174
8. Mishra J, Dent C, Tarabishi R, et al (2005) Neutrophil gelatinase-associated lipocalin (ngal) as a biomarker for acute renal injury after cardiac surgery. Lancet 365: 1231–1238
9. Dent CL, Ma Q, Dastrala S, et al (2007) Plasma neutrophil gelatinase associated lipocalin predicts acute kidney injury, morbidity and mortality after pediatric cardiac surgery: a prospective uncontrolled cohort study. Crit Care 11: R127
10. Parikh CR, Devarajan P, Zappitelli M, et al (2011) Postoperative Biomarkers Predict Acute Kidney Injury and Poor Outcomes after Pediatric Cardiac Surgery. J Am Soc Nephrol 22: 1737–1747
11. Parikh CR, Coca SG, Thiessen-Philbrook H, et al (2011) Postoperative biomarkers predict acute kidney injury and poor outcomes after adult cardiac surgery. J Am Soc Nephrol 22: 1748–1757
12. Perry TE, Muehlschlegel JD, Liu KY, et al (2010) Plasma neutrophil gelatinase-associated lipocalin and acute postoperative kidney injury in adult cardiac surgical patients. Anesth Analg 110: 1541–1547
13. McIlroy DR, Wagener G, Lee HT (2010) Neutrophil gelatinase-associated lipocalin and acute kidney injury after cardiac surgery: the effect of baseline renal function on diagnostic performance. Clin J Am Soc Nephrol 5: 211–219
14. Liangos O, Tighiouart H, Perianayagam MC, et al (2009) Comparative analysis of urinary biomarkers for early detection of acute kidney injury following cardiopulmonary bypass. Biomarkers 14: 423–431
15. Haase-Fielitz A, Bellomo R, Devarajan P, et al (2009) Novel and conventional serum biomarkers predicting acute kidney injury in adult cardiac surgery--a prospective cohort study. Crit Care Med 37: 553–560
16. Koyner JL, Vaidya VS, Bennett MR, et al (2010) Urinary Biomarkers in the Clinical Prognosis and Early Detection of Acute Kidney Injury. Clin J Am Soc Nephrol 5: 2154–2165
17. Shlipak MG, Coca SG, Wang Z, et al (2011) Presurgical serum cystatin C and risk of acute kidney injury after cardiac surgery. Am J Kidney Dis 58: 366–373
18. Zappitelli M, Krawczeski CD, Devarajan P, et al (2011) Early postoperative serum cystatin C predicts severe acute kidney injury following pediatric cardiac surgery. Kidney Int 80: 655–662
19. Haase M, Bellomo R, Devarajan P, et al (2009) Novel biomarkers early predict the severity of acute kidney injury after cardiac surgery in adults. Ann Thorac Surg 88: 124–130

20. Han WK, Wagener G, Zhu Y, et al (2009) Urinary biomarkers in the early detection of acute kidney injury after cardiac surgery. Clin J Am Soc Nephrol 4: 873–882
21. Shaw A, Swaminathan M, Stafford-Smith M (2008) Cardiac surgery-associated acute kidney injury: putting together the pieces of the puzzle. Nephron Physiol 109: 55–60
22. Xin C, Yulong X, Yu C, et al (2008) Urine neutrophil gelatinase-associated lipocalin and interleukin-18 predict acute kidney injury after cardiac surgery. Ren Fail 30: 904–913
23. Han WK, Waikar SS, Johnson A, et al (2008) Urinary biomarkers in the early diagnosis of acute kidney injury. Kidney Int 73: 863–869
24. Eijkenboom JJA, van Eijk LTGJ, Pickkers P (2005) Small increases in the urinary excretion of glutathione S-transferase A1 and P1 after cardiac surgery are not associated with clinically relevant renal injury. Intensive Care Med 31: 664–667
25. Wagener G, Minhaz M, Mattis FA, et al (2011) Urinary neutrophil gelatinase-associated lipocalin as a marker of acute kidney injury after orthotopic liver transplantation. NDT 26: 1717–1728
26. Portal AJ, McPhail MJ, Bruce M, et al (2010) Neutrophil gelatinase-associated lipocalin predicts acute kidney injury in patients undergoing liver transplantation. Liver Transplant 16:1257–1266
27. Hall IE, Yarlagadda SG, Coca SG, et al (2010) IL-18 and urinary NGAL predict dialysis and graft recovery after kidney transplantation. J Am Soc Nephrol 21: 189–197
28. Cruz DN, de Cal M, Garzotto F, et al (2010) Plasma neutrophil gelatinase-associated lipocalin is an early biomarker for acute kidney injury in an adult ICU population. Intensive Care Med 36: 444–451
29. Constantin JM, Futier E, Perbet S, et al (2010) Plasma neutrophil gelatinase-associated lipocalin is an early marker of acute kidney injury in adult critically ill patients: a prospective study. J Crit Care 25: 176e1-e6
30. Endre ZH, Pickering JM, Walker RJ, et al (2011) Improved performance of urinary biomarkers of acute kidney injury in the critically ill by stratification for injury duration and baseline renal function. Kidney Int 79: 1119–1130
31. de Geus HRH, Woo JG, Wang Y, et al (2011) Urinary NGAL measured on admission to the intensive care unit accurately discriminates between sustained and transient acute kidney injury in adult critically ill patients. Nephron Extra 1: 9–23
32. Nickolas TL, O'Rourke MJ, Yang J, et al (2008) sensitivity and specificity of a single emergency department measurement of urinary neutrophil gelatinase-associated lipocalin for diagnosing acute kidney injury. Ann Intern Med 148: 810–819
33. Shapiro NI, Trzeciak S, Hollander JE, et al (2010) The diagnostic accuracy of plasma neutrophil gelatinase-associated lipocalin in the prediction of acute kidney injury in emergency department patients with suspected sepsis. Ann Emerg Med 56: 52–59
34. Tuladhar SM, Puntmann VO, Soni M, Punjabi PP, Bogle RG (2009) Rapid detection of acute kidney injury following cardiopulmonary bypass. J Cardiovasc Pharmacol 53: 261–266
35. Wagener G, Gubitosa G, Wang S, et al (2008) Urinary neutrophil gelatinase-associated lipocalin and acute kidney injury after cardiac surgery. Am J Kidney Dis 52: 425–433
36. Wagener G, Jan M, Kim M, et al (2006) Association between increases in urinary neutrophil gelatinase-associated lipocalin and acute renal dysfunction after adult cardiac surgery. Anesthesiology 105: 485–491
37. Haase-Fielitz A, Bellomo R, Devarajan P, et al (2009) The predictive performance of plasma neutrophil gelatinase-associated lipocalin (NGAL) increases with grade of acute kidney injury. Nephrol Dial Transplant 24: 3349–3354
38. Makris K, Markou N, Evodia E, et al (2009) Urinary neutrophil gelatinase-associated lipocalin (NGAL) as an early marker of acute kidney injury in critically ill multiple trauma patients. Clin Chem Lab Med 47: 79–82
39. Ling W, Zhaohui N, Ben H, et al (2008) Urinary IL-18 and NGAL as early predictive biomarkers in contrast-induced nephropathy after coronary angiography. Nephron 108: c176–181
40. Bachorzewska-Gajewska H, Malyszko J, Sitniewska E, et al (2007) Could neutrophil gelatinase-associated lipocalin and cystatin C predict the development of contrast-induced nephropathy after percutaneous coronary interventions in patients with stable angina and normal serum creatinine values? Kidney Blood Press Res 30: 408–415

XV

41. Bagshaw SM, Bennett M, Haase M, et al (2010) Plasma and urine neutrophil gelatinase-associated lipocalin in septic versus non-septic acute kidney injury in critical illness. Intensive Care Med 36: 452–461
42. Martensson J, Bell M, Oldner A, et al (2010) Neutrophil gelatinase-associated lipocalin in adult septic patients with and without acute kidney injury. Intensive Care Med 36: 1333–1340
43. Siew ED, Ware LB, Gebretsadik T, et al (2009) Urine neutrophil gelatinase-associated lipocalin moderately predicts acute kidney injury in critically ill adults. J Am Soc Nephrol 20: 1823–1832
44. Metzger J, Kirsch T, Schiffer E, et al (2010) Urinary excretion of twenty peptides forms an early and accurate diagnostic pattern of acute kidney injury. Kidney Int 78: 1252–1262
45. Hall IE, Yarlagadda SG, Coca SG, et al (2010) IL-18 and urinary NGAL predict dialysis and graft recovery after kidney transplantation. J Am Soc Nephrol 21: 189–197
46. Yang HN, Boo CS, Kim MG, et al (2010) Urine neutrophil gelatinase-associated lipocalin: an independent predictor of adverse outcomes in acute kidney injury. Am J Nephrol 31: 501–509
47. Kumpers P, Hafer C, Lukasz A, et al (2010) Serum neutrophil gelatinase-associated lipocalin at inception of renal replacement therapy predicts survival in critically ill patients with acute kidney injury. Crit Care 14: R9
48. Singer E, Elger A, Elitok S, et al (2011) Urinary neutrophil gelatinase-associated lipocalin distinguishes pre-renal from intrinsic renal failure and predicts outcomes. Kidney Int 80: 405–414
49. Shapiro NI, Trzeciak S, Hollander JE, et al (2010) The diagnostic accuracy of plasma neutrophil gelatinase-associated lipocalin in the prediction of acute kidney injury in emergency department patients with suspected sepsis. Ann Emerg Med 56: 52–59
50. Bolignano D, Lacquaniti A, Coppolino G, et al (2008) Neutrophil gelatinase-associated lipocalin reflects the severity of renal impairment in subjects affected by chronic kidney disease. Kidney Blood Press Res 31: 255–258

XV

Possible Role of NGAL as an Early Renal Biomarker

S. Kokkoris, S. Nanas, and P. Andrews

Introduction

The incidence of acute kidney injury (AKI) in critically ill patients is currently increasing [1]. Even though serum creatinine (sCr) is currently used for AKI diagnosis, it is an insensitive and unreliable marker during acute alterations of renal function [2]. The lack of an early biomarker is an obstacle for the development of new preventive strategies and timely interventions against AKI [2]. Recent research for novel biomarkers with early diagnostic and/or prognostic value has revealed several candidates, including neutrophil gelatinase-associated lipocalin (NGAL) [3, 4], cystatin C (CysC) [5, 6], kidney injury molecule 1 (KIM-1) [7], and interleukin 18 (IL-18) [8–11], with NGAL being the most promising so far.

The purpose of the present article is to review the studies that have tested the prognostic ability of NGAL (in either urine and/or blood) for early AKI development in the heterogeneous population of adult critically ill patients, in whom AKI insult(s) and timing are unclear. This has not been studied systematically to date.

Acute Kidney Injury in the Intensive Care Unit

Definitions

The term 'acute renal failure' was first introduced by Homer Smith in 1951, by which he referred to kidney dysfunction related to traumatic injuries. Since then, this term has been extensively used in the medical literature to describe an abrupt and sustained decrease in renal function. However, until recently there was no clear definition of acute renal failure. A recent study found that there were at least 35 definitions in the literature [12], leading to wide variation in the reported incidence and outcomes of acute renal failure. The need for a consensus definition for AKI was evident. Therefore, the Acute Dialysis Quality Initiative (ADQI) workgroup developed the RIFLE classification [Risk-Injury-Failure-Loss-End-stage kidney disease (ESKD)] (**Table 1**) [13]. For further refinement of the definition of AKI, the Acute Kidney Injury Network (AKIN) proposed a modified version of the RIFLE classification, also known as the AKIN criteria (**Table 1**) [14].

XV

J.-L. Vincent (ed.), *Annual Update in Intensive Care and Emergency Medicine 2012*
DOI 10.1007/978-3-642-25716-2 © Springer-Verlag Berlin Heidelberg 2012

Table 1. RIFLE and AKIN criteria for diagnosis of acute kidney injury (AKI)

RIFLE criteria		
Class	**GFR criteria**	**Urine output criteria**
Risk (R)	Increased creatinine x 1.5 or GFR decrease > 25 %	Urine output < 0.5 ml/kg/h x 6 h
Injury (I)	Increased creatinine x 2 or GFR decrease > 50 %	Urine output < 0.5 ml/kg/h x 12 h
Failure (F)	Increased creatinine x 3 or GFR decrease > 75 % or creatinine ≥4 mg/dl (acute rise of ≥0.5 mg/dl)	Urine output < 0.3 ml/kg/h x 24 h or anuria x 12 h
Loss (L)	Persistent AKI = complete loss of renal function > 4 weeks	
ESKD (E)	End-stage kidney disease > 3 months	
AKIN classification		
Stage	**Serum creatinine criteria**	**Urine output criteria**
1	Increase in serum creatinine of ≥0.3 mg/dl or increase to ≥150 to 200 % from baseline	Urine output < 0.5 ml/kg/h x 6 h
2	Increase in serum creatinine to > 200 to 300 % from baseline	Urine output < 0.5 ml/kg/h x 12 h
3	Increase in serum creatinine to > 300 % from baseline (or serum creatinine of ≥4.0 mg/dl with an acute increase of at least 0.5 mg/dl)	Urine output < 0.3 ml/kg/h x 24 h or anuria x 12 h

RIFLE = Risk-Injury-Failure-Loss-End-stage kidney disease; AKIN = Acute Kidney Injury Network; GFR = glomerular filtration rate

Epidemiology

There are several epidemiological studies so far that have studied the incidence of AKI in critically ill patients. In a study from north-east Italy, AKI occurred in 10.8 % of all intensive care unit (ICU) patients when RIFLE criteria were applied at the time of admission [15]. Hoste et al. performed a retrospective study on 5,383 patients admitted during a one year period to the 7 ICUs of a single center and found that AKI occurred in 67.2 % of ICU patients when RIFLE criteria were applied at peak creatinine during the ICU stay [16]. Uchino et al. [17] performed a prospective observational study of ICU patients who either were treated with renal replacement therapy (RRT) or fulfilled at least 1 of the predefined criteria for acute renal failure at 54 hospitals in 23 countries. Of 29,269 critically ill patients admitted during the study period, 1,738 (5.7 %) had acute renal failure during their ICU stay, including 1,260 who were treated with RRT. The most common contributing factor to acute renal failure was septic shock (47.5 %). A recent study by Ostermann and Chang [18] analyzed 41,972 patients admitted to 22 ICUs in the United Kingdom and Germany between 1989 and 1999 as part of the Riyadh Intensive Care Program database. AKI defined by RIFLE occurred in 15,019 (35.8 %) patients: 7,207 (17.2 %) with R, 4,613 (11 %) I, and 3,199 (7.6 %) with F. Hospital mortality rates were RIFLE R 20.9 %, I 45.6 %, and F 56.8 %, compared with 8.4 % among patients without AKI. Bagshaw and colleagues [19] studied 120,123 patients admitted to 57 ICUs across Australia for at least 24 h from January 2000 to December 2005. AKI occurred in 36.1 %, with a maximum category R in 16.3 %, I in 13.6 %, and F in 6.3 %. The crude hospital mortality by RIFLE category was 17.9 % for R, 27.7 % for I, and 33.2 % for F.

Complications

Various studies have reported on the increased mortality of ICU patients with AKI. Ympa et al. [20], in a systematic review of the literature from 1970 to 2004, observed an unchanged mortality of around 50 % from 80 studies. Uchino et al. reported a hospital mortality rate of 60.3 % [17]. Hoste et al. [16] found that patients with maximum RIFLE class R, class I and class F had hospital mortality rates of 8.8 %, 11.4 % and 26.3 %, respectively, compared with 5.5 % for patients without AKI. A multicenter evaluation of RIFLE criteria by Bagshaw et al. [19] showed a crude hospital mortality of 17.9 % for R, 27.7 % for I and 33.2 % for F criteria of the RIFLE classification. AKI, defined by any RIFLE category, was associated with an increase in hospital mortality (OR 3.29, 95 % confidence interval [CI] 3.19–3.41), whereas by multivariable analysis, each RIFLE category was independently associated with hospital mortality (odds ratios [OR]: R 1.58, I 2.54, and F 3.22). In another systematic review, Ricci et al. [21] found a stepwise increase in relative risk for death with increasing AKI severity (R 2.40, I 4.15, F 6.37) compared with non-AKI patients. Finally, another study reported that increasing severity of AKI was also associated with increased 1-month and 1-year mortality compared with non-AKI patients [22]. Development of AKI is also associated with longer ICU and hospital stays. In a study by Hoste et al. [16], patients with AKI had a longer hospital stay (RIFLE class R 8 days, I 10 days, F 16 days) compared to the patients without AKI (6 days).

Limitations of Creatinine and the Need for Novel AKI Biomarkers

To date, sCr has typically been used for diagnosis of AKI. However, it is an insensitive and unreliable biomarker during acute changes in kidney function and there are several limitations to its use as an AKI biomarker [23]. First, its release varies with age, gender, diet, muscle mass, drugs and vigorous exercise. Second, tubular secretion accounts for 10–40 % of creatinine clearance, which could mask a decrease in glomerular filtration rate (GFR). Third, creatinine becomes abnormal when more than 50 % of GFR has been lost. Therefore, there is a delay between injury and the subsequent increase in sCr and it may require up to 24 hours before sufficient increases in blood concentration are detectable.

It is assumed that biological damage at a cellular or molecular level precedes the clinical spectrum of AKI. For instance, injured tubular cells secrete various molecules many hours before the functional decline that is evident by creatinine increase. However, so far the lack of an early AKI biomarker has hampered the development of preventive strategies against AKI. Recent studies in humans have established the need for timely intervention for successful AKI prevention or treatment [24]. Consequently, with the incidence of AKI reaching epidemic dimensions, the need for novel biomarkers is imperative.

XV

NGAL Biology and Pathophysiology

NGAL belongs to the lipocalin superfamily of > 20 structurally related secreted proteins that are thought to transport a variety of ligands within a β-barreled calyx [25]. Human NGAL was originally identified as a 25-kDa protein covalently bound to gelatinase (matrix metalloproteinase [MMP]-9) from human neutrophils, where it represents one of the neutrophil secondary granule proteins [26, 27]. NGAL is expressed at very low levels in other human tissues, including kidney, trachea, lungs, stomach, and colon [28]. NGAL expression is markedly induced in stimulated epithelia. For example, it is upregulated in colonic epithelial cells in areas of inflammation or neoplasia but is absent from intervening uninvolved areas or within metastatic lesions [29]. NGAL concentrations are elevated in the serum of patients with acute bacterial infections [30], which is consistent with NGAL's proposed function as an endogenous bacteriostatic protein that scavenges bacterial siderophores (sidereophore is a small molecule which binds iron and in bacteria it is called enterochelin), the sputum of subjects with asthma or chronic obstructive pulmonary disease (COPD) [31], and the bronchial fluid from the emphysematous lung [32]. In all of these cases, NGAL induction is postulated to be the result of interactions between inflammatory cells and the epithelial lining, with upregulation of NGAL expression being evident in both neutrophils and the epithelium [29–32]. Goetz et al. [33] showed that NGAL binds siderophore-iron and, therefore, it could participate in iron transport. In mammals, a siderophore has not been identified so far. These data were obtained by x-ray crystallography and molecular modeling. By binding iron, NGAL could mediate various physiologic functions, such as bacteriostatic and antioxidant effects. Alternatively, it could act as a growth factor, regulating apoptosis or cell differentiation. There are data supporting a role for NGAL as a regulator of the epithelial phenotype, inducing the formation of kidney epithelia in embryos and adults [34].

NGAL as a Novel Renal Biomarker

Preclinical Studies

Supavekin et al. [35] identified NGAL as one of the most upregulated genes in the early post-ischemic mouse kidney, by using a cDNA microarray technique. Mishra et al. [36] used a transcriptome-wide interrogation strategy to identify renal genes that are induced early after renal ischemia and found that NGAL induction represents a novel intrinsic response of the kidney proximal tubule cells to ischemic injury. More specifically, by microarray analysis of mice with unilateral renal ischemia, NGAL mRNA was markedly induced in the early postischemic kidney, while NGAL protein was markedly overexpressed in the proximal tubules of early ischemic mouse kidneys. Moreover, NGAL protein was easily detected in the urine immediately after induction of acute renal failure in mice.

Another study [3], using a mouse model of severe renal failure through ischemia-reperfusion injury, showed that a single dose of NGAL introduced during the initial phase of the disease, dramatically protected the kidney and mitigated azotemia, implying that endogenous NGAL might also play a protective role. Its action was mediated by upregulation of heme oxygenase-1 (a protective enzyme), preservation of proximal tubule N-cadherin, and inhibition of cell death. Current data suggest that induction of NGAL under harmful conditions is a compensatory response to ameliorate oxidative stress-mediated toxicity [37].

NGAL in AKI

Preliminary Clinical Studies

The aforementioned findings have initiated a number of translational studies to evaluate NGAL as a novel biomarker in human AKI. In a landmark prospective study of children undergoing cardiopulmonary bypass (CPB), AKI diagnosis using sCr was only possible 1–3 days after surgery [4]. In contrast, NGAL measurements by Western blotting and by ELISA revealed a 10-fold or more increase in the urine and plasma, within 2–6 h of the surgery in patients who subsequently developed AKI. Both urine and plasma NGAL (at a cut-off value of 50 μg/l) were excellent independent predictors of AKI, with an area under the receiver operating characteristics curve (AUROC) of 0.998 for the 2-h urine NGAL (uNGAL) and 0.91 for the 2-h plasma NGAL (pNGAL) concentration [4]. These findings have now been confirmed in prospective studies of children and adults who developed AKI after cardiac surgery, in whom urinary and/or plasma NGAL were significantly elevated by 1–3 h after the operation. However, the AUROCs for the prediction of AKI in adult patients have been rather disappointing when compared with those of pediatric studies, and have ranged widely from 0.61 to 0.96. This could be attributed to various confounding factors, such as older age, comorbidities or prolonged by-pass time. A recent meta-analysis of published studies in all patients after cardiac surgery revealed an overall AUROC of 0.78 for prediction of AKI, when NGAL was measured within 6 h of initiation of CPB and AKI was defined as a > 50 % increase in serum creatinine [38]. Apart from cardiac surgery, NGAL has shown promising results as a predictive biomarker for AKI development in various other conditions, such as after kidney or liver transplantation as well as after exposure to contrast materials. However, we will focus on the studies that included adult patients admitted to general ICUs.

The Role of NGAL in a General Adult ICU

Studies published so far have many methodological inconsistencies that should be taken into consideration, namely differences in study design, AKI definition, baseline creatinine definition and percentage of patients already suffering from AKI on admission. Generally, the definition of baseline sCr value is crucial because it will determine whether a patient has AKI or not. Among studies, there is great heterogeneity about this definition. In most of them, whenever an sCr value prior to ICU admission was not available, a value based on the Modification of Diet in Renal Disease-estimated GFR (MDRD-eGFR) equation solution (taking an arbitrary value of 75 ml/kg/m^2 for eGFR) was used. This resulted in a high percentage of patients having already developed AKI at admission. **Table 2** contains information about all these components for better comparison among the studies. Moreover, adult patients of a general ICU constitute an extremely heterogeneous population with much comorbidity, various disease severities and multiple interventions. In such patients, AKI could be attributed to multiple insults, each occurring at different time point, which could explain why NGAL has better performance in homogeneous populations with predictable forms of AKI, such as pediatric or cardiac surgery populations.

Table 2. Studies on neutrophil gelatinase-associated lipocalin (NGAL) in adult general intensive care unit (ICU) patients

Ref.	Sample size	AKI definition	AKI on entry (% out of total)	Primary outcome	Baseline or peak value of NGAL used	AUROC for pNGAL	AUROC for uNGAL
[39]	632	RIFLE	16	AKI prediction within first week post-admission	baseline	0.77	0.80
[40]	301	RIFLE	30	AKI prediction within 48 h post-admission	baseline	0.78	NA
[41]	451	AKIN	14	AKI prediction within 24 and 48 h post-admission	baseline	NA	0.64[*]
[42]	88	RIFLE	36	Association between pNGAL and AKI	baseline	0.92[#]	NA
[43]	65	AKIN	0	AKI detection in patients with septic shock	peak	0.67[§]	0.86[§]
[44]	83	RIFLE	100	Discrimination between septic and non-septic AKI within 48 h	peak	0.77	0.70
[45]	109	RIFLE	100	28-day mortality after RRT initiation	pNGAL at inception of RRT	0.74	NA

AKI: acute kidney injury; AUROC: area under receiver-operating characteristic curve; pNGAL: plasma NGAL; uNGAL: urine NGAL; NA: not available; RRT: renal replacement therapy. [*]AKI within 48 h post-admission; [#]AKI within the first week post-admission; [§]AKI within 12 h post-admission.

There are only four studies, so far, that have prospectively examined the prognostic ability of NGAL for AKI development in the mixed adult ICU population. de Geus et al. [39] conducted a large prospective study including 632 consecutive patients, of whom 16 % had AKI on entry. The percentage of patients with more severe AKI (RIFLE F) was 9 %. A steady state level 4 weeks before admission was used as a baseline value for sCr and if it was not available, then the admission value was used as a surrogate baseline. The AUROCs for AKI prediction one week after admission were 0.77 for baseline pNGAL and 0.80 for baseline uNGAL, whereas the AUROCs for RRT need were 0.88 for baseline pNGAL and 0.89 for baseline uNGAL. Cruz et al. [40] performed a prospective observational study with 301 consecutive patients, of whom 30 % had AKI on admission. The AUROCs for baseline pNGAL regarding AKI prediction within 48 h post-admission and continuous RRT (CRRT) need during the ICU stay were 0.78 and 0.82, respectively. The lowest known value during the preceding 3 months was used as baseline sCr value; if not available, it was estimated by solving the MDRD-eGFR equation. Siew et al. [41], in a prospective cohort study including 451 patients, of whom 14 % had AKI on entry, found poor performance for baseline uNGAL regarding AKI diagnosis within 48 h post-admission, with an AUROC of 0.64. uNGAL remained independently associated with AKI development after adjustment for other confounding factors included in a clinical model, but addition of uNGAL only marginally improved the predictive performance of the clinical model alone. Moreover, baseline uNGAL independently predicted RRT initiation during the ICU stay (hazard ratio [HR]: 2.60 [95 % CI: 1.55 – 4.35]), when included in a multivariate Cox proportional hazards model. This study had some particularities compared with the other studies. For instance, in

XV

52 % of patients, baseline sCr was unavailable, multiple imputations methodology was used to define baseline sCr values, and AKIN instead of RIFLE criteria for AKI were used. Lastly, Constantin et al. [42] reported excellent diagnostic ability for baseline pNGAL regarding AKI development within the first week after admission (AUROC = 0.92). The AUROC for RRT need was 0.78. The study included 88 patients, 36 % of whom had AKI on admission. Baseline sCr was defined by recent medical history and, if not available, by solving the MDRD-eGFR equation.

The Role of NGAL in Septic AKI

The impact of sepsis on NGAL levels in plasma and urine of critically ill adult patients is controversial. Martensson et al. [43] conducted a study in 65 septic patients, none of whom had AKI on entry, and evaluated the predicted ability of pNGAL and uNGAL for the early detection of AKI. The AUROCs for AKI within 12 h post-admission in patients with septic shock were 0.86 for peak uNGAL and 0.67 for peak pNGAL. These authors also found that uNGAL was a more robust marker of AKI than pNGAL in patients with septic shock, since uNGAL levels remained within normal limits even when pNGAL increased in patients without AKI. On the other hand, Bagshaw et al. [44] performed a prospective observational study in 83 patients with AKI and either sepsis or not, and sought to determine whether there were unique patterns to pNGAL and uNGAL in septic compared with non-septic AKI. However, there was no septic non-AKI control group for comparison. Septic AKI was associated with significantly higher baseline pNGAL and uNGAL compared with non-septic AKI. The AUROCs for septic AKI prediction within 48 h after admission were 0.77 and 0.70 for peak pNGAL and peak uNGAL, respectively. Furthermore, the AUROCs for CRRT need prognosis were 0.78 and 0.70, for peak pNGAL and peak uNGAL, respectively. In contrast, Cruz et al. [40] found no significant difference in pNGAL among patients with and without sepsis or systemic inflammatory response syndrome (SIRS). Lastly, Kumpers et al. [45] conducted a prospective study in 109 critically ill patients with AKI at inception of RRT and identified pNGAL as a strong independent predictor for 28-day survival (HR: 1.6 [95 %CI: 1.15 – 2.23]). The extent to which AKI *per se* contributes to pNGAL levels could be confounded by the release of NGAL into the bloodstream in septic conditions; therefore, larger studies in septic patients are required to elucidate the role of NGAL in sepsis.

Conclusion

To date, NGAL seems to be the most promising novel biomarker for AKI development even in the mixed population of a general ICU. However, the question is whether a single biomarker is sufficient for AKI prediction or if a panel of such markers would perform better. Early AKI detection by novel biomarkers (or a combination) could lead to timely interventions (e.g., avoidance of nephrotoxic drugs, early RRT initiation) to prevent the detrimental effects of AKI in critically ill patients. With the incidence of AKI in the ICU currently increasing, it is strongly suggested that large randomized studies be performed to validate the role of NGAL (or a panel of renal biomarkers) in clinical decision making processes about earlier implementation of more aggressive interventions, for example CRRT, when those markers are elevated, before irreversible renal damage has occurred.

XV

References

1. Kellum JA (2008) Acute kidney injury. Crit Care Med 36: S141–S145
2. Devarajan P (2008) Neutrophil gelatinase-associated lipocalin (NGAL): a new marker of kidney disease. Scand J Clin Lab Invest (Suppl) 241: 89–94
3. Mori K, Lee HT, Rapoport D, et al (2005) Endocytic delivery of lipocalin-siderophore-iron complex rescues the kidney from ischemia-reperfusion injury. J Clin Invest 115: 610–621
4. Mishra J, Dent C, Tarabishi R, et al (2005) Neutrophil gelatinase-associated lipocalin (NGAL) as a biomarker for acute renal injury after cardiac surgery. Lancet 365: 1231–1238
5. Herget-Rosenthal S, Marggraf G, Husing J, et al (2004) Early detection of acute renal failure by serum cystatin C. Kidney Int 66: 1115–1122
6. Villa P, Jimenez M, Soriano MC, Manzanares J, Casasnovas P (2005) Serum cystatin C concentration as a marker of acute renal dysfunction in critically ill patients. Crit Care 9: R139–R143
7. Han WK, Bailly V, Abichandani R, Thadhani R, Bonventre JV (2002) Kidney Injury Molecule-1 (KIM-1): A novel biomarker for human renal proximal tubule injury. Kidney Int 62: 237–244
8. Parikh CR, Abraham E, Ancukiewicz M, Edelstein CL (2005) Urine IL-18 is an early diagnostic marker for acute kidney injury and predicts mortality in the intensive care unit. J Am Soc Nephrol 16: 3046–3052
9. Parikh CR, Jani A, Melnikov VY, Faubel S, Edelstein CL (2004) Urinary interleukin-18 is a marker of human acute tubular necrosis. Am J Kidney Dis 43: 405–414
10. Parikh CR, Jani A, Mishra J, et al (2006) Urine NGAL and IL-18 are predictive biomarkers for delayed graft function following kidney transplantation. Am J Transplant 6: 1639–1645
11. Parikh CR, Mishra J, Thiessen-Philbrook H, et al (2006) Urinary IL-18 is an early predictive biomarker of acute kidney injury after cardiac surgery. Kidney Int 70: 199–203
12. Kellum JA, Levin N, Bouman C, Lameire N (2002) Developing a consensus classification system for acute renal failure. Curr Opin Crit Care 8: 509–514
13. Bellomo R, Ronco C, Kellum JA (2004) The ADQI Workgroup: Acute renal failure – definition, outcome measures, animal models, fluid therapy and information technology needs: The Second International Consensus Conference of the Acute Dialysis Quality Initiative (ADQI) Group. Crit Care 8: R204–R212
14. Mehta RL, Kellum JA, Shah SV, et al (2007) Acute Kidney Injury Network: Report of an initiative to improve outcomes in acute kidney injury. Crit Care 11: R31
15. Cruz DN, Bolgan I, Perazella MA, et al (2007) North-East Italian Prospective Hospital Renal Outcome Survey on Acute Kidney Injury (NEIPHROS-AKI): Targeting the problem with the rifle criteria. Clin J Am Soc Nephrol 2: 418–425
16. Hoste EA, Clermont G, Kersten A et al (2006) RIFLE criteria for acute kidney injury is associated with hospital mortality in critical ill patients: a cohort analysis. Crit Care 10: R73
17. Uchino S, Kellum JA, Bellomo R, et al (2005) Acute renal failure in critically ill patients: a multinational, multicenter study. JAMA 294: 813–818
18. Ostermann M, Chang RW (2007) Acute kidney injury in the intensive care unit according to RIFLE. Crit Care Med 35: 1837–1843
19. Bagshaw SM, George C, Dinu I, Bellomo R (2008) A multi-centre evaluation of the rifle criteria for early acute kidney injury in critically ill patients. Nephrol Dial Transplant 23: 1203–1210
20. Ympa YP, Sakr Y, Reinhart K, Vincent JL (2005) Has mortality from acute renal failure decreased? A systematic review of the literature. Am J Med 118: 827–832
21. Ricci Z, Cruz D, Ronco C (2008) The RIFLE criteria and mortality in acute kidney injury: a systematic review. Kidney Int 73: 538–546
22. Bagshaw SM, Mortis G, Doig CJ, Godinez-Luna T, Fick GH, Laupland KB (2006) One-year mortality in critically ill patients by severity of kidney dysfunction: a population-based assessment. Am J Kidney Dis 48: 402–409
23. Bagshaw SM, Gibney RT (2008) Conventional markers of kidney function. Crit Care Med 36: S152–158
24. Schrier RW (2004) Need to intervene in established acute renal failure. J Am Soc Nephrol 15: 2756–2758

XV

25. Flower DR, North AC, Sansom CE (2000) The lipocalin protein family: Structural and sequence overview. Biochim Biophys Acta 1482: 9–24
26. Kjeldsen L, Cowland JB, Borregaard N (2000) Human neutrophil gelatinase-associated lipocalin and homologous proteins in rat and mouse. Biochim Biophys Acta 1482: 272–283
27. Xu S, Venge P (2000) Lipocalins as biochemical markers of disease. Biochim Biophys Acta 1482: 298–307
28. Cowland JB, Borregaard N (1997) Molecular characterization and pattern of tissue expression of the gene for neutrophil gelatinase-associated lipocalin from humans. Genomics 45: 17–23
29. Nielson BS, Borregaard N, Bundgaard JR, Timshel S, Sehested M, Kjeldsen L (1996) Induction of NGAL synthesis in epithelial cells of human colorectal neoplasia and inflammatory bowel diseases. Gut 38: 414–420
30. Xu SY, Pauksen K, Venge P (1995) Serum measurements of human neutrophil lipocalin (HNL) discriminate between acute bacterial and viral infections. Scand J Clin Lab Invest 55: 125–131
31. Keatings VM, Barnes PJ (1997) Granulocyte activation markers in induced sputum in comparison between chronic obstructive pulmonary disease, asthma, and normal subjects. Am J Respir Crit Care Med 155: 449–453
32. Betsuyaky T, Nishimura M, Takeyabu K et al (1999) Neutrophil granule proteins in bronchoalveolar lavage fluid from subjects with subclinical emphysema. Am J Respir Crit Care Med 159: 1985–1991
33. Goetz DH, Holmes MA, Borregaard N, Bluhm ME, Raymond KN, Strong RK (2002) The neutrophil lipocalin NGAL is a bacteriostatic agent that interferes with siderophore-mediated iron acquisition. Mol Cell 10: 1033–1043
34. Yang J, Goetz D, Li JY (2002) An iron delivery pathway mediated by a lipocalin. Mol Cell 10: 1045–1056
35. Supavekin S, Zhang W, Kucherlapati R, Kaskel FJ, Moore LC, Devarajan P (2003) Differential gene expression following early renal ischemia/reperfusion. Kidney Int 63: 1714–24.
36. Mishra J, Ma Q, Prada A, et al (2003) Identification of neutrophil gelatinase-associated lipocalin as a novel early urinary biomarker for ischemic renal injury. J Am Soc Nephrol 14: 2534–2543
37. Roudkenar M, Halabian R, Bahmani P, Roushandeh A, Kuwahara Y, Fukumoto M (2011) Neutrophil gelatinase-associated lipocalin: A new antioxidant that exerts its cytoprotective effect independent on Heme Oxygenase-1. Free Radic Res 45: 810–819
38. Haase M, Bellomo R, Devarajan P, et al (2009) Accuracy of neutrophil gelatinase-associated lipocalin (NGAL) in diagnosis and prognosis in acute kidney injury: A systematic review and meta-analysis. Am J Kidney Dis 54: 1012–1024
39. de Geus H, Bakker J, Lesaffre E, Noble L (2011) Neutrophil gelatinase-associated lipocalin at ICU admission predicts for acute kidney injury in adult patients. Am J Respir Crit Care Med 183: 907–914
40. Cruz DN, de Cal M, Garzotto F, et al (2010) Plasma neutrophil gelatinase-associated lipocalin is an early biomarker for acute kidney injury in an adult ICU population. Intensive Care Med 36: 444–451
41. Siew ED, Ware LB, Gebretsadik T, et al (2009) Urine neutrophil gelatinase-associated lipocalin moderately predicts acute kidney injury in critically ill adults. J Am Soc Nephrol 20: 1823–1832
42. Constantin JM, Futier E, Perbet S, et al (2010) Plasma neutrophil gelatinase-associated lipocalin is an early marker of acute kidney injury in adult critically ill patients: a prospective study. J Crit Care 25: 176.e1–e6
43. Martensson J, Bell M, Oldner A, Xu S, Venge P, Martling CR (2010) Neutrophil gelatinase-associated lipocalin in adult septic patients with and without acute kidney injury. Intensive Care Med 36: 1333–1340
44. Bagshaw SM, Bennett M, Haase M, et al (2010) Plasma and urine neutrophil gelatinase-associated lipocalin in septic versus non-septic acute kidney injury in critical illness. Intensive Care Med 36: 452–461
45. Kumpers P, Hafer C, Lukasz A, et al (2010) Serum neutrophil gelatinase-associated lipocalin at inception of renal replacement therapy predicts survival in critically ill patients with acute kidney injury. Crit Care 14: R9

XV

NGAL Curve for the Early Diagnosis of AKI in Heart Failure Patients

C. Ronco and B. Noland

Introduction

There has been increasing interest of clinicians in the high frequency of acute kidney injury (AKI) in acute heart failure (AHF). The most important mechanism behind cardiorenal syndrome type 1 is frequently an iatrogenic derangement caused by inappropriate use of diuretics or other strategies to alleviate congestion such as extracorporeal ultrafiltration [1]. In the attempt to remove fluid overload, severe hemodynamic consequences may lead to renal hypoperfusion and AKI.

In these circumstances, the importance of sensitive, specific, but most of all, early criteria to diagnose AKI has clearly emerged. The main issue is to characterize the type of renal injury, separating functional disorders from tubular damage. In this field, creatinine has been proven useful as a biomarker for AKI although it represents a late diagnostic tool serving as a surrogate marker for a fall in glomerular filtration rate (GFR) [2]. By the time GFR is declining, the damage has often already occurred and very little can be done to prevent or to protect the kidney from further damage. In this area, several molecules have proved useful diagnostic tools to detect the presence of early kidney damage and to describe the level of its severity [3]. Among them, neutrophil gelatinase-associated lipocalin (NGAL) is the most carefully and extensively studied molecule. Because of its ability to discriminate between volume responsive functional changes and true kidney damage, NGAL has emerged as the most attractive and reliable candidate biomarker [4]. Potential applications for biomarkers can thus be matched to different phases of the AKI continuum (**Fig. 1**).

In some studies however, the area under the receiver operating characteristic curve (AUROC) has been suboptimal compared to other reports in the literature [5, 6]. Because of the dynamic nature of the marker kinetics, uncertainties remain pertaining to the optimal cut-off point and the timing at which the measurement should be made, despite some interesting results [7, 8], and it may be that in certain settings the predictive capacity of a single NGAL measurement could be somewhat limited. Furthermore, when AKI is in its early phases, the levels of NGAL in blood may still be quite low and difficult to discriminate with a single absolute cut-off value across individual patients. For these reasons, an approach may be required that includes a clear definition of a continuous scale of NGAL values in the low range and a repeated series of measurements as the clinical situation is evolving. In this chapter, we present a new way to utilize NGAL for the early diagnosis of AKI and a new expanded range plasma assay capable of discrete measurement even in the range below the classic lower limit of detection.

J.-L. Vincent (ed.), *Annual Update in Intensive Care and Emergency Medicine 2012*
DOI 10.1007/978-3-642-25716-2 © Springer-Verlag Berlin Heidelberg 2012

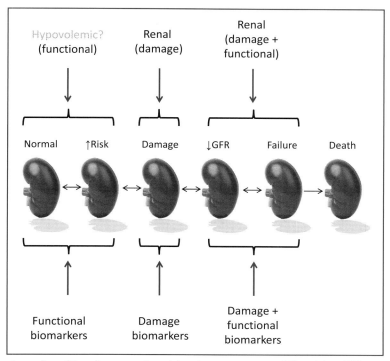

Fig. 1. The spectrum of conditions from normal renal function to severe acute kidney injury (AKI) represents a continuum in which, in the early phases, functional, hypovolemic AKI may be detected by a rise in serum creatinine not related to damage. In this condition, neutrophil gelatinase-associated lipocalin (NGAL) has been shown to remain unaffected. In the subsequent steps of the continuum, parenchymal damage may occur and biomarkers, such as NGAL, may rise even in the presence of normal functional biomarkers, such as creatinine. In the later phases of AKI, functional biomarkers, such as creatinine, rise due to a significant decrease in glomerular filtration rate (GFR). NGAL may remain high, increase or even decrease depending on the presence or absence of an ongoing insult.

NGAL and its Current Applications

NGAL was first characterized as a protein complexed with matrix metallopeptidase (MMP)-9 isolated from neutrophils in response to specific stimuli [9]. NGAL is also known as lipocalin-2 and siderocalin, and is known to play a role in fighting bacterial infections through specific binding of siderophore-chelated iron earmarked for bacterial importation [10]. The association between NGAL and kidney injury was first identified using the ischemia/reperfusion model in rodents, in which NGAL mRNA increased markedly with resultant NGAL protein increases in the plasma and urine within a few hours following ischemia/reperfusion injury, 24–48 hours preceding serum creatinine (sCr) elevation [11]. Similar results with early rise in NGAL ahead of creatinine were obtained using cisplatin nephrotoxic injury models in animals [11, 12].

NGAL is, therefore, one of the most reliable early biomarkers for ischemic and nephrotoxic kidney injury (acute tubular necrosis [ATN], contrast-induced

XV

nephropathy [CIN] and intensive care unit [ICU] settings). NGAL levels increase significantly in AKI patients, but not in controls, 24–48 h before the rise of creatinine [13]. NGAL levels on the day of transplant predict delayed graft function and dialysis requirement (2–4 days later) [14]. NGAL predicts the severity of AKI and dialysis requirement in children and in adults [13, 15–18]. This biomarker has been shown to be useful in several clinical settings especially after cardiopulmonary bypass (CPB) in children and adults, in pediatric and adult ICU patients, in trauma patients, in CIN and in toxic AKI [13–23]. Measurements of NGAL may be influenced by coexisting variables, such as systemic or urinary tract infections, and pre-existing renal diseases, but nevertheless, NGAL has been shown to have remarkable specificity and sensitivity [24–26]. Recently, one important study has demonstrated that NGAL allows early diagnosis of AKI, distinguishing between kidney damage AKI and functional volume responsive renal disorders [4].

Cardiorenal Syndrome Type 1

Cardiorenal syndrome type 1 is defined by an acute heart disease (e.g., acute heart failure) leading to AKI [1]. The clinical importance of AKI as far as outcome is concerned has emerged clearly in recent years. AKI diagnosed by RIFLE (Risk-Injury-Failure-Loss-End-stage kidney disease) or Acute Kidney Injury Network (AKIN) criteria is associated with adverse clinical outcome. Worsening of renal function in patients with heart failure represents an extremely important risk factor and often results in an accelerated decline in the clinical picture [27]. For this reason, questions that need to be answered in the immediate future are: Is it possible to prevent AKI in patients with acute heart failure, or is it at least possible to make the diagnosis in the very early stages when mitigation of the severe consequences is still conceivable? How can we manage heart failure patients without harming their kidneys? Why have our previous attempts to prevent AKI failed even in the presence of promising experimental results? In order to answer these questions one must analyze the pathophysiology of renal damage in cardiorenal syndrome. First, in contrast to experimental models of AKI, in clinical practice AKI is diagnosed quite late so interventions that have seemed to have a beneficial and protective action in the experimental setting may not give similar results in the real world because they are probably applied too late. If we had an earlier indicator of kidney damage, protective molecules might be able to be applied earlier within a window of potential clinical benefit. If we could diagnose AKI early enough, we could likely completely rewrite the chapter of renal prevention/protection with new or pre-existing drug molecules. Second, in acute heart failure, many mechanisms play an important role in the development of AKI and the most important among them should be addressed and considered in a more timely fashion. We may identify hemodynamic changes, neuro-hormonal derangements, associated exogenous factors and toxic effects, embolic episodes and important immunomediated effects, such as inflammation-derived necrosis and apoptosis, in the target organ. Even assuming the coexistence of risk factors such as obesity, subclinical inflammation, endothelial dysfunction and accelerated atherosclerosis, anemia and previous chronic kidney disease (CKD), we cannot neglect the paramount importance of two main factors, renal hypoperfusion and renal congestion.

NGAL Curve in the Diagnosis of Cardiorenal Syndrome

Most patients admitted to the hospital for acute heart failure present with a status of congestion and are definitely fluid overloaded [27]. In such patients, the renin-angiotensin-aldosterone (RAA) axis is activated and a non-osmotic release of vasopressin determines inappropriate renal vasoconstriction mediated by the V1 receptors and significant free water reabsorption mediated by the V2 receptors present in the distal segment of the nephrons. These hemodynamic and patho-physiological changes are worsened by significant venous congestion, which in the presence of decreased perfusion of the glomerular tuft leads to a marked decrease in the glomerular trans-capillary pressure gradient. This results in severe oliguria, water and sodium retention, worsening congestion and peripheral edema. In these circumstances, in addition to pharmacological therapy and the often overlooked dietary recommendations, the cornerstone of immediate management is represented by diuretics. Patients are squeezed with loop diuretics often at very high doses since a 'status of diuretic resistance' often occurs with limited poliuric response to increasing doses of the drug. In some cases, diuretics become ineffective and the only method to resolve the clinical impasse is the use of extracorporeal ultrafiltration. In all cases however, the clinician has little or no idea of the level of over hydration, and especially of the target body weight and hydration that the patient should reach. In recent studies, the use of bioimpedance vectorial analysis (BIVA) has been advocated as a tool to be used in conjunction with B-natriuretic peptide (BNP) to modulate therapy and to define criteria for hospital discharge [28]. In particular, although BNP is useful in identifying when the patient should be discharged, BNP + BIVA may help to optimize fluid status of the patient at discharge, reducing the number of subsequent rehospitalizations for acute heart failure. These two parameters do not, however, contribute to understanding the renal response to diuretic and fluid removal strategies and especially do not allow detection of possible renal insults because of excessive fluid removal and iatrogenic renal hypoperfusion. In fact, over a third of these patients display a significant increase in creatinine 48 to 72 hours after the beginning of intensive diuretic or ultrafiltration therapy [29, 30]. In these circumstances, we suggest use of NGAL determination in blood as a biomarker of early renal damage. NGAL has been shown to predict AKI 24 to 48 hours before a creatinine increase is observed. However, since the management of acute heart failure patients may often be carried out over several days, it is unclear when the NGAL should be measured. We believe that an 'NGAL curve' could be a useful tool and could be created by taking blood samples every 12–24 hours as has been done in the past for other biomarkers, such as troponin, myoglobin etc. To support this approach, we report our experience in several cases.

In **Figure 2**, we describe a typical case of a patient hospitalized for acute heart failure. The patient displayed high values of BNP at admission and severe fluid overload. The BIVA analysis suggested a moderate status of over-hydration with a slight condition of malnutrition. The patient presented typical signs of congestion with shortness of breath and oliguria. Treatment with high-dose diuretics produced a significant increase in diuresis already after 24 hours, with partial relief of symptoms. On subsequent days, the progressive increase in diuresis was coupled with a parallel reduction in BNP levels (wet BNP) until both diuresis and BNP stabilized (dry BNP level). By day 3, BIVA, which is serially performed in these patients, displayed a moderate status of dehydration whereas creatinine

XV

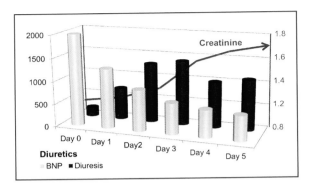

Fig. 2. Didactic representation of the time course of B-natriuretic peptide (BNP), diuresis and creatinine over several days after hospitalization for acute decompensated heart failure and the beginning of a high dose diuretic regime.

started to rise, reaching the condition of AKI (RIFLE R). Further increase in creatinine over subsequent days led to RIFLE I class of AKI. The diagnosis of such conditions is typically cardiorenal syndrome type 1.

In **Figure 3**, a similar patient was hospitalized for acute heart failure and a pharmacological approach similar to the previous case was undertaken. However, in this case, close monitoring of plasma NGAL was performed together with BNP, diuresis and BIVA. After 24 hours, NGAL values had more than doubled compared to baseline. At 48 hours, BIVA showed a significant reduction of the overhydration with values close to normal, whereas NGAL was more than 4 times higher than baseline value at hospital admission. The NGAL warning triggered the treating physician to stop the diuretic therapy and stabilize the patient for the days that followed. Diuresis and BNP values remained stable whereas NGAL showed a trend towards reduction. The values of creatinine remained stable throughout the hospital admission. In this case, we may speculate that a type 1 cardiorenal syndrome was prevented by modifying the treatment strategy based on the NGAL warning. This approach is only possible if a series of NGAL measurements are made. In particular, the use of the 'NGAL curve' may allow the treating physician to overcome the limitations because of uncertainties about the cut-off value, and may create a more personalized evaluation in individual patients considering baseline values and subsequent changes in NGAL values over time. However, a potential limitation to this approach in the acute heart failure population may be the relatively low NGAL levels expected in these patients in light of the lower limit of detection of the first generation plasma NGAL assay and the expected variation at the extreme low end of competitive immunoassays. For this reason, we can speculate that the novel extended range plasma NGAL assay may allow for better use of the potential of the NGAL curve offering quantitative determinations of NGAL levels even in the low ranges. As in the case for C-reactive protein (CRP) and troponin, we can consider that NGAL values in a single subject are a continuum in which significant variations within the low range or even below the previous assay detection limit, represent a significant event from the clinical point of view. For this reason development of the extended range assay represents a step forward for the early diagnosis of AKI in patients with acute heart failure, especially if used in conjunction with the 'NGAL curve' concept.

XV

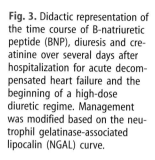

Fig. 3. Didactic representation of the time course of B-natriuretic peptide (BNP), diuresis and creatinine over several days after hospitalization for acute decompensated heart failure and the beginning of a high-dose diuretic regime. Management was modified based on the neutrophil gelatinase-associated lipocalin (NGAL) curve.

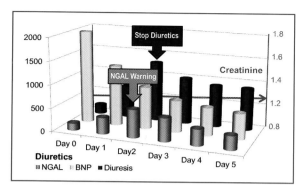

Extended Range NGAL Tests

The extended range competitive NGAL test (Triage®, Biosite Inc, Waltham, MA) measures NGAL from the median of normal endogenous NGAL (ca. 60 ng/ml) to 1,300 ng/ml. As is typical of all immunoassays, at the extremes of the NGAL dose response curve, assay imprecision increases. Nevertheless, the zone where the best concentration precision is achieved is aligned with the intended use as an aid for diagnosis of AKI in ICU patients.

However, many other indications where NGAL may prove useful, such as CIN, worsening renal function in the background of heart failure, and AKI in CKD require improved precision within the apparently healthy, NGAL concentration range. Toward this aim, attempts were made to extend the quantifiable range of NGAL. The final design was a sandwich format immunoassay that utilizes two antibodies distinct of the one used in the competitive format as well as a different sized detection particle (**Fig. 4**, Panels **a** and **d**).

In the initial competitive format, immunization, antibody selection, capture chemistry, and calibration material were all derived from recombinant NGAL cloned and expressed in bacteria. The re-designed sandwich assay used the same NGAL construct but expressed in mammalian cells which impart post-translational modifications in the form of glycosylations. This mammalian cell-expressed NGAL was used for immunization, antibody selection, and final calibration. In addition, the antibodies employed in the sandwich immunoassay have been selected to target the 'free' form of NGAL, not NGAL that is in the covalent homodimeric form or heterodimeric complexes with MMP-9. It is believed that this 'free' form of NGAL is more closely associated with AKI [31].

This design lowered the lower limit of NGAL detection from 60 ng/ml in the competitive format to 15 ng/ml in the sandwich immunoassay. As such, the new sandwich assay can provide quantitative measurements of NGAL over the entire range of expected NGAL values from a non-diseased apparently healthy population.

The properties cited above taken together give rise to a broader dynamic range in the sandwich NGAL immunoassay as compared to the competitive format (**Fig. 4**, Panels **c** and **e**). This, in turn, yields a much broader range over which relatively lower concentration coefficients of variation can be obtained (**Fig. 4**, Panels **b** and **d**). This becomes important as the concentration of NGAL

XV

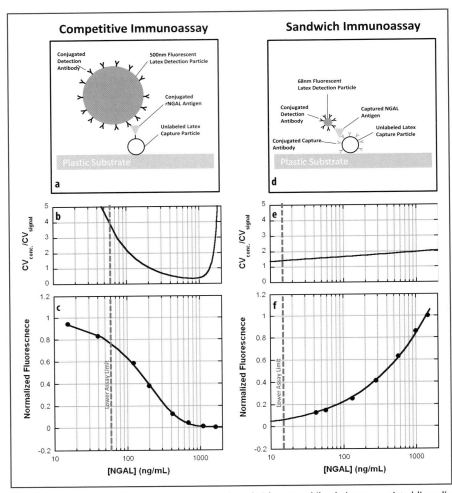

Fig. 4. Comparison of attributes of competitive and sandwich neutrophil gelatinase-associated lipocalin (NGAL) immunoassays on the Triage platform. Panels **a** and **d** show a cartoon representation of the competitive and sandwich Triage NGAL immunoassays respectively. Panels **b** and **e** show the dependence of signal-to-concentration percentage coefficient of variation (%CV) conversion factors as a function of NGAL concentration for the competitive and sandwich formats respectively. Panels **c** and **f** show the normalized dose response characteristics for the competitive and sandwich immunoassay formats, respectively. The filled circles represent averaged measurements from multiple Triage device replicates. The solid black line through the measured points is a non-linear least-squares fit of those data to a 5-parameter asymmetric sigmoid model. The vertical dashed blue line represents the lower assay cut-off as per the product package inserts.

approaches the endogenous NGAL levels observed in apparently healthy, normal patient samples and in the additional indications of interest cited previously. The effect can be demonstrated if one considers an example where both assays measure an NGAL concentration of 80 ng/ml with a fluorescence signal coefficient of variation of 7 %. At 80 ng/ml, the signal-to-concentration conversion factors are

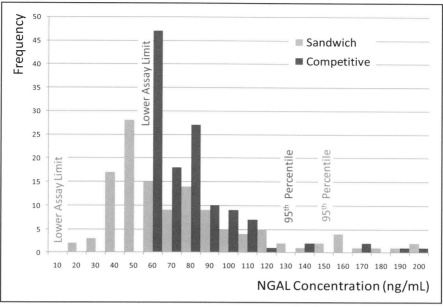

Fig. 5. Comparison of the competitive and sandwich assays in different samples at different concentrations. This demonstrates that the new extended range sandwich immunoassay for plasma NGAL is capable of quantitatively measuring the full range of expected values from apparently healthy donor populations.

2.8 and 1.6 for the competitive and the sandwich immunoassays respectively, **Fig. 4**, Panels **b** and **e**). The 7 % signal coefficient of variation then corresponds to an NGAL concentration coefficient of variation of 19.6 % and 11.2 % for the competitive and sandwich formats, respectively.

To characterize the lower limits of the measurable range of the two assay formats, plasma samples from apparently healthy donors were tested side-by-side on the sandwich and competitive NGAL test devices. The extended detection range of the sandwich immunoassay allowed for quantitative measurement of all apparently healthy donor samples and identified a minimum sample NGAL concentration of 18 ng/ml. In 40 % of these samples, the NGAL concentration measured on the extended range sandwich immunoassay was less than the lower limit of detection of the competitive immunoassay, i.e., 60 ng/ml. In the case of samples at or above 60 ng/ml NGAL, the distribution of assay results for the two immunoassays was comparable, as can be seen in **Figure 5**.

Conclusion

Cardiorenal syndrome is a complex clinical condition with potentially severe consequences. AKI in heart failure patients is often caused by iatrogenic hemodynamic derangement following inappropriate fluid status assessment and management. Based on current knowledge, we can use early biomarkers, such as NGAL, for early diagnosis of AKI. However, differences in individual response and uncertainties about cut-off values may limit the application of these new biomarkers. We suggest that the usefulness of plasma NGAL in the diagnosis and prevention of cardiorenal syndrome may increase if a curve of plasma values rather than a single plasma measurement is determined. Even when a curve is used, however, limitations of the first generation assay in measuring lower range values may affect the meaning of results. For this reason, the new high sensitivity assay for plasma NGAL may contribute to an improvement in the sensitivity of diagnosis leading to more effective intervention strategies.

Acknowledgements: The authors would like to kindly thank Fred Sundquist PhD and Gillian Parker for their contributions to this manuscript.

References

1. Ronco C, McCullough PA, Anker SD, et al (2010) Cardiorenal syndromes: an executive summary from the consensus conference of the Acute Dialysis Quality Initiative (ADQI). Contrib Nephrol 165: 54–67
2. Ronco C, Grammaticopoulos S, Rosner M, et al (2010) Oliguria, creatinine and other biomarkers of acute kidney injury. Contrib Nephrol 164: 118–127
3. Coca SG, Yalavarthy R, Concato J, Parikh CR (2008) Biomarkers for the diagnosis and risk stratification of acute kidney injury: a systematic review. Kidney Int 73: 1008–1016
4. Paragas N, Qiu A, Zhang Q, et al (2011) The Ngal reporter mouse detects the response of the kidney to injury in real time. Nat Med 17: 216–222
5. Koyner JL, Bennett MR, Worcester EM, et al (2008) Urinary cystatin C as an early biomarker of acute kidney injury following adult cardiothoracic surgery. Kidney Int 74: 1059–1069
6. Aghel A, Shrestha K, Mullens W, Borowski A, Tang WH (2010) Serum neutrophil gelatinase-associated lipocalin (NGAL) in predicting worsening renal function in acute decompensated heart failure. J Card Fail 16: 49–54
7. Nickolas TL, O'Rourke MJ, Yang J, et al (2008) Sensitivity and specificity of a single emergency department measurement of urinary neutrophil gelatinase-associated lipocalin for diagnosing acute kidney injury. Ann Intern Med 148: 810–819
8. Alvelos M, Pimentel R, Pinho E, et al (2011) Neutrophil gelatinase-associated lipocalin in the diagnosis of type 1 cardiorenal syndrome in the general ward. Clin J Am Soc Nephrol 6: 476–481
9. Kjeldsen L, Johnsen AH, Sengeløv H, Borregaard N (1993) Isolation and primary structure of NGAL, a novel protein associated with human neutrophil gelatinase. J Biol Chem 268: 10425–10432
10. Flo TH, Smith KD, Sato S, et al (2004) Lipocalin 2 mediates an innate immune response to bacterial infection by sequestrating iron. Nature 432: 917–921
11. Mishra J, Ma Q, Prada A, et al (2003) Identification of neutrophil gelatinase-associated lipocalin as a novel early urinary biomarker for ischemic renal injury. J Am Soc Nephrol 14: 2534–2543
12. Mishra J, Mori K, Ma Q, Kelly C, Barasch J, Devarajan P (2004) Neutrophil gelatinase-associated lipocalin: a novel early urinary biomarker for cisplatin nephrotoxicity. Am J Nephrol 24: 307–315
13. Mishra J, Dent C, Tarabishi R, et al (2005) Neutrophil gelatinase-associated lipocalin (NGAL) as a biomarker for acute renal injury after cardiac surgery. Lancet 365: 1231–1238
14. Kusaka M, Kuroyanagi Y, Mori T, et al (2008) Serum neutrophil gelatinase-associated lipocalin as a predictor of organ recovery from delayed graft function after kidney transplantation from donors after cardiac death. Cell Transplant 17: 1–100
15. Dent C, Ma Q, Dastrala S, et al (2007) Plasma neutrophil gelatinase-associated lipocalin predicts acute kidney injury, morbidity and mortality after pediatric cardiac surgery: a prospective uncontrolled cohort study. Crit Care 11: R127

16. Zappitelli M, Washburn KK, Arikan AA, et al (2007) Urine neutrophil gelatinase associated lipocalin is an early marker of acute kidney injury in critically ill children: a prospective cohort study. Crit Care 11: R84

17. Cruz DN, de Cal M, Garzotto F, et al (2010) Plasma neutrophil gelatinase-associated lipocalin is an early biomarker for acute kidney injury in an adult ICU population. Intensive Care Med 36: 444–451

18. de Geus HR, Bakker J, Lesaffre EM, le Noble JL (2011) Neutrophil gelatinase-associated lipocalin at ICU admission predicts for acute kidney injury in adult patients. Am J Respir Crit Care Med 183: 907–914

19. Shapiro NI, Trzeciak S, Hollander JE, et al (2010) The diagnostic accuracy of plasma neutrophil gelatinase-associated lipocalin in the prediction of acute kidney injury in emergency department patients with suspected sepsis. Ann Emerg Med 56: 52–59

20. Haase-Fielitz A, Bellomo R, Devarajan P, et al (2009) Novel and conventional serum biomarkers predicting acute kidney injury in adult cardiac surgery--a prospective cohort study. Crit Care Med 37: 553–560

21. Makris K, Markou N, Evodia E, et al (2009) Urinary neutrophil gelatinase-associated lipocalin (NGAL)as an early marker of acute kidney injury in critically ill multiple trauma patients. Clin Chem Lab Med 47: 79–82

22. Malyszko J, Bachorzewska-Gajewska H, Poniatowski B, Malyszko JS, Dobrzycki S (2009) Urinary and serum biomarkers after cardiac catheterization in diabetic patients with stable angina and without severe chronic kidney disease. Renal Failure 31: 910–919

23. Wasilewska A, Zoch-Zwierz W, Taranta-Janusz K, Michaluk-Skutnik J (2010) Neutrophil gelatinase-associated lipocalin (NGAL): a new marker of cyclosporine nephrotoxicity? Pediatr Nephrol 25: 889–897

24. Yilmaz A, Sevketoglu E, Gedikbasi A, et al (2009) Early prediction of urinary tract infection with urinary neutrophil gelatinase associated lipocalin. Pediatr Nephrol 24: 2387–2392

25. Bagshaw SM, Bennett M, Haase M, et al (2010) Plasma and urine neutrophil gelatinaseassociated lipocalin in septic versus non-septic acute kidney injury in critical illness Intensive Care Med 36: 452–461

26. Haase M, Bellomo R, Devarajan P, Schlattmann P, Haase-Fielitz A; NGAL Meta-analysis Investigator Group (2009) Accuracy of neutrophil gelatinase-associated lipocalin (ngal) in diagnosis and prognosis in acute kidney injury: A systematic review and meta-analysis. Am J Kidney Dis 54: 1012–1024

27. Damman K, Voors AA, Hillege HL, et al (2010) Congestion in chronic systolic heart failure is related to renal dysfunction and increased mortality. Eur J Heart Fail 12: 974–982

28. Valle R, Aspromonte N, Milani L, et al (2011) Optimizing fluid management in patients with acute decompensated heart failure (ADHF): the emerging role of combined measurement of body hydration status and brain natriuretic peptide (BNP) levels. Heart Fail Rev 16: 519–529

29. Gottlieb SS, Abraham W, Butler J, et al (2002) The prognostic importance of different definitions of worsening renal function in congestive heart failure. J Card Fail 8: 136–141

30. Costanzo MR, Guglin ME, Saltzberg MT, et al (2007) Ultrafiltration versus intravenous diuretics for patients hospitalized for acute decompensated heart failure. J Am Coll Cardiol 49: 675–683

31. Cai L, Rubin J, Han W, Venge P, Xu S (2010) The origin of multiple molecular forms in urine of HNL/NGAL. Clin J Am Soc Nephrol 5: 2229–2235

Urine Output and the Diagnosis of Acute Kidney Injury

J.R. Prowle and R. Bellomo

Introduction

Prevention and management of organ dysfunction are central to the practice of critical care medicine. To this end, physiological monitoring is used to assess organ function and the effects of treatment in real time. One of the foremost challenges for the intensive care specialist is to understand how to relate physiological variables, such as oxygenation, blood pressure and cardiac output, to underlying organ function. These relationships are complex and reflect interdependence of organ function, treatment, disease and comorbid conditions. Nevertheless, in search of patterns to guide clinical management, we commonly relate certain measurements to the function of particular organs, such as blood pressure and cardio-circulatory function. In the case of the kidneys, maintenance of urine output is a continuous manifestation of organ function and urine production is both monitored as an index of organ function and targeted as a therapeutic goal. However, in common with other continuously monitored physiological variables, the relationship between urine output and underlying kidney function is complex and there are many pitfalls to its interpretation in isolation.

Driven by attempts to better define kidney dysfunction and standardize treatment, research has recently been focused on the significance of urine output during critical illness. Here we discuss the pathophysiology of changes in urine flow during acute illness, the role of urine output in the definition of renal dysfunction, and recent evidence relating reductions in urine output to clinical outcomes and biochemical measures of kidney function.

What We Understand by Acute Kidney Injury

Acute kidney injury (AKI) is characterized by a sudden and sustained decrease in glomerular filtration (GFR) leading to clinical manifestations of renal dysfunction. The term 'acute kidney injury' encompasses a spectrum of pathophysiological processes, which may cause renal dysfunction. Whereas a small number of cases of AKI in intensive care are related to urinary obstruction or intrinsic renal disease, the majority of episodes in the intensive care unit (ICU) are due to a combination of global hemodynamic changes, systemic inflammatory responses and exogenous nephrotoxic insults. Discussion of AKI in critical care, therefore, focuses on the occurrence of renal dysfunction secondary to these insults. A normal GFR is dependent on the ultrafiltration pressure gradient, determined by the glomerular capillary-Bowman's space hydrostatic pressure gradient and rate of

J.-L. Vincent (ed.), *Annual Update in Intensive Care and Emergency Medicine 2012*
DOI 10.1007/978-3-642-25716-2 © Springer-Verlag Berlin Heidelberg 2012

renal plasma flow. During ultrafiltration, development of an opposing colloid osmotic pressure gradient limits the GFR, which is normally 20 % of renal plasma flow. Consequently reduced cardiac output (resulting in lower renal plasma flow) and/or systemic hypotension (reducing glomerular capillary pressure) can generally be expected to cause a hemodynamically mediated, reversible, fall in GFR – so called pre-renal azotemia. Commonly, however, reduction in GFR is not rapidly reversible after correction of hemodynamic abnormalities, reflecting progression of AKI to renal cellular injury or sustained neurohormonal changes. AKI occurring in the context of acute illness typically involves tubular cellular injury [1], principally in the late proximal convoluted tubule and distal loop of Henle, which is characterized by cellular dedifferentiation, disruption of intercellular tight junctions, shedding of cytoskeletal debris into the tubular lumen and loss of polarized expression of transmembrane ion channels [2] and may culminate in shedding of viable tubular cells or cellular apotosis. Local inflammatory responses [1] play an important role in the pathogenesis of this process and a primary physiological consequence of tubular injury is a failure to actively reabsorb salt and water from the ultrafiltrate because of disruption of the polarized tubular epithelium [2]. A number of mechanisms then go on to decrease actual or effective glomerular filtration including elevated intra-tubular pressure, activation of tubulo-glomerular feedback (causing pre-glomerular vasoconstriction) and unselective back-leak of ultrafiltrate.

The etiology of tubular cellular injury is complex and multifactorial. Absolute renal ischemia and reperfusion is common in experimental models of AKI. However, such extreme reductions in renal blood flow are uncommon clinically; experimentally near, but not complete, reduction of renal blood flow in the absence of other insults is not followed by sustained AKI [3]. Cellular injury in AKI complicating critical illness is probably the result of complex interactions between the borderline oxygen supply-demand relationship at the renal corticomedullary junction, microcirculatory dysfunction in systemic inflammation and the effects of nephrotoxins [4]. Of note, as loss of tubular integrity precedes reduction in GFR, any effect of this reduction on urine output can be blunted by the loss of urinary concentrating capacity.

How AKI is Diagnosed and Defined

Diagnosis of AKI has traditionally been reliant on the accumulation of nitrogenous products of metabolism, such as creatinine, in the bloodstream, reflecting a reduction in their excretion via the glomerular ultrafiltrate. Historically, a wide variety of biochemical and clinical criteria have been used to define renal dysfunction. More recently, consensus definitions of AKI have been developed reflecting the reciprocal relationship between an increase in serum creatinine (sCr) to a new steady state and the underlying decrease in GFR. In the RIFLE (Risk-Injury-Failure-Loss-End-stage kidney disease) classification of AKI [5], sequentially greater classes of renal dysfunction (RIFLE class R, I or F) are defined by increases in sCr to 1.5, 2 or 3 times the baseline level (**Table 1**). Subsequently the AKI Network (AKIN) [6] (**Table 1**) modified the RIFLE definitions by including an absolute creatinine increase of 27 µmol within 48 h, which has been associated with adverse patient outcomes [7], to widen the criteria for the least severe category of renal injury (AKIN 1). Additionally the AKIN criteria remove the need for an estimated

Table 1: Consensus definitions of acute kidney injury (AKI)

	RIFLE [5]			AKIN [6]*	
Criteria	Creatinine definition	Urine definition	Criteria	Creatinine definition	Urine definition
Risk	≥ 1.5-fold increase from reference sCr[‡] *or decrease in GFR ≥ 25 %***	< 0.5 ml/kg/h for > 6 consecutive hours	Stage 1	≥ 26 μmol/l increase within 48 h or ≥ 1.5 fold increase[†] from reference sCr[‡]	< 0.5 ml/kg/h for > 6 consecutive hours
Injury	≥ 2 fold increase[†] from reference sCr[‡] *or decrease in GFR ≥ 50 %***	< 0.5 ml/kg/h for > 12 h	Stage 2	≥ 2 fold increase[†] from reference sCr[‡]	< 0.5 ml/kg/h for > 12 hours
Failure	≥ 3 fold increase[†] from reference sCr[‡] or ≥ 354 μmol/l increase *or decrease in GFR ≥ 75 %***	< 0.3 ml/kg/h for > 24 hr or anuria for 12 h	Stage 3	≥ 3 fold increase[†] from reference sCr[‡] or ≥ 354 μmol/l increase or commenced on RRT	< 0.3 ml/kg/h for > 24 h or anuria for 12 h

Only one criterion (creatinine or urine output) has to be fulfilled to qualify for a stage.
sCr: serum creatinine; RIFLE – Risk Injury Failure Loss End-stage kidney disease; AKIN: Acute Kidney Injury Network; GFR: glomerular filtration rate; RRT: renal replacement therapy
* AKIN definition assumes that diagnosis based on the urine output criterion alone will require exclusion of urinary tract obstructions that reduce urine output or other easily reversible causes of reduced urine output and that AKIN criteria should be used in the context of the clinical presentation and following adequate fluid resuscitation when applicable.
** In practice GFR definitions in the RIFLE criteria have not been widely employed.
[†] In both definitions, change in SCr is presumed to have occurred within one week.
[‡] Reference creatinine is lowest recorded creatinine value in last 3 months. In absence of a reference value, RIFLE criteria suggest calculation of a theoretical baseline serum creatinine value for a given patient assuming a low-normal GFR (75 ml/min/1.73m^2), whereas AKIN criteria suggest daily determination of creatinine and use of lowest creatinine within a 7-day timeframe as reference.

baseline creatinine if none is available, and stipulate that adequate acute resuscitation has been given before assessment of criteria. Finally, the AKIN definition also categorizes all patients receiving renal replacement therapy (RRT) to the most severe category of AKI (AKIN 3). Most recently these definitions have been incorporated into the latest Kidney Disease: Improving Global Outcomes (KDIGO) [8] recommendations on the diagnosis and treatment of AKI.

Although these biochemical classifications of AKI have immeasurably strengthened AKI research by standardizing approaches, they are intrinsically limited by the dynamic nature of renal injury, since a steady state of serum biochemistry is rarely obtained and creatinine changes can considerably lag acute changes in GFR. Furthermore, decreases in creatinine generation rate during acute illness and increases in volume of distribution with fluid therapy can act counter to rises in plasma creatinine after a fall in GFR, potentially masking the severity of renal dysfunction that has occurred. Concerns about the speed and accuracy with which changes in plasma creatinine reflect real-time changes in GFR led to the adoption of urine output criteria to additionally identify AKI within the consensus definitions. In the RIFLE criteria, a urine output of less than 0.5 ml/kg/h for 6 consecutive hours is diagnostic of RIFLE-R and for 12 consecu-

XV

tive hours of RIFLE I, whereas 24 hours of more severe oliguria (< 0.3 ml/kg/h) or 12 h of complete anuria fulfil the criteria for RIFLE F. The choice of these cut-off values was based on expert opinion only and these values were subsequently transferred unchanged to the AKIN stages 1, 2 and 3 respectively (although with the explicit requirement that adequate fluid resuscitation has occurred prior to assessment).

What Physiological Processes Cause Oliguria and How They Relate To AKI

The quantity of urine output is dependent on the GFR and the subsequent rate of water and solute reabsorption along the nephron. In normal physiology, a high GFR is required to effectively maintain a low concentration of products of metabolism in the plasma by unselective convective clearance in the glomerular ultrafiltrate. The composition of the ultrafiltrate is then modified in the tubules to maintain salt, water and extracellular volume homeostasis. Given that a healthy adult with a GFR of ~100 ml/min can stably excrete less than 1000 ml of urine a day, much less than 1 % of the ultrafiltrate volume can appear as urine. Depending on the body's salt and water balance, urinary osmolality may vary from less than 100 to over 1200 milliosmoles and urinary sodium concentration from less than 10 to over 100 millimoles. The composition of the urine is governed by local and systemic neuroendocrine mechanisms principally the renin/angiotensin/aldosterone system (RAAS) and the hypothalamic-pituitary antidiuretic hormone (ADH) axis. Thus, in healthy adults subjected to water deprivation, urine output falls to a physiological minimum and hormonal mechanisms attempt to maintain plasma osmolality and extracellular volume. It has been known since the 1940s that, if water deprivation is maintained, maximal urinary concentrating capacity will result in an obligatory minimum urine output of around 500 ml/day [9,10]. Urine output falling below this level thus implies that a reduction in GFR must have occurred. These early studies underlie the concept that severe oliguria is indicated by a sustained urine output of approximately < 15 ml/h or 0.3–0.4 ml/kg/h – reflected in the RIFLE F/AKIN 3 definition. Crucially, however, the ability to excrete such a concentrated urine is critically dependent on intact tubular function – in the setting of chronic kidney disease or diuretic therapy more modest decreases in urine volume, which might be entirely physiological for a healthy adult, will not occur without an acute fall in GFR. Furthermore, if concentrating capacity is significantly limited, very large decreases in GFR (>> 50 %) may be required for clinical oliguria to occur. Thus, oliguria in the presence of biochemical renal dysfunction has traditionally been regarded as indicative of more severe AKI, associated with greater need for RRT and higher risk of death. In summary, oliguria can be regarded either as an early sign of hemodynamic instability, in which the kidney may be intact but at risk, or a late sign of severity of renal dysfunction, a dual role that can confuse its clinical interpretation without considering the underlying mechanism of oliguria.

Mechanistically, in acute illness, actual or effective hypovolemia may trigger salt and water retention and oliguria by neuroendocrine physiological responses even when cardiac output and blood pressure are maintained by vasoconstriction and tachycardia. Additionally, pain and surgical stress can trigger these neuroendocrine responses resulting in transient oliguria even in the absence of circula-

XV

tory compromise. In early illness, even though renal plasma flow and GFR may be preserved, renal oxygen consumption can be increased and the kidney may be at risk from circulating nephrotoxins or changes in intrarenal blood flow. With more severe illness, or in the presence of comorbid conditions, the patient's cardiovascular reserve may become exhausted and hypotension and/or reduction in cardiac output may occur. At this renal blood flow point, GFR will decrease, but, in addition, ADH-, sympathetic- and RAAS-mediated urinary concentration will also contribute to oliguria. Significantly, the exact mechanisms of hemodynamically-mediated reduction in GFR may vary in differing clinical contexts. In hypovolemic or cardiogenic shock, reduction in cardiac output and ability to auto-regulate renal blood flow may be most important. Conversely, in sepsis, renal vasodilation, systemic hypotension and intrarenal shunting may abolish ultrafiltration even though renal blood flow might be increased [11]. In this context, while global renal ischemia may not occur, circulating inflammatory mediators, endothelial injury and microvascular blood flow changes can cause renal (tubular) injury [4]. Finally, irrespective of the nature of the insult, if it is sustained, tubular injury will progressively occur and reduction in GFR will become the primary driver of oliguria. Thus, clinical interpretation of oliguria requires understanding of the disease process involved.

Consider four scenarios: First, an adequately resuscitated patient with postoperative pain; second, a healthy individual with 25 % blood loss after trauma; third, a patient with chronic heart failure and low grade sepsis; and fourth, a young patient with abdominal sepsis and hyperdynamic shock. All these patients are likely to be oliguric, and might recover urine output with timely appropriate treatment, but may benefit from different clinical approaches – particularly with regard to fluid management. Thus, while adequate resuscitation is essential in true hypovolemia, several lines of evidence have linked fluid overload to adverse outcomes and AKI [12], both observationally in mixed critically ill patients [13, 14], and prospectively in elective surgery [15]. Additionally, because of the speed of onset of illness, therapy or co-morbid conditions, it is not uncommon for patients to develop sustained AKI without a prior 'pre-renal' phase of oliguria so that reduction in urine output is, from the outset, a direct manifestation of a (non-rapidly reversed) decrease in GFR when hemodynamic intervention will not be likely to restore urine output; here, continued fluid administration risks systemic edema and worsening organ dysfunction [12]. Conversely, whereas decreased GFR has been described as a protective response in tubular injury, by limiting renal work and preventing further ischemic injury, recent evidence in AKI after cardiopulmonary bypass (CPB) has shown that oxygen consumption relative to the amount of sodium reabsorption is actually increased in AKI [16], suggesting that unless GFR is near zero, tubular metabolic demand may be higher than expected and that maintaining renal oxygen delivery is of importance even if AKI is established.

Historically, indices of urinary concentration and tubular function, such as fractional excretion of sodium or urea have been employed to distinguish the underlying nature of renal injury in oliguria. In practice, little evidence exists to support their clinical utility [17, 18]. Whereas production of very concentrated urine implies relatively intact tubular function, multiple acute and chronic conditions can cause failure of concentration capacity. Furthermore, the transition to tubular injury is unlikely to be abrupt, but instead progressive so that in most cases in the ICU the interpretation of a snapshot urinary electrolyte assay is likely to be of limited value.

XV

The Rationale for the Oliguria Criteria in the Consensus Definitions of AKI

The most severe RIFLE F or AKIN 3 definition of AKI requires a sustained level of urine output below that achievable with the maximal renal concentrating capacity and intact renal function and thus implies that a reduction in GFR has occurred. This is useful given the lag that may occur before the rise in plasma creatinine fully reflects the fall in GFR and because plasma creatinine is generally only determined on a daily basis. Urine output definitions of less severe renal dysfunction, RIFLE R or I and AKIN 1 or 2, require shorter durations (6–12 or > 12 h) and a less stringent definition of oliguria (< 0.5 ml/kg/h), which probably lies on the borderline of maximal urinary concentration. These definitions probably capture two groups: First, patients with intact concentrating capacity and physiological oliguria who are at risk of AKI; and second, a group with chronically or acutely impaired concentrating capacity who have mild to moderate acute reduction in GFR. Of course, reduction in GFR may occur without any decrease in urine output meeting these criteria. Thus, these less severe urine output criteria represent a heterogeneous mix of clinical circumstances. Furthermore, nothing in the formulation of these definitions confirmed that urine criteria were comparable to their equivalent creatinine-based criteria in terms of clinical course and outcomes despite their interchangeability in the definitions; neither is any additional significance ascribed to fulfilment of both urine and creatinine criteria. Finally shorter periods of oliguria – that commonly trigger clinical interventions – were not examined in these definitions.

Validation of AKI Definitions

Since their inception, the association between RIFLE or AKIN-defined AKI and risk of death has been examined in a number of retrospective and prospective observational studies. Increasing severity of AKI has been associated with increasing mortality both in ICU [19–30] and general hospital populations [31]. Comparison of the RIFLE and AKIN definitions has not clearly favored one above the other [24, 27, 29, 30], although in some studies, differing grades of the AKIN definition have not clearly defined differing risk of death, suggesting loss of precision with use of the AKIN definition [28, 30, 32, 33]. A number of studies have examined large patient databases; inclusion of a large number of patient episodes has demonstrated robust relationships between severity of AKI and outcome although only creatinine criteria were employed as incomplete urine output data was available [23, 28, 31]. Reports that did include some form of urine output criteria when relating AKI definition to survival are shown in **Table 2**.

XV

Studies have varied in their ability to accurately incorporate urinary output into the definitions, depending on the datasets available. The association between severity of AKI and higher risk of death remains when employing combined definitions; however, for urine output criteria in isolation, there are significant inconsistencies in the reported ability to predict survival, with some studies suggesting that urinary criteria alone are inferior to creatinine-based or combined definitions [22, 27, 29, 30], others suggesting they perform equally [25, 26] and one recent large study suggesting that urinary changes could be a better predictor of outcome [33]. Of course oliguria, occurring as a sign of hemodynamic compro-

Table 2. Studies including urine output criteria when examining association between acute kidney injury (AKI) diagnosis and clinical outcomes.

Author, year [ref]	Setting	Number with AKI	Criteria used	Urine output criteria	Relationship between AKI and outcome	Effect of urine output criteria versus creatinine criteria
Abosaif, 2005 [19]	Mixed ICU admissions	183	RIFLE score on ICU admission day	RIFLE in first 24 h ICU only	Increased mortality for RIFLE F vs R or I	Not assessed
Cruz, 2006 [22]	Mixed ICU admissions	234	RIFLE	RIFLE during ICU stay	Independent increase in risk of death with increasing RIFLE category	Independent association with mortality remained when considering creatinine criteria alone but was not seen when urine output was examined in isolation
Hoste, 2006 [20]	Mixed ICU admissions	3617	RIFLE	RIFLE (2 h urine measurements during ICU stay)	Independent association between RIFLE classes I or F with hospital mortality	Patients with RIFLE F on creatinine criteria had somewhat higher hospital mortality than class F on urine output criteria
Kuitunen, 2006 [21]	Post cardiothoracic surgery	156	RIFLE	RIFLE during ICU stay	RIFLE classification was an independent risk factor for 90-day mortality	Not assessed
Bagshaw, 2008 [24, 25]	Mixed ICU	44553 (AKIN) 43395 (RIFLE)	AKIN and RIFLE	Modified: < 840 ml/day R/1 < 504 ml/day I/2 < 96 ml/day F/3	Crude mortality was higher for higher AKI class in both definitions No statistical difference in mortality by AKI definition	Similar finding of increased odds ratio for death when analysis restricted to RIFLE by only serum creatinine or only urine output criteria
Barrantes, 2008 [26]	Medical ICU admissions	213	Any AKIN (AKIN 1–3)	AKIN during ICU stay	Presence of AKI (AKIN 1–3) was an independent predictor of hospital mortality	Odds ratios for death were not significantly different when using creatinine, urine output or the presence of both criteria to diagnose AKI
Lopes, 2008 [27]	Mixed ICU admissions	334 (AKIN) 290 (RIFLE)	AKIN and RIFLE	AKIN/RIFLE during ICU stay	Mortality was significantly higher for AKI defined by any of the AKIN or RIFLE criteria. There were no statistical differences in mortality by the AKI definition	Serum creatinine criteria was a better predictor of mortality than urine output. Increase in creatinine was an earlier sign of worsening renal function than oliguria

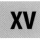

XV

Table 2. (continued)

Author, year [ref]	Setting	Number with AKI	Criteria used	Urine output criteria	Relationship between AKI and outcome	Effect of urine output criteria versus creatinine criteria
Haase, 2009 [29]	Post cardiothoracic surgery	127(AKIN) 130(RIFLE)	AKIN and RIFLE	AKIN/RIFLE during ICU stay	Worsening RIFLE or AKIN stage was associated with increasing in-hospital mortality with no significant difference between definitions	Serum creatinine–based classes were the strongest predictors of in-hospital mortality whereas urine output criteria showed the lowest predictive value although RIFLE F/AKIN 3 on urine output criteria predicted higher hospital mortality, LOS and need for RRT
Joannidis, 2009 [30]	Mixed ICU admissions	4093(AKIN) 5093(RIFLE)	AKIN and RIFLE	All patients with urine output < 12 ml/kg/day assigned to AKIN stage 2 or RIFLE	AKI by RIFLE or AKIN was associated with increased hospital mortality RIFLE showed higher detection rate of AKI in the first 48 h.	Mortality rates by criteria defined by worst urine output were consistently lower than when defined by worst serum creatinine.
Morgan, 2010 [35]	Mixed ICU admissions	228 (RIFLE-F)	RIFLE F only	RIFLE F urine output criteria during ICU stay	Increased risk of death	Oliguric RIFLE-F AKI was associated with a significantly higher risk of requiring acute dialysis, long-term dialysis and hospital mortality compared with creatinine defined RIFLE-F alone.
Mandelbaum, 2011 [33]	Mixed ICU admissions	8272	AKIN	AKIN during ICU stay	AKIN-defined AKI was independently associated with mortality, risk associated with classes 1 and 2 did not significantly differ	Urine output criteria alone was a better predictor of mortality than creatinine alone or a combination of both at each stage of AKI

RIFLE – Risk Injury Failure Loss End stage; AKIN – Acute Kidney Injury Network; LOS: length of stay; RRT: renal replacement therapy

XV

mise, could be associated with an increased risk of death, without implying actual renal injury; however, the same concerns might also apply to analysis of more rapidly reversed changes in sCr, which are still associated with adverse outcomes [34] even though overt tubular injury is unlikely to have occurred and it is likely that both urine and creatinine criteria will identify heterogeneous patient populations.

Oliguria may have additional significance when considering more severe renal dysfunction. In a study specifically examining this question [35], RIFLE F defined by oliguria (with or without creatinine criteria) was associated with worse outcomes when compared with RIFLE F defined by creatinine criteria in isolation. This finding is further supported by the poor outcomes in oliguria-defined RIFLE F reported by Haase et al. [29]; however, it is in contradiction to the outcomes reported by Hoste et al. [20], which showed that creatinine-defined RIFLE F was associated with modestly worse survival than oliguria-defined RIFLE F.

Recent Evidence Relating Oliguria-defined AKI to Clinical Outcomes

Although evidence relating creatinine-based and combined definitions of AKI to outcomes is robust, there is conflicting evidence on the specific value of oliguria in these definitions. The complexity of the physiology of oliguria and study-specific differences may account for these discrepancies. These issues have recently been specifically explored in prospective studies of oliguria in AKI diagnosis.

Macedo et al. [36] prospectively examined urine output in 75 admissions to a US medical ICU over a two-month period. A digital continuous urine flow meter was used to accurately and continuously monitor urine flow. These investigators employed different definitions of AKI based on the time interval for evaluation of oliguria: < 0.5 ml/kg/h for 6 consecutive hours (the AKIN 1/RIFLE R standard), < 3 ml/kg total during any 6 hour period and < 3 ml/kg during fixed six hour blocks based on nursing shifts. Fifty-five percent of patients had an episode of oliguria and there was no significant difference among the three methods of assessment. Overall, 21 patients (28 %) were diagnosed with AKI based on AKIN creatinine criteria and as many again (24, 32 %) were diagnosed by urine criteria in the absence of creatinine changes. Patients with AKI diagnosed exclusively by urine output criteria had non-significantly higher mortality than non-AKI patients, and patients with urine output < 6 ml/h over a 12 h block (approximates AKIN 2) had a significantly greater risk of death (7 vs. 33 % p = 0.004). Finally, the total number of hours of oliguria and total number of episodes of oliguria during the ICU stay were incrementally associated with increasing risk of death.

In another study, Han et al. [32] assessed 1625 critically ill patients over the first seven days of ICU admission. Fifty-seven percent of patients were diagnosed with AKI, 25.7 % on urine output criteria alone. More severe AKI, defined by urine output, was associated with incrementally greater hazard ratios for hospital mortality (hazard ratios, 1.81, 2.96, 4.17 for AKIN stages 1 to 3 respectively), comparable to those observed using creatinine or combined criteria. Adjustment for diuretic administration did not affect these results. In this study, creatinine criteria did not distinguish AKIN stages 2 and 3 as of differing risk of death – again suggesting a possible role for oliguria in risk stratification of more severe AKI.

Recently, Macedo and co-workers reported a second study [37] examining hourly urine output in 317 critically ill patients. Adding urine output criteria to AKIN creatinine definitions increased the diagnosis of AKI from 24 % to 52 %. In this cohort, oliguric patients without a change in sCr had significantly higher ICU mortality than patients without AKI (8.8 % vs. 1.3 %), comparable to mortality in patients with sCr-defined AKI (10.4 %). Addition of urine output to the sCr criteria also significantly increased the area under the curve to predict death. Oliguric patients were diagnosed more swiftly than patients with non-oliguric AKI, although this may have been associated with the frequency with which creatinine was measured. Again, increasing number of hours of oliguria or number of 6 h blocks of low urine output were similarly associated with increased risk of death, suggesting that assessment of urine output may be simplified into blocks of 6 hours without loss of discrimination. Finally, the authors examined the ability of different oliguria definitions to predict sCr-defined AKIN stage 1. Increasing duration of oliguria was associated with high specificity for excluding creatinine-defined AKI, but with marked loss of sensitivity, reflecting the occurrence of non-oliguric AKI.

How Shorter Periods of Oliguria Relate to Subsequent Renal Dysfunction

Given the interest in prediction of AKI and clinical use of oliguria, we have recently examined the ability of consecutive periods of oliguria to predict subsequent biochemical AKI. In a multinational, multicenter study [38], we chose RIFLE I defined AKI as a measure likely to represent parenchymal renal injury and not merely hemodynamically-related AKI. We did not seek to assess the association of oliguria with survival or other outcomes. Despite studying 239 patients over 723 patient days, only 22 patients developed creatinine-defined RIFLE I in the ICU. We found that all durations of consecutive oliguria (defined as < 0.5 ml/kg/h) from 1 h to 12 h were significantly associated with RIFLE I AKI in the next 24 or 48 hrs. Receiver-operator characteristic (ROC) analysis demonstrated an area under the curve for oliguria to predict RIFLE-I AKI on the next day of 0.75 (**Fig. 1**) with episodes of 4 h or more of oliguria, the optimal cut-off, having a sensitivity of 52 % and sensitivity of 86 %. Although this initially appears a fairly good performance, in our population AKI was infrequent whereas episodes of oliguria were common, so that the positive predictive value for 4 h episodes of oliguria was only 11 % and the likelihood ratio 3.8, implying that oliguria has poor utility as a diagnostic test for AKI. However, episodes of oliguria preceding AKI were associated with higher heart rate, lower mean blood pressure, higher central venous pressure and greater need for vasopressors or inotropes. In addition, clinicians were far more likely to intervene with fluid or diuretics in oliguria preceding AKI, despite no significant difference between duration of the episodes. This suggests that oliguria may be a more useful predictor of AKI when interpreted in the wider clinical context; and that physicians probably incorporate these considerations into their normal decision-making. Finally, in our study, more patients arrived in the ICU with biochemical RIFLE-I AKI (32) than those who developed AKI in the ICU (22). As urine output is unlikely to be accurately monitored in the pre-ICU environment, it will not be useful in the diagnosis of AKI in a large number of patients. However, in these patients, presence of oliguria might still be useful in risk stratification of biochemically defined AKI.

XV

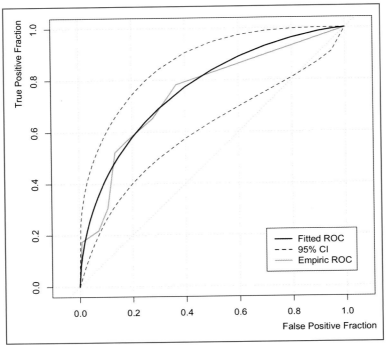

Fig. 1. Receiver-operating characteristic (ROC) curve analysis of the ability of episodes of varying duration of consecutive oliguria (1 – 12 h) in the ICU to predict new RIFLE Injury (I) or more by creatinine criteria the next day. ROC area under the curve = 0.75, 95 % confidence interval (CI) 0.64 – 0.85. Reproduced from [38].

Conclusion

The relationship between urine output and renal dysfunction is a complex one, which makes oliguria difficult to interpret in isolation. Nevertheless, definitions of oliguria have been incorporated in consensus definitions of AKI and oliguria is associated with an increased risk of death in the ICU, albeit with some inconsistencies between studies. Evidence also supports the concept that sustained oliguria occurring in the context of significant biochemical AKI is associated with worse outcomes than when urine output is maintained. However, while shorter periods of oliguria are statistically associated with the development of biochemical renal dysfunction, ability to accurately predict subsequent increases in sCr on an individual patient basis is limited. Further studies, perhaps incorporating hemodynamic data, examination of urinary sediment or novel biomarkers of renal dysfunction are required to help better interpret this widely measured, but ill understood, physiological measurement.

XV

References

1. Sharfuddin AA, Molitoris BA (2011) Pathophysiology of ischemic acute kidney injury. Nat Rev Nephrol 7: 189–200
2. Alejandro VS, Nelson WJ, Huie P, et al (1995) Postischemic injury, delayed function and Na+/K(+)-ATPase distribution in the transplanted kidney. Kidney Int 48: 1308–1315
3. Saotome T, Ishikawa K, May CN, Birchall IE, Bellomo R (2010) The impact of experimental hypoperfusion on subsequent kidney function. Intensive Care Med 36: 533–540
4. Ishikawa K, May CN, Gobe G, Langenberg C, Bellomo R (2010) Pathophysiology of septic acute kidney injury: A different view of tubular injury. Contrib Nephrol 165: 18–27
5. Bellomo R, Ronco C, Kellum JA, Mehta RL, Palevsky P (2004) Acute renal failure – definition, outcome measures, animal models, fluid therapy and information technology needs: the Second International Consensus Conference of the Acute Dialysis Quality Initiative (ADQI) Group. Crit Care 8: R204–212
6. Mehta RL, Kellum JA, Shah SV, et al (2007) Acute Kidney Injury Network: report of an initiative to improve outcomes in acute kidney injury. Crit Care 11: R31
7. Chertow GM, Burdick E, Honour M, Bonventre JV, Bates DW (2005) Acute kidney injury, mortality, length of stay, and costs in hospitalized patients. J Am Soc Nephrol 16: 3365–3370
8. Kidney Disease: Improving Global Outcomes (KDIGO) Available at: http://www.kdigo.org Accessed Nov 2011
9. Chesley LC (1938) Renal excretion at low urine volumes and the mechanism of oliguria. J Clin Invest 17: 591–597
10. Gamble JL (1946) Physiological information gained from studies of the life raft ration. Harvey Lect 42: 247–278
11. Langenberg C, Wan L, Egi M, May CN, Bellomo R (2006) Renal blood flow in experimental septic acute renal failure. Kidney Int 69: 1996–2002
12. Prowle JR, Echeverri JE, Ligabo EV, Ronco C, Bellomo R (2010) Fluid balance and acute kidney injury. Nat Rev Nephrol 6: 107–115
13. Payen D, de Pont AC, Sakr Y, et al (2008) A positive fluid balance is associated with a worse outcome in patients with acute renal failure. Crit Care 12: R74
14. Bouchard J, Soroko SB, Chertow GB, et al (2009) Fluid accumulation, survival and recovery of kidney function in critically ill patients with acute kidney injury. Kidney Int 76: 422–427
15. Brandstrup B, Tønnesen H, Beier-Holgersen R, et al (2003) Effects of intravenous fluid restriction on postoperative complications: comparison of two perioperative fluid regimens: a randomized assessor-blinded multicenter trial. Ann Surg 238: 641–648
16. Redfors B, Bragadottir G, Sellgren J, Swärd K, Ricksten SE (2010) Acute renal failure is NOT an "acute renal success"--a clinical study on the renal oxygen supply/demand relationship in acute kidney injury. Crit Care Med 38: 1695–1701
17. Bagshaw SM, Langenberg C, Bellomo R (2006) Urinary biochemistry and microscopy in septic acute renal failure: a systematic review. Am J Kidney Dis 48: 695–705
18. Bagshaw SM, Langenberg C, Wan L, May CN, Bellomo R (2007) A systematic review of urinary findings in experimental septic acute renal failure. Crit Care Med 35: 1592–1598
19. Abosaif NY, Tolba YA, Heap M, Russell J, El Nahas AM (2005) The outcome of acute renal failure in the intensive care unit according to RIFLE: model application, sensitivity, and predictability. Am J Kidney Dis 46: 1038–1048
20. Hoste EAJ, Clermont G, Kersten A, et al (2006) RIFLE criteria for acute kidney injury are associated with hospital mortality in critically ill patients: a cohort analysis. Crit Care 10: R73
21. Kuitunen A, Vento A, Suojaranta-Ylinen R, Pettila V (2006) Acute renal failure after cardiac surgery: evaluation of the RIFLE classification. Ann Thorac Surg 81: 542–546
22. Cruz DN, Bolgan I, Perazella MA, et al (2007) North East Italian Prospective Hospital Renal Outcome Survey on Acute Kidney Injury (NEiPHROS-AKI): targeting the problem with the RIFLE Criteria. Clin J Am Soc Nephrol 2: 418–425
23. Ostermann M, Chang RW (2007) Acute kidney injury in the intensive care unit according to RIFLE. Crit Care Med 35: 1837–1843

XV

24. Bagshaw SM, George C, Bellomo R, ANZICS Database Management Committe (2008) A comparison of the RIFLE and AKIN criteria for acute kidney injury in critically ill patients. Nephrol Dial Transplant 23: 1569–1574
25. Bagshaw SM, George C, Dinu I, Bellomo R (2008) A multi-centre evaluation of the RIFLE criteria for early acute kidney injury in critically ill patients. Nephrol Dial Transplant 23: 1203–1210
26. Barrantes F, Tian J, Vazquez R, Amoateng-Adjepong Y, Manthous CA (2008) Acute kidney injury criteria predict outcomes of critically ill patients. Crit Care Med 36: 1397–1403
27. Lopes JA, Fernandes P, Jorge S, et al (2008). Acute kidney injury in intensive care unit patients: a comparison between the RIFLE and the Acute Kidney Injury Network classifications. Crit Care 12: R110
28. Ostermann M, Chang R (2008) Correlation between the AKI classification and outcome. Crit Care 12: R144
29. Haase M, Bellomo R, Matalanis G, Calzavacca P, Dragun D, Haase-Fielitz A (2009) A comparison of the RIFLE and Acute Kidney Injury Network classifications for cardiac surgery-associated acute kidney injury: a prospective cohort study. J Thorac Cardiovasc Surg 138: 1370–1376
30. Joannidis M, Metnitz B, Bauer P, et al (2009) Acute kidney injury in critically ill patients classified by AKIN versus RIFLE using the SAPS 3 database. Intensive Care Med 35: 1692–1702
31. Uchino S, Bellomo R, Goldsmith D, Bates S, Ronco C (2006) An assessment of the RIFLE criteria for acute renal failure in hospitalized patients. Crit Care Med 34: 1913–1917
32. Han SS, Kang KJ, Kwon SJ, et al (2012) Additional role of urine output criterion in defining acute kidney Injury. Nephrol Dial Transplant (in press)
33. Mandelbaum T, Scott DJ, Lee J, et al (2011) Outcome of critically ill patients with acute kidney injury using the Acute Kidney Injury Network criteria. Crit Care Med 39: 2659–2664
34. Uchino S, Bellomo R, Bagshaw SM, Goldsmith D (2010) Transient azotaemia is associated with a high risk of death in hospitalized patients. Nephrol Dial Transplant 25: 1833–1839
35. Morgan DJ, KM Ho (2010) A comparison of nonoliguric and oliguric severe acute kidney injury according to the risk injury failure loss end-stage (RIFLE) criteria. Nephron Clin Pract 115: c59–65
36. Macedo E, Malhotra R, Claure-Del Granado R, Fedullo P, Mehta RL (2011) Defining urine output criterion for acute kidney injury in critically ill patients. Nephrol Dial Transplant 26: 509–515
37. Macedo E, Malhotra R, Bouchard J, Wynn SK, Mehta RL (2011) Oliguria is an early predictor of higher mortality in critically ill patients. Kidney Int 80: 760–767
38. Prowle JR, Liu YL, Licari E, et al (2011) Oliguria as predictive biomarker of acute kidney injury in critically ill patients. Crit Care 15: R172

XV

XVI Management of AKI

Fluid Overload in Heart Failure and Cardiorenal Syndrome: The "5 B" Approach

C. Ronco and W.F. Peacock

Introduction

Fluid overload is a common result of cardiovascular disease (especially heart failure) and kidney disease. The diagnosis, objective quantification, and management of this problem are integral in attempting to improve clinical outcomes, including mortality, and quality of life. Many clinical conditions lead to fluid overload, including decompensated heart failure and acute kidney injury (AKI) following the use of contrast media, the administration of nephrotoxic drugs (e.g., amphotericin B), drugs associated with precipitation of crystals (e.g., methotrexate, acyclovir), or shock due to cardiogenic, septic, or traumatic causes. Thus, the clinical challenge becomes the utilization of all currently available methods for objective measurement to determine the patient's volume status.

The term cardiorenal syndrome is used to include the vast array of interrelated derangements between the heart and kidney, and to stress the bidirectional nature of their interactions. Generally, cardiorenal syndrome is defined as a pathophysiologic disorder of either organ system, in which acute or chronic dysfunction of one may induce acute or chronic dysfunction of the other. Cardiorenal syndrome can be categorized into five subtypes that reflect the pathophysiology, time-frame, and nature of concomitant cardiac and renal dysfunction (**Table 1**). Cardiorenal syndromes are, therefore, typical conditions in which fluid overload may occur and may require specific diagnosis and management.

Table 1. Cardiorenal syndrome types

CRS Type	Pathophysiologic description
1	Abrupt worsening of cardiac function (e.g., acute cardiogenic shock or decompensated congestive heart failure) leads to acute kidney injury.
2	Chronic abnormalities in cardiac function (e.g., chronic congestive heart failure) causing progressive chronic kidney disease
3	Abrupt worsening of renal function (e.g., acute kidney ischemia or glomerulonephritis) causes acute cardiac dysfunction (e.g., heart failure, arrhythmia, ischemia)
4	Chronic kidney disease (e.g., chronic glomerular disease) contributes to decreased cardiac function, cardiac hypertrophy, and/or increased risk of adverse cardiovascular events
5	A systemic condition (e.g., sepsis) causes both cardiac and renal dysfunction

XVI

J.-L. Vincent (ed.), *Annual Update in Intensive Care and Emergency Medicine 2012*
DOI 10.1007/978-3-642-25716-2 © Springer-Verlag Berlin Heidelberg 2012

For cardiorenal syndrome type 1, the hemodynamic mechanisms underlying heart failure represent the etiologic event and compensatory mechanisms can be divided into two phases: Vasoconstriction or vasodilation. First, activation of the sympathetic nervous system, renin angiotensin aldosterone system (RAAS), vasopressin and endothelin result in decreased water and sodium excretion and, depending on the degree of renal functional impairment, increased urine concentration. To compensate, vasodilatation occurs via natriuretic peptide release, activation of the kinin-kallikrein system develops, vasodilatory prostaglandins are secreted, and endothelin relaxation factor is expressed, thus increasing water and sodium excretion. However, this second phase may be inadequate to counter the initial vasoconstrictor effects, and disease progression may occur.

When cardiac disease (or heart failure) results in renal hypoperfusion, renal medullary ischemia is the consequence. Initially functional, it ultimately results in tissue damage. Further hypoperfusion and sustained tubular-glomerular feedback will often sustain the hemodynamic effect. In such clinical situations, the important objective is the maintenance of renal blood flow. This may be accomplished by acting on cardiac output, thus maintaining intravascular volume and renal perfusion pressure. Efficient management of cardiac output requires optimization of heart rate, rhythm, preload, afterload, myocardial contractility, and if required, surgical intervention in the instance of anatomical instability. Left ventricular assist devices are considered when these approaches fail. Ultimately, knowledge of the degree of cardiac output is vital as there is no scientific case for fluid administration when the cardiac output exceeds 2.5 l/min/m^2 in patients not receiving inotropes. If the cardiac output is high and the patient is hypotensive, vasopressors, rather than fluids, are required, irrespective of central venous pressure (CVP), pulmonary artery occlusion pressure (PAOP), or right ventricular end-diastolic volume (RVEDV) levels. Vasopressors, such as norepinephrine (and dobutamine, especially in sepsis), are required. If heart failure is present, diuretics and/or extracorporeal ultrafiltration must be considered.

The "5 B" Approach

The following are five aspects of the approach to fluid overload in the context of cardio-renal syndromes, a mnemonic termed '5 B' (**Fig. 1**).

Balance of Fluids

Body volume and fluid composition must be considered. Assessment of volume status requires knowledge of all subdivisions of total body water, particularly the intravascular compartment (arterial, venous and capillary) and the interstitial compartment. Composition of the body fluid, i.e., total osmolality, the concentration of specific electrolytes, and the acid-base status must also be known. When patients first present, clinical examination, particularly of the jugular venous pressure, may help discriminate between fluid overload and hypovolemia.

Blood pressure, lying and standing if possible, hepatic enlargement, the observation of pulmonary rales or pleural effusion, and examination for peripheral edema are useful physical signs. Urinary excretion rate, its osmolality, sodium concentration, and microscopic examination may help to differentiate dehydration and AKI in the oliguric patient. Invasive monitoring, including CVP, pulmo-

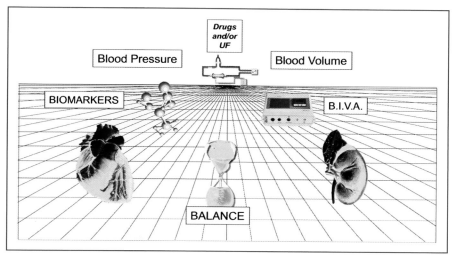

Fig. 1. The five factors included in the '5B' approach. **B**alance of fluids (reflected by body weight), **B**lood pressure, **B**iomarkers, **B**ioimpedance vector analysis (BIVA), and **B**lood volume. UF: ultrafiltration

nary arterial pressure, cardiac output, volume responsiveness, and use of echocardiography and bioimpedance contribute diagnostic information. Although the chest x-ray is useful to exclude various pathologies, and may be diagnostic in severe presentations, overall it is a blunt tool with poor sensitivity and specificity, and is even less reliable when a portable technique is used.

Whatever the initial estimate of volume is in the patient with potential or recognized AKI, continued knowledge of fluid balance is essential for successful fluid management. An accurate measure of body weight is an excellent starting point. A major benefit of the ICU environment is the ability to obtain reasonably accurate estimates of fluid balance. Challenges in obtaining vital information are obvious, even in the best circumstances. Much fluid balance information may be available only in a research environment (examples include fluid loss by respiration, insensible loss, and fecal electrolyte excretion). In the critically ill patient, accurate measurement of oral, intravenous, and fluid intake during extracorporeal therapy is countered by insensate losses, and those from the gastrointestinal tract and wound drainage are required but seldom obtained. Further, volume administration is often mismanaged by the use of a routine intravenous line through which the combination of maintenance fluids, fluids for drug administration, nutritional requirements, and therapeutic or diagnostic boluses may amount to large daily volumes. Whereas urinary excretion can usually be measured accurately, all other fluid losses are subject to gross error. 'Balance' may often be replaced by estimates of body fluid compartments. This also is difficult since much excess fluid may be in non-communicating pools ('third spacing', not directly related to the circulation). New methods of assessing tissue hydration may be useful in this context.

In practice, the approach to fluid balance is to do no harm while maintaining perfusion. In many instances, a gradual reduction in administered fluid volumes is appropriate, coupled with careful observation of vital signs. The use of diuretics to test renal responsiveness requires that the patient is at least normally

XVI

hydrated. With decreasing blood pressures in the septic patient, it may be difficult to have confidence in the volume assessment. As a consequence, large fluid volumes are often administered quickly. Although achieving a positive balance, this approach carries the potential for harm. Alternatively, excessive use of diuretics is associated with worsening renal function, as shown by creatinine increases in heart failure patients, with little clinical improvement [1]. The Ultrafiltration versus IV Diuretics for Patients Hospitalized for Acute Decompensated Congestive Heart Failure (UNLOAD) Trial [2] compared diuretic use with ultrafiltration in the management of heart failure. Ultrafiltration resulted in greater weight loss and an initial, but not later, increase in serum creatinine and fewer hospital readmissions. These data suggest that ultrafiltration results in more effective fluid removal and improvement in cardiac function. Importantly, ultrafiltration can be controlled more tightly than the use of diuretics. Diuretic administration has the defect of intermittent stimulation of the sympathetic nervous system; this effect is less with the more controllable use of ultrafiltration.

Evidence that diuretics actually improve mortality is poor, but any increase in urine production clearly facilitates fluid management. Registry data have demonstrated that earlier diuretic use decreases mortality in severe acute decompensated heart failure [3], but also the presence of a relationship between increased loop diuretic dosing and mortality [4]. Felker et al. clearly showed in patients with decompensated heart failure that use of boluses or continuous infusions of diuretics at high doses did not improve outcomes [1]. In cardiorenal syndrome type 1, the use of diuretics at inappropriate doses or frequencies, even in the less acutely ill patient, can cause sympathetic stimulation and RAAS activation that results in decreased cardiac and renal perfusion, and concomitant increases in sodium reabsorption. With the sicker patient, the hemodynamic effects of diuretics may precipitate acute cardiac ischemic insult and AKI.

The benefits of prompt action to replace fluid based on CVP and oxygen control have been emphasized. However, fluid overload in the oliguric patient can easily occur with consequent endothelial damage and added cardiac risk. In the absence of diuretic responsiveness, techniques available for fluid removal are ultrafiltration, hemofiltration, hemodialysis and hemodiafiltration. These can all be used intermittently, and the first two continuously. What are the special indications? Continuous slow ultrafiltration and hemofiltration permit the dissociation of water and salt removal by varying the combination of different removal and replacement fluids. Intermittent hemodialysis, with inappropriate choices of dialysate electrolyte concentrations or ultrafiltration rates, can result in blood volume reduction, hypotension, but paradoxically sodium loading. The response to fluid removal is dependent on rate of removal, blood volume refilling into the vascular space, cardiovascular compensation, and the initial state of body hydration. Potential errors in the estimation of fluid balance can vary from catastrophic to negligible.

XVI

An interesting approach to potential errors with the use of continuous renal replacement therapy (CRRT) machines is the prevention of a fluid balance error by altering flow. Most machines continue treatment after multiple over-ridings of the fluid balance alarm, thus creating the risk of severe injury. By analyzing the times taken for alarm occurrence, and the threshold value for fluid balance error after the alarm has been overridden, changes in software now prevent the accumulated error from exceeding 200–250 ml before the treatment is automatically stopped.

Blood Pressure

Blood pressure, as a measure of volume status, is a poor and late changing indicator. Since pressure and perfusion are linked in the physiologic range, a myriad of compensatory responses hold blood pressure constant, despite wide fluctuations in volume status. The consequences of administered medications further obscure the relationship, as does the impact of co-existing underlying pathologies. Thus, while an isolated blood pressure measurement in the expected range does not exclude the possibility of volume perturbations, an abnormal blood pressure suggests that the patient's volume status is significantly disturbed, and of a severity of sufficient magnitude to overwhelm endogenous counterbalances.

Orthostatic vital signs combine dynamic gravity-induced changes in pulse and blood pressure that occur as a consequence of volume movement resulting from postural change. Easily obtained, rapidly performed, commonly used, and non-invasive, significant changes are defined as a blood pressure decrease in excess of 10 mmHg, or a heart rate increase exceeding 20 beats per minute. Unfortunately, the results do not withstand scientific validation. In a prospective study of 132 euvolemic patients, using the standard definition of a significant change, 43 % would have been considered 'positive' [5]. In another study of 502 hospitalized geriatric patients with orthostatic vital signs obtained 3 times daily, 68 % had significant changes documented daily [6]. Clearly, orthostatic vital signs changes are non-specific. Conversely, in a systematic review [7] evaluating blood loss, the most helpful findings were postural dizziness to the extent that it prevented upright vital signs, or a postural pulse increase exceeding 30 beats/min. Unfortunately, the sensitivity for moderate blood loss with either of these predictors was only 22 %. Only when blood loss exceeded 1 liter did the sensitivity and specificity improve to 97 and 98 %, respectively.

Biomarkers

There are many contenders for diagnostic and prognostic biomarker indicators of acute and chronic injury occurring in cardiorenal syndrome type 1. The most frequently used heart failure markers are the natriuretic peptides. Knowledge of the B-type natriuretic peptide (BNP) level, a hormone produced by the myocardium in response to pressure or volume stress, can assist in differentiating heart failure from other causes of dyspnea [8] Natriuretic peptides are initially synthesized as the precursor protein, pro-BNP, which is then cleaved by the enzyme, corin, into the inactive metabolite N-terminal, proBNP (NTproBNP), and the biologically active BNP that causes both vasodilation and natriuresis.

Natriuretic peptides can be measured clinically. If elevated (> 900 pg/ml NTproBNP, or > 400 pg/ml BNP), early treatment may be considered as the positive predictive value for acute heart failure is in the range of 90 %. Alternatively, a low natriuretic peptide level (< 300 pg/ml NTproBNP, or 100 pg/ml BNP) suggests an alternative diagnosis, as the negative predictive values approximate 90 %. Levels between the paired cutpoints define a gray zone (300 to 900 pg/ml for NTproBNP, and 100 to 400 pg/ml for BNP) in which diagnostic certainty is unclear and additional testing is suggested [9] (Fig. 2).

Natriuretic peptides have several limitations. As any myocardial stress (e.g., myocardial infarction) may cause elevated natriuretic peptides, it is important to consider the clinical scenario when interpreting results. Furthermore, non-heart

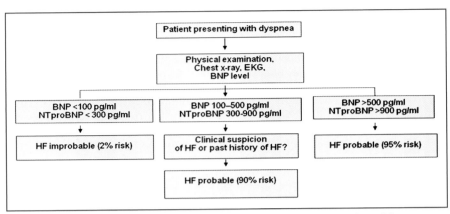

Fig. 2. B-natriuretic peptide (BNP) Consensus Guidelines. Adapted from [9]. HF: heart failure

failure elevations of natriuretic peptide occur with renal insufficiency, where levels increase in proportion to the severity of renal injury [10]. Even with the absence of heart failure, natriuretic peptide levels are 8 to 40-fold higher in chronic kidney disease (CKD) than in normal individuals [11, 12]. Some researchers have suggested that the BNP cut-off point for heart failure should be doubled in the setting of renal insufficiency. Finally, another natriuretic peptide confounder is obesity, as an inverse relationship between natriuretic peptide levels and body mass exists [13]. It has been suggested that if the body mass index (BMI) is > 35, the measured BNP should be doubled to improve the sensitivity for heart failure.

The clinical impact of BNP testing has been evaluated in the 1586 patient prospective Breathing Not Properly study [14], which found that the accuracy of clinical judgment without BNP was 74 %, improving to 81.5 % if BNP results were also considered. Similar findings have been demonstrated with NTproBNP [15].

In addition to diagnostic utility, BNP has prognostic ability to identify patients with a heart failure mortality risk. In a 50,000 patient analysis of the Acute Decompensated Heart Failure Registry (ADHERE), an elevated BNP was associated with a marked increase in acute mortality [16]. Acute mortality was 6 % in patients with a BNP in the highest quartile at presentation (BNP > 1730 pg/ml) versus 2.2 % in those in the lowest quartile (BNP < 430 pg/ml).

Kidney injury biomarkers have been clearly divided into those useful as indicators for diagnosis of AKI, for cell damage, and for the diagnosis of cell death (serum creatinine and blood urea nitrogen [BUN] increase). Unfortunately, BUN and creatinine are extremely late indicators of renal injury. Neutrophil gelatinase–associated lipocalin (NGAL), combined with BNP, is probably the indicator for which there is the most evidence of successful use in the diagnosis of acute cardio-renal syndrome type 1. NGAL is a member of the lipocalin protein family. Normally produced by kidney tubule cells, it is secreted into the urine and serum at low levels. However, the synthesis of NGAL increases dramatically after ischemic, septic, or toxic injury of the kidneys [17–23]

Evidence from experimental and human studies indicates that urinary NGAL is derived from increased synthesis and release from the distal nephron as a rapid response to AKI, previously referred to as acute renal failure [4–7]. The utility of

XVI

NGAL as a novel serum or urine biomarker of AKI has been studied in post-cardiac surgery [7], cardiac catheterization, after contrast-induced nephropathy (CIN) [6], hemolytic uremic syndrome, and kidney transplantation [17, 24–28], CKD secondary to autoimmune disease [29], polycystic and proteinuric diseases [30–32]. In these areas, NGAL has been shown to be a useful, sensitive, specific, non-invasive, and highly predictive biomarker for AKI.

BNP levels may provide early evidence of fluid overload, followed by NGAL as indicating renal damage. Both measurements can be performed at the bedside, using point of care equipment.

Bioimpedance

Bioimpedance vector analysis (BIVA) is a non-invasive beside volume assessment technique that can be performed within minutes. BIVA is based on the electrical principle that the body is a circuit with a given resistance (opposition of current flow through intra- and extracellular solutions) and reactance (the capacitance of cells to store energy). With BIVA, total body water (TBW) may be measured by placing a pair of electrodes on the dorsum of the wrist and ipsilateral ankle, then applying a 50 kHz current to the body. BIVA is graphically displayed so that relative hydration is depicted as vector length. Shorter vectors are associated with volume overload, while longer vectors equate to volume depletion.

BIVA is an excellent indicator of total body water. Reports indicate it has a strong correlation with the gold standard volume assessment technique of deuterium dilution (r > 0.99) [33]. Clinically, BIVA has been used to determine both volume depletion [34] and volume overload in heart failure [35], kidney failure [36], and liver disease [37]. It is superior for diagnosing volume overload as compared to anthropometric measurements, with a sensitivity of 88 % and specificity of 87 % for detecting edema [38]. Further, BIVA is able to identify volume overloaded states in diverse populations. In 217 renal patients, BIVA accurately differentiated edematous and normovolemic populations [39].

BIVA is not confounded by obesity, a common challenge for volume assessment. In 540 obese (BMI > 31 kg/m^2), 726 non-obese (BMI< 31 kg/m^2) and 50 edematous renal patients, BIVA was 91 % accurate for discriminating between edematous and obese patients [40]. Subsequent caloric restriction for 1 month found no vector change, but volume removal was associated with vector lengthening. Ultimately, in critical care environments, where rapid accurate and objective results are needed, BIVA's ease and speed may provide opportunities for improved patient care.

Clinically, BIVA has been used to diagnose and guide therapy. In one study, BIVA was used to determine the adequacy of ultrafiltration in > 3000 hemodialysis patients [41]. Short vector lengths corresponded to greater soft tissue hydration (less adequate ultrafiltration). Defining a vector length of 300–350 ohm/m as the reference category, the risk of death was approximately 50 % and 180 % higher for those with inadequate volume removal as reflected by BIVA vector lengths of 200–250 and < 200 ohm/m, respectively.

Combining BIVA with a natriuretic peptide may provide both biomarker and physical evidence concerning fluid overload. One prospective study evaluated the diagnostic value of the use of BIVA and BNP measurements in 292 dyspneic patients [42]. Regression analysis found that while whole body BIVA was a strong predictor of acute decompensated heart failure (area under the receiver operating

XVI

characteristic curve [AUROC] 0.934, SE 0.016), with similar accuracy to BNP (AUROC 0.970, SE 0.008). The most accurate volume status determination was with a combination of BIVA and BNP (AUROC 0.989, SE 0.005), for which the combined accuracy exceeded that of either BNP or BIVA alone.

The combination of BNP and BIVA may assist in guiding acute heart failure therapy. In 186 hospitalized heart failure patients [43], serial BNP and BIVA were used to monitor diuretic induced body fluid changes. The combination of improved BIVA parameters and a discharge BNP of < 250 pg/ml predicted successful management. A follow-up study then demonstrated that in 166 hospitalized heart failure patients discharged by a BNP level and BIVA, there was improved morbidity compared to 149 patients discharged based on clinical acumen alone [44]. Patients assessed with BNP and BIVA had lower 6-month readmissions (23 % vs. 35 %, p = 0.02) and lower overall cost of care. Thus, the combination of clinical acumen and objective measures may improve outcomes compared to clinical impression alone.

Blood Volume

Because RRT may result in large volume changes, concomitant blood pressure measurement during the use of convective removal techniques, in addition to BIVA and BNP, increases safety. Reduction in blood volume with ultrafiltration continuing at the same rate throughout the therapy results in hypotension with the possibility of myocardial stunning and increases the potential for arrhythmia. Continuous blood volume assessment indicates the need to slow ultrafiltration rates to reduce marked changes in blood volume. Although there are uncertainties, there is little evidence that changes in blood pressure provide the same accuracy of information concerning degree of fluid load as does BIVA.

Conclusion

Consideration of the 5 B approach presents a pathway for assessing the appropriate degree of hydration and the determination of a neutral fluid balance in patients with cardioenal syndromes. This approach combines clinical judgment, biomarkers, technology, and precise nursing to achieve the best outcome for patients in heart failure associated with fluid overload and varying degrees of renal dysfunction.

Acknowledgement: We are grateful to Nathan Levin and Linda Donalds for the precious help in the preparation of the manuscript.

References

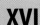

1. Felker GM, Lee KL, Bull DA, et al (2011) Diuretic strategies in patients with acute decompensated heart failure. N Engl J Med 364: 797–805
2. Costanzo MR, Guglin ME, Saltzberg MT, et al (2007) Ultrafiltration vs intravenous diuretics for patients hospitalized for acute decompensated heart failure. J Am Coll Cardiol 49: 675–683
3. Maisel AS, Peacock WF, McMullin N, et al (2008) Timing of immunoreactive B-type Natriuretic Peptide levels and treatment delay in acute decompensated heart failure. J Am Coll Cardiol 52: 534–540

4. Peacock WF, Costanzo MR, DeMarco T, et al (2009) Impact of intravenous loop diuretics on outcomes of patients hospitalized with acute decompensated heart failure: Insights from the ADHERE Registry. Cardiology 113: 12–19
5. Koziol-McLain J, Lowenstein S, Fuller B (1991) Orthostatic vital signs in emergency department patients. Ann Emerg Med 20: 606–610
6. Weiss A, Grossman E, Beloosesky Y, Grinblat J (2002) Orthostatic hypotension in acute geriatric ward – is it a consistent finding? Arch Intern Med 162: 2369–2374
7. McGee S, Abernethy WB III, Simel DL (1999) Is this patient hypovolemic? JAMA 281: 1022–1029
8. Dao Q, Krishnaswamy P, Kazanegra R, et al (2001) Utility of B-type natriuretic peptide in the diagnosis of congestive heart failure in an urgent-care setting. J Am Coll Cardiol 37: 379–385
9. Silver MA, Maisel A, Yancy CW, et al (2004) A clinical approach for the diagnostic, prognostic, screening, treatment monitoring, and therapeutic roles of natriuretic peptides in cardiovascular disease. Congestive Heart Fail 10 (5 Suppl 3): 1–30
10. McCullough PA, Duc P, Omland T, et al (2003) B-type natriuretic peptide and renal function in the diagnosis of heart failure: an analysis from the Breathing Not Properly Multinational Study. Am J Kidney Dis 41: 571–519
11. Buckley MG, Sethi D, Markandu ND, et al (1992) Plasma concentrations and comparisons of brain natriuretic peptide and atrial natriuretic peptide in normal subjects, cardiac transplant recipients and patients with dialysis-independent or dialysis-dependent chronic renal failure. Clin Sci (Lond) 83: 437–444
12. Kohse KP, Feifel K, Mayer-Wehrstein R (1993) Differential regulation of brain and atrial natriuretic peptides in hemodialysis patients. Clin Nephrol 40: 83–90
13. McCord J, Mundy BJ, Hudson MP, et al (2004) Relationship between obesity and B-type natriuretic peptide levels. Arch Intern Med 164: 2247–2252
14. Maisel AS, Krishnaswamy P, Nowak RM, et al (2002) Rapid measurement of B-type natriuretic peptide in the emergency diagnosis of heart failure. N Engl J Med 347: 161–167
15. Januzzi JL, Camargo CA, Anwaruddin S, et al (2005) The N-terminal Pro-BNP Investigation of Dyspnea in the Emergency department (PRIDE) study. Am J Cardiol 95: 948–954
16. Fonarow GC, Peacock WF, Phillips CO, Givertz MM, Lopatin M, for the ADHERE Scientific Advisory Committee and Investigators (2007) Admission B-type natriuretic peptide levels and in-hospital mortality in acute decompensated heart failure. J Am Coll Cardiol 49: 1943–1950
17. Supavekin S, Zhang W, Kucherlapati R, Kaskel FJ, Moore LC, Devarajan P (2003) Differential gene expression following early renal ischemia/reperfusion. Kidney Int 63: 1714–1724
18. Mishra J, Mori K, Ma Q, Kelly C, Barasch J, Devarajan P (2004) Neutrophil gelatinase-associated lipocalin: a novel early urinary biomarker for cisplatin nephrotoxicity. Am J Nephrol 24: 307–315
19. Mori K, Lee HT, Rapoport D, et al (2005) Endocytic delivery of lipocalin-siderophore-iron complex rescues the kidney from ischemia-reperfusion injury. J Clin Invest 115: 610–621
20. Schmidt-Ott KM, Mori K, Li JY, et al (2007) Dual action of neutrophil gelatinase-associated lipocalin. J Am Soc Nephrol 18: 407–413
21. Mori K, Nakao K (2007) Neutrophil gelatinase-associated lipocalin as the real-time indicator of active kidney damage. Kidney Int 71: 967–970
22. Hirsch R, Dent C, Pfriem H, et al (2007) NGAL is an early predictive biomarker of contrast-induced nephropathy in children. Pediatr Nephrol 22: 2089–2095
23. Mishra J, Dent C, Tarabishi R, et al (2005) Neutrophil gelatinase-associated lipocalin (NGAL) as a biomarker for acute renal injury after cardiac surgery. Lancet 365: 1231–1238
24. Kusaka M, Kuroyanagi Y, Mori T, et al (2008) Serum neutrophil gelatinase-associated lipocalin as a predictor of organ recovery from delayed graft function after kidney transplantation from donors after cardiac death. Cell Transplant 17: 129–134
25. Bachorzewska-Gajewska H, Malyszko J, Sitniewska E, Malyszko JS, Dobrzycki S (2006) Neutrophil-gelatinase-associated lipocalin and renal function after percutaneous coronary interventions. Am J Nephrol 26: 287–292
26. Bachorzewska-Gajewska H, Malyszko J, Sitniewska E, et al (2008) NGAL (neutrophil gelatinase-associated lipocalin) and cystatin C: are they good predictors of contrast nephropa-

thy after percutaneous coronary interventions in patients with stable angina and normal serum creatinine? Int J Cardiol 127: 290–291

27. Trachtman H, Christen E, Cnaan A, et al (2006) Urinary neutrophil gelatinase-associated lipocalcin in D+HUS: a novel marker of renal injury. Pediatr Nephrol 21: 989–994

28. Wagener G, Jan M, Kim M, et al (2006) Association between increases in urinary neutrophil gelatinase-associated lipocalin and acute renal dysfunction after adult cardiac surgery. Anesthesiology 105: 485–491

29. Brunner HI, Mueller M, Rutherford C, et al (2006) Urinary neutrophil gelatinase-associated lipocalin as a biomarker of nephritis in childhood-onset systemic lupus erythematosus. Arthritis Rheum 54: 2577–2584

30. Bolignano D, Coppolino G, Campo S, et al (2007) Neutrophil gelatinase-associated lipocalin in patients with autosomal-dominant polycystic kidney disease. Am J Nephrol 27: 373–378

31. Bolignano D, Coppolino G, Campo S, et al (2008) Urinary neutrophil gelatinase-associated lipocalin (NGAL) is associated with severity of renal disease in proteinuric patients. Nephrol Dial Transplant 23: 414–416

32. Ding H, He Y, Li K, et al (2007) Urinary neutrophil gelatinase-associated lipocalin (NGAL) is an early biomarker for renal tubulointerstitial injury in IgA nephropathy. Clin Immunol 123: 227–234

33. Kushner RF, Schoeller DA, Fjeld CR, et al (1992) Is the impedance index (ht2/R) significant in predicting total body water? Am J Clin Nutr 56: 835–839

34. Ackland GL, Singh-Ranger D, Fox S, et al (2004) Assessment of preoperative fluid depletion using bioimpedance analysis. Br J Anaesth 92: 134–136

35. Uszko-Lencer NH, Bothmer F, van Pol PE, et al (2006) Measuring body composition in chronic heart failure: a comparison of methods. Eur J Heart Fail 8: 208–214

36. Piccoli A, Rossi B, Pillon L, et al (1994) A new method for monitoring body fluid variation by bioimpedance analysis: the RXc graph. Kidney Int 46: 534–539

37. Panella C, Guglielmi FW, Mastronuzzi T, et al (1995) Whole-body and segmental bioelectrical parameters in chronic liver disease: effect of gender and disease stages. Hepatology 21: 352–358

38. Piccoli A (2004) Bioelectric impedance vector distribution in peritoneal dialysis patients with different hydration status. Kidney Int 65: 1050–1063

39. Piccoli A, Rossi B, Pillon L, et al (1996) Body fluid overload and bioelectrical impedance analysis in renal patients. Miner Electrolyte Metab 22: 76–78

40. Piccoli A, Brunani A, Savia G, et al (1998) Discriminating between body fat and fluid changes in the obese adult using bioimpedance vector analysis. Int J Obes Relat Metab Disord 22: 97–104

41. Pillon L, Piccoli A, Lowrie EG, et al (2004) Vector length as a proxy for the adequacy of ultrafiltration in hemodialysis. Kidney Int 66: 1266–1271

42. Parrinello G, Paterna S, Di Pasquale P, et al (2008) The usefulness of bioelectrical impedance analysis in differentiating dyspnea due to decompensated heart failure. J Card Fail 14: 676–686

43. Valle R, Aspromonte N, Giovinazzo P, et al (2008) B-type natriuretic Peptide-guided treatment for predicting outcome in patients hospitalized in sub-intensive care unit with acute heart failure. J Card Fail 14: 219–224

44. Valle R, Aspromonte N, Carbonieri E, et al (2008) Fall in readmission rate for heart failure after implementation of B-type natriuretic peptide testing for discharge decision: a retrospective study. Int J Cardiol 126: 400–406

Coupled Plasma Filtration-adsorption

G. Berlot, A. Tomasini, and A. Agbedjro

Introduction

In the past 25 years, various techniques have been developed to remove endo-toxin and/or the sepsis mediators produced and released during the interaction between the host and the infecting agent [1]. The rationale of this approach is based on the hypothesis that a reduction in the blood concentration of these compounds should determine a gradient favoring the elimination of these sub-stances from the target cells [2]. All the techniques used so far are based on the passage of the blood through an extracorporeal circuit containing one or more filters that are supposed to exert their depurative effects either via the elimination of these substances or by sticking them on their surface. The first approach takes advantage of the membranes normally used during continuous renal replacement treatment (CRRT) for the treatment of acute kidney injury (AKI), the cut-off val-ues of which are high enough to allow elimination of medium-high molecular weight (MW) mediators; to this aim, different blood flows (Qb) and ultrafiltrate flows (Qf) have been and are currently used. A second approach consists of use of plasma exchange, aimed at removing of one or more volumes of plasma, which is replaced with colloids, albumin or fresh frozen plasma (FFP) [3]. The third option uses some physico-chemical properties of the membranes, which can adsorb endotoxin or other substances on their surface: A typical example is the binding of polymixin B or other substances with elevated affinity for endotoxin to a membrane inserted in an extracorporeal circuit [4]; the elimination of endo-toxin from the bloodstream and from the tissues is supposed to blunt the over-whelming inflammatory response associated with Gram -ve infections.

A more recent approach is coupled plasma filtration-adsorption (CPFA) [5], which represents a combination of the three techniques described above, being

Box 1. Substances that are/are not adsorbed by coupled plasma filtration-adsorption (CPFA). (Source: Bellco Laboratories, Mirandola, Italy)

Adsorbed by CPFA
Interleukin (IL)-1α, IL-5, IL-6, IL-7, IL-8, IL-10, IL-12, IL-16, IL-18, macrophage inflammatory protein (MIP)-α, MIP-β, TNF-α, monocyte chemotactic protein-1, C-reactive protein (CRP), vascular endo-thelial growth factor

Not Adsorbed by CPFA
Procalcitonin, heparin, citrate, endotoxin

Unknown
Drotrecogin alfa activated (DAA), immunoglobulins

J.-L. Vincent (ed.), *Annual Update in Intensive Care and Emergency Medicine 2012*
DOI 10.1007/978-3-642-25716-2 © Springer-Verlag Berlin Heidelberg 2012

based on: (a) The removal of plasma by a plasma filter; (b) its subsequent processing inside a cartridge containing a synthetic resin (Amberchrome®) able to adsorb different sepsis mediators (**Box 1**); and (c) its final reinfusion upstream of a CRRT filter (**Figs. 1** and **2**). During CPFA, the adsorptive capabilities of the resin are time-limited, but the CRRT can continue even beyond their exhaustion with no need to change the extracorporeal circuit. In contrast to plasma exchange, the patient's plasma is not discarded, thus making transfusion of FFP unnecessary and abolishing the risk of transmissible diseases, fluid overload or transfusional reactions. CPFA is increasingly used in many intensive care units (ICU) on the basis of experimental and clinical evidence of its effectiveness in the treatment of critically ill septic patients.

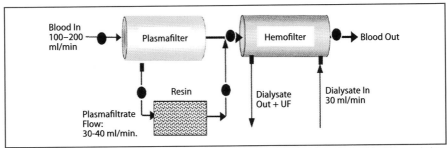

Fig. 1. Scheme of the coupled plasma filtration and adsorption (CPFA) system. From [5] with permission

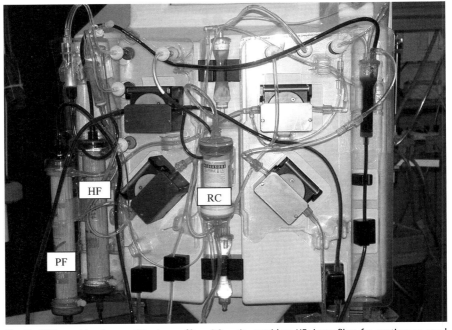

Fig. 2. CPFA machine in use. PF: plasma filter; RC: resin cartridge; HF: hemofilter for continuous renal replacement therapy (CRRT)

XVI

Experimental Studies

Several experimental studies have been performed to address the effects of CPFA in terms of types and amount of mediators removed and amelioration of sepsis-induced changes of biological variables. A preliminary *in vitro* study [6], using outdated blood challenged with *Escherichia coli* endotoxin, evaluated the blood purification capabilities of different sorbents compared with ultrafiltration alone and demonstrated that: (a) the sorbents were superior to ultrafiltration in terms of removal of several cytokines, including tumor necrosis factor-α (TNF-α), interleukin-1β (IL-1), IL-1 receptor antagonist (IL-1ra) and IL-8; (b) these effects persisted at different Qb; and (c) the decrease in the considered cytokines was related to the sorbent used, being better with the Amberchrome® than with the others.

As demonstrated by Tetta et at. [7], rabbits given intravenous lipopolysaccharide (LPS) and treated with CPFA had better outcomes compared to animals in whom the plasma was removed and subsequently reinfused downstream without passing through the resin; moreover, although there were no significant differences in blood LPS levels between treated and control rabbits, survivors of both groups had reduced peak LPS levels at 60 minutes after the infusion. This effect appears particularly surprising, as LPS is not absorbed by the resin used in CPFA. In the CPFA group, TNF-α bioactivity measured in the blood before and after the cartridge decreased sharply already after one hour of treatment although this decrease was highly variable among different animals. However, other investigators failed to demonstrate a beneficial effect of CPFA. Sykora et al. [8] randomly assigned a group of pigs to CPFA or to control 12 hours after the onset of septic shock caused by peritoneal injection of a feces solution: in contrast with the other study, the authors did not observe any beneficial effect of this procedure on the different variables considered, which included renal and intestinal mucosal microcirculations and markers of endothelial injury and of systemic inflammation.

Clinical Experience

A small number of investigations involving a limited number of patients have evaluated the effects of CPFA on some relevant clinical variables. In a randomized cross-over study, a group of septic shock patients needing norepinephrine to maintain an adequate arterial pressure were treated alternatively with CPFA or continuous veno-venous hemodiafiltration (CVVHDF): The authors observed a decrease in the administration of norepinephrine, which was used as a proxy of hemodynamic improvement, during CPFA but not during CVVHD [9]. Moreover, CPFA was associated with some immunological changes, since (a) normal monocytes challenged with LPS and incubated with plasma drawn upstream of the cartridge produced less TNF than when they were incubated with healthy plasma, and (b) leukocytes of patients treated with CPFA had restored immune capabilities, which were severely depressed before the treatment. Lentini et al. [10] also observed a marked reduction in vasopressor needs in a group of septic shock patients treated with CPFA alternated with continuous pulse high-volume hemofiltration (CHVHF), but there were no significant changes between the two treatments in terms of percentage of change in the administration of vasopressors. Improvement in cardiovascular and respiratory functions has also been described

XVI

in a multicenter study involving 55 severe sepsis and septic shock patients treated with CPFA [11]. Interestingly, the hemodynamic improvement seems to at least partly vanish during CPFA off-time. In a group of 12 septic shock patients, Formica et al. [12] observed an improvement in the cardiac index and the PaO_2/FiO_2 ratio during CPFA; however, both variables tended to return to the baseline during inter-treatment intervals, indicating that the beneficial effects of the procedure tend to fade between treatments. This saw-tooth attitude was also described by Berlot et al. [13], who, using the orthogonal polarization spectral (OPS) imaging technique, observed similar changes in the sublingual microvascular network in a septic shock patient undergoing CPFA: The improvement in blood flow in the absence of any change in hemodynamic support was evident from the first hours after initiation of the procedure but it declined without reaching the initial values after its termination. This pattern of change of the sublingual microvascular blood flow strictly resembles the picture described by De Backer et al. [14] in a group of patients with severe sepsis treated with recombinant human activated protein C (drotrecogin-α activated, DAA): In this study, an improvement in the sublingual microvascular perfusion demonstrated with the OPS was present already 4 hours after the initiation of the DAA but decreased after the end of the infusion.

Unresolved Issues

Not dissimilar to what happened for the multiple modalities of CRRT used for renal and non-renal indications in critically ill patients, use of CPFA raises several relevant clinical questions. First, when should it be initiated? The guidelines of the Surviving Sepsis Campaign (SSC) [15] cast much emphasis on the relative narrow window of opportunity for most treatments to be maximally effective, including the early administration of antibiotics, hemodynamic stabilization, etc. Probably because of the lack of studies fulfilling evidence-based medicine (EBM) criteria, in the same guidelines only a few words are dedicated to the non-renal indications of CRRT, limiting their use to the treatment of AKI. However, despite the relative paucity of large, randomized controlled trials, a recent meta-analysis [16] demonstrated that early initiation of RRT in patients with AKI was associated with a better outcome. Similar considerations apply for other measures adopted in septic patients which are not yet included in the SSC recommendations. Administration of an immunoglobulin M (IgM) preparation has been demonstrated to be associated with a reduction in mortality of patients with severe sepsis and septic shock and to be cost-effective [17, 18]; moreover, its efficacy is maximal if given in the first hours after the occurrence of severe sepsis and septic shock [19]. It is likely that the same consideration applies for CPFA but the number of published studies so far does not allow for an occlusive indication.

XVI

Second, how should the efficacy of CPFA be monitored? In the published clinical studies, the initiation of this procedure has been associated with a reduced need for vasopressors. This seems be an easy-to-perform practical approach, because the measurement of other markers, including C-reactive protein (CRP) and procalcitonin (PCT) is unreliable, as the former is removed by the sorbent and the latter is eliminated through the CRRT filter because of its low MW [20]. To overcome this problem, in our center we measure blood PCT concentrations immediately before the initiation of the next CPFA session, after a 12-hour treatment-free interval. The same variables may also be suited to indicate how many sessions are required; in our practice, fast-responding patients are treated for three days whereas five procedures are performed in those subjects whose blood PCT values or cardiorespiratory conditions do not improve in this interval.

Third, CPFA is only a part of the multifaceted treatment of septic patients: The above quoted negative results presented by Sykora et al. [8] who observed a detrimental effect of CPFA in fecal peritonitis-induced septic shock pigs must be likely ascribed to the delay in the treatment, which was initiated as long as twelve hours after the onset of peritonitis, and to the failure to drain the peritonitis. In other terms, neither CPFA nor other sophisticated procedures can replace an appropriate surgical approach when indicated.

Finally, how can CPFA influence other treatments commonly used in critically ill septic patients, including the administration of DAA and IgM? Presently there is no information concerning the binding of these substances to the sorbent used. In our center, in which IgM preparations are part of the standard approach to the treatment of septic patients, they are administered during the interval between two consecutive procedures.

Conclusion

Despite the relatively few experimental and clinical studies that have been published, CPFA is increasingly used in the treatment of patients with severe sepsis and septic shock. Its use has been associated with the improvement of several variables deranged by the action of sepsis mediators. Its beneficial effects can likely be ascribed to this removal, as these changes tend to worsen during CPFA-free intervals. Optimal timing of initiation, monitoring and the number of sessions remain unclear.

References

1. Rimmelè T, Kellum JA (2011) Clinical review: blood purification for sepsis. Crit Care 15: 205–215
2. Honorè PM (2004) Extracorporeal removal for sepsis: acting at the tissue level: the beginning of a new era for this treatment modality in septic shock. Crit Care Med 32: 896–897
3. Berlot G, Di Capua G, Nosella P, Rocconi S, Thomann C (2004) Plasmapheresis in sepsis. Contr Nephrol 144: 387–394
4. Davies B, Davies J (2010) Endotoxin removal devices for the treatment of sepsis and septic shock. Lancet Infect Dis 11: 65–71
5. Bellomo R, Tetta C, Ronco C (2003) Coupled plasma filtration adsorption. Intensive Care Med 29: 1222–1228
6. Tetta C, Cavaillon JM, Schulze M, et al (1998) Removal of cytokines and complement componenst in experimental model of continuous plasma filtration coupled with sorbent adsorption. Nephrol Dial Transplant 13: 1458–1464
7. Tetta C, Gianotti L, Cavaillon JM, et al (2000) Coupled plasmafiltration-adsorption in a rabbit model of endotoxic shock. Crit Care Med 28: 1526–1533
8. Sykora R, Chvojka J, Krouzecky A, et al (2009) Coupled plasma filtration and adsorption in experimental peritonitis-induced septic shock. Shock 31: 473–480
9. Ronco C, Brendolan A, Lonneman NG, et al (2002) A randomized cross-over study of coupled plasmafiltration-with adsorption in septic shock. Crit Care Med 30: 1250–1255
10. Lentini P, Cruz D, Nalesso F, et al (2009) [A pilot study comparing pulse high volume hemofiltration (pHVHF) and coupled plasma filtration adsorption (CPFA) in septic shock patients]. G Ital Nefr 26: 695–703

XVI

11. Turani F, Falco M, Natoli S, Leonardis F, et al (2010) Coupled plasma filtration and adsorption in septic shock: a multicentric experience. Crit Care 14 (Suppl 1): P412 (abst)
12. Formica M, Olivieri C, Livigni S, et al (2003) Hemodynamic response to coupled plasma-filtration-adsorption in human septic shock. Intensive Care Med 29: 703–708
13. Berlot G, Bianco N, Tomasini A, Vassallo MC, Bianco F (2011) Changes in microvascular blood flow during couple plasma filtration and adsorption. Anesth Intensive Care 39: 687–689
14. De Backer D, Verdant C, Chierego M, Gullo A, Vincent JL (2006) Effects of drotrecogin alpha activated on microcirculatory alteration in patients with severe sepsis. Crit Care Med 34: 1919–1924
15. Dellinger RP, Levy MM, Carlet JM, et al (2008) Surviving Sepsis Campaign: International guidelines for management of severe sepsis and septic shock: 2008. Intensive Care Med 34: 17–60
16. Karvellas CJ, Farhat MR, Sajjad I, Morgensen SS, leuna AA, Wald R, Bagshaw SM (2011) A comparison of early versus late initiation of renal replacement therapy in critically ill patients with acute kidney injury: a systematic review and meta-analysis. Crit Care 15: R72
17. Turgeon AF, Hutton B, Fergusson DA, et al (2007) Meta-analysis: intravenous immunoglobulin in critically ill adult patients with sepsis. Ann Intern Med 146: 193–203
18. Neilson AR, Burchardi H, Schneider H (2005) Cost-effectiveness of immunoglobulin M-enriched immunoglobulin (Pentaglobin) in the treatment of severe sepsis and septic shock. J Crit Care 20: 239–250
19. Berlot G, Vassallo MC, Busetto N, et al (2012) Relationship between the timing of administration of IgM and IgA-enriched immunoglobulins in patients with severe sepsis and septic shock and the outcome: a retrospective analysis. J Crit Care (in press)
20. Dahaba AA, El-Awadi GA, Rehak PH, List WF (2002) Procalcitonin and proinflammatory cytokine clearance during continuous venovenous haemofiltration in septic patients. Anaesth Intensive Care 30: 269–274

XVI

XVII Nutrition

Best Timing for Energy Provision during Critical Illness

M.M. Berger and C. Pichard

Introduction

Malnutrition is a persistent problem in hospitals and intensive care units (ICUs) worldwide. Critically ill patients quickly develop malnutrition or aggravate a pre-existing malnutrition because of the inflammatory response, metabolic stress and bed rest, which all cause catabolism [1, 2]. The persistence of this problem despite existing guidelines, is partly explained by the absence of immediately visible consequences of acute malnutrition: Deleterious consequences are not easily measurable and become obvious only after 7 – 14 days, i.e., frequently after discharge from the ICU. Nevertheless, after a week already, new infections may be attributable to incipient malnutrition [3, 4]. In contrast, the biological consequences of insufficient oxygen delivery are immediate, requiring the ICU team's rapid attention. This longer time constant between event and consequence is one of the important reasons why nutritional therapy is so frequently forgotten early on, resulting in progression of energy deficits, in turn associated with impaired outcome.

Confusion has arisen in recent years among ICU specialists because of the publication of conflicting results about the respective merits of hypo- and hypercaloric feeding [5]. Indeed, some studies suggest that feeding the critically ill patient is deleterious in terms of glycemic control and clinical outcome [6 – 8], whereas other trials confirm that acute malnutrition causes complications and increases mortality at levels of energy deficit that are current in clinical practice [2, 3, 9 – 11].

The principal issue appears to be the need to be able to prescribe within the first 24 – 48 hours an optimal and individualized energy and protein target, and to monitor achievement of this goal.

How Do We Define Nutritional Requirements?

Prediction of the optimal energy target is relatively difficult in critically ill patients because of the high variability in resting energy expenditure during the course of severe illness as a result of alterations induced by shock, sedation, fever, reduction of lean body mass, surgical procedures, etc. A reasonable prediction requires knowledge of the accurate pre-illness weight and body height, but this information is frequently missing. When an actual body weight is available, it is generally inaccurate as a result of fluid accumulation following resuscitation. The actual weight is also frequently increased by excess fat mass, which nobody wants to feed (**Fig. 1**).

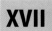

XVII

J.-L. Vincent (ed.), *Annual Update in Intensive Care and Emergency Medicine 2012*
DOI 10.1007/978-3-642-25716-2 © Springer-Verlag Berlin Heidelberg 2012

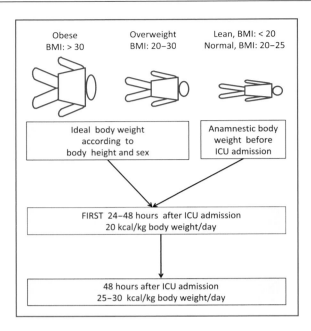

Fig. 1. Actual body weight is usually artificially increased by the expansion of body water (i.e., fluid administration, stress-related water retention). Therefore, it is recommended that energy requirements are calculated based on the anamnestic body weight for lean or normal weight patients (body mass index [BMI] = [body weight/(body height)²]) and the ideal body weight for overweight and obese patients (BMI ≥ 20).

Guidelines recommend that energy expenditure be measured on an individual basis by indirect calorimetry. The underlying physiological principle is that calculation of energy expenditure from the measurement of oxygen consumption (VO₂) and carbon dioxide production (VCO₂) reflects the energy needs at the cellular level. The essential assumption is that under steady state conditions, respiratory gas exchange is in equilibrium with gas exchange within the mitochondria, thus indirectly measuring oxidative phosphorylation. Energy requirements are then extrapolated using the Weir equation [12]:

Total energy = 3.9 liters of O_2 used + 1.1 liters CO_2 produced

The limitations and obstacles to measurements in clinical settings are those impeaching stable conditions: Change in vasoactive drugs, an inspired oxygen fraction (FiO₂)> 60 %, fever with shivering, an abnormal pH, CO_2 retention, patient movement, leaks in the system, and the use of nitric oxide (NO) [13].

This technique is relatively time-consuming and expensive. Indirect calorimetry, despite being the gold standard for determination of energy expenditure, remains unavailable in the vast majority of ICUs [14]. Inclusion of an indirect calorimeter in modern ventilators would represent a major technical advance. Another problem is that energy expenditure varies over time. Measurement at one time point can be very different from total 24-hour energy expenditure; the latter can be measured using the double-labeled water method [15–17]. This technique is based on the assumption that ingested double-labeled water (^2H_2O and $H_2^{18}O$) is distributed rapidly and homogeneously within the body water pool and more importantly that oxygen atoms in exhaled CO_2 and water are in isotopic equilibrium. By giving a dose of $H_2^{18}O$, both the water and CO_2 pool will be labeled, whereas when ^2H_2O is given, only the water pool will be labeled. Total energy expenditure measured by this technique is 1.4 times the energy expenditure measured by indirect calorimetry in critically ill in septic and trauma patients [15]. This method is only applicable in research settings.

What Should We Do While Waiting For Clever 'Metabolic' Ventilators?

The above technical problems, along with the limited availability of indirect calorimetry, have led to the development of predictive equations as surrogates, most of which have been shown to be inaccurate [18]. The Harris & Benedict equation (adjusted or not for ideal body weight), and equations of Owen, Mifflin, the American College of Chest Physicians (ACCP), Ireton-Jones 1992 and 1997, Penn State 1998 and 2003, and Swinamer 1990 are the most commonly used. These equations have all repeatedly been shown to be poorly correlated with the results of indirect calorimetry in critically ill patients [16, 18, 19]. Further, these equations are open to misinterpretation, as they often include a subjective 'stress factor' varying between 110 and 200 %.

Two equations have been developed for critically ill patients based on regression analysis of multiple variables collected during indirect calorimetry: The Toronto equation for major burns [20] and the Faisy-Fagon equation for patients on mechanical ventilation [21]. The latter equation calculates resting energy expenditure on the basis of body weight, height, minute ventilation, and body temperature and is clinically more accurate than the other predictive equations for metabolically stable, mechanically ventilated patients [21].

Consequences of Under- and Over-feeding

Both extremes of feeding have well defined adverse effects and should be avoided [22].

Overfeeding: More Is Worse ...

In the 1980s, the concept of parenteral hyperalimentation prevailed. This new therapy indeed saved multiple lives, but simultaneously caused serious complications. Further the concept of counting only non-protein calories, but not including the energy from proteins, contributed to overfeeding. This way to calculate energy intake should definitively be banned: All energy sources should be included in the total energy counts [23, 24]. Finally, a computerized information system is needed to be aware of the rather important amounts of energy infused for non-nutritional purpose, including glucose 5 % solutions and fat soluble sedatives [25]. Such inaccuracies have been responsible for systematic overfeeding in several studies.

Hypercaloric feeding has well known deleterious consequences on glycemic control, liver function, infections, and outcome. Detailed analysis of several papers supporting the negative effects of feeding [6, 26] show that the authors were actually overfeeding their isocaloric groups, with the expected deleterious clinical consequences, which invalidates the interpretation of the results. In a study including 200 ICU patients receiving parenteral nutrition, Dissanaike et al. showed that increased parenteral caloric intake was an independent risk factor

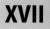

for blood stream infections [6]: Three groups out of four received more than 26 kcal/kg per day, with the mean energy intake in the group with blood stream infections being 35 kcal/kg! This study should have been called the 'effects of overfeeding'.

An important characteristic of ICU patients, is their poor tolerance to overfeeding. In a large multicenter study conducted in 40 Spanish ICUs and including 725 patients receiving either enteral or parenteral nutrition, Grau et al. showed that overfeeding (> 27 kcal/kg) was one of the determinants of altered hepatic function [22]. The problem started at values as low as 110–120 % of true requirements, with early increases in the liver enzymes AST and ALT after 3–4 days, followed by increased cholestasis or a combination of both [22].

The consequence of this high liver susceptibility to overfeeding is that an accumulated energy deficit cannot be recovered by giving 120–130 % of requirements for a few days. The 'gavage' causes hepatic steatosis, the 'foie gras' of geese. In cases of early insufficient energy delivery, the patients get a 'double hit': First by the complications of underfeeding, followed by those of overfeeding. The only strategy is, therefore, to prevent development of a relevant energy deficit by starting enteral feeding early.

Underfeeding and Pseudo-underfeeding

In reaction to trials that showed the deleterious effects of overfeeding, a few investigators hypothesized that semi-starvation might be the solution. Ahrens et al. randomized 40 surgical patients to receive either 'low-calorie' parenteral nutrition (20 non-protein kcal/kg/day) or standard parenteral nutrition (30 non-protein kcal/kg/day) [26]: To this, the investigators added lipid emulsions 3 times weekly, resulting in an additional 3 × 1000 = 3000 kcal for all patients. The authors concluded that the administration of 'low-calorie' parenteral nutrition resulted in fewer (0 % versus 33 %) and less-severe hyperglycemic events, with reduced insulin requirements. The problem is that all patients were overfed, the pseudo-low-calorie group being less overfed than the other, so of course doing better! As previously stated, all substrates must be included in the calculations [24]!

After a study by Fong et al. in volunteers given endotoxin [27], parenteral nutrition became considered a poison, because its delivery had primed a stronger inflammatory response compared with enteral nutrition. Over the subsequent two decades, the pendulum shifted towards predominance of enteral feeding with the appearance of malnutrition. The earliest study to show worsening of outcome related to growing negative energy balances came from the UK and was conducted in 57 critically ill patients [28]: With targets set by calorimetry, the authors showed that a cumulated energy deficit above -10000 kcal was associated with increased mortality.

Negative energy balances and low feeding supply have since been shown to prevail across diagnostic categories [2, 10, 29, 30]. Two prospective studies conducted in ICUs with feeding protocols and using indirect calorimetry and the same computerized information system customized for nutritional monitoring (Metavision, iMDsoft, Tel Aviv) [10, 11] showed a proportionality between an increasing energy debt and clinical complications, particularly infection rates. Energy deficit developed in respectively 55 % and 60 % of the patients. The cutoff for increasing complication rates in both studies was between −4000 and

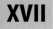

–8000 kcal of cumulated energy balance corresponding to -50 to -110 kcal/kg. The same type of impact on infectious complications was observed in a neuro-ICU after subarachnoid hemorrhage in which the mean cumulative energy balance over the first 7 days was -117 kcal/kg [31].

Rubinson et al. showed in 138 patients that the incidence of bacteremia was directly related to energy delivery with a steep increase in those patients receiving less than 25 % of that recommended by the ACCP [3]: The difference appeared already by day 7 after admission. Using the same ACCP recommendations, another American study, including 187 medical ICU patients, showed that unintentional hypocaloric feeding occurred on 51 % of ICU days [7]. A randomized British study including 277 patients and testing enteral immunonutrition ended up delivering a median intake of 14 kcal/kg/day to both groups [32], which compromised the interpretation of their trial. In a French study, including 38 medical ICU consecutive adult patients intubated for at least 7 days on early exclusive enteral feeding, the patients with a mean energy deficit of -1,200 kcal/day had a higher ICU mortality rate than patients with lower deficit after two weeks (p = 0.01) [33]. The same authors showed recently that the level of energy deficit was also a determinant of the type of microbial agents causing the infectious complications, *Staphylococcus aureus* being predominant in ventilator-associated pneumonia in patients with the largest energy deficits [34]. This phenomenon is worldwide as shown by Alberda et al. in 2,772 mechanically ventilated patients [2]: The level of energy intake averaged 14 kcal/kg/day across countries with a mean delivery of 1,034 kcal/day and 47 g protein/day. Of note, an increase of 1,000 kcal per day was associated with a progressive mortality reduction.

Energy requirements are pathology dependent. It is, therefore, not surprising that the level of energy intake required to prevent problems is higher in patients with major burns as shown by a prospective Finnish study: The intake cut-off separating patients with and without nutrition-related complications was shown to be about 30 kcal/kg/day [35]; the lower delivery was associated with a 32.6 % death rate versus a rate of 5.3 % (p < 0.01) in those receiving adequate feeding; the pneumonia rate doubled, sepsis rate increased 1.8-fold (p < 0.05), and the length of stay was prolonged by 12.6 days (p = 0.01).

A recent ICU study from the Netherlands showed that protein delivery is another player in outcome because optimal intake further reduces mortality when the energy target is reached: Achievement of the guideline levels (1.2 g/kg/day) should be monitored [36].

In summary, semi-starvation may possibly be tolerated in young patients who are not too severely ill, although nobody knows yet exactly how long fasting is tolerable in acute illness without deleterious consequences. Data in healthy subjects show that the duration is probably shorter than previously believed [37], with mitochondrial alterations already detectable after 18 hours. But current ICU populations are older and more severely ill than ever, and often stay for prolonged periods of time. Inappropriate feeding jeopardizes recovery. As long as we have no laboratory determinations available for clinical settings, the calculation of energy deficit probably constitutes a good surrogate for detection of complications: The cut-off for appearance of biological consequences of underfeeding is probably somewhere between -50 and -60 kcal/kg body weight.

Clinical Evidence from Intervention Studies

Optimizing energy delivery by individualizing and adapting it to a patient's daily status is a new concept [38]. Combined nutrition, with parenteral nutrition to top up insufficient enteral nutrition is a tool to prevent a growing energy deficit while using the gut. Several recent interventional trials are now delivering results.

The TICACOS Trial

Recently, a prospective controlled randomized trial including 112 critically ill patients, tested the clinical impact of two strategies on outcome [39] while closely monitoring energy expenditure using indirect calorimetry. In the study group, energy target was adapted daily to these results (TIght CAlorie COntrol Study = TICACOS) whereas in the control group, the target was fixed at 25 kcal/kg/d. The authors observed a significant difference in energy delivery (+ 600 kcal/day) and in protein delivery (+13 g/day) between the groups, in favor of the calorimetry group. As a consequence, daily and cumulated energy balances were positive in the intervention group, versus negative in the control group. Unfortunately, non-nutritional energy was not taken into account for feeding prescription, which led to modest systematic overfeeding with prolonged mechanical ventilation and more infections. This tighter energy management was nevertheless associated with a significant reduction in post-ICU mortality. The study has weaknesses, but is the first to show that individualized nutritional support brings clinical benefit.

The EPaNIC Trial

This large study, Early Parenteral Nutrition to supplement insufficient enteral nutrition in Intensive Care patients (EPaNIC), randomized patients on admission to early (day 2) versus late (day 8) parenteral nutrition and concluded that early hypercaloric parenteral nutrition was deleterious [40]. This is no surprise, and confirmed what we have known for 20 years, since the Veterans' study published in the same journal [41].

This study has several limitations and was not at all in line with the European Society for Clinical Nutrition and Metabolism (ESPEN) guidelines [42], which the study claims to have followed for the early parenteral nutrition group. The patients of the early parenteral nutrition group did not have a clear indication for this technique. Patients were fed intravenously even though they had no clinical indication for this therapy because of a very short stay (39.1 % of the studied population had left the ICU by day 3, and > 50 % by day 5) or conditions that rarely need parenteral nutrition, such as elective heart surgery (61 % of the population). Large and numerous studies have shown the advantage of the enteral route over the intravenous route in ICU patients. This misinterpretation raises an ethical question as the guidelines state that no parenteral nutrition should be initiated unless enteral nutrition has been tested.

Energy delivery was elevated early on during the most acute phase of illness, with the delivery of glucose 20 % to the parenteral nutrition group. Further there was no confirmation of the energy targets by indirect calorimetry. Early elevated intravenous energy delivery has been shown to result in increased morbidity. The

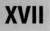

study certainly included patients who merited parenteral nutrition but these were hidden by the forest of patients without an indication. Patients with severe malnutrition (body mass index [BMI] < 18.5), who may have benefited from parenteral nutrition, were excluded. This study confirms that parenteral nutrition should not be considered on admission.

The SPN Trial

The latest study to investigate timing of feeding is the Supplemental Parenteral Nutrition (SPN) trial [43]. This Swiss bi-center, randomized trial enrolled 305 patients who stayed for at least 5 days in the ICU in whom enteral nutrition was initiated but clearly insufficient (< 60 % of energy target on day 3). Supplemental parenteral nutrition was delivered to cover 100 % of target, measured mostly by indirect calorimetry, from day 4 to day 8, whereas enteral feeding was pursued in all patients, in line with ESPEN guidelines (indication for parenteral nutrition was enteral nutrition failure)[42]. The authors applied a glucose control strategy (target < 8 mmol/l), and glucose control was not compromised by the supplementary parenteral nutrition [44]. Isoenergetic feeding improved outcome, with a significant reduction in new infections, an increase in antibiotic free days, and reduced time on mechanical ventilation.

Timing and Tools

The answer to the wide persistence of malnutrition consists of a bundle of measures:

- Teaching about nutrition
- Application of guidelines
- Systematic target calculation with insertion in the medical order sheets
- Daily monitoring of nutrition delivery.

Teaching basic nutritional knowledge in medical schools is a big priority, and its absence in curricula is a worldwide problem [5, 45]. Among the mnemotechnic tools, the "FAST HUG" strategy [46], where "F" stands for feeding, has only partially penetrated into the critical care milieu.

Guidelines provide standard targets for route, timing and energy targets. Timing is essential: Starting enteral nutrition within 24 hours in patients on mechanical ventilation is a very efficient way to reduce energy deficit [47]. Early enteral nutrition has a second advantage, which is to keep the gut working, particularly in the sickest patients. Prokinetics may help restore motility, and acupuncture may be even more effective than standard promotility medications [48]. Early feeding does not mean 'force feeding' though [49]; the sick gut is telling us something important, that we should listen too. Persistent gastric intolerance on day 3 automatically selects patients who will require supplemental parenteral nutrition.

In the absence of calorimetry, guideline targets should be applied, with a cautious initial 20–25 kcal/kg/day target increasing thereafter in the recovery phase. Importantly, when prescribing these targets one should integrate the existence of inadvertent non-nutritional energy intakes (see above). Monitoring energy balance to detect a growing energy debt is essential: This can be easily achieved with some computerized systems. Computer assisted nutritional support has been

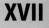

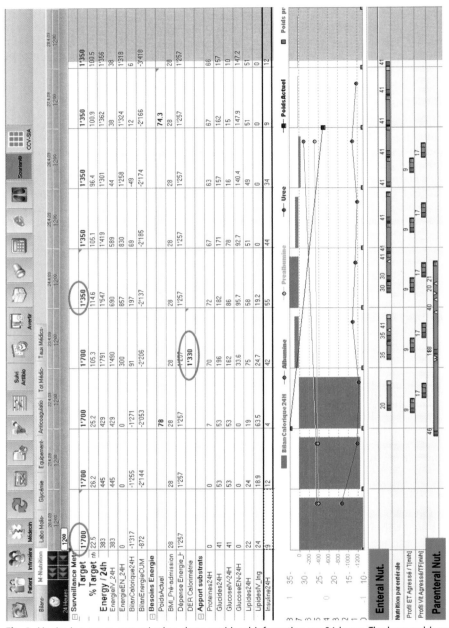

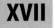

XVII

Fig. 2. Monitoring screen customized to show nutritional information per 24 hours. The large red bars reflect negative balances (here present the 3 first days) or over-feeding: The closer the patient is to target, the thinner the bar. The tabular data provide information about energy delivery by intravenous and enteral routes, and about exact protein, glucose and fat delivery. The table also shows insulin requirements.

show to be more efficient in achieving energy targets [25, 50]. Indeed, visualization of real-time energy delivery is an important tool to obtain a rapid response. **Figure 2** shows the case of an elderly patient who was deemed 'nil per os' by the surgeon, with parenteral nutrition started on day 3 (some energy came from glucose 5 % solution and propofol). The initial target was 1700 kcal and was reset to 1350 kcal on day 4 after calorimetry control. Discussion with the surgeons then enabled initiation of slow enteral nutrition on day 3, resulting in combined feeding for 3 days. Computerized information systems (CIS), also called Patient Data Management Systems (PDMS), are expensive, however, much more so than calorimeters. As an alternative, it is easy to create an Excel file (available worldwide) and to customize tables enabling rapid check of protein, glucose, lipid and calorie delivery per 24 hours: The precise (ml) delivery of feeding solution and of drug solutions should be entered, including the sedative propofol (lipid) and other glucose containing solutions. Some applications for smartphones from the industry may also be helpful. Evidence is accumulating that the development of energy deficits > -4000 kcal should be prevented: Early enteral nutrition and the use of combined enteral and parenteral nutrition (in case of enteral nutrition failure) seem the best ways to achieve this target [51].

Conclusion

Nutrition is a medical therapy and basic rules need to be followed, such as respect of indications, contraindications and dose adaptation, timing of initiation, and monitoring. Timing has proven important in the prevention of malnutrition-related complications. Early enteral nutrition remains the best tool to prevent problems. We now know that combined feeding introduced around day 4 in those patients not achieving their targets is a second-line tool. Indeed, interventional trials that have respected these basic rules have achieved improved clinical outcomes. It is also important to check the target: Ventilators with integrated calorimeters would be a great help. Finally, as any therapy, under- and over-dosage must be avoided, which implies monitoring nutritional delivery in order to identify a growing energy gap or excess administration.

References

1. Thibault R, Chikhi M, Clerc A, et al (2011) Assessment of food intake in hospitalised patients: A 10-year comparative study of a prospective hospital survey. Clin Nutr 30: 289–296
2. Alberda C, Gramlich L, Jones N, et al (2009) The relationship between nutritional intake and clinical outcomes in critically ill patients: results of an international multicenter observational study. Intensive Care Med 35: 1728–1737
3. Rubinson L, Diette GB, Song X, Brower RG, Krishnan JA (2004) Low caloric intake is associated with nosocomial bloodstream infections in patients in the medical intensive care unit. Crit Care Med 32: 350–357
4. Braga M, Gianotti L, Constantini E, et al (1994) Impact of enteral nutrition on intestinal bacterial translocation and mortality in burned mice. Clin Nutr 13: 256–261
5. Möwe M, Bosaeus I, Rasmussen HH et al (2008) Insufficient nutritional knowledge among health care workers? Clin Nutr 27: 196–202
6. Dissanaike S, Shelton M, Warner K, O'Keefe GE (2007) The risk for bloodstream infections is associated with increased parenteral caloric intake in patients receiving parenteral nutrition. Crit Care 11: R114

7. Krishnan JA, Parce PB, Martinez S, Diette GB, Brower RG (2003) Caloric intake in medical ICU patients: Consistency of care with guidelines and relationship to clinical outcomes. Chest 124: 297–305

8. McCowen KC, Friel C, Sternberg J, et al (2000) Hypocaloric total parenteral nutrition: effectiveness in prevention of hyperglycemia and infectious complications--a randomized clinical trial. Crit Care Med 28: 3606–3611

9. Berger MM, Mechanick JI (2010) Continuing controversy in the intensive care unit: why tight glycemic control, nutrition support, and nutritional pharmacology are each necessary therapeutic considerations. Curr Opin Clin Nutr Metab Care 13: 167–169

10. Dvir D, Cohen J, Singer P (2005) Computerized energy balance and complications in critically ill patients: An observational study. Clin Nutr 25: 37–44

11. Villet S, Chioléro RL, Bollmann MD, et al (2005) Negative impact of hypocaloric feeding and energy balance on clinical outcome in ICU patients. Clin Nutr 24: 502–509

12. Weir JB (1949) New methods for calculating metabolic rate with special reference to protein metabolism. J Physiol 109: 1–9

13. Weekes EC (2007) Controversies in the determination of energy requirements. Proc Nutr Soc 66: 367–377

14. Stapleton RD, Jones N, Heyland DK (2007) Feeding critically ill patients: what is the optimal amount of energy? Crit Care Med 35: S535–S540

15. Plank LD, Hill GL (2003) Energy balance in critical illness. Proc Nutr Soc 62: 545–552

16. Reid CL (2007) Poor agreement between continuous measurements of energy expenditure and routinely used prediction equations in intensive care unit patients. Clin Nutr 26: 649–657

17. Koea JB, Wolfe RR, Shaw JH (1995) Total energy expenditure during total parenteral nutrition: ambulatory patients at home versus patients with sepsis in surgical intensive care. Surgery 118: 54–62

18. Frankenfield DC, Coleman A, Alam S, Cooney RN (2009) Analysis of estimation methods for resting metabolic rate in critically ill adults. JPEN J Parenter Enteral Nutr 33: 27–36

19. Walker RN, Heuberger RA (2009) Predictive equations for energy needs for the critically ill. Respir Care 54: 509–521

20. Allard JP, Pichard C, Hoshino E, et al (1990) Validation of a new formula for calculating energy requirements of burn patients. JPEN J Parenter Enteral Nutr 14: 115–118

21. Faisy C, Guerot E, Diehl JL, Labrousse J, Fagon JY (2003) Assessment of resting energy expenditure in mechanically ventilated patients. Am J Clin Nutr 78: 241–249

22. Grau T, Bonet A, Rubio M, et al (2007) Liver dysfunction associated with artificial nutrition in critically ill patients. Crit Care 11: R10

23. Biolo G, Ciocchi B, Stulle M, et al (2007) Calorie restriction accelerates the catabolism of lean body mass during 2 wk of bed rest. Am J Clin Nutr 86: 366–372

24. Biolo G, Agostini F, Simunic B, et al (2008) Positive energy balance is associated with accelerated muscle atrophy and increased erythrocyte glutathione turnover during 5 wk of bed rest. Am J Clin Nutr 88: 950–958

25. Berger MM, Revelly JP, Wasserfallen JB, et al (2006) Impact of a computerized information system on quality of nutritional support in the ICU. Nutrition 22: 221–229

26. Ahrens CL, Barletta JF, Kanji S, et al (2005) Effect of low-calorie parenteral nutrition on the incidence and severity of hyperglycemia in surgical patients: a randomized, controlled trial. Crit Care Med 33: 2507–2512

27. Fong Y, Marano MA, Braber A, et al (1989) Total parenteral nutrition and bowel rest modify the metabolic response to endotoxin in humans. Ann Surg 210: 449–457

28. Bartlett RH, Dechert RE, Mault JR, Ferguson SK, Kaiser AM, Erlandson EE (1982) Measurement of metabolism in multiple organ failure. Surgery 92: 771–779

29. Villet S, Chiolero RL, Bollmann MD, et al (2005) Negative impact of hypocaloric feeding and energy balance on clinical outcome in ICU patients. Clin Nutr 24: 502–509

30. Doig GS, Simpson F, Finfer S, et al (2008) Effect of evidence-based feeding guidelines on mortality of critically ill adults: a cluster randomized controlled trial. JAMA 300: 2731–2741

31. Badjatia N, Fernandez L, Schlossberg MJ, et al (2010) Relationship between energy balance and complications after subarachnoid hemorrhage. JPEN J Parenter Enteral Nutr 34: 64–69

XVII

32. Atkinson S, Sieffert E, Bihari D (1998) A prospective, randomized, double-blind controlled clinical trial of enteral immunonutrition in the critically ill. Crit Care Med 26: 1164–1172
33. Faisy C, Lerolle N, Dachraoui F, et al (2009) Impact of energy deficit calculated by a predictive method on outcome in medical patients requiring prolonged acute mechanical ventilation. Br J Nutr 101: 1079–1087
34. Faisy C, Llerena M, Savalle M, Mainardi JL, Fagon JY (2011) Early ICU energy deficit is a risk factor for Staphylococcus aureus ventilator-associated pneumonia. Chest 140: 1254–1260
35. Rimdeika R, Gudaviciene D, Adamonis K, Barauskas G, Pavalkis D, Endzinas Z (2006) The effectiveness of caloric value of enteral nutrition in patients with major burns. Burns 32: 83–86
36. Weijs PJM, Stapel SN, de Groot SDW, et al (2012) Optimal protein and energy nutrition decreases mortality in mechanically ventilated, critically ill patients: A prospective observational cohort study. JPEN J Parenter Enteral Nutr (in press)
37. Awad S, Stephenson MC, Placidi E, et al (2010) The effects of fasting and refeeding with a 'metabolic preconditioning' drink on substrate reserves and mononuclear cell mitochondrial function. Clin Nutr 29: 538–544
38. Wernerman J (2011) Individualized ICU nutrition for a better outcome. Intensive Care Med 37: 564–565
39. Singer P, Anbar R, Cohen J, et al (2011) The tight calorie control study (TICACOS): a prospective, randomized, controlled pilot study of nutritional support in critically ill patients. Intensive Care Med 37: 601–609
40. Casaer MP, Mesotten D, Hermans G, et al (2011) Early versus late parenteral nutrition in critically ill adults. N Engl J Med 365: 506–517
41. The Veterans Affairs Total Parenteral Nutrition Cooperative Study Group (1991) Perioperative total parenteral nutrition in surgical patients. N Engl J Med 325: 525–532
42. Singer P, Berger MM, Van den Berghe G, et al (2009) ESPEN Guidelines on Parenteral Nutrition: Intensive care. Clin Nutr 28: 387–400
43. Heidegger CP, Graf S, Thibault R, Darmon P, Berger MM, Pichard C (2012) Supplemental parenteral nutrition (SPN) in intensive care unit (ICU) patients for optimal energy coverage: improved clinical outcome. Clin Nutr (in press)
44. Berger MM, Brancato V, Graf S, Heidegger CP, Darmon P, Pichard C (2011) SPN study: supplemental aprenteral nutrition (PN) to reach energy target does not compromise glucose control. Clin Nutr (in press)
45. McClave SA, Mechanick JI, Kushner RF, et al (2010) Compilation of recommendations from summit on increasing physician nutrition experts. JPEN J Parenter Enteral Nutr 34: 123S–132S
46. Vincent JL (2005) Give your patient a fast hug (at least) once a day. Crit Care Med 33: 1225–1229
47. Artinian V, Krayem H, DiGiovine B (2006) Effects of early enteral feeding on the outcome of critically ill mechanically ventilated medical patients. Chest 129: 960–967
48. Pfab F, Winhard M, Nowak-Machen M, et al (2011) Acupuncture in critically ill patients improves delayed gastric emptying: a randomized controlled trial. Anesth Analg 112: 150–155
49. Heyland DK, Cahill NE, Dhaliwal R, et al (2010) Enhanced protein-energy provision via the enteral route in critically ill patients: a single center feasibility trial of the PEP uP protocol. Crit Care 14: R78
50. van Schijndel RJ, de Groot SD, Driessen RH, et al (2009) Computer-aided support improves early and adequate delivery of nutrients in the ICU. Neth J Med 67: 388–393
51. Heidegger CP, Romand JA, Treggiari MM, Pichard C (2007) Is it now time to promote mixed enteral and parenteral nutrition for the critically ill patient? Intensive Care Med 33: 963–969

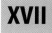

XVII

Pharmaconutrition with Selenium in ICU Patients

W. Manzanares, I. Hardy, and G. Hardy

Introduction

Critical illness is characterized by hyperinflammation, oxidative stress, mitochondrial and cellular immune dysfunction. Oxidative stress is defined as a state in which the level of toxic reactive oxygen species (ROS) overcomes the endogenous antioxidant defenses of the host. It is recognized as a major promoter and mediator of the systemic inflammatory response syndrome (SIRS) and multiple organ dysfunction syndrome (MODS), which can result from either excessive ROS production, or depletion of antioxidant defenses. During critical illness, antioxidant capacity is drastically decreased due to an excessive production of ROS and reactive nitrogen-oxygen species (RNOS) [1].

Selenium is an essential micronutrient with antioxidant, immunological and anti-inflammatory properties for animals and humans [2]. Evidence suggests that selenium status affects the cell-mediated and humoral aspects of immune function, which are linked to inflammatory processes involving the production of ROS and redox control processes. ROS production increases expression of pro-inflammatory cytokines through up-regulation of nuclear factor-kappa B (NF-κB) activity. Conversely, when incorporated into the various selenoenzymes, selenium acts as an antioxidant, influencing the inflammatory signaling pathways that modulate ROS by inhibiting activation of the NF-κB cascade and thus suppressing the production of pro-inflammatory cytokines [3].

Severe sepsis is characterized by an increase in ROS and low endogenous antioxidative capacity. Many patients with severe sepsis exhibit profound selenium depletion, which correlates with higher mortality and morbidity. Thus, repletion of selenium status should be able to reduce illness severity, reduce infectious complications, improve clinical outcome, and decrease mortality [2]. In the last two decades, several clinical trials have evaluated the role of seleno-compounds (especially sodium selenite) as part of an antioxidant strategy for critically ill SIRS-MODS patients. However, the results have sometimes been contradictory and inconclusive, partly because selenium has been studied not only as a single pharmaconutrient but frequently in combination with other antioxidants (trace elements and vitamins) in enteral or parenteral 'antioxidant cocktails' [2]. Current guidelines for nutrition therapy recommend a combination of antioxidant vitamins and trace elements (specifically including selenium) for all critically ill patients requiring enteral or parenteral nutrition [4,5]. However, the consensus view is that inducing a beneficial antioxidant and/or anti-inflammatory response necessitates a much higher 'pharmaconutritional' dose than the 'normal' requirement for restoration of nutrient deficiency. Notwithstanding, the optimal dose,

XVII

J.-L. Vincent (ed.), *Annual Update in Intensive Care and Emergency Medicine 2012*
DOI 10.1007/978-3-642-25716-2 © Springer-Verlag Berlin Heidelberg 2012

the best mode of administration and the duration of this intervention for ICU patients are still unknown [2].

Biological Role of Selenium

Selenium exerts its biological role largely through its presence in selenoproteins where selenium is incorporated into selenocysteine, the 21st amino acid. So far, more than 25 genes for selenoproteins have been identified in the human genome [6]. The many selenoproteins have numerous biological functions, especially related to redox signaling, antioxidant defense systems, thyroid hormone metabolism, and immune responses [5]. The most extensively characterized selenoproteins are the glutathione peroxidase (GPx) family of selenoenzymes [7], consisting of eight isoforms that catalyze the reduction of various hydroperoxides but differ in their substrate specificity; namely cytosolic GPx1, gastrointestinal GPx2, plasma GPx3, and phospholipid/cholesterol hydroperoxides GPx4. Extracellular or plasma GPx (also named GPx3) acts as a functional parameter for selenium status and deficiencies have been associated with cardiovascular disease, SIRS, and severe sepsis. Selenoprotein P, produced in the liver contains up to 10 selenocysteine per protein, indicative of a high antioxidant potential. A key characteristic of selenoprotein P is its ability to bind to the endothelium, which may be a mechanism for selenoprotein P recruitment to the site of inflammation. Selenoprotein P is the major selenoenzyme, accounting for up to 60 % of selenium in plasma and has been shown to be responsive to changes in dietary intake. A further 30 % is measurable as GPx-3 with a normal value of 0.72 ± 0.16 U/ml and approximately 6 – 10 % is bound to albumin, with less than 1 % existing as free selenium [8].

Selenium also has an important role in thyroid hormone metabolism. Thioredoxin reductases (TRxR), and iodothyronine deiodinases are selenoenzymes, also involved in redox reactions, and it has been shown that low plasma selenium levels in critically ill patients correlate with low T3 levels [9]. Moreover, selenium supplementation leads to an earlier normalization of plasma T3 levels compared with controls but selenium repletion has no direct effect on the activity of free and total thyroid hormones.

Selenium and Inflammation in the Critically Ill

There is considerable evidence to support anti-inflammatory effects of selenium through different mechanisms and pathways. In critically ill patients, especially those with severe sepsis, low plasma selenium levels have been found to be associated with more extensive tissue damage, systemic inflammation and organ failure [10]. Decreased serum selenium levels in patients with SIRS have been associated with high levels of C-reactive protein (CRP). Recently, Valenta et al. [11] showed that high-dose selenite supplementation was able to reduce CRP levels, demonstrating its anti-inflammatory effect. In a very elegant review, Duntas [10] proposed other key mechanisms of the anti-inflammatory action of selenium, namely its effect on immune cells, particularly macrophage signal transduction pathways, inhibition of NF-κB and the pro-inflammatory genes for tumor necrosis factor (TNF)-α and cyclooxygenase-2, which was demonstrated by Zamamiri-

Davis and coworkers [12], as well as upregulation of the normal half-life of the NF-κB inhibitor alpha (IκBα). Therefore, by inhibiting TNF-α, selenium limits the production of adhesion molecules, such as intercellular adhesion molecule-1 (ICAM-1), vascular cell adhesion molecule-1 (VCAM-1), and endothelial leukocyte adhesion molecule-1 (E-selectin) [13], which are responsible for recruiting leukocytes across the endothelium during the inflammatory response.

Selenium Status in ICU Patients

Critical illness with systemic inflammation and organ failure is characterized by low selenium status [14], which can be assessed by determining the selenium concentration of whole blood, plasma, serum or erythrocytes, although plasma selenium concentration is the parameter most frequently used to determine selenium status. In a meta-analysis of 14 selenium supplementation/depletion studies, Ashton et al. [15] confirmed that plasma or serum levels were the most commonly used and reasonably accurate biomarkers of selenium status, responding to short-term changes in intake. Expression of individual selenoproteins may be a more accurate measure. Selenoprotein P responds to selenium supplementation in a dose-dependent way, and is more sensitive to deficiency than GPx, but is still difficult to analyze [16].

During critical illness, trace element and vitamin availability is substantially modified. SIRS is associated with redistribution of vitamins and trace elements from the circulating compartment to those tissues involved in protein synthesis and immune cell proliferation, which could explain the finding of an early decrease in selenium and selenoenzymes in SIRS patients [17]. Like other micronutrients, selenium escapes to the interstitial compartment by capillary leakage, but the causes and underlying mechanisms have yet to be elucidated. In addition,

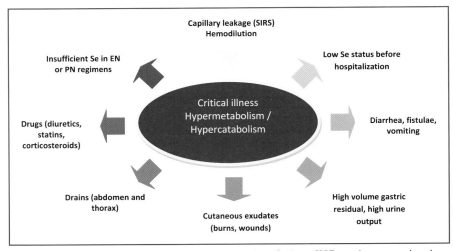

 XVII

Fig. 1. Etiology of selenium deficiency in ICU patients. Se: selenium; CRRT: continuous renal replacement therapy; ICU: intensive care unit; SIRS: systemic inflammatory response syndrome; EN: enteral nutrition; PN: parenteral nutrition

losses through biological fluids, hemodilution, previous insufficient intake and continuous renal replacement therapies (CRRT) contribute to selenium depletion [18] (**Fig. 1**). Forceville et al. [19] investigated 134 consecutive ICU patients and showed that plasma selenium levels were decreased by up to 40 %, especially in septic shock. Furthermore, selenium concentrations less than 0.7 µmol/l were associated with a 4-fold increase in mortality and a 3-fold increase in new organ failure and ventilator-associated pneumonia (VAP). More recently, the same group reported an early 70 % decrease in selenoprotein P plasma levels in severe sepsis and septic shock, whereas GPx-3 activity remained unchanged [20]. In 92 % (55/60) of surgical patients at ICU admission, Sakr et al. [21] showed that plasma selenium levels were lower than in healthy controls (74 µg/l), and further decreased during the ICU stay for SIRS patients, and those with organ failure as a result of severe sepsis. In Uruguay, we have found that selenium and GPX-3 levels were significantly decreased in SIRS and MODS patients (p = 0.0001 and p = 0.002, respectively) [22] (**Fig. 2**). In addition, univariate analysis showed that plasma selenium had a relatively good predictive value for ICU mortality (p = 0.034) but GPx-3 did not (p = 0.056). However, multivariate analysis of our data shows that, independently of the Simplified Acute Physiology Score II (SAPS II),

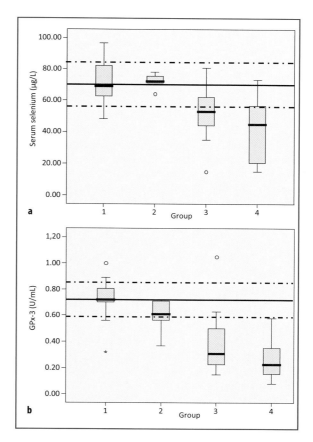

Fig. 2. Serum selenium **a** and glutathione peroxidase-3 (GPx-3) activity **b** in healthy volunteer subjects: (1) critically ill non-SIRS patients, (2) SIRS patients, (3) and SIRS-MODS patients (4). The solid and broken lines represent the mean ± SD normal serum selenium and GPx-3 in a Uruguayan control group (72.8 ± 13.1 µg/l and 0.72 ± 0.16 U/ml, respectively). P values refer to differences between groups using the Mann–Whitney U test. For serum selenium: p 1–2 = 0.787; p 1–3 = 0.002; p 1–4 = 0.0001; p 2–3 = 0.008; p 2–4 = 0.001; p 3–4 = 0.153. For GPx-3: p 1–3 = 0.0001; p 1–4 = 0.0001; p 2–3 = 0.014; p 2–4 = 0.0001. MODS: multiple organ dysfunction syndrome, SIRS: systemic inflammatory response syndrome. From [22] with permission

creatinine and leukocyte count, a low serum selenium within the first 24–48 h after admission to the ICU was not associated with mortality and was not an independent predictor of death [22].

The selenium cut-off value of 60 µg/l and the GPx-3 cut-off value of 0.5 U/ml have high specificity for severity of critical illness. Furthermore, the areas under the curves (AUC) of GPx-3 and selenium demonstrate that these are excellent predictors of SIRS: GPx-3 yielded the highest discriminative value, with an AUC of 0.921 (CI 95 % 0.844 to 0.999) [22]. Wereszczynska-Siemiatkowska et al. [23] similarly reported significantly lower plasma selenium and GPx-3 activity in severe acute pancreatitis and this had a high prognostic accuracy for severity. Further confirmation is provided by a recent study showing that selenium blood levels were significantly reduced during cardiopulmonary bypass (CPB) surgery when compared to preoperative values (89.05 ± 12.65 to 70.84 ± 10.46 µg/l) [24]. Additionally, low selenium levels at the end of surgery were independently associated with postoperative MODS (OR 0.8479, 95 % CI 0.7617 to 0.9440, p = 0.0026). On the basis of all these data we propose that early assessment of selenium status should be mandatory for all patients on admission to the ICU [22].

Molecular Effects and Pharmacokinetic Profile of Selenite in ICU Patients

In addition to the different chemical forms of selenium, the mode of administration appears to influence the pharmacokinetics of selenium therapy and hence may account for the conflicting results of different supplementation studies. Most intervention trials in the ICU have been performed using the parenteral route and we lack comparative data between enteral and parenteral selenium supplementation. Inorganic selenocompounds (sodium selenite or selenious acid) are the most effective parenteral forms of selenium supplementation for optimizing GPx-3 activity and have been evaluated in several clinical and animal studies. Organic selenium compounds, such as selenomethionine, are not available for intravenous use. The following parenteral options are available: Single nutrient monotherapy; separate infusion in combination with other micronutrients; bolus versus continuous infusion; bolus plus continuous infusion; in combination with other trace elements in a parenteral nutrition regimen [2].

The optimum safe dose and method of administration remains controversial but the best clinical outcomes in SIRS, with no apparent adverse effects, have been reported from very high selenium doses, administered first by bolus followed by continuous infusion. Selenite is postulated to have a biphasic action, initially as a pro-oxidant and then as an antioxidant. Depending on intracellular conditions, such as peroxide tone and redox potential, it can potentially have a toxic effect at very high dosages [25]. Nevertheless, the early transient pro-oxidant effect of selenite might be a useful therapeutic strategy for some ICU patients. A loading dose given as a bolus in the early phase of septic shock and SIRS could have the following effects: a) Direct reversible inhibition of NF-κB binding to DNA through a rupture of the disulfide bridging bond controlling gene expression and thus downregulating the synthesis of pro-inflammatory cytokines (at selenium concentrations > 5 µmol/l) [26, 27]; b) induction of apoptosis and cytotoxicity in activated pro-inflammatory circulating cells at the microcirculation level; and c) a direct virucidal and bactericidal effect [25]. Unfortunately, this transient pro-oxidant effect of a sele-

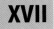

Fig. 3. Pharmacodynamic profile of two high doses of selenite assessed by glutathione peroxidase (GPx-3) activity in SIRS patients. Only the very high dose (loading dose as an intravenous bolus of 2000 μg in 30 min and, thereafter, an intravenous infusion of 1600 μg/day during 10 days) achieved physiologic levels (0.72 ± 0.16 U/ml) from day 2. After day 7, GPx-3 decreased in both groups, but only the very high-dose group maintained physiologic levels until day 10. From [29] with permission

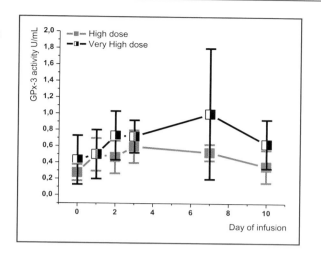

nium bolus loading dose has never been confirmed in SIRS patients. The antioxidant action of high doses of selenium is secondary to its incorporation into selenocysteine residues at the active site of the selenoenzymes. In septic shock patients, the combined effect of an intravenous bolus followed by continuous infusion is thought to stimulate the synthesis of selenoprotein P, which protects against endothelial dysfunction leading to decreased organ failure. Using a sheep model of severe peritoneal sepsis and septic shock, Wang et al. [28] investigated the effects of a large selenium bolus (as sodium selenite 2000 μg) into the right atrium, followed by a continuous intravenous infusion of 0.06 μg/kg/h for the remainder of the study. A second group of animals received the same dose of sodium selenite but only by continuous infusion (4 μg/kg/h) without the initial bolus. Only bolus-injected animals, but not the continuous infusion group, reached a transient peak plasma selenium concentration (7.7 ± 2.7 μmol/l, 4 – 14 μmol/l). In addition, interleukin-6 (IL-6) decreased significantly, but only in the bolus group ($p < 0.05$). These metabolic improvements were associated with a better hemodynamic status – blood pressure, cardiac index, stroke volume index and response to fluid replacement ($p < 0.05$) – suggesting that in an inflammatory condition, such as severe sepsis/septic shock, the pro-oxidant effect of a large selenium bolus may be pivotal to the anti-inflammatory process and hence outcome improvement [28].

Our own dosing study, performed in 20 critically ill SIRS patients, compared and analyzed the pharmacokinetic profile of two high doses of selenite (as selenious acid) [29]. The first group received a bolus loading dose of 1200 μg (15.18 μmol) over 2 h, and thereafter 800 μg/d (10.12 μmol/d) as a continuous infusion for 10 days. The second group received a loading dose of 2000 μg (25.3 μmol) and thereafter 1600 μg/day (20.24 μmol) as a continuous infusion for the same time period. Data analysis showed that the concentration/time curves for selenium overlapped and were independent of dose. However, the pharmacodynamic profile of GPx-3 showed that optimal GPx-3 levels were only achieved with the higher dose of selenious acid (1600 μg/day selenium) (**Fig. 3**). In both groups, GPx–3 decreased after day 7 of supplementation independent of the selenium dose. Clinical outcomes were similar in both groups. This suggests that despite continued selenium supplementation, GPx-3 inhibition or saturation occurs as a result of insufficient synthesis of precursors such as hydrogen selenide or selenocysteine, and/or limitation of glutathione (GSH) synthesis due to lack of glutamine or cysteine. We, therefore, hypothesize that depleted GSH or precursor stores need to be replenished in addition to selenium, to maintain GPx-3 intracellular levels in SIRS [29]. Combined supplementation of high dose selenite with glutamine and/or cysteine could potentially avoid the observed GPx-3 decrease after day 7, thus further optimizing the pharmacodynamic profile and efficacy of the therapy [2, 29].

Studies on Intravenous Selenium Supplementation in the Critically Ill

Selenium Monotherapy

In the 1990s, some German and Swiss trials first evaluated different doses of parenteral selenium, as sodium selenite, in ICU patients (**Table 1**). Zimmermann et al. [30] showed that a high dose of 1000 μg sodium selenite given over 30 minutes on the first day followed by a continuous infusion of 1000 μg/day for 14 days after surgery or trauma improved multiorgan function scores with a 2.6-fold reduction in mortality. Angstwurm et al. [31] used a novel protocol in SIRS patients with APACHE II >15, involving an initial intravenous bolus followed by a stepwise reduction in dosage of sodium selenite (535 μg from day 1–3, 285 μg from day 4–6 and 160 μg from day 7–9) as continuous infusions and, thereafter, 35 μg sodium selenite in the parenteral nutrition. Selenium supplementation reduced the severity index and need for hemodialysis, but the reduction in mortality (52 % to 33.5 %) did not reach statistical significance (p = 0.13) [31].

The most important prospective randomized controlled trial (RCT) on selenium supplementation as monotherapy so far is the 'Selenium in Intensive Care' (SIC) [32] study in patients with severe SIRS, sepsis and septic shock with an APACHE III > 70. Initially, 249 patients were randomized to receive either a 1000 μg bolus of sodium selenite on day 1 followed by a daily continuous infusion of a further 1000 μg for 14 days or a saline placebo. Of these, 11 patients were excluded for various reasons, leaving 238 patients for the intention-to-treat analysis. Subsequently a further 49 patients had to be excluded due to protocol deviations bringing the total number of patients in the per-protocol analysis down to 189. Although the reduction in 28-day mortality for selenium-supplemented patients failed to reach statistical significance in the intention-to-treat analysis (50.0 % vs. 39.7 %; p = 0.109), in the per protocol analysis, mortality was significantly lower in the selenium group (56.7 % vs. 42.6 %, p = 0.049) [32]. No toxicity or adverse effects from the high dose of selenium were observed. It is very encouraging that the mortality rate was significantly reduced in the subgroup of patients with severe sepsis and disseminated intravascular coagulation (p = 0.018) and also in patients with more than three organ dysfunctions (p = 0.039) as well as in the most severely ill (APACHE III > 102) patients (p = 0.04) [32].

A smaller, prospective RCT evaluated the effect of approximately half this selenium dose on biochemical markers and clinical outcome in 40 septic ICU patients [33]. Patients were randomized to receive intravenous sodium selenite supplementation, providing 474, 316, 158 μg/day selenium, for each of 3 consecutive days, followed by a standard infusion of 31.6 μg (0.4 μmol)/day for a total duration of two weeks. Although selenium supplementation did not reduce mortality or oxidative stress (as measured by F2 isoprostanes), there was a significant reduction in

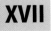
XVII

Table 1. Summary of the most relevant studies on parenteral pharmaconutrition using selenite as monotherapy

Reference	Patient population and characteristics	Selenium daily dose (as monotherapy)	Clinical outcome
Angstwurm et al. (1999) [31]	Sepsis APACHE II > 15 (n = 42)	535 µg/day 3 days; 285 µg/day 3 days; 155 µg/day 3 days, and then 35 µg/day	APACHE II was significantly lower (day 7, p = 0.018; and day 14, p = 0.045). CRRT was less necessary in the selenite group (p = 0.035)
Angstwurm et al. (2007) [32]	Severe sepsis, septic shock. APACHE III > 70 (n = 249)	Day 1: loading bolus 1000 µg in 30 min and then continuous infusion 1000 µg/day for 14 days	28-day mortality was lower (39.7 vs. 50 %, p = 0.109). In the per-protocol analysis (n = 189), the decrease was significant (p = 0.049)
Mishra et al. (2007) [33]	Severe sepsis APACHE II > 18 (n = 40)	Day 1–3: 474 µg/day, day 4–6:316 µg/day, day 7–9:158 µg/day, day 9–14: 31.6 µg/day by continuous infusion	Negative correlation between plasma Se and SOFA (r = -0.36, p= 0.03). No difference in 28-day mortality (p = 0.95) CRRT requirement no different between groups (p = 0.99)
Forceville et al. (2007) [34]	Severe sepsis/septic shock APACHE II > 25 (n = 60)	Day 1: loading infusion 4000 µg/24 h and then 1000 µg/day for 9 days	No effect on clinical outcome: time to vasopressor withdrawal, hospital and ICU LOS, duration of mechanical ventilation and 28-day mortality (p = 0.59)
Valenta et al. (2011) [11]	Severe sepsis/SIRS APACHE II > 30 (n = 150)	Day 1: loading bolus 1000 µg in 30 min and thereafter 30 min infusion 500 µg/day for days 2 to 14	Negative correlations between plasma Se: CRP (p = 0.035), PCT (p = 0.022) and SOFA (p = 0.001) at admission but not on days 7 or 14.
Manzanares et al (2011) [35]	Severe sepsis/SIRS APACHE II > 23 (n = 35)	Day 1: loading bolus: 2000 µg in 2 h and thereafter continuous infusion 1600 µg/day for 10 days	SOFA score decreased significantly (1.3 ± 1.2 versus 4.6 ± 2.0, p = 0.0001). Early VAP rate was lower (6.7 % versus 37.5 %, p = 0.04). HAP was lower after ICU discharge (p = 0.03)

APACHE II, Acute Physiology and Chronic Health Evaluation II; CRP: C-reactive protein; CRRT: continuous renal replacement therapy ; HAP: hospital-acquired pneumonia; ICU: intensive care unit; LOS: length of stay; PCT: procalcitonin; RRT, renal replacement therapy; SIRS: systemic inflammatory response syndrome; SOFA: sequential organ failure assessment; VAP: ventilator-associated pneumonia; Se: selenium

sequential organ failure assessment (SOFA) score with a significant negative correlation between plasma selenium and SOFA (r = –0.36, p = 0.03) [33].

In contrast, in a multicenter prospective RCT, Forceville et al. [34] enrolled 60 patients with septic shock and safely infused the therapeutic group (n = 31) with a very high initial dose of sodium selenite (4000 µg [50.6 µmol] selenium) as a continuous infusion in the first 24 hours (without an initial bolus loading dose), followed by 1000 µg/day for an additional 9 days (total selenium 13,000 µg [156

XVII

μmol per treatment]). However, there was no improvement in clinical outcome. Mortality rates did not differ significantly between the groups at any time point (45 % vs. 45 % on day 28, p = 0.59; 59 % vs. 68 % at 6 months, p = 0.32, and 66 % vs. 71 % at 1 year, p= 0.43) [34]. These findings differ from the previous achievements of these authors and the SIC study [32], leading to speculation that the unimproved outcome results are due to the omission of the initial pro-oxidant and anti-inflammatory intravenous bolus-loading dose of sodium selenite. Animal data from the same French group added further weight to this hypothesis [28]. In our own phase II prospective RCT in adult SIRS patients with APACHE II ≥ 8.5 ± 15 [35], we investigated high-dose selenious acid, administered first as a bolus, providing 2,000 µg (25.3 µmol) selenium over 2 h, and thereafter 1,600 µg/day (20.24 µmol) selenium as a continuous infusion. After 10 days of therapy, SOFA scores decreased significantly in the selenite group (1.3 ± 1.2 versus 4.6 ± 2.0, p = 0.0001). The rates of early VAP (6.7 % versus 37.5 %, p = 0.04), and hospital-acquired pneumonia after ICU discharge were lower (p = 0.03) in the selenite group [35]. Additionally, selenium was not associated with a higher incidence of adverse events during 28 days' follow-up. Similarly to our findings, Valenta et al. [11] reported a decrease in whole-blood GPx from day 10 onwards. In this study, patients received an initial selenite bolus of 1,000 µg selenium on day 1 followed by 500 µg on days 2 to 14 as a 30-min rapid infusion, rather than as a prolonged continuous infusion. Despite the late decrease in whole blood GPx, which was not discussed by the authors, they demonstrated that this approach was able to significantly increase selenium and GPx-3 levels (p < .001) [11]. Biomarkers of systemic inflammation decreased similarly in both groups and a negative correlation was demonstrated between low plasma selenium and CRP (p = 0.035), procalcitonin (PCT) (p = 0.022), and SOFA score (p = 0.001) at ICU admission, but not at day 7 or day 14. The 28-day mortality was slightly, but not significantly, lower in the selenium group (25 % vs. 32 %), and there was no significant reduction in mortality in the sub-group analysis by severity of illness either, but the authors admitted that their study was not sufficiently powered to determine this. There was however a trend towards reduced mortality in the most severely ill patients (APACHE II > 28) [11].

Selenium in Antioxidant Cocktails

In many prospective RCTs, selenite has been combined with other trace elements and vitamins in antioxidant cocktails. Interesting data were reported by Berger et al. [36] who aggregated two RCTs published in 1998 and 2004 and involving 41 burned patients. The intervention groups received parenteral antioxidant cocktails including selenium 315–380 µg/day (2.9–4.8 µmol/day) plus copper 2.5–3.1 mg/day and zinc 26.2–31.4 mg/day for 8 to 21 days. In these patients, plasma selenium and GPx levels in plasma and skin increased. Additionally, there was a reduction in nosocomial pneumonia compared to controls (33 % vs. 80 %, p < 0.001) and fewer episodes of VAP (13 vs. 6, p = 0.023) [36]. The same group also evaluated the effect of high dose enteral glutamine (30 g/day) plus antioxidants (including selenium) in 86 critically ill, burned and major trauma patients [37]. Enteral selenium supplementation was 300 µg/day, and burned patients received an additional 485.5 µg/day intravenous selenite for a maximum of 10 days. This combination of enteral glutamine plus parenteral micronutrients was reportedly safe but did not significantly improve clinical outcome. A similar parenteral anti-

XVII

oxidant cocktail (zinc, vitamins C and B1 and selenium 270 μg/day) given as a double loading dose on the first two days to 200 patients with organ failure after complicated cardiac surgery, major trauma and subarachnoid hemorrhage significantly reduced the inflammatory response in the intervention group (n = 102) [38]. In a retrospective analysis of 4294 trauma patients, half of whom had received an antioxidant mixture of parenteral vitamin C, enteral α-tocopherol and selenium (200 μg as a bolus over 2 hours) for 7 days, Collier et al. [39] showed a significantly shorter hospital and ICU length of stay (p < 0.001 and p = 0.001, respectively) as well as lower mortality (6.1 % vs. 8.5 %, p = 0.001) in the antioxidant group, which the authors translated into a 28 % relative risk reduction for mortality [39]. A phase I dose-ranging study by Heyland et al. [40] demonstrated that high dose glutamine (0.35 g/kg parenterally plus 30 g enterally daily) and parenteral selenium (500 μg) in combination with an enteral antioxidant cocktail including selenium 300 μg was associated with an improvement in mitochondrial function. Currently, the Reducing Deaths due to Oxidative Stress (REDOXS study) [41], a multicenter prospective double-blind randomized trial in 1200 ICU patients is investigating the effect of this high-dose glutamine and antioxidant combination on mortality. A different combination of glutamine and selenium incorporated into a standard parenteral nutrition regimen was investigated in the multicenter Scottish Intensive care Glutamine or seleNium Evaluative Trial (SIGNET) [42]. Four groups of patients were randomized to receive: a) glutamine 0.2 g/kg/day; b) selenium (as sodium selenite) 500 μg/day; c) glutamine 0.2 g/kg/day plus selenium 500 μg/day; or d) parenteral nutrition with no additional glutamine or selenium. None of the parenteral nutrition regimens had any effect on new infections or on mortality. However, there was a reduced incidence of new infections (odds ratio 0.53, 95 % CI 0.30 to 0.93) in the subgroup of patients who received parenteral nutrition supplemented with high dose sodium selenite for at least 5 days [42].

Current Evidence on Selenium Supplementation

In 2005, the first meta-analysis on antioxidants in ICU patients was published [43]. Moderate to low doses of selenium (less than 500 μg/day) were not associated with a decrease in mortality (RR 1.47, 95 % CI 0.20 – 10.78, p = 0.70), whereas studies that used doses higher than 500 μg/day showed a tendency towards a decrease in mortality (RR 0.52, 95 % CI 0.24 – 1.14, p = 0.10) [43]. More recently, the same Canadian group finished a large updated meta-analysis on the same topic including a total of 20 RCTs, and demonstrated that, overall, antioxidants including selenium are associated with a significant reduction in mortality (RR = 0.81, 95 CI 0.71 – 0.93, p = 0.003) [44]. Of the studies included, 15 (n = 1411) have evaluated selenium alone or combined with other micronutrients in antioxidants cocktails. Selenium, administered either by the enteral or parenteral route, was associated with a trend toward a reduction in mortality (RR = 0.88, 95 % CI 0.76 – 1.02, p = 0.10). Furthermore, when aggregated, trials using selenium demonstrated a significant reduction in infections (RR = 0.86, 95 % CI 0.74 – 1.00, p = 0.05), whereas trials not using selenium manifested a non-significant trend toward an increase in infectious complications [44]. In 9 studies including 1120 patients, selenium was given as monotherapy, which was associated with a trend toward reduction in mortality (RR = 0.85, 95 % CI 0.72 – 1.01, p = 0.06). Finally, the effect of parenteral selenium via bolus infusion on mortality

XVII

was evaluated in 4 RCTs and showed a trend toward mortality reduction (RR = 0.63, 95 % CI 0.32 – 1.23, p = 0.17) [44].

Safety of Selenium Supplementation in the Critically Ill

The complex mechanisms underlying selenium toxicity in humans were investigated in the 1970s and 80s but are still not fully understood. In our recent review of selenium supplementation in the critically ill [45], we concluded from these early published data that toxicity probably involves a pro-oxidant effect from replacement of a sulfur with a selenium atom in key molecules, leading to neurotoxicity, anemia, liver dysfunction and pancreatic changes, at an oral dose of selenite above 0.05 mg/kg (or 3500 μg/70 kg human). This led to the establishment of a lowest adverse events level (LOAEL) for clinical symptoms of selenosis at 900 – 1000 μg selenium/day. No selenosis has been recorded in individuals with blood selenium concentrations below 1000 μg/l, (corresponding to an approximate daily intake of 850 μg), and this has been taken as a NOAEL (no observed adverse effect level) for clinical selenosis. In 2000, the Scientific Committee on Food, deliberating on the Tolerable Upper Intake Level (TUIL) [46] of selenium established an upper limit for dietary selenium of 300 μg/day in adults, including pregnant and lactating women. Selenium concentrations increase in a dose-dependent manner and a risk of toxicity exists at the highest levels of supplementation. Nevertheless, most of the published human toxicity data relate to chronic oral intakes and cannot necessarily be extrapolated to the situation in the ICU, where selenium is not normally administered for more than 1 to 2 weeks to already depleted patients.

What then is the optimum therapeutic but safe posology for critically ill patients? It has been suggested that parenteral selenium doses greater than 400 μg/day could be harmful [46] but this seems to be based on the recommended TUIL for daily oral intake of at least three months and is actually less than half the World Health Organization (WHO) toxic level of 900 μg/day [47]. Heyland [48] in turn suggested that doses greater than 1000 μg/day could be harmful but proposed that a dose less than 800 μg/day is probably inadequate and ineffective for selenium deficient ICU patients. On the other hand, Vincent and Forceville [25] proposed that any dose below the TUIL may be used in the critically ill, but doses above 800 μg/day need to be researched further. However, all these suggestions are speculative and not sustained by strong toxicological evidence. Taking into account total parenteral and enteral selenium, the various protocols from Germany and Uruguay have supplemented a total selenium dose ranging up to 19,000 μg (19 mg) during 10 – 14 days [45]. Neither group of investigators reported any selenium-specific adverse events due to the high acute dose selenium supplementation, but demonstrated improvements in certain clinical end points [2, 45]. This finding supports a recommended posology of 1000 – 1600 μg/day.

XVII   Conclusion

We currently know that SIRS is characterized by low selenium status, which is associated with poor prognosis. The optimum safe dose and method of administration remains controversial but greatest efficacy in critically ill SIRS patients has been reported from very high selenium doses, administered by bolus followed by continuous infusion. Daily doses of sodium selenite providing between 1000 – 1600 µg for 10 to 14 days, after an initial intravenous bolus, appear to be safe without side effects. Selenium supplementation has been shown to improve clinical outcomes, such as illness severity and infectious complications. Further studies should aim to confirm the benefit of high dose intravenous selenite, alone or in combination, on antioxidant capacity and mortality in the critically ill.

References

1. Berger MM, Chiólero R (2007) Antioxidant supplementation in sepsis and systemic inflammatory response syndrome. Crit Care Med 35 (Suppl): S584-S590
2. Manzanares W, Hardy G (2009) Selenium supplementation in the critically ill: posology and pharmacokinetics. Curr Opin Clin Nutr Metab Care 12: 273 – 280
3. Steinbrenner H, Sies H (2009) Protection against reactive oxygen species by selenoproteins. Biochim Biophys Acta 1790: 1478 – 1485
4. Martindale RG, McClave SA, Vanek VW, et al (2009) Guidelines for the provision of nutrition support therapy in the adult critically ill patient: Society of Critical Care Medicine and A.S.P.E.N: Crit Care Med 37: 1757 – 1761
5. Singer P, Berger M, Van den Berghe G, et al (2009) ESPEN guidelines on parenteral nutrition: intensive care. Clin Nutr 28: 387 – 400
6. Lu J, Holmgren A (2009) Selenoproteins. J Biol Chem 284: 723 – 727
7. Moghadaszadeh B, Beggs AH (2006) Selenoproteins and their impact on human health through diverse physiological pathways. Physiology 21: 307 – 315
8. Fairweather-Tait SJ, Bao Y, Broadley M, et al (2011) Selenium in Human Health and Disease. Antioxid Redox Signal 14: 1337 – 1383
9. Angstwurm MW, Schopohl J, Gaertner R (2004) Selenium substitution has no direct effect on thyroid hormone metabolism in critically ill patients. Eur J Endocrinol 151: 47 – 54
10. Duntas LH (2009) Selenium and inflammation: underlying anti-inflammatory mechanisms. Horm Metab Res 41: 443 – 447
11. Valenta J, Brodska H, Drabek T, Hendl J, Kazda A (2011) High-dose selenium substitution in sepsis: a prospective, randomized clinical trial. Intensive Care Med 37: 808 – 815
12. Zamamiri-Davis F, Lu Y, Thompson JT, et al (2002) Nuclear factor-kappa B mediates overexpression of cyclooxygenase-2 during activation of RAW 264.7 macrophages in selenium defi ciency. Free Radic Biol Med 32: 890 – 897
13. Zhang F, Yu W, Hargrove JL, et al (2002) Inhibition of TNF-alpha induced ICAM-1, VCAM-1 and E-selectin expression by selenium. Atherosclerosis 161: 381 – 386
14. Geoghegan M, McAuley D, Eaton S, Powell-Tuck J (2006) Selenium in critical illness. Curr Opin Crit Care 12: 136 – 141
15. Ashton K, Hooper L, Harvey LJ, Hurst R, Casgrain A, Fairweather-Tait SJ (2009) Methods of assessment of selenium status in humans: a systematic review. Am J Clin Nutr 89: 2025S – 2039S
16. Burk RF, Hill KE (2005) Selenoprotein P: an extracellular protein with unique physical characteristics and role in selenium homeostasis. Ann Rev Nutr 25: 2125 – 235
17. Maehira F, Luyo GA, Miyagy I, et al (2002) Alterations of serum selenium concentration in the acute phase of pathological conditions. Clin Chim Acta 316: 137 – 146
18. Berger MM (2006) Antioxidant micronutrients in major trauma and burns: evidence and practice. Nutr Clin Pract 21: 438 – 449
19. Forceville X, Vitoux D, Gauzit R, Combes A, Lahilaire P, Chappuis P (1998) Selenium, systemic immune response syndrome, sepsis and outcome in critically ill patients. Crit Care Med 26: 1536 – 1544
20. Forceville X, Mostert V, Pierantoni A, et al (2009) Selenoprotein P, rather than glutathione peroxidase, as a potential marker of septic shock and related syndromes. Eur Surg Res 43: 338 – 347

XVII

21. Sakr Y, Reinhart K, Bloos F, et al (2007) Time course and relationship between plasma selenium concentrations, systemic inflammatory response, sepsis and multiorgan failure. Br J Anaesth 98: 775–784

22. Manzanares W, Biestro A, Galusso F, et al (2009) Serum selenium and glutathione peroxidase-3 activity: biomarkers of systemic inflammation in the critically ill. Intensive Care Med 35: 882–889

23. Wereszczynska-Siemiatkowska U, Mroczko B, Siemiatkowskia A, Szmitkowski M, Borawska M, Kosel J (2004) The importance of interleukin 18, glutathione peroxidase, and selenium concentration changes in acute pancreatitis. Dig Dis Sci 49: 642–650

24. Stoppe C, Shalte G, Rossaint R, et al (2011) The intraoperative decrease of selenium is associated with the postoperative development of multiorgan dysfunction in cardiac surgical patients Crit Care Med 39: 1879–1885

25. Vincent JL, Forceville X (2008) Critically elucidating the role of selenium. Curr Opin Anesthesiol 21: 148–154

26. Jeong DW, Yoo MH, Kim TS, Kim IY (2002) Protection of mice from allergen-induced asthma by selenite: prevention of eosinophil infiltration by inhibition of NF-kappa B activation. J Biol Chem 277: 17871–17876

27. Stewart MS, Spallholz JE, Neldner KH, Pence BC (1999) Selenium compounds have disparate abilities to impose oxidative stress and induce apoptosis. Free Radic Biol Med 26: 42–48

28. Wang Z, Forceville X, Van Antwerpen P, et al (2009) A large bolus, but not a continuous infusion, of sodium selenite improves outcome in peritonitis. Shock 32: 140–146

29. Manzanares W, Biestro A, Galusso F, et al (2010) High-dose selenium for critically ill patients with systemic inflammation: a pilot study. Nutrition 26: 634–640

30. Zimmermann T, Albrecht S, Kuhne H, Vogelsang U, Grutzmann R, Kopprasch S (1997) Selenium administration in patients with sepsis syndrome: a prospective randomized study. Med Klin 92: 3–4

31. Angstwurm MA, Schottdorf J, Schopohl J, Gaertner R (1999) Selenium replacement in patients with severe systemic inflammatory response syndrome improves clinical outcome. Crit Care Med 27: 1807–1813

32. Angstwurm MW, Engelmann L, Zimmermann T, et al (2007) Selenium in Intensive Care (SIC): results of a prospective randomized, placebo-controlled, multiple-center study in patients with severe systemic inflammatory response syndrome, sepsis, and septic shock. Crit Care Med 35: 118–126

33. Mishra V, Baines M, Perry SE, et al (2007) Effect of selenium supplementation on biochemical markers and outcome in critically ill patients. Clin Nutr 26: 41–50

34. Forceville X, Laviolle B, Annane D, et al (2007) Effects of high doses of selenium, as sodium selenite, in septic shock: a placebo-controlled, randomized, double-blind, phase II study. Crit Care 11: R73

35. Manzanares W, Biestro A, Torre MH, Galusso F, Facchín G, Hardy G (2011) High dose selenium reduces ventilator associated pneumonia and illness severity in critically ill patients with systemic inflammation. Intensive Care Med 37: 1120–1127

36. Berger MM, Eggimann P, Heyland DK, et al (2006) Reduction of nosocomial pneumonia after major burns by trace element supplementation: aggregation of two randomised trials. Crit Care 10: R153

37. Soguel L, Chiólero RL, Ruffieux C, Berger MM (2008) Monitoring the clinical introduction of a glutamine and antioxidant solution in critically ill trauma and burn patients. Nutrition 24: 1123–1132

38. Berger MM, Soguel L, Shenkin A, et al (2008) Influence of early antioxidant supplements on clinical evolution and organ function in critically ill cardiac surgery, major trauma and subarachnoid hemorrhage patients. Crit Care 12: R101

39. Collier BR, Giladi A, Dosset LA, Dyer L, Fleming SB, Cotton BA (2008) Impact of high-dose antioxidants on outcomes in acutely injured patients. JPEN J Parent Enteral Nutr 31: 384–388

40. Heyland DK, Dhaliwal R, Day A, Drover J, Cote H, Wischmeyer P (2007) Optimizing the dose of glutamine dipeptides and antioxidants in critically ill patients: a phase I dose-finding study. JPEN J Parenter Enteral Nutr 31: 109–118

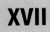

41. Heyland DK, Dhaliwal R, Day AG, et al (2006) REducing Deaths due to OXidative Stress (The REDOXS Study): rationale and study design for a randomized trial of glutamine and antioxidant supplementation in critically ill patients. Proc Nutr Soc 65: 250–263
42. Andrews PJD, Avenell A, Noble DW, et al (2011) Randomised trial of glutamine, selenium, or both to supplement parenteral nutrition for critically ill patients. BMJ 342: d1542
43. Heyland DK, Dhaliwal R, Suchner U, Berger MM (2005) Antioxidants nutrients: a systematic review of trace elements and vitamins in the critically ill patient. Intensive Care Med 31: 327–337
44. Canadian Clinical Practice Guidelines. Available at http://www.criticalcarenutrition.com. Accessed November 2011
45. Hardy G, Hardy IJ, Manzanares W (2012) Selenium supplementation in the critically ill. Nutr Clin Pract 27 (in press)
46. Shenkin A. Selenium in intravenous nutrition (2009) Gastroenterology 137: S61–S69.
47. World Health Organization (1987) Selenium, Environmental Health Criteria 58. WHO, Geneva
48. Heyland DK (2007) Selenium supplementation in critically ill patients: can too much of a good thing be a bad thing? Crit Care 11: 153

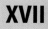

XVIII Trauma

A New Understanding of Coagulopathy in Trauma

M.C. READE and A.D. HOLLEY

Introduction

Exsanguination is the second commonest cause of death in trauma after central nervous system (CNS) injury [1]. Admission coagulopathy in trauma is associated with multiple organ failure, longer intensive care unit (ICU) stay, and mortality [2]. If this association is causative, prevention, rapid identification and appropriate management of coagulopathy may improve outcome. Until recently, the pathogenesis of the coagulopathy of trauma was thought to be a 'triad' of loss and dilution of procoagulant clotting factors, hypothermia and acidemia [3, 4], perhaps along with disseminated intravascular coagulation (DIC) [5]. However, there is emerging evidence that tissue hypoperfusion accompanying major trauma also causes hypo- (and later, hyper-) coagulation, as do endothelial dysfunction, inflammation, and possibly platelet dysfunction. More specific focus on these factors may be useful therapeutic targets in trauma. Here, we review evidence for and against the traditional model of traumatic coagulopathy and explore what is known of the interaction between traumatic coagulopathy and hypoperfusion, inflammation, and endothelial and platelet dysfunction. We conclude by suggesting potential therapeutic avenues to exploit these relationships.

Traditional 'Extrinsic' Models of the Coagulopathy of Trauma

Traditional understanding of the coagulopathy of trauma rests on observed associations between the extrinsically imposed triad of acidemia, dilution of clotting factors and hypothermia, and abnormalities of clotting tests and greater blood loss [3, 4, 6]. To this pathogenic triad is sometimes added DIC [5], such as occurs in other forms of critical illness. The extent to which these associations are causative is, however, speculative.

Hypothermia

Severe hypothermia (core temperature less than 32°C) is occasionally seen in postoperative and critically ill patients, but is rarely present in trauma cases [7]. Severe hypothermia directly interferes with hemostasis by slowing the activity of reactions catalyzed by coagulation enzymes, and by reducing fibrinogen synthesis [8]. However, most shocked trauma patients have only mild hypothermia (35 to 33°C), which has little effect on coagulation proteases or clinical bleeding [9, 10]. Platelet aggregation and adhesion are more sensitive to hypothermia, being

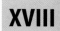

XVIII

J.-L. Vincent (ed.), *Annual Update in Intensive Care and Emergency Medicine 2012*
DOI 10.1007/978-3-642-25716-2 © Springer-Verlag Berlin Heidelberg 2012

decreased by 40 % in the moderate hypothermic range. However, these *in vitro* platelet effects do not appear to contribute to clinical bleeding [10]. Lack of an important effect of mild hypothermia is well known to cardiac surgeons, whose patients on cardiopulmonary bypass (CPB) are often maintained at around 34 °C without clinically significant adverse effects. Therefore, although the severity of both coagulopathy and hypothermia increase with the severity of trauma, lack of a causal relationship suggests attention to core temperature alone will not reduce coagulopathic bleeding in the majority of patients.

Dilution

Initial resuscitation of hemorrhagic shock is often achieved with crystalloid or colloid solutions containing no clotting factors. Dilution of remaining factors has logically been assumed by many authors [11] to contribute to an acute coagulopathy. This argument ignores the homeostatic balance between procoagulant and anticoagulant factors immediately prior to trauma, and the consequent proportional dilution of anticoagulant factors as well [11]. Indeed, the effect of loss of procoagulant factors may be proportionately less important than loss of anticoagulant factors, because the endothelium can release factor XIII and von Willebrand factor in major trauma [11]. Notwithstanding this theoretical argument, dilution does indeed appear to contribute at least a little to coagulopathy. A European study of 8724 patients found that more than 50 % of patients who had received more than 3 l fluid in the prehospital phase were coagulopathic, compared to only 10 % of patients who had received less than 500 ml [2]. Early administration of plasma rather than crystalloid or colloid to patients requiring more than 10 units of packed red cells appears [12, 13] (although not yet conclusively [14]) to improve outcome. This is probably because dilutional coagulopathy is avoided, although as noted elsewhere in this chapter, modulation of inflammation is another possible explanation. Dilutional coagulopathy is, however, not the only cause of the coagulopathy of trauma. In a seminal paper that led to re-examination of much traditional teaching, Brohi et al. [15] demonstrated that the incidence of coagulopathy was determined more by severity of injury than by volume of intravenous fluid administered. These authors showed that coagulopathy was present on hospital admission in 25 % of trauma patients who had received minimal or no prehospital fluid administration. This finding was replicated in a larger database study of 7638 patients [16]. As with hypothermia, there must be an explanation other than dilution for the coagulopathy of trauma.

Acidemia

Metabolic acidosis in trauma is primarily due to hyperlactatemia resulting from tissue hypoperfusion and hypoxia. Multiple studies have demonstrated that mortality and morbidity in trauma and critical illness correlate with the severity of metabolic acidosis [17]. At least at extremes of pH, this association is plausibly causative. Metabolic acidosis impairs cardiac contractility, is arrhythmogenic, and precipitates vasodilatory hypotension with decreased hepatic and renal blood flow [18]. Acidosis directly reduces the activity of the coagulation cascade proteases as assayed by prothrombin time (PT) and partial thromboplastin time (PTT), and diminishes platelet aggregation [19, 20]. However, separating the independent effect of acidemia from that of illness severity is difficult in observa-

XVIII

tional clinical studies. Experimentally-induced severe acidosis in animals, using infusions of hydrochloric acid to achieve pH down to 7.1, inhibits the propagation phase of thrombin generation in a cell-based model of coagulation and accelerates fibrinogen degradation by nearly two-fold [21]. With more modest manipulations of pH, into the range more often encountered in trauma, however, the effect is less marked [19]. A clinically significant effect of acidemia on coagulopathy is, therefore, unlikely until the pH decreases below 7.2. Only a minority of trauma patients become this acidemic. Moreover, hydrogen ion concentration *per se* appears unlikely to be the mechanism of traumatic coagulopathy, as correction of pH using buffer has little effect on bleeding [8]. It appears that acidemia is a marker for cellular stress and severity of illness, rather than a quantitatively important direct cause for coagulopathy. Therapy for the coagulopathy of trauma should, therefore, be targeted elsewhere.

An Alternative, 'Intrinsic', Pathogenesis of the Coagulopathy of Trauma?

The three proposed 'extrinsic' explanations for the coagulopathy of trauma appear inadequate to explain a substantial proportion of the observed abnormalities of laboratory tests and clinical bleeding in severely injured patients. At one level this is disappointing, as normalization of body temperature, pH and clotting factor concentration can be relatively easy to achieve in adequately equipped hospitals. However, identification of an endogenous pathophysiological mechanism would open the possibility of entirely new therapeutic approaches, and so warrants exploration.

Is 'Consumption Coagulopathy' a Feature of Major Trauma?

If the above 'triad' is not a major pathophysiological mechanism for trauma-induced coagulopathy, explanations must be sought elsewhere. In other forms of critical illness, consumption of clotting factors (DIC) with as an underlying mechanism of coagulopathy because of shock has long been recognized [22]. However, there is debate over whether DIC commonly occurs in the acute phase of trauma. In trauma patients with preserved systemic perfusion, Brohi et al. [23] found that coagulation parameters, including PT and PTT, were typically not prolonged, regardless of the amount of thrombin generated. If consumption was the mechanism accounting for the acute coagulopathy of hemorrhagic shock, then increasing thrombin genesis would imply factor consumption and subsequent derangement of measures of clotting, but this was not the case. Furthermore, this group also showed that platelets and fibrinogen levels were within normal ranges in patients with acute traumatic coagulopathy in the absence of hypoperfusion [24]. The clear conclusion is that the acute coagulopathy of trauma is not caused by disseminated consumption of clotting factors. In contrast, others have pointed to observations of reduced fibrinogen, fibrinolysis, thrombin and plasmin activity in trauma patients on arrival to hospital as evidence of a consumptive coagulopathy and microvascular thrombosis [25]. Debate on this point would be resolved if microvascular thrombosis could be demonstrated in patients dying in the acute phase of trauma, which to date has not occurred. Of interest, later in this chapter

XVIII

we argue that acute trauma is a pro-inflammatory state. If the inflammation of trauma does not cause DIC, the manner in which traumatic inflammation differs from that of other forms of critical illness remains open to question.

The Modern Cell-based Model of Coagulation

Before exploring evidence for an endogenous or 'intrinsic' pathogenesis of acute traumatic coagulopathy, it is useful to briefly review the modern understanding of the initiation, propagation and resolution of blood clotting. The classic extrinsic and intrinsic coagulation cascade was proposed in 1905 by Morawitz [26], based on four known coagulation factors, and postulated the conversion of fibrinogen to fibrin by thrombin. This theory was replaced by the cascade or waterfall model in 1964 to accommodate the discovery of additional coagulation factors [27]. The cascade model proposed that coagulation consisted of an activating sequence in which proenzymes were converted into active enzymes with associated amplification. Although this model is intellectually appealing, more recently it has been understood that the major quantitative *in vivo* elements of coagulation are not just the soluble clotting factors, but cells bearing exposed tissue factor (TF) tightly integrated with anticoagulant and fibrinolytic systems. Discovery of cellular surface receptors and TF-bearing cells required development of a cell-based model of coagulation [28]. The endothelium and platelets occupy central roles as active drivers of these processes [29, 30]. This model is characterized in three overlapping phases: Initiation, amplification and propagation [31].

Initiation

Endothelial disruption through illness or injury exposes TF to the circulation. TF is a receptor for circulating factor (F) VII, which on binding undergoes a conformational change to become enzymatically active (FVIIa). The TF/FVIIa complex catalyzes conversion of prothrombin to thrombin. During this phase the TF/FVIIa complex also activates FIX and FX. FIXa migrates and binds to platelet surfaces, whereas FXa remains bound to the TF-bearing cell. The small quantity of thrombin generated during this phase is critical to subsequent thrombin and fibrin production [28, 31].

Amplification

Thrombin generated during the initiation phase activates platelets, FV, FVIII and FXI. The amplification phase predominantly occurs on the platelet surface. Thrombin activates FVIII by cleaving and liberating it from von Willebrand factor (vWF) [28] and also activates FV, FVIII and FXI allowing for the generation of large quantities of thrombin in the propagation phase. The amplification phase terminates with FVa and activated FVIII (FVIIIa) bound to the surface of the activated platelets.[31]

Propagation

In the propagation phase, tenase (FVIIIa/FIXa) and prothrombinase (FVa/FXa) complexes are generated on the platelet surface. The tenase complex then activates FX, which binds its cofactor, FVa. The platelet bound prothrombinase initiates a burst of thrombin resulting in the conversion of fibrinogen to fibrin. Thrombin produced in this phase also activates factor XIII, which stabilizes the fibrin clot by catalyzing covalent crosslinkages [28].

The coagulation response is tightly modulated to ensure timely thrombus formation without an overshoot of fibrin formation. Once the injured or diseased endothelium is isolated, fibrin formation not only ceases but is subsequently removed by fibrinolysis. This process involves the breakdown of fibrin clots by plasmin to D-dimer fragments, so named because they contain two linked 'D' fragments of fibrinogen protein. Plasmin is formed from plasminogen by tissue plasminogen activator. The principle inhibitor of plasminogen activator is plasminogen activator inhibitor (PAI)-1, which is produced by the endothelium. The protein C system is a second important regulator of both hemostasis and inflammation. Protein C is synthesized in the liver and is turned into activated protein C (APC) by thrombin bound to the endothelial cell membrane. APC then serves as an anticoagulant by inhibiting activated coagulation factors VIII and V (together with a cofactor, protein S). APC also exhibits profibrinolytic function by inhibiting PAI-1 [32].

Mechanisms of 'Intrinsic' Trauma-induced Coagulopathy ('Acute Traumatic Coagulopathy'[33] Or 'Endogenous Acute Coagulopathy' [34])

Two recent studies of 1088 and 7638 patients have found acute coagulopathy is already present on arrival to the emergency department in around 25 % of patients with major trauma [15, 16]. This observation cannot be explained solely on the basis of acidemia, hypothermia or dilutional coagulopathy. There are only two possible logical explanations for this finding: Either the cell-based procoagulant processes referred to above have become dysfunctional; or the counter-regulatory anti-inflammatory processes have become abnormally amplified. There is little evidence that procoagulant factors become acutely deficient. In contrast, there is emerging evidence that the thrombomodulin-protein C pathway is responsible for the activation of anticoagulant and fibrinolytic pathways [24].

Tissue Hypoperfusion as an Initiator of Acute Traumatic Coagulopathy via Activated Protein C

Tissue hypoperfusion in hemorrhagic shock due to trauma is a likely mechanism for the development of acute traumatic coagulopathy (**Fig. 1**). In the presence of tissue hypoperfusion, the endothelium expresses thrombomodulin which complexes with thrombin. The thrombin-thrombomudulin complex activates protein C to APC [34]. APC subsequently deactivates cofactors V and VIII potentiating the anticoagulated state. Interestingly, APC in excess can effectively consume PAI-1 and thus lead to a 'de-repression' of fibrinolytic activity and systemic hyperfibrinolysis [35]. In binding to thrombomodulin, less thrombin is available to catalyze the conversion of fibrinogen to fibrin. Similarly activation of fibrinolysis may occur as tissue plasminogen activator (tPA) is released from the endothelium following injury or ischemia in the setting of hypoperfusion. In a prospective cohort study of 208 patients, an increasing base deficit (indicative of tissue hypoperfu-

XVIII

sion) was associated with high soluble thrombomodulin, low protein C levels [23], and reduced fibrinogen utilization [24]. Reduced (quiescent) protein C was taken to indicate an increase of APC, and therefore inhibition of coagulation, a hypothesis confirmed by preliminary data [34].

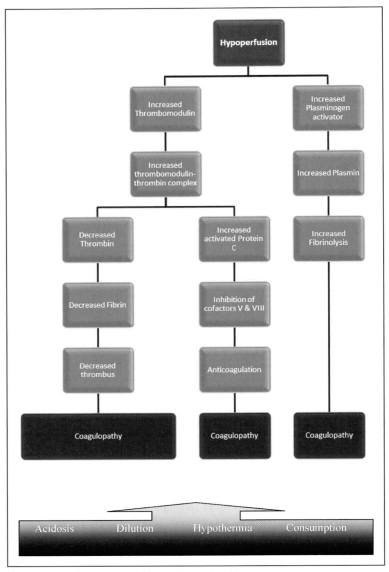

Fig. 1. Hypoperfusion as the initiator of coagulopathy

Inflammation as a Modulator of Hypercoaguability Following on From Acute Traumatic Coagulopathy

Even before the 2001 demonstration of improved mortality with pharmacologically administered recombinant APC in patients with severe sepsis [36], the interaction between inflammation and coagulopathy was widely appreciated [37]. Inflammation is a clear consequence of major tissue trauma [38]. In other forms of critical illness, such as sepsis, inflammatory mediators downregulate protein C and antithrombin [39], leading to a procoagulant state [34]. Major trauma patients are particularly prone to developing venous thromboembolic disease during the subacute phase of their illness [40]. Depletion of APC is a possible mechanism for this effect, along with downregulation of thrombomodulin expression [34, 41], but the full explanation has not yet been characterized.

Platelet Dysfunction

In the cell-based coagulation model described above, amplification of clotting takes place on the platelet membrane. Despite this central place in coagulation, whether or not platelet dysfunction contributes to acute traumatic coagulopathy is unclear [42]. Platelet counts are usually normal despite the initial presence of acute traumatic coagulopathy, in part due to their release from the spleen and lungs [11], suggesting any major defect must be with their function. *In vivo* platelet function is difficult to assess, but what evidence there is suggests increased platelet activation (characterized by circulating platelet microparticles, P-selectin and activated platelet receptor glycoprotein IIb–IIIa expression) and function (measured using collagen/epinephrine closure time) in the early response to trauma [43]. However, patients who did not survive had significantly lower platelet function, suggesting a defect in platelet function is a pathological response in the most unwell patients. Whether transfused platelets, or activators of platelet adhesion, such as desmopressin [44], might improve coagulation (and perhaps outcome) in such patients remains speculative.

Tests of Coagulopathy Inadequate in Trauma

As is the case with derangements in many physiological parameters, initial abnormal PT and PTT were significantly independently associated with an increased risk of death in 7638 patients in a trauma registry [16]. PT is the more greatly affected. However, these two tests of coagulation in common clinical use poorly reflect *in vivo* hemostasis [45], principally because they do not assess the *in vivo* interactions with platelets and endothelium. They also remain prolonged even if coagulation is improved by reductions in antithrombin or APC, and give no measure of clot stability. Lastly, they take 45–60 minutes to assay, which may be too long to guide therapy in an exsanguinating patient. Therefore, they are not the optimal measures of the efficacy of coagulation therapy in trauma. Alternative point-of-care tests still establishing their place in clinical practice, thromboelastography (TEG) and thromboelastometry (ROTEM), rely on the viscoelastic properties of a clot formed *in vitro* in the presence of activators and inhibitors. Deficiencies in platelet function and fibrinogen are identified by maximal clot strength (and distinguished from one another by additional testing in the presence of cytochalasin D to inhibit platelet adhesion), and in coagulation factors by the clotting time. Fibrinolysis (and therefore the indication for anti-fibrinolytic therapy) is indicated by the premature lysis of the clot. The ROTEM system is currently used to guide coagulation therapy in massive transfusion in military [46] and civilian hospitals, albeit without convincing data demonstrating an impact on patient outcome.

Therapeutic Implications of a Unified Model of Endothelial Hypoperfusion, Coagulopathy and Inflammation

There are a number of therapeutic implications to the pathophysiological mechanisms proposed above that go beyond the simple (but still most likely useful) conventional strategies to avoid hypothermia, tissue hypoperfusion and dilution of clotting factors. First, aggressive resuscitation with plasma as well as red blood cells is theoretically warranted not only to replace lost (or perhaps consumed) clotting factors, but to restore peripheral perfusion and so reduce the endothelial contribution to coagulopathy. Second, whether augmentation of peripheral perfusion using vasodilators can improve acute traumatic coagulopathy is an attractive question; conversely it is not surprising that use of vasopressors in traumatic shock is associated with higher mortality [47]. Third, a normal platelet count is not sufficient reassurance that a platelet function defect does not exist. Whether the best response to platelet dysfunction is platelet transfusion or a medication to 'activate' platelets is not yet known. Fourth, as inflammation and coagulation are tightly linked, therapy that impacts on one of these may have beneficial or detrimental effects on the other. The effect of hypoperfusion on the development of acidosis in trauma might be improved by strategies that reduce metabolism and inflammation [48, 49], but such strategies may (or may not) worsen acute coagulopathy by increasing APC. Fifth, the transition between hypo- and hyper-coagulable state in trauma is neither well characterized nor clinically readily detected. Better understanding of this transition may allow more specific and better timed thromboprophylaxis. Last and most importantly, it is clear that the pathophysiological mechanisms at play are only just starting to be understood, and that acute traumatic coagulopathy (including clinical methods for its characterization) is a promising field of acute care research.

Conclusion

It is increasingly apparent that whereas acidemia, hypothermia and dilution are common 'extrinsic' accompaniments to severe trauma, they cannot explain all the coagulopathy observed. Equally valid if not better therapeutic targets are, therefore, the increasingly understood 'intrinsic' drivers of acute traumatic coagulopathy: Hypoperfusion-induced endothelial dysfunction, inflammation, and the activation of protein C. At least some of these factors will plausibly be targeted in clinical trials in the next few years. With its beginnings in the renewed interest in trauma-induced coagulopathy resulting from systematic observations in military hospitals during the wars in Iraq and Afghanistan, improvement in medical science may be one of the few positive legacies of these armed conflicts.

XVIII

References

1. Sauaia A, Moore FA, Moore EE, et al (1995) Epidemiology of trauma deaths: a reassessment. J Trauma 38: 185–193
2. Maegele M, Lefering R, Yucel N, et al (2007) Early coagulopathy in multiple injury: an analysis from the German Trauma Registry on 8724 patients. Injury 38: 298–304
3. Kashuk JL, Moore EE, Millikan JS, Moore JB (1982) Major abdominal vascular trauma--a unified approach. J Trauma 22: 672–679
4. Moore EE (1996) Thomas G. Orr Memorial Lecture. Staged laparotomy for the hypothermia, acidosis, and coagulopathy syndrome. Am J Surg 172: 405–410
5. Hess JR, Lawson JH (2006) The coagulopathy of trauma versus disseminated intravascular coagulation. J Trauma 60: S12–S19
6. Mitra B, Cameron PA, Mori A, Fitzgerald M (2012) Acute coagulopathy and early deaths post major trauma. Injury 43: 22–25
7. Martin RS, Kilgo PD, Miller PR, Hoth JJ, Meredith JW, Chang MC (2005) Injury-associated hypothermia: an analysis of the 2004 National Trauma Data Bank. Shock 24: 114–118
8. Martini WZ (2009) Coagulopathy by hypothermia and acidosis: mechanisms of thrombin generation and fibrinogen availability. J Trauma 67: 202–208
9. Martini WZ, Pusateri AE, Uscilowicz JM, Delgado AV, Holcomb JB (2005) Independent contributions of hypothermia and acidosis to coagulopathy in swine. J Trauma 58: 1002–1009
10. Wolberg AS, Meng ZH, Monroe DM, III, Hoffman M (2004) A systematic evaluation of the effect of temperature on coagulation enzyme activity and platelet function. J Trauma 56: 1221–1228
11. Bolliger D, Gorlinger K, Tanaka KA (2010) Pathophysiology and treatment of coagulopathy in massive hemorrhage and hemodilution. Anesthesiology 113: 1205–1219
12. Borgman MA, Spinella PC, Perkins JG, et al (2007) The ratio of blood products transfused affects mortality in patients receiving massive transfusions at a combat support hospital. J Trauma 63: 805–813
13. Holcomb JB, Wade CE, Michalek JE, et al (2008) Increased plasma and platelet to red blood cell ratios improves outcome in 466 massively transfused civilian trauma patients. Ann Surg 248: 447–458
14. Snyder CW, Weinberg JA, McGwin G Jr, et al (2009) The relationship of blood product ratio to mortality: survival benefit or survival bias? J Trauma 66: 358–362
15. Brohi K, Singh J, Heron M, Coats T (2003) Acute traumatic coagulopathy. J Trauma 54: 1127–1130
16. MacLeod JB, Lynn M, McKenney MG, Cohn SM, Murtha M (2003) Early coagulopathy predicts mortality in trauma. J Trauma 55: 39–44
17. Eberhard LW, Morabito DJ, Matthay MA, et al (2000) Initial severity of metabolic acidosis predicts the development of acute lung injury in severely traumatized patients. Crit Care Med 28: 125–131
18. Wildenthal K, Mierzwiak DS, Myers RW, Mitchell JH (1968) Effects of acute lactic acidosis on left ventricular performance. Am J Physiol 214: 1352–1359
19. Engstrom M, Schott U, Romner B, Reinstrup P (2006) Acidosis impairs the coagulation: A thromboelastographic study. J Trauma 61: 624–628
20. Meng ZH, Wolberg AS, Monroe DM, III, Hoffman M (2003) The effect of temperature and pH on the activity of factor VIIa: implications for the efficacy of high-dose factor VIIa in hypothermic and acidotic patients. J Trauma 55: 886–891
21. Frith D, Goslings JC, Gaarder C, et al (2010) Definition and drivers of acute traumatic coagulopathy: clinical and experimental investigations. J Thromb Haemost 8: 1919–1925
22. Schreiber MA (2005) Coagulopathy in the trauma patient. Curr Opin Crit Care 11: 590–597
23. Brohi K, Cohen MJ, Ganter MT, Matthay MA, Mackersie RC, Pittet JF (2007) Acute traumatic coagulopathy: initiated by hypoperfusion: modulated through the protein C pathway? Ann Surg 245: 812–818
24. Brohi K, Cohen MJ, Ganter MT, et al (2008) Acute coagulopathy of trauma: hypoperfusion induces systemic anticoagulation and hyperfibrinolysis. J Trauma 64: 1211–1217

XVIII

25. Gando S, Sawamura A, Hayakawa M (2011) Trauma, shock, and disseminated intravascular coagulation: lessons from the classical literature. Ann Surg 254: 10–19
26. Beck EA (1977) The chemistry of blood coagulation: a summary by Paul Morawitz (1905) Thromb Haemost 37: 376–379
27. Macfarlane RG (1964) An enzyme cascade in the blood clotting mechanism, and its function as a biochemical amplifier. Nature 202: 498–499
28. Hoffman M, Monroe DM III (2001) A cell-based model of hemostasis. Thromb Haemost 85: 958–965
29. Roberts HR, Hoffman M, Monroe DM (2006) A cell-based model of thrombin generation. Semin Thromb Hemost 32 (Suppl 1): 32–38
30. Verhamme P, Hoylaerts MF (2006) The pivotal role of the endothelium in haemostasis and thrombosis. Acta Clin Belg 61: 213–219
31. Hoffman M (2003) Remodeling the blood coagulation cascade. J Thromb Thrombolysis 16: 17–20
32. Knoebl P (2010) Blood coagulation disorders in septic patients. Wien Med Wochenschr 160: 129–138
33. Brohi K (2009) Trauma induced coagulopathy. J R Army Med Corps 155: 320–322
34. Cohen MJ, West M (2011) Acute traumatic coagulopathy: from endogenous acute coagulopathy to systemic acquired coagulopathy and back. J Trauma 70:S47-S49
35. Rezaie AR (2001) Vitronectin functions as a cofactor for rapid inhibition of activated protein C by plasminogen activator inhibitor-1. Implications for the mechanism of profibrinolytic action of activated protein C. J Biol Chem 276: 15567–15570
36. Bernard GR, Vincent JL, Laterre PF, et al (2001) Efficacy and safety of recombinant human activated protein C for severe sepsis. N Engl J Med 344: 699–709
37. Opal SM (2000) Phylogenetic and functional relationships between coagulation and the innate immune response. Crit Care Med 28: S77–S80
38. Cohen MJ, Brohi K, Calfee CS, et al (2009) Early release of high mobility group box nuclear protein 1 after severe trauma in humans: role of injury severity and tissue hypoperfusion. Crit Care 13: R174
39. Fukudome K, Esmon CT (1994) Identification, cloning, and regulation of a novel endothelial cell protein C/activated protein C receptor. J Biol Chem 269: 26486–26491
40. Geerts WH, Code KI, Jay RM, Chen E, Szalai JP (1994) A prospective study of venous thromboembolism after major trauma. N Engl J Med 331: 1601–1606
41. Esmon CT (2003) The protein C pathway. Chest 124: 26S–32S
42. Davenport RA, Brohi K (2009) Coagulopathy in trauma patients: importance of thrombocyte function? Curr Opin Anaesthesiol 22: 261–266
43. Jacoby RC, Owings JT, Holmes J, Battistella FD, Gosselin RC, Paglieroni TG (2001) Platelet activation and function after trauma. J Trauma 51: 639–647
44. Ng KF, Cheung CW, Lee Y, Leung SW (2011) Low-dose desmopressin improves hypothermia-induced impairment of primary haemostasis in healthy volunteers. Anaesthesia 66: 999–1005
45. Levi M, Opal SM (2006) Coagulation abnormalities in critically ill patients. Crit Care 10: 222
46. Doran CM, Woolley T, Midwinter MJ (2010) Feasibility of using rotational thromboelastometry to assess coagulation status of combat casualties in a deployed setting. J Trauma 69 (Suppl 1): S40–S48
47. Collier B, Dossett L, Mann M, et al (2010) Vasopressin use is associated with death in acute trauma patients with shock. J Crit Care 25: 173–114
48. Cotton BA (2011) Alternative fluids for prehospital resuscitation: "pharmacological" resuscitation fluids. J Trauma 70: S30–S31
49. Letson HL, Dobson GP (2011) Ultra-small intravenous bolus of 7.5 % NaCl/Mg2+ with adenosine and lidocaine improves early resuscitation outcome in the rat after severe hemorrhagic shock in vivo. J Trauma 71: 708–719

Diagnosis of Occult Bleeding in Polytrauma

F. Corradi, C. Brusasco, and P. Pelosi

Introduction

Traumatic injury is the most prevalent cause of death among persons aged 5–44 years and accounts for 10 % of all deaths worldwide [1]. Approximately, one third of trauma-related deaths are the result of uncontrolled bleeding, which may occur early after hospital admission [2]. Massive hemorrhage may be associated with either severe hypovolemia, in which blood volume decreases with no changes in hemoglobin concentration, or isovolemic anemia, in which extreme decreases in hemoglobin concentration occur with normal or even increased blood volume [3].

Massive bleeding after blunt trauma is often preventable by timely intervention. A challenge to the clinician is presented by the fact that shock may be masked by compensatory mechanisms, particularly in young otherwise healthy subjects. In addition, even small increments in intravascular volume, as in the case when crystalloid fluid boluses are given, may results in a near normal systolic blood pressure (SBP) despite continued hemorrhage. All the above may lead to delayed diagnosis and treatment with increased morbidity and mortality [4]. Currently, most emergency practitioners continue to rely on mental status, pulse character, and hypotension (SBP < 90 mmHg) as indicators of the need for life-saving interventions.

Parameters suggested for the initial assessment of blood loss in otherwise hemodynamically stable patients include the mechanism of injury, focused-assessment sonography for trauma (FAST), computed tomography (CT) scan, advanced trauma life support (ATLS) grading system [5], hematocrit level [6], markers of hypoperfusion (e.g., serum lactate level and base deficits), central venous oxygen saturation (ScvO$_2$), central venous pressure (CVP), and inferior vena cava (IVC) diameter. The major limitation of all these suggested markers of early hemorrhagic shock is that they have shown poor sensitivity and specificity [6–9].

In the present chapter, we will discuss: a) methods to diagnose the source and extent of bleeding; b) markers of tissue hypoperfusion and hypovolemia; c) possible new methods for early detection of occult bleeding and cryptic shock in hemodynamically stable polytrauma patients.

Diagnosing the Source of Bleeding

The 'high-risk' mechanism of injury is defined, according to the American College of Surgeons' (ACS) classification, as a fall from a height > 6 m, blunt trauma mechanism, or high-energy deceleration impact [5]. Together with the site of

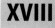

J.-L. Vincent (ed.), *Annual Update in Intensive Care and Emergency Medicine 2012*
DOI 10.1007/978-3-642-25716-2 © Springer-Verlag Berlin Heidelberg 2012

injury (e.g., unstable pelvic fractures), this definition represents an important screening method, enabling those patients who are potentially at risk for major post-traumatic bleeding to be identified. However, only a few studies have addressed the relationship between mechanism and type of injury and the risk of bleeding, and none of them was a randomized prospective trial with a high level of evidence. In blunt trauma with high-energy injury, several organs are involved but pelvis and abdominal organs are the most frequently damaged. None of these studies demonstrated greater effectiveness of one mechanism of injury over another as a useful early screening method for bleeding. Among sites of injury, unstable pelvic fractures are associated with massive hemorrhage [10], which is the leading cause of death in these patients who therefore require more transfusion units [11] and for this reason require closer monitoring and follow-up, even if apparently stable at admission [12].

Sonography

FAST has been defined by consensus conference as designating an expeditious, focused screening of the pericardial and peritoneal space looking for free fluid as a marker of injury [13]. Early FAST has been established as the primary screening examination for blunt trauma patients in the emergency department (ED) [14, 15] and its use is therefore recommended for patients with suspected torso trauma [16]. However, FAST is less reliable for localization of visceral injury compared to CT scan [12, 17, 18] and rarely shows rupture of hollow viscera [19, 20]. Regardless of FAST findings, hemodynamically stable polytrauma patients without free intra-abdominal fluid will almost always undergo CT scanning before they are transferred to the intensive care unit (ICU) [21]. This approach is reasonable because negative sonography does not decrease a high pre-test probability of intra-abdominal injury.

Some polytrauma patients who present with free intra-abdominal fluid on FAST can safely wait for CT scanning provided they are hemodynamically stable [22].

CT Scan

Regardless of sonography and clinical findings, all hemodynamically stable patients with suspected bleeding after high-energy injuries undergo CT scanning [16, 23], the role of which in imaging of acute trauma patients is well documented [24, 25]. Immediate CT scanning of polytrauma patients allows for faster diagnosis, thus shortening ED, operating room and ICU stays [25]. Compared with CT, all traditional diagnostic criteria, including imaging techniques, have limitations. In contrast with FAST, contrast-enhanced CT evaluation can yield information regarding organ-specific injury, intraperitoneal, intrathoracic or intraparenchymal pooling of blood, as well as the presence of retroperitoneal injury. But CT cannot provide information on the amount of blood already lost or the speed of ongoing hemorrhage.

Therefore, FAST is the primary screening examination for all blunt polytrauma patients with a major mechanism of injury and is always followed by CT scan regardless of whether or not there is intra-abdominal free fluid in the presence of stable hemodynamics. CT scan remains the gold standard but its main limitation is the need to move the patient to the radiology rooms with consequent waste of time and the risks of moving patients with potentially unstable fractures.

Monitoring the Extent of Bleeding

ATLS Grading System

On admission to the ED, the extent of traumatic hemorrhage should be clinically assessed by a grading system, such as the classification established by the ACS [5], which may be useful in the initial assessment of bleeding. To better assess the optimal amount of volume replacement, hemorrhage can be divided into four classes ranging from Class I, which represents a non-shock state (such as the case of blood donors of 1 unit of blood), to Class IV, representing a pre-terminal state requiring immediate therapy. However, this tool has been proposed to quantify the magnitude of shock and is, therefore, not very useful in hemodynamically stable patients, because of the low sensitivity of the parameters on which it is based (pulse rate, SBP, respiratory rate, urine output, mental status).

Hematocrit

Single hematocrit (Hct) measurements are not recommended as a sole marker of bleeding [15], because their diagnostic value is very poor for detecting occult bleeding sources [26] probably due to the confounding influence of resuscitative measures, such as fluid administration [27].

Markers of Tissue Hypoperfusion

Uncorrected microcirculatory alterations that occur after polytrauma may result in inadequate oxygen transport to achieve sufficient oxidative phosphorylation and ultimately cause tissue hypoxia and organ dysfunction [28]. Tissue hypoxia after injury is largely responsible for subsequent respiratory complications and multiple organ failure [29]. In this section, we discuss serum lactate, base deficit and $ScvO_2$ as potential markers of increased anaerobic metabolism and tissue hypoxia.

Serum lactate

Initial serum lactate is a reliable indicator of morbidity and mortality following trauma [9]. Changes in serial lactate measurements provide an early and objective evaluation of a patient's response to therapy and represent a reliable prognostic index for patients with circulatory shock [30]. In general, lactate levels have proved to be useful in predicting mortality and operative intervention rates, but not bleeding or transfusion requirements [31]. Moreover, most of these studies did not stratify patients based on hemodynamic stability and for this reason conclusions cannot be generalized.

Base deficit

Base deficit values provide an indirect estimation of global tissue acidosis due to impaired perfusion [32], and initial base deficit was an independent single predictor of post-traumatic mortality and transfusion requirements within the first 24 h [33]. As in the case of lactate, neither of these studies stratified patients based on their hemodynamic stability at admittance; thus their effectiveness in hemodynamically stable patients cannot be evaluated. Furthermore, elevated initial lactate levels and base deficit are not direct reflections of tissue hypoxia and are affected by numerous non-hypoxic causes of metabolic acidosis, such as infu-

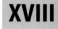

XVIII

sions of saline solutions or lactate Ringer's solution, hypothermia, agitation with polypnea, stress-increased glycolysis, catecholamine response to trauma, drug toxicity (e.g., cocaine and ethanol consumption), liver/renal dysfunction and ethanol intoxication, which often co-exist during critical illness, thus limiting the utility of these measures.

Neither base deficit nor lactate measurements give an indication of acute hypovolemia in hemodynamically stable patients. Current theories emphasize the gut as the first target to suffer from hypoperfusion during acute hypovolemia [34]. If lactate production or localized acidosis occurs in this region, it will be subjected to a large dilution factor when distributed in the body volume during measurements of whole body arterial lactate or base deficit. Also lactate is metabolized largely by the liver; thus, as long as perfusion to this organ is preserved, local changes in gut lactate production will be masked until production outweighs hepatic metabolism.

Central venous oxygenation
In a study of initially hemodynamically stable patients after trauma, an $ScvO_2 < 65\%$ enabled patients who suffered from blood loss and required blood transfusion to be identified [35]. This finding suggests that low $ScvO_2$ in hemodynamically stable patients is associated with a poor outcome and may represent a potential endpoint of resuscitation in trauma patients [36]. However, in a similar study, only lactate and arterial base deficit but not $ScvO_2$ were able to differentiate between patients with or without delayed occult bleeding prior to surgery [37].

Markers of Hypovolemia

Potential markers for hypovolemia, easily obtained at the bedside in the ED are CVP and sonographic assessment of IVC diameter as well as the collapsibility index.

Central venous pressure
Central venous pressure monitoring has already been demonstrated to be unreliable as an indicator of volume status in conditions of increased vascular tone, such as under high catecholamine stimulation [38]. In addition to this, central catheter placement is not avoid of morbidity and is time consuming.

Inferior vena cava diameter and collapsibility index
Previous studies have shown that, in patients treated for trauma, IVC diameter and collapsibility index are good indicators of blood loss despite normal vital signs on ED admission. These findings suggest that IVC diameter is better correlated to circulating blood volume than blood pressure. In retrospective studies, a collapsed IVC [39], or a flattened IVC (< 9 mm) [40] indicated hypovolemia attributable to a major blood in trauma patients. It has also been reported that CT evidence of a flat IVC is an accurate predictor of incipient hemodynamic instability in polytrauma patients with blunt solid organ injuries [41]. Similar results have been reported with ultrasonography [42, 43]. The main limitations of these studies that reported a high accuracy of IVC to detect occult bleeding early, were the lack of stratification at ED admission based on hemodynamic status and levels of hemoglobin as well as the CVP. Moreover, in most studies values of lac-

XVIII

tate and base deficit were not reported. We were not able to confirm these results in a selected population of patients who were initially hemodynamically stable and without biochemical signs of hypoperfusion at ED admission [44]. In fact, no significant differences in IVC diameter or collapsibility index have been found between patients with active bleeding and incipient hemodynamic instability and patients with persistent hemodynamic stability.

A Future Perspective: Renal and Splenic Doppler Resistive Indexes

Renal Doppler Resistive Index

Marked increments of renal vascular resistance have been demonstrated in animal models of hemorrhagic shock [45], mainly owing to cortical vasoconstriction [46]. In humans, renal blood flow can be reduced by > 1 l/min during initial hemorrhagic shock, thereby acting as a reservoir against severe hypoperfusion of other vital organs [45]. Various quantitative and semi-quantitative Doppler parameters have been proposed to quantify renal blood flow. Among these, the Doppler resistive index of an intrarenal artery is the most frequently used for clinical investigations, because it does not require estimations of Doppler angle or vessel cross-sectional area [47]. In a series of studies in this area, we have shown that in multitrauma patients, the renal Doppler resistive index was closely related to arterial lactate as a marker of organ hypoperfusion [48, 49] (**Fig. 1**) and had a better diagnostic accuracy than either base deficit or serum lactate (**Fig. 2**). Furthermore, renal Doppler resistive index was clinically useful, as it was identified by multivariate analysis as the only independent predictor of hemorrhagic shock in the first 24 h of hospitalization [44].

In this study, we also showed that more than half the polytrauma patients who were hemodynamically stable at ED admission developed complications because of early unrecognized occult bleeding during the first 24 h. In addition, renal Doppler resistive index at ED admission was lower in patients who did not develop hemorrhagic shock. Therefore, renal Doppler resistive index showed that early changes in renal cortical blood flow even in normotensive patients may represent a clinically useful non-invasive method for the early detection of

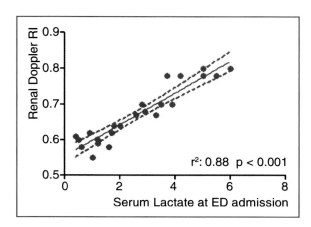

Fig. 1. Correlation between renal Doppler resistive index (RI) and arterial lactate on admission to the emergency department.

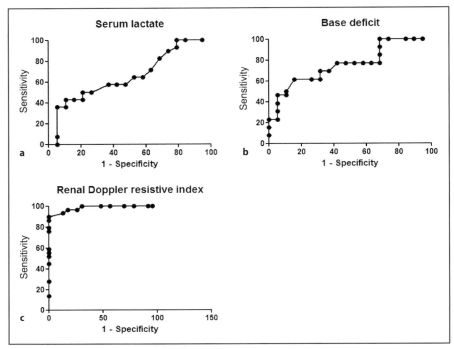

Fig. 2. Sensitivity and specificity expressed as receiver operating characteristic (ROC) curve of renal Doppler resistive index to detect occult hemorrhagic shock early of: Serum lactate (Panel **a**); standard base excess (Panel **b**); and renal Doppler resistive index (Panel **c**). Data from [44].

occult hemorrhagic shock and occult hypoperfusion in polytrauma patients (**Fig. 3**).

Splenic Doppler Resistive Index

Over the past several years, our understanding of the role of the spleen in physiology and pathophysiology has expanded to include regulation of intravascular volume and arterial pressure. This regulation may occur through microvascular control of intrasplenic fluid extravasation, or reflex modulation of the renal and splanchnic microvascular beds, or both [50]. In humans, a reduction in splenic size has been reported to occur within individuals after trauma, probably reflecting reduced vascularization due to marked adrenergic stimulation [51].

Preliminary data from our laboratory show that acute adjustments in splenic perfusion also occur after trauma. Thus, splenic Doppler resistive index may be a valid alternative to renal resistive index for the detection of occult bleeding, with the advantage of being easier to measure and less time consuming [52].

In **Table 1**, the advantages and disadvantages of different methods that have been proposed to predict occult hemorrhage are shown.

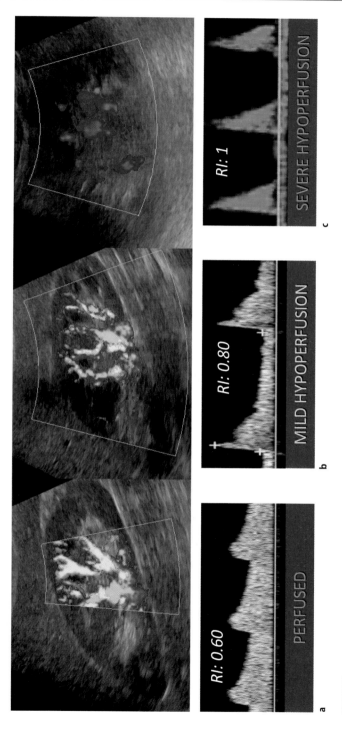

Fig. 3. Doppler resistive index (RI) of an intra-renal artery does not require estimations of Doppler angle or vessel cross-sectional area and is dependent on the perfusion (diastolic) pressure. The figure represents the three principal patterns of parenchymal perfusion with the corresponding pulsed Doppler traces. Pattern **a** = perfused with a well represented diastolic phase and low Doppler RI value; pattern **b** = hypoperfused with a reduced diastolic phase between systolic peaks and higher Doppler RI value; pattern **c** = vascularized but not perfused in the absence of the diastolic phase within systolic peaks.

Table 1. Advantages and disadvantages of methods to predict occult hemorrhage

	Available at bed-side	Operator depen-dent	Time consum-ing	Predictor of bleeding	Predictor of transfusion require-ments	Predictor of occult hypoper-fusion	Predictor of hospital mortality
FAST	+	+	–	–	–	–	–
CT scan	–	+	+	–	–	–	–
ATLS GS §	+	–	–	–	+	–	–
Hematocrit	+	–	–	–	–	–	–
Serum lactate §	+	–	–	+	–	+	+
Base deficit §	+	–	–	–	+	+	–
ScvO₂ #	+	–	+	–	+	+	–
CVP	+	–	+	–	–	–	–
IVC #	+	–	+	–	–	–	–
RDRI	+	+	+	+	+	+	+
SDRI	+	+	+	+	+	+	+

FAST: focused assessment with sonography for trauma; CT: computed tomography; ATLS GS: advanced trauma life support grading system; ScvO₂: central venous oxygen saturation; CVP: central venous pressure; IVC: inferior vena cava diameter or collapsibility index; RDRI: renal Doppler resistive index; SDRI: splenic Doppler resistive index; §: not validated in hemodynamically stable patients; #: conflicting results

Stepwise Approach to Early Detect Occult Bleeding: A Proposal

Based on these observations, we propose a new stepwise approach to detect occult bleeding early in trauma patients (**Fig. 4**). This approach includes a CT scan in all hemodynamically stable patients regardless of the outcome of FAST, if the CT is within the emergency department and readily available. In cases with a

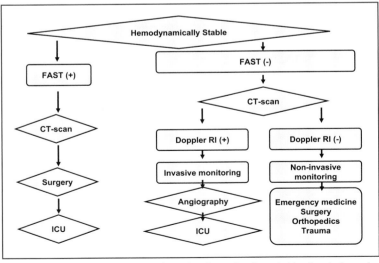

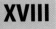

Fig. 4. A proposed stepwise approach to the diagnosis of occult bleeding in hemodynamically stable blunt polytrauma patients.

positive FAST, the patient should be transported to the operating room immediately after the CT. In cases with a negative FAST, subsequent management will be based on the assessment of the presence or absence of organ hypoperfusion by renal or splenic Doppler resistive index of the highly vascularized parenchymatous organs, such as kidney and spleen, or biochemical parameters, such as pH, lactic acid, base deficit. When signs of organ hypoperfusion are present, we propose invasive monitoring and possibly angiography targeted on the basis of CT results. In the absence of signs of splanchnic hypoperfusion, data in our possession seem to suggest less aggressive monitoring by non-invasive parameters, such as urine output, systolic blood pressure, hemoglobin, and lactacidemia in medical, orthopedic or traumatology wards.

Conclusion

Occult hemorrhagic shock if not promptly diagnosed can be associated with high morbidity and mortality in trauma patients. Different methods are available for early detection of occult bleeding but none of them is sufficiently sensitive and specific. The use of renal and splenic Doppler resistive indexes might be included in physiologically-based resuscitative protocols. Prospective randomized controlled trials are warranted to better define the role of sonography in the emergency setting.

References

1. Murray CJ, Lopez AD (1997) Mortality by cause for eight regions of the world: Global Burden of Disease Study. Lancet 349: 1269–1276
2. Sauaia A, Moore FA, Moore EE, et al (1995) Epidemiology of trauma deaths: a reassessment. J Trauma 38: 185–193
3. Gutierrez G., Reines HD, Wulf-Gutierrez ME (2004) Clinical review: Hemorrhagic shock. Crit Care 8: 373–381
4. Clarke JR, Trooskin SZ, Doshi PJ, Greenwald L, Mode CJ (2002) Time to laparotomy for intra-abdominal bleeding from trauma does affect survival for delays up to 90 minutes. J Trauma 52: 420–425
5. American College of Surgeons Committee on Trauma (2004) Advanced trauma life support, 7th ed. American College of Surgeons, Chicago
6. Zehtabchi S, Sinert R, Goldman M, Kapitanyan R, Ballas J (2006) Diagnostic performance of serial haematocrit measurements in identifying major injury in adult trauma patients. Injury 37: 46–52
7. Wilson M, Davis DP, Coimbra R (2003) Diagnosis and monitoring of hemorrhagic shock during the initial resuscitation of multiple trauma patients: a review. J Emerg Med 24: 413–422
8. Abramson D, Scalea TM, Hitchcock R, Trooskin SZ, Henry SM, Greenspan J (1993) Lactate clearance and survival following injury. J Trauma 35: 584–589
9. Baron BJ, Scale TM (1996) Acute blood loss. Emerg Med Clin North Am 14: 35–55
10. Cryer HM, Miller FB, Evers BM, Rouben LR, Seligson DL (1988) Pelvic fracture classification: correlation with hemorrhage. J Trauma 28: 973–980
11. Burgess AR, Eastridge BJ, Young JW, et al (1990) Pelvic ring disruptions: effective classification system and treatment protocols. J Trauma 30: 848–856
12. Sirlin CB, Brown MA, Deutsch R, et al (2003) Screening US for blunt abdominal trauma: Objective predictors of false-negative findings and missed injuries. Radiology 229: 766–774
13. Scalea TM, Rodriguez A, Chiu WC, et al (1999) FAST results from an international consensus conference. J Trauma 46: 466–472

14. Brown MA, Casola G, Sirlin CB, Patel NY, Hoyt DB (2001) Blunt abdominal trauma: screening us in 2,693 patients. Radiology 218: 352–358
15. Rozycki GS, Newman PG (1999) Surgeon-performed ultrasound for the assessment of abdominal injuries. Adv Surg 33: 243–259
16. Rossaint R, Bouillon B, Cerny V, et al (2010) Management of bleeding following major trauma: an update European guideline. Crit Care 14: R52
17. Brown MA, Sirlin CB, Hoyt DB, Casola G (2003) Screening ultrasound in blunt abdominal trauma. J Intensive Care Med 18: 253–260
18. Sirlin CB, Brown MA, Andrade-Barreto OA, et al (2004) Blunt abdominal trauma: clinical value of negative screening US scans. Radiology 230: 661–668
19. Allen TL, Mueller MT, Bonk RT, Harker CP, Duffy OH, Stevens MH (2004) Computed tomographic scanning without oral contrast solution for blunt bowel and mesenteric injuries in abdominal trauma. J Trauma 56: 314–322
20. Hawkins AE, Mirvis SE (2003) Evaluation of bowel and mesenteric injury: role of multidetector CT. Abdom Imaging 28: 505–514
21. Stengel D, Bauwens K, Rademacher G, Mutze S, Ekkernkamp A (2005) Association between compliance with methodological standards of diagnostic research and reported test accuracy: Meta-analysis of focused assessment of US for trauma. Radiology 236: 102–111
22. Rozycki GS, Ballard RB, Feliciano DV, Schmidt JA, Pennington SD (1998) Surgeon-performed ultrasound for the assessment of truncal injuries: lessons learned from 1540 patients. Ann Surg 228: 557–567
23. Spahn DR, Cerny V, Coats TJ, et al (2007) Management of bleeding following major trauma: a European guideline. Crit Care 11: R17
24. Becker CD, Poletti PA (2005) The trauma concept: the role of MDCT in the diagnosis and management of visceral injuries. Eur Radiol 15 (Suppl 4): D105–109
25. Weninger P, Mauritz W, Fridrich P, et al (2007) Emergency room management of patients with blunt major trauma: evaluation of the 'MSCT protocol' exemplified by an urban trauma center. J Trauma 62: 584–591
26. Zehtabchi S, Sinert R, Goldman M, Kapitanyan R, Ballas J (2006) Diagnostic performance of serial haematocrit measurements in identifying major injury in adult trauma patients. Injury 37: 46–52
27. Kass LE, Tien IY, Ushkow BS, Snyder HS (1997) Prospective crossover study of the effect of phlebotomy and intravenous crystalloid on hematocrit. Acad Emerg Med 4: 198–201
28. Vollmar B, Menger MD (2004) Volume replacement and microhemodynamic changes in polytrauma. Langenbecks Arch Surg 389: 485–491
29. Blow O, Magliore L, Claridge JA, Butler K, Young JS (1999) The golden hour and the silver day: detection and correction of occult hypoperfusion within 24 hours improves outcome from major trauma. J Trauma 47: 964–969
30. Vincent JL, Dufaye P, Berre J, Leeman M, Degaute JP, Kahn RJ (1983) Serial lactate determinations during circulatory shock. Crit Care Med 11: 449–451
31. Lavery RF, Livingston DH, Tortella BJ, Sambol JT, Slomovitz BM, Siegel JH (2000) The utility of venous lactate to triage injured patients in the trauma center. J Am Coll Surg 190: 656–664
32. Davis JW, Kaups KL, Parks SN (1998) Base deficit is superior to pH in evaluating clearance of acidosis after traumatic shock. J Trauma 44: 114–118
33. Davis JW, Parks SN, Kaups KL, Gladen HE, O'Donnell-Nicol S (1996) Admission base deficit predicts transfusion requirements and risk of complications. J Trauma 41: 769–774
34. Price HL, Deutsch S, Marshall BE (1966) Hemodynamic and metabolic effects of hemorrhage in man with particular reference to the splanchnic circulation. Circ Res 18: 469–474
35. Scalea TM, Hartnett RW, Duncan AO, et al (1990) Central venous oxygen saturation: a useful clinical tool in trauma patients. J Trauma 30: 1539–1543
36. Rady MY, Rivers EP, Martin GB, et al (1992) Continuous central venous oximetry and shock index in the emergency department: use in the evaluation of clinical shock. Am J Emerg Med 10: 538–541
37. Bannon MP (1995) Central venous oxygen saturation, arterial base deficit and lactate concentration in trauma patients. Am Surg 61: 738–745

XVIII

38. Perko G, Perko MJ, Jansen E (1995) Thoracic impedance as an index of body fluid balance during cardiac surgery. Acta Anaesthesiol Scand 35: 568–571
39. Jeffrey RB Jr, Federle MP (1988) The collapsed IVC: CT evidence of hypovolemia. AJR Am J Roentgenol 150: 431–432
40. Mirvis SE, Shanmuganathan K, Erb R (1994) Diffuse small bowel ischemia in hypotensive adults after blunt traumatic (shock bowel): CT findings and clinical significance. AJR Am J Roentgenol 163: 1375–1379
41. Liao YY, Lin HJ, Lu YH, Foo NP, Guo HR, Chen KT (2011) does ct evidence of a flat inferior vena cava indicate hypovolemia in blunt trauma patients with solid organ injuries? J Trauma 70: 1358–1361
42. Yanagawa Y, Nishi K, Sakamoto T, Okada Y (2005) Early diagnosis of hypovolemic shock by sonographic measurement of inferior vena cava in trauma patients. J Trauma 58: 825–829
43. Sefidbakht S, Assadsangabi R, Abbasi HR, Nabavizadeh A (2007) Sonographic measurement of the inferior vena cava as a predictor of shock in trauma patients. Emerg Radiol 14: 181–185
44. Corradi F, Brusasco C, Vezzani A, et al (2011) Hemorrhagic shock in polytrauma patients: early detection with renal Doppler resistive measurements. Radiology 260: 112–118
45. Sondeen JL, Gonzaludo GA, Loveday JA, et al (1990) Renal responses to graded hemorrhage in conscious pig. Am J Physiol 259: R119–R125
46. Hardaker WT Jr, Graham TC, Wechsler AS (1975) Renal intracortical blood flow during hemorrhage: role of adrenergic mechanisms. Am J Physiol 229: 178–184
47. Rivers BJ, Walter PA, Polzin DJ, King VL (1997) Duplex doppler estimation of intrarenal pourcelot resistive index in dogs and cats with renal disease. J Vet Intern Med 11: 250–260
48. Corradi F, Vezzani A, Palermo S, Altomonte F, Moscatelli P, Brusasco C (2009) Renal Doppler resistance index: early marker of splanchic hypoperfusion and bleeding in major trauma with a borderline hemodynamic status. Intensive Care Med 35: s257 (abst)
49. Corradi F, Brusasco C, Vezzani A, Mergoni M, Palermo S, Launo C (2010) Measurement of renal cortical blood flow for detection of early haemorrhagic shock after trauma. Minerva Anestesiol 76: 45 (abst)
50. Hamza SM, Kaufman S (2009) Role of spleen in integrated control of splanchnic vascular tone: physiology and pathophysiology. J Physiol Pharmacol 87: 1–7
51. Goodman LR, Aprahamian C (1990) Changes in splenic size after abdominal trauma. Radiology 176: 629
52. Corradi F, Brusasco C, Vezzani A, Altomonte F, Moscatelli P (2010) Measurement of splenic Doppler resistance index for detection of early hemorrhagic shock after trauma. Intensive Care Med 36: s120 (abst)

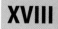

Mitochondrial Dysfunction after Traumatic Brain Injury

J. SAHUQUILLO, M.-A. MERINO, and C. AIRADO

> *"The lessons to be learnt, in both science and the law,*
> *are to question your assumptions, to be open to new evidence,*
> *and not to accept statements from witnesses*
> *until their reliability has been verified"*
> (Ekert and Vaux, 2005) [1]

Introduction

Traumatic brain injury (TBI) is the leading cause of death and disability in the world's population under 45 years of age. About 10 % of cases of TBI are severe (Glasgow Coma Scale [GCS] score ≤ 8 points); in this subgroup, the incidence of poor neurological outcome (severe disability, vegetative state or death) still exceeds 55 % in many centers [2]. The endpoints in the early treatment of TBI are adequate and aggressive resuscitation and patient management in the neuro-intensive care unit is focused on the avoidance and treatment of high intracranial pressure (ICP). To date, no neuroprotective therapy has proven effective in controlled clinical trials involving severe TBI and the International Mission for Prognosis and Analysis of Clinical Trials inTBI (IMPACT) study showed that despite a significant reduction in mortality, neurological sequelae in TBI survivors have not changed significantly in the last 25 years [3].

Significant advances in the treatment of TBI have been limited, at least in part, by a lack of knowledge of the biochemical, cellular and molecular changes involved in its pathophysiology. These obstacles have been overcome to a certain degree by new monitoring tools – cerebral microdialysis and monitoring of partial pressure of oxygen in the brain ($PbtO_2$) – that have allowed clinicians to explore the metabolic disturbances of the injured brain with unprecedented detail. The data gathered by these monitoring tools in the past two decades have provided an opportunity to take a second look at the pathophysiology of TBI, motivating clinical researchers to redefine some of the unchallenged traditional concepts. The hypothesis that mitochondrial dysfunction is at the core of many acute metabolic disorders observed in acute TBI is one of the old concepts that deserves a second look and is the focus of this chapter.

Cerebral Ischemia: An Overvalued Factor in the Pathophysiology of TBI?

In the past two decades, cerebral ischemia has been, for clinicians and researchers, the protagonist of most secondary lesions occurring after TBI. The clinical relevance of ischemia was based on the influential neuropathological studies of the Glasgow group. In the 1970s, these investigators reported a high frequency of ischemic lesions in patients who died of TBI, and in the late 1980s, they observed that ischemic lesions remained highly prevalent in these patients [4, 5]. These studies were later supported by clinical research published in the 1990s showing

XVIII

J.-L. Vincent (ed.), *Annual Update in Intensive Care and Emergency Medicine 2012*
DOI 10.1007/978-3-642-25716-2 © Springer-Verlag Berlin Heidelberg 2012

that cerebral blood flow (CBF) was significantly reduced very early after TBI and that this finding was an independent predictor of poor neurological outcome. This evidence fueled the now commonly accepted idea that modulation of CBF is an important therapeutic target [6, 7]. In addition, the consequences of early extracranial systemic insults (hypotension, hypoxemia, anemia, etc.) are widely believed to have devastating effects on the damaged and already vulnerable brain.

Modern neuromonitoring has focused on designing systems capable of quickly detecting early reductions in CBF and oxygen supply to allow clinicians time to reverse them. New neuromonitoring techniques, including $PbtO_2$ and microdialysis monitoring, are widely used in neurocritical care units, allowing for the *quasi*-continuous profiling of brain oxygen supply and brain metabolism [8, 9]. Data provided by these tools have cast doubt on the predominant role of ischemia in

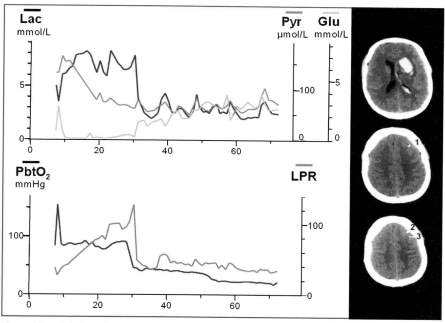

Fig. 1. Microdialysis and partial pressure of oxygen in the brain ($PbtO_2$) monitoring of a 31-year-old male injured in a bike accident. The Glasgow Coma Scale score upon admission to our center was 8. The initial computed tomography (CT) scan (right inset) showed a left frontal hematoma open to the ventricles. An intraparenchymal intracranial pressure probe (2), a microdialysis catheter (1) and a Licox $PbtO_2$ probe (3) were inserted in the patient. Both probes were placed in the penumbral brain, the tips being 18 mm from the highest part of the hematoma. In this figure (lower panel), an episode of high lactate/pyruvate ratio is observed, starting at 9 hours after injury and reaching levels above 100. $PbtO_2$ is markedly increased during this period, reflecting an adequate brain tissue oxygenation (84.1 ± 9.7 mmHg). Mean intracranial pressure (ICP) during the same period was 12.5 ± 2.7 mmHg and mean cerebral perfusion pressure (CPP) 71.7 ± 4.9 mmHg. This episode lasted 21 hours and spontaneously reverted 30 hours after injury. During the same period (upper panel) lactate was very high (7.0 ± 0.8 mmol/l), whereas glucose and pyruvate were low. This episode would have been considered a typical pattern of ischemia were the information regarding $PbtO_2$ not available. This case is a good example of the shortcomings of interpreting microdialysis data with no additional information on the state of oxygenation in the brain.

the pathophysiology of TBI. Many studies have found that the injured brain may experience severe alterations in energy metabolism in the presence of CBF and oxygen supply well above the ischemic range [10–12]. Vespa et al. found that ischemia (reduced CBF uncoupled with cerebral metabolic rate of oxygen [$CMRO_2$]) was uncommon in positron emission tomography (PET) and microdialysis measurements taken during the early period after injury [12]. In a cohort of 19 severe TBI patients monitored using strict criteria – defined by microdialysis and PET studies – the frequency of ischemia was found to be only 2.4 % by microdialysis criteria and less than 1 % when using PET criteria [12]. The same scenario was observed by our group in a cohort of patients in whom both microdialysis and $PbtO_2$ were monitored. We observed that patients with an adequate oxygen supply may present severe metabolic disturbances with an increase in lactate and in the lactate/pyruvate ratio [13] (**Fig. 1**). Several lines of evidence support the idea that cellular energetics are deranged in TBI not because of an inadequate brain oxygen supply, but rather on the basis of impaired mitochondrial respiration, either in isolation or in combination with other causes of brain hypoxia.

Non-Ischemic Causes of Brain Metabolic Dysfunction

As noted by Vespa et al. in their seminal paper, TBI results in "...primary cellular death in a limited region of the brain directly involved in the insult, while creating a more widespread state of metabolic dysfunction in remote areas of the brain" [12]. Both clinical and experimental studies show that aerobic metabolism is consistently impaired in many patients shortly after TBI [12–14]. Some authors have reported that macroscopically normal brain tissue with normal or high $PbtO_2$ in patients with no detectable intracranial or systemic insults may have severe metabolic alterations. Vilalta et al. described a cohort of severe and moderate TBI patients of whom 45 % had brain lactate levels above 3 mmol/l, even when the probe was placed in macroscopically non-injured brain tissue [13]. Furthermore, the largest single-center retrospective study published so far showed that a lactate/pyruvate ratio above 25 was a significant independent predictor of unfavorable outcome in TBI [15].

Accumulating evidence in recent years shows that brain metabolism is impaired not only because the delivery of oxygen is impaired, but also because the cells are unable to use the available oxygen. The term 'cytopathic hypoxia' was coined in 1997 to define these changes in mitochondrial respiratory function [16], a type of disorder equivalent to the 'histotoxic hypoxia' defined previously by Siggäard-Andersen et al. [17]. New experimental and clinical data support this early hypothesis and indicate that metabolic failure in the brain is not necessarily mediated by ischemia but may often represent the consequence of mitochondrial damage and disruption in the electron transport chain [13, 14].

Nelson et al. found a high incidence of perturbed energetic metabolism in TBI using machine-learning algorithms and time-series analysis applied to datamining microdialysis data. However, the relationships between microdialysis, ICP and/or cerebral perfusion pressure (CPP) were found to be weak and did not explain the metabolic disturbances observed, suggesting that factors other than pressure and/or flow variables were the main cause of the metabolic dysfunction [18].

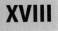
XVIII

The Siggäard-Andersen Classification of Tissue Hypoxia Revisited

Connett et al. stated in 1990 that in the discussion of oxygen-limited function it was important that "...both the vocabulary used to discuss the adequacy of oxygen supply and the criteria used to detect an inadequate supply be unambiguous and consistent" [19]. The previously discussed evidence reflects an urgent need for a consensus-based classification system that includes all types of brain tissue hypoxia, including failures in the mitochondrial respiratory chain or even more complex situations, such as mitochondrial dysfunction characterized by the uncoupling of the respiratory chain with the production of ATP through the ATPase complex.

Such a comprehensive and unambiguous classification system has been available since Siggäard-Andersen et al. first described it in 1995 [17, 20]. These authors described and mathematically modeled all the possible causes of tissue hypoxia and their corresponding pathophysiology, including histotoxic, hypermetabolic and uncoupling hypoxia [17, 20]. A disappointing paradox is that this pivotal classification system has not received enough attention in intensive care literature or in the framework of brain hypoxia; to date, this seminal paper has received only 44 citations, amounting to 2.59 citations per year, according to Harzing's *Publish and Perish* citation software [21]. The different types of tissue hypoxia described provide the theoretical framework for the characterization of all types of brain hypoxia found in the clinical setting.

The Siggäard-Andersen classification system stratifies tissue hypoxia into 7 basic types: 1) Ischemic hypoxia; 2) low extractivity hypoxia; 3) shunt hypoxia; 4) dysperfusion hypoxia; 5) histotoxic hypoxia; 6) uncoupling hypoxia; and 7) hypermetabolic hypoxia [17, 20]. It is beyond the scope of this review to examine this classification in detail, but some elements should be highlighted. Low extractivity hypoxia was a new concept introduced by the authors, who defined a new variable, the oxygen extraction tension (P_x), which allows the detection of the three potential causes of low extractivity: Hypoxemia, anemia, and low half-saturation tension (high-affinity hypoxia). The use of measured variables (hemoglobin content, PaO_2, mixed venous oxygen tension, etc.) and calculated variables (P_{50} and P_x) simplify the differential diagnosis of the different types of hypoxia and facilitate a pathophysiologically based approach to their management.

An additional contribution of this system was the non-intuitive concept that modest alterations in more than one of the variables involved in oxygen transport and delivery can contribute to tissue hypoxia. This is especially relevant in what was described as "low extractivity hypoxia"; mathematical modeling shows that moderate respiratory alkalosis combined with hypothermia and moderate anemia – a frequent scenario in the acute phase of TBI – can contribute significantly to the impairment of oxygen delivery to the brain [17, 20, 22, 23].

According to Connett et al., energy production by mitochondria has three stages of control: 1) The phosphorylation state; 2) the redox state; and 3) the concentration of dissolved oxygen $[O_2]$ [19]. The phosphorylation state, the concentration of ATP, ADP, AMP, PCr and inorganic phosphate (P_i), is believed to be the main regulated variable in most circumstances [19]. Modern neuromonitoring tools, such as microdialysis and $PbtO_2$ monitoring and direct or indirect measurements of global and regional CBF, already allow the implementation of diagnostic algorithms to establish a step-by-step approach to the diagnosis of brain metabolic disturbances and hypoxia [24–26]. Microdialysis allows clinicians to

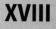

XVIII

Table 1. Proposal to adapt the Siggäard-Andersen classification of brain tissue hypoxia using microdialysis and partial pressure of oxygen in the brain ($PbtO_2$)

	Cause	$PbtO_2$	Glucose	Lactate	Pyruvate	Lactate/pyruvate ratio
Pattern I	Normal metabolism	≥ 20	Normal	Normal	Normal	Normal
Pattern II	Ischemic/low extractivity hypoxia/shunt/dysperfusion	< 20	Low	High	Low	High
Pattern III	Hyperglycolysis	≥ 20	Normal/Low	High	High	Normal
Pattern IV	Mitochondrial dysfunction	≥ 20	Normal/Low	High	Low	High

estimate the redox state of the cytosol though the lactate/pyruvate ratio, whereas Clark-type polarographic electrodes, which measure the dissolved oxygen in the brain interstitium ($PbtO_2$), can allow them to accurately measure brain oxygen levels.

A potential adaptation of the system using both $PbtO_2$ and microdialysis data is shown in **Table 1**. The use of global measurements of brain oxygen extraction, such as the arteriojugular differences of oxygen in the measurement of oxyhemoglobin saturation in the jugular bulb (SjO_2), may increase the accuracy of the diagnosis. This idea has been discussed previously [24–26].

Mitochondrial Dysfunction after TBI: An Elusive Target

Mitochondria may be at the core of some alterations found in TBI, in addition to initiating the major pathways implicated in secondary cell death, especially in injury-induced apoptosis. TBI is characterized by a gamut of complex temporal events evolving over hours or even days. Autoregulation impairment, reductions in CBF, low ATP levels and energy stores, severe ionic shifts, alterations in the permeability of the blood-brain barrier, and metabolic impairment frequently co-exist in the early phases after injury. Experimental models have shown that mitochondria sustain considerable structural and functional damage at this time and that brain survival is closely linked to mitochondrial homeostasis [27]. Clausen et al. have reported some lines of evidence to support the theory regarding the mitochondrion's crucial involvement in the pathophysiology of severe TBI. Some of the most relevant points are discussed below [28].

1. The $CMRO_2$ is consistently low after severe TBI. In the 1980s, Obrist et al. showed that oxidative metabolism, and therefore $CMRO_2$, was reduced to half normal levels in severe TBI and that the degree of depression was related to the depth of coma, and therefore to the GCS score [29]. It has been proposed that the origin of this metabolic depression could be an injury-induced mitochondrial inhibition. In cardiac ischemia, it has been shown that a reversible shutdown inhibition of mitochondrial metabolism is a physiological mechanism of cardioprotection [30]. It has been established experimentally that the reversible inhibition of the proximal respiratory chain by blocking mitochondrial complex I – NADH ubiquinone oxidoreduc-

XVIII

tase, a regulator of NADH/NAD$^+$ redox balance – is a very effective strategy for cardioprotection [30].

2. Increased levels of the cerebral extracellular lactate concentrations and in the lactate/pyruvate ratio have been observed in severe TBI, even when both CBF and PbtO$_2$ are within the normal range (**Fig. 1**). This suggests that even in the absence of brain ischemia, the brain might experience a "metabolic crisis", a term coined by Vespa et al. These authors identified mitochondrial dysfunction as the probable cause of this crisis [12, 31]. Experimental evidence has confirmed that mitochondria have a pivotal role in metabolic dysfunction after TBI and contribute to post-traumatic neuronal death [10, 11].

3. Mitochondrial swelling has been observed in the early stages of TBI, both in experimental models and in brain specimens explanted from human TBI patients [32]. Both oxidative stress and Ca^{2+} overload of the mitochondrial matrix causes permeabilization of the mitochondrial membranes. This phenomenon, termed the mitochondrial permeability transition (MPT), dissipates the proton electrochemical gradient that drives many mitochondrial functions, leading to ATP depletion, further production of reactive oxygen species (ROS), and, ultimately, swelling and mitochondrial rupture.

4. Significantly decreased respiratory rates and ATP production have been observed in mitochondria isolated from both experimental models and TBI patients [33, 34].

The above mentioned evidence indicates that mitochondria are an important etiological factor involved in the alterations in brain energy substrate metabolism and in the apoptotic cell death occurring after TBI. However, the causes and consequences of these abnormalities remain poorly understood and require clarification.

What are the Causes of Mitochondrial Failure?

The causes of mitochondrial dysfunction underlying histotoxic hypoxia may be numerous, although blockage of the respiratory chain and reduced delivery of pyruvate into the Krebs cycle are the most established mechanisms. How these abnormalities occur is not yet evident, although Ca^{2+} overload is known to be an indiscriminate killer of brain cells in ischemia, brain injury, and hypoglycemia. The main buffer for cytosolic Ca^{2+} is mitochondria, but membrane permeability is significantly increased by changes in what is known as the MPT pore (MPTP), a protein complex antagonized by cyclosporin-A [48]. The opening of the MPTP uncouples respiration from ATP synthesis (uncoupling hypoxia), induces mitochondrial swelling, disrupts the outer membrane and allows the release of different pro-apoptotic factors into the cytosol, such as cytochrome-c, apoptosis-inducing factors (AIF), and pro-caspases [48]. Some of the most well identified mechanisms involved in mitochondrial dysfunction are discussed below.

Inhibition of Mitochondrial Enzymes of the Respiratory Chain

Accidental exposure to cyanide – from inhalation of fire smoke, ingestion of toxins, etc – prevents cells from using oxygen and induces a rapid shift from aerobic to anaerobic metabolism, with a rapid increase in plasma lactate levels to above 8 mmol/l [35]. Cytochrome c oxidase is the primary intracellular target of cyanide

XVIII

poisoning. In an experimental model in cats, Clausen et al. were able to reproduce selective mitochondrial block in the brain through the local application of a cyanide solution via a microdialysis probe [28]. In this model, the local $CMRO_2$ was moderately reduced and a consistent metabolic pattern of increased $PbtO_2$, a five-fold increase in the extracellular levels of lactate, and no changes in pyruvate were observed [28]. A similar pattern has been frequently observed in the acute phase of TBI. The causes of respiratory chain inhibition are highly speculative and based on data from experimental models, but many authors believe nitric oxide (NO) to be the main suspect.

TBI is associated with an increase in inducible NO synthase (iNOS) and a consequent increased production of NO, a pluripotent signaling and effector molecule, and an endogenous free radical formed in many cell types by the enzymatic oxidation of L-arginine. In addition to its function as a signal-transducing molecule, NO is implicated in cytotoxic processes due to its ability to interfere in cell energy metabolism by reversible inhibition of the enzymatic activity of the terminal complex of the mitochondrial electron transport chain – complex IV or cytochrome a,a3 – [36]. NO-mediated inhibition of mitochondria is the result of competition with oxygen for the same binding site on complex IV. In addition, NO reacts rapidly with superoxide radicals to form peroxynitrite, a very powerful oxidizing and nitrosating agent that causes irreversible inhibition of mitochondrial respiration by blocking complexes I, III and V[36]. NO may also lower cellular ATP via the poly-ADP-ribose polymerase (PARP)-1 route in neurons as discussed below [37].

Inhibition of Pyruvate Dehydrogenase (PDH)

Pyruvate is the end-product of glycolysis and is reduced to lactate or enters the Krebs cycle inside the mithocondrion to be oxidized to CO_2 and H_2O. PDH catalyzes the reaction in which pyruvate is converted to acetyl-coenzyme A. This enzyme is tightly regulated by both end-product inhibition and reversible phosphorylation. Inactivation of PDH, even with sufficient oxygen, limits the flux of the substrate through the Krebs cycle and causes pyruvate to accumulate, leading to an increased production of lactate.

Activation of the Enzyme PARP-1

PARP-1 is a nuclear enzyme that participates in the repair of breaks in nuclear DNA [36]. ROS can induce breaks in nuclear DNA, thus activating PARP-1. PARP-1 activation depletes $NAD^+/NADH$ stores and impairs the utilization of oxygen to support ATP synthesis, producing a form of histotoxic hypoxia. The exposure of cultured cells to physiologically relevant concentrations of peroxynitrite-activated PARP-1 results in impaired mitochondrial respiration [38]. *In vitro* studies support the importance of PARP-1-dependent $NAD^+/NADH$ depletion as a mechanism of histotoxic hypoxia caused by inflammatory mediators. The incubation of cells with cytomix (a cocktail of three pro-inflammatory cytokines: tumor necrosis factor [TNF]-α, interleukin [IL]-1β, and interferon [IFN]γ) was associated with a more than 50 % decrease in cellular oxygen consumption. This phenomenon was reversible if the cells were washed free of the cytokines and incubated in normal culture medium, indicating that the cytokine-induced decrease in oxygen consumption is not caused by cell death, but rather a sublethal process that impairs normal cellular respiration.

XVIII

It is important to emphasize that many other mechanisms apart from the three described above may be involved in the metabolic disturbances and mitochondrial dysfunction observed after TBI, but to discuss them in detail is beyond the scope of this review.

The MPTP: The Common Etiopathogenic Factor

Many of the cascades that damage mitochondria converge into the already described MPTP, a non-specific channel formed by a complex of proteins, the architecture of which is still poorly understood [10, 39]. Mitochondria are made up of a matrix surrounded by a folded inner membrane, an outer membrane and the intermembrane space. ATP is produced by the ATPase complex using a proton gradient created by the electron transport chain across the inner mitochondrial membrane. This produces an electrochemical potential known as the transmembrane mitochondrial potential ($\Delta\psi$) [10, 39]. Under physiological conditions, the inner membrane is almost impermeable to solutes except for transient increases in permeability to selected ions and metabolites with a molecular weight less than 1.5 kDa [40].

It was thought that the MPTP, having low conductance under physiological conditions, spanned both mitochondrial membranes communicating the mitochondrial matrix with the cytosol. In experimental models, it has been shown that a reduction in $\Delta\psi$ is an early step in apoptosis [1]. Recent evidence suggests that the MPTP is located only in the inner membrane, although its components have yet to be clarified and are the topic of intense debate [39]. The molecular identity of the MPTP has been reviewed by Halestrap and may be described as a structure formed by four types of proteins: 1) Cyclophilin-D (CyP-D); 2) adenine nucleotide translocase (ANT); 3) mitochondrial phosphate carrier (PiC); and 4) other structural or regulatory proteins. The best characterized protein is CyP-D, which was purified by Halestrap and Davidson in 1990 and is the known target for the cyclosporin-inhibited pore [41].

The MPTP controls the permeability of the mitochondrial membranes to ions, metabolites and proteins. The MPTP is regulated by the redox state of the cell, by oxidative stress, Ca^{2+}, voltage, phosphorylation status, and pH [1–3]. After TBI, numerous processes, such as oxidative stress and Ca^{2+} accumulation, induce an increase in the permeability and structural integrity of the MPTP, resulting in an influx of water and electrolytes with dissipation of the $\Delta\psi$, loss of mitochondrial functions, and outer membrane disruption. Once the outer membrane is disrupted, mitochondrial pro-apoptotic proteins are passed to the cytosol – cytochrome c, Smac/DIABLO, and endonuclease-G – and activate caspase-dependent and caspase-independent aptoptosis [10, 39].

Independent of its molecular architecture, the opening of the MPTP in isolated mitochondria produces a population of mitochondria that are either 'normal' or massively swollen, but never in an intermediate state [41]. In experiments conducted *in vitro*, the pore is opened by adding calcium and rapidly closed by calcium chelators [41]. The calcium paradox is such that high cytosolic Ca^{2+} induces mitochondrial swelling, while at the same time mitochondria function as a Ca^{2+} buffer for the cell.

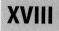

XVIII

Making Translational Research Work: Defining New Therapeutic Targets

The absence of suitable biomarkers to act as surrogates for drug efficacy in human TBI is a fundamental research problem. The validation of new biomarkers for histotoxic hypoxia detectable by microdialysis would dramatically improve the early detection, diagnosis, and treatment of some metabolic disorders in TBI patients.

The early diagnosis of mitochondrial dysfunction is crucial to design therapeutic strategies to target mitochondria within an as-yet-unknown window of opportunity. Potential therapies for this situation have recently been tested. One strategy already tested in a variety of models of TBI and in pilot clinical trials is normobaric or hyperbaric hyperoxia. Normobaric hyperoxia is easily achieved in mechanically ventilated patients and could be used as a potential treatment to improve brain oxygenation and the metabolic disorders resulting from TBI. However, there is significant controversy regarding this treatment due to contradictory clinical results [42, 43]. In a recent study by our group, normobaric hyperoxia significantly increased $PbtO_2$ and decreased the lactate/pyruvate ratio in patients in whom baseline brain lactate levels were increased, suggesting that normobaric hyperoxia improved the brain redox state. In patients with normal brain lactate levels, we did not find any significant change in the metabolic variables after normobaric hyperoxia. This suggests that the baseline metabolic state should be taken into account when applying normobaric hyperoxia [13].

An additional therapeutic strategy would be to enhance substrate delivery to the tissue by enhancing the diffusion of substrates through the plasma boundary layer and the brain tissue. Recently, trans-sodium crocetinate (TSC), a synthetic carotenoid, has been developed as a treatment for enhancing the oxygenation of hypoxic tissue [44]. TSC can facilitate the diffusivity of other small molecules, including glucose [45]. Manabe et al. showed that the administration of TSC in a permanent murine ischemia model reduced infarct volume in a dose-dependent manner. Indeed, several drugs have been shown to improve mitochondrial bioenergetics in many respiratory chain diseases, with the MPTP being one of the most attractive targets for neuroprotection. There are drugs that inhibit the MPTP directly, such as sanglifehrin A, cyclosporine, and its non-immunosuppressive analogues –6-MeAla-CsA, NIM811 and Debio-025 – , some of which show preliminary evidence of efficacy in cardioprotection [41]. Another drug that works well in experimental models of TBI is Ro5–4864. This drug has been shown to be effective not only in reducing the loss of mitochondrial transmembrane potential, but also in reducing mitochondrial ultrastructure alterations, improving cerebral metabolism (lactate and lactate/pyruvate ratio), and significantly reducing the amount of brain edema. Ro5–4864 also has a robust effect on ICP and neurological recovery [14].

Although some drugs have a promising profile in experimental models, they may only be effective for use in TBI if the target population is clearly defined and the drugs are tested *in vitro* and in experimental models before proceeding to clinical trials. The therapeutic window for mitochondrial dysfunction has not been defined yet, although it is most likely narrow after TBI. Once tissues are damaged beyond a critical point, cell death is inevitable despite the restoration of ATP levels [46]. Future research with new experimental models, such as organotypic cultures of the adult human brain, should help to analyze and clarify some of these important issues.

XVIII

Conclusion

There is increasing evidence that the classical 'ischemic' interpretation of micro-dialysis values in TBI is partially flawed; the metabolic derangements found in the early phases of TBI often reflect metabolic states unrelated to ischemia or an inadequate oxygen supply. Accumulating evidence shows that brain metabolism is impaired, not only because the delivery of oxygen is impaired but also because the cells are unable to use the available oxygen. Mitochondrial dysfunction is at the core of many metabolic disorders and needs to be incorporated into the differential diagnosis of metabolic impairment. Although the site of ATP generation is known to be in the mitochondria, the way in which energy requirements and mitochondrial oxidative phosphorylation are regulated in the cell is not yet fully understood. In the clinical setting, microdialysis can be used to monitor the metabolic effects of reduced oxygen delivery and identify the frequent histotoxic hypoxia profiles, thus allowing the early diagnosis of this type of metabolic dysfunction, a necessary preliminary step before designing new therapeutic strategies. With modern neuromonitoring systems and an adequate classification of brain hypoxia, it is already possible to define the various metabolic patterns in TBI and search for potential therapeutic strategies. We suggest the Siggäard-Andersen classification as the theoretical framework for implementing clinical diagnostic algorithms. It can be implemented at the bedside using already-available monitoring tools, such as microdialysis and PbtO$_2$ monitoring. The mitochondrion is a pathophysiological target with therapeutic potential. It is our hope that new clinical and experimental findings about the crucial role of mitochondria in TBI will spur new research and insight into the important role for this organelle in the pathophysiology of TBI.

Acknowledgements: The authors' research unit has been supported by grants from the Fondo de Investigación Sanitaria (Instituto de Salud Carlos III), numbers PI080480 and PI10/00302 which were cofinanced by the European Regional Development Fund (ERDF) and granted to Dr. J. Sahuquillo and Dr. MA. Poca. This work has also been partially supported by the Mutua Madrileña Grant (FMM-2010–10) given to Dr. J. Sahuquillo. M.A. Merino received an AGAUR grant 2008FI00747 from 2008 to 2011. We thank Sabrina Voss for editorial assistance.

References

1. Ekert PG, Vaux DL (2005) The mitochondrial death squad: hardened killers or innocent bystanders? Curr Opin Cell Biol 17: 626–630
2. Gomez PA, Lobato RD, Gonzalez P, et al (1999) Severe head injury. Hospital 12 de Octubre data base. Description of the data and analysis of the final outcome. Neurocirugía 10: 297–308
3. Marmarou A, Lu J, Butcher I, et al (2007) IMPACT database of traumatic brain injury: design and description. J Neurotrauma 24: 239–250
4. Graham DI, Adams JH, Doyle D (1978) Ischaemic brain damage in fatal non-missile head injuries. J Neurol Sci 39: 213–234
5. Graham DI, Ford DI, Adams JH, et al (1989) Ischaemic brain damage is still common in fatal non-missile head injury. J Neurol Neurosurg Psychiatry 52: 346–350
6. Marion DW, Darby J, Yonas H (1991) Acute regional cerebral blood flow changes caused by severe head injuries. J Neurosurg 74: 407–414

7. Bouma GJ, Muizelaar JP, Stringer WA, et al (1992) Ultra-early evaluation of regional cerebral blood flow in severely head-injured patients using xenon-enhanced computerized tomography. J Neurosurgery 77: 360–368

8. Bellander BM, Cantais E, Enblad P, et al (2004) Consensus meeting on microdialysis in neurointensive care. Intensive Care Med 12: 2166–2169

9. Hillered L, Vespa PM, Hovda DA (2005) Translational neurochemical research in acute human brain injury: the current status and potential future for cerebral microdialysis. J Neurotrauma 22: 3–41

10. Soustiel JF, Larisch S (2010) Mitochondrial damage: a target for new therapeutic horizons. Neurotherapeutics 7: 13–21

11. Soustiel JF, Sviri GE (2007) Monitoring of cerebral metabolism: non-ischemic impairment of oxidative metabolism following severe traumatic brain injury. Neurol Res 29: 654–660

12. Vespa P, Bergsneider M, Hattori N, et al (2005) Metabolic crisis without brain ischemia is common after traumatic brain injury: a combined microdialysis and positron emission tomography study. J Cereb Blood Flow Metab 25: 763–774

13. Vilalta A, Sahuquillo J, Merino MA, et al (2011) Normobaric hyperoxia in traumatic brain injury. Does brain metabolic state influence the response to hyperoxic challenge? J Neurotrauma 28: 1139–1148

14. Soustiel JF, Vlodavsky E, Milman F, Gavish M, Zaaroor M (2011) Improvement of cerebral metabolism mediated by Ro5–4864 is associated with relief of intracranial pressure and mitochondrial protective effect in experimental brain injury. Pharm Res 28: 2945–2953

15. Timofeev I, Carpenter KL, Nortje J, et al (2011) Cerebral extracellular chemistry and outcome following traumatic brain injury: a microdialysis study of 223 patients. Brain 134: 484–494

16. Fink M (1997) Cytopathic hypoxia in sepsis. Acta Anesthesiol Scand (Suppl) 110: 87–95

17. Siggäard-Andersen O, Ulrich A, Gothgen IH (1995) Classes of tissue hypoxia. Acta Anaesthesiol Scand 39: 137–142

18. Nelson DW, Thornquist B, Maccallum RM, et al (2011) Analyses of cerebral microdialysis in patients with traumatic brain injury: relations to intracranial pressure, cerebral perfusion pressure and catheter placement. BMC Med 9: 21

19. Connett RJ, Honig CR, Gayeski TE, Brooks GA (1990) Defining hypoxia: a systems view of VO_2, glycolysis, energetics, and intracellular PO_2. J Appl Physiol 68: 833–842

20. Siggäard-Andersen O, Fogh-Andersen N, Gothgen IH, Larsen VH (1995) Oxygen status of arterial and mixed venous blood. Crit Care Med 23: 1284–1293

21. Harzing AW (2007) Publish or Perish. Available at http://www.harzing.com/pop.htm. Accessed Nov 2011

22. Siggäard-Andersen O, Gothgen IH (1995) Oxygen and acid-base parameters of arterial and mixed venous blood, relevant versus redundant. Acta Anaesthesiol Scand 39: 21–27

23. Siggaard-Andersen M, Siggaard-Andersen O (1995) Oxygen status algorithm, version 3, with some applications. Acta Anaesthesiol Scand 39: 13–20

24. Sahuquillo J, Poca MA, Amoros S (2001) Current aspects of pathophysiology and cell dysfunction after severe head injury. Curr Pharm Des 7: 1475–503

25. Marin-Caballos AJ, Murillo-Cabezas F, Dominguez-Roldan JM, et al (2008) [Monitoring of tissue oxygen pressure (PtiO2) in cerebral hypoxia: diagnostic and therapeutic approach.] Med Intensiva 32: 81–90

26. Poca MA, Sahuquillo J, Mena MP, Vilalta A, Riveiro M (2005) [Recent advances in regional cerebral monitoring in the neurocritical patient: brain tissue oxygen pressure monitoring, cerebral microdialysis and near-infrared spectroscopy.] Neurocirugía (Astur) 16: 385–410

27. Gilmer LK, Roberts KN, Joy K, Sullivan PG, Scheff SW (2009) Early mitochondrial dysfunction after cortical contusion injury. J Neurotrauma 26: 1271–1280

28. Clausen TF, Zauner AF, Levasseur Je FAU, Rice Ac FAU, Bullock R (2001) Induced mitochondrial failure in the feline brain: implications for understanding acute post-traumatic metabolic events. Brain Res 908: 35–48

29. Obrist WD, Langfitt TW, Jaggi JL, Cruz J, Gennarelli TA (1984) Cerebral blood flow and metabolism in comatose patients with acute head injury.Relationship to intracranial hypertension. J Neurosurg 61: 241–253

XVIII

30. Burwell LS, Nadtochiy SM, Brookes PS (2009) Cardioprotection by metabolic shut-down and gradual wake-up. J Mol Cell Cardiol 46: 804–810
31. Vespa PM, McArthur D, O'Phelan K, et al (2003) Persistently low extracellular glucose correlates with poor outcome 6 months after human traumatic brain injury despite a lack of increased lactate: a microdialysis study. J Cereb Blood Flow Metab 23: 865–877
32. Bullock R, Maxwell WL, Graham DI, Teasdale GM, Adams JH (1991) Glial swelling following human cerebral contusion: an ultrastructural study. J Neurol Neurosurg Psychiatry 54: 427–434
33. Verweij BH, Muizelaar JP, Vinas FC, et al (1997) Mitochondrial dysfunction after experimental and human brain injury and its possible reversal with a selective N-type calcium channel antagonist (SNX-111). Neurol Res 19: 334–339
34. Xiong Y, Peterson PL, Verweij BH, et al (1998) Mitochondrial dysfunction after experimental traumatic brain injury: combined efficacy of SNX-111 and U-101033E. J Neurotrauma 15: 531–544
35. Geller RJ, Barthold C, Saiers JA, Hall AH (2006) Pediatric cyanide poisoning: causes, manifestations, management, and unmet needs. Pediatrics 118: 2146–2158
36. Fink MP (2002) Bench-to-bedside review: Cytopathic hypoxia. Crit Care 6: 491–499
37. Zhang J, Dawson VL, Dawson TM, Snyder SH (1994) Nitric oxide activation of poly(ADP-ribose) synthetase in neurotoxicity. Science 263: 687–689
38. Szabó C, Zingarelli B, O'Connor M, Salzman AL (1996) DNA strand breakage, activation of poly (ADP-ribose) synthetase, and cellular energy depletion are involved in the cytotoxicity of macrophages and smooth muscle cells exposed to peroxynitrite. Proc Natl Acad Sci USA 93: 1753–1758
39. Baines CP (2009) The molecular composition of the mitochondrial permeability transition pore. J Mol Cell Cardiol 46: 850–857
40. Kroemer G, Reed JC (2000) Mitochondrial control of cell death. Nat Med 6: 513–519
41. Halestrap AP (2009) What is the mitochondrial permeability transition pore? J Mol Cell Cardiology 46: 821–831
42. Magnoni S, Ghisoni L, Locatelli M, et al (2003) Lack of improvement in cerebral metabolism after hyperoxia in severe head injury: a microdialysis study. J Neurosurgery 98: 952–958
43. Menzel M, Doppenberg EM, Zauner A, et al (1999) Increased inspired oxygen concentration as a factor in improved brain tissue oxygenation and tissue lactate levels after severe human head injury. J Neurosurgery 91: 1–10
44. Manabe H, Okonkwo DO, Gainer JL, Clarke RH, Lee KS (2010) Protection against focal ischemic injury to the brain by trans-sodium crocetinate. Laboratory investigation. J Neurosurg 113: 802–809
45. Stennett AK, Dempsey GL, Gainer JL (2006) Trans-Sodium crocetinate and diffusion enhancement. J Phys Chem B 110: 18078–18080
46. Lo EH, Dalkara T, Moskowitz MA (2003) Mechanisms, challenges and opportunities in stroke. Nat Rev Neurosci 4: 399–415

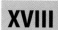

The First 24 Hours after Severe Head Trauma

B. Vigué B, C. Ract, and K. Tazarourte

"One gram of first-hour treatment can avoid kilograms of treatment,
later, in the intensive care unit"
Paul E. Pepe, Oral presentation, ISICEM, 2011

Introduction

Severe traumatic brain injury (TBI) is defined by a Glasgow Coma Scale (GCS) score of 8 or less during the first post-trauma day. It is recognized as a devastating pathology in terms of mortality and morbidity. Long-term recovery is poor with only 10 to 20 % patients returning to work after 1 year [1, 2]. If all severe TBI patients are taken into account (including those deceased before arrival at hospital), one-year mortality ranges between 35 to 45 % [3–6]. Mortality is dramatic in the first days with more than 40 % of all deaths occurring within the first 24 hours [1, 6].

Numbers of studies have demonstrated the importance of the initial hours after severe head trauma. After trauma, physiologic mechanisms against ischemia in cerebral tissue are impaired and traumatized brain highly vulnerable to ischemic injuries [7]. And the more recent the trauma, the more the brain is vulnerable [8]. Moreover, ischemic injuries are frequent during the first post-traumatic hours, notably in cases of multiple trauma. These ischemic injuries, even for a few minutes, have a dramatic negative impact on long-term outcomes. Thus, amelioration of initial care should greatly improve outcome.

Control of Arterial Pressure before Hospital Admission

Hypoxia and arterial hypotension, the "lethal duo" [9], decreasing oxygen and glucose transport, have been identified as major prognosis factors since the early nineties [10, 11]. Just one episode of arterial hypotension during the pre-hospital period increases mortality rates two- to four-fold [5, 10]. Ventilation and circulation control should thus be the two central axes of immediate management.

Whereas pre-hospital intubation decreases mortality when performed by trained teams [4, 5], the frequency of pre-hospital arterial hypotension, observed in about one third of patients, has not decreased since the early nineties, even with pre-hospital medical teams [5, 12–14]. Given the dramatic effect of hypotension during this period, control of arterial pressure must be a major goal of pre-hospital medical teams. Causes of hypotension are multiple and interconnected: Hypovolemia related to extra cerebral hemorrhages, decreased venous return because of positive intrathoracic pressure during controlled ventilation [15], but also deep sedation [14, 16].

During the pre-hospital period, mechanical ventilation of severe TBI patients is recommended to prevent inhalation and hypoxic events, and to control PCO_2.

J.-L. Vincent (ed.), *Annual Update in Intensive Care and Emergency Medicine 2012*
DOI 10.1007/978-3-642-25716-2 © Springer-Verlag Berlin Heidelberg 2012

Sedation is needed to limit causes of increased intrathoracic pressure, such as pain, cuff and ventilator asynchrony. All of these recommendations are aimed to limit risks of increased intracranial pressure (ICP). But if induction of anesthesia for tracheal intubation and sedation induce arterial hypotension, the net benefit on cerebral perfusion pressure (CPP) is lost (**Fig. 1**). Control of arterial pressure requires first efficient monitoring, which is not available during the pre-hospital period. Non-invasive techniques should be used to measure arterial pressure every 2 minutes, with particular attention during dangerous phases, such as the induction of anesthesia and sedation. Second, sedation must be cautiously titrated. Norepinephrine infusion (or phenylephrine bolus) should be used liberally, notably during induction of anesthesia to *prevent* hypotension.

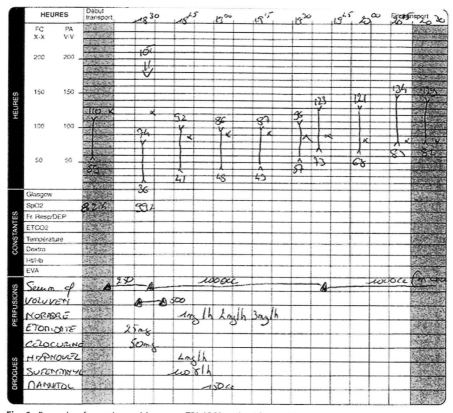

Fig. 1. Example of a patient with severe TBI (GCS = 7) with a moderate scalp hemorrhage during the pre-hospital period. Induction of anesthesia, sedation and controlled ventilation induced a prolonged decrease in systolic arterial pressure (< 90 mmHg) for nearly one hour despite fluid resuscitation and norepinephrine (NORADRE) infusion.

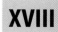

Immediate Care at Hospital Admission

As for the pre-hospital period, the most important goal on arrival at the hospital is control of peripheral events, such as hypoxia and hypotension [17]. Severe TBI patients must be admitted to a dedicated area by a team trained in polytrauma care. As for all multiple trauma patients, admission to hospital has therapeutic and diagnostic periods that allow ventilation and pressure control [18]. All polytrauma patients are managed following the same rules (**Fig. 2**):

- Respiratory control with SaO_2 and end-tidal CO_2 ($EtCO_2$) monitoring, bedside chest x-ray and sonography; chest tube insertion if necessary.
- Arterial and 3-line venous femoral catheters for arterial monitoring, blood samples, fluid resuscitation and norepinephrine infusion.
- Circulation control: Close monitoring of invasive arterial pressure, fluid resuscitation and transfusion (with particular attention to coagulation abnormalities), search for occult blood loss, bedside chest and pelvis x-rays, and FAST (focused assessment with sonography for trauma). Surgical control of massive hemorrhage is, of course, an absolute priority [19]. Coagulation abnormalities are a major cause of worsening of even minor cerebral lesions. In cases of severe TBI, mean arterial pressure (MAP) should ideally be adjusted using transcranial Doppler (TCD) measurements to normalize cerebral blood flow (CBF) as soon as possible [20] (please see below).
- Information and coordination of surgical and radiological teams.

Many patients with severe TBI now benefit from standardized care in specialized trauma centers [21] and this is most probably related to the strong prognostic influence of hypotension and hypoxia events.

Early Transcranial Doppler

The first step in the resuscitation of a patient with severe TBI is, thus, the standardized protocol of care for all multiple trauma patients; however severe TBI patients also require control of CBF. CBF is maintained in normal ranges by variations in cerebrovascular resistance above 50 mmHg of CPP (CPP = MAP – ICP). After trauma, autoregulatory responses are depressed and higher CPP levels are needed to maintain CBF in normal ranges (**Fig. 3**). Thus, most experts recommend maintaining MAP at 80 mmHg. But, even with a mean MAP at 80 mmHg, up to 40 % of severe TBI patients have ischemic injuries at the time of implementation of invasive monitoring (CPP < 60 mmHg or jugular venous oxygen saturation [SjO_2] < 55 %) [20, 22]. Given that the mean reported delay before availability of invasive cerebral monitoring is about 7 hours after trauma [22, 23], we need other ways to evaluate and correct CBF earlier.

   TCD permits rapid and non-invasive estimation of CBF and is particularly accurate at detecting low CBF [24]. Temporal windows are used for insonation of mean cerebral arteries that account for 70 % of the homolateral internal carotid flow. Peak systolic (Vs), end-diastolic (Vd) and time-averaged mean (Vm) velocities are measured and the pulsatility index (PI) calculated as: PI = (Vs – Vd)/Vm. It has been shown, in experimental and clinical studies, that below the autoregulation range (i.e., when CBF decreases), Vd decreases with CPP more rapidly than Vm and Vs, with the strongest correlation observed between CPP and PI [24]

XVIII

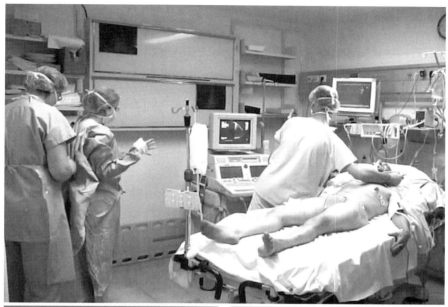

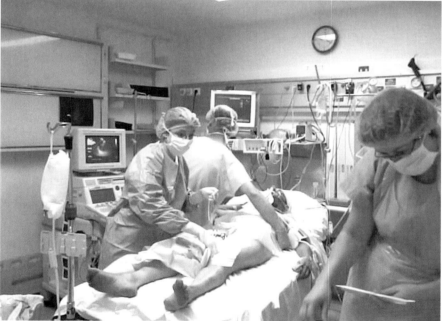

Fig. 2. Admission of a multiple trauma patient at our institution: A junior physician is responsible for arterial and venous catheterization, while, at the same time, the trauma leader performs FAST including, systematically, transcranial Doppler.

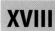

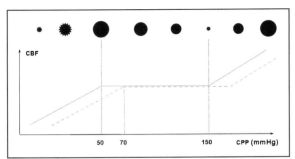

Fig. 3. Cerebral autoregulation: In normal conditions, cerebral blood flow (CBF) is maintained over a wide range of CPP (from 50 to 150 mmHg) by changes in cerebral vascular resistance. After traumatic head injury, autoregulatory responses are depressed and the autoregulation curve shifted to the right. This partially explains the importance of hypotension after TBI and the vulnerability of brain tissue. The state of vascular tonicity is symbolized by blue circles at the top of the figure. Small arteries are empty at low pressure and dilated when autoregulation begins. They then constrict progressively to maintain CBF constant. Vessels are stretched for high CPP after the plateau.

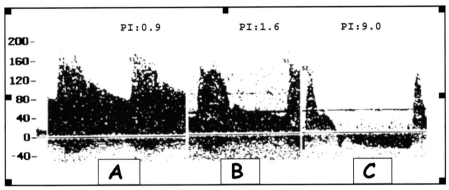

Fig. 4. Successive transcranial Doppler measurements during a progressive decrease in cerebral blood flow (CBF). A: normal. B: The pulsatility index (PI) is abnormally high (> 1.2), indicating decreased CBF. C: Oscillating flow, cessation of cerebral perfusion has been reached when forward and reverse flow are nearly equal. Note that end-diastolic velocity (Vd) decreases far more than the peak systolic velocity (Vs) when CBF decreases, i.e., pulsatility increases.

(Fig. 4). Thus, an increase in PI (> 1.4) is the first sign of decreased CBF, whatever the cause: Hypocapnia [25] or low CPP (because of high ICP and/or low MAP) [24]. The thresholds of PI and Vd have not yet been fully elucidated. It has been shown that, in severe TBI patients, a PI > 1.4 coupled with a Vd < 20cm/sec identifies patients with the highest ICP and lowest SjO_2 at admission [20] and is significantly correlated with poor outcome [26].

When CBF is impaired as diagnosed on TCD measurements, $PaCO_2$ must first be controlled because hypocapnia decreases CBF by a direct vasoconstrictive effect. Cerebral perfusion may then be restored by increasing MAP and/or use of osmotherapy [20]. Osmotherapy usually increases CBF in 15 minutes [24] for 4 hours. If necessary, it provides time for a computed tomography (CT) scan to be performed, then other indicated therapies (such as hypothermia or surgery) with restored cerebral perfusion.

Given the ease of use of TCD, it may even be considered before hospital admission to further reduce the duration of cerebral ischemic injuries. The feasibility of TCD measurements in pre-hospital settings has been demonstrated [27, 28].

Computed Tomography Scans

CT scans are central to diagnosis of surgical situations. About 10 % of patients with severe TBI need neurosurgery [3, 6, 13]. The timing of a CT scan is important, because hemorrhagic lesions increase in the first post-trauma hours. When the CT scan is done in the first 2 hours after trauma, Oertel et al. observed growing lesions in 50 % of cases with neurosurgery indicated in 30 % [29] (**Fig. 5**). Major factors of progressive lesions were age and coagulation abnormalities. Some studies have also shown that the second CT scan is more predictive of outcome than the first [30]. Nevertheless, a CT scan does not give us a real view of ischemic risks. Although CT scan classification from a "trauma data bank" was related to cerebral hypertension [31], ICP cannot be estimated based on CT scan results [32].

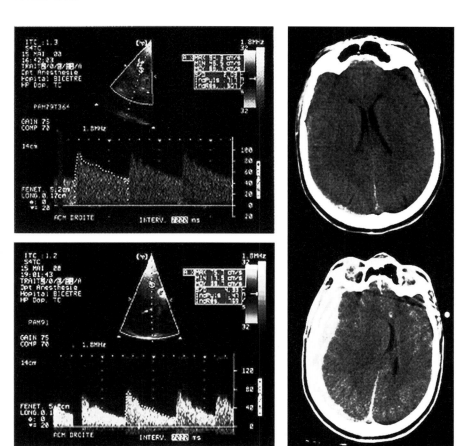

Fig. 5. Example of a 32-year old man with head trauma after a traffic accident. One hour after trauma, he was conscious with a normal transcranial Doppler (pulsatility index [PI] = 0.72). CT scan showed a minor subdural hematoma. After 3 hours, the patient became unconscious (Glasgow Coma Scale [GCS] = 5) with an abnormal transcranial Doppler (PI = 1.45, end-diastolic velocity [Vd] = 19 cm/s). Osmotherapy was performed before a second CT scan, which demonstrated an urgent surgical situation.

XVIII

Intracranial Monitoring

Guidelines for ICP monitoring are clear [17]. Insertion of an intracranial monitoring device for continuous ICP is recommended for severe TBI (GCS≤8) in all
cases when the CT scan is abnormal, and also when the vulnerability of the brain
is suspected (age more than 40, hypotension or local signs) even with a normal
CT scan [17]. ICP monitoring is urgent for rapid control of ischemic risks. However, it is first important to have a real evaluation of the GCS without any sedation or intoxication (alcohol can be present in 60 % of TBI patient [33]). Moreover, insertion of an intracranial monitoring device also requires hemostasis correction (international normalized ratio [INR] ≤ 1.5 [34], platelet count ≥ 100000).
Therefore, intraparenchymal ICP monitoring, implemented by neurosurgeons or
intensivists at the bedside, is not available until several hours after trauma [6, 23].
Intraventricular catheters must be placed in the operating room by neurosurgeons and are at risk of becoming infected.

A jugular catheter has been proposed to measure SjO_2 on admission [22] but
insertion load and technical difficulties have limited expansion of this method.
Brain tissue oxygen monitoring ($PbtO_2$) could be an elegant additional monitoring technique. $PbtO_2$ probes can be inserted through the same burr-hole as an
ICP probe and secured with a multiple-lumen bolt. $PbtO_2$-guided management
seems to be more informative than CPP monitoring alone [35] with some promising results on outcome [36].

Discussion about Intracranial Monitoring

Several studies have shown that use of invasive monitoring greatly reduces mortality and morbidity of severe TBI patients using historical comparisons [37] or
invasive versus non-invasive centers comparisons [38]. However, these results
have been debated because of the lack of randomized studies and the conflicting
results observed these last ten years [39]. Some publications, excluding patients
who died during the first 48 hours, found a better outcome and shorter ICU stay
without ICP monitoring [40].

We conducted an observational study including all patients with severe TBI in the
Paris area during a 22-month period, and following them from field to hospital discharge (Paris-TBI study). An ICP device was placed in 51 % of the 504 severe TBI
patients included. This rate is similar to or higher than that published in other countries (28 % [3] to 45 % [13]). We observed that ICP was less often inserted in patients
older than 45 years or those with a GCS score of 3. Multivariate analysis with a propensity score analysis of ICP monitoring at admission showed a two-fold increase in early
mortality (one week) for patients without ICP monitoring [6]. Other parameters independently associated with increased early mortality, with or without ICP monitoring,
were: At least one episode of areactive mydriasis (odds ratio [OR]=2.8 [1.9–4.2]) or
hypotension (OR = 2.8 [1.9–4.1], hemorrhagic shock (OR = 1.9 [1.1–3.1]), age more
than 75 years (OR = 2.9 [1.5–5.2]) and GCS score less than 6 (OR = 2.1 [1.3–4.0]).
Admission to a specialized center was an independent factor for favorable outcome
(OR = 0.6 [0.4–0.9]). Early mortality was significantly increased in patients aged
more than 45 years or with GCS at 3 *only* in the absence of ICP monitoring.

These results show that patients with some factors of poor prognosis benefit
less from invasive monitoring and that the decision to use ICP monitoring inde-

pendently increases their early mortality two-fold. This problem, also known as 'self-fulfilling prophecies', has been extensively described in neurological situations. For example, an early 'do not resuscitate (DNR) in case of cardiac arrest' decision after intracerebral hemorrhage is associated with a two-fold increase in mortality rate when adjusted for other factors of bad outcome [41]. How statistical analyses are biased after early DNR orders has been studied, and showed that the induced bias is so strong that an accurate evaluation of a treatment effect is not really possible [42]. This and exclusion of early deaths (i.e., more than 50 % of all deaths) may explain the negative outcome in patients with ICP monitoring compared to patients without [40]. This aspect is one of the causes for uncertainty and debate about ICP monitoring and, perhaps, one of the reasons for the stagnation in mortality rates of patients with TBI.

Conclusion

The first post-trauma hours are crucial for the long-term outcome of patients with severe TBI. As in all acute pathologies, quality of care depends to a great extent on the determination to treat. Organization of transport to specialized centers should be reinforced and guidelines respected. Ethical issues are important but should be discussed only after a few days of care and dialogue with relatives [43, 44]. These facets are the conditions needed for progress and to organize clinical studies free of prejudice and, perhaps, ameliorate the immediate critical survival and long-term outcomes.

References

1. Cooper DJ, Myles PS, McDermott FT, et al (2004) Pre-hospital hypertonic saline resuscitation of patients with hypotension and severe traumatic brain injury. A randomized controlled trial. JAMA 291: 1350–1357
2. Nakase-Richardson R, Yablon SA, Sherer M (2007) Prospective comparison of acute confusion severity with duration of post-traumatic amnesia in predicting employment outcome after traumatic brain injury. J Neurol Neurosurg Psychiatry 78: 872–876
3. Bulger EM, May S, Brasel KJ, et al (2010) Out-of-hospital resuscitation following severe traumatic brain injury: a randomized controlled trial. JAMA 304: 1455–1464
4. Bernard SA, Nguyen V, Cameron P, et al (2010) Pre-hospital rapid sequence intubation improves functional outcome for patients with severe traumatic brain injury. A randomized controlled trial. Ann Surg 252: 959–965
5. Davis DP, Koprowicz KM, Newgard CD, et al (2011) The relationship between out-of-hospital airway management and outcome among trauma patients with Glasgow Coma Scale scores of 8 or less. Pre-hospital Emergency Care 15: 184–192
6. Vigué B, Matéo J, Ghout I, et al (2011) Influence de la pose de la PIC dans la mortalité immédiate des patients TCG, étude PariS-TBI. SFAR R169 (abst)
7. DeWitt DS, Jenkins LW, Prough DS (1995) Enhanced vulnerability to secondary ischemic insults after experimental traumatic brain injury. New Horiz 3: 376–383
8. Geeraerts T, Friggeri A, Mazoit X, Benhamou D, Duranteau J, Vigué B (2008) Post-traumatic brain vulnerability to hypoxia-hypotension. The importance of the delay between brain trauma and secondary insult. Intensive Care Med 34: 551–560
9. Stahel PF, Smith WR, Moore EE (2008) Hypoxia and hypotension, the "lethal duo" in traumatic brain injury: implications for pre-hospital care. Intensive Care Med 34: 402–404
10. Chesnut RM, Marshall LF, Klauber MR, et al (1993) The role of secondary brain injury in determining outcome from severe head injury. J Trauma 34: 216–222

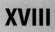

XVIII

11. Jones PA, Andrew PJD, Midgley S, et al (1994) Measuring the burden of secondary insults in head-injured patient during intensive care. J Neurosurg Anesthesiol 6: 4–14
12. Butcher I, Maas AIR, Lu J, et al (2007) The prognostic value of admission blood pressure in TBI: results from the IMPACT study. J Neurotrauma 24: 293–302
13. Myburgh JA, Cooper J, Finfer SR, et al (2008) Epidemiology and 12-month outcomes from traumatic brain injury in Australia and New Zeeland. J Trauma 64: 854–862
14. Tazarourte K, Ghout I, Matéo J, et al (2011) L'hypotension préhospitalière reste en 2011 un facteur prédictif majeur de mortalité des traumatisés crâniens graves, étude PariS-TBI. SFAR R247 (abst)
15. Pepe P, Raedler C, Lurie KG, Wigginton JG (2003) Emergency ventilatory management in hemorrhagic states: elemental or detrimental? J Trauma 54: 1048–1055
16. Rouxel JM, Tazarourte K, Le Moigno S, Ract C, Vigué B (2004) Prise en charge pré-hospitalière des traumatisés crâniens. Ann Fr Anesth Reanim 23: 6–14
17. Bratton SL, Chestnut RM, Ghajar J, et al (2007) Guidelines for the management of severe traumatic brain injury. J Neurotrauma 27: S1–S117
18. Peytel E, Menegaux E, Cluzel P, Langeron O, Coriat P, Riou B (2001) Initial imaging assessment of severe blunt trauma. Intensive Care Med 27: 1756–1761
19. Wisner DH, Victor NS, Holcroft JW (1993) Priorities in the management of multiple trauma. Intracranial pressure versus intraabdominal injury. J Trauma 35: 271–278
20. Ract C, Le Moigno S, Bruder N, Vigué B (2007) Early Transcranial Doppler ultrasound goal-directed therapy for the early management of severe traumatic brain injury. Intensive Care Med 33: 645–651
21. MacKenzie EJ, Rivara FP, Jurkovich GJ, et al (2006) A national evaluation of the effect of trauma-center care on mortality. N Engl J Med 354: 366–378
22. Vigué B, Ract C, Benayed M, et al (1999) Early SvjO$_2$ in patients with severe brain trauma. Intensive Care Med 25: 445–451
23. Struchen MA, Hannay HJ, Contant CF, Robertson CS (2001) The relation between acute physiological variables and outcome on the Glasgow Outcome Scale and Disability Rating Scale following severe traumatic brain injury. J Neurotrauma 18: 115–125
24. Kirkpatrick PJ, Chan KH (1997) Transcranial Doppler. In: Reilly P, Bullock R (eds) Head Injury. National Neurotrauma Society Guest Book, London, pp 244–259
25. Coles JP, Fryer TD, Coleman MR, et al (2007) Hyperventilation following head injury: effect on ischemic burden and cerebral oxidative metabolism. Crit Care Med 35: 568–578
26. Trabold F, Meyer PG, Blanot S, Carli PA, Orliaguet GA (2004) The prognostic value of transcranial Doppler studies in children with moderate and severe head injury. Intensive Care Med 30: 108–112
27. Tazarourte K, Atchabahian A, Tourtier JP, et al (2011) Pre-hospital Transcranial Doppler in severe brain injury: a pilot study. Acta Anaesthesiol Scand 55: 422–428
28. Knudsen L, Sandberg M (2011) Ultrasound in pre-hospital care. Acta Anaesthesiol Scand 55: 377–378
29. Oertel M, Kelly DF, McArthur D, et al (2002) Progressive hemorrhage after head trauma: predictors and consequences of evoluting injury. J Neurosurg 96: 109–116
30. Lobato RD, Gomez PA, Alday R, et al (1997) Sequential computerized tomography changes and related final outcome in severe head injury patients. Acta Neurochir (Wien) 139: 385–391
31. Eisenberg HM, Gary HE Jr, Aldrich EF, et al (1990) Initial CT findings in 753 patients with severe head injury. A report from the NIH Traumatic Coma Data Bank. J Neurosurg 73: 688–698
32. Poca MA, Sahuquillo J, Baguena M, Pedraza S, Gracia RM, Rubio E (1998) Incidence of intracranial hypertension after severe head injury: a prospective study using the Traumatic Coma Data Bank classification. Acta Neurochir Suppl (Wien) 71: 27–30
33. Clifton GL, Valadka A, Zygun D, et al (2011) Very early hypothermia induction in patients with severe brain injury (the national acute brain injury study: hypothermia II): a randomized trial. Lancet Neurol 10: 131–139
34. Bauer DF, McGwin G, Malton SM, George RL, Markert JM (2011) The relationship between between INR and development of hemorrhage with placement of ventriculostomy. J Trauma 70: 1112–1117

XVIII

35. Chang JJ, Youn TS, Benson D, et al (2009) Physiologic and functional outcome correlates of brain tissue hypoxia in traumatic brain injury. Crit Care Med 37: 283–290

36. Spiotta AM, Stiefel MF, Gracias VH, et al (2010) Brain tissue oxygen–directed management and outcome in patients with severe traumatic brain injury. J Neurosurg 113: 571–580

37. Tilford JM, Aitken ME, Anand KJ, et al (2005) Hospitalizations for critically ill children with traumatic brain injuries: a longitudinal analysis. Crit Care Med 33: 2074–2081

38. Bulger EM, Nathens AB, Rivara FP, et al (2002) Brain Trauma Foundation. Management of severe head injury: institutional variations in care and effect on outcome. Crit Care Med 30: 1870–1876

39. Lavinio A, Menon DK (2011) Intracranial pressure: why we monitor it, how to monitor it, what to do with the number and what's the future? Curr Opin Anaesthesiol 24: 117–123

40. Shafi S, Diaz-Arrastia R, Madden C, Gentilello L (2008) Intracranial pressure monitoring in brain-injured patients is associated with worsening of survival. J Trauma 64: 335–340

41. Zahuranec DB, Brown DL, Lisabeth LD, et al (2007) Early care limitations independently predict mortality after intracerebral hemorrhage. Neurology 68: 1651–1657

42. Creutzfeldt CJ, Becker KJ, Weinstein JR, et al (2011) Do-not-attempt-resuscitation orders and prognostic models for intraparenchymal hemorrhage. Crit Care Med 39: 158–162

43. Finley Caulfield A, Gabler L, Lansberg MG, et al (2010) Outcome prediction in mechanically ventilated neurologic patients by junior neurointensivists Neurology 74: 1096–1101

44. Rabinstein AA, Hemphill JC III (2010) Prognosticating after severe acute brain disease. Science, art and biases. Neurology 74: 1086–1087

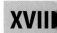

XVIII

XIX Neurological Aspects

Brain Tissue Oxygen Monitoring in Neuro-critical Care

P. Geukens and M. Oddo

Introduction

Avoidance of secondary cerebral hypoxia/ischemia is a mainstay of therapy in neurocritical care. On-line monitoring of brain tissue oxygen tension ($PbtO_2$) enables detection of secondary brain hypoxic/ischemic insults and targeting of therapeutic interventions, such as intracranial pressure (ICP) control, cerebral perfusion pressure (CPP) augmentation, blood transfusion, and ventilation. Emerging evidence shows that compared to standard ICP/CPP management, $PbtO_2$-directed therapy may improve outcomes of selected populations of brain-injured patients. Larger prospective multicenter trials are underway to further evaluate the potential benefit of $PbtO_2$-directed therapy.

In light of recent important advances in this topic, the aim of this review is to summarize the physiology underlying $PbtO_2$ monitoring, its main indications and clinical utility, and the potential benefit of $PbtO_2$-directed therapy on outcome.

The Physiology Underlying $PbtO_2$ Monitoring

Definition

$PbtO_2$ is defined as the partial pressure of oxygen in the interstitial space of the brain and reflects the availability of oxygen for oxidative energy production. $PbtO_2$ represents the balance between oxygen delivery and oxygen consumption, and is influenced by changes in cerebral capillary perfusion.

Technology

The technique involves the insertion of a fine catheter (approximately 0.5 mm in diameter) into the brain parenchyma for the continuous monitoring of $PbtO_2$ at the bedside (**Fig. 1**). Catheters can be inserted through a single or multiple lumen bolt via a burr hole or by tunneling, and can be placed in the operating room or at the beside in the intensive care unit (ICU). Probes are generally placed in the sub-cortical white matter adjacent to an ICP catheter and measure $PbtO_2$ locally, in an area of about $15-20$ mm^2 around the probe. Two devices for $PbtO_2$ monitoring are available (the Licox® system from Integra and the Neurovent® system from Raumedic), which utilize polarographic Clark-type cell with reversible electrochemical electrodes. Post-insertion non-contrast head computed tomography (CT) confirmation of probe position in the brain parenchyma is important for interpretation of readings. A 'run-in' or equilibration time of up to one hour is

J.-L. Vincent (ed.), *Annual Update in Intensive Care and Emergency Medicine 2012*
DOI 10.1007/978-3-642-25716-2 © Springer-Verlag Berlin Heidelberg 2012

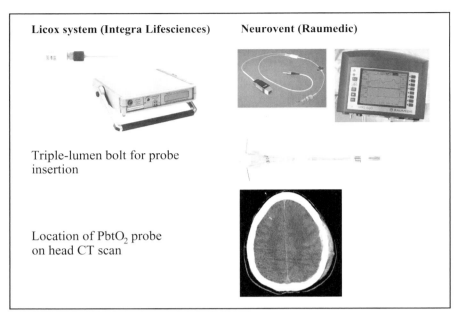

Licox system (Integra Lifesciences)   **Neurovent (Raumedic)**

Triple-lumen bolt for probe insertion

Location of PbtO$_2$ probe on head CT scan

Fig. 1. Figure illustrating the technology underlying brain tissue oxygen tension (PbtO$_2$) monitoring. Insertion of PbtO$_2$ probes into sub-cortical white matter is generally realized via a single or multiple (triple in the example illustrated here) lumen bolt, that can be inserted in the ICU or operating room. Correct catheter placement is controlled with a non-contrast head CT scan. For additional details see text.

required before readings are stable. At the beginning of monitoring, and daily thereafter, an 'oxygen challenge' is performed to evaluate the function and the responsiveness of the PbtO$_2$ probe. The oxygen challenge involves increasing the FiO$_2$ from baseline to 1.0 for approximately 20 minutes in order to evaluate the probe's responsiveness (defined by an increase of about 2 times of baseline PbtO$_2$). PbtO$_2$ monitoring is safe, causing a small iatrogenic hematoma in less than 2 % of patients, this number comparing favorably with the rate reported with intraparenchymal ICP monitoring, and being much smaller than that associated with external ventricular drains [1]. No catheter-related infections have been reported [2]; technical complication (dislocation or defect) rates may reach 13.6 %, with the greatest PbtO$_2$ display errors measured in the first 4 days [1].

Probe Location

The PbtO$_2$ value is highly dependent on oxygen diffusion from the vasculature to a small amount of tissue [3, 4]. Location of the probe is of critical importance for the interpretation of PbtO$_2$. Most centers have measured PbtO$_2$ in the right 'normal appearing' frontal sub-cortical white matter, particularly in conditions of diffuse brain injury. PbtO$_2$ probes can be placed around focal injuries (e.g., hemorrhagic contusions or hematomas in patients with head trauma, and areas perfused by the artery where the ruptured aneurysm has been secured and are at higher risk of delayed ischemia in patients with subarachnoid hemorrhage

[SAH]). In such areas surrounding brain lesions, $PbtO_2$ values may be lower than those measured in normal appearing tissue [5]. Although considered as regional monitoring, $PbtO_2$ has been shown to be a good indicator of global brain oxygenation, particularly in conditions of diffuse injury [6].

Interpretation of Measured Values

In agreement with recent data indicating that the venous fraction within the cortical microvasculature exceeds 70 %, it is suggested that $PbtO_2$ predominantly reflects venous PO_2 [7]. Among the factors affecting $PbtO_2$, the effects of decreased CPP and cerebral blood flow (CBF) have been studied most [8]. $PbtO_2$ appears to correlate well with regional CBF and the relationship follows the autoregulation curve regulating CBF along a wide range of mean arterial pressures (MAPs) [9]. CPP and MAP augmentation might significantly increase $PbtO_2$ [10] further supporting the notion that $PbtO_2$ can be a good marker of CBF and cerebral ischemia in certain conditions.

$PbtO_2$ is, however, more than a marker of ischemia. Rosenthal and colleagues, using parenchymal thermal diffusion CBF and $PbtO_2$ monitoring, showed that $PbtO_2$ more appropriately reflects the product of CBF and arterio-venous oxygen tension difference ($AVTO_2$) [4]:

$$PbtO_2 = CBF \cdot AVTO_2$$

where $AVTO_2 \approx CaO_2 - CvO_2 \approx [(SaO_2 \cdot 1.34 \cdot [hemoglobin] + (0.003 \cdot PaO_2)] - [(SvO_2 \cdot 1.34 \cdot [hemoglobin]) + (0.003 \cdot PvO_2)]$.

The very close association of $PbtO_2$ with the product of CBF and $AVTO_2$ implies a relationship between the amount of dissolved plasma oxygen passing through a given volume of brain per unit time and the steady-state oxygen concentration in brain tissue. Based on the formula $PbtO_2 = CBF \cdot AVTO_2$, reduced $PbtO_2$ occurs frequently because of low CBF. However, PaO_2 is also an important determinant of $PbtO_2$ [11] and additional pathological events (e.g., impaired lung function [12] or reduced oxygen extraction due to increased gradients for oxygen diffusion in injured brain tissue [3]) might decrease $PbtO_2$, in the absence of reduced CBF. $PbtO_2$ is therefore more a marker of cellular function than simply an 'ischemia monitor', which suggests that it may be an appropriate target for therapy.

PbtO₂ Thresholds for Therapy

In stable conditions, $PbtO_2$ averages 35–50 mmHg, with lower values observed after acute brain injury (25–35 mmHg). There has been intense debate about the thresholds for physiologic abnormality that should guide therapeutic interventions (**Table 1**). A $PbtO_2$ < 20 mmHg has been generally accepted as the threshold for compromised brain oxygen or *moderate* brain hypoxia [5, 13, 14]. *Severe* brain hypoxia has been defined as a $PbtO_2$ < 10 mmHg [2]. Recently the Brain Trauma Foundation defined the threshold for *critical* brain hypoxia as a $PbtO_2$ < 15 mmHg, representing the lower threshold to initiate therapy [15]. Trends over time and the duration and the magnitude of brain hypoxia are of outmost importance from the clinical standpoint since they have a great influence on prognosis [2, 13, 14].

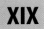

Table 1. Physiological and pathological brain tissue oxygen tension (PbtO$_2$) thresholds in humans.

Condition	Values
PbtO$_2$ ranges:	
Neurosurgical patients, stable conditions	35 – 50 mmHg
Neurosurgical patients, acute injury (SAH, TBI)	25 – 35 mmHg
PbtO$_2$ thresholds of brain hypoxia:	
Moderate brain hypoxia (compromised brain oxygen)	20 mmHg
Critical brain hypoxia	15 mmHg*
Severe brain hypoxia	10 mmHg

* PbtO$_2$ threshold to initiate therapy according to Brain Trauma Foundation guidelines (2007).
SAH: subarachnoid hemorrhage; TBI: traumatic brain injury.

Indications for PbtO$_2$ Monitoring

The two major conditions in which PbtO$_2$ monitoring has been applied and might have clinical utility are severe traumatic brain injury (TBI) and poor-grade SAH (**Table 2**).

Table 2. Indications for brain tissue oxygen tension (PbtO$_2$) monitoring

Pathology	Therapeutic interventions that may be targeted to PbtO$_2$
Traumatic brain injury (TBI)	
Severe TBI	*Management of CPP*
	• Identification of optimal CPP threshold
	ICP control
	• Evaluate the efficacy of osmotherapy
	• Aggressive management of ICP (e.g., decompressive craniectomy) if high ICP/ low PbtO$_2$ pattern
	Blood transfusion
	Lung-protective strategy
Subarachnoid hemorrhage (SAH)	
Poor grade/ comatose SAH	*Prevention of DCI*
	• Identify patients at high risk of DCI
	Treatment of DCI
	• Optimal MAP/CPP threshold for medical therapy of DCI (induced hypertension)
	Blood transfusion

CPP: cerebral perfusion pressure; DCI: delayed cerebral ischemia; ICP: intracranial pressure; MAP: mean arterial pressure

Traumatic Brain Injury

Low PbtO$_2$ is associated with poor outcome after severe TBI [2]. Importantly, it has been demonstrated that secondary brain hypoxic insults may go unnoticed when therapy is guided by ICP/CPP alone and that brain hypoxia can occur despite ICP and CPP being within normal thresholds [13, 14]. Monitoring and management of PbtO$_2$ has been included in international guidelines to complement ICP/CPP guided care of patients with severe TBI [15].

Subarachnoid Hemorrhage

Recent international consensus guidelines have included $PbtO_2$ monitoring as a useful tool to detect delayed cerebral ischemia in comatose/poor-grade SAH patients [16]. In this setting, $PbtO_2$ monitoring might identify patients at high risk for delayed cerebral ischemia [17] and is a valid complement to transcranial Doppler (TCD) and radiographic monitoring. Results from $PbtO_2$ monitoring after SAH also led to questions about the efficacy of triple H therapy in the treatment of delayed cerebral ischemia [18] (see below). In SAH patients, an association between low $PbtO_2$ and outcome has been reported by some [19] but not all [20, 21] authors.

$PbtO_2$-directed therapy

$PbtO_2$ monitoring and management is a good complement to ICP/CPP standard care. Referring to the equation $PbtO_2 = CBF \cdot AVTO_2$ provides valuable information about how to integrate $PbtO_2$ in clinical practice and to direct therapy of brain hypoxia.

Management of Cerebral Perfusion Pressure

The most studied role of $PbtO_2$ in guiding therapy, and possibly the one with greatest clinical utility, is in CPP management. Increased CPP is often associated with increased $PbtO_2$, thereby allowing a CPP threshold to be set to prevent brain hypoxia [10].

The response of $PbtO_2$ to changes in MAP/CPP has been explored in patients with severe TBI [22] and poor-grade SAH [17], in whom the aim was to identify the optimal CPP level above which secondary brain ischemia could be prevented. Interestingly, when using this approach in selected populations of patients with severe TBI, the CPP threshold needed to avoid brain hypoxia was variable (60–100 mmHg) across subjects and on average lay between 70–75 mmHg, suggesting that optimal CPP may be higher in some TBI patients [23]. Use of $PbtO_2$ monitoring is of value for the continuous surveillance and detection of delayed cerebral ischemia in patients with SAH [17, 20].

In patients with SAH, $PbtO_2$ monitoring has proved helpful to tailor the so-called triple H therapy. Based on evidence showing that the first component of triple H (induced hypertension) improves CBF and $PbtO_2$, whereas the other two components (hemodilution and hypervolemia) have no or even a negative effect on both physiological endpoints [18], induced hypertension alone is now preferred to triple H therapy for the treatment of delayed cerebral ischemia [16].

Control of Intracranial Pressure

Sustained pathological elevations of ICP may translate into reduced CPP and secondary brain hypoxia/ischemia. A recent study showed that when elevated ICP occurs together with low $PbtO_2$, outcome is worse than when ICP is elevated but $PbtO_2$ is normal [14]. Recent studies have shown that $PbtO_2$ monitoring has the potential to improve management of intracranial hypertension. First, the simultaneous occurrence of a pattern of high ICP/low $PbtO_2$ may direct therapy towards

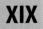

more aggressive management of brain edema, e.g., decompressive craniectomy [24]. Second, recent studies found that hypertonic saline was superior to mannitol in achieving effective and long-lasting reduction of ICP while at the same time improving $PbtO_2$ [25, 26]; thus, $PbtO_2$ may help monitor the efficacy of osmotherapy. Third, since moderate hyperventilation might reduce $PbtO_2$ substantially [27], brain oxygen monitoring can help target optimal $PaCO_2$ during ICP control and prevent further cerebral ischemia.

Additional Interventions

Anemia-induced brain hypoxia has been observed in brain-injured patients and can be corrected by blood transfusion [28, 29]. Monitoring of $PbtO_2$ can thus be used to guide transfusions in patients at risk for brain hypoxia.

Impaired lung function with subsequent reduction in SaO_2, PaO_2 and PaO_2/FiO_2 ratio correlates strongly with brain hypoxia [12]. This argues in favor of lung-protective strategies (positive end-expiratory pressure [PEEP], lung recruitment) guided by $PbtO_2$ in order to improve brain oxygenation and at the same time reduce secondary brain hypoxic insults.

Standardized Algorithm for PbtO₂-directed Therapy

A proposed algorithm for $PbtO_2$-directed therapy is illustrated in **Figure 2**. As with all ICU monitoring tools, verification and interpretation of measured values is of outmost importance. Also, despite its potential utility, monitoring of $PbtO_2$ should not be used alone to direct therapy, but rather as part of a multimodal approach. Over-interpretation or aggressive treatment may result in treatment-related complications, which will negate potential outcome benefits [30]. Thus, the importance of monitoring $PbtO_2$ trends over time and examining on-line response to therapeutic trials must be emphasized. For example, in some patients, CPP augmentation [23] or blood transfusion [29] may fail to improve $PbtO_2$, which should then lead to discontinuation of such therapies.

How to treat low $PbtO_2$ is still debated. As for ICP therapy, a stepwise management approach has been proposed, starting when $PbtO_2$ is < 20 mmHg [31]. This strategy includes: (1) give an 'oxygen challenge' (FiO_2 100 % for 2 minutes, to restore $PbtO_2$ temporarily, check functioning of the probe and ensure adequate control of elevated ICP (> 20 mmHg) if necessary; (2) test $PbtO_2$ response to MAP/CPP increase with vasopressors; (3) improve pulmonary function (increase FiO_2 up to 60 %, add PEEP if needed, aspirate pulmonary secretions); (4) reduce excessive metabolic demand (analgesia, sedation, temperature < 37 °C, rule out non-convulsive seizures); (5) administer blood transfusion if hemoglobin concentration is < 9 g/dl. In a recent retrospective study by Bohman and colleagues, the most frequently employed interventions were respiratory manipulations, CPP augmentation and sedation, with an improvement of compromised $PbtO_2$ in about two-thirds of treated episodes and a better outcome in $PbtO_2$ responders [31].

> **VENTILATION/OXYGENATION**
> ➤ ↑ FiO_2 to 100% transiently (2 min)
> ➤ check CXR for atelectasis, pulmonary infiltrate, ALI/ARDS
>> • physiotherapy
>> • ↑ PEEP by steps of 2-4 cmH_2O (under strict ICP control)
>> • FiO_2 60%
> ➤ check $PaCO_2$
>> • if $PaCO_2$ 30-35 mmHg, and ICP < 20 mmHg, ↑ $PaCO_2$ 35-40 mmHg

> **CEREBRAL PERFUSION PRESSURE**
> ➤ test $PbtO_2$ response to MAP augmentation
>> • ↑ MAP by > 10 mmHg (norepinephrine, phenylephrine)
> ➤ if ICP > 20-25 mmHg
>> • treat elevated ICP

> **OXYGEN CONSUMPTION**
> ➤ ↑ sedation and analgesia
> ➤ ↓ body temperature if > 37°C
> ➤ rule out seizures

> **OXYGEN TRANSPORT**
> ➤ check [Hb]
>> • test response of $PbtO_2$ to blood transfusion
> ➤ optimize cardiac output, hemodynamic status

Fig. 2. Stepwise algorithm for brain tissue oxygen tension ($PbtO_2$)-directed therapy (threshold to start therapy: $PbtO_2$ < 15 – 20 mmHg). As with all ICU monitoring tools, verification and interpretation of measured values is of utmost importance. In addition to target thresholds, the importance of monitoring $PbtO_2$ trends over time and carefully evaluating $PbtO_2$ response to therapeutic interventions must be emphasized. Monitoring of $PbtO_2$ should not be used alone to direct therapy, but rather as part of a multimodal approach. CXR: chest x-ray; ALI: acute lung injury; ARDS: acute respiratory distress syndrome; PEEP: positive end-expiratory pressure; ICP: intracranial pressure; MAP: mean arterial pressure; Hb: hemoglobin

$PbtO_2$-directed Therapy and Outcome

A large body of evidence shows that reduced $PbtO_2$ is associated with worse outcome after severe TBI [2, 13, 14]. In particular, longer duration of brain hypoxia, irrespective of ICP and CPP levels, is a strong and independent outcome predictor after severe TBI [14]. Given that $PbtO_2$ is an important physiological predictor of outcome it is reasonable to test the hypothesis that $PbtO_2$-directed therapy – aimed to prevent/treat brain hypoxia – might translate into better outcome. This issue has been examined by several studies, all performed in patients with severe TBI, and comparing the effect of $PbtO_2$-directed therapy versus ICP/CPP standard care on patient outcome (**Table 3**). Stiefel and colleagues, in a small retrospective historical control study (n = 53 patients; 27 $PbtO_2$ vs. 26 ICP/CPP therapy), showed that $PbtO_2$-directed therapy (with a threshold of 25 mmHg) reduced mortality from 44 % to 25 % [32]. Meixensberger and colleagues, in a similar histori-

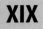

Table 3. Studies comparing the effect of brain tissue oxygen tension (PbtO$_2$)-directed therapy vs. standard intracranial pressure/cerebral perfusion pressure (ICP/CPP) care on the outcome of patients with severe traumatic brain injury.

First author [ref]	Study type	PbtO$_2$ therapy	ICP/CPP therapy	PbtO$_2$ threshold for therapy	Outcome endpoint	Effect on outcome of PbtO$_2$ vs. ICP/CPP therapy
Meixensberger et al. 2003 [33]	R, historical control	n = 52	n = 39	10 mmHg	6-month GOS	Trend towards better outcome (65 % vs. 54 %, p = 0.27)
Stiefel et al. 2005 [32]	R, historical control	n = 28	n = 25	25 mmHg	Mortality at hospital discharge	Reduced mortality (25 % vs. 44 %, p< 0.05)
Martini et al. 2009 [30]	R, cohort	n = 123	n = 506	20 mmHg	FIM at hospital discharge	Worse outcome (FIM 7.6 ± 3.0 vs. 8.6 ± 2.8, p< 0.01). After adjustment for injury severity, − 0.75 point difference (95 % CI − 1.41 to − 0.09) in mean FIM score with PbtO$_2$ vs. ICP/CPP therapy
McCarthy et al. 2009 [34]	P	n = 63	n = 48	20 mmHg	3-month GOS	Trend towards better outcome (79 % vs. 61 %, p = 0.09)
Narotam et al. 2009 [35]	R, historical control	n = 127	n = 39	20 mmHg	6-month GOS	Better outcome (GOS score 3.55 ± 1.75 vs. 2.71 ± 1.65, p < 0.01; OR of good outcome 2.09, 95 % CI 1.03 – 4.24) Reduced mortality (26 % vs. 41.5 %; RR reduction 37 %)
Spiotta et al. 2010 [36]	R, historical control	n = 70	n = 53	20 mmHg	3-month GOS	Better outcome (64 % vs. 40 %, p = 0.01)

FIM: Functional Independence Measure; GOS: Glasgow Outcome Score; MAP: mean arterial pressure; OR: odds ratio; P: prospective; R: retrospective; RR: relative risk

cal control study (n = 93 patients; 52 PbtO$_2$ vs. 39 ICP/CPP therapy, using a much lower PbtO$_2$ threshold for intervention of 10 mmHg) found that more patients assigned to PbtO$_2$-directed therapy achieved favorable neurological outcome at 6 months than those treated with ICP/CPP care, although this difference was not statistically significant [33]. More recently, four additional studies have measured the benefit of PbtO$_2$-directed therapy in severe TBI patients [30, 34–36], and the findings of these studies were conflicting (**Table 3**). McCarthy et al. (n = 145 patients, 81 PbtO$_2$ vs. 64 ICP/CPP therapy) found a trend towards better 6-month outcome with PbtO$_2$-directed therapy (PbtO$_2$ threshold 25 mmHg) versus ICP/CPP care (p = 0.08) [34]. Importantly, although not randomized, this was the only true prospective study. In a historical control study (n = 180 patients; 139 PbtO$_2$

vs. 41 ICP/CPP care, PbtO$_2$ threshold for therapy 20 mmHg), Narotam and colleagues observed similar benefits of PbtO$_2$-directed therapy, in terms of both a significant reduction in mortality rate and a higher proportion of good neurological recovery at 6 months [35]. Similar to their previous study [32], the Philadelphia group more recently reported better 3-month outcome with PbtO$_2$-directed therapy compared to ICP/CPP care [36].

In contrast to these studies however, using a large cohort of 629 severe TBI patients, Martini et al. found worse neurological outcome in the PbtO$_2$-treated group (n = 123 patients, PbtO$_2$ threshold for therapy 20 mmHg) versus the ICP/CPP-treated group (n = 506 patients), and more complications and greater resource consumption [30]. Although patients assigned to PbtO$_2$-directed therapy were more severely injured, these associations remained significant after adjusting for initial cerebral and systemic injury severity, thus questioning the validity and potential outcome benefit of PbtO$_2$-directed therapy. These conflicting results also underline the complexity of such therapy, which furthermore concerns a heterogeneous group of patients, such as those suffering from TBI. In addition, all studies reported until now and summarized in **Table 3** were single-center, most of them (except one [34]) were retrospective historical control or case-matched series, and they used variable PbtO$_2$ thresholds for intervention. Finally, few reported a standardized approach for PbtO$_2$-directed therapy. Given these limitations, a multicenter randomized study comparing PbtO$_2$-directed therapy to ICP/CPP standard care may be of value to test the potential benefit on outcome of this intervention.

Conclusion

The increasing use of PbtO$_2$ monitoring has contributed to ameliorate our understanding of the pathophysiology of acute cerebral conditions, such as TBI and SAH. The integration of PbtO$_2$ as an additional physiological target for therapy has the potential to improve the management of brain-injured patients and to optimize several interventions routinely employed in neurocritical care, such as the management of CPP. As for ICP control, PbtO$_2$-directed therapy is a stepwise multi-interventional approach that needs further standardization and consensus guidelines. Careful management of PbtO$_2$-directed therapy is mandatory to avoid treatment-related complications and to optimize its potential benefit on outcome.

References

1. Dings J, Meixensberger J, Jager A, Roosen K (1998) Clinical experience with 118 brain tissue oxygen partial pressure catheter probes. Neurosurgery 43: 1082–1095
2. van den Brink WA, van Santbrink H, Steyerberg EW, et al (2000) Brain oxygen tension in severe head injury. Neurosurgery 46: 868–876
3. Menon DK, Coles JP, Gupta AK, et al (2004) Diffusion limited oxygen delivery following head injury. Crit Care Med 32: 1384–1390
4. Rosenthal G, Hemphill JC 3rd, Sorani M, et al (2008) Brain tissue oxygen tension is more indicative of oxygen diffusion than oxygen delivery and metabolism in patients with traumatic brain injury. Crit Care Med 36: 1917–1924
5. Longhi L, Pagan F, Valeriani V, et al (2007) Monitoring brain tissue oxygen tension in brain-injured patients reveals hypoxic episodes in normal-appearing and in peri-focal tissue. Intensive Care Med 33: 2136–2142

6. Gupta AK, Hutchinson PJ, Al-Rawi P, et al (1999) Measuring brain tissue oxygenation compared with jugular venous oxygen saturation for monitoring cerebral oxygenation after traumatic brain injury. Anesth Analg 88: 549–553

7. Scheufler KM, Rohrborn HJ, Zentner J (2002) Does tissue oxygen-tension reliably reflect cerebral oxygen delivery and consumption? Anesth Analg 95: 1042–1048

8. Doppenberg EM, Zauner A, Bullock R, Ward JD, Fatouros PP, Young HF (1998) Correlations between brain tissue oxygen tension, carbon dioxide tension, pH, and cerebral blood flow – a better way of monitoring the severely injured brain? Surg Neurol 49: 650–654

9. Hemphill JC 3rd, Smith WS, Sonne DC, Morabito D, Manley GT (2005) Relationship between brain tissue oxygen tension and CT perfusion: feasibility and initial results. AJNR Am J Neuroradiol 26: 1095–1100

10. Johnston AJ, Steiner LA, Coles JP, et al (2005) Effect of cerebral perfusion pressure augmentation on regional oxygenation and metabolism after head injury. Crit Care Med 33: 189–195

11. Nortje J, Coles JP, Timofeev I, et al (2008) Effect of hyperoxia on regional oxygenation and metabolism after severe traumatic brain injury: preliminary findings. Crit Care Med 36: 273–281

12. Oddo M, Nduom E, Frangos S, et al (2010) Acute lung injury is an independent risk factor for brain hypoxia after severe traumatic brain injury. Neurosurgery 67: 338–344

13. Chang JJ, Youn TS, Benson D, et al (2009) Physiologic and functional outcome correlates of brain tissue hypoxia in traumatic brain injury. Crit Care Med 37: 283–290

14. Oddo M, Levine JM, Mackenzie L, et al (2011) Brain hypoxia is associated with short-term outcome after severe traumatic brain injury independent of intracranial hypertension and low cerebral perfusion pressure. Neurosurgery 69: 1037–1045

15. Bratton SL, Chestnut RM, Ghajar J, et al (2007) Guidelines for the management of severe traumatic brain injury. X. Brain oxygen monitoring and thresholds. J Neurotrauma 24 (Suppl 1): S65–70

16. Diringer MN, Bleck TP, Claude Hemphill J 3rd, et al (2011) Critical care management of patients following aneurysmal subarachnoid hemorrhage: Recommendations from the Neurocritical Care Society's Multidisciplinary Consensus Conference. Neurocrit Care 15: 211–240

17. Jaeger M, Schuhmann MU, Soehle M, Nagel C, Meixensberger J (2007) Continuous monitoring of cerebrovascular autoregulation after subarachnoid hemorrhage by brain tissue oxygen pressure reactivity and its relation to delayed cerebral infarction. Stroke 38: 981–986

18. Muench E, Horn P, Bauhuf C, et al (2007) Effects of hypervolemia and hypertension on regional cerebral blood flow, intracranial pressure, and brain tissue oxygenation after subarachnoid hemorrhage. Crit Care Med 35: 1844–1851

19. Ramakrishna R, Stiefel M, Udoetuk J, et al (2008) Brain oxygen tension and outcome in patients with aneurysmal subarachnoid hemorrhage. J Neurosurg 109: 1075–1082

20. Kett-White R, Hutchinson PJ, Al-Rawi PG, Gupta AK, Pickard JD, Kirkpatrick PJ (2002) Adverse cerebral events detected after subarachnoid hemorrhage using brain oxygen and microdialysis probes. Neurosurgery 50: 1213–1221

21. Meixensberger J, Vath A, Jaeger M, Kunze E, Dings J, Roosen K (2003) Monitoring of brain tissue oxygenation following severe subarachnoid hemorrhage. Neurol Res 25: 445–450

22. Jaeger M, Schuhmann MU, Soehle M, Meixensberger J (2006) Continuous assessment of cerebrovascular autoregulation after traumatic brain injury using brain tissue oxygen pressure reactivity. Crit Care Med 34: 1783–1788

23. Jaeger M, Dengl M, Meixensberger J, Schuhmann MU (2010) Effects of cerebrovascular pressure reactivity-guided optimization of cerebral perfusion pressure on brain tissue oxygenation after traumatic brain injury. Crit Care Med 38: 1343–1347

24. Strege RJ, Lang EW, Stark AM, et al (2003) Cerebral edema leading to decompressive craniectomy: an assessment of the preceding clinical and neuromonitoring trends. Neurol Res 25: 510–515

25. Oddo M, Levine JM, Frangos S, et al (2009) Effect of mannitol and hypertonic saline on cerebral oxygenation in patients with severe traumatic brain injury and refractory intracranial hypertension. J Neurol Neurosurg Psychiatry 80: 916–920

26. Al-Rawi PG, Tseng MY, Richards HK, et al (2010) Hypertonic saline in patients with poor-grade subarachnoid hemorrhage improves cerebral blood flow, brain tissue oxygen, and pH. Stroke 41: 122–128
27. Rangel-Castilla L, Lara LR, Gopinath S, Swank PR, Valadka A, Robertson C (2010) Cerebral hemodynamic effects of acute hyperoxia and hyperventilation after severe traumatic brain injury. J Neurotrauma 27: 1853–1863
28. Leal-Noval SR, Rincon-Ferrari MD, Marin-Niebla A, et al (2006) Transfusion of erythrocyte concentrates produces a variable increment on cerebral oxygenation in patients with severe traumatic brain injury: a preliminary study. Intensive Care Med 32: 1733–1740
29. Smith MJ, Stiefel MF, Magge S, et al (2005) Packed red blood cell transfusion increases local cerebral oxygenation. Crit Care Med 33: 1104–1108
30. Martini RP, Deem S, Yanez ND, et al (2009) Management guided by brain tissue oxygen monitoring and outcome following severe traumatic brain injury. J Neurosurg 111: 644–649
31. Bohman LE, Heuer GG, Macyszyn L, et al (2011) Medical management of compromised brain oxygen in patients with severe traumatic brain injury. Neurocrit Care 14: 361–369
32. Stiefel MF, Spiotta A, Gracias VH, et al (2005) Reduced mortality rate in patients with severe traumatic brain injury treated with brain tissue oxygen monitoring. J Neurosurg 103: 805–811
33. Meixensberger J, Jaeger M, Vath A, Dings J, Kunze E, Roosen K (2003) Brain tissue oxygen guided treatment supplementing ICP/CPP therapy after traumatic brain injury. J Neurol Neurosurg Psychiatry 74: 760–764
34. McCarthy MC, Moncrief H, Sands JM, et al (2009) Neurologic outcomes with cerebral oxygen monitoring in traumatic brain injury. Surgery 146: 585–590
35. Narotam PK, Morrison JF, Nathoo N (2009) Brain tissue oxygen monitoring in traumatic brain injury and major trauma: outcome analysis of a brain tissue oxygen-directed therapy. J Neurosurg 111: 672–682
36. Spiotta AM, Stiefel MF, Gracias VH, et al (2010) Brain tissue oxygen-directed management and outcome in patients with severe traumatic brain injury. J Neurosurg 113: 571–580

Quantitative EEG for the Detection of Brain Ischemia

B. FOREMAN and J. CLAASSEN

Introduction

Monitoring in most intensive care units (ICUs) is limited to continuous assessments of cardiopulmonary function, whereas brain monitoring has traditionally been limited to serial neurological examinations and infrequent imaging studies. Increasingly it is becoming clear that secondary neurological complications, such as seizures and brain ischemia, are also seen in the medical-surgical ICU population and are not limited to patients with primarily neurological injury. Electroencephalography (EEG) offers a continuous, real-time, non-invasive measure of brain function. Originally developed for the characterization of seizures and epilepsy, continuous EEG monitoring (cEEG) has been used for seizure detection in the ICU. Additionally, cEEG has been used as a method of identifying subclinical brain injury during neurosurgical procedures, such as carotid endarterectomy, and for ischemia detection, global function assessment, medication titration, and prognostication [1].

In the ICU, ischemia detection in particular has been under-utilized, but the potential to diagnose ischemia as it occurs is tremendous (e.g., monitoring after high risk vascular or cardiac surgery, during refractory hypotension, or in the context of sepsis-associated encephalopathy). When cerebral blood flow (CBF) becomes compromised, changes occur in both the metabolic and electrical activity of cortical neurons, with associated EEG changes [2]. In the operating room, EEG has an established role in identifying ischemia prior to the development of infarction during carotid endarterectomy [3]. In acute ischemic stroke, the primary injury has typically occurred prior to presentation, but EEG may be able to detect patterns to suggest severity, prognosis, and secondary injury (e.g., reocclusion, edema, or hemorrhagic transformation) [4]. Delayed cerebral ischemia from vasospasm after subarachnoid hemorrhage (SAH) illustrates an application in which early detection may prevent the development of permanent damage by triggering appropriate interventions such as angioplasty or intra-arterial administration of vasodilator therapy [5, 6]. Serial neurological exams and imaging are only capable of detecting delayed cerebral ischemia once the damage becomes clinically or radiographically apparent. In this case, EEG may be a useful way to detect and subsequently treat ischemia before the injury becomes irreversible [7–10].

EEG Changes in Ischemia

Brain function is represented on EEG by oscillations of certain frequencies. Slower frequencies (typically delta [0.5–3 Hz] or theta [4–7 Hz]) are generated

J.-L. Vincent (ed.), *Annual Update in Intensive Care and Emergency Medicine 2012*
DOI 10.1007/978-3-642-25716-2 © Springer-Verlag Berlin Heidelberg 2012

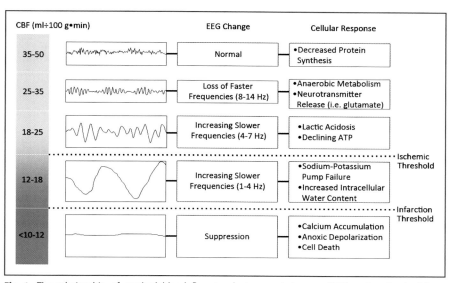

Fig. 1. The relationship of cerebral blood flow to electroencephalogram (EEG) and pathophysiology. ATP: adenosine triphosphate (CBF). Data from [2, 4]

by the thalamus and by cells in layers II-VI of the cortex. Faster frequencies (or alpha, typically 8–12 Hz) derive from cells in layers IV and V of the cortex [11]. All frequencies are modulated by the reticular activating system, which corresponds to the observation of reactivity on the EEG [12]. Pyramidal neurons found in layers III, V, and VI are exquisitely sensitive to conditions of low oxygen, such as ischemia, thus leading to many of the abnormal changes in the patterns seen on EEG [4].

EEG changes are closely tied to CBF (**Fig. 1**) [3]. When normal CBF declines to approximately 25–35 ml/100 g/min, the EEG first loses faster frequencies, then as the CBF decreases to approximately 17–18 ml/100 g/min, slower frequencies gradually increase. This represents a crucial ischemic threshold at which neurons begin to lose their transmembrane gradients, leading to cell death (infarction). In the setting of carotid clamping, CBF that decreases instantaneously to the ischemic threshold leads to rapid and reversible changes in the EEG (within 20 seconds) [3]. Infarction may not occur for hours at this degree of flow limitation [2] and some electrical activity (mostly delta frequencies) may be seen, but as the CBF continues to decrease toward the infarction threshold (10–12 ml/100 g/min and below), the EEG becomes silent and cellular damage becomes irreversible [2–4]. Some EEG patterns, such as regional attenuation of faster frequencies without delta (RAWOD), may reflect early severe loss of CBF (mean 8.6 ml/100 g/min) as seen during large occlusive infarcts, leading to complications such as edema and herniation [13].

Studies of CBF and cerebral rate of oxygen metabolism (CMRO$_2$) using Xenon computed tomography (CT) and positron emission tomography (PET) in ischemic stroke have demonstrated that regional EEG changes also reflect the coupling of CBF and metabolism [14]. In early subacute ischemic stroke, the EEG correlates well with CBF as the oxygen extraction fraction increases to preserve CMRO$_2$, a period termed "misery perfusion" or stage 2 hemodynamic failure [14,

15]. Later, the EEG appears to correlate less well with CBF and instead begins to correlate with $CMRO_2$ during a period of "luxury perfusion" or stage 3 hemodynamic failure [14, 15]. Early in this dynamic relationship, the threshold for cellular damage is shifted such that neuronal loss and decreased protein metabolism may in fact precede changes related to critical CBF, particularly in peri-infarct areas [2]. These areas are also complicated by abnormal glutamate release (between 20–30 ml/100 g/min) or peri-infarct depolarizations [2, 16].

The transition from ischemia to infarct occurs over a range of CBF, potentially providing a window of opportunity to treat and reverse impending neuronal cell death. Diffusion-weighted magnetic resonance images (DWI MRI) are capable of detecting changes at CBF 35–40 ml/100 g/min within 30 minutes [17]. In contrast, EEG detects changes at the same CBF within seconds and allows for continuous monitoring of these changes over time. This can be crucial to detect evolving ischemic changes after treatment with tissue plasminogen activator (tPA), when the CT is negative during early infarction, or when there is a mismatch between DWI MRI and the clinical examination. Additionally, EEG may assist in guiding treatment, to rapidly reverse the region at risk if it has not reached the infarction threshold. Examples include shunt placement in carotid endarterectomy [3], tPA in acute ischemic stroke [18, 19], and augmentation of blood pressure or CBF after acute ischemic stroke [20].

There are some data suggesting that EEG may help with prognostication in patients with acute ischemic stroke. Because cortical changes are modulated by brainstem reticular formations, global changes, such as loss of reactivity [21] and lack of sleep-wake cycles [22], may portend poor prognosis (and indicate possible brainstem involvement). Regional changes, including a lack of delta or the presence of faster frequencies within 24 hours, correlate with a good outcome [23] while the persistence of unilateral prominent, continuous delta slowing or decreased alpha adds significantly to clinical predictions of poor outcome [24]. Other specific patterns may also indicate poor prognosis, such as RAWOD (with up to 67 % mortality) [13] or periodic lateralized epileptiform discharges (PLEDs) [25].

A Need for Quantitative EEG

Despite the potential to detect ischemia, there are a number of limitations that need to be overcome before using this technique for automated event detection in ICU practice. Early obstacles, such as data acquisition, remote access, and data storage have been largely overcome by technological advances. Nonetheless, raw EEG requires interpretation by trained experts, ideally with experience in continuous monitoring for critically ill patients. Subtle changes over time (hours to days) may be missed and visual analysis can be extraordinarily time-consuming. To achieve the goal of real-time detection of critical brain events, raw EEG would require continuous expert review. Although telemedicine has become a prominent tool in acute stroke, centralized EEG monitoring with access to around-the-clock neurophysiology experts is not currently available and would be extremely expensive.

The most pressing limitation to cEEG remains its interpretation, which is ultimately subjective. By applying a Fourier transformation, EEG can be quantified in terms of its amplitude, power, frequency, and rhythmicity in order to generate numerical values, ratios, or percentages; graphically display arrays or trends; and set thresholds for alarms. A variety of quantitative EEG (qEEG) measures have been used clinically to quantify slowing or attenuation of faster frequencies in the EEG, specifically: The calculation of power within different frequency bands (i.e., delta, theta, alpha, and beta); ratios or percentages of power in specific frequency bands; and spectral edge frequencies (based on the frequency under which x% of the EEG resides). These discrete values can then be compared between different regions (between hemispheres, for instance, or between electrode-pair channels). Time-compressed spectral arrays were developed to incorporate both power and frequency spectrum data and are reconstructed using color to represent power at different frequencies (a so-called 'spectrogram'). These spectrograms have the highest pixel-to-data ratio, yielding easy-to-digest color representations of large amounts of data within a single screen (compared with the raw EEG) [26]. Additional measures include amplitude integrated EEG, which was developed to continuously monitor comatose patients via average ranges of peak-to-peak amplitudes displayed using a logarithmic scale, and the commercial Bispectral Index, often used to monitor the depth of anesthesia (Aspect Medical Systems, Inc., Newton, MA). Other nonparametric methods exist beyond Fourier transformation, including interval or period analysis and alternative transformation techniques. Parametric, mimetic, and spatiotemporal analyses are also available using a variety of computational methods that are beyond the scope of this review [27]. For now, fast Fourier transformation appears to be the most suitable for quantifying the EEG [28] but future algorithms may also incorporate ICU-specific EEG feature recognition and waveform analysis based on machine learning approaches trained on ICU EEG recordings.

It is important to emphasize that there are a large number of confounders to be considered when evaluating EEG signals. Both raw EEG and qEEG can be altered in response to the presence of seizures or periodic discharges, changes in intracranial pressure (ICP, e.g., acute hydrocephalus), or in the setting of systemic illness such as ventilator-acquired pneumonia (VAP). In addition, sedatives, narcotics, antipsychotics, and other medications may have varying effects on the EEG. Even normal state changes, such as slow wave sleep, appear similar to changes seen during ischemia. Moreover, the ICU is contaminated with a variety of artifacts: Chest percussion, bed movement, condensation in ventilator tubing, and electrical (50Hz or 60Hz) artifact from other monitoring devices. Ultimately, the raw EEG remains the gold standard for the assessment of brain function. Any algorithm based on qEEG should include raw EEG for review by staff familiar with EEG – either on site or remotely [9, 26].

Quantitative EEG in Ischemia

Like raw EEG, qEEG is capable of reflecting changes in blood flow and metabolism in as little as 28 – 104 seconds [29]. However, different quantitative parameters may have their own strengths for a given clinical situation. Intraoperative spectral edge frequencies, for example, detect ischemic changes in carotid endarterectomy patients receiving isoflurane anesthesia, whereas changes in the relative delta percentage (that is, delta power/total power) are accurate in patients receiving propofol [29]. In acute ischemic stroke, hemispheric relative delta percentage, spectral edge frequencies 25 % and 75 %, and the overall mean frequency correlated well with CBF [28]. Cerebral perfusion pressure (CPP), related to CBF and to ICP, correlates with decreases in mean frequency as CPP falls below 60 mmHg, even in comatose or sedated patients [30]. Finally, increased power in slower frequency bands (delta and theta) and decreased power in faster frequency bands (alpha and beta) are seen with reductions in brain metabolism ($CMRO_2$) [14]. Overall, the relative delta percentage appears to provide the most robust correlation with CBF and metabolism during focal ischemia.

Clinically, qEEG correlates with stroke severity, radiographic findings, and response to treatment. Several parameters correlate with initial stroke severity as measured by the National Institutes of Health Stroke Scale (NIHSS) in both the acute (brain symmetry index [BSI]) [19, 31] and subacute periods (relative alpha percentage, relative alpha-beta percentage, relative delta-theta percentage, delta/alpha ratio, delta-theta/alpha-beta ratio, and global pairwise derived BSI [pdBSI]) [32–34]. qEEG parameters correlate with the volume of infarction on MRI, such as the acute delta change index [35], global pdBSI [32], relative alpha percentage, relative alpha-beta percentage, relative delta-theta percentage, delta/alpha ratio, and delta-theta/alpha-beta ratio [36]. In the case of subcortical infarcts, both the delta-theta/alpha-beta ratio and the pdBSI correlate surprisingly well with infarct volumes, possibly related to the consequences of diaschisis on CBF in lacunar brainstem infarcts [33, 36]. qEEG may be more sensitive than raw EEG to subtle changes [37, 38], and some parameters may even detect improvement prior to improvement in the clinical exam. For example, after tPA, a decrease in delta power was documented 100 minutes prior to the start of functional improvement [18] and in a series of 16 patients with moderate stroke, one patient had an improvement in BSI a few minutes prior to clinical improvement after the administration of tPA [19].

qEEG may also provide a method of quantifying short-term and long-term prognosis. At one year, functional outcome after stroke in one series was predicted correctly by clinical criteria 60 % of the time. The addition of EEG data improved the predictive value to 85 % (for both raw and quantitative EEG) [24]. The acute delta change index correlates with 30-day NIHSS as accurately as initial mean transit time on MRI and actually better than initial DWI volume (emphasizing the link between qEEG parameters and blood flow) [35]; other parameters such as the delta/alpha ratio and the relative alpha percentage also correlate with the 30-day NIHSS [34]. As early as 6 hours after stroke, the pdBSI correlates with the 1-week NIHSS. Subacute abnormalities in pdBSI and, particularly, the delta-theta/alpha-beta ratio are associated with the 6-month modified Rankin score [39]. For deeper infarcts, pdBSI and the delta-theta/alpha-beta ratio correspond to 1-week outcome [33]. Extremely elevated pdBSI may even predict early neuro-deterioration from other complications at 1 week [36].

The ability to infer CBF patterns, quantify the severity of brain ischemia, and objectively monitor the response to treatment may be useful across critically ill patient populations. Ischemia detection could alert intensivists to acute ischemia after cardiac valve replacement, for example, and could prompt intra-arterial thrombectomy and prevention of stroke. Titration of vasopressors may be influenced by the detection of ischemic changes despite an otherwise appropriate mean arterial pressure (MAP) goal. Although recent studies of EEG in patients with sepsis have focused on seizure detection and other abnormal epileptiform patterns [40], quantification of cerebral perfusion in these patients could be an invaluable measure of end-organ perfusion to guide pressor management, particularly in patients with sepsis-associated encephalopathy, which may be related to impaired perfusion of the small vessels [41]. SAH provides a useful example to illustrate the need for and potential of existing data related to qEEG techniques in the ICU.

Clinical Scenario: Delayed Cerebral Ischemia after Subarachnoid Hemorrhage

SAH has an incidence of 6–15/100,000 and is associated with high morbidity and mortality [42]. Much of the outcome is determined by secondary complications many of which are treatable if diagnosed in a timely fashion. Between 20–40 % of SAH patients either clinically deteriorate or have evidence of new ischemia on repeat brain imaging from vasospasm, together termed delayed cerebral ischemia [5, 42, 43]. Delayed cerebral ischemia is associated with worse outcome [5], but may be particularly challenging to diagnose in the comatose patient [6].

The effects of vasospasm-mediated delayed cerebral ischemia can be mitigated with pressure and volume augmentation (so-called triple-H therapy), intra-arterial vasodilators, such as verapamil, or angioplasty. The benefit of these measures relies on the earliest possible detection – before neuronal damage becomes irreversible. Serial neurological exams and radiological confirmation of ischemia offer *post hoc* diagnosis, but do not adequately detect pre-clinical events. Currently, the only serial detection method in routine use is transcranial Doppler ultrasonography (TCD). Although mean blood flow velocities of > 120 cm/s are around 60–70 % sensitive to changes in the proximal middle cerebral artery (MCA), this cut-off is less reliable (and less well studied) for other territories and does not include the distal vasculature [42]. When used daily, TCDs have been 60–70 % sensitive for delayed cerebral ischemia with limited predictive value; they also exhibit frequent false negatives or false positives [44].

EEG Changes in Subarachnoid Hemorrhage

SAH produces a wide variety of abnormalities on EEG. Even before the onset of vasospasm, EEG may detect disorganization or slowing, disruption of the normal posterior dominant rhythm, seizures (6 %), periodic discharges (16 %), a lack of reactivity (14 %), or a lack of sleep transients (in up to 85 %) [45, 46]. In a serial EEG study of 151 patients with SAH, the authors found that even on day 1, certain patterns predicted later vasospasm, including the presence of very brief frontally predominant biphasic delta waves ('axial bursts'), focal polymorphic delta overlying an area of clot, or a predominance of unreactive delta frequency slowing. By day 5, the development of continuous polymorphic, rhythmic, or unreactive delta predicted vasospasm 100 % of the time. These patterns correlated well with CT grades of SAH severity and 40 % of patients with abnormal EEG on day 5 had neurodeterioration [47]. As predicted by the EEG's close correlation with CBF and metabolism, raw EEG was capable of detecting developing ischemia up to 78 % of the time in one study of poor-grade SAH patients [9].

The use of qEEG for ischemia detection in SAH has been examined systematically in a total of 89 patients over 4 studies since 1991 (**Table 1**). In the first of these studies, EEG was found to detect ischemia earlier and better than clinical

Table 1. Clinical summary of quantitative EEG in subarachnoid hemorrhage

First author [ref]	N	SAH Grade	Clinical Criteria	Outcome	qEEG Results
Labar [7]	11	HH I: 2 HH III: 8 HH IV: 1	1) Focal neurological deficit 2) Global cortical dysfunction 3) Encephalopathy	Ischemic events (n = 18)	5 silent infarcts detected by qEEG alone 4 qEEG changes prior to clinical changes
Vespa [8]	32	Awake (HH I-III)	1) Angiographic vasospasm 2) TCD vasospasm (> 120 cm/s or Lindegaard ratio > 3)	Vasospasm (n = 19)	All vasospasm with qEEG changes. 10/19 qEEG changed mean 2.9 days prior to vasospasm confirmation.
Claassen [9]	34	Comatose (HH IV-V)	DCI 1) Clinical deterioration 2) New infarct on CT	DCI (n = 9)	Raw EEG changed in 78 %; qEEG sensitive to a 10 % change in 6 post-stimulation minutes or 50 % change in only 1 post-stimulation minute.
Rathakrishnan [10]	12	mF 3–4 HH I: 1 HH II: 5 HH III: 2 HH IV: 3 HH V: 1	DCI 1) Clinical deterioration 2) New infarct on CT	DCI (n = 8)	qEEG sensitivity with clinical data is 67 %. 3/8 qEEG changed more than 24 hours prior to clinical change.

DCI: delayed cerebral ischemia; HH: Hunt-Hess Grade; mF: Modified Fisher Grade; qEEG: quantitative EEG; SAH: subarachnoid hemorrhage; TCD: transcranial Doppler ultrasonography

exam alone [7] in 11 patients, most of whom were Hunt-Hess grade 3. Total power, the alpha/delta-theta ratio, and the relative delta percentage were performed in only six patients, but were in aggregate 100 % sensitive to detect infarcts if the changes were sustained over a 24-hour period. Total power specifically detected 100 % of the silent infarcts seen on CT; compressed spectral array on the other hand, was 67 % sensitive for ischemia. Four ischemic events had qEEG changes prior to the development of clinical deficits and five ischemic events had changes in total power that predicted silent infarcts when the clinical exam did not. There were only two false positives reported during 62 days of monitoring.

qEEG and xenon CT measures of CBF were used simultaneously in 32 awake SAH patients (Hunt-Hess 1–3) to detect vasospasm, which was confirmed by angiography or TCD [8]. The relative alpha percentage, defined uniquely as 6–14Hz frequency power divided by the total power (1–20Hz), was calculated over 2 minute windows to generate a histogram periodically throughout the day. The variability of this histogram was then qualitatively scored from 1 to 4. Decreased variability trended toward decreased CBF. Overall, 19 of 32 patients developed vasospasm, all of whom had decreased variability of the relative alpha percentage. Seven patients without vasospasm had decreased variability, largely due to stroke or increased ICP. Changes in variability occurred in 4 or more of the 6 electrode channels monitored, suggesting this measure reflects a more global change. Importantly, decreased variability occurred a mean of 2.9 days prior to the development of TCD or angiographic vasospasm.

Using a standard electrode array divided into vascular distributions (anterior circulation and posterior circulation), 34 comatose SAH patients (Hunt-Hess 4–5) were evaluated to detect delayed cerebral ischemia; angiography and TCD data were not required to confirm the clinical or radiological diagnosis [9]. Rather than utilizing continuously generated data, 10 sixty-second clips were obtained both at baseline and between days 4 and 6. The strength of this particular analysis is that each clip was obtained after stimulation – thereby eliminating the variability associated with state changes or sleep. Total power and power in each frequency band were measured in addition to relative alpha, relative delta, the alpha/delta ratio, and the alpha-beta/delta ratio. The coherence of each hemisphere was calculated for both alpha and delta frequencies and a total average frequency was also determined. Different cut-offs were used to determine whether a change was significant: 10, 20, or 50 % changes from baseline. In predicting the 9 of 34 patients with delayed cerebral ischemia, the post-stimulation alpha/delta ratio correlated best when anterior and posterior regions were considered together, followed by relative delta, alpha-beta/delta ratio, and relative alpha (**Fig. 2**). For region specific parameters, only the relative delta percentage and the alpha/delta ratio correlated with delayed cerebral ischemia and only in the anterior derivations; however, only one patient had a posterior circulation event. When six minutes of EEG were used, a 10 % change in the alpha/delta ratio was 100 % sensitive and 76 % specific for delayed cerebral ischemia. When just one minute was used, a 50 % or more change from baseline yielded a sensitivity of 89 % and specificity of 84 %. Overall, relative rather than absolute parameters appeared to be more sensitive to changes. Despite indications that hemispheric indices are predictive of clinical events in acute ischemic stroke, coherence performed only modestly well in this study, perhaps because of the background changes associated with SAH in general. Similarly, although spectral edge frequencies correlate with ischemia in acute ischemic stroke [28] and carotid endarterectomy [29] and mean frequency changes correlate with improvements in CBF [20], frequency measures were not predictive of delayed cerebral ischemia in poor-grade SAH, potentially because of lower overall frequencies at baseline. These parameters have not been adequately studied in better grade SAH, and may still hold some promise.

A recent study used a standard electrode array, excluding the posterior derivations to avoid the impact of the frequent (albeit normal) asymmetry of the posterior dominant rhythm on qEEG values [10]. Twelve patients with modified Fisher grades 3–4, corresponding to highest risk for vasospasm [43], were evaluated using the total power of the alpha frequency band (defined as 8–15Hz). Each 30 seconds, an alpha frequency value was calculated and averaged over 30 minutes. The standard deviation and the mean alpha power were then multiplied to create a 'composite alpha index'. Overall, 8 of 12 patients developed delayed cerebral ischemia. Three patients with delayed cerebral ischemia developed worsening trends in the composite alpha index more than 24 hours prior to neurodeterioration. Predictions of neurodeterioration made exclusively on clinical data were 40 % sensitive, whereas the addition of qEEG data increased this to 67 % with a specificity of 73 %.

XIX

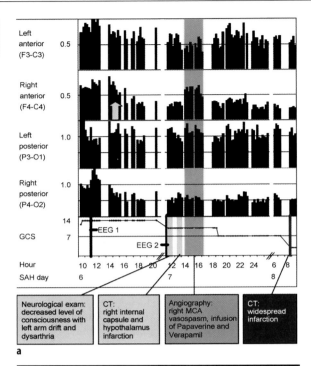

Neurological exam: decreased level of consciousness with left arm drift and dysarthria	CT: right internal capsule and hypothalamus infarction	Angiography: right MCA vasospasm, infusion of Papaverine and Verapamil	CT: widespread infarction

a

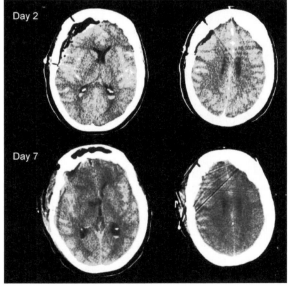

b

Fig. 2. Alpha/delta ratio (ADR) calculated every 15 min and Glasgow Coma Score (GCS), shown for days 6–8 of continuous EEG (cEEG) monitoring (**Fig. 2a**). A 57-year old woman admitted for acute subarachnoid hemorrhage (admission Hunt-Hess grade 4) from a right posterior communicating aneurysm. Admission angiography did not show vasospasm. The aneurysm was clipped on SAH day 2. No infarcts were seen on postoperative computed tomography (CT) scan (**Fig. 2b**). Postoperatively she had a GCS of 14. cEEG monitoring was performed from SAH days 3 to 8. The ADR progressively decreased after day 6, particularly in the right anterior region (blue arrow), to settle into a steady trough level later that night, reflecting loss of fast frequencies and increased slowing over the right hemisphere in the raw cEEG (**Fig. 2c**, EEG2 compared with EEG1). On SAH day 6, flow velocities in the right MCA were marginally elevated (144 cm/s), but the patient remained clinically stable with hypertensive, hypervolemic therapy (systolic blood pressure >180 mmHg). On day 7, the GCS dropped from 14 to 12 and a CT scan showed a right internal capsule and hypothalamic infarction (**Fig. 2b**, Day 7). Angiography demonstrated severe distal right MCA and left vertebral artery spasm; however, due to the marked tortuosity of the parent vessels and the location of vasospasm, a decision was made not to perform angioplasty, but to infuse verapamil and papaverine. This resulted in a marked, but transient increase of the right anterior and posterior alpha/delta ratios (blue shaded area). Later that day the patient further deteriorated clinically to a GCS of 7, with a new onset left hemiparesis, and died on SAH day 9 from widespread infarction due to vasospasm. From [9] with permission

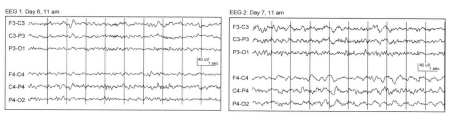

Fig. 2c

Future Directions

Both the relative alpha variability and the composite alpha indices were derived in an effort to generate a discrete trending value accessible to other members of the patient care team. Unfortunately, both measures require artifact detection based on visual inspection by electroencephalographers. While post-stimulation clips can be easily evaluated for artifact at the time of the stimulation, this may be labor intensive and does not provide a continuous measure. Future studies of ischemia detection should focus on discrete and easily interpretable values generated in real-time, accessible to the neurophysiologist, intensivists, and the nursing staff.

Based on qEEG data in ischemia, it appears that regional power values may be more specific to the nature and size of the underlying lesion and, therefore, correlate with later functional outcome; however, they may not be sensitive enough to use alone in ischemia detection [9]. Hemispheric power differences highlight acute ischemic changes, but correlate less well with the subtle, multifocal, and more gradual changes seen in SAH. qEEG frequency values (such as spectral edge frequencies) may be useful to detect changes in relatively healthy brain [29], but it is not clear that these are helpful in more widespread pathology such as SAH. Some values (such as global increases in theta range frequency) may have a relationship to the penumbra and, therefore, be useful in the pre-infarct stage of ischemia in good-grade SAH [36] but this has not been adequately studied. To develop a rational approach to the detection of ischemia, a combination of regional, hemispheric, and total measures of both power and frequency may be needed.

An attempt should be made to integrate qEEG parameters into the multimodal monitoring infrastructure available in some ICUs. Electrophysiological changes should be interpreted in the context of blood pressure, systemic oxygenation, intracranial or cerebral perfusion pressures, cerebral measures of oxygen tension, or microdialysis. More recently, intra-cortical electroencephalography has provided valuable information on both seizure and ischemia detection: In a series of 5 patients who had intra-cortical electroencephalography, a change in the alpha/delta ratio of 25 % sustained over 4 hours was the most accurate parameter in detecting vasospasm between 1 and 3 days prior to confirmation with angiography [48]. Subdural electrodes have detected peri-infarct depolarizations and cortical spreading depression [16], phenomena invisible to scalp EEG but that might play a role in delayed cerebral ischemia after SAH. Interestingly, using subdural electrodes these researchers were also able to detect an abnormal hemodynamic response when analyzing the cortical spreading depression signal in relation to ischemia from vasospasm [16].

Ultimately, ischemia detection requires real-world validation. Software currently exists that allows real-time quantification of qEEG parameters. The numerical values generated by qEEG can be used to set threshold alarms such that when a specified value is reached for more than a specified period of time (e.g., to avoid confusion with artifact), an alert is sent to a treating member of the ICU team. This should be done in the context of a prospective and randomized trial that compares integrating qEEG into a novel algorithm versus best clinical practice, for example comparing different triggers to obtain established confirmatory assessments of vasospasm-associated delayed cerebral ischemia, such as CT angiography, CT perfusion, or conventional angiography.

Conclusion

EEG is a very promising tool for monitoring brain function in real-time in the ICU. There are characteristic changes that occur on EEG in response to brain ischemia, correlating with CBF and brain metabolism. Although raw EEG evaluations are time consuming, quantification of EEG features in real-time has been incorporated into many of the standard EEG software packages. Some of these quantitative parameters have also been found to correspond to physiologic changes associated with ischemia. Sensitive techniques are needed to detect cerebral ischemia, for example, in vasospasm-associated delayed cerebral ischemia after SAH. Early evidence suggests that qEEG may be sensitive enough to allow pre-clinical detection of delayed cerebral ischemia from vasospasm. This approach may be utilized to widen the window of opportunity in order to prevent permanent neuronal damage in a variety of clinic scenarios.

References

1. Friedman D, Claassen J, Hirsch LJ (2009) Continuous electroencephalogram monitoring in the intensive care unit. Anesth Analg 109: 506–523
2. Hossmann KA (1994) Viability thresholds and the penumbra of focal ischemia. Ann Neurol 36: 557–565
3. Sharbrough FW, Messick JM Jr, Sundt TM Jr (1973) Correlation of continuous electroencephalograms with cerebral blood flow measurements during carotid endarterectomy. Stroke 4: 674–683
4. Jordan KG (2004) Emergency EEG and continuous EEG monitoring in acute ischemic stroke. J Clin Neurophysiol 21: 341–352
5. Frontera JA, Fernandez A, Schmidt JM, et al (2009) Defining vasospasm after subarachnoid hemorrhage: what is the most clinically relevant definition? Stroke 40: 1963–1968
6. Schmidt JM, Wartenberg KE, Fernandez A, et al (2008) Frequency and clinical impact of asymptomatic cerebral infarction due to vasospasm after subarachnoid hemorrhage. J Neurosurg 109: 1052–1059
7. Labar DR, Fisch BJ, Pedley TA, Fink ME, Solomon RA (1991) Quantitative EEG monitoring for patients with subarachnoid hemorrhage. Electroencephalogr Clin Neurophysiol 78: 325–332
8. Vespa PM, Nuwer MR, Juhasz C, et al (1997) Early detection of vasospasm after acute subarachnoid hemorrhage using continuous EEG ICU monitoring. Electroencephalogr Clin Neurophysiol 103: 607–615
9. Claassen J, Hirsch LJ, Kreiter KT, et al (2004) Quantitative continuous EEG for detecting

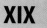

delayed cerebral ischemia in patients with poor-grade subarachnoid hemorrhage. Clin Neurophysiol 115: 2699–2710

10. Rathakrishnan R, Gotman J, Dubeau F, Angle M (2011) Using continuous electroencephalography in the management of delayed cerebral ischemia following subarachnoid hemorrhage. Neurocrit Care 14: 152–161

11. Amzica F, Lopes da Silva FH (2010) Cellular substrates of brain rhythms. In: Niedermeyer E, Schomer DL, Lopes da Silva FH (eds) Niedermeyer's Electroencephalography : Basic Principles, Clinical Applications, and Related Fields. 6th edn. Wolters Kluwer/Lippincott Williams & Wilkins Health, Philadelphia, pp 33–64

12. Evans BM (1976) Patterns of arousal in comatose patients. J Neurol Neurosurg Psychiatry 39: 392–402

13. Schneider AL, Jordan KG (2005) Regional attenuation without delta (RAWOD): a distinctive EEG pattern that can aid in the diagnosis and management of severe acute ischemic stroke. Am J Electroneurodiagnostic Technol 45: 102–117

14. Nagata K, Tagawa K, Hiroi S, Shishido F, Uemura K (1989) Electroencephalographic correlates of blood flow and oxygen metabolism provided by positron emission tomography in patients with cerebral infarction. Electroencephalogr Clin Neurophysiol 72: 16–30

15. Powers WJ (1991) Cerebral hemodynamics in ischemic cerebrovascular disease. Ann Neurol 29: 231–240

16. Dreier JP, Major S, Manning A, et al (2009) Cortical spreading ischaemia is a novel process involved in ischaemic damage in patients with aneurysmal subarachnoid haemorrhage. Brain 132: 1866–1881

17. Kohno K, Hoehn-Berlage M, Mies G, Back T, Hossmann KA (1995) Relationship between diffusion-weighted MR images, cerebral blood flow, and energy state in experimental brain infarction. Magn Reson Imaging 13: 73–80

18. Finnigan SP, Rose SE, Chalk JB (2006) Rapid EEG changes indicate reperfusion after tissue plasminogen activator injection in acute ischaemic stroke. Clin Neurophysiol 117: 2338–2339

19. de Vos CC, van Maarseveen SM, Brouwers PJ, van Putten MJ (2008) Continuous EEG monitoring during thrombolysis in acute hemispheric stroke patients using the brain symmetry index. J Clin Neurophysiol 25: 77–82

20. Wood JH, Polyzoidis KS, Epstein CM, Gibby GL, Tindall GT (1984) Quantitative EEG alterations after isovolemic-hemodilutional augmentation of cerebral perfusion in stroke patients. Neurology 34: 764–768

21. Bricolo A, Turazzi S, Faccioli F (1979) Combined clinical and EEG examinations for assessment of severity of acute head injuries. Acta Neurochir Suppl (Wien) 28: 35–39

22. Bergamasco B, Bergamini L, Doriguzzi T, Sacerdote I (1968) The sleep cycle in coma: prognostic value. Electroencephalogr Clin Neurophysiol 25: 87

23. Burghaus L, Hilker R, Dohmen C, et al (2007) Early electroencephalography in acute ischemic stroke: prediction of a malignant course? Clin Neurol Neurosurg 109: 45–49

24. Cillessen JP, van Huffelen AC, Kappelle LJ, Algra A, van Gijn J (1994) Electroencephalography improves the prediction of functional outcome in the acute stage of cerebral ischemia. Stroke 25: 1968–1972

25. Pohlmann-Eden B, Hoch DB, Cochius JI, Chiappa KH (1996) Periodic lateralized epileptiform discharges--a critical review. J Clin Neurophysiol 13: 519–530

26. Scheuer ML, Wilson SB (2004) Data analysis for continuous EEG monitoring in the ICU: seeing the forest and the trees. J Clin Neurophysiol 21: 353–378

27. Lopes da Silva FH (2010) EEG analysis: theory and practice. In: Niedermeyer E, Schomer DL, Lopes da Silva FH (eds) Niedermeyer's Electroencephalography : Basic Principles, Clinical Applications, and Related Fields. 6th edn. Wolters Kluwer/Lippincott Williams & Wilkins Health, Philadelphia, pp 1147–1178

28. Tolonen U, Sulg IA (1981) Comparison of quantitative EEG parameters from four different analysis techniques in evaluation of relationships between EEG and CBF in brain infarction. Electroencephalogr Clin Neurophysiol 51: 177–185

29. Laman DM, Wieneke GH, van Duijn H, Veldhuizen RJ, van Huffelen AC (2005) QEEG changes during carotid clamping in carotid endarterectomy: spectral edge frequency parameters and relative band power parameters. J Clin Neurophysiol 22: 244–252

30. Diedler J, Sykora M, Bast T, et al (2009) Quantitative EEG correlates of low cerebral perfusion in severe stroke. Neurocrit Care 11: 210–216

31. van Putten MJ, Tavy DL (2004) Continuous quantitative EEG monitoring in hemispheric stroke patients using the brain symmetry index. Stroke 35: 2489–2492

32. Sheorajpanday RV, Nagels G, Weeren AJ, van Putten MJ, De Deyn PP (2009) Reproducibility and clinical relevance of quantitative EEG parameters in cerebral ischemia: a basic approach. Clin Neurophysiol 120: 845–855

33. Sheorajpanday RV, Nagels G, Weeren AJ, De Deyn PP (2011) Quantitative EEG in ischemic stroke: correlation with infarct volume and functional status in posterior circulation and lacunar syndromes. Clin Neurophysiol 122: 884–890

34. Finnigan SP, Walsh M, Rose SE, Chalk JB (2007) Quantitative EEG indices of sub-acute ischaemic stroke correlate with clinical outcomes. Clin Neurophysiol 118: 2525–2532

35. Finnigan SP, Rose SE, Walsh M, et al (2004) Correlation of quantitative EEG in acute ischemic stroke with 30-day NIHSS score: comparison with diffusion and perfusion MRI. Stroke 35: 899–903

36. Sheorajpanday RV, Nagels G, Weeren AJ, De Surgeloose D, De Deyn PP (2010) Additional value of quantitative EEG in acute anterior circulation syndrome of presumed ischemic origin. Clin Neurophysiol 121: 1719–1725

37. Nuwer MR, Jordan SE, Ahn SS (1987) Evaluation of stroke using EEG frequency analysis and topographic mapping. Neurology 37: 1153–1159

38. Murri L, Gori S, Massetani R, Bonanni E, Marcella F, Milani S (1998) Evaluation of acute ischemic stroke using quantitative EEG: a comparison with conventional EEG and CT scan. Neurophysiol Clin 28: 249–257

39. Sheorajpanday RV, Nagels G, Weeren AJ, van Putten MJ, De Deyn PP (2011) Quantitative EEG in ischemic stroke: correlation with functional status after 6 months. Clin Neurophysiol 122: 874–883

40. Oddo M, Carrera E, Claassen J, Mayer SA, Hirsch LJ (2009) Continuous electroencephalography in the medical intensive care unit. Crit Care Med 37: 2051–2056

41. Taccone FS, Su F, Pierrakos C, et al (2010) Cerebral microcirculation is impaired during sepsis: an experimental study. Crit Care 14: R140

42. Washington CW, Zipfel GJ (2011) Detection and monitoring of vasospasm and delayed cerebral ischemia: A review and assessment of the literature. Neurocrit Care 15: 312–317

43. Claassen J, Bernardini GL, Kreiter K, et al (2001) Effect of cisternal and ventricular blood on risk of delayed cerebral ischemia after subarachnoid hemorrhage: the Fisher scale revisited. Stroke 32: 2012–2020

44. Carrera E, Schmidt JM, Oddo M, et al (2009) Transcranial Doppler for predicting delayed cerebral ischemia after subarachnoid hemorrhage. Neurosurgery 65: 316–323

45. Claassen J, Hirsch LJ, Frontera JA, et al (2006) Prognostic significance of continuous EEG monitoring in patients with poor-grade subarachnoid hemorrhage. Neurocrit Care 4: 103–112

46. Tettenborn B, Niedermeyer E, Schomer DL (2011) Cerebrovascular diseases and EEG. In: Niedermeyer E, Schomer DL, Lopes da Silva FH (eds) Niedermeyer's Electroencephalography : Basic Principles, Clinical Applications, and Related Fields. 6th edn. Wolters Kluwer/Lippincott Williams & Wilkins Health, Philadelphia, pp 351–374

47. Rivierez M, Landau-Ferey J, Grob R, Grosskopf D, Philippon J (1991) Value of electroencephalogram in prediction and diagnosis of vasospasm after intracranial aneurysm rupture. Acta Neurochir (Wien) 110: 17–23

48. Stuart RM, Waziri A, Weintraub D, et al (2010) Intracortical EEG for the detection of vasospasm in patients with poor-grade subarachnoid hemorrhage. Neurocrit Care 13: 355–358

Transitory Vegetative State/unresponsive Wakefulness Syndrome: Does it Exist?

M.-A. Bruno, D. Ledoux, and S. Laureys

Introduction

Since the invention of the artificial respirator in the 1950s, many patients who previously did not survive their severe traumatic or hypoxic-ischemic brain damage and coma can now be artificially ventilated and their cardiac circulation sustained. This has led to the redefinition of death based on neurological criteria (i.e., brain death) and the notion of therapeutic obstinacy (i.e., continuation or start of treatment in the absence of any hope of recovery). It has also led to an increasing number of patients who have awakened from coma (i.e., showed eye opening, incompatible with the diagnosis of coma) yet remain unresponsive (i.e., showed reflex movements with no sign of voluntary interaction with the environment – also observed in coma). In Europe, this clinical syndrome was initially termed "apallic syndrome" [1] or "coma vigil" [2] but is currently known in the medical community as "vegetative state (VS)", a term first coined by Jennett and Plum in 1972 [3]. The name 'vegetative state' was chosen in reference to the preserved vegetative nervous functioning – meaning that these patients have (variably) preserved sleep-wake cycles, respiration, digestion or thermoregulation. The term 'persistent' was added to denote that the condition remained for at least one month after insult. In 1994, a Multi-Society Task Force on Persistent Vegetative State defined the temporal criteria for irreversibility (i.e., more than one year for traumatic and three months for non-traumatic (anoxic) etiology) and introduced the notion of "permanent vegetative state" [4]. Over the last three decades, it appears, however, that some healthcare workers, members of the media and lay public continue to feel some unease regarding the unintended denigrating 'vegetable-like' connotation seemingly intrinsic to the term 'vegetative state' [5–7], resulting in a number of papers reiterating the intellectual justification of the origins and choice of the term [8]. Recently the European Task Force on Disorders of Consciousness has proposed a more descriptive and neutral term for VS: "Unresponsive Wakefulness Syndrome" (UWS) [9]. 'Unresponsive' was chosen to illustrate that these patients only show reflex movements without response to commands; 'wakefulness' refers to the presence of eye opening – spontaneous or stimulation induced – never observed in coma; 'syndrome' stresses that we are assessing a series of clinical signs. In contrast to coma, which is an acute condition lasting no more than a few days or weeks, VS/UWS is often considered as a chronic condition and is generally viewed as a poor clinical state with limited recovery potential. However, VS/UWS is a disorder of consciousness that can be acute and reversible. The aim of the present chapter is to provide a description of VS/UWS patients at the acute stage by analyzing data collected in intensive care

J.-L. Vincent (ed.), *Annual Update in Intensive Care and Emergency Medicine 2012*
DOI 10.1007/978-3-642-25716-2 © Springer-Verlag Berlin Heidelberg 2012

units (ICUs) at Liège University Hospital, Belgium, and to examine the available literature concerning the prognosis of these patients. We will show that VS/UWS is not only a chronic or even permanent condition but may also be encountered in the acute or subacute setting as a transitional state on the way to recovery.

Prognosis for Recovery and Survival: A Five-year Follow-Up

A patient's recovery can be considered in three dimensions: Survival/mortality, recovery of consciousness, and functional recovery. The mortality of patients with disorders of consciousness is conditioned by several factors: i) a Glasgow motor score less than or equal to 2 [10]; ii) an absence of pupillary and/or corneal reflexes; iii) status epilepticus; iv) a flat or an isoelectric electroencephalogram (EEG); v) absence of somatosensory evoked potentials (N20); and vi) serum neuron-specific enolase (NSE) concentration of > 33 µg/l [11]. Medical complications such as hypotension, hyperthermia, hyperglycemia, infection or prolonged mechanical ventilation also decrease the chances of survival [11–13]. The most common causes of mortality for patients with VS/UWS in the ICU and rehabilitation center are urinary and pulmonary infections, heart failure and cachexia, sudden death and organ failure [4, 14]. Once a patient's medical condition is stabilized, physicians need to estimate the chances of recovery of consciousness and/or of useful function. Recovery of consciousness is reflected by the presence of clear-cut signs of self- or environmental awareness (fluctuating voluntary responses to an oral and/or a written request, visual tracking, context-specific emotional responses, etc., – i.e., criteria of the minimally conscious state [MCS]) [15]. Functional recovery is characterized by the reappearance of functional communication and/or a functional use of objects and an ability to learn and perform new tasks as well as to participate in personal, professional or recreational activities (emergence from MCS) [15, 16]. Sometimes, restoration of consciousness can occur without functional recovery. VS/UWS patients may recover consciousness and evolve into a MCS and then may present functional recovery reflecting emergence from the MCS with or without physical, psychological or neuropsychological disorders (**Fig. 1**).

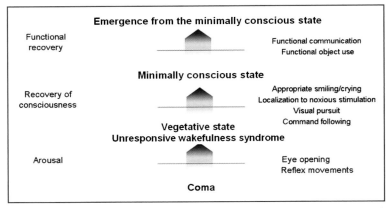

Fig. 1. Behaviorally progressive transitions from coma, to vegetative state/unresponsive wakefulness syndrome, to minimally conscious state, to emergence from the minimally conscious state

Table 1. Hospital outcome assessed separately for traumatic (TBI) and non-traumatic (NTBI) brain injuries

Total admissions		5908	Traumatic	Non-traumatic	p-value
Impaired consciousness on day 1		631 (11 %)	203 (32 %)	428 (68 %)	
Vegetative state during stay in ICU (sustained or transient)		356 (56 %)	129 (36 %)	227 (64 %)	
ICU outcome	Died in ICU	99 (28 %)	16 (12 % of TBI)	83 (37 % of NTBI)	< 0.001
	Remained VS on ICU discharge	60 (17 %)	23 (18 % of TBI)	37 (16 % of NTBI)	0.7694
	Conscious on ICU discharge	195 (55 %)	90 (70 % of TBI)	105 (47 % of NTBI)	< 0.0001
	Missing data	2 (0.6 %)			

XIX

Over a 5-year period, we prospectively collected and analyzed data on all consecutive admissions in 26 ICU beds at the University Hospital of Liège. During that period of time, the best Glasgow Coma Score (GCS) [10] was recorded daily. Patients with a GCS < 15 during the first 24-hours of ICU stay were included for further analysis. Among these patients, VS/UWS was defined according to the Multi Society Task Force criteria: Eye opening (spontaneously or induced by intense auditory or noxious stimulation); no verbal response or incomprehensible sounds or groaning or not assessable; ventilated and no motor response or stereotyped response or normal flexion in response to painful stimulus [4]. We looked at ICU outcome separating traumatic from non-traumatic etiologies. Over the 5-year period, 5908 patients were admitted to the ICU. Among them, 11 % (n = 631) suffered from impaired consciousness on admission. During their ICU stay, 56 % (n = 356) of the studied patients with impaired consciousness were diagnosed as VS/UWS of whom 129 (36 %) were of traumatic etiology and 227 (64 %) were non-traumatic. Out of the 356 VS/UWS patients, 99 (28 %) patients died in the ICU, 60 (17 %) remained VS/UWS on ICU discharge and 195 (55 %) patients left the ICU having recovered consciousness or minimal consciousness (2 missing data [1 %]). On ICU discharge, 90 (70 %) of the trauma patients as compared to 105 (47 %) non-trauma patients recovered some level of consciousness (p< 0.001). Median ICU stay was 10 days – IQR 5–18 days. Data were analyzed using Stata 10.0 (Stata, 2007) (**Table 1**). Our study is the first to assess the outcome during ICU hospitalization. These data were thus compared to the available literature on prognosis of traumatic (TBI) and non-traumatic brain injury VS/UWS patients.

Mortality Rates

Among 356 VS/UWS patients, 28 % (n = 99) died in the ICU. Sixteen patients had TBI (12 % of the TBI group) and 83 patients had non-TBI (37 % of the non-trauma group). The mortality rate on ICU discharge was higher in the non-trauma group than in the TBI group. Previous studies, showing rates ranging from 10 % to 20 % in TBI VS/UWS patients 1 year post-onset, are in line with our results [17, 18]. However, others showed rates ranging from 30 to 50 % [16, 19–21]. In 1980, Bricolo and colleagues studied the prognosis of 135 patients who

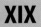

Table 2. Mortality and recovery rates of traumatic vegetative state/unresponsive wakefulness syndrome (VS/UWS) patients

First author [ref]	n	Delay post-onset	Follow-up	Results
Hygashi [14, 25]	38	3 months	1–5 years	3-year cumulative mortality rate: 55 %, 5-year: 66 %
Bricolo [21]	135	2 weeks	1 year	30 % dead, 8 % VS/UWS, 31 % severe disability, 18 % moderate recovery, 13 % good recovery
Braakman [20]	140	1 month	1 year	51 % dead, 11 % VS/UWS, 26 % severe disability, 10 % moderate disability or recovery, 2 % unknown. Mortality rate: 30 % of after 3 months, 40 % after 6 months. Duration of unconsciousness was negatively correlated with the functional recovery.
Sazbon [32]	55	1 month	1 year	51 % recovery of consciousness
Sazbon [12]	134	1 month	1 year	54 % recovery of consciousness, 46 % VS/UWS (69 % of them did not survive the 1st year)
Sazbon [19]	134	1 month	1 year	3, 6 and 12 month cumulative mortality rate: 7 %, 19 % and 32 %. 5-year cumulative mortality rate: 68 %
Multi Society Task Force [16]	434	1 month	1 year	33 % dead, 15 % VS/UWS, 52 % recovery of consciousness: 28 % severe disability, 17 % moderate disability, 7 % good recovery.
Danze [17]	522	1 month	1 year	19 % dead, 20 % VS/UWS, 61 % recovery of consciousness: 47 % severe disability, 12 % moderate disability, 2 % good recovery.
Dubroja [31]	19	1 month	2 years	68 % recovery of consciousness (58 % after 1 year, 5 % after 2 years): 58 % moderate disability, 42 % severe disability.
Giacino [18]	30	11±5 weeks	1 year	10 % dead, 60 % extremely severe disability or VS/UWS, 30 % moderate to severe disability, 0 % partial or good recovery.
Estraneo [23]	18	11 months	28 ± 12 months	39 % dead, 17 % VS/UWS, 44 % recovery of consciousness and functional recovery (17 % MCS).

stayed in a "non-responsive state" for at least 2 weeks post-onset and showed a mortality rate of 30 % after 1 year [21]. Braakman and colleagues followed 140 VS/UWS patients and observed a mortality rate of 51 % [20]. Finally, the Multi Society Task Force on Persistent VS studied 434 patients and reported a mortality rate of 33 % 1 year post-TBI [16] (**Table 2**).

Regarding the mortality rate of non-trauma VS/UWS patients, we reported a rate of 37 % whereas previous studies showed rates ranging from 50 to 70 %. Whereas in 1978, Levy and colleagues reported a mortality rate of more than 70 % 1 year post-onset (n = 25) [22], the Multi Society Task Force [16], Estraneo and colleagues [23] and Sazbon and colleagues [24] showed mortality rates of 53 % (n = 169), 43 % (n = 32) and 46 % (n = 100), respectively (**Table 3**). Such differences in results could be explained by the limited number of patients included

Table 3. Mortality and recovery rates of non-traumatic vegetative state/unresponsive wakefulness syndrome (VS/UWS) patients

First author [ref]	N	Etiology	Delay since onset	Follow-up	Results
Levy [22]	25	Non-traumatic	1 month	1 year	72 % dead, 8 % intelligible words but no command following, 12 % visual pursuit or localization to sounds. None of the patients can live independently
Sazbon [32]	118	Non-traumatic	1 month	1 year	21 % recovery of consciousness
Sazbon [24]	100	Anoxic	1 month	1–5 years	1 year post-onset: 46 % dead, 20 % conscious (13 % after 3 months, 20 % after 6 months, 17 % tetraparetic, 19 % cognitive disability, 15 % dysphasic and 13 % psychological disability), 33 % unconscious, 1 % unknown. 5 years post-onset: 68 % dead, 20 % conscious, 7 % unconscious, 5 % unknown. Cumulative mortality rate: 15 % at 3 months, 31 % at 6 months. After 5 months of VS/UWS, no recovery of consciousness.
Multi Society Task Force [16]	169	Non-traumatic	1 month	1 year	53 % dead, 32 % VS/UWS, 11 % severe disability, 3 % moderate disability, 1 % good recovery.
Giacino [18]	34	Non-traumatic	11 ± 5 weeks	1 year	7 % dead, 87 % extremely severe disability or VS, 6 % severe to moderate disability, 0 % partial or total recovery
Estraneo [23]	50	Hemorragic Anoxic	12 months 9 months	26 ± 13 months 23 ± 12 months	4 % dead, 50 % VS, 6 % recovery of consciousness (6 % MCS). 43 % dead, 36 %VS/UWS, 20 % recovery of consciousness and functional recovery (7 % MCS).

in these studies [22, 23], the inclusion criteria (delay post-onset, ranging from 1 month [22] to 1 year [23]) and the time elapsed to follow-up (ICU discharge or 1 year follow-up). Finally, as showed by our results and previous studies, non-trauma patients had higher mortality rates than TBI patients [12, 14, 16, 23–26] (**Tables 2** and **3**).

VS/UWS as a Chronic Condition

Of our 356 VS/UWS patients studied, 60 (17 %) remained VS/UWS at ICU discharge; 23 had TBI (18 % of the TBI group) and 37 were non-trauma (16 % of the non-trauma group). Similar results are available from previous studies. Bricolo and colleagues studied 134 TBI VS/UWS patients and showed that 8 % (n= 11) remained in a "non-responsive state" 1 year post-onset [21]. Similarly, Braakman and colleagues followed 140 VS/UWS patients and observed that 11 % remained unconscious after 1 year [20]. The Multi Society Task Force [16] and Danze and collaborators [17] showed that 15 % (n = 434) and 20 % (n = 522) of their studied VS/UWS patients remained unconscious 1 year post-TBI, respectively. Estraneo and colleagues, who followed, over a period of 2 years, 18 TBI VS/UWS patients who had been in that state for 11 months, noted that 17 % of their studied population remained in a VS/UWS [23] (**Table 2**). Concerning prolonged VS/UWS in non-trauma patients, our results are in contradiction to previous studies. We observed that only 16 % of our patients were still unconscious on ICU discharge, whereas Sazbon and colleagues observed that, 1 year post-onset, 33 % of their patients were unconscious [24]. Similar results were reported by the Multi Society Task Force (34 % of unconscious patients) (**Table 3**).

The question of long-term survival in VS/UWS has been studied by several authors. Usually, once the first year is survived, many VS/UWS patients become quite stable. A review of the available literature showed that mean survival after acute brain damage ranged from 2 to more than 10 years [16, 26]. Walshe and Leonard observed 21 institutionalized VS/UWS patients and showed mean survival rates of 3.5 to 7 years, with some surviving 16 years [27]. Occasional reports appear of exceptionally long survivals, e.g., 18 years [28], 37 years [29] and 41 years [30]. Predictions of long-term survival are of most interest in those who have already survived a year or more in a VS/UWS state.

Recovery of Consciousness

Recovery of consciousness and functional recovery in VS/UWS patients could be considered as a single category (as in our study). We then use the general term "recovery". We showed that 55 % of our 356 VS/UWS patients recovered consciousness by ICU discharge based on the CGS assessment (VS/UWS patients progressing to or emerging from a MCS; i.e., GCS subscores showing spontaneous or stimulation-induced eye opening E ≥ 1; presence of verbalization V ≥ 3; and presence of localization of pain M ≥ 5). Ninety patients were TBI (70 % of the TBI group) and 105 patients were non-TBI (47 % of the non-trauma group). For the TBI patients, our study agrees with the literature showing recovery rates ranging from 40 to 60 %. Results obtained by Braakman and colleagues (n = 140) [20] and Estraneo and colleagues (n = 18) [23] showed recovery rates of 36 % and 44 %, respectively. Sazbon and colleagues showed a rate of 54 % 1 year post-TBI (n = 134) [12], the Multi Society Task Force a rate of 52 % (n = 434) [16], Giacino and Kalmar of 56 % (n = 30) [18], Dubroja and colleagues of 58 % after 2 years (n = 19) [31] and Bricolo and colleagues observed a recovery rate of 62 % 1 year post-onset (n = 135) [21]. Our results on non-trauma VS/UWS patients showed higher recovery rates compared to previous studies (47 % versus rates ranging from 0 to 21 % 1 year post-onset) [16, 22, 24, 32]. The variability observed between our results and the literature could be explained by the inclusion criteria (**Table 2** and 3).

Functional Recovery

Previous results on TBI VS/UWS patients (n = 135) showed, 1 year post-TBI, severe disability in 31 %, moderate recovery in 18 %, and good recovery in 13 % [21]. This study is line with that by Braakman and colleagues showing, 1 year post-onset, 26 % severe disability and 10 % moderate or complete recovery (patients able to live independently) (n = 140). In 1994, out of 522 patients, Danze and colleagues reported that 14 % of their patients recovered cognitive and motor capacities allowing them to live independently [17]. Giacino and Kalmar [18] noted a recovery rate of 30 % (n = 30) and the Multi Society Task Force found that 28 % of their studied patients presented severe deficits, 17 % moderate deficits and 7 % had good recovery 1 year post-onset (n = 434) [16].

Regarding non-trauma VS/UWS patients, out of their 25 studied patients, Levy and colleagues [22] observed that no patient recovered a functional state permitting independent living. The Multi-Society Task Force showed that out of the 169 studied patients, 3 % presented moderate deficits, and only 1 % showed a good recovery [16]. Also note that late recovery (more than a year post-injury) is always possible, occurring more frequently for traumatic patients [14, 16, 33–35].

The results of these studies are difficult to compare because of the different criteria and/or different scales used to assess the functional recovery of patients. Indeed, some studies estimated recovery using the Glasgow Outcome Scale (GOS) [36] whereas others used the Disability Rating Scale (DRS) [37]. The GOS includes five categories: A score of 5 corresponds to a good recovery (independent daily life with or without neurological deficit), a score of 4 to 5 is given to patients with moderate disability (independent daily life with moderate neurological and/or intellectual deficit), a score of 3 corresponds to severe disability (conscious patient but totally dependent in daily living activities), a score of 2 characterizes VS/UWS patients and finally a score of 1 is assigned to dead patients. The DRS assesses the level of functioning of patients by scoring their level of ability. A total score of 30 is assigned to dead patients, a score between 25 and 29 corresponds to patients who are "extremely vegetative", 22–24 for VS/UWS patients, 17–21 characterizes patients with extreme severe deficits, 12–16 characterizes patients with severe deficits, 7–11 moderate to severe deficits, 4–6 moderate deficits, 2–3 partial or light deficits, and finally a score of 0 is given to patients with no deficit. Note that for these two scales, patients with an MCS and patients who have emerged from MCS are classified in the same category (total score of 3 at the GOS, total score between 17 and 21 at the DRS). This obviously raises many problems in the quantification, interpretation and generalization of functional recovery rate. Although these results are difficult to generalize, we can conclude that the rate of functional recovery of TBI VS/UWS patients ranges from 10 to 30 % and that the proportion of patients who live independently is very limited ranging from 0 to 14 %. Note also that functional recovery occurs more frequently in TBI patients compared to patients with non-TBI.

Conclusion

Regarding the negative connotation inherent in the term 'vegetative state' and its possible effect on vulnerable patients awakening from coma, who sometimes never recover any voluntary responsiveness but may (probably more often than initially believed) recover minimal signs of consciousness, the European Task Force on Disorders of Consciousness has passed a proposal to change the name to "Unresponsive Wakefulness Syndrome" or UWS. Physicians can now use this neutral descriptive term to refer to patients who, as the name indicates, show a number of clinical signs (hence the use of 'syndrome') of unresponsiveness (meaning they fail to show non-reflex behavior or command following) in the presence of wakefulness (meaning they open their eyes spontaneously or upon stimulation). Our study showed that acute VS/UWS is far from being a rare clinical entity in the ICU. The prognosis of patients who are or transit through an acute VS/UWS depends greatly on the nature of the brain damage (with higher rates of recovery in patients with traumatic as compared to non-traumatic etiologies). Reliable prognostication in patients with an altered state of consciousness is a fundamental aspect of care, from the ICU to the long-term life institution. Surgical, medical or ethical decisions will depend on this information. Although scientific advances allow a better understanding of the mortality rates and the degree of recovery of VS/UWS patients, great caution should be taken concerning ethical decisions by medical staff and families because of the heterogeneity of the results obtained in the literature. Studies must be undertaken to better characterize the functional recovery of patients who have emerged from an MCS and quantify the cognitive impairment with specific neuropsychological testing. The challenge is now to identify paraclinical prognostic markers for these devastating neurological conditions.

Acknowledgements: This research was funded by the Belgian National Funds for Scientific Research (FNRS), the European Commission (Mindbridge, DISCOS, Marie-Curie Actions, DECODER & COST), the James McDonnell Foundation, the Mind Science Foundation, the French Speaking Community Concerted Research Action (ARC-06/11 – 340), the Fondation Médicale Reine Elisabeth and the University of Liège.

References

1. Kretschmer E (1940) Das apallische Syndrom. Z ges Neurol Psychiat 169: 576 – 579
2. Calvet J, Coll J (1959) Meningitis of sinusoid origin with the form of coma vigil. Rev Otoneuroophtalmol 31: 443 – 445
3. Jennett B, Plum F (1972) Persistent vegetative state after brain damage. A syndrome in search of a name. Lancet 1: 734 – 737
4. The Multi-Society Task Force on PVS (1994) Medical aspects of the persistent vegetative state (1). N Engl J Med 330: 1499 – 1508
5. Shewmon DA (2004) A critical analysis of conceptual domains of the vegetative state: sorting fact from fancy. NeuroRehabilitation 19: 343 – 347
6. Kotchoubey B (2005) Apallic syndrome is not apallic: Is vegetative state vegetative? Neuropsychol Rehabil 15: 333 – 356
7. Schoenle PW, Witzke W (2004) How vegetative is the vegetative state? Preserved semantic processing in VS patients – evidence from N 400 event-related potentials. NeuroRehabilitation 19: 329 – 334
8. Jennett B (2005) Thirty years of the vegetative state: clinical, ethical and legal problems. Prog Brain Res 150: 537 – 543
9. Laureys S, Celesia G, Cohadon F, et al (2010) Unresponsive wakefulness syndrome: a new name for the vegetative state or apallic syndrome. BMC Med 8: 68
10. Teasdale G, Jennett B (1974) Assessment of coma and impaired consciousness. A practical scale. Lancet 2: 81 – 84
11. Wijdicks EF, Hijdra A, Young GB, et al (2006) Practice parameter: prediction of outcome in comatose survivors after cardiopulmonary resuscitation (an evidence-based review): report of the Quality Standards Subcommittee of the American Academy of Neurology. Neurology 67: 203 – 210
12. Sazbon L, Groswasser Z (1990) Outcome in 134 patients with prolonged posttraumatic unawareness. Part 1: Parameters determining late recovery of consciousness. J Neurosurg 72: 75 – 80

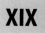

13. Jennett B, Teasdale G, Braakman R, et al (1976) Predicting outcome in individual patients after severe head injury. Lancet 1: 1031–1034
14. Higashi K, Sakata Y, Hatano M, et al (1977) Epidemiological studies on patients with a persistent vegetative state. J Neurol Neurosurg Psychiatry 40: 876–885
15. Giacino JT, Ashwal S, Childs N, et al (2002) The minimally conscious state: Definition and diagnostic criteria. Neurology 58: 349–353
16. The Multi-Society Task Force on PVS (1994) Medical aspects of the persistent vegetative state (2). N Engl J Med 330: 1572–1579
17. Danze F, Veys B, Lebrun T, et al (1994) [Prognostic factors of post-traumatic vegetative states: 522 cases]. Neurochirurgie 40: 348–357
18. Giacino J, Kalmar K (1997) The vegetative and minimally conscious state: a comparison of clinical features and functional outcome. J Head Trauma Rehabil 12: 36–51
19. Sazbon L, Groswasser Z (1991) Medical complications and mortality of patients in the postcomatose unawareness (PC-U) state. Acta Neurochir (Wien) 112: 110–112
20. Braakman R, Jennett WB, Minderhoud JM (1988) Prognosis of the posttraumatic vegetative state. Acta Neurochir 95: 49–52
21. Bricolo A, Turazzi S, Feriotti G (1980) Prolonged posttraumatic unconsciousness: therapeutic assets and liabilities. J Neurosurg 52: 625–634
22. Levy DE, Knill-Jones RP, Plum F (1978) The vegetative state and its prognosis following nontraumatic coma. Ann N Y Acad Sci 315: 293–306
23. Estraneo A, Moretta P, Loreto V, et al (2010) Late recovery after traumatic, anoxic, or hemorrhagic long-lasting vegetative state. Neurology 75: 239–245
24. Sazbon L, Zagreba F, Ronen J, et al (1993) Course and outcome of patients in vegetative state of nontraumatic aetiology. J Neurol Neurosurg Psychiatry 56: 407–409
25. Higashi K, Hatano M, Abiko S, et al (1981) Five-year follow-up study of patients with persistent vegetative state. J Neurol Neurosurg Psychiatry 44: 552–554
26. Luaute J, Maucort-Boulch D, Tell L, et al (2010) Long-term outcomes of chronic minimally conscious and vegetative states. Neurology 75: 246–252
27. Walshe TM, Leonard C (1985) Persistent vegetative state. Extension of the syndrome to include chronic disorders. Arch Neurol 42: 1045–1047
28. Field RE, Romanus RJ (1981) A decerebrate patient: eighteen years of care. Conn Med 45: 717–723
29. Cranford RE (1984) Termination of treatment in the persistent vegetative state. Semin Neurol 4: 36–44
30. Sibbison JB (1991) USA: right to live, or right to die? Lancet 337: 102–103
31. Dubroja I, Valent S, Miklic P, et al (1995) Outcome of post-traumatic unawareness persisting for more than a month. J Neurol Neurosurg Psychiatry 58: 465–466
32. Sazbon L (1985) Prolonged coma. Prog Clin Neurosci 2: 65–81
33. Avesani R, Gambini MG, Albertini G (2006) The vegetative state: a report of two cases with a long-term follow-up. Brain Inj 20: 333–338
34. Childs NL, Mercer WN (1996) Late improvement in consciousness after post-traumatic vegetative state. N Engl J Med 334: 24–25
35. Voss HU, Uluc AM, Dyke JP, et al (2006) Possible axonal regrowth in late recovery from the minimally conscious state. J Clin Invest 116: 2005–2011
36. Jennett B, Bond M (1975) Assessment of outcome after severe brain damage. Lancet 1: 480–484
37. Rappaport M, Hall KM, Hopkins K, et al (1982) Disability rating scale for severe head trauma: coma to community. Arch Phys Med Rehabil 63: 118–123

XX Sedation

Comparative Efficacy and Safety of Sedative Agents in Severe Traumatic Brain Injury

D.J. Roberts and D.A. Zygun

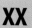

Introduction

Sedative agents are commonly used to manage adults in the intensive care unit (ICU) with severe traumatic brain injury (TBI) [1–3]. These drugs prevent or treat agitation, permit manipulation of artificial ventilation, and induce and maintain anxiolysis and amnesia [1–3]. Moreover, sedative agents may diminish cerebral metabolic rate and, through flow-metabolism coupling, reduce brain blood flow, intracranial blood volume, and ultimately intracranial pressure (ICP) [4]. Boluses or infusions of sedatives possibly also reduce the prolonged and marked increases in ICP produced by endotracheal suctioning or bronchoscopy [3, 5]. Unfortunately, however, sedative agents may also lower mean arterial pressure (MAP), hinder the neurological examination, and prolong the length of ventilatory support or ICU stay [3]. This chapter reviews regulation of brain blood flow and metabolic rate in TBI, relevant sedative neuropharmacology, and the comparative efficacy and safety of propofol, ketamine, etomidate, and agents from the opioid, benzodiazepine, α_2-agonist (i.e., clonidine and dexmedetomidine), and antipsychotic drug classes for management of adults in the ICU with severe TBI.

Brain Blood Flow and Metabolic Rate in TBI

Brain blood flow is determined by cerebral perfusion pressure (CPP), cerebrovascular resistance, and blood viscosity [6]. CPP is approximately the difference between MAP and ICP (CPP = MAP − ICP) while cerebrovascular resistance is directly proportional to the length of cerebral arterioles and inversely proportional to their radius to the fourth power [6]. Cerebral arteriolar radius is increased by heightened arterial partial pressures of carbon dioxide ($PaCO_2$) and possibly by arterial partial pressures of oxygen (PaO_2) below 60 mmHg [6]. In patients without TBI, cerebral arterioles vasoconstrict or vasodilate in response to increases or decreases in CPP through a process known as cerebral autoregulation [6]. A second regulatory process, known as flow-metabolism coupling, increases regional brain blood flow in response to concomitant increases in brain function and metabolic rate [6].

Cerebral autoregulation is significantly impaired or abolished and brain blood flow and cerebral metabolic rate are frequently reduced following TBI [4, 7]. With cerebral autoregulatory impairment, alterations in MAP produce proportionate and possibly detrimental changes in CPP [6]. Although severe brain blood flow

J.-L. Vincent (ed.), *Annual Update in Intensive Care and Emergency Medicine 2012*
DOI 10.1007/978-3-642-25716-2 © Springer-Verlag Berlin Heidelberg 2012

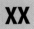

restrictions often occur throughout the brain following TBI, injured brain regions exhibit lower brain blood flow than non-injured regions, and a gradual return to baseline flow occurs hours to days after injury [4, 7]. Cerebral oxidative rate and metabolism are also reduced in patients with TBI, although not always in proportion to brain blood flow as variable degrees of flow-metabolism uncoupling may occur [4, 7].

Neuropharmacology of Sedative Agents in Severe TBI

Sedative agents exert several potentially beneficial pharmacodynamic effects in adults with severe TBI. These drugs may produce metabolic suppression by reducing cerebral oxygen demand and metabolic rate [4, 8]. This action is largely dependent on the post-head injury cerebral metabolic rate and would be unexpected in a patient with an already isoelectric or burst-suppressed elentroencephalogram (EEG) [4]. Sedative-induced reductions in cerebral metabolic rate may, in turn, result in cerebral vasoconstriction and lowered brain blood flow if flow-metabolism coupling is intact [4, 8, 9]. Ultimately, lowered brain blood flow may decrease overall intracranial blood volume and, therefore, ICP, which will increase CPP as long as MAP remains constant [4]. However, this mechanism appears variably effective as propofol-induced metabolic suppression resulted in a decrease in ICP of more than 20 % in only 48.8 % of critically ill adults with moderate or severe TBI in one case series [9].

Other potentially beneficial sedative effects in adults with TBI include their ability to curb agitation and increase seizure threshold [8]. Agitation alone may increase intrathoracic pressure through a reduction in jugular venous outflow from the intracranial compartment and a consequent rise in ICP [8]. Although benzodiazepines increase and propofol has mixed effects on seizure threshold [8], the influence of sedative agents on seizure incidence in patients with TBI are complex and beyond the scope of this review.

Comparative Sedative Agent Efficacy and Safety

In order to compare the relative efficacy and safety of available sedative agents for management of adults with severe TBI, we expanded upon our recent systematic review of randomized controlled trials (RCTs) [3]. The 158 full-text citations that had been retrieved for this systematic review were re-examined and observational studies and previously excluded RCTs relevant to this article were included herein. We excluded one RCT as few (16 %) of the included participants had severe TBI [10] and 82 observational studies as three addressed a different intervention [11–13], three investigated an outcome irrelevant to this review [14–16], and 76 studied a patient population that did not comprise adults in the ICU with severe TBI. A total of 16 interventional trials, including 15 RCTs [17–31] and one 'pseudo-randomized' trial [3, 32], as well as 15 observational studies were ultimately included in this review [5, 33–46]. Outcomes of the 16 interventional trials are summarized in **Table 1** while those of the 15 observational studies are displayed in **Table 2**. Notable limitations of the findings in many of these trials included inadequate descriptions of relevant baseline TBI prognostic factors and frequent and unregulated use of co-sedatives and ICP-lowering co-interventions

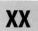

Table 1. Randomized controlled trials of sedation for adults in the intensive care unit with severe traumatic brain injury (TBI)

First author, year [ref]	Diagnoses (No. patients)	Sedatives	Mean or median dosage or infusion rate	Mean change in ICP, MAP, and CPP from baseline (mmHg)*†
Opioid vs. Opioid(s), Other Drugs, or Placebo				
White, 1982 [17]	Severe TBI (15)	Fentanyl Thiopental i.v./IT Lidocaine Succinylcholine Normal saline	1 µg/kg 3 mg/kg 1.5 mg/kg 1 mg/kg 2 ml	A bolus of fentanyl vs. saline ↓ the ICP ↑ produced by endotracheal suctioning by 8
Sperry, 1992 [19]	Severe TBI (9)	Sufentanil Fentanyl	0.6 µg/kg 3 µg/kg	Max ICP ↑ of 6 and 8; MAP ↓ of 10 and 10; and CPP ↓ of 10 and 13 after bolus of sufentanil or fentanyl (ICP returned to baseline by ~ 25-min and MAP by ~ 60-min)
Lauer, 1997 [21]	Severe TBI (15)	Morphine Fentanyl Sufentanil	0.03±0.02 mg/kg/h 1.63±0.48 µg/kg/h 0.33±0.16 µg/kg/h	No ICP or CPP change after a short infusion of morphine, fentanyl, or sufentanil at a dose predetermined to produce a max 5 % ↓ in MAP; MAP ↓ at 10- and 45- min for sufentanil
Albanèse, 1999 [23]	Severe TBI (6)	Sufentanil Alfentanil Fentanyl	0.005 mg/kg/min 0.75 mg/kg/min 0.075 mg/kg/min	ICP ↑ of 9, 8, and 5.5; MAP ↓ of 21, 24, and 26; and CPP ↓ of 30, 31, and 34 after sufentanil, alfentanil, or fentanyl (ICP returned to baseline by 15-min)
de Nadal, 2000 [25]	Severe TBI (30)	Morphine Fentanyl	0.2 mg/kg 2 µg/kg	ICP ↑ and MAP and CPP ↓ after a bolus of either opioid
Propofol vs. Midazolam, Morphine, or Midazolam and Morphine				
McArthur, 1995 [30]	TBI (8), ICH/SAH (11), or postoperative cerebral edema (2) with mean GCS 6	Propofol Morphine + midazolam	3.1 mg/kg/h 0.076 mg/kg/h + 0.076 mg/kg/h	No difference in ICP, incidence of intracranial hypertension, or use of NMB between agents
Sanchez-Izquierdo-Riera, 1998 [22]	Severe TBI (59) or multisystem trauma without head injury (41)	Propofol Midazolam	1.5 – 5 mg/kg/h 0.1 – 0.3 mg/kg/h	No ICP, MAP, or CPP change for either agent
Kelly, 1999 [24]	Severe (39) or moderate (3) TBI	Propofol Morphine	55±42 µg/kg/h 10±6.7 mg/h	ICP ↓ of 4 for propofol versus morphine on day 3; CSF drainage ↓ on day 2 and 3 as well as ↓ overall use of NMB, BZPs, and pentobarbital
Sandiumenge Camps, 2000 [26]	Severe TBI (43) or multisystem trauma without head injury (20)	Propofol Midazolam	3.7 mg/kg/h 0.16 mg/kg/h	No ICP, MAP, or CPP change for either agent

Table 1. (continued)

First author, year [ref]	Diagnoses (No. patients)	Sedatives	Mean or median dosage or infusion rate	Mean change in ICP, MAP, and CPP from baseline (mmHg)*†
Ghori, 2007 [29]	Severe TBI (28)	Propofol / Midazolam	1.5 – 5 mg/kg/h / 0.1 – 0.3 mg/kg/h	No ICP change for either agent
Ketamine vs. Fentanyl or Sufentanil				
Kolenda, 1996¶ [32]	Severe (13), moderate (1), mild (6), or unknown severity (4) TBI	Ketamine / Fentanyl	104 µg/kg/day / 100 µg/kg/day	ICP and MAP ↑ for ketamine vs. fentanyl on days 8 and 10 and 3 and 7
Bourgoin, 2003 [27]	Severe TBI (25)	Ketamine / Sufentanil	82 ± 25 µg/kg/min / 0.008 ± 0.002 µg/kg/min	No ICP, MAP, or CPP change for either agent
Bourgoin, 2005 [28]	Severe TBI (30)	Ketamine / Sufentanil	↑ [target] from 2.6- to 5.5 µg/ml / ↑ [target] from 0.4- to 0.7 ng/ml	No ICP, MAP, or CPP change for either agent
Schmittner, 2007 [31]	Severe TBI (10) or aneurysmal SAH (14)	S(+)-Ketamine / Fentanyl	Loading dose then infusion up to 2 mg/kg/h / Loading dose then infusion up to 10 µg/kg/h	No ICP or CPP difference between agents
Etomidate vs. Althesin or Pentobarbital				
Dearden, 1985 [18]	Severe TBI (10)	Etomidate / Althesin	20 – 50 µg/kg/min / 0.2 to 0.5 mL/kg/h	ICP ↓ at 10- and 30-min for etomidate and at 30-, 50-, and 70-min for althesin with no change in CPP; MAP ↓ at 50-min for etomidate
Levy, 1995 [20]	Severe TBI (4) or vascular brain injury (3)	Etomidate / Pentobarbital	Loading dose then 0.02 mg/kg/min / Loading doses then 1.5 mg/kg/h	ICP ↓ of 12 and 9 for etomidate and pentobarbital with no change in CPP (no statistics)

BZP: benzodiazepines; CPP: cerebral perfusion pressure; CSF: cerebrospinal fluid; GCS: Glasgow Coma Scale; ICH: intracranial hemorrhage; ICP: intracranial pressure; ICU: intensive care unit; i.v.: intravenous; IT: intrathecal; LOS: length of hospital or ICU stay; MAP: mean arterial pressure; min: minute; NMB: neuromuscular blocking agents; SAH: subarachnoid hemorrhage

* Unless otherwise stated, only differences with a p-value of ≤ 0.05 are presented.

† Changes in ICP, MAP, and CPP are presented in respective order unless stated otherwise.

¶ This trial was 'pseudo-randomized' as patients were allocated to "receive either ketamine or fentanyl according to their administrative patient number which they received after they arrived as emergencies ..." [32].

Table 2. Observational studies of sedation for adults in the intensive care unit with severe traumatic brain injury (TBI).

First author, year [ref]	Diagnoses (No. patients)	Design	Sedative(s) (mean or median dosage or infusion rate)	Mean or median change in ICP, MAP, and CPP from baseline (mmHg)*†
Opioid Alone or Opioid vs. No Drugs or an Opioid with Vecuronium				
Albanese, 1993 [33]	Severe TBI (10)	Case series	Sufentanil (1 µg/kg loading dose then infusion of 0.005 µg/kg/min)	Max ICP ↑ of 9 and MAP and CPP ↓ of 19 and 28 5-min after bolus (all values returned to baseline by 15-min)
Scholz, 1994 [34]	Severe TBI (10)	Case series	Sufentanil (2 µg/kg loading dose then infusion of 150 µg/h + midazolam at 9.0 mg/h)	ICP and MAP ↓ of 5 each within 15-min with no change in CPP after bolus
Kerr, 1998 [5]	Severe TBI (71)	Prospective cohort	No drugs vs. fentanyl (90.8 µg/h) or morphine (4.7 mg/h) vs. vecuronium + fentanyl (108.3 µg/h) or morphine (10.4 mg/h)	ICP ↑ produced by endotracheal suctioning reduced by vecuronium plus an opioid vs. an opioid alone
Tipps, 2000 [35]	Severe TBI (6)	Case series	Remifentanil (0.68 µg/kg loading dose then infusion of 0.01 to 0.26 µg/kg/min)	Endotracheal suctioning and bronchoscopy was performed without a large ↑ in ICP or ↓ in CPP
Engelhard, 2004 [36]	Severe TBI (20)	Case series	Remifentanil (0.5 µg/kg loading dose then infusion of 0.25 µg/kg/min)	No ICP, MAP, or CPP change
Propofol Alone or Propofol vs. Morphine and Midazolam				
Herrogods, 1988 [37]	Severe TBI (6)	Case series	Propofol (1 µg/kg)	ICP, MAP, and CPP ↓ of 14, 40, and 42 after bolus
Farling, 1989 [38]	Severe (9) or moderate (1) TBI	Case series	Propofol (2.88 mg/kg/h)	ICP ↓ of 2 at 2-h and CPP ↑ of 10 at 24-h with no change in MAP
Stewart, 1994 [39]	Severe (12) or moderate (3) TBI	Prospective or retrospective cohort	Propofol (232 mg/h) vs. morphine (2.3 mg/h) and midazolam (2.8 mg/h)	No ICP, MAP, or CPP change for either propofol or morphine and midazolam

XX

Table 2. (*continued*)

First author, year [ref]	Diagnoses (No. patients)	Design	Sedative(s) (mean or median dosage or infusion rate)	Mean or median change in ICP, MAP, and CPP from baseline (mmHg)*†
Etomidate Alone				
Cohn, 1983 [40]	Severe TBI (20) and vascular- (20) or tumor-related (12) brain injury	Case series	Etomidate (0.2 mg/kg loading dose then infusion of 20 to 100 µg/kg/min)	Only small or brief ICP elevations occurred during bronchial toilet; decreased frequency of ventricular tapping and mannitol administration (no statistics)
Prior, 1983 [41]	Severe TBI (10)	Case series	Etomidate (infusion of 5 to 25 µg/kg/min with prn 0.2 mg/kg boluses)	ICP and MAP ↑ produced by endotracheal suctioning prevented or limited by a bolus of etomidate
Bingham, 1985 [42]	Severe TBI (8)	Retrospective cohort	Etomidate (infusion of 5 to 25 µg/kg/min with prn boluses)	ICP ↓ and CPP ↑ more following an etomidate bolus in patients with a minimum voltage on the cerebral function monitor > 5 µV vs. ≤ 5 µV with no change in MAP
Midazolam, Clonidine, Ketamine, or Loxapine Alone				
Papazian, 1993 [43]	Severe TBI (12)	Case series	Midazolam (0.15 mg/kg)	MAP and CPP ↓ following bolus with no change in ICP
ter Minassian, 1997 [44]	Severe TBI (12)	Case series	Clonidine (2.5 µg/kg)	MAP and CPP ↓ of 11 and 14 at 5-min following bolus with no overall change in ICP
Albanese, 1997 [45]	Severe TBI (8)	Case series	Ketamine (bolus doses of 1.5, 3, and 5 mg/kg)	ICP↓ at 2-min for the 1.5 and 5 mg/kg dose and ICP ↑ at 5-, 20-, and 30-min and 30-min for the 1.5 and 5 mg/kg dose with no change in MAP or CPP
Lescot, 2007 [46]	Severe (6) or moderate (1) TBI	Case series	Loxapine (10 mg)	ICP ↓ of 1 with no change in MAP following bolus

CPP: cerebral perfusion pressure; ICP: intracranial pressure; ICU: intensive care unit; LOS: length of hospital or ICU stay; MAP: mean arterial pressure; prn: as needed.
* Unless otherwise stated, only differences with a p-value of ≤ 0.05 are presented.
† Changes in ICP, MAP, and CPP are presented in respective order unless stated otherwise.

[3]. Many trials also enrolled small patient samples and, therefore, may have been underpowered to detect differences in mortality and neurological outcome [3].

Effect of Sedative Agents on Clinical Outcomes:

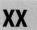

Seven RCTs [22, 24, 26, 27, 29, 31, 32] and one cohort study [39] examined the effects of prolonged sedative infusions on mortality, neurological outcome, or length of hospital or ICU stay amongst adults with predominantly severe TBI. Two RCTs comparing propofol and midazolam [22, 26] found no difference in length of ICU stay while another [29] reported no difference in neurological outcome [3]. Moreover, our recent systematic review found no difference in mortality between propofol and midazolam when mortality estimates from two RCTs [22, 29] were combined in meta-analysis (relative risk [RR], 1.07; 95 % confidence interval [CI], 0.51 to 2.3) [3]. A similar mortality rate and neurological outcome were also observed in a prospective cohort study comparing propofol to midazolam and morphine [39]. In the only available multicenter RCT, no difference in mortality or subsequent neurological outcome was observed amongst patients randomized to propofol or morphine [24]. Although authors of this study reported that high ($\geq$ 100 mg/kg for $\geq$ 24 hours and beginning within 48-hours of injury) versus low dose propofol resulted in a significantly higher rate of favorable neurological outcomes at 6-months, a recalculation of this finding in our recent systematic review revealed a RR of 1.82 and a 95 % CI that included one (0.81 to 4.05) [3]. Ketamine and either fentanyl or sufentanil were compared in three of the seven RCTs [27, 28, 31] and the one 'pseudo-randomized' trial (**Table 2**) [32]. Two of these four trials reported no change in mortality [27, 32], and three found no difference in neurological outcome [27, 31, 32].

Effect of Sedative Agents on ICP, CPP, and MAP
Opioids Alone or Versus Opioid(s), Other Drugs, or Placebo

As opioids confer analgesia, they are commonly administered in conjunction with propofol or midazolam and afford additive sedation for adults with severe head injury [2, 4]. The influence of a bolus dose or short infusion of an opioid on cerebral and systemic hemodynamics in patients with severe TBI has been investigated by five RCTs [3], four before-and-after case series [33–36], and one prospective cohort study [5].

Three of the four RCTs that administered an often large bolus dose (up to 3 µg/kg of fentanyl) (**Table 1**) or short infusion of an opioid agent [19, 23, 25], as well as one of the three case series [33], observed an increase in ICP ranging from 5.5 to 9 mmHg above baseline following morphine, fentanyl, and sufentanil [3]. Only one of these four RCTs [21] and two of the three case series [34, 36] found no change or a small decrease in ICP (by 5 mmHg) versus baseline after morphine, fentanyl, sufentanil, or remifentanyl. Moreover, the one RCT that found no effect on ICP administered an opioid dose predetermined by the investigators to produce a maximum 5 % decrease in MAP, potentially limiting generalizability of this study's findings [3, 21]. ICP increases in two RCTs [19, 23] and one observational study [33] were transient and returned to baseline after approximately 15 to 25 minutes. One RCT [17] and two observational studies [5, 35] found that ICP increases produced by endotracheal suctioning were limited by a dose or short infusion of either fentanyl or remifentanil.

MAP decreased in all four RCTs [19, 21, 23, 25] that administered a bolus or short infusion of morphine, fentanyl, sufentanil, or alfentanil and two of four observational investigations [33, 34] after sufentanil (combined range across all opioid studies, 5 to 26 mmHg). This translated into a decrease in CPP in three of four RCTs [19, 23, 25] and one case series [33], which altogether collectively ranged from 10 to 34 mmHg. Although decreases in MAP and CPP were transient in one RCT [19] and another case series [33], one investigation found that although there was a gradual increase in CPP toward baseline after the initial reduction, CPP values remained somewhat depressed throughout the study [3, 23].

In sum, the above evidence suggests that opioids, in large bolus doses, may result in transient (approximately 15 to 25 minutes), yet clinically significant, increases in ICP and decreases in MAP and CPP amongst adults with severe TBI [3]. Increases in ICP may occur through central opioid accumulation following acute neurological injury [47] with decreased cerebral arteriolar resistance or MAP, increased $PaCO_2$, or disturbed cerebral autoregulation [3], and possibly may be avoided by several measures. These include slow and cautious opioid administration, prevention of hypotension through volume resuscitation or vasopressors, and ventilatory titration to prevent hypercarbia [3]. However, we support that clinicians should closely monitor ICP, MAP, and CPP following an opioid bolus or rapid infusion in a patient with severe TBI for deleterious cerebral and systemic hemodynamic changes and treat these appropriately [3].

Propofol Alone or Versus Midazolam or Midazolam and Morphine

Propofol and midazolam are two of the most commonly used sedative agents among critically ill adults with severe TBI given their rapid onset and often short duration of action, which permits serial neurological examination [3]. The effect of propofol on cerebral and systemic hemodynamics in patients with predominantly severe TBI has been examined by four RCTs [22, 26, 29, 30], two before-and-after case series [37, 38], and one cohort study [39].

Two of the four RCTs, which also included multisystem trauma patients without head injury [22, 26], allocated patients to propofol or midazolam and found no difference in ICP, MAP, or CPP between agents or versus baseline. No difference in ICP was found in an additional RCT comparing propofol to midazolam [29] or in an RCT [30] or cohort study [39] that compared propofol to midazolam and morphine. Propofol decreased ICP in two case series (range, 2 to 14 mmHg) [37, 38] and improved CPP in one [38]. However, a large respective decrease in MAP and CPP of 40 and 42 mmHg was noted after propofol in another case series [37].

Aside from the more reliable rapid on-off pharmacokinetic profile associated with propofol versus midazolam [3, 8], preferential use of propofol for management of critically ill adults with TBI may be supported by the findings of a multicenter trial [24]. This investigation observed a reduced requirement for neuromuscular blocking agents, benzodiazepines, and pentobarbital as well as reduced ventriculostomy cerebrospinal fluid (CSF) drainage amongst patients with severe TBI versus morphine [3, 24]. However, no randomized evidence exists to support a significant benefit for any of these three therapies for improving patient-centered outcomes, ICP, or CPP [48]. Moreover, this trial was limited by its comparison of propofol with morphine (rather than midazolam), an agent which, as mentioned above, has been observed to have untoward effects on ICP and CPP.

Ketamine Alone or Versus Opioids

As ketamine has historically been linked with increases in ICP, this agent is uncommonly used in hemodynamically stable patients with severe TBI [1–3]. Two RCTs [27, 31] and one 'pseudo-randomized' trial [32] allocated patients with moderate or severe TBI and subarachnoid hemorrhage (SAH) to infusions or bolus doses of ketamine, sufentanil, or fentanyl. An additional RCT studied the effect of a transient doubling of the plasma concentration of ketamine or sufentanil [28]. Although one [27] of the four trials noted an increase in heart rate and another [32] observed an increase in ICP and MAP for ketamine versus fentanyl, three [27, 28, 31] found no difference in ICP, MAP, or CPP between agents or versus baseline. In the only identified case series, boluses of varying ketamine dosage produced a biphasic cerebral hemodynamic response with ICP decreasing slightly at 2 minutes and then increasing between 5 and 30 minutes [45].

Etomidate Alone or Versus Althesin or Pentobarbital

Etomidate and althesin or pentobarbital infusions of varying length were compared in two RCTs of patients with severe TBI and vascular or ischemic brain injury [18, 20]. Although statistics were not given for one of the RCTs [20], both trials reported a decrease in ICP and no change in CPP or consistent alteration in MAP [3]. An etomidate infusion was also examined by two case series and one retrospective cohort study of patients with severe TBI and vascular- or tumor-related brain injury [40–42]. In both of these series, the increase in ICP (and MAP in one trial) produced by endotracheal suctioning was diminished by a bolus or infusion of etomidate [40, 41]. The retrospective cohort study further demonstrated that larger decreases in ICP occurred in severe TBI patients without a dramatic reduction in cortical electrical activity, and that these decreases were often linked with increases in CPP [42].

Midazolam, Clonidine, and Loxapine Alone

A bolus of midazolam or clonidine resulted in a decrease in MAP and CPP without a change in ICP in two case series of adults with severe TBI [43, 44]. In the only series involving antipsychotics in patients with moderate or severe TBI, a bolus of loxapine resulted in a marginal 1 mmHg ICP reduction with no change in MAP [46].

Non-Hemodynamic Adverse Drug Events of Sedative Agents

Apart from the untoward changes in ICP, MAP, and CPP observed following certain sedative agents that were described above, several additional adverse effects were noted in identified RCTs and observational studies. In the multicenter RCT comparing propofol and morphine, a trend towards an increased rate of uncontrollable intracranial hypertension was observed for the morphine group [24]. Moreover, although no cases of propofol infusion syndrome occurred, hypertriglyceridemia developed following use of propofol in two RCTs [3, 22, 26]. Propofol infusion syndrome, originally reported in children and later in adults with head injury receiving prolonged, high dose intravenous propofol infusions (> 5 mg/kg/hour for > 58 hours), is characterized by metabolic acidosis, rhabdomyolysis, hyperkalemia, lipemia, and cardiac dysrhythmias and failure [4, 49]. The odds of developing propofol infusion syndrome in adults with head injury have been observed to be 1.93 times greater for every mg/kg/hour increase in mean propofol dose above 5 mg/kg/hour [49]. Propylene glycol toxicity, characterized by increased serum osmolality and renal failure, occurred in all seven patients with acute neurological injury treated with etomidate versus pentobarbital in another RCT [20, 3]. Several other sedative-related adverse events, including etomidate-induced adrenal suppression, were not reported in interventional trials [3], but should be recognized as possible outcomes of certain sedative agents.

Conclusion

Although no sedative agent is associated with an improvement in mortality, neurological outcome, or length of hospital or ICU stay, existing agents vary in their effects on ICP, CPP, and MAP [3]. Large bolus doses of opioids have been observed to result in transient (approximately 15 to 25 minutes), yet clinically significant, increases in ICP and decreases in MAP and CPP in both RCTs and observational studies [3]. In contrast, infusions of propofol and midazolam have been demonstrated to have neutral and equal effects on ICP, MAP, and CPP [3]. Although ketamine may increase heart rate and MAP [3], most evidence from randomized trials suggests that this agent also has neutral effects on ICP, MAP, and CPP in the severe TBI population. While etomidate and pentobarbital may have similar effects on ICP, MAP, and CPP [3], clonidine, dexmedetomidine, and antipsychotics have a largely unknown effect on cerebral hemodynamics. As sedatives are commonly used to manage adults in the ICU with severe TBI, appropriately designed and adequately-powered RCTs addressing the comparative efficacy and safety of these agents are urgently required [3].

References

1. Jeevaratnam DR, Menon DK (1996) Survey of intensive care of severely head injured patients in the United Kingdom. BMJ 312: 944–947
2. Matta B, Menon D (1996) Severe head injury in the United Kingdom and Ireland: a survey of practice and implications for management. Crit Care Med 24: 1743–1748
3. Roberts DJ, Hall RI, Kramer AH, Robertson HL, Gallagher CN, Zygun DA (2011) Sedation for critically ill adults with severe traumatic brain injury: a systematic review of randomized controlled trials. Crit Care Med 39: 2743–2751
4. Urwin SC, Menon DK (2004) Comparative tolerability of sedative agents in head-injured adults. Drug Saf 27: 107–133
5. Kerr ME, Sereika SM, Orndoff P, et al (1998) Effect of neuromuscular blockers and opiates on the cerebrovascular response to endotracheal suctioning in adults with severe head injuries. Am J Crit Care 7: 205–217
6. Kramer AH, Zygun DA (2009) Anemia and red blood cell transfusion in neurocritical care. Crit Care 13: R89
7. Coles JP, Cunningham AS, Salvador R, et al (2009) Early metabolic characteristics of lesion and nonlesion tissue after head injury. J Cereb Blood Flow Metab 29: 965–975
8. Citerio G, Cormio M (2003) Sedation in neurointensive care: advances in understanding and practice. Curr Opin Crit Care 9: 120–126

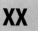

9. Oertel M, Kelly DF, Lee JH, et al (2002) Efficacy of hyperventilation, blood pressure elevation, and metabolic suppression therapy in controlling intracranial pressure after head injury. J Neurosurg 97: 1045–1053

10. Karabinis A, Mandragos K, Stergiopoulos S, et al (2004) Safety and efficacy of analgesia-based sedation with remifentanil versus standard hypnotic-based regimens in intensive care unit patients with brain injuries: a randomised, controlled trial [ISRCTN50308308]. Crit Care 8: R268–R280

11. Chiolero RL, Ravussin P, Anderes JP, Ledermann P, de Tribolet N (1988) The effects of midazolam reversal by RO 15–1788 on cerebral perfusion pressure in patients with severe head injury. Intensive Care Med 14: 196–200

12. McCall M, Jeejeebhoy K, Pencharz P, Moulton R (2003) Effect of neuromuscular blockade on energy expenditure in patients with severe head injury. JPEN J Parenter Enteral Nutr 27: 27–35

13. Huang SJ, Shieh JS, Fu M, Kao MC (2006) Fuzzy logic control for intracranial pressure via continuous propofol sedation in a neurosurgical intensive care unit. Med Eng Phys 28: 639–647

14. Bullock R, Stewart L, Rafferty C, Teasdale GM (1993) Continuous monitoring of jugular bulb oxygen saturation and the effect of drugs acting on cerebral metabolism. Acta Neurochir Suppl (Wien) 59: 113–118

15. Steiner LA, Johnston AJ, Chatfield DA, et al (2003) The effects of large-dose propofol on cerebrovascular pressure autoregulation in head-injured patients. Anesth Analg 97: 572–576

16. Payen D, Quintin L, Plaisance P, Chiron B, Lhoste F (1990) Head injury: clonidine decreases plasma catecholamines. Crit Care Med 18: 392–395

17. White PF, Schlobohm RM, Pitts LH, Lindauer JM (1982) A randomized study of drugs for preventing increases in intracranial pressure during endotracheal suctioning. Anesthesiology 57: 242–244

18. Dearden NM, McDowall DG (1985) Comparison of etomidate and althesin in the reduction of increased intracranial pressure after head injury. Br J Anaesth 57: 361–368

19. Sperry RJ, Bailey PL, Reichman MV, Peterson JC, Petersen PB, Pace NL (1992) Fentanyl and sufentanil increase intracranial pressure in head trauma patients. Anesthesiology 77: 416–420

20. Levy ML, Aranda M, Zelman V, Giannotta SL (1995) Propylene glycol toxicity following continuous etomidate infusion for the control of refractory cerebral edema. Neurosurgery 37: 363–369

21. Lauer KK, Connolly LA, Schmeling WT (1997) Opioid sedation does not alter intracranial pressure in head injured patients. Can J Anaesth 44: 929–933

22. Sanchez-Izquierdo-Riera JA, Caballero-Cubedo RE, Perez-Vela JL, Ambros-Checa A, Cantalapiedra-Santiago JA, Alted-Lopez E (1998) Propofol versus midazolam: safety and efficacy for sedating the severe trauma patient. Anesth Analg 86: 1219–1224

23. Albanese J, Viviand X, Potie F, Rey M, Alliez B, Martin C (1999) Sufentanil, fentanyl, and alfentanil in head trauma patients: a study on cerebral hemodynamics. Crit Care Med 27: 407–411

24. Kelly DF, Goodale DB, Williams J, et al (1999) Propofol in the treatment of moderate and severe head injury: a randomized, prospective double-blinded pilot trial. J Neurosurg 90: 1042–1052

25. de Nadal M, Munar F, Poca MA, Sahuquillo J, Garnacho A, Rossello J (2000) Cerebral hemodynamic effects of morphine and fentanyl in patients with severe head injury: absence of correlation to cerebral autoregulation. Anesthesiology 92: 11–19

26. Sandiumenge Camps A, Sanchez-Izquierdo Riera JA, Toral Vazquez D, Sa Borges M, Peinado Rodriguez J, Alted Lopez E (2000) Midazolam and 2 % propofol in long-term sedation of traumatized critically ill patients: efficacy and safety comparison. Crit Care Med 28: 3612–3619

27. Bourgoin A, Albanese J, Wereszczynski N, Charbit M, Vialet R, Martin C (2003) Safety of sedation with ketamine in severe head injury patients: comparison with sufentanil. Crit Care Med 31: 711–717

28. Bourgoin A, Albanese J, Leone M, Sampol-Manos E, Viviand X, Martin C (2005) Effects of sufentanil or ketamine administered in target-controlled infusion on the cerebral hemodynamics of severely brain-injured patients. Crit Care Med 33: 1109–1113

29. Ghori KA, Harmon DC, Elashaal A, et al (2007) Effect of midazolam versus propofol sedation on markers of neurological injury and outcome after isolated severe head injury: a pilot study. Crit Care Resusc 9: 166–171
30. McArthur CJ, Gin T, McLaren IM, Critchley JA, Oh TE (1995) Gastric emptying following brain injury: effects of choice of sedation and intracranial pressure. Intensive Care Med 21: 573–576
31. Schmittner MD, Vajkoczy SL, Horn P, et al (2007) Effects of fentanyl and S(+)-ketamine on cerebral hemodynamics, gastrointestinal motility, and need of vasopressors in patients with intracranial pathologies: a pilot study. J Neurosurg Anesthesiol 19: 257–262
32. Kolenda H, Gremmelt A, Rading S, Braun U, Markakis E (1996) Ketamine for analgosedative therapy in intensive care treatment of head-injured patients. Acta Neurochir (Wien) 138: 1193–1199
33. Albanese J, Durbec O, Viviand X, Potie F, Alliez B, Martin C (1993) Sufentanil increases intracranial pressure in patients with head trauma. Anesthesiology 79: 493–497
34. Scholz J, Bause H, Schulz M, et al (1994) Pharmacokinetics and effects on intracranial pressure of sufentanil in head trauma patients. Br J Clin Pharmacol 38: 369–372
35. Tipps LB, Coplin WM, Murry KR, Rhoney DH (2000) Safety and feasibility of continuous infusion of remifentanil in the neurosurgical intensive care unit. Neurosurgery 46: 596–601
36. Engelhard K, Reeker W, Kochs E, Werner C (2004) Effect of remifentanil on intracranial pressure and cerebral blood flow velocity in patients with head trauma. Acta Anaesthesiol Scand 48: 396–399
37. Herregods L, Verbeke J, Rolly G, Colardyn F (1988) Effect of propofol on elevated intracranial pressure. Preliminary results. Anaesthesia 43 Suppl: 107–109
38. Farling PA, Johnston JR, Coppel DL (1989) Propofol infusion for sedation of patients with head injury in intensive care. A preliminary report. Anaesthesia 44: 222–226
39. Stewart L, Bullock R, Rafferty C, Fitch W, Teasdale GM (1994) Propofol sedation in severe head injury fails to control high ICP, but reduces brain metabolism. Acta Neurochir Suppl (Wien) 60: 544–546
40. Cohn BF, Rejger V, Hagenouw-Taal JC, Voormolen JH (1983) Results of a feasibility trial to achieve total immobilization of patients in a neurosurgical intensive care unit with etomidate. Anaesthesia 38 Suppl: 47–50
41. Prior JG, Hinds CJ, Williams J, Prior PF (1983) The use of etomidate in the management of severe head injury. Intensive Care Med 9: 313–320
42. Bingham RM, Procaccio F, Prior PF, Hinds CJ (1985) Cerebral electrical activity influences the effects of etomidate on cerebral perfusion pressure in traumatic coma. Br J Anaesth 57: 843–848
43. Papazian L, Albanese J, Thirion X, Perrin G, Durbec O, Martin C (1993) Effect of bolus doses of midazolam on intracranial pressure and cerebral perfusion pressure in patients with severe head injury. Br J Anaesth 71: 267–271
44. ter Minassian A, Beydon L, Decq P, Bonnet F (1997) Changes in cerebral hemodynamics after a single dose of clonidine in severely head-injured patients. Anesth Analg 84: 127–132
45. Albanese J, Arnaud S, Rey M, Thomachot L, Alliez B, Martin C (1997) Ketamine decreases intracranial pressure and electroencephalographic activity in traumatic brain injury patients during propofol sedation. Anesthesiology 87: 1328–1334
46. Lescot T, Pereira AR, Abdennour L, et al (2007) Effect of loxapine on electrical brain activity, intracranial pressure, and middle cerebral artery flow velocity in traumatic brain-injured patients. Neurocrit Care 7: 124–127
47. Roberts DJ, Goralski KB, Renton KW, et al (2009) Effect of acute inflammatory brain injury on accumulation of morphine and morphine 3- and 6-glucuronide in the human brain. Crit Care Med 37: 2767–2774
48. Roberts I, Schierhout G, Alderson P (1998) Absence of evidence for the effectiveness of five interventions routinely used in the intensive care management of severe head injury: a systematic review. J Neurol Neurosurg Psychiatry 65: 729–733
49. Cremer OL, Moons KG, Bouman EA, Kruijswijk JE, de Smet AM, Kalkman CJ (2001) Long-term propofol infusion and cardiac failure in adult head-injured patients. Lancet 357: 117–118

'Cooperative Sedation': Optimizing Comfort while Maximizing Systemic and Neurological Function

H.E. Goodwin, J.J. Lewin III, and M.A. Mirski

Introduction

Common indications for sedation in the intensive care unit (ICU) include patient comfort, management of agitation, pain, ventilator dysynchrony, and intracranial hypertension. Current trends in ICU care, however, have shifted towards sedation strategies that provide the minimally effective amount of sedation, to improve patient autonomy and preserve both the neurological exam and neurocognitive function.

Long Term Cognitive Effects of Critical Illness

Perhaps the earliest investigations to realize severe cognitive deficits following ICU care were studies that evaluated patients post-coronary artery bypass graft (CABG) surgery [1]. The investigators of one study found that 53 % of such patients demonstrated cognitive dysfunction at hospital discharge, and 42 % exhibited continued cognitive dysfunction at the five-year follow-up visit [2]. Patients with acute respiratory distress syndrome (ARDS) have also received significant attention as relates long-term outcomes following ICU discharge and, notably, such patients have not had a surgical intervention that may have independently resulted in neurological sequelae. One study reported that 100 % of ARDS patients had cognitive impairments at hospital discharge and, at the one-year follow-up visit, 78 % had at least one persistent impairment relating to cognition [3]. Other reported data support that patients with general medical problems often experience cognitive impairments following ICU discharge [1]. Although clinical review suggests that the mechanism of cerebral dysfunction following critical illness may most often be related to hypoxia and hypoperfusion, other factors, such as metabolic encephalopathy, delirium, and embolic phenomena, have also been implicated [1, 3]. Regardless of the etiology of neurocognitive deficits, strategies that target a lighter, 'cooperative' depth of sedation would allow the primary team to identify changes in mental status and cognition in the early phase of critical illness when the condition may still be reversible.

Daily Awakenings

The initial therapeutic intervention that evaluated the benefit of reducing the depth or interval of sedation was in the context of introducing daily prescribed

J.-L. Vincent (ed.), *Annual Update in Intensive Care and Emergency Medicine 2012*
DOI 10.1007/978-3-642-25716-2 © Springer-Verlag Berlin Heidelberg 2012

awakenings or brief 'off-periods' for sedative medications. The hypothesis entertained was that such interval off-periods, even if for only a brief period, would enhance the ability of the ICU team to assess and accelerate ventilator weaning, and thus may lead to a reduction in mean duration of mechanical ventilation and a shorter ICU length of stay (LOS). Hence, the primary outcome measure has typically been time to extubation as compared to a controlled ICU ventilated population.

The first trial evaluating the daily interruption of sedation was performed as a single center study by Kress and colleagues [4]. The investigators of this important study randomized patients to either a daily interruption of sedation (n = 68) or standard practice (n = 60). In both groups, sedative agents were titrated by nurses based on standard protocols to achieve a Ramsey Score of 3–4 (responsive to commands or wake briskly to the sound of a loud noise). In the intervention group, sedation was stopped daily, beginning on the 3rd ventilated day, until the patient could perform at least three of the following activities: Open eyes in response to voice, track the investigator with eyes, squeeze hand or stick out tongue upon request. Kress and colleagues found that this practice of daily sedation interruption led to fewer days requiring mechanical ventilation and shorter LOS in the ICU. In addition, as a secondary outcome measure, patients in the intervention group required fewer imaging studies to investigate poor neurologic function. Despite the positive findings, the study was too small and not sufficiently powered to rigorously assess the effect on patient safety. In addition, patients in this study were managed solely in the medical ICU, so the role of daily interruption of sedation in other ICU populations remained unclear. [4]

A second study was published in 2008 that coupled spontaneous awakening trials to a spontaneous breathing trial (SBT) [5]. All patients in the trial were screened for SBT, but only the intervention group paired the latter with the spontaneous awakening trials. This trial also demonstrated the positive effects of daily interruption of sedation, which included increased ventilator-free days and reduced ICU and hospital LOS. Although there were more self-extubations in the intervention group compared to the control group, the rate of re-intubation was similar between groups. In addition, this study demonstrated a statistically significant 32 % reduction in deaths at one year [5].

In 2010, a group of investigators took the concept of daily awakenings one step further, in fact challenging the need to routinely offer continuous sedation [6]. One hundred and twenty-eight patients were randomized to receive either sedation with a combination of propofol and midazolam or no sedation at all. In the sedation group, patients participated in daily awakening trials similar to those described in a previous study [4]. The group receiving no sedation required significantly fewer days of mechanical ventilation, in addition to shorter ICU and hospital LOS [6].

One concern for limiting sedation is the psychological impact it may have on the survivors of intensive care. The development of post-traumatic stress disorder (PTSD) has been reported to varying degrees after discharge from an ICU [7]. In order to evaluate the effect of daily awakenings on the development of PTSD, patients were evaluated for the presence of PTSD by a clinical psychologist [8]. Some of the patients included were in the trial evaluating the daily interruption of sedation mentioned earlier in this chapter [4]. Although chronic anxiety and mild depression were found in both the control and daily interruption groups, PTSD was identified in 6 of 19 patients in the control group. None of the 13 patients in the daily interruption group developed PTSD. Interestingly, no patient in the daily interruption group even recalled any of the awakened periods [8]. These data suggest that daily interruption of sedation does not have a detrimental effect on the long-term psychological outcome of patients and may even have a protective effect, though that could not be determined solely based on this report.

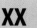

Early Mobilization

In addition to the long-term neurocognitive effects, it is well known that critical illness can cause a variety of neuromuscular sequelae, including muscle wasting from inactivity, critical illness myopathy and polyneuropathy [9]. These disorders contribute to prolonged functional disability after ICU discharge [9]. In one study of 87 survivors of ARDS who were evaluated at the one-year mark [10], only 49 % had returned to work, and patients reported muscle weakness and chronic fatigue as reasons for unemployment. In addition, at one year, patients were only able to walk 66 % of the predicted distance during a 6-minute walk test [10], further supporting the long lasting impact of critical illness.

Prolonged inactivity is thought to be a contributor to neuromuscular illness in the intensive care unit. In order to refute the concept that immobility is required for mechanically ventilated patients, a group in Salt Lake City conducted a feasibility trial for early mobility in 103 ventilated patients [11]. Early mobility was measured by the ability of the patient to sit on the edge of the bed, sit in a chair, and ambulate with or without assistance. The investigators demonstrated that 69.4 % of patients were able to walk a minimum of 200 feet, with less than 3 % being incapable of activity during their ICU admission. This impressive level of mobilization was achieved at the expense of very few adverse events; a total of 14 occurred over 1,449 activity events, including falls to the knees without injury, acute desaturation, changes in systolic blood pressure, and removal of feeding tube [11].

After the feasibility study had been conducted, other studies followed providing further evidence in support of early patient mobilization prior to liberation from mechanical ventilators [12–14]. One randomized controlled trial demonstrated that early mobilization was associated with more frequent return to independent functional status at hospital discharge and more frequent discharge home [14]. In addition, mobility was associated with a reduction in the duration of delirium during hospitalization.

In each of the above studies, the intervention involved a multidisciplinary team. Members included respiratory, physical, and occupational therapists, a nurse and a critical care technician [11–14]. In addition to the team, it was concluded that a coordinated sedation strategy was important to the success of the early mobilization intervention. One of the clinical studies specifically combined the intervention of early mobilization with daily interruption of sedation [14], although clearly such effort placed to coordinate such activities may not be readily translated to usual ICU practice. In all these trials, it was noted that lower depth of sedation was a significant predictor for success. Hence, minimizing the use of sedation, or eliminating it completely may increase the ability to successfully involve an interdisciplinary team in mobilizing mechanically ventilated patients.

Neurological Monitoring

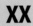

As more patients are admitted to the ICU and survive the experience, more attention is being given to the neurologic complications of critical illness, especially persistent neurocognitive dysfunction as it may occur even following admission for a non-neurological condition. Despite the brain being widely recognized as the most important organ, it often receives little attention during critical care management. This is likely due to several factors. One, the primary admission diagnosis to the ICU is non-neurologic, thus the primary focus lies initially elsewhere. Second, often the true neurologic status of the patient is unclear, as it may be masked by desirable or necessary sedation, alone or together with the addition of pharmacological paralysis, rendering neurological evaluation difficult or impossible.

Fortunately, the common-held belief in ICU practice that patient sedation *de facto* leads to an un-examinable patient is now fully in jeopardy. Previously cited studies have confirmed both the capability and safety of reducing the depth of sedation for the benefits of systemic physiology. There is also evidence that sedation need not be incompatible with preservation of intellectual capacity. Mirski and colleagues demonstrated in the Acute Neurological ICU Sedation Trial (ANIST) that anxious or agitated ventilator-dependent patients tolerated well a light plane of continuous sedation – 'cooperative sedation' – and were able to participate in neurocognitive evaluations [15]. Important to this fundamental acknowledgement, it was observed that neurocognitive capacity could be maintained or even improved during active continuous sedation as the disruptive influences of anxiety and agitation on concentration were eliminated. Dexmedetomidine, specifically, was shown not to reduce intellectual capacity during periods of cooperative sedation in contrast to low-dose infusion of propofol [15]. Other sedatives may also be effective in low doses.

The use of minimal to no sedation may have many benefits that have yet to be discovered. In addition to reduction in days requiring mechanical ventilation, shorter durations of stay, fewer diagnostic scans, and less PTSD, awake and cooperative patients should be able to be more engaged in their own care and decision making, and play a more significant role in their own recovery.

Monitoring Sedation

Sedation scales play an enormous role in the evaluation and communication of sedating therapies in the ICU. For patients requiring sedation, there are many validated scales available to assess the levels of consciousness and arousal. Perhaps the most widely used scale is the Richmond Agitation-Sedation Scale (RASS) [16, 17]. Other scales available include the Riker Sedation-Agitation Scale (SAS) [18], the Motor Activity Assessment Scale [19], the Adaptation to the Intensive Care Environment (ATICE) [20], and the Nursing Instrument for the Communication of Sedation (NICS) [21]. Although each scale is unique, the over-all objective of the sedation scales is to allow for the assessment of goal-directed sedation for each patient. Although phrased differently, each scale has a value that represents calm and alert. Whereas the optimum level of sedation may be 'awake and cooperative', needs may vary greatly among ICU patients. Sedatives are often administered for therapeutic reasons other than sedation. Examples include reduction of cerebral metabolic rate of oxygen consumption and subsequent lowering of intracranial pressure (ICP), ventilator dysynchrony, or withdrawal syndromes. Thus, it is imperative to use a scale that can represent many levels of sedation, as targets may differ depending on the therapeutic intent.

Other objective tools have been studied for the assessment of sedation in critically ill patients. One that has perhaps received the most attention is the bispectral index, a cerebral function monitor that uses data based on the raw electroencephalograph (EEG) to quantify a patient's level of arousal. The bispectral index allows for continuous monitoring of sedation with the benefit of assigning an ordinal score to relative EEG wave form activity that lacks the subjectivity of the sedation scales. This technology has been used to assess depth of anesthesia in the operating room and has been shown, in that arena, to have reduced the number of episodes of intraoperative awareness [22]. The bispectral index has also been studied in the ICU in several populations of patients including medical, brain-injured and cardiac surgery patients and has been tested against several different sedation scales, including the visual analog scales, the Ramsey scale, RASS and SAS [23–26]. Although the bispectral index correlates to varying degrees with validated sedation scales, the wide-spread use of bispectral index for ICU sedation has not been adopted for monitoring in the ICU, predominantly because of motor artifacts in non-paralyzed patients, and the lack of data demonstrating improved outcomes when bispectral index technology is used over standard sedation scales. Bispectral index monitors have found a unique niche in patients requiring sedation with concurrent neuromuscular blockers, in whom other validated sedation scales would not apply.

Monitoring Cognition

Because of increased awareness of the neurocognitive complications of critical illness, evaluating and maintaining cognition in the ICU has also received considerable recent attention. Cognitive dysfunction can occur as a result of primary neurological disorders (e.g., stroke, head injury), or secondary neurologic complications resulting from critical illness (e.g., delirium, encephalopathy, hypoxia). Delirium, perhaps the best studied etiology of ICU-related neurocognitive dysfunction, is defined by the Diagnostic and Statistical Manual for Mental Disorders as the following: A disturbance of consciousness with reduced ability to focus, sustain or shift attention; a change in cognition or the development of a perceptual disturbance; a disturbance with a rapid onset and fluctuating nature; evidence that the disruption is caused by either a general medical condition, intoxication or drug-withdrawal [27]. The Confusion Assessment Method for the ICU (CAM-ICU) is a validated tool developed to screen patients for delirium, including patients who are unable to communicate verbally because of intubation [27, 28]. CAM-ICU uses the following to identify delirium: Acute onset or fluctuating mental status, inattention, disorganized thinking, and an altered level of consciousness [27, 28]. Not only is CAM-ICU a validated assessment of delirium, but it has also been shown to be a predictor of outcomes in ventilated and non-ventilated patients [29, 30]. Other validated delirium screening tools include the Intensive Care Delirium Screening Checklist (ICDSC) [31]. One potential advantage of the ICDSC compared to the CAM-ICU is that it permits a continuous or graded assessment of delirium (score 0 to 8), as opposed to a categorical assignment, thus offering the advantage of identifying patients with subsyndromal delirium, who are also at risk of poor neurocognitive outcomes. Although studies have shown that delirium is a predictor of poor outcome, it remains unknown whether prevention or appropriate treatment will result in improved outcomes, and this important issue is worthy of further research. Whereas validated tools exist to detect the presence or absence of delirium in the ICU (one potential cause of cognitive dysfunction), limited tools are available at present outside of a formal neurological exam to monitor or quantify cognition itself in the critically ill.

One standard tool that offers a rapid assessment of cognition over a period of 5 to 10 minutes is the Mini Mental State Exam (MMSE), which divides cognition into 5 domains: Orientation, registration, attention and calculation, recall and language [32]. This scale was developed primarily as a screening tool for the presence of dementia in outpatients, and application of this instrument in the ICU is difficult given the requirement for verbal responses. The Adapted Cognitive Exam (ACE) is a scale that has recently been developed and validated to evaluate cognition in the critically ill [33]. It was modeled on the MMSE using the same five domains, but tailored to critically ill patients in such a way that it could be performed in patients who were non-verbal. Like the MMSE, it evaluates cognition on a numerical scale. The ACE has many potential clinical applications, and is an important measurement tool that can be applied to help better understand the continuum of neurocognitive sequelae starting at entry to the ICU through recovery and long-term follow up. This scale was utilized in the ANIST study to assess the differential effects on cognition of two different sedatives (dexmedetomidine and propofol) administered to achieve the same level of sedation. [15].

Sedative Agents

Many agents have been used for sedation, analgesia, and anxiolysis in the ICU. The most frequently used agents include members of the following drug or drug classes: Opioid, benzodiazepines, propofol and dexmedetomidine. When choosing an agent for ICU sedation, multiple factors must be taken into consideration. Typical considerations include indication for sedation, onset of action, duration of action, route of elimination, drug interactions, and adverse effects. We submit that another (perhaps less commonly considered) criteria be considered: The potential impact of the sedative on cognition and neurological sequelae, and the likelihood of the agent (appropriately dosed) to achieve a state of 'cooperative sedation'. A comprehensive review of the pharmacokinetics and dynamics of these medications is beyond the scope of this review; however, details for individual agents can be found in **Table 1** [34].

Comparative Trials

Despite the many options for sedative agents, no one agent has been identified as superior in all cases. There are, however, several important trials comparing agents. The Maximizing Efficacy of Targeted Sedation and Reducing Neurological Dysfunction (MENDS) trial was the first randomized, double-blind trial evaluating the effect of sedative agents on delirium-free and coma-free days [35]. The two agents compared in this trail were lorazepam and dexmedetomidine. For the primary outcome, use of dexmedetomidine was associated with a greater number

Table 1. Key characteristics of agents commonly used for sedation in intensive care unit (ICU) patients

Drug	Type of medication	Sedation	Analgesia	Mechanism of action	Advantages	Adverse effects
Fentanyl	Opioid	+	+++	Mu receptor agonist	Reversible, rapid onset, short duration	Respiratory depression, chest wall rigidity, gastric dysmotility, hypotension
Remi-fentanil	Opioid	+	+++	Mu receptor agonist	Reversible, rapid onset, short duration	Respiratory depression, chest wall rigidity, gastric dysmotility, hypotension
Morphine sulfate	Opioid	+	+++	Mu receptor agonist	Reversible	Respiratory depression, gastric dysmotility, hypotension, hallucinations
Diazepam	Benzodiazepine	+++	+	GABA$_a$ receptor agonist	Reversible	Respiratory depression, hypotension, confusion
Lorazepam	Benzodiazepine	+++	–	GABA$_a$ receptor agonist	Reversible	Respiratory depression, hypotension, confusion
Midazolam	Benzodiazepine	+++	–	GABA$_a$ receptor agonist	Reversible, shorter duration, and titratable	Respiratory depression, hypotension, confusion
Dexmedetomidine	Alpha-2 agonist	++	++	Alpha-2 receptor agonist (pre- and post-synaptic	Maintains cognitive function	Dry mouth, bradycardia, hypotension, adrenal suppression, atrial fibrillation
Propofol		+++	–	Unclear	Very short duration, easy to titrate	Hypotension, respiratory depression, metabolic acidosis, rhabdomyolysis, anaphylaxis, sepsis, pain at injection site

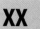

of delirium-free and coma-free days; however, this difference was driven by the number of coma-free days, as the number of delirium-free days was similar between groups. No differences in outcomes, including duration of mechanical ventilation, ICU LOS, or 28-day mortality were seen. One major limitation of the trial was the depth of sedation, which was chosen by the primary team. Baseline RASS scores for the dexmedetomidine and lorazepam groups were -3 and -4 respectively [35]. Had lighter or 'cooperative' sedation goals been achieved (closer to 0 to -1), the incidence of drug-induced coma would likely have been less (particularly with lorazepam), and results may have differed. Another recent randomized, double-blind trial, the Safety and Efficacy of Dexmedetomidine Compared with Midazolam (SEDCOM) trial, compared midazolam to dexmedetomidine [36], requiring daily awakening trials and a targeted RASS score of -2 to +1. The primary outcome was percent time within RASS goal and secondary outcomes included assessment of delirium, duration of mechanical ventilation and ICU LOS. Whereas there was no difference in the primary outcome, patients in the dexmedetomidine group had a lower prevalence of delirium and a larger number of delirium-free days. In addition, patients sedated with dexmedetomidine had a shorter time to extubation [36].

A final study that further highlights the additional cognitive benefits of dexmedetomidine was conducted as a double blind, cross-over trial that compared dexmedetomidine to propofol [15]. The primary endpoint of the ANIST trial was the change in cognition (as measured by the 100-point ACE test) with dexmedetomidine as compared to propofol. Patients were randomized to either dexmedetomidine or propofol to start, and after an appropriate washout period, switched to the other agent. Cognitive assessments were performed at baseline, after the washout phase, and on each drug (RASS = 0 to -1) [15]. Sedation with propofol diminished ACE scores on average by 12.4 points, whereas dexmedetomidine improved patient cognition by 6.8 points (difference in cognitive score = 19.2 [95 % CI 12.3–26.1, p < 0.001]). These results are important, and illustrate the differential impact of two different sedative agents (titrated to the same level of sedation) on cognition.

In general, benzodiazepines are thought to be the most closely associated with delirium, as supported by the SEDCOM trial [36], although other data have linked benzodiazepines and opioids to the onset and increased duration of delirium [37]. Although propofol is not associated with delirium, it does affect cognition as shown in the ANIST study [15]. Dexmedetomidine is superior to the alternatives when preservation of cognition and avoidance of delirium is necessary. Low dose opioid infusions may also be able to achieve this in certain patients.

Practical Considerations

Despite recommendations for daily interruption of sedation and protocol-driven sedation, survey data suggest that clinical practice lags behind the evidence. The use of daily interruption for patients receiving continuous infusions occurs inconsistently, with surveys reporting 40 to 62 % rates of compliance [38–41]. In addition, despite the perception that sedation scales are beneficial, only 47 – 60 % of ICUs had implemented sedation protocols at the time of the survey [39–41], and 85.6 % of physicians in a Brazilian survey indeed believed their patients were usually over-sedated [41]. The same survey reported sedation levels being assessed 2 times or less per day in over 50 % of patients.

Nursing support of sedation strategies is crucial since they are the providers implementing the sedation plan. According to a survey, most critical care nurses believe that sedation is necessary when patients are intubated, and some reported feeling influenced by family members of patients as it relates to sedation practices [42]. The impact of staffing and the pressure of performing other nursing functions were identified as influences for one-third of nurses [42]. Nurses are at the patient end of a caring and compassionate group of health care providers, so the reason behind light sedation, and the likely greater nursing effort involved, must be appropriately communicated at the time the plan is made.

Although light or 'cooperative' sedation necessitates an increased level of vigilance, the heightened awareness and intellectual capacity promotes patient autonomy. Despite the potential need for restraints in some circumstances, reduction in sedation may permit patients to be more involved in decision-making as it relates to their own healthcare. Some patients in fact may be appropriate candidates for the no-sedation strategies that showed improved outcome in one study [6]; but it is important to evaluate the safety measures of that group before implementing such a protocol. For example, Strom and colleagues [6] implemented the protocol of no-sedation in a unit where all patients had 1:1 nursing care, plus an additional person in the ICU to 'calm patients'. Some units may have to increase staffing in order to accommodate this practice; however, it may yet be a cost effective strategy considering the improved outcomes observed. Another intervention, early mobilization, requires a multidisciplinary team to execute safely and effectively, yet some investigators have found that implementing strategies for early mobilization is feasible without increase ICU staffing [11].

As far as which sedatives to consider, dexmedetomidine has been shown to be beneficial for general cognition, as measured by the ACE, and for minimizing delirium, although more costly than other sedative agents. As with any agent, careful consideration of a drug usage policy must consider cost-effectiveness, ensuring optimal use of the drug to maximize drug-related outcomes.

Conclusion

Despite data suggesting significant improvements with daily awakening trials and early mobilization, these practices are far from being universally adopted in critical care units. Implementation of these interventions into standard practice in individual ICUs takes the effort of a multidisciplinary team and in some cases increases expenditures for institutions. However, with the potential improvement in outcomes, these interventions have the potential to be cost-effective and have a positive impact on patient outcomes above and beyond ICU survival. The neurocognitive effects of critical illness continue to gain recognition and represent an area ripe for continued research. Existing data suggest that the choice of sedative and sedation strategy can have an impact on cognition, duration of ventilation, and outcomes in acute illness. Further research is needed to identify whether active strategies to minimize or treat cognitive abnormalities during the ICU stay will translate to better neurocognitive outcomes in the long term.

References

1. Hopkins RO, Brett S (2005) Chronic neurocognitive effects of critical illness. Curr Opin Crit Care 11: 369–375
2. Newman MF, Kirchner JL, Phillips-Bute B, et al (2001) Longitudinal assessment of neurocognitive function after coronary-artery bypass surgery. N Engl J Med 344: 395–402
3. Hopkins RO, Weaver LK, Pope D, Orme JF, Bigler ED, Larson-Lohr V (1999) Neuropsychological sequelae and impaired health status in survivors of severe acute respiratory distress syndrome. Am J Respir Crit Care Med 160: 50–56
4. Kress JP, Pohlman AS, O'Connor MF, Hall JB (2000) Daily interruption of sedative infusions in critically ill patients undergoing mechanical ventilation. N Engl J Med 342: 1471–1477
5. Girard TD, Kress JP, Fuchs BD, et al (2008) Efficacy and safety of a paired sedation and ventilator weaning protocol for mechanically ventilated patients in intensive care (Awakening and Breathing Controlled trial): a randomized controlled trial. Lancet 371: 126–134
6. Strom T, Martinussen T, Toft P (2010) A protocol of no sedation for critically ill patients receiving mechanical ventilation: a randomized trial. Lancet 375: 475–480
7. Jackson JC, Hart RP, Gordon SM, Hopkins RO, Girard TD, Ely EW (2007) Post-traumatic stress disorder and post-traumatic stress symptoms following critical illness in medical intensive care unit patients: assessing the magnitude of the problem. Crit Care 11: R27

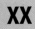

8. Kress JP, Gehlback B, Lacy M, Pliskin N, Pohlman AS, Hall JB (2003) The long-term psychological effects of daily sedative interruption on critically ill patients. Am J Respir Crit Care Med 168: 1457–1461

9. Rochester CL (2009) Rehabilitation in the intensive care unit. Semin Respir Crit Care Med 30: 656–669

10. Herridge MS, Cheung AM, Tansey CM, et al (2003) One year outcomes in survivors of the acute respiratory distress syndrome. N Engl J Med 348: 683–693

11. Bailey P, Thomsen GE, Spuhler VJ, et al (2007) Early activity is feasible and safe in respiratory failure patients. Crit Care Med 35: 139–145

12. Thomsen GE, Snow GL, Rodriguez L, Hopkins RO (2008) Patients with respiratory failure increase ambulation after transfer to an intensive care unit where early activity is a priority. Crit Care Med 36: 1119–1124

13. Morris PE, Goad A, Thompson C, et al (2008) Early intensive care unit mobility therapy in the treatment of acute respiratory failure. Crit Care Med 36: 2238–2243

14. Schweikert WD, Pohlman MC, Pohlman AS, et al (2009) Early physical and occupational therapy in mechanically ventilated, critically ill patients: a randomized controlled trial. Lancet 373: 1874–1882

15. Mirski MA, Lewin JJ, LeDroux S, et al (2010) Cognitive improvement during continuous sedation in critically ill, awake and responsive patients: the Acute Neurological ICU Sedation Trial (ANIST). Intensive Care Med 36: 1505–1513

16. Sessler CN, Gosnell MS, Grap MJ, et al (2002) The Richmond Agitation-Sedation Scale: validity and reliability in adult intensive care unit patients. Am J Respir Crit Care Med 166: 1338–1344

17. Ely EW, Truman B, Shintani A, et al (2003) Monitoring sedation status over time in ICU patients: reliability and validity of the Richmond Agitation-Sedation Scale (RASS). JAMA 289: 2983–2991

18. Riker RR, Picard JT, Fraser GL (1999) Prospective evaluation of the Sedation-Agitation Scale for the adult critically ill patients. Crit Care Med 27: 1325–1329

19. Devlin JW, Boleski G, Mlynarek M, et al (1999) Motor Activity Assessment Scale: avalid and reliable sedation scale for use with mechanically ventilated patients in an adult surgical intensive care unit. Crit Care Med 27: 1271–1275

20. De Jonghe B, Cook D, Griffith L, et al (2003) Adaptation to the intensive care environment (ATICE): development and validation of a new sedation assessment instrument. Crit Care Med 31: 2344–2354

21. Mirski MA, LeDroux SN, Lewin JJ, Thompson CB, Mirski KT, Griswold M. (2010) Validity and reliability of an intuitive conscious sedation scoring tool: The nursing instrument for the communication of sedation. Crit Care Med 38: 1674–1684

22. Myles PS, Leslie K, McNeil J, et al (2004) Bispectral index monitoring to prevent awareness during anaesthesia: the B-Aware randomized controlled trial. Lancet 363: 1757–1763

23. Deogaonkar A, Gupta R, DeGorgia M, et al (2004) Bispectral index monitoring correlates with sedation scales in brain-injured patients. Crit Care Med 32: 2403–2406

24. Olson DM, Thoyre SM, Peterson ED, Graffagnino C. (2009) A randomized evaluation of bispectral index-augmented sedation assessment in neurological patients. Neurocrit Care 11: 20–27

25. Riker RR, Fraser GL, Simmons LE, Wilkins ML (2001) Validating the sedation-agitation scale with the bispectral index and visual analog scale in adult ICU patients after cardiac surgery. Intensive Care Med 27: 853–858

26. Karachandani K, Rewari V, Trikha A, Batra RK (2010) Bispectral index correlates well with Richmond agitation sedation scale in mechanically ventilated critically ill patients. JAnesth 24: 394–398

27. Ely EW, Margolin R, Francis J, et al (2001) Evaluation of delirium in critically ill patients: validation of the confusion assessment method for the intensive care unit (CAM-ICU). Crit Care Med 29: 1370–1379

28. Ely EW, Inouye SK, Bernard GR, et al (2001) Delirium in mechanically ventilated patients: validity and reliability of the confusion assessment method for the intensive care unit (CAM-ICU). JAMA 286: 2703–2710

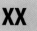

29. Ely WE, Shintani A, Truman B, et al (2004) Delirium as a predictor of mortality in mechanically ventilated patients in the intensive care unit. JAMA 291: 1753–1762

30. Thomason JWW, Shintani A, Peterson JF, Pun BT, Jackson JC, Ely WE (2005) Intensive care unit delirium is an independent predictor of longer hospital stay: a prospective analysis of 261 non-ventilated patients. Crit Care 9: R375–R381

31. Ouimet S, Riker R, Bergeron N, Cossette M, Kavanagu B, Skrobik Y (2007) Subsyndromal delirium in the ICU: evidence for a disease spectrum. Intensive Care Med 33: 1007–1013

32. Folstein MF, Folstein SE, McHugh PR (1975) Mini-Mental State: a practical method for grading the cognitive state of patients for the clinician. J Psychiat Res 12: 189–198

33. Lewin JJ, LeDroux SN, Shermock KM, et al (2012) Validity and reliability of The Johns Hopkins Adapted Cognitive Exam for critically ill patients. Crit Care Med 40: 139–144

34. Mirski MA, Lewin JJ (2007) Sedation and analgesia for the critically ill patient. Contemp Crit Care 4: 1–12

35. Pandharipande PP, Pun BT, Herr DL, et al (2007) Effect of sedation with dexemedetomidine vs lorazepam on acute brain dysfunction in mechanically ventilated patients: the MENDS randomized controlled trial. JAMA 298: 2644–2653

36. Riker RR, Shehabi Y, Bokesch PM, et al (2009) Dexmedetomidine vs midazolam for sedation of critically ill patients. JAMA 301: 489–499

37. Pisani MA, Murphy TE, Araujo KL, Slattum P, Van Ness PH, Inouye SK (2009) Benzodiazepine and opioid use and the duration of intensive care unit delirium in an older population. Crit Care Med 37: 177–183

38. Mehta S, Burry L, Fischer S, et al (2006) Canadian survey of the use of sedatives, analgesics, and neuromuscular blocking agents in critically ill patients. Crit Care Med 34: 374–380

39. O'Connor M, Bucknall T, Manias E (2010) Sedation management in Australian and New Zealand intensive care units: doctors' and nurses' practices and opinions. Am J Crit Care 19: 285–295

40. Salluh JIF, Dal-Pizzol F, Mello PVC, et al (2009) Delirium recognition and sedation practices in critically ill patients: a survey on the attitudes of 1015 Brazilian critical care physicians. J Crit Care 24: 556–562

41. Tanios MA, de Wit M, Epstein SK, Devlin JW (2009) Preceived barriers to the use of sedation protocols and daily interruptions: a multidisciplinary survey. J Crit Care 24: 66–73

42. Guttormson JL, Chlan L, Weinert C, Savik K (2010) Factors influencing nurse sedation practices with mechanically ventilated patients: a US national survey. Intensive Crit Care Nurs 26: 44–50

XXI Management, Method and Morale

Pre-hospital Care and Orientation of Critically Ill Geriatric Patients

J. Mantz, F.-X. Duchateau, and A. Burnod

Introduction

The pre-hospital emergency medical service (EMS) is often the first to intervene in life-threatening events in elderly persons. Elderly persons are defined by the World Health Organization (WHO) as patients aged > 75 years. However, emergency calls for patients aged 80 years or greater are very common in Western countries. This patient subpopulation is a high-risk one and requires particularly close attention in healthcare management. These patients are characterized by a decrease in functional organ reserve and a higher susceptibility to insult, which make them at particularly high risk of mortality or disability. A particularly important point that should be taken into account at the very early stage of resuscitation is the ability of these patients not only to survive, but also to achieve a sufficient level of autonomy after recovery which enables an acceptable quality of life. This fact raises complex and interesting issues related to ethics, economy, medical and social environments. Therefore, the possibility of limitation of aggressive therapy should be kept in mind during all EMS medical interventions for geriatric critically ill patients. In this brief review, we will discuss the management and the elements of decision-making that enable appropriate pre-hospital and in-hospital orientation of critically ill patients. We will pay particular attention to frequent situations encountered with elderly patients, i.e., cardiac arrest, coronary artery disease and trauma.

A Physician-based Pre-hospital EMS for Critically Ill Geriatric Persons

Unlike the situation in the US, French EMSs are characterized by the presence of physicians on scene at the early stage of resuscitation. This organization allows intensive care strategies (tracheal intubation, non-invasive or invasive mechanical ventilation, central venous access, administration of vasoactive agents...) to be delivered on-scene. However, whether this medical organization of pre-hospital emergency care has a positive impact on patient outcome (elderly patients or not) compared to a paramedic-based one remains to be established.

There is general agreement in the French emergency medical community that medicalized mobile intensive care units (ICUs) should be the first response to a life-threatening situation in the pre-hospital setting, and that age should not be a limitation to this strategy [1]. One of the main reasons for this accord is the difficulty in rapidly obtaining sufficient information during emergency calls to determine whether or not an emergency physician is required on scene. This task is

J.-L. Vincent (ed.), *Annual Update in Intensive Care and Emergency Medicine 2012*
DOI 10.1007/978-3-642-25716-2 © Springer-Verlag Berlin Heidelberg 2012

assigned on scene to the medical emergency team. Sometimes, the pathological context of the patient is available (e.g., an elderly patient being handled in a palliative care network), which should theoretically facilitate a decision not to undertake resuscitation maneuvers. Except in these specific situations, the presence of the EMS on scene allows both a medical evaluation of the context and an immediate therapeutic response to the life-threatening event [2]. Telemedicine offers a promising approach for the future in this regard.

These considerations support and justify a principle of early and full involvement of the EMS in out-of-hospital life-threatening situations, independent of age. A growing body of recent work suggests that on-scene medical intervention by the EMS in patients > 80 years presenting with a life-threatening situation (except cardiac arrest) has a positive impact on outcome. Three-month mortality in such patients was not significantly different from a control elderly patient population. Moreover, rapid return to the place of residence and recovery of satisfactory autonomy were observed in those patients who survived the initial episode [3, 4]. Of note, autonomy and functional capacity represent the cornerstones of quality of life in elderly subjects [5]. Interestingly, medical intervention by the EMS was found to be a predictor of survival at 3 months, which supports the role of medicalized pre-hospital emergency care in older persons [3, 4]. In some specific acute diseases, such as acute pulmonary edema, the in-hospital mortality rate in patients having undergone pre-hospital emergency tracheal intubation and mechanical ventilation was not increased in patients aged 75 years or more in comparison with younger patients (26 %) [6]. Interestingly, in this study, not only survival, but also functional recovery, was found to be satisfactory at distance from the acute event [6].

Chest pain related to coronary artery disease is a major cause of EMS calls in the elderly. However, elderly patients are frequently excluded from randomized controlled trials (RCTs) and specific data in this area can be obtained from prospective cohorts only. The higher mortality rates from acute coronary artery disease in older patients is related in part to poor access to reperfusion techniques [7]. Nevertheless, after adjustment for the delay in reperfusion, age remains a predictor of mortality in patients undergoing early coronary revascularization (3.5 % < 65 years, 9.2 % from 65 to 74 years, 15.2 % from 75 to 84 years, 28.9 % ≥ 85 years; p < 0.0001) [8]. Early management of out-of-hospital elderly persons requiring coronary revascularization by the EMS improves access to reperfusion techniques within the delays recommended by the guidelines [9]. This reasoning applies to the situation of acute stroke as well. Age is no longer an absolute contraindication to reperfusion, at least until 3-hours post-stroke onset [10]. In patients who are not eligible for early reperfusion, a positive impact on outcome has been demonstrated from specialized care at the early stage of stroke [11].

In-hospital Orientation of Elderly Critically Ill Patients

There is no reason to believe that geriatric patients requiring emergency admission into a specialized unit should be oriented differently simply because of their age. Further supporting this statement, it has been recently demonstrated that in selected patients aged > 80 years with good functional status who were directly admitted to an emergency cardiology unit for acute heart disease, the mortality rate remained remarkably low (13 %) [12]. Interestingly, no decrease in autonomy was observed in this study [12]. The real life situation, however, remains somewhat different. In many cases, intensivists remain reluctant to admit elderly patients into the ICU immediately after management by the pre-hospital EMS, simply because of their age [13]. This is noticeable for patients aged 70 years or more, particularly when ICU beds are overbooked [14]. The main argument supporting this behavior is that elderly patients exhibit a higher in-ICU mortality rate than younger ones [15]. It should be acknowledged that not all elderly persons presenting with life-threatening organ failure should be admitted to an ICU. The role of the EMS in evaluating the patient's previous functional status and autonomy, cognitive functions and comorbidities is crucial, because it may help to make the 'correct' decision whether or not to admit the patient to an ICU [16]. This goal can be achieved only when clear information on the patient's autonomy and previous health status is delivered to the EMS.

XXI

The ADL (Activity of Daily Living) index consists of simple items of daily life, which are generally easily available (**Table 1**) [17]. Use of the ADL index has become increasingly popular in the context of pre-hospital emergency medicine because it appears to be highly reproducible [4]. In contrast, reliable evaluation of a patient's cognitive status in the context of an out-of-hospital emergency intervention is particularly difficult. Most of the usual cognitive tasks used for this purpose in the geriatric population are simply not usable in the context of a life-threatening emergency situation. Therefore, the only available information is generally a binary yes/no response to the question "Did the patient exhibit alterations of his/her cognitive functions before?" [12]. It is important that the decision to admit to an ICU should be considered with caution in elderly patients in whom a complete ICU process appears unreasonable. Such patient subpopulations are those patients in whom cumulative comorbidities markedly increase the risk of ICU mortality, patients with early signs of pejorative outcome, or patients (such as those with end-stage cancer) in whom initiation of invasive critical care can be considered as unreasonable according to the French law of April 22, 2005 [18]. Contact with the attending physician in charge of the patient may be helpful in collecting reliable information on the patient's previous health status. In some cases, patients themselves may have clearly stated whether or not they would be willing to undergo invasive critical care.

Similar to a decision of limitation of care in the ICU, the decision whether or not to admit a geriatric critically ill patient to the ICU should never be taken on a single physician's opinion. This is a challenging issue in the context of out-of-hospital emergency situations, particularly when the patient's physician cannot

Table 1. The items of the Activity of Daily Living (ADL) scale [17].

Item	No autonomy (0 point)	Partial dependency (0.5 point)	Total dependency (1 point)
Body care			
Dressing			
Go to the bathroom			
Transfer			
Continence			
Eating			

The maximum score is 6 (full autonomy), the minimum is zero (no autonomy).

be reached at the moment of decision. The senior physician responsible for the regulation of emergency medical calls, or the intensivist contacted to manage the patient once admitted into the ICU, represent valuable alternatives for this purpose [19]. In cases where there is a consensus not to undertake resuscitation maneuvers or not to admit the patient to the ICU, active limitation of healthcare may be acceptable in the pre-hospital setting. Nevertheless, when such a decision remains unclear, an interesting strategy consists of using non-invasive, reversible maneuvers by the EMS, such as non-invasive ventilation, which can help maintain vital functions during transportation to the hospital where a collective discussion of cessation of these life-sustaining treatments can be initiated with more available information, including response to the first resuscitation maneuvers [20].

Specific Situations

Acute Cardiac Failure

It is remarkable that in elderly patients with good prior autonomy and health status who are directly admitted to an ICU for an acute life-threatening disease of cardiac origin, survival rate and functional outcome are excellent [12]. This observation provides strong support for these patients to receive optimal cardiologic intensive care at the early stage of their disease. We, therefore, share the view that no difference in the pre-hospital orientation of these patients should be made on the basis of age. This strategy seems to have gained popularity among physicians of French EMSs. In a recent study, patients aged 80 and more with pre-hospital acute coronary syndrome had similar reperfusion delays and treatments to younger patients [9].

Severe Trauma

Severe trauma represents an increasing cause of transfer to the ICU in elderly persons. Unlike the younger population, fall is the main cause of trauma in elderly patients (84 % of accidents after 65 years of age) [21]. Several lines of evidence support that mortality and functional outcome are worse in elderly trauma patients than in younger ones, after adjustment for the mechanisms of injury [22–27]. There are several explanations for this detrimental impact of aging on outcome in the context of trauma: Pre-existing comorbidities have been shown to significantly contribute to increased mortality rates in this patient subpopulation. In addition, aging is associated with a decrease in physiological organ reserve and compensatory mechanisms involved in stress situations: A decrease in heart rate, cardiac output and sympathetic reactivity as well as an increase in baseline vascular resistances and altered oxygen delivery account for poor compensation to acute hemorrhage [28–30]. This effect emphasizes the importance of maintaining normovolemia and optimal tissue oxygen delivery at the early stage of trauma hemorrhagic shock [31]. Moreover, elderly patients often receive polymedication, and their liver metabolism and glomerular filtration are decreased. This factor makes elderly patients more prone than younger subjects to develop drug toxicity. When management of severe trauma at the early stage is successful, a precise evaluation of the former autonomy and ability to walk of the patient (number of falls/month) is needed to optimize healthcare of rehabilitation.

Cardiac Arrest

The prognosis of out-of-hospital cardiac arrest in elderly patients is poor, as is the case in younger patient populations. Of note, however, the increase in the mortality rate of cardiac arrest attributable to aging is not of major importance. The main predictors of survival are, as in younger populations, rapidity of initiation of resuscitation maneuvers, quality of chest compression, and the nature of the initial rhythm [32, 33]. In a previous study conducted in elderly patients with cardiac arrest, age > 80 was a reason for not undertaking resuscitation maneuvers. However, when resuscitation was undertaken, results were encouraging, because recovery of spontaneous cardiac activity was obtained in 39 % of the patients, and 6 % of these patients survived without sequelae [34].

XXI

Conclusion

Older persons represent a growing patient subpopulation. There is no justification that age *per se* should be a cut-off for limitation of healthcare, and particularly critical care. A large body of recent work supports that older patients should benefit from the same standard of care as younger ones. The key issue of correct patient selection is particularly complex in the context of pre-hospital emergency medicine, because the decision to admit to an ICU for a life-threatening acute disorder or to limit active therapeutics requires a large panel of information, which is often not available in such a short period of time. Such decisions should not be based on an individual physician's opinion.

References

1. Lapandry C (2003) Décision de réanimation préhospitalière chez le sujet âgé. In: Gueugniaud PY (ed) Médecine d'Urgence 2003. 45e Congrès National d'Anesthésie et de Réanimation. Elsevier, Paris, pp 21–28
2. Burnod A, Lenclud G, Ricard-Hibon A, Juvin P, Mantz J, Duchateau FX (2012) Collaboration between emergency medical teams and palliative networks allows a better respect of a patient's will. Eur J Emerg Med 19: 46–47
3. Duchateau FX, Burnod A, Dahmani S, Delpierre S, Ricard-Hibon A, Mantz J (2008) Out-of-hospital interventions by the French Emergency Medical Service are associated with a high survival in patients aged 80 year or over. Intensive Care Med 34: 1544–1545
4. Duchateau FX, Burnod A, Josseaume J, Pariente D, Mantz J (2010) The benefits of out-hospital Advanced life support in elderly persons. J Am Geriat Soc 58: 606–608
5. Matsubayashi K, Okumiya K, Osaki Y, Fujisawa M, Doi Y (1997) Quality of life of old people living in the community. Lancet 350: 1521–1522
6. Adnet F, Le Toumelin P, Leberre A, et al (2001) In-hospital and long-term prognosis of elderly patients requiring endotracheal intubation for life-threatening presentation of cardiogenic pulmonary edema. Crit Care Med 29: 891–895
7. Schuler J, Maier B, Behrens S, Thimme W (2006) Present treatment of acute myocardial infarction in patients over 75 years--data from the Berlin Myocardial Infarction Registry (BHIR). Clin Res Cardiol 95: 360–367
8. Newell MC, Henry JT, Henry TD, et al (2011) Impact of age on treatment and outcomes in ST-elevation myocardial infarction. Am Heart J 161: 664–672
9. Duchateau FX, Ricard-Hibon A, Devaud ML, Burnod A, Mantz J (2006) Does age influence quality of care in acute myocardial infarction in the prehospital setting. Am J Emerg Med 24: 512
10. Lees KR, Bluhmki E, von Kummer R, et al (2010) Time to treatment with intravenous alteplase and outcome in stroke: an updated pooled analysis of ECASS, ATLANTIS, NINDS, and EPITHET trials. Lancet 375: 1695–1703

11. Wahlgren N, Ahmed N, Eriksson N, et al (2008) Multivariable analysis of outcome predictors and adjustment of main outcome results to baseline data profile in randomized controlled trials: Safe Implementation of Thrombolysis in Stroke MOnitoring STudy (SITS-MOST). Stroke. 39: 3316–3322

12. Josseaume J, Duchateau FX, Burnod A, et al (2011) Observatoire du sujet âgé de plus de 80 ans pris en charge en urgence par le service mobile d'urgence et de réanimation. Ann Fr Anesth Réanim 30: 553–558

13. Duchateau FX, Pasgrimaud L, Devoir C, Ricard-Hibon A, Mantz J (2006) L'âge influence-t-il l'admission des patients en réanimation après une prise en charge par le Smur ? Ann Fr Anesth Réanim 25: 1011–1018

14. Nucton TJ, List D. Age as a factor in critical care unit admission (1995). Arch Intern Med 155: 1087–1092

15. Chelluri L, Pinsky MR, Grevik A (1992) Outcome of intensive care of the « oldest-old » critically ill patients. Crit Care Med 20: 757–761

16. Muller L, Lenfant JY, Gache A, de La Coussaye JE (2003). Critères d'admission du sujet âgé en réanimation. In: Gueugniaud PY (ed) Médecine d'Urgence. 45e Congrès National d'Anesthésie et de Réanimation. Elsevier, Paris, pp 29–37

17. Katz S, Ford AB, Moskowitz RW, Jackson BA, Jaffe MW (1963). Studies of illness in the aged. The index of ADL: a standardized measure of biological and psychosocial function. JAMA 185: 914–919

18. Loi n°2005–370 du Code de la Santé Publique du 22 avril 2005 relative aux droits des malades et à la fin de vie. Available at: http://www.legifrance.gouv.fr/affichTexte.do?cidTexte=JORFTEXT000000446240&dateTexte Accessed Nov 2011

19. Duchateau FX, Burnod A, Ricard-Hibon A, Mantz J, Juvin P (2007) Withholding advanced cardiac life support in out-of-hospital cardiac arrest: A prospective study. Resuscitation 76: 134–136

20. Duchateau FX, Beaune S, Ricard-Hibon A, Mantz J, Juvin P (2010) Prehospital noninvasive ventilation can help in management of patients with limitations of life-sustaining treatments. Eur J Emerg Med 17: 7–9

21. Taylor MD, Tracy JK, Meyer W, Pasquale M, Napolitano LM (2002) Trauma in the elderly: intensive care unit resource use and outcome. J Trauma 53: 407–414

22. Baker SP, O'Neil B, Haddon W Jr, Long WB (1974) The injury severity score: a method for describing patients with multiple injuries and evaluating emergency care. J Trauma 14: 187–196

23. Pellicane J, Byrne K, DeMaria E (1992) Preventable complications and death from multiple organ failure among geriatric trauma victims. J Trauma 33: 440–444

24. Lonner J, Koval K (1995) Polytrauma in the elderly. Clin Orthop Relat Res 318: 136–143

25. Smith D, Enderson B, Maull K (1990) Trauma in the elderly: determinants of outcome. South Med J 83: 171–177

26. McCoy GF, Johnston RA, Duthie RB (1989) Injury to the elderly in road trafic accidents. J Trauma 29: 494–497

27. Champion HR, Copes WS, Buyer D, Flanagan ME, Bain L, Sacco WJ (1989) Major trauma in geriatric patients. AM J Public Health 79: 1278–1282

28. Bessereau J, Elikessikian A, Querellou E, et al (2010) Traumatisme grave du sujet âgé. Maximaliste d'emblée...ou pas ! Revue de Gériatrie 35: 25–31

29. Horst HM, Obeid FN, Sorensen VJ, Bivins BA (1986) Factors influencing survival of elderly trauma patients. Crit Care Med 14: 681–684

30. Broos PL, Stappaerts KH, Rommens PM, Louette LK, Gruwez JA (1988). Polytrauma in patients of 65 and over. Injury patterns and outcome. Int Surg 73: 119–122

31. Broos PL, D'Hoore A, Vanderschot P, Rommens PM, Stappaerts KH (1993). Multiple trauma in elderly patients. Factors influencing outcome: importance of aggressive care. Injury 24: 365–388

32. Wuerz RC, Holliman CJ, Meador SA, et al (1995). Effect of age on prehospital cardiac resuscitation outcome. Am J Emerg Med 13: 389–391

33. Bonnin MJ, Pepe PE, Clark PS Jr (1993) Survival in the elderly after out-of-hospital cardiac arrest. Crit Care Med 11: 1645–1651

34. Duchateau FX, Burnod A, Josseaume J, Pariente D, Mantz J (2011) Cardiopulmonary resuscitation for very elderly patients. Eur J Emerg Med 18: 127–129

XXI

Total Rehabilitation of the Critically Ill

R.D. Griffiths, C. Jones, and A. Gilmore

Introduction

Total rehabilitation of critically ill patients requires a strategy in which the goal is to help recover the lives of patients and to return their well-being to the best that is possible [1]. The key lesson over the last 25 years, supported by the testimony of patients and their carers, is that the strategy must appreciate the myriad factors that impact physically, psychologically, emotionally and socially on the pathway back to health. Rehabilitation must start early within the intensive care unit (ICU) and involve the family and carers, because the effects of a critical illness are not merely experienced by the patient but have a deep impact on the family and the environment to which they will return. This underlines the fundamental difference between rehabilitation versus follow-up (**Table 1**); the latter is an inclusive but passive observational process of information gathering that may inform general outcome. Experience during and after an ICU stay shows that to recover lives one needs a distinct early active and selective decision-making process with a therapeutic strategy that starts within the ICU to optimize the recovery of the patient and the family following what most likely has been their most challenging life experience [2].

Table 1. Rehabilitation is not follow-up

ICU rehabilitation	ICU follow-up
Starts early within the ICU	Starts after the ICU stay
Primarily for individual patient benefit	For the benefit of future patients
Involves family and carers	Rarely involves families
Assessment for risk avoidance	Assessment of complications
Highly selective and specific	Inclusive and general
Screens to filter out and exclude	Screens to include
Highly pathology dictated	Generally pathology independent
Step-wise longitudinally	Cross-sectional and serial
Patient dictated, no set time points	Set time points, patient independent
Involves specific therapies as required	No therapy role, primarily observational

Recognizing the Need

Within the ICU, processes should be in place that can identify those most at risk of later problems and so allow planning to help and support recovery. It is not

J.-L. Vincent (ed.), *Annual Update in Intensive Care and Emergency Medicine 2012*
DOI 10.1007/978-3-642-25716-2 © Springer-Verlag Berlin Heidelberg 2012

difficult to recognize prolonged critical illness, major systemic sepsis, severe pulmonary dysfunction, profound weakness, coma and confusion. Similarly, patients who have required prolonged and heavy use of sedative drugs and those in whom early physiotherapy and mobilization have proved impractical and their illness has been characterized by immobility are easily identified. The same assessment process must also recognize that many ICU patients, especially those only having a brief stay in the ICU, are likely to need no additional rehabilitation support. Therefore, awareness and a clinical screening process within the ICU that recognizes those with persistent delirium (and other acute brain dysfunction), drug dependency or drug withdrawal issues or a history of anxiety or prior psychiatric illness and those lacking family or social support can be helpful. The full clinical assessment of depression and anxiety within the ICU can only be made once patients can verbalize again and obviously only once delirium is excluded. In contrast it is not difficult to recognize stress in their relatives; this can manifest in many patterns including avoidance, withdrawal and depression, sleep disturbance or overt anxiety and anger. Importantly, this assessment indicates whether relatives are coping or not with a devastating life experience. UK clinical guidelines suggest a clinical risk assessment and screening process should be maintained during an ICU stay and be formalized on leaving the ICU to plan for the physically immediately apparent (e.g., muscle weakness) and start screening for later developments (e.g., acute anxiety state) [3].

Acting Early

Prevention is always preferable and therapeutic measures shown to have profound effects on long-term recovery should start during the ICU stay. The immediacy of critical illness and its complex management has tended to obscure the perspective of critical care practitioners and marginalize those factors that impinge on long term well-being. Fortunately, there is an increasing emphasis on new sedation paradigms, drug avoidance, and reduced sedation, waking and weaning protocols, and early mobilization and delirium management.

Acting early by anticipating rehabilitation needs prepares the ground to which the patient will return. This means early handling of a relative's stress and the delivery of coping support to bring them into a 'culture of recovery and rehabilitation therapy'. The experienced ICU nurse both recognizes and can deliver valued coping support but must also promote this rehabilitation culture. Such a culture helps the family to understand, and even where appropriate, assist with physical, psychological and emotional support at all stages of recovery. As discussed later even when the patient is ventilated and unaware involvement of relatives or carers using a patient diary record not only delivers a tool that can be used later but may in itself be of benefit to relatives as something they can contribute to.

Strategic Management Within and After Intensive Care

The fundamental cultural change over the last 25 years has been the move to avoid immobility and an active program of mobilization within and after intensive care. The traditional model that a critically ill patient was ventilated, paralyzed and sedated and, therefore, immobilized until they left the ICU to then recover with 'bed rest' is fortunately now in the past. This change has come about by a better understanding of the harmful consequences of immobility and bed rest and benefits of maintaining activity. Sadly, also, the legacy of profound weakness and debility was not seen by ICU practitioners unless it directly impacted on weaning from the ventilator; rather it was left to ill-informed general ward staff and distressed relatives to cope with. With no discussion or strategy to assess its severity or any idea of the timescales of recovery, the patient and family had unrealistic expectations and disappointment ensued. Fortunately, understanding of ICU-acquired weakness [4] has matured with the recognition that muscle wasting can be ameliorated by passive [5] and active movement [6] and that preservation of neuromuscular activity and mobility has wider benefits on metabolism, immune function and cognitive function.

With the average age of the general population increasing, so the proportion of patients admitted to ICUs who are elderly and suffering from significant cardio-respiratory co-morbidity is also increasing [7]. Elderly patients will typically have less physical reserve and reduced muscle mass before ICU admission, and are subsequently more functionally debilitated by critical illness and immobility than younger patients. Although there is growing evidence that early mobilization and physical therapy within the intensive care setting is beneficial, there are few data supporting specific methods and these currently vary significantly between and even within countries [8]. Other evidence supporting post-ICU rehabilitation has tended to focus on pulmonary function and exercise capacity. Safety of mobilization and physical therapy strategies in ICU patients has thus far concentrated on the effects on hemodynamic and respiratory function [9].

The profound loss of muscle mass these patients experience is a major risk factor for subsequent falls [10], but there is currently a lack of physiological data demonstrating how these patients regain balance and gait control. The risk of falls occurring and their potential for significant morbidity is further increased by factors including neurocognitive disturbance, drug side effects and immobilized bone loss. If we are going to continue to improve our understanding of how to help patients regain mobility and function after critical illness as effectively and safely as possible, we need further research examining the relationship between intensive care-associated weakness and gait and balance recovery.

The culture of new sedation and waking protocols in ICU should be combined with early and active physiotherapy that continues as the patient leaves the ICU. This culture of rehabilitation therapy must transfer and be seen as important to the subsequent carers and relatives over the whole course of their recovery. To give a patient and relatives a realistic timescale of recovery, experience suggests, and in keeping with how muscle recovers, that a simple aid memoir on the time scale of recovery is that for a young patient each day in the ICU will need 1 week of recovery and for the older patient 2 weeks is needed for every day spent ill in the ICU.

Why Amnesia and Memory Matter

When planned, short-term amnesia for an unpleasant event is appropriate for elective surgery during which the recipient has a desire to be pain free, not distressed and holds an understanding of why and how long the duration will be, even if for 24 h. However, for the majority of emergency ICU patients, in particular sicker and longer-stay patients, memory disturbance and amnesia present a serious and under-appreciated problem. The impact of brain dysfunction during intensive care means that the intensive care experience is a mixture of amnesia or profound distortion in time, place and content, where even the reason for admission is not remembered. There are some patients who, despite having apparently been awake and aware while on the ICU, in later stages subsequently fail to maintain any memory of intensive care. Patients have been known to vigorously deny ever being in the ICU despite the assertion of their relatives. Any significant periods of amnesia have consequences later and are associated with an impact on well-being during recovery [11]. The most direct consequence of simple amnesia is the loss of the patient's own ability to place the changes that have occurred to them (e.g., wasting and weakness) into context and allow them to have an understanding of why it has happened and how they will recover [12]. Whereas this lack of understanding can be addressed by information and timescale discussion, poor memory retention in patients and stress in the relatives means it must be repeated many times.

The impact of the memory and experiences of the ICU stay are not merely academic but have an impact on subsequent recovery. Patient memories are highly abnormal because of acute brain dysfunction, most commonly manifesting as delirium and, apart from amnesia for real early ICU events, some patients have an experience dominated by frank delusions and later by highly distorted interpretations of events. It had been assumed that unpleasant ICU experiences may trigger acute stress reactions and lead to post-traumatic stress disorder (PTSD); however research has suggested that frightening delusional experiences, particularly associated with early amnesia are a strong predictor of PTSD and the relationship with real ICU experiences as a responsible factor is less distinct [13]. Earlier retrospective studies had associated unpleasant ICU experiences as a factor but subsequent prospective studies confirmed that the strongest direct associations with the development of PTSD were frightening delusional experiences followed by heavy sedation use [14]. Delusions are an important manifestation of acute brain dysfunction and result in an incidence of new PTSD in patients who stay more than a few days of about 10 %. For all patients, delusional experiences are vivid and strongly retained in memory over real events. To appreciate the significance of delusions, it is important to understand that for some they are not troubling but for others they are life-threatening in nature and where amnesic may be the only memory consistently retained of the critical illness.

General Principles

At its simplest level, the 'culture of recovery and rehabilitation therapy' needs to be continued as the patient progresses through intensive care, the hospital ward and home. A patient specific program that focuses on personal needs and goals should be established and incorporate review processes to recognize any evolving need using a combination of information, setting realistic goals and timescales, positive reinforcement, normalizing issues of distress and supporting effective coping mechanisms, and encouraging physical rehabilitation.

To allow patients to regain control psychologically, an initial watch and wait approach allied to reassurance is advocated for psychological issues using review and screening to identify those not coping (e.g., screen for acute anxiety/PTSD symptoms). For practical purposes, it is best to assume memory is impaired initially in most patients and that memory processing and decision making is poor or abnormal. This impacts directly on how information is given, patient decisions made and patient autonomy protected. This is why a patient-centered, multi-modality self-help program provides support to rehabilitation and allows the patient, and importantly the relative, to engage with and regain ownership of their recovery.

XXI

Evidence and Challenges for Specific Approaches

In longer stay patients (e.g., median ICU stay 14 days) a six-week multi-modal program delivered as a patient-centered and self-guided rehabilitation manual (ICU Recovery Manual) started while in hospital has been shown to aid physical recovery [15]. Directed at physical, psychological and social aspects it combines information on recovery from critical illness, weekly exercise diaries and a self-directed exercise program. Based on educational principles, the design allows patients to tailor the program to their individual needs with the information available to share with their family and so returns control of recovery back to the patient and their family. Although also having a short-term positive impact on psychological recovery when assessed at 8 weeks after ICU discharge, this benefit was not consistently sustained to the end of the study at six months for all patients. Subsequent *post hoc* analysis suggested this was because the program had not adequately treated those patients with unpleasant delusional experiences nor prevented the development of PTSD. The 'diary study' discussed below is an attempt to address this particularly challenging issue.

Continuing physiotherapy into outpatient based rehabilitation programs once the patient has returned home has been adapted from that used in pulmonary rehabilitation programs. At the Manchester Royal Infirmary (UK) the program design follows on after early ICU mobilization and intensive in-patient exercise physiotherapy [16] with a subsequent two hours of supervised outpatient exercise and education sessions each week and two unsupervised home exercise sessions each week for 6 weeks. After six weeks, the distance patients walked in 6 minutes improved by 160 meters (p < 0.001), and there were significant improvements in anxiety (p = 0.001) and depression (p = 0.001) scores [17].

The wide heterogeneity of ICU patients means the timescales and rates of recovery are highly variable in the first six months. Younger and shorter stay patients will make a rapid recovery in a few weeks whereas older and longer stay patients may take many months. Being able to detect the efficacy of any intervention will require a sufficiently large enough functional deficit to exist, which is also able to respond to therapy and show recovery rates during the observation period significantly beyond the normal recovery rate that occurs naturally. This is a tall order and it is not surprising, therefore, that some studies have been unable to demonstrate a benefit if they recruited patients too late following intensive care and, especially, included many short-stay patients. A large study centered on a nurse-led three month follow-up clinic recruited patients with a median ICU stay of only 2.9 days [18]. With so many staying such a short time, it is unlikely that the added benefit of any therapy could be detected by the outcome measures employed. Similarly, in another study involving relatively shorter-stay patients (median 6 days) in whom therapy was started only after hospital once the patients were at home was unable to show any benefits [19]. The piloting of other models of multi-component rehabilitation with a focus on physical, functional and cognitive training is occurring and includes using new communication technologies but will suffer from these problems of interpreting change from a highly variable recovery baseline if efficacy has any chance of being established [20].

XXI

Our experience suggests that any recovery program will likely fail if it does not address in some patients the lack of autographical memory for the period of critical illness coupled with the presence of frightening delusional memories. For the patient, these problems can make it difficult to make sense of what has happened to them when they were at their sickest. The use of an ICU diary is becoming increasingly popular to address this challenge. The diary is a daily account of the stay in ICU, written in everyday language, which the relatives are encouraged to contribute to and is complimented with appropriate photographs at points of change in the patients' treatment or condition. It can be used by the patient later to fill in gaps in their memory and put any delusional memories into context [21, 22]. Two recent randomized, controlled trials have also demonstrated that the provision of an ICU diary can have an impact on anxiety and depression [23] and, in a large multicenter European study, it reduced by half the incidence of new onset PTSD [24]. Because this approach is a therapy for the family, it is encouraging that in addition to benefiting the patient there was an associated reduction in the level of PTSD-related symptoms in family members of patients who had an ICU diary [25].

Specific Psychological Support and Practical Observations

It is recognized that following critical illness, early and milder reactive psychological distress may resolve spontaneously in the first month without any intervention. However, in some patients, high levels of early anxiety, depression or PTSD symptoms may not resolve without formal therapy. The key is to recognize at an early stage, including within the ICU, those patients and/or families who are not coping with their symptoms and then offer appropriate and timely help, without interfering unnecessarily [26]. In some carefully identified patients, counseling/therapy services following critical illness may be needed for severe anxiety, depression and PTSD and are effective in helping both patients and their relatives get back to normal functioning [27]. Cognitive behavioral therapy and eye movement desensitization and reprocessing (EDMR) are recommended effective treatments for significant psychological distress. Cognitive behavioral therapy uses a goal-oriented, systematic procedure to change individuals' feelings and thoughts about their present difficulties [28]. EMDR was developed to resolve traumatic disorders [29] caused, for example, by exposure to the distressing events of rape. A traumatic experience may overwhelm the individual's normal coping mechanisms and the inadequately processed memories. EMDR aims to help process these distressing memories, allowing individuals to develop more adaptive coping mechanisms.

Feedback from patients and their families reports various tricks that they develop to help them cope with memory problems and other issues. To help a patient not to forget or muddle a large number of hospital appointments, the habit of sticking the appointment cards onto the front of the fridge in date order was adopted and on making her breakfast coffee she would check if she had an appointment that day. The habit of routinely filling a diary with anything patients need to remember, including lists of questions they need to ask their doctor, is a helpful tip. UK hospitals, to improve outpatient attendance, send a text to the patient the day before an appointment as a helpful reminder, but this has to be done consistently as patients become reliant on them and when the text is missed the patient may not attend having believed they must have confused the date!

XXI

Conclusion

Do not confuse follow-up with rehabilitation. The former is the observation of patients to inform future care and by definition occurs after the event whereas the latter is an early active process to avoid anticipated problems. The heterogeneity of our ICU population in diagnosis, severity and biological age means that recovery pathways and timescales are highly individual and varied. Although there are some common aspects to recovery (physical and behavioral) there is no unique post-ICU pattern of pathology so the approach needs to be measured, selective and appropriate to each patient and hence it is a mistake to treat everyone the same and expect the same trajectory of recovery. It is reassuring that only a proportion of patients need rehabilitation and hence it is a burdensome mistake to assume *all* patients need rehabilitation when there are many short-stay patients who have well developed coping mechanisms, family support and personal motivation that comfortably exceed any external provision.

Over the last few decades, we have learnt much by listening to patients and relatives, so failing to include either of them in the recovery process is a serious mistake. Not listening to your patients and using a preformed questionnaire approach used in 'follow-up' dangerously assumes that problems are understood and much may be missed. Our experience suggests that the greatest contribution to improve rehabilitation care and understanding of the unexpected (for example the impact of delusions) has come through frequent enquiring dialog with patients and relatives. The development of rehabilitation of the critically ill requires a caring attitude and an early 'culture of recovery and rehabilitation therapy' combined with an open minded diagnostic problem-solving approach. Remember, we are merely the interim guardians; ultimate recovery involves rejoining the patient with their family and social network.

References

1. Griffiths RD, Jones C (2011) Recovering lives: The follow-up of ICU survivors. Am J Respir Crit Care Med 183: 833–844
2. Griffiths RD, Jones C (2007) Seven lessons from 20 years of follow up of intensive care unit survivors. Curr Opin Crit Care 13: 508–513
3. National Institute for Health and Clinical Excellence (2009) Rehabilitation after critical illness: NICE clinical guideline 83. Available from: www.nice.org.uk/CG83 Accessed November 2011
4. Griffiths RD, Hall J (2010) Intensive care unit-acquired weakness. Crit Care Med 38: 779–787
5. Griffiths RD, Palmer TEA, Helliwell T, Maclennan P, Macmillan RR (1995) Effect of passive stretching on the wasting of muscle in the critically-ill. Nutrition 11: 428–432
6. Burtin C, Clerckx B, Robbeets C, et al (2009) Early exercise in critically ill patients enhances short-term functional recovery. Crit Care Med 37: 2499–2505

7. Carson SS. (2003) The epidemiology of critical illness in the elderly. Crit Care Clin 19: 605–617
8. Clini E, Ambrosino N (2005) Early physiotherapy in the respiratory intensive care unit. Respir Med 99: 1096–1104
9. Stiller K, Phillips A (2003) Safety aspects of mobilising acutely ill inpatients. Physiotherapy Theory Pract 19: 239–257
10. Wolfson L, Judge J, Whipple R, King M (1995) Strength is a major factor in balance, gait, and the occurrence of falls. J Gerontol 50: 64–67
11. Granja C, Lopes A, Moreira S et al (2005) Patients' recollections of experiences in the intensive care unit may affect their quality of life. Crit Care 9: R96–R109
12. Griffiths RD, Jones C (2001) Filling the intensive care memory gap? Intensive Care Med 27: 344–346
13. Jones C, Griffiths RD, Humphris G, Skirrow PM (2001) Memory, delusions, and the development of acute posttraumatic stress disorder-related symptoms after intensive care. Crit Care Med 29: 573–580
14. Jones C, Bäckman C, Capuzzo M, Flaatten H, Rylander C, Griffiths RD (2007) Precipitants of post traumatic stress disorder following intensive care: a hypothesis generating study of diversity in care. Intensive Care Med 33: 978–985
15. Jones C, Skirrow P, Griffiths RD, et al (2003) Rehabilitation after critical illness: A randomised, controlled trial. Crit Care Med 31: 2456–2461
16. McWilliams DJ, Westlake EV, Griffiths RD (2011) Weakness on the intensive care unit: current therapies. Br J Intensive Care 21: 23–27
17. McWilliams DJ, Atkinson D, Carter A, Foe BA, Benington S, Conway DH (2009) Feasibility and impact of a structured, exercise-based rehabilitation programme for intensive care survivors. Physiother Theory Prac 25: 566–571
18. Cuthbertson BH, Rattray J, Campbell MK, et al (2009) The PRaCTICaL study of nurse led, intensive care follow-up programmes for improving long term outcomes from critical illness: a pragmatic randomised controlled trial. BMJ 339: b3723–3731
19. Elliott D, McKinley S, Alison J, et al (2011) Health-related quality of life and physical recovery after a critical illness: a multi-centre randomised controlled trial of a home-based physical rehabilitation program. Crit Care 15: R142–52
20. Jackson JC, Ely EW, Morey MC, et al (2012) Cognitive and physical rehabilitation of ICU survivors: results of the RETURN randomized, controlled pilot investigation. Crit Care Med (in press)
21. Bäckman CG, Walther SM (2001) Use of a personal diary written on the ICU during critical illness. Intensive Care Med 27: 426–429
22. Bergbom I, Svensson C, Berggren E, Kamsula M (1999) Patients' and relatives' opinions and feelings about diaries kept by nurses in an intensive care unit: pilot study. Intensive Crit Care Nurs 15: 185–191
23. Knowles RE, Tarrier N (2009) Evaluation of the effect of prospective patient diaries on emotional well-being in intensive care unit survivors: A randomized controlled trial. Crit Care Med 37: 184–191
24. Jones C, Bäckman C, Capuzzo M, et al (2010) Intensive care diaries reduce new onset PTSD following critical illness: a randomised, controlled trial. Crit Care 14: R168
25. Jones C, Bäckman C, Griffiths R D (2012) Intensive care diaries reduce PTSD-related symptom levels in relatives following critical illness: a pilot study. Am J Crit Care (in press)
26. Jones C, Griffiths RD (2007) Patient and caregiver counselling after the intensive care unit: what are the needs and how should they be met? Curr Opin Crit Care 13: 503–507
27. Jones C, Hall S, Jackson S. (2008) Benchmarking a nurse-led ICU counselling initiative. Nursing Times 104: 32–34
28. Foa E, Rothbaum, B, Furr J (2011) Augmenting exposure therapy with other CBT procedures. Psychiatr Ann 33: 47–56
29. Shapiro F (2002) EMDR as an Integrative Psychotherapy Approach: Experts of Diverse Orientations Explore the Paradigm Prism. Washington, DC: American Psychological Association, pp 3–26

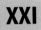
XXI

Psychological Burnout in Acute Care Medicine: "Physician Heal Thyself"

P.G. Brindley, B. Patel, and P.A. Farnan

"In a culture where work is a religion,
burnout is its crisis of faith" [1]

Introduction

In 1964, during an obscenity trial, US Supreme Court Justice, Potter Stewart, famously opined that although he could not define pornography, he "knew it when he saw it" [2]. 'Burnout' is, no doubt, a less titillating topic, but the reference to Justice Potter is useful. For example, 'burnout' may also be difficult to define, but with a little insight, we can learn to recognize it (**Box 1**). This should not be surprising; after all, studies suggest that physicians (and other healthcare workers) have amongst the highest percentage of self-reported burnout [3–9]. Because of its prevalence and its consequences (see below), it is reasonable to expect the modern physician-leader to appreciate the basics of burnout, to screen for burnout, and to be a non-judgmental resource (**Box 2**). Fortunately, practical strategies do exist and a few are outlined. The goal is to build up resilience, retain staff, and protect patients. Regardless, efforts must be deliberate and sustained. After all, a medical career- while privileged and rewarding- can also be exhausting and stressful.

Just What Is Burnout and Why Should I Care?

'Burnout' as a term in psychology appears to have originated in the 1970s [7]. It is usually attributed to Freudenberger, Maslach and Leiter [10, 11], and before that to the 1960 novel *"A Burnt-Out Case"* by Graham Greene [7]. Burnout is commonly described as an emotional condition encompassing mental fatigue and physical fatigue, frustration and aggravation, and a reduced sense of personal accomplishment (**Box 1**) [3–11]. It typically results when dedication to a cause fails to produce the hoped-for results. Studies typically rely upon self-reporting and, therefore, the incidence may be underestimated. Regardless, over 30 % of American surgeons were found to be burned out [3]; as were greater than 40 % of

Box 1. What is burnout?

- Mental and physical fatigue
- Loss of ideals; cynicism
- Sense of purposeless ("what's the point")
- Insensitivity towards others
- Sense that you are underappreciated
- Loss of respect/concern for others

J.-L. Vincent (ed.), *Annual Update in Intensive Care and Emergency Medicine 2012*
DOI 10.1007/978-3-642-25716-2 © Springer-Verlag Berlin Heidelberg 2012

Dutch general practitioners [4], and approximately 50 % of all types of Canadian physicians [5, 6].

Some ideas are best described by what they are not. For example, burnout is not just 'tiredness'. Instead, it has been described as an erosion of ideals and commitment [12]. Burnout is also not just depression, even if there is overlap. Sufferers of burnout report not just decreased energy and effort, but also a loss of concern or respect for others. This can manifest as insensitivity and scorn [1]. Burnout is also more than just boredom, and more than just a 'mid-life crisis' [13]. Burnout has been described in all levels of medical practitioners (including trainees) [3, 9]. The aforementioned study of burnout in American surgeons actually suggested a higher incidence in younger rather than older practitioners, a finding attributed to unrealistic expectations amongst the young [3]. Burnout is also not clearly associated with particular specialties, or solely with physically taxing work. However, there is a strong correlation with whether the work is valued, both by others and personally [14].

Burnout can deteriorate to the point of derogatory or dehumanizing views about both colleagues and patients [3–11]. In fact, physicians can ultimately 'loathe' the very people they set out to help [1]. Burnout can also cause resentment, hopelessness and powerlessness ("what's the point... I can't change the system") [1]. For those seeking a simple mnemonic, four Cs of burnout commonly occur. These include callousness, the tendency to cut corners, intense cynicism, and even contempt. Regardless, for a profession that relies upon dedication, innovation, volunteerism and empathy, burnout should not be ignored.

It is difficult to accurately quantify the cost of burnout to employers. However, a New York Times article of 2004 suggested $300 billion is expended each year in stress-related healthcare and missed work [1, 15]. It is also difficult to measure its effect upon patient safety. However, physician burnout may be the nexus at which a deficient hospital culture and insufficient resources are most likely to affect quality of care [8]. Overall, mounting evidence suggests that professional burnout is probably associated with lower productivity, less caring practitioners, and lower retention. On a system level, burnout probably stifles progress while entrenching old habits. On a personal level burnout can impair relationships, and contribute to substance abuse and suicidal ideation [3–11].

Why do Doctors Burnout?

Many professions are apt to burnout, especially given the accelerated pace of the modern workplace [1]. In fact, Boudreau et al. estimated that approximately 40 % of all Canadian workers were burned out [6]. Therefore, this is certainly not an affliction unique to physicians. However, we might be (to use a medical analogy) the "poster children" [16], and the best group to bring attention to the problem. Burnout is common in the 'caring professions', and in individuals who are educated, self-motivated and attracted to demanding jobs where risks and rewards are high [3–11]. Burnout sufferers are also the types of person who originally enjoy promoting change, and prior to their burnout added significantly to the productivity and morale of the workplace [7]. Interestingly, it has also been argued that burnout does not happen to 'wimps' because it requires individuals who are initially eager, engaged and concerned; before, that is, they deteriorate to the point of disillusionment [11].

We should accept a few 'inconvenient truths' about medical practice (and medical practitioners). First, even the most challenging cases become routine over time. As such, it is unreasonable to expect every day to be fascinating. Once the novelty has gone, we risk simply being left with the stress and long-hours. In addition, medical science has changed more rapidly than medical culture. In other words, although we may still expect a single physician to know and do 'everything', the complexity of medicine makes this impossible [17]. For example, it has been estimated that intensive care necessitates approximately 180 steps per patient, per day [17]. In addition, there are now over 13,000 listed diseases and syndromes, over 6,000 drugs and over 4,000 procedures [17]. There are also over 5500 medical journals indexed by Medline alone [18]. In short, physicians need to accept that it is impossible to be up to date in all areas.

The same personality traits that may be well suited to the clinical arena can become vulnerabilities when it comes to interpersonal and domestic relationships [19]. For example, physicians are known for our need for control; our competitiveness; our dedication; and our emotional remoteness. We are also quite used to postponing gratification [20] ("graduate on a Sunday; begin work on a Monday") [21]. This trait may have maintained us through the years of long-hours and low pay. However, assuming that we can also postpone attending to our personal relationships may be dangerous. After all, interpersonal relationships can be a prime source of happiness and resilience. If taken for granted, or mismanaged, they can also be an additional source of frustration and despondency [20].

Although physicians are lauded for their perfectionism, this is often accompanied by an intense need for external validation [22]. Too often we buy into the 'myth of invincibility' ("my patients get sick... I don't get sick") [23]. This attitude discourages physicians from seeking help. In addition, we rarely say 'no', and, just as importantly, we rarely encourage others to say 'no'. In fact, medicine commonly follows the ethos of 'the better we do, the better we are expected to do' [24, 25]. For example, high performing clinicians are expected to teach (also a high burnout pursuit), and then to research, and then to administer... and frequently all at the same time. We also share the 'myth of the imposter', believing that whereas others have got their lives under control, we are underperforming or we are not intelligent enough... and that we will soon be 'found out' [26]. Most people react to this fear by trying still harder and striving to achieve still more; this can in turn result in further exhaustion and resentment.

We often compare our insides (i.e., how we really feel) with our colleagues' outsides (i.e., how they appear). We also have a profession where overwork is the norm, and where our identity or definition of self, comes primarily from being a physician (rather than, say, a parent or spouse). Many of us may feel 'out of place' when outside of work. We are also used to carrying pagers and being on-call and, therefore, used to blurring the lines between work-life and home-life. In short, we live with an unfortunate combination of compulsiveness, self-doubt, guilt, and an exaggerated sense of responsibility [19, 20]. Add to this the increasing pace of life, and the advent of email and blackberries (aka 'crackberries'). This means that we are always 'on', and always aware that we could 'do more' [1]. Perhaps it is surprising that rates of burnout are not higher.

Can Burnout Be Measured?

Some ideas are also best described, and measured, by their opposite. For example, Maslach and Leiter described burnout as the opposite of "engagement" [11]. Therefore, if engagement equals 'energy', 'involvement' and 'efficacy', then burnout can be measured in terms of 'emotional exhaustion', 'depersonalization' and 'lack of personal accomplishment' [27]. These dimensions are captured in the Maslach Burnout Inventory [27]. There is also a non-validated but shorter test for "compassion fatigue" (typically described as a gradual lessening of compassion over time) [28]. Excellent internet links exist for those concerned enough to screen others... or brave enough to self-test [29, 30].

In order to recognize the natural history of burnout, Freudenberger and Richelson suggested 12 phases [10]. These include: 1) Compulsion to prove oneself; 2) efforts to work harder; 3) neglect of one's own needs; 4) displacement of conflict (i.e., the person does not realize the root cause of his/her distress); 5) alteration of values (friends, family and hobbies are neglected); 6) denial of emerging problems (for example, cynicism and aggression); 7) withdrawal (reduction in social contacts); 8) behavioral changes (which may include substance abuse); 9) depersonalization (life becomes 'mechanical' or routine); 10) inner emptiness; 11) depression; and 12) frank 'burnout' syndrome. All 12 steps are not experienced by all sufferers, and they do not always occur sequentially. However, this construct allows individuals to see how far along they are, or what might happen without corrective action.

Burnout develops gradually. However, its speed and severity is likely worsened by stress; inadequate support; insufficient respect; long and irregular hours; sleep deprivation, a sense of overwhelming responsibility, and disillusionment resulting from the difference between the realities and expectations of the job ('love the work; hate the job!') [3–12]. Accordingly, Maslach and colleagues postulated that burnout results from a 'disconnect' between an individual and an organization in one or more of six areas: Workload, control, reward, community, fairness, and values [11, 27]. As a result, efforts to combat burnout should focus on these areas. These efforts should also include the individual and the organization within which they work (**Box 2**).

Box 2. Strategies to reduce burnout

Organizational Strategies
Stress management/counseling
Increase work-place socializing
Time-off/sabbaticals
Programs in self-awareness/mindfulness

Individual Strategies
Setting deliberate/realistic goals
Dividing career into thirds (learning; earning; returning)
Accept your limitations ("you can't know everything")
Strive for balance/"purposeful imbalance" [21]

Organizational Strategies to Reduce Burnout

Maslach has stated that burnout says as much about the employer as about the employee, and reportedly went as far as to write: "Imagine investigating the personality of cucumbers to discover why they had turned into sour pickles, without analyzing the vinegar barrels in which they'd been submerged!" [1]. Bakker et al. also argued that burnout can be become contagious if ignored [31]. Accordingly, those that wish to become the best organizations (and retain the best staff) should have the best burnout strategies.

Chronic stress is intrinsic to burnout [1–11]. As such, non-discriminatory stress management classes, confidential counseling, life-coaches, and time-off might help. Physician-leaders can also trial no-meeting weeks and no email weekends. After all, getting the *most* out of staff does not always mean getting the *best* out of the staff [1]. Many physicians work alone, or feel either isolated or in competition to those in close proximity. Therefore, bolstering social support is one of the best ways to reduce stress and burnout. Unfortunately, nowadays, where workplace socializing does occur it is often 'sanitized'. Perhaps this is in an effort to be inclusive, but it ends up diminishing spontaneity. When socializing is forced it risks becoming another chore rather than much-needed stress relief.

An intensive program of self-awareness, communication and mindfulness can be associated with both short- and long-term improvements in burnout, wellbeing, psychological distress, conscientiousness and empathy [9]. Burnout also appears to be lessened whenever employees and employers share common values, and where leadership is seen to be supportive and collegial. The concept of 'fairness' is particularly important, as is the chance to resolve perceived inequities, and a sense that management is 'sharing the load'. [1, 9–11]

Sabbatical (whether from the Greek 'sabbatikos', the Latin 'sabbaticus', or the Hebrew 'shabbat/sabbath') [32] refers to taking a break from work or altering work's focus ('a change is as good as a rest'). Traditionally, sabbaticals last no less than two months and more commonly a year. Although these authors claim no authority in religious matters, multiple biblical references to sabbaticals exist (including Genesis, Leviticus, Exodus and Deuteronomy...for those that wish to check!) [32]. This observation illustrates that the idea has existed for thousands of years and is, therefore, well established. Therefore, those that apply for time off should be supported rather than being made to feel inferior, lazy or guilty. However, we might go further. After all, the Sabbath was universal: Jew and Gentile, slaves and free men, even 'beasts of burden' [32]. Therefore, the sabbatical could be usual rather than exceptional, and, given our poor insight, it could simply be mandated. Regardless, if we can schedule parental leave then we can do the same for sabbatical leave.

Individual Strategies to Reduce Burnout

If, as stated by Sylvia Boorstein "happiness truly is an inside job" [33] then we also need to focus on internal strategies. We need self-awareness and self-care. In a similar vein, Alden Cass argued "happiness is reality divided by expectations" [1]. This means we also need to set *realistic* goals. If expectations are unrealistic then we leave no room for failure, and this encourages burnout. Physicians are often quick to admonish patients for having unrealistic goals. Presumably this is one area where we should heal ourselves first. In addition, we need to set *deliberate* goals. After all, how can we be surprised if we are not where we wanted to be if we never planned where we wanted to go.

We often pursue "money rather than memories", and "professional growth rather than personal growth" [21]. We often neglect what we enjoy or what is

XXI

meaningful and devote our limited energy into being noticed- rather than being ful-filled [19]. Solutions include learning to set limits (e.g., "if I must take work home then it has to be enjoyable work") [34] or simply saying 'no'. We could also try 'reframing' [35], namely trying to see things in a different light ("that patient was rude to me, but he's probably more scared than angry"). Perhaps it sounds trite, but physicians can also simply decide each morning that they are going to be happy that day. If this is too fanciful, then when faced with negative triggers, we can at least take a moment to modify our response, even if we cannot completely step away.

'Maslow's Hierarchy' is a useful psychological construct for combating burn-out. It argues that after we secure our basic needs, and then satisfy our material wants, we also need to pursue greater meaning in our lives [21]. Similarly, Carl Jung wrote of the need to address all parts of our personalities: The need to achieve, but also to find meaning [1]. If these ideas fail to resonate with physi-cians, then we can still convey the same idea by dividing our careers into thirds: Learning, earning and returning [36, 37] (where the last third represents 'giving back'). Many other professions accept that career changes are typical, and per-haps even desirable. Instead, we often stay in the same jobs because of money or prestige, a fear of the unknown, or even an exaggerated sense of our importance [21]. When we do contemplate career change, there is a tendency to pick another altruistic (or high stress) pursuit. Of course, this is laudable, but is the same approach that led to burnout in the first place [1].

Managing Burnout

It may be better to conceptualize burnout as a chronic rather than an acute condi-tion. This construct is useful as it means that we should not be looking for a quick fix. As healthcare workers well know, chronic conditions require a multidi-mensional approach and substantial life-change. This chronic construct also emphasizes that the goal is often long-term symptom management- or prevention of 'flare-ups'- rather than outright cure. This aspect is important for those physi-cians used to solving problems rapidly, or by 'buckling down' and simply 'trying harder' [24–26]. Unfortunately, burnout is rarely that simple. This is also why the relief gained from a short vacation (for example) is unlikely to last after we return to the same old stresses and triggers. If this is not understood then the sufferer merely amplifies their unhappiness with additional shame (i.e., disappointment that they cannot easily shake their burnout) or with resignation (i.e., that this is how they will feel for the rest of their career). In addition, when we do take a break, we paradoxically multitask: Taking work on vacation; running on a tread-mill while listening to podcasts; cooking while watching the news; or walking while making calls [1]. If leisure is to be restorative, then we need to learn that doing *less* really can achieve *more*.

'Work/life balance' [21] offers a key strategy to revitalize, to rediscover joy, to maintain perspective, and to 'blow-off steam'. This can mitigate burnout, build up resilience, and extend our working life. However, 'balance' is difficult to define and, therefore, easier to ignore (at least in the short-term). The analogy of the tightrope (as presented by Todd Duncan in "Life on the Wire") may be useful [21]. After all, we all feel the pressure to perform, do not always have an adequate safety net, and rarely feel completely in balance. However, perfect balance may be elusive. Instead we could strive for "purposeful imbalance" [21]. Like a tightrope walker, we are constantly making back and forth adjustments. Furthermore, it is actually those adjustments that keep you balanced, whereas standing still is when you risk falling [21]. In medicine, there are times when work will dominate; this means that we must discipline ourselves in order that later on family can also (unashamedly) dominate. As Duncan emphasizes this "purposeful imbalance" [21] might be the best chance of achieving a satisfying career without sacrificing family, and a happy family without giving up on career. The analogy also reminds us that balance requires effort and deliberate strategies: You rarely achieve it by accident... or on the first try.

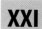

Conclusion

It may seem ironic to add burnout as an issue for the busy physician. After all, he or she is already overtaxed. However, the field of physician-health has expanded and, therefore, this topic now falls within our bailiwick. For example, we might once have trivialized burnout as a 'noble infliction', and only intervened in obvious substance-abuse or mental illness. Recently, physician-health has expanded to include collegiality, disruptive behavior, and our personal relationships [22]. Therefore, screening for burnout and being a non-judgmental resource is a natural evolution. As outlined, practical strategies are available at both the organization and individual level. In addition, we may have to accept that burnout is better 'managed' rather than 'cured'. Either way, dedicated resources and dedicated time are needed. If not, then efforts will be little more than an additional imposition on our limited time and patience. It remains to be seen if we truly have the insight and humility to heal ourselves. However, burnout is not a problem that we should continue to ignore.

References

1. Jennifer Senior (2006) New York Magazine November 26, 2006. Available at http://nymag.com/news/features/24757/Accessed November 2011
2. Justice Potter Stewart (1964) Available at http://en.wikipedia.org/wiki/Potter_Stewart. Accessed November 2011
3. Campbell DA Jr, Sonnad SS, Eckhauser FE, Campbell KK, Greenfield L (2001) Burnout among American Surgeons. Surgery 130: 696–702
4. Bakker AB, Schaufeli WB, Sixma HJ, Bosweld W, van Dierendonck D (2000) Patient demands, lack of reciprocity and burnout: a five-year longitudinal study. J Organ Behav 21: 425–441
5. Boudreau RA, Grieco RL, Cahoon SL, Robertson RC, Wede RJ (2006) The pandemic from within: two surveys of physician burnout in Canada. Can J Commun Ment Health 25: 71–88
6. Executive Summary Physician and Family Support Program (2002) Alberta physician stress and burnout research study. Available at http://www.albertadoctors.org/bcm/ama/ama-website.nsf/AllDoc/87256D8000705C3F87256E0500552925/$File/Executive_summary_burnout_study_2002.pdf. Accessed November 2011
7. Burnout Psychology (2011) Available at http://en.wikipedia.org/wiki/Burnout_(psychology) Accessed November 2011
8. Montgomery A, Panagopoulou E, Kehoe I, Valkanos E (2011) Connecting organisational culture and quality of care in the hospital: is job burnout the missing link?" J Health Organ Manag 25: 108–123
9. Krasner MS., Epstein RM, Beckman H, et al (2009) Association of an educational program in mindful communication with burnout, empathy, and attitudes among primary care physicians. JAMA 302: 1284–1293

XXI

10. Freudenberger H, Richelson G (1980) Burnout: The High Cost of High Achievement. What it is and How to Survive it. Bantam Book/Random House, New York
11. Maslach C, Leiter MP (1997) The truth about burnout: how organizations cause personal stress and what to do about It. San Francisco, Jossey-Bass
12. Cole TR, Carlin N (2009) The suffering of physicians. Lancet 374: 1414–1415
13. Kirwan M, Armstrong D (1995) Investigation of burnout in a sample of British general practitioners. Br J Gen Pract 45: 259–260
14. Fields AI, Cuerdon TT, Brasseux CO, et al (1995) Physician burnout in pediatric critical care medicine. Crit Care Med 23: 1425–1429
15. John Swartz (2004) Always on the job: employees pay with health. New York Times Sept 5, 2004. Available at: http://www.nytimes.com/2004/09/05/health/05stress.html. Accessed November 2011
16. Poster Child (2011) Available at: http://en.wikipedia.org/wiki/Poster_child. Accessed November 2011
17. Gawande A (2009) The problem of extreme complexity. In: Gawande A (ed) The Checklist Manifesto. Henry Holt and Company, New York, pp 15–31
18. Collections of the National Library of medicine (2011) Available at: http://www.ncbi.nlm.nih.gov/sites/entrez?Db=journals&Cmd=DetailsSearch&Term=currentlyindexed%5BAll%5D. Accessed November 2011
19. Gabbard GO (1985) The role of compulsiveness in the normal physician. JAMA 254: 2926–2929
20. Gabbard GO, Menninger RO (1989) The psychology of postponement in the medical marriage. JAMA 261: 2378–2381
21. Duncan T (2010) Life on the Wire: Avoid Burnout and Succeed in Work and Life. Thomas Nelson, Nashville
22. Hewitt PL, Flett GL (1991) Perfectionism in the self and social contexts: conceptualization, assessment and association with psychopathology. J Pers Soc Psychol 60: 456–470
23. McKevitt C, Morgan M (1997) Illness doesn't belong to us. J R Soc Med 90: 491–495
24. Myers MF, Gabbard GO (2008) The Physician as Patient: A Clinical Handbook for Mental Health Professionals. American Psychiatric Publishing Inc, Arlington
25. Flett GL, Hewitt PL (2002) Perfectionism: Theory, Research and Treatment. American Psychological Association, Washington
26. Clance PR, Imes SA (1978) "The impostor phenomenon among high achieving women: dynamics and therapeutic intervention". Psychotherapy Theory, Research and Practice 15: 241–244
27. Maslach C. Jackson S (1981) The measurement of experienced burnout. Journal of Occupational Behaviour 2: 99–113
28. Compassion fatigue (2011) Available at: http://en.wikipedia.org/wiki/Compassion_fatigue. Accessed November 2011
29. Burn out self-test. Stress Management From Mind Tools (1996–2011) Available at http://www.mindtools.com/stress/Brn/BurnoutSelfTest.htm. Accessed November 2011
30. Pfefferling J-H, Gilley K (2000) Overcoming compassion fatigue. Available at http://www.aafp.org/fpm/2000/0400/p39.html. Accessed November 2011
31. Bakker AB, Schaufeli WB, Sixma HJ, Bosweld W (2001) Burnout contagion among general practitioners. J Soc Clin Psychol 20: 82–98
32. Sabbatical (2011) Availble at: http://en.wikipedia.org/wiki/Sabbatical. Accessed November 2011
33. Boorstein S (2007) Happiness is an inside job: practicing for a joyful life. Ballantine Books, New York
34. Angus D (2011) The quest for leadership and striking the perfect work/life balance: An interview with Dr Derek Angus. ICU Management 11: 38–40
35. St Pierre M, Hofinger G, Buerschaper C (2008) Crisis management in acute care settings: human factors and team psychology in a high stakes environment. Springer, New York
36. Dietrich D (2011) Learn, earn, return. Available at: http://www.ler3.com/. Accessed November 2011
37. Skoll J (2009) Learning, Earning and Dreaming. Available at: http://www.hksef.org/files/files/newsletter/Social_Entrepreneurs_Newsletter_No_56.pdf Accessed November 2011

Designing a Safer Intensive Care Unit

M. Ferri and H.T. Stelfox

Introduction

The purpose of this article is to introduce the discipline of human factors as it can be applied to critical care medicine and designing a safer intensive care unit (ICU). Organizations including ICUs have recently been challenged with reducing the incidence and severity of adverse events and improving the quality and safety of care. We will illustrate how critical care medicine has begun to adopt human factor methods such as standardization of communication, checklists, and incident analysis from high-risk industries outside of healthcare.

Patient Safety

Healthcare appears to be far behind other high-risk industries in ensuring basic safety. Awareness of patient safety problems in medicine has been growing since 1991 with publication of the Harvard Medical Practice Study [1, 2]. This retrospective review of 30,000 medical records studied the incidence and nature of adverse events in hospitalized patients in New York State. It revealed that about 4 % of the patients experienced an adverse event, and that two-thirds of these events were deemed preventable. Subsequent publication of the Institute of Medicine report, *To Err is Human* [3], turned patient safety into a general public concern, stimulating broad research and discussion [3, 4]. The report stated that errors caused between 44,000 and 98,000 deaths every year in American hospitals, and over one million injuries. Studies from around the world have corroborated these findings [5, 6].

An adverse event is defined as an unintended injury or complication resulting in a prolonged hospital stay, disability or death as a result of health care management rather than the patient's underlying disease process [1, 5]. Error, as defined by James Reason, is a generic term to encompass occasions in which a planned sequence of mental or physical actions fails to be completed as intended, either because planning or execution were inadequate [7]. Both definitions are widely accepted, do not ascribe provider intent and highlight a subtle yet important difference between failure and consequence.

The Institute of Medicine report highlighted that adverse events are rarely the result of careless, undertrained and incompetent providers, but rather a consequence of complex interactions of system failures with the individual provider and patient at the sharp-end of the organizational process [3, 8]. Despite considerable efforts in recent years, many institutions still react to adverse events with

J.-L. Vincent (ed.), *Annual Update in Intensive Care and Emergency Medicine 2012*
DOI 10.1007/978-3-642-25716-2 © Springer-Verlag Berlin Heidelberg 2012

a person-based approach, identifying the most responsible individual, determining their culpability, scheduling retraining and advertising a corrective disciplinary action. New operational procedures are then implemented with a reassurance to society that workers will be better trained and more careful in the future. Such a reaction fits the medical analogy of treating only the symptoms while failing to address the underlying disease process. Adverse events are not the disease, but symptoms of the disease [9]. Understanding this principle allows healthcare organizations to adopt the systems-based management approach successfully used by other high-risk industries.

Human Factors

Most healthcare providers have experienced situations of suboptimal individual or collective performance. If human capabilities and limitations are not taken into account in the design process, behaviors, devices and work environments can be unsafe. Human factors is a discipline of applied research that describes, and seeks to optimize, the interaction of people, devices and environments [10]. Also called cognitive ergonomics, it applies concepts from a diverse range of sciences including psychology, management, anatomy, physiology, industrial engineering and social sciences. Human factors activities in healthcare have expanded considerably since the publication of *To Err is Human* (**Table 1**). Applications of human factors in healthcare are frequently reported as an extension of aviation principles and practices, and include standardization of interfaces and communication, checklists for complex processes, and simplification of information [11].

Table 1. Sample human factors interventions for common patient safety targets in the ICU.

ICU Safety Target	Human Factors Interventions
Communication Failure	
1. Clinical rounds	Standardized structure: location, duration, composition [38, 39] Standardized process: Daily goals sheet [18]
2. Patient Handover	Standardized structures and process [17, 19] Tool assisted [19, 20]
3. Teamwork	Explicit team member roles [17, 36, 37]
Complex Task Completion	
4. Complex procedures	Central line insertion checklist [24] Surgical checklist and time-out [25, 26]
Learning from Failure	
5. Incident reporting systems	Confidential, voluntary, independent [28, 33] Local and multicenter [28, 31, 32, 33] Performance feedback to providers [28, 33]

XXI

Framework

James Reason's "Swiss cheese" model is a well-recognized human factors conceptual framework in healthcare. Reason's model is routinely used to approach human error and provides an explanation for the apparent random nature of adverse events (**Fig. 1**) [12, 13]. It proposes two root causes for errors: Active failures and latent conditions.

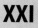

Active failures are unsafe acts committed by people who are in direct contact with the patient. They can be classified as slips, lapses, mistakes, and procedural violations [13, 14]. Active failures have a direct and usually short-lived impact on the integrity of system defenses [13]. Traditionally, healthcare has ascribed adverse events to active failures. For example, aspiration pneumonitis may be attributed to provider failure to identify an incorrectly placed feeding tube on chest x-ray. However, Reason's model demonstrates that virtually all active failures have a causal history that extends back in time and through the various levels of the process [13]. It also explains the many intrinsic defensive layers (e.g., alarms, protocols, skilled workers) of most systems, each represented by a slice of Swiss cheese with the holes corresponding to latent conditions. The model illustrates that an adverse event is a consequence of multiple active failures and latent conditions aligned through the successive layers of system defense (**Fig. 1**).

Latent conditions are resident pathogens within the system that affect the rate providers execute active failures and potentiate the associated risks. They can include provider staffing, communication methods, adherence to procedures, equipment choices and room design, amongst others. Latent conditions occur when individuals make decisions that have unintended consequences in the future – they lie in wait. For example, organizations that use staffing models that depend on providers to routinely perform clinical duties above and beyond their regular responsibilities may introduce time pressures, fatigue and distractions that increase the risk of active failures.

We will discuss the application of human factors to three interconnected domains of patient safety in the ICU: Human interactions (communication), completion of complex tasks (checklists), and incident reporting (learning from failure) (**Table 1**).

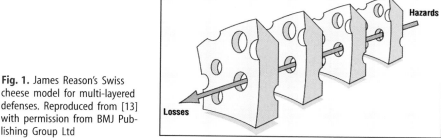

Fig. 1. James Reason's Swiss cheese model for multi-layered defenses. Reproduced from [13] with permission from BMJ Publishing Group Ltd

Application of Human Factors To ICU Design

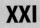

ICUs receive vulnerable patients with high illness severity and little physiological reserve into a complex, tightly coupled system comprised of multiple providers, sophisticated technologies and frequent time-sensitive interventions. The average ICU patient experiences over 100 healthcare related activities (e.g., laboratory tests, medications, procedures, etc) per day, one to two errors per day [15], and one serious adverse event during their stay [16]. Although human factor methods may be applied in any healthcare setting, the ICU offers many potential opportunities.

Designing Standardized Communication

Healthcare providers may be well trained and highly skilled in their individual roles, but are not necessarily trained in teamwork. Communication failure is the number one human error resulting in airplane crashes. Evidence suggests that communication failures are similarly important in critical care medicine [15, 17].

The deadliest accident in aviation history happened at Tenerife North Airport in 1977, when Pan Am and KLM Jumbo jets collided on the runway causing 583 fatalities. The initial investigation identified the active failure responsible for the crash to be one of the pilots initiating takeoff without clearance from the control tower. However, further analysis also revealed latent conditions related to communication within the cockpit team and between the cockpit and the control tower. In response, the aviation industry implemented measures directed at improving cockpit teamwork. This package of interventions evolved into crew resource management, a tool to foster leadership, mutual support, and situation awareness skills as well as development of shared mental models and achievement of task coordination so as to make full use of the cognitive resources available [8]. The Tenerife disaster exemplifies how a high-risk industry redesigned human interactions to improve communication and team management by using the strengths of the team (cockpit crew) and addressing the limitations of human performance.

Peter Pronovost applied the principles of crew resource management in developing a "Daily Goals Sheet" to improve communication and team performance during ICU rounds [18]. The "Daily Goals Sheet" was designed to prompt and document explicit review of the day's planned tasks and care goals prior to completion of each patient's bedside discussion. The main objectives of the exercise were to create an explicit care plan for each patient and to ensure all team members understood the plan. Pronovost et al. demonstrated in a single surgical ICU that before "Daily Goals Sheet" implementation, residents and nurses understood less than 10 % of the daily goals for patients, but this increased to more than 95 % after the 16 week study. Although more research on the adoption of ICU tools based on crew resource management principles is needed, the results highlight the potential for designing human interactions in the ICU.

Formula One racing provides an illustrative example of multi-professional human interaction in a time-constrained fashion. At least once during a race, drivers are required to pit stop. Soon after the car enters the pit lane, the 'lollipop man' directs the driver with a paddle sign (situation awareness), while mechanics execute a pre-established sequence of actions to change tires and refuel the car (task allocation and standardized verbal and non-verbal language). Formula One teams practice pit stop routines to ensure maximum safety and efficiency. A British healthcare team applied the pit stop model along with crew resource management principles to standardize handover of pediatric cardiac surgery patients to the ICU [19]. The team's objective was to promote seamless transfer of care (monitors, support devices, clinical knowledge about the patient gained in the operation room) by standardizing human interactions previously documented as being unstructured, inconsistent, and frequently resulting in incomplete transfer of information. These problems are widely recognized as root causes of communication failures during handover [20]. Formula One racing and crew resource management provide potential guides for developing interventions to address similar communication failures in critical care medicine.

XXI

Designing Checklists For Complex Tasks

Classical studies of human memory have found that most individuals can only recall about seven pieces of information accurately (hence the common use of seven digit telephone numbers). Our memory becomes increasingly unreliable with complex tasks, stress, and fatigue [21]. Checklists are cognitive tools designed to standardize processes by facilitating the systematic execution of multi-step procedures in error-prone contexts [21, 22].

In 1935, the United States Army Air Corps sponsored an airplane demonstration at Wright Air Field in Dayton, Ohio, to choose the next generation of long-range bombers. A Boeing prototype, Model 299, was the favorite. However, within seconds of takeoff the airplane crashed. The subsequent investigation identified no mechanical problems, but highlighted pilot error in a brand new complex airplane. The American press described the prototype as "too much airplane for one man to fly". The United States Army Air Corps response to the crash changed the course of aviation safety. They developed a checklist containing step-by-step checks for taxiing, takeoff, flight and landing procedures. B-17 Flying Fortresses (model 299) subsequently flew 1.8 million miles without accident, providing a strategic weapon for American operations in World War II [23].

The first large study to investigate checklists in the ICU was the Keystone ICU project [24]. The objective was to evaluate the effect of a multilayered intervention to reduce catheter-related blood stream infections in patients admitted to ICUs in Michigan. The authors included five evidence-based procedures for central line insertion recommended by the Centers for Disease Control: Hand washing, use of chlorhexidine, full-barrier precautions, avoiding femoral sites, and removing unnecessary catheters. To ensure clinician adherence to these safety procedures, a checklist was developed and applied. The bedside nurse managing the checklist was empowered to abort a procedure if the physician inserting the catheter was not adhering to the proposed safety measures. The median rate of catheter-related blood stream infections decreased from 2.7 per 1000 catheter-days at baseline to zero cases three months and 18 months after implementation of the checklist [24]. Subsequently, the Safe Surgery Checklist was developed to reduce perioperative adverse events from non-cardiac surgery [25]. The checklist was designed to facilitate operating room communication and ensure that all steps in the complex operative process were successfully performed to the satisfaction of all providers. The World Health Organization (WHO) sponsored an evaluation of the checklist in a multinational, randomized controlled trial of more than 3000 patients in eight centers representing diverse global populations and

XXI

economic circumstances [25]. The checklist was used before anesthesia induction, incision, and patient transfer to the recovery room. It included a patient verification section (name, procedure, site and allergies), a team preparedness section (availability of necessary equipment, imaging tests required, etc) and a debriefing section (review of case upon completion). Following implementation of the Safe Surgery Checklist, complications decreased from 11 % to 7 % and in-hospital mortality from 1.5 % to 0.8 %. Implementation of a surgery checklist in hospitals in the Netherlands yielded significant reductions in complications and morbidity [26]. These studies have stimulated increased implementation of healthcare checklists, although opportunities exist for further evaluation and implementation.

Designing Incident Reporting Systems (Learning From Failure)

Reprimand and punishment for failure are commonly practiced in many societies. Blaming individuals is easier and emotionally more satisfying than changing systems [13]. Paradoxically, this tradition hinders efforts to prevent similar failures in the future. It is widely accepted that successful organizations learn from failure.

Up to the mid 1970s, the Federal Aviation Administration (FAA) office operated both the reporting system of near misses and the regulatory and enforcement system for individuals and organizations that had experienced failures. As a result, reporting rates for near misses were very low, since individuals and organizations were afraid of being punished for their mistakes. In 1976, an independent agency called Aviation Safety Reporting System (ASRS) was created to prospectively collect confidential and voluntary reports of near misses from airline personnel and air traffic controllers. This resulted in a large increase in reporting rates and greatly facilitated safety efforts by the aviation industry [27].

Reporting critical incidents has been increasingly implemented in healthcare with mixed results. Critical incidents are any events that could have reduced, or did reduce, the patient safety margin [16, 28]. Therefore, they encompass adverse events and near misses. Near misses are particularly important, since they are defined as lower level incidents that may not be otherwise identified, and can provide invaluable insight into human behavior and error prevention strategies.

The Australian Incident Monitoring Study in Intensive Care (AIMS-ICU) and the ICU Safety Reporting System (ICUSRS) represent two national multicenter critical incident reporting systems for ICUs [29, 30]. Both systems were designed to improve the quality and number of incident reports by encouraging staff engagement through anonymous, voluntary, and nonpunitive reporting. Increased safety climate and safety culture have been demonstrated to increase reporting rates, whereas lack of regular feedback of incident reports to providers has been demonstrated to be one of the greatest deterrents to reporting [31–33]. It is unknown whether electronic or paper-based reporting mechanisms impact reporting rates, but many institutions incorporate incident reporting within their computer systems

Transforming incident reports into safer care is not straightforward. Reporting of itself does not improve patient safety or outcomes. Rather, incident reporting can only bring substantial improvement if coupled with comprehensive analysis of active failures and latent conditions. One approach that has been successfully used is based on a 'critical incident technique'. This approach comprises a set of principles to guide human behavior observation and interviews so as to find common causes to a cluster of incidents, or provide in-depth information about a single event [34]. For example, in 1978 a Harvard based group performed one of the first published evaluations of patient safety by interviewing 47 anesthesiologists to identify and analyze near misses and adverse events. The authors demonstrated the feasibility of using a modified critical incident technique to identify incidents (e.g., medication syringe swaps resulting in administration of the incorrect medication), describe factors associated with incidents (e.g., haste, distraction, fatigue etc.) and propose potential interventions to prevent future incidents (e.g., standardized color coded labeling of syringes) [35]. Many tools, such as the critical incident technique, have been incorporated into reporting systems, but the gap between knowledge and action remains large in many institutions.

XXI

Conclusion

Patient safety is an important healthcare issue because of the consequences of iatrogenic injuries. Adverse events in critical care are frequent, serious, and predictable. Until recently, the healthcare industry has applied a person-based approach to patient safety, ascribing errors and adverse events as individual provider failures. Human factors offers a different perspective, attributing adverse events to a combination of active failures and latent conditions. Evidence from high-risk industries, including healthcare, suggests that demanding greater vigilance from healthcare providers will not result in meaningful safety improvement. Instead, incorporating human factors principles and methods to learn from failure and to develop simple, focused, and evidence-based interventions that can be locally adapted to revise faulty systems is more promising.

Acknowledgement: We thank Dr Jeff Caird for his comments on earlier versions of the manuscript.

References

1. Brennan TA, Leape LL, Laird N, et al (1991) Incidence of adverse events and negligence in hospitalized patients: results from the Harvard Medical Practice Study I. N Engl J Med 324: 370–376
2. Leape LL, Brennan TA, Laird NM, et al (1991) The nature of adverse events in hospitalized patients: Results of the Harvard Medical Practice Study II. N Engl J Med 324: 377–384
3. Kohn LT, Corrigan JM, Donaldson MS (2000) To Err is Human: Building a safer health System. Institute of Medicine, National Academy Press, Washington
4. Stelfox HT, Palmisani S, Scurlock C, Orav EJ, Bates DW (2006) The "To Err is Human" report and the patient safety literature. Qual Saf Health Care 15: 174–178
5. de Vries EN, Ramrattan MA, Smorenbury SM, Gouma DJ, Boermeester MA (2008) The incidence and nature of in-hospital adverse events: A systematic review. Qual Saf Health Care 17: 216–223
6. Baker GR, Norton PG, Flintoft V, et al (2004) The Canadian Adverse Events Study: the incidence of adverse events among hospital patients in Canada. Can Med Assoc J 170: 1678–1686
7. Reason J (1990) Human Error, 1st edn. Cambridge University Press, Cambridge
8. St. Pierre M, Hofinger G, Buerschaper C (2008) The human factor: Errors and skills. In: St Pierre M, Hofinger G, Buerschaper C (eds) Crisis Management in Acute Care Settings:

Human Factors and Team Psychology in a High Stakes Environment. Springer. Berlin, pp 4–15

9. Leape LL (2004) Errors are not diseases: they are symptoms of diseases. Laryngoscope 114: 1320–1321

10. Chapanis A (1996) Human Factors In Systems Engineering. Wiley-Interscience, New York

11. Leape LL, Berwick DM, Bates DW (2002) What practices will most improve safety? Evidence-based medicine meets patient safety. JAMA 288: 501–507

12. Camiré E, Moyen E, Stelfox HT. (2009) Medication errors in critical care: risk factors, prevention and disclosure. CMAJ 180: 936–943

13. Reason J (2000) Human error: Models and management. BMJ 320: 768–770

14. Armitage G (2009) Human error theory: relevance to nurse management. J Nurs Manag 17: 193–202

15. Donchin Y, Gopher D, Olin M, et al (1995) A look into the nature and causes of human errors in the intensive care unit. Crit Care Med 23: 294–300

16. Pronovost PJ, Thompson DA, Holzmueller CG, Lubomski LH, Morlock LL (2005) Defining and measuring patient safety. Crit Care Clin 21: 1–19

17. Brindley PG, Reynolds SF. (2011) Improving verbal communication in critical care medicine. J Crit Care 26: 155–159

18. Pronovost P, Berenholtz S, Dorman T, Lipsett PA, Simmonds T, Haraden C (2003) Improving communication in the ICU using daily goals. J Crit Care 18: 71–75

19. Catchpole KR, De Laval MR, McEwan A, et al (2007) Patient handover from surgery to intensive care: using Formula 1 pit stop and aviation models to improve safety and quality. Paediatr Anaesth 17: 470–478

20. Nagpal K, Arora S, Abboudi M, et al (2010) Postoperative handover: problems, pitfalls, and prevention of error. Ann Surg 252: 171–176.

21. Winters BD, Gurses AP, Lehmann H, Sexton JB, Rampersad CJ, Pronovost PJ (2009) Checklists – translating evidence into practice. Crit Care 13: 210–219

22. Degani A, Wiener EL (1990) Human Factors Of Flight-Deck Checklists: The Normal Checklist (Tech. Rep. 177549). National Aeronautics and Space Administration (NASA), Moffett Field

23. Gawande A (2007). The checklist: If something so simple can transform intensive care, what else can it do? The New Yorker Dec 10, pp 86–95

24. Pronovost P, Needham D, Berenholtz S, et al (2006) An intervention to decrease catheter-related bloodstream infections in the ICU. N Engl J Med 355: 2725–2732

25. Haynes AB, Weiser TG, Berry WR, et al (2009) A surgical safety checklist to reduce morbidity and mortality in a global population. N Engl J Med 360: 491–499

26. de Vries EN, Prins HA, Crolla R, et al (2010) Effect of comprehensive surgical safety system on patient outcomes. N Engl J Med 363: 1928–1937

27. Vicente K (2003) The Human Factor. Revolutionizing The Way People Live With Technology. Alfred A. Knopf, Toronto, pp 195–203

28. Frey B, Schwappach D (2010) Critical incident monitoring in paediatric and adult critical care: from reporting to improved patient outcomes? Curr Opin Crit Care 16: 649–653

29. Beckmann U, West LF, Groombridge GJ, et al (1996) The Australian Incident Monitoring Study in Intensive Care: AIMS-ICU. The development and evaluation of an incident reporting system in intensive care. Anaesth Intensive Care 24: 314–319

30. Needham DM, Thompson DA, Holzmueller CG, et al (2004) A system factors analysis of airway events from the Intensive Care Unit Safety Reporting System (ICUSRS). Crit Care Med 32: 2227–2233

31. Hutchinson A, Young TA, Cooper KL, et al (2009) Trends in healthcare incident reporting and relationship to safety and quality data in acute hospitals: results from the National Reporting and Learning System. Qual Saf Health Care 18: 5–10

32. Snijders C, Kollen BJ, van Lingen RA, et al (2009) Which aspects of safety culture predict incident reporting behaviour in neonatal intensive care units? A multilevel analysis. Crit Care Med 37: 61–66

33. Mahajan RP (2010) Critical incident reporting and learning. Br J Anaesth 105: 69–75

34. Woloshynowych M, Rogers S, Taylor-Adams S, Vincent C (2005) The investigation and analysis of critical incidents and adverse events in healthcare. Health Technol Assess 9: 1–143

XXI

35. Cooper JB, Newbower RS, Long CD, McPeek B (1978) Preventable anesthesia mishaps: a study of human factors. Anesthesiology 49: 399–406
36. Reader TW, Flin R, Mearns K, Cuthbertson BH (2009) Developing a team performance framework for the intensive care unit. Crit Care Med 37: 1787–1793
37. Dodek PM, Raboud J (2003) Explicit approach to rounds in an ICU improves communication and satisfaction of providers. Intensive Care Med 29: 1584–1588
38. Landry MA, Lafrenaye S, Roy MC, Cyr C (2007) A randomized, controlled trial of bedside versus conference-room case presentation in a pediatric intensive care unit. Pediatrics 120: 275–280
39. Kim MM, Barnato AE, Angus DC, Fleisher LF, Kahn JM (2010) The effect of multidisciplinary care teams on intensive care unit mortality. Arch Intern Med 170: 369–376

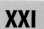

Challenges in Implementing Evidence-based Medicine

A.C. Kajdacsy-Balla Amaral and G.D. Rubenfeld

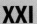

Introduction

Medical knowledge increases rapidly, making it difficult for clinicians to update their practice to allow the incorporation of new advances in care. Arguably the largest deficiency in modern health care is the frequent failure to adhere to evidence-based best practices [1]. These are practices related to the prevention, diagnosis and treatment of disease that have been demonstrated to improve clinically relevant outcomes. Effective interventions fostering best practices are particularly important in critical care services. Progress in most areas of healthcare is leading to a large number of patients living longer and with increasingly complex combinations of diseases and new treatments. Within hospitals, intensive care units (ICUs) are one of the most costly types of care offered, with medical-surgical ICUs accounting for 45 % of admissions to special care units [2].

However, both the government [3] and the healthcare industry allocate the majority of their resources towards the discovery of new interventions. In the United States, the annual budget of the Agency for Healthcare Research and Quality, the federal agency responsible for research devoted to improve fidelity, is 1 % of the budget for the National Institutes of Health [4], where the majority of money is allocated to research towards the discovery of new and more effective interventions. The assumption that new interventions are effectively adopted by healthcare systems may partially explain this disparity. However, studies have shown that as many as 30 – 50 % of patients do not get recommended evidence-based care and 20 – 30 % of patients receive unnecessary interventions [1, 5]. The consistent and reliable translation of knowledge into practice has eluded clinical practice to date. Recent trials and meta-analyses demonstrate only modest, or even a lack of improvement, in evidence-based practices through the use of multifaceted programs to improve quality, including educational efforts, 'bundle' tools, and audit and feedback [6 – 10]. Filling this gap in the implementation of evidence that is already known can be a better opportunity to improve care than investigating for more effective interventions [11].

Challenges abound when it comes to the timely adoption of, and ongoing adherence to, evidence-based practices known to improve care for critically ill patients. This has resulted in inappropriate use of drugs and devices; and in some situations, an increased risk of morbidity and mortality among these vulnerable patients, and inappropriate healthcare resource utilization. For example, acute lung injury (ALI) is one of the most common syndromes observed in critically ill patients [12]. The use of lung-protective ventilation, which consists of applying lower tidal volumes, leads to an impressive 9 % absolute reduction in mortality

J.-L. Vincent (ed.), *Annual Update in Intensive Care and Emergency Medicine 2012*
DOI 10.1007/978-3-642-25716-2 © Springer-Verlag Berlin Heidelberg 2012

[13]. It is a simple and free intervention, with a large effect size, which we would expect to be rapidly and largely adopted. However, in an observational cohort in the US, only 6 % of patients with ALI were being treated with this intervention, and there was more than two-fold variation in its use by center [14]. Clearly, we have not met the expectation that evidence-based interventions will be easily incorporated into clinical practice.

Factors that Modulate Adoption of a New Intervention

The science of implementation involves changing behavior of patients, clinicians and organizations. Changing behavior of clinicians involves a framework of factors related to the intervention, the clinicians and the healthcare organizations (**Table 1**):

Table 1. Factors influencing adoption of evidence-based processes

Factor	Barriers	Solutions	Examples
Intervention			
Level of evidence	Guidelines or protocols that are not based on evidence are less likely to be followed	• Focus on implementing processes that are evidence-based	• DVT prophylaxis • Sedation vacation • Spontaneous breathing trials
Simplicity	Complex interventions are more likely to fail	• Simplifying processes	• 'Default' orders for 6 ml/kg in mechanical ventilation • 'Shock bags' with 1 dose of broad-spectrum antibiotics for initial resuscitation
Frequency	In situations that occur infrequently, clinicians are less likely to learn new processes	• Assembling teams for special situations	• Cardiac and post-cardiac arrest teams • Massive bleeding teams
Persons			
Time	Time-consuming processes are less likely to be followed	• Simplifying processes	• Alarm clock to prompt reassessments in the initial 6-hours of sepsis
Knowledge	Lack of awareness and familiarity with guidelines	• Using protocols and pre-printed orders • Using multiple forms of education	• Protocolized care • Internet-based education • Education at the point-of-care
Inertia	Clinicians have to overcome inertia to acquire a new behavior	• Using protocols and pre-printed orders	• Protocolized care
Social Structure	Larger groups have complex social networks. If influential stakeholders do not adhere to the intervention, it is more likely to fail	• Mapping the social network	• Providing a more in-depth training to influential nodes in a network

Table 1. (*continued*)

Factor	Barriers	Solutions	Examples
Memory	The multitude of problems in a single patient may lead clinicians to forget routine processes	• Memory aids	• Use of checklists • Electronic reminders
Organization			
Resources	Unavailability of required resources	• Involving decision makers in the implementation	• Acquisition of electronic medical record • Budget for physiotherapists to implement early mobility
Culture	Some organizations may not have cultures that are conducive to the adoption of new behaviors	• Mapping the social network	• Using the existing social network to influence behavior change • Changing the current social network by adding or removing influential members
Leadership	Style and involvement of leaders influences the adoption of new behaviors	• Recruiting leaders who support continuous improvement	• Quality walk rounds

Nature of the Intervention

- Evidence-based. Not unexpectedly, interventions based on sound scientific evidence are more likely to be accepted [15]. Evidence-based guidelines have compliance rates that are 14 % higher than those lacking evidence (71 % vs 57 %) [16], whereas controversial guidelines are associated with a 23 % lower compliance (68 % vs 35 %) [16].
- Simplicity. Simpler interventions have a lower threshold for adoption. Simpler interventions allow clinicians to easily understand their meaning and the rationale behind them. Also, clinicians perceive simple interventions to reduce their workload, which clinicians identify as an important barrier for implementation [17]. Almost 40 % of physicians classified specific guidelines as 'inconvenient' or difficult to use [18]. A systematic review identified guideline complexity, defined as when the average clinician perceives the guideline to be difficult to understand or to acquire the necessary skills, as responsible for 30 % of the variation in compliance [19].
- Although simplicity is desired, medical interventions are often complex in their nature. For example, some medical interventions require a stepwise approach, where the patient's response to one intervention changes the decision in the next step. For example, deep-venous thrombosis (DVT) prophylaxis is an example of an evidence-based intervention that can be considered simple: There are few steps in the decision to provide it or not and, once decided that a patient has no contraindications, the intervention requires minimal or no customization to the individual patient. On the other hand, achieving high rates of compliance with early antibiotics for patients who are in septic shock is more complex as it involves a timely decision and a cognitive task to decide whether a patient has septic shock or not. One of the

ways to improve time to antibiotic delivery is to promote a program with clinician education, pre-printed order sets, and early lactate measurements. A simpler intervention would simply rely on 'shock-bags' in which the first liter of fluid resuscitation for hypotensive patients already includes one dose of a broad-spectrum antibiotic. It is likely that the latter would be more effective in reducing time to antibiotic delivery.

- Frequency. Interventions can also be classified on how frequently they occur. Interventions that are more frequent increase the clinician's opportunity to experiment with the intervention. Some tasks can be performed daily in the ICU, such as daily interruption of sedation [20], whereas others are less frequent and require specific training, such as hypothermia after cardiac arrest. Variations in frequency of the intervention were responsible for 14 % of the variation in compliance with guidelines [19]. Implementation of strategies that are infrequent may be successful by using teams assembled and trained to these specific situations. Training smaller groups may be more effective, and these teams will benefit from a greater exposure to the procedure.

Persons

- Time. Clinicians dedicate the majority of their practice time to patient care. Although empiric evidence does not support the hypothesis that clinicians with a higher workload have lower compliance with guidelines [21] (e.g., physicians with high workload do not provide less evidence-based medicine than physicians with a lower workload), the perceived effect of a guideline on workload does: When a clinician perceives that a new process may lead to increased workload the likelihood of adoption is lower. Some evidence-based recommendations may save time, whereas others may increase the time required for completion of activities during usual care. Not surprisingly, interventions that reduce the amount of patient care time are more easily adopted [21]. For example, guiding hemodynamic resuscitation in the early phase of septic shock by either central venous oxygen saturation ($ScvO_2$) [22] or serial lactate measurements [23] may lead to reduced mortality. However, inserting a central venous catheter quickly may not always be feasible to measure $ScvO_2$ and drawing blood for lactate measurement every 2 hours may also be time-consuming. Interestingly, in the lactate study [23], there was no difference in serial lactate levels between the two-groups. Could the difference in outcomes be simply related to frequent physician re-assessment rather than specific guidance by lactate levels? If that is the case, an alarm-clock that prompts frequent clinical reassessments may be a simpler, less time-consuming strategy than frequent laboratory tests, to deliver better care [24].

- Knowledge. Different clinician characteristics, such as type of practice, age, time devoted to continuing medical education, may influence learning. Indeed, lack of awareness of clinical guidelines is reported by 54 % of clinicians [18], and lack of familiarity with recommendations may be an even greater problem. The use of protocols or pre-printed order sets may help because they provide a practical summary of the evidence-based intervention. Clinicians may choose to read this summary when they do not have time to read the complete guideline. Therefore, clinicians can at least become aware of the guideline, removing knowledge as a barrier. Targeting the type of knowledge delivery to the type of learner is a key strategy to overcome these barriers.

- Inertia. The inertia of previous practice may influence adoption, even when there is knowledge and awareness of the new evidence. A survey of physicians on cancer screening demonstrated that more than half of them were in a "pre-contemplative" phase and not ready to change their practice, even though they were aware and in agreement with the guidelines [25]. The use of protocols may be helpful when there is inertia. In the treatment of dyslipidemia, therapeutic inertia was defined as failure to modify treatment based on high cholesterol levels. The presence of protocols for clinical management was associated with a reduction in inertia of 40 % [26].

- Social structure. The types of relationships – or social networks – among healthcare workers may also influence adoption of evidence-based practice. For example, if an intervention is adopted by a clinician who is a 'role model' for others, the intervention may be more quickly adopted [27]. In more 'competitive' networks, clinicians may adopt practices that their peers are already using to avoid being perceived as outdated [28]. In the near future, one of the strategies to facilitate implementation may be the mapping of the social networks of an ICU and targeting specific individuals who function as nodes in a network when starting a process, as opposed to the whole team, therefore simplifying the implementation and possibly gaining time.

- Memory. Even when all resources are in place and clinicians are aware of recommendations, they may forget to provide evidence-based interventions. A good example of this is the use of DVT prophylaxis. This is an intervention where there is robust evidence, with no disagreement. It is simple, not time consuming, and clinicians are aware of its importance and willing to use it. However, they may still forget to prescribe it. A randomized-controlled trial of electronic reminders demonstrated a greater than two-fold increase in the use of DVT prophylaxis in hospitalized patients [29].

Organization

- Resources. Organizations play a significant role as they provide the resources necessary for the intervention, such as personnel, equipment, and structure [30]. For example, unavailability of physiotherapists in an ICU may interfere with ability to provide early mobilization [31]. Also, the lack of a computerized system with automatic reminders may decrease compliance with DVT prophylaxis [29].

- Culture. The values and attitudes shared amongst the members of an organization may facilitate the adoption and implementation of new practices, with some organizations having cultures that are more conducive to innovation [32]. When culture is a barrier for implementation, most other efforts may be doomed to fail. Despite extensive research, effective cultural change is seen in only a minority of corporations and it may take a decade to be accomplished [33]. Since culture comes from the members of the organization, effective cultural change can only occur by changing the members (by either removing personnel that work against the expected culture, or introducing new personnel that may act positively towards the expected culture) or by providing opportunity for members to change their behavior.

- Leadership. Both the style [34] and involvement [15] of the leaders in the organization influence the adoption of a new practice. Outside healthcare, successful implementation of quality programs will occur in settings where the leadership perceives the program as relevant and needed [35]. In ICUs, involvement of the leadership is perceived by clinicians as a key-component of successful implementation [15]. An example on how leaders can help support the adoption of new behavior is the use of quality rounds. Having the ICU director or quality improvement officer discuss new processes of care directly with the clinicians at the bedside is a strategy that shows commitment to the implementation. It may also help these decision-makers to learn about what is working or not in an informal way that may disclose problems in implementation.

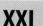

The Evidence for Implementing Evidence-Based Interventions

Promoting behavior change in such a complex environment is not simple, and a multitude of tools and theories are available [36], including the formation of teams to lead implementation [37], education [38], audit and feedback tools [15], informatics [39], reminders [29], interventions aimed at changing culture [40] and leadership [41]. However, there is insufficient evidence to support these tools and theories. A large meta-analysis across all fields in healthcare looked at the evidence on the type and number of interventions used for guideline implementation. The author observed modest effects (close to 10 % improvement in process of care) for the majority of single interventions, such as educational efforts, audit and feedback, reminders, or for multiple interventions [8]. A more recent meta-analysis, focusing specifically on complex quality improvement interventions for glycemic control for type 2 diabetes, synthesized data from 66 different trials in the outpatient setting and failed to demonstrate significant improvements [38].

In critical care, there is a paucity of data to support strategies that effectively lead to successful implementation. A large multicenter educational program was targeted to decrease mortality in sepsis by improving compliance with the Surviving Sepsis Campaign guidelines in 59 Spanish ICUs [7]. Although institution of the program was associated with an increased compliance with both the 6-hour and the 24-hour sepsis bundles, caution must be exerted when interpreting these results because there were no contemporary controls in this study, therefore we cannot exclude the possibility of a secular trend in compliance with the guidelines [42] and, most strikingly, although a statistically significant association was observed, the effect size of the intervention was minimal – compliance increased from 5 to 10 % in the 6-hour bundle and from 10 to 15 % in the 24-hour bundle [7]. In particular, the components of the bundle for which there is better evidence for improved outcomes had minimal changes – A 2 % increase in early antibiotics, a 3 % decrease in maintaining plateau pressures below 30 cmH_2O, a 1 % decrease in the administration of activated protein C, and a 5 % increase in $ScvO_2$ above 70 %. Clearly, there is still an enormous opportunity to improve compliance.

Conclusion

Research has focused in past decades on the generation of new knowledge to improve quality of care. However, a significant number of evidence-based interventions are not applied to the majority of critically ill patients. Several factors are responsible for the lack of success in translating this evidence into practice. Organizations, clinicians and the nature of the intervention all act to facilitate or hinder the widespread adoption of practices and to date there is no evidence to guide intensivists on how to safely and quickly adopt new processes of care. A local strategy may be to adopt clinicians devoted to implementation and quality improvement [43], but even these individuals will need more information on how to focus their efforts as the current practice of education, although necessary, is not enough. Future research will need to focus on alternative strategies to facilitate implementation and, to support this research, funding agencies will need to change the current allocation of resources, which is mainly directed to the generation of new knowledge, and increase resources to implementation science.

XXI

References

1. Chassin MR, Galvin RW (1998) The urgent need to improve health care quality. Institute of Medicine National Roundtable on Health Care Quality. JAMA 280: 1000–1005
2. Leeb K, Jokovic A, Sandhu M, Zinck G (2006) Intensive care in Canada. Healthc Q 9: 32–33
3. Sung NS, Crowley WF, Genel M, et al (2003) Central Challenges Facing the National Clinical Research Enterprise. JAMA 289: 1278–1287
4. Clancy CM (2004) AHRQ's FY 2005 Budget request: New mission, new vision. Health Serv Res 39: 11–18
5. Schuster MA, McGlynn EA, Brook RH (2005) How good is the quality of health care in the United States? Milbank Q 83: 843–895
6. Hsu DJ, Stone RA, Obrosky DS, et al (2010) Predictors of timely antibiotic administration for patients hospitalized with community-acquired pneumonia from the cluster-randomized EDCAP trial. Am J Med Sci 339: 307–313
7. Ferrer R, Artigas A, Levy MM et al. (2008) Improvement in process of care and outcome after a multicenter severe sepsis educational program in Spain. JAMA 299: 2294–2303
8. Grimshaw JM, Thomas RE, MacLennan G et al. (2004) Effectiveness and efficiency of guideline dissemination and implementation strategies. Health Technol Assess 8: 3–72
9. Saint S, Hofer TP, Rose JS, Kaufman SR, McMahon LF Jr (2003) Use of critical pathways to improve efficiency: a cautionary tale. Am J Manag Care 9: 758–765
10. Walsh JM, McDonald KM, Shojania KG, et al (2006) Quality improvement strategies for hypertension management: a systematic review. Med Care 44: 646–657
11. Woolf SH, Johnson RE (2005) The break-even point: when medical advances are less important than improving the fidelity with which they are delivered. Ann Fam Med 3: 545–552
12. Rubenfeld GD, Caldwell E, Peabody E, et al (2005) Incidence and outcomes of acute lung injury. N Engl J Med 353: 1685–1693
13. The Acute Respiratory Distress Syndrome Network (2000) Ventilation with lower tidal volumes as compared with traditional tidal volumes for acute lung injury and the acute respiratory distress syndrome. N Engl J Med 342: 1301–1308
14. Treggiari MM, Martin DP, Yanez ND, Caldwell E, Hudson LD, Rubenfeld GD (2007) Effect of intensive care unit organizational model and structure on outcomes in patients with acute lung injury. Am J Respir Crit Care Med 176: 685–690
15. Sinuff T, Cook D, Giacomini M, Heyland D, Dodek P (2007) Facilitating clinician adherence to guidelines in the intensive care unit: A multicenter, qualitative study. Crit Care Med 35: 2083–2089

16. Grol R, Dalhuijsen J, Thomas S, Veld C, Rutten G, Mokkink H (1998) Attributes of clinical guidelines that influence use of guidelines in general practice: observational study. BMJ 317: 858–861

17. Toma A, Bensimon CM, Dainty KN, Rubenfeld GD, Morrison LJ, Brooks SC (2010) Perceived barriers to therapeutic hypothermia for patients resuscitated from cardiac arrest: a qualitative study of emergency department and critical care workers. Crit Care Med 38: 504–509

18. Cabana MD, Rand CS, Powe NR, et al (1999) Why don't physicians follow clinical practice guidelines? A framework for improvement. JAMA 282: 1458–1465

19. Grilli R, Lomas J (1994) Evaluating the message: the relationship between compliance rate and the subject of a practice guideline. Med Care 32: 202–213

20. Girard TD, Kress JP, Fuchs BD, et al (2008) Efficacy and safety of a paired sedation and ventilator weaning protocol for mechanically ventilated patients in intensive care (Awakening and Breathing Controlled trial): a randomised controlled trial. Lancet 371: 126–134

21. van den Berg MJ, de Bakker DH, Spreeuwenberg P, et al (2009) Labour intensity of guidelines may have a greater effect on adherence than GPs' workload. BMC Fam Pract 10: 74–85

22. Rivers E, Nguyen B, Havstad S, et al (2001) Early goal-directed therapy in the treatment of severe sepsis and septic shock. N Engl J Med 345: 1368–1377

23. Jansen TC, Van Bommel J, Schoonderbeek FJ, et al (2010) Early lactate-guided therapy in intensive care unit patients: a multicenter, open-label, randomized controlled trial. Am J Respir Crit Care Med 182: 752–761

24. de Ruiter J, Zijlstra JG, Ligtenberg JJ (2011) Does lactate-guided therapy really improve outcome? Am J Respir Crit Care Med 183: 680–680

25. Main DS, Cohen SJ, DiClemente CC (1995) Measuring physician readiness to change cancer screening: preliminary results. Am J Prev Med 11: 54–58

26. Lazaro P, Murga N, Aguilar D, Hernandez-Presa MA (2010) Therapeutic inertia in the outpatient management of dyslipidemia in patients with ischemic heart disease. The inertia study. Rev Esp Cardiol 63: 1428–1437

27. Meltzer DO (2009) Social science insights into improving workforce effectiveness: examples from the developing field of hospital medicine. J Public Health Manag Pract 15: S18–S23

28. Keating NL, Ayanian JZ, Cleary PD, Marsden PV (2007) Factors affecting influential discussions among physicians: a social network analysis of a primary care practice. J Gen Intern Med 22: 794–798

29. Kucher N, Koo S, Quiroz R, et al (2005) Electronic alerts to prevent venous thromboembolism among hospitalized patients. N Engl J Med 352: 969–977

30. Resnicow KA, Schorow M, Bloom HG, Massad R (1989) Obstacles to family practitioners' use of screening tests: determinants of practice? Prev Med 18: 101–112

31. Schweickert WD, Pohlman MC, Pohlman AS, et al (2009) Early physical and occupational therapy in mechanically ventilated, critically ill patients: a randomised controlled trial. Lancet 373: 1874–1882

32. Baer M, Frese M (2003) Innovation is not enough: Climates for initiative and psychological safety, process innovations, and firm performance. J Organ Behav 24: 45–68

33. Kotter JP, Heskett JL (1992) Corporate Culture and Performance. Free Press, New York

34. Ogbonna E, Harris LC (2000) Leadership style, organizational culture and performance: empirical evidence from UK companies. International Journal of Human Resource Management 11: 766–788

35. Elenkov DS, Manev IM (2005) Top management leadership and influence on innovation: The role of sociocultural context. J Manage 31: 381–402

36. Michie S, Abraham C, Eccles MP, Francis JJ, Hardeman W, Johnston M (2011) Strengthening evaluation and implementation by specifying components of behaviour change interventions: a study protocol. Implement Sci 6: 10–17

37. Curtis JR, Cook DJ, Wall RJ, et al (2006) Intensive care unit quality improvement: a "how-to" guide for the interdisciplinary team. Crit Care Med 34: 211–218

38. Shojania KG, Ranji SR, McDonald KM, et al (2006) Effects of quality improvement strategies for type 2 diabetes on glycemic control: a meta-regression analysis. JAMA 296: 427–440

39. Cheng CH, Goldstein MK, Geller E, Levitt RE (2003) The Effects of CPOE on ICU Workflow: An Observational Study. Proc AMIA Symp 150–154
40. Huang DT, Clermont G, Kong L, et al (2010) Intensive care unit safety culture and outcomes: a US multicenter study. Int J Qual Health Care 22: 151–161
41. Scott TE, Mannion R, Davies HTO, Marshall MN (2003) Implementing culture change in health care: theory and practice. Int J Qual Health Care 15: 111–118
42. Ramsay CR, Matowe L, Grilli R, Grimshaw JM, Thomas RE (2003) Interrupted time-series designs in health technology assesment: lessons from two systematic reviews of behavior change strategies. Int J Technol Assess Health Care 19: 613–623
43. Shojania KG, Levinson W (2009) Clinicians in quality improvement: A new career pathway in academic medicine. JAMA 301: 766–768

Subject Index

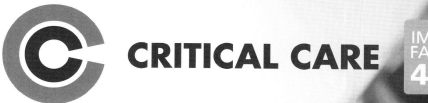
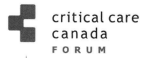

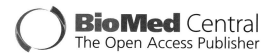